W9-CCK-547

Surgery for Cerebrovascular Disease

Surgery for Cerebrovascular Disease

SECOND EDITION

WESLEY S. MOORE, M.D.
Professor of Surgery
Chief, Section of Vascular Surgery
Department of Surgery
UCLA Center for Health Sciences
Los Angeles, California

W.B. SAUNDERS COMPANY
A Division of Harcourt Brace & Company
Philadelphia   London   Toronto   Montreal   Sydney   Tokyo

W.B. SAUNDERS COMPANY
A Division of Harcourt Brace & Company

The Curtis Center
Independence Square West
Philadelphia, Pennsylvania 19106

Library of Congress Cataloging-in-Publication Data

Surgery for cerebrovascular disease / [edited by] Wesley S. Moore.—2nd ed.

    p.   cm.

Includes bibliographical references and index.

ISBN 0–7216–3624–1

1. Cerebrovascular disease—Surgery.   I. Moore, Wesley S.
   [DNLM: 1. Cerebrovascular Disorders—surgery. WL 355 S9598 1996]

RD594.2.S867 1996   617.4′81059—dc20

DNLM/DLC   94–43381

Surgery for Cerebrovascular Disease, second edition   ISBN 0–7216–3624–1

Printed in the United States of America.

Last digit is the print number: 9   8   7   6   5   4   3   2   1

Contributors

SAMUEL S. AHN, M.D.
Associate Clinical Professor of Surgery, University of California at Los Angeles, Center for the Health Sciences, Los Angeles, California; Chief of Vascular Surgery, Olive View Medical Center, Sylmar, California.
Computed Electroencephalographic Topographic Brain Mapping

JOSEPH ALPERT, M.D.
Clinical Professor of Surgery, Retired, University of Medicine and Dentistry of New Jersey–New Jersey Medical School; Past Director of Vascular Surgery, Newark Beth Israel Medical Center, Newark, New Jersey.
The Management of Patients Requiring Coronary Bypass and Carotid Endarterectomy

CHARLES M. ANDERSON, M.D., Ph.D.
Associate Professor of Radiology, University of California at San Francisco; Chief of Magnetic Resonance Imaging, San Francisco VA Medical Center, San Francisco, California.
Magnetic Resonance Angiography of Cerebrovascular Disease

ROBERT G. ATNIP, M.D.
Associate Professor of Surgery, Pennsylvania State University College of Medicine; Chief of Vascular Surgery, The Milton S. Hershey Medical Center, Hershey, Pennsylvania.
Immediate and Long-Term Results of Brachiocephalic Repair: Direct Versus Extrathoracic Operations

ALLEN W. AVERBOOK, M.D., F.A.C.S.
Fellow, Vascular Surgery, Harbor General Hospital–St. Mary's, Long Beach, California.
Intraoperative Assessment of the Technical Results of Carotid Endarterectomy: Angiography

J. DENNIS BAKER, M.D.
Professor of Surgery, University of California at Los Angeles School of Medicine; Vascular Surgeon, V.A. Medical Center, Los Angeles, California.
Transcranial Doppler Ultrasonography; Preoperative and Postoperative Management of Patients Undergoing Carotid Endarterectomy; Recurrent Stenosis of the Carotid Artery: Incidence, Diagnosis, Prognosis, and Management

WILLIAM H. BAKER, M.D.
Professor of Surgery, Head, Section of Peripheral Vascular Surgery, Loyola University, Stritch School of Medicine, May Wood, Illinois; Consultant, Hines VA Hospital, Hines, Illinois.
Justification for Routine Nonshunting of the Carotid Artery; Carotid Endarterectomy for Global or Nonfocal Symptoms: Indications and Results

JEFFREY L. BALLARD, M.D.
Assistant Professor of Surgery, Division of Vascular Surgery, Loma Linda University School of Medicine, Loma Linda, California.
Carotid Artery Shunt: Argument for its Routine Use; Carotid Body Paragangliomas: Diagnosis, Prognosis, and Surgical Management

PETER BARKER, Ph.D.
Senior Bioscientific Staff, Department of Neurology, Henry Ford Hospital, Detroit, Michigan.
Magnetic Resonance Techniques in the Investigation and Management of Acute Ischemic Stroke

WILEY F. BARKER, M.D.
Professor Emeritus (Surgery), University of California at Los Angeles, Los Angeles, California.
The History of Surgery for Cerebrovascular Disease

HENRY J. M. BARNETT, O.C., M.D., F.R.C.P.(C)
Professor Emeritus, University of Western Ontario Clinical Neurological Sciences, University of Western Ontario; Scientist and Principal Investigator, North American Symptomatic Carotid Endarterectomy Trial, The John P. Robarts Research Institute, London, Ontario, Canada.
The Importance of Symptoms in Predicting Risk for Subsequent Stroke Following an Initial Transient Ischemic Attack or Minor Stroke; Prospective Randomized Trial of Symptomatic Patients: Results from the NASCET Study

HUGH G. BEEBE, M.D.
Adjunct Professor of Surgery, University of Michigan, Ann Arbor, Michigan; Director, Jobst Vascular Center, Toledo, Ohio.
The Natural History and Current Status of Carotid Endarterectomy for Stroke Secondary to Acute Carotid Occlusion; Upper Limit of Risk for Performance of Carotid Endarterectomy: Position Statement of the Stroke Council of the American Heart Association

JOHN R. BENTSON, M.D.
  Professor of Radiology, Chief of Neuroradiology,
  University of California at Los Angeles Medical Center,
  Los Angeles, California.
  Computed Tomography of Stroke

RAMON BERGUER, M.D., Ph.D.
  Professor of Surgery, Wayne State University; Chief,
  Section of Vascular Surgery and Director, Acute Stroke
  Unit, Harper Hospital, Detroit, Michigan.
  *Indications for Vertebral Artery Repair; Surgical
  Exposure and Methods of Vertebral Artery Repair*

EUGENE F. BERNSTEIN, M.D., Ph.D., F.A.C.S.
  Senior Consultant, Division of Vascular and Thoracic
  Surgery, Scripps Clinic and Research Foundation, La
  Jolla, California.
  The CHAT Classification

DAVID R. BLATT, M.D.
  Neurosurgeon, Baptist Hospital, Nashville, Tennessee.
  *Traumatic Dissection of the Internal Carotid Artery:
  Conservative Versus Surgical Management*

RICHARD W. BOCK, M.D.
  Vascular Surgeon, Memorial Mission Hospital, Asheville,
  North Carolina.
  *Lesions, Dynamics, and Pathogenetic Mechanisms
  Responsible for Ischemic Events in the Brain; Arguments
  in Favor of the Routine Patch Angioplasty of the Carotid
  Artery*

NATAN M. BORNSTEIN, M.D.
  Associate Professor, Sackler School of Medicine, Tel-
  Aviv University; Director, Stroke Unit, Department of
  Neurology, Tel-Aviv Medical Center, Tel-Aviv, Israel.
  *The Natural History of Patients With Asymptomatic
  Carotid Stenosis*

BRUCE J. BRENER, M.D.
  Clinical Professor of Surgery, University of Medicine
  and Dentistry of New Jersey–New Jersey Medical
  School; Chief, Vascular Surgery, Newark Beth Israel
  Medical Center, Newark, New Jersey.
  *The Management of Patients Requiring Coronary Bypass
  and Carotid Endarterectomy*

DAVID C. BREWSTER, M.D.
  Clinical Professor of Surgery, Massachusetts General
  Hospital and Harvard Medical School, Boston,
  Massachusetts.
  *Transthoracic or Transmediastinal Repair of the
  Brachiocephalic Trunks; Immediate and Long-Term
  Results of Brachiocephalic Repair: Direct versus
  Extrathoracic Operations*

DONALD K. BRIEF, M.D.
  Clinical Professor of Surgery, University of Medicine
  and Dentistry of New Jersey–New Jersey Medical
  School; Director of Surgery, Newark Beth Israel Medical
  Center, Newark, New Jersey.
  *The Management of Patients Requiring Coronary Bypass
  and Carotid Endarterectomy*

JOSEPH P. BRODERICK, M.D.
  Associate Professor of Neurology, University of
  Cincinnati College of Medicine, Cincinnati, Ohio.
  Medical Management of Acute Cerebral Ischemic Stroke

THOMAS BROTT, M.D.
  Professor of Neurology, University of Cincinnati College
  of Medicine, Cincinnati, Ohio.
  *Medical Management of Acute Cerebral Ischemic Stroke;
  Risk of Carotid Endarterectomy Based on Community
  Audit*

RONALD W. BUSUTTIL, M.D.
  Professor of Surgery, Dumont Chair in Transplantation
  Surgery, and Director, Dumont–UCLA Transplant Center,
  University of California at Los Angeles, Los Angeles,
  California.
  *Surgical Repair of Coils, Kinks, and Redundancy of the
  Carotid Artery: Indications, Techniques, and Results*

ALLAN D. CALLOW, M.D., Ph.D.
  Research Professor of Surgery and Medicine, Boston
  University School of Medicine and the Whitaker
  Cardiovascular Institute; Attending Staff, University
  Hospital and Boston City Hospital, Boston,
  Massachusetts.
  *The Social, Economic, and Personal Impact of Stroke
  and Its Prevention*

YUE CAO, Ph.D.
  Assistant Professor in Medical Physics, Oakland
  University, Rochester, Minnesota; Senior Bioscientific
  Staff, Henry Ford Hospital, Detroit, Michigan.
  *Magnetic Resonance Techniques in the Investigation and
  Management of Acute Ischemic Stroke*

LOUIS R. CAPLAN, M.D.
  Professor and Chairman, Neurology, Tufts University;
  Neurologist-in-Chief, New England Medical Center,
  Boston, Massachusetts.
  *Transient Ischemic Attacks and Stroke in the Distribution
  of the Vertebrobasilar System: Clinical Manifestations;
  Medical Management of Vertebrobasilar Disease; The
  Rand Study Positions Concerning Carotid
  Endarterectomy*

STANLEY N. COHEN, M.D.
  Professor of Neurology, University of California at Los
  Angeles, School of Medicine; Assistant Chief of
  Neurology and Director, Stroke Service, West Los
  Angeles VA Medical Center, Los Angeles, California.
  Intellectual Function Following Carotid Endarterectomy

DEBRA CREIGHTON, B.A.
  Research Associate, Newark Beth Israel Medical Center,
  Newark, New Jersey.
  *The Management of Patients Requiring Coronary Bypass
  and Carotid Endarterectomy*

ARTHUR L. DAY, M.D.
   Professor, Department of Neurosurgery, University of
   Florida College of Medicine, Gainesville, Florida.
   *Traumatic Dissection of the Internal Carotid Artery:
   Conservative Versus Surgical Management*

FERNANDO G. DIAZ, M.D., Ph.D.
   Professor and Chairman, Department of Neurosurgery,
   Wayne State University, Detroit, Michigan.
   Technique for Extracranial–Intracranial Bypass Grafting

STEVEN W. DIBERT, B.S., M.D.
   Adult Neurologist, Coastal Neurological Associates, New
   Bern, North Carolina.
   *Transient Ischemic Attacks and Stroke in the Distribution
   of the Carotid Artery: Clinical Manifestations*

MARK L. DYKEN, M.D.
   Professor Emeritus, Indiana University, Indianapolis,
   Indiana.
   Risk Factors Predisposing to Stroke

J. DONALD EASTON, B.S., M.D.
   Professor and Chairman, Department of Clinical
   Neurosciences, Brown University School of Medicine;
   Neurologist-in-Chief, Rhode Island Hospital, Providence,
   Rhode Island.
   Spectrum of Pathology Responsible for Ischemic Stroke

DAVID J. EFFENEY, M.B.,B.S., F.R.A.C.S.
   Dean, Faculty of Medicine, The University of
   Queensland, Herston, Queensland, Australia.
   *Surgery for Fibromuscular Dysplasia of the Carotid
   Artery: Indications, Technique, and Results*

DAVID E. EISENBUD, M.D.
   Director and Founder, Newark Beth Israel Center for
   Wound Management, Newark, New Jersey, and Union
   Hospital Center for Wound Management, Union, New
   Jersey.
   *The Management of Patients Requiring Coronary Bypass
   and Carotid Endarterectomy*

BRUCE A. EVANS, M.D.
   Assistant Professor of Neurology, Mayo Medical School;
   Consultant in Neurology, Mayo Clinic and St. Marys
   Hospital, Rochester, Minnesota.
   *The Importance of Symptoms in Predicting Risk for
   Subsequent Stroke Following an Initial Transient
   Ischemic Attack or Minor Stroke*

RICHARD L. FEINBERG, M.D.
   Clinical Assistant Professor of Surgery, George
   Washington University Medical Center, Washington,
   District of Columbia.
   *Immediate and Long-Term Results of Carotid
   Endarterectomy in Reducing Recurrent Stroke Risk in
   Patients With Prior Hemispheric Stroke; Cost-Benefit
   Analysis of Carotid Endarterectomy: A Surgical
   Perspective*

WILLIAM M. FEINBERG, M.D.
   Associate Professor, Department of Neurology,
   University of Arizona College of Medicine, Tucson,
   Arizona.
   *Medical Management of Carotid Territory Transient
   Ischemic Attacks*

D. PRESTON FLANIGAN, M.D.
   Clinical Professor of Surgery, University of California,
   Irvine, California; Visiting Professor of Surgery,
   University of Illinois, Chicago, Illinois.
   *Assessment of the Technical Results of Carotid
   Endarterectomy Using Real-Time Intraoperative
   Ultrasonography; Tandem Lesions of the Extracranial
   and Intracranial Carotid Artery: Management and
   Results*

MAX R. GASPAR, M.D., F.A.C.S.
   Emeritus Clinical Professor of Surgery, University of
   Southern California School of Medicine, Los Angeles,
   California.
   *Intraoperative Assessment of the Technical Results of
   Carotid Endarterectomy: Angiography*

WILLIAM GEE, M.D.
   Medical Director, Vascular Laboratory, Lehigh Valley
   Hospital, Allentown, Pennsylvania.
   Ocular Pneumoplethysmography

HUGH A. GELABERT, M.D.
   Assistant Professor of Surgery, Vascular Surgery Section,
   University of California at Los Angeles, School of
   Medicine, Los Angeles, California.
   *Arguments in Favor of the Routine Use of Primary
   Closure of the Carotid Artery*

GEORGE GEROULAKOS, M.D., F.R.C.S., D.I.C.,
Ph.D.
   Lecturer in Surgery, Professorial Surgical Unit, St.
   Bartholomew's Hospital Medical School, London,
   England; Fellow, Division of Vascular Surgery, Ohio
   State University Hospital, Columbus, Ohio.
   *The Importance of Carotid Plaque Characteristics as
   Independent Variables in Predicting Stroke Risk*

MARK S. GOLD, M.D.
   Assistant Professor of Anesthesiology, Department of
   Anesthesiology, New York University Medical Center;
   Director of Vascular Anesthesia, New York University
   Medical Center, New York, New York.
   *Alternatives to General Anesthesia for Carotid
   Endarterectomy*

ROBERT J. GOLDENKRANZ, M.D.
   Assistant Clinical Professor of Surgery, University of
   Medicine and Dentistry of New Jersey, New Jersey
   Medical School; Chief, Division of General Surgery,
   Newark Beth Israel Medical Center, Newark, New
   Jersey.
   *The Management of Patients Requiring Coronary Bypass
   and Carotid Endarterectomy*

JERRY GOLDSTONE, M.D.
Professor of Surgery and Chief, Division of Vascular Surgery, University of California at San Francisco, San Francisco, California.
Emergency Surgery for Stroke in Evolution and Crescendo Transient Ischemic Attacks

ANTOINETTE S. GOMES, M.D.
Associate Professor of Radiology and Medicine, University of California at Los Angeles, School of Medicine and Medical Center, Los Angeles, California.
Aortic Arch Studies and Selective Arteriography

GARY J. HARPOLD, M.D.
Assistant Professor of Neurology, University of Virginia, Charlottesville, Virginia; Veterans Affairs Medical Center, Salem, Virginia.
Transient Ischemic Attacks and Stroke in the Distribution of the Carotid Artery: Clinical Manifestations

E. JOHN HARRIS, JR., M.D.
Assistant Professor of Surgery, Stanford University School of Medicine; Attending Surgeon, Stanford University Hospital, Stanford, California; Staff Vascular Surgeon, Palo Alto VA Medical Center, Palo Alto, California.
External Carotid Endarterectomy: Indications, Techniques, and Results

ROBERT S. HEPLER, M.D.
Professor Emeritus of Ophthalmology, School of Medicine, University of California at Los Angeles; Active Staff, Department of Ophthalmology, Jules Stein Eye Institute, School of Medicine, University of California at Los Angeles, Los Angeles, California.
Ophthalmic Manifestations of Cerebrovascular Disease

HOWARD HERMANS, M.D.
Associate Staff Surgeon, Ellis Hospital, Schenectady, New York.
The Management of Patients Requiring Coronary Bypass and Carotid Endarterectomy

NORMAN R. HERTZER, M.D.
Chairman, Department of Vascular Surgery, The Cleveland Clinic Foundation, Cleveland, Ohio.
Early Complications of Carotid Endarterectomy: Incidence, Diagnosis, and Management

ROBERT W. HOBSON II, M.D.
Professor of Surgery and Chief, Section of Vascular Surgery, University of Medicine and Dentistry of New Jersey–New Jersey Medical School, Newark, New Jersey.
Carotid Endarterectomy for Asymptomatic Carotid Stenosis: Review of the Veterans Administration Cooperative Clinical Trial

VIRGINIA J. HOWARD, M.S.P.H.
Research Assistant Professor of Neurology, Bowman Gray School of Medicine of Wake Forest University, Winston-Salem, North Carolina.
Design and Current Status of the Asymptomatic Carotid Atherosclerosis Study

KATE T. HUNCKE, M.D.
Assistant Clinical Professor, University of California at Los Angeles, Medical Center, Department of Anesthesia, Attending Physician, Center for Health Sciences, Los Angeles, California.
Anesthetic Considerations for Carotid Endarterectomy

JAN HUSTON, M.D.
Director of Laparoscopic Surgery, Newark Beth Israel Medical Center, Newark, New Jersey.
The Management of Patients Requiring Coronary Bypass and Carotid Endarterectomy

ANTHONY M. IMPARATO, M.D.
Professor of Surgery, Department of Surgery, Division of Vascular Surgery, New York University Medical School, New York, New York.
Surgery of the Vertebral Artery: Overview and Results; Indications for Repair of The Brachiocephalic Trunks

ANNE M. JONES, B.S.N., R.V.T.
Lecturer, Department of Neurology, Bowman Gray School of Medicine, Winston-Salem, North Carolina.
Transcranial Doppler Ultrasonography

SHELDON E. JORDAN, M.D.
Assistant Clinical Professor of Neurology, University of California at Los Angeles, Center for the Health Sciences, Los Angeles, California.
Clinical Evaluation and Differential Diagnosis of Patients with Cerebrovascular Disease; Computed Electroencephalographic Topographic Brain Mapping

KATHLEEN S. KAGAN-HALLET, B.S., M.D.
Associate Professor, Neuropathology and Pediatric Pathology, University of Texas Health Sciences Center, San Antonio, Texas.
Spectrum of Pathology Responsible for Ischemic Stroke

RICHARD F. KEMPCZINSKI, M.D.
Professor of Surgery and Chief, Division of Vascular Surgery, University of Cincinnati Medical Center, Cincinnati, Ohio.
Risk of Operation as a Function of Indication: Retrospective Institution and Individual Surgeon Reviews; Rationale and Method for Auditing Individual Surgeons: Relationship to Hospital Privileges

J. DAVID KILLEEN, M.D.
Chief, Vascular Surgery, Associate Professor, Loma Linda University School of Medicine, Loma Linda, California.
Standard and Extensile Exposure of the Carotid Artery

TED R. KOHLER, M.D.
Associate Professor of Surgery, University of Washington School of Medicine; Chief, Vascular Surgery Section, VA Medical Center, Seattle, Washington.
Duplex Scanning and Spectral Analysis

LOUIS KOZLOFF, M.D.
Clinical Professor of Surgery, George Washington University Medical Center; Consultant, National Institutes of Health, Bethesda, Maryland.
Cost-Benefit Analysis of Carotid Endarterectomy: A Surgical Perspective

JOSEPH LIPSCOMB, Ph.D.
Associate Professor, Public Policy Studies and Community and Family Medicine, Duke University, Durham, North Carolina.
A Health Policy Perspective on Carotid Endarterectomy: Cost, Effectiveness, and Cost-Effectiveness

JOHN R. LITTLE, M.D., F.A.C.S., F.R.C.S.(C)
Chief of Neurosurgery, Naples Community Hospital, Naples, Florida.
Indications for Extracranial–Intracranial Bypass Surgery; Immediate and Late Results of Extracranial–Intracranial Bypass Surgery

PAUL E. LIZOTTE, D.O.
Fellow, Nuclear Medicine, University of California at San Francisco, San Francisco, California.
SPECT Scanning in Cerebrovascular Disease

ROBERT J. LULL, M.D.
Clinical Professor of Radiology and Laboratory Medicine, University of California at San Francisco School of Medicine; Director, Nuclear Medicine Department, San Francisco General Hospital Medical Center, San Francisco, California.
SPECT Scanning in Cerebrovascular Disease

ROBERT J. LUSBY, M.D., F.R.C.S., F.R.A.C.S.
Professor of Surgery, University of Sydney; Visiting Surgeon, Mater Hospital, Auburn District Hospital and Ryde Hospital, Sydney, New South Wales, Australia; Head, Department of Vascular Surgery, Concord Repatriation General Hospital, Concord, New South Wales, Australia; Consultant Vascular Surgeon, Royal Australian Army Medical Corps.
Lesions, Dynamics, and Pathogenetic Mechanisms Responsible for Ischemic Events in the Brain

WILLIAM C. MACKEY, M.D.
Associate Professor of Surgery, Tufts University School of Medicine; Attending Vascular Surgeon, New England Medical Center, Boston, Massachusetts.
The Social, Economic, and Personal Impact of Stroke and Its Prevention

ALICE E. MADDEN, R.N.
Director, Vascular Laboratory, Lehigh Valley Hospital, Allentown, Pennsylvania.
Ocular Pneumoplethysmography

CHRISTINE BROWN MAHONEY, Ph.D., M.S., B.S., R.N.
Assistant Professor, Metropolitan State University, College of Management, Minneapolis, MN; Adjunct

Faculty, School of Public Health, University of Minnesota, Minneapolis, Minnesota.
The Management of Patients Requiring Coronary Bypass and Carotid Endarterectomy

JAMES M. MALONE, M.D.
Chairman, Department of Surgery, Maricopa Medical Center; Professor of Surgery, University of Arizona College of Medicine, Phoenix, Arizona.
Carotid Artery Shunt: Argument for its Routine Use

DAVID B. MATCHAR, M.D.
Director, Center for Health Policy Research and Education, Duke University; Associate Professor, Department of Medicine, Duke University Medical Center, Durham, North Carolina.
A Health Policy Perspective on Carotid Endarterectomy: Cost, Effectiveness, and Cost-Effectiveness

MARC R. MAYBERG, M.D.
Associate Professor, Department of Neurological Surgery, University of Washington School of Medicine, Seattle, Washington.
Veterans Affairs Cooperative Studies Program Trial for Carotid Endarterectomy in Patients with Symptomatic Carotid Stenosis

JOHN C. MAZZIOTTA, M.D.
Vice Chairman and Professor, Neurological and Radiological Sciences, University of California at Los Angeles, Center for Health Sciences, Los Angeles, California.
Positron Emission Tomography

LESLIE MEMSIC, M.D., F.A.C.S.
Attending Surgeon, Cedars-Sinai Medical Center, Los Angeles, California.
Surgical Repair of Coils, Kinks, and Redundancy of the Carotid Artery: Indications, Techniques, and Results

JORDAN D. MILLER, M.D.
Associate Professor of Anesthesiology, University of California at Los Angeles School of Medicine; Attending Physician, Center for Health Sciences, Los Angeles, California.
Anesthetic Considerations for Carotid Endarterectomy

MAX B. MITCHELL, M.D.
Resident, Cardiothoracic Surgery, University of Colorado Medical School; Chief Resident, General Surgery, University Hospital, Denver, Colorado.
The Importance of Percent Stenosis as an Independent Variable for Predicting Stroke Risk in Symptomatic and Asymptomatic Patients

J. P. MOHR, M.D.
Sciarra Professor of Clinical Neurology, College of Physicians and Surgeons of Columbia University, New York, New York.
Morbidity and Mortality of Stroke

WESLEY S. MOORE, M.D.
Professor of Surgery and Chief, Section of Vascular Surgery, University of California at Los Angeles, Center for Health Sciences, Los Angeles, California.
Role of the Vascular Laboratory in the Diagnosis and Management of Patients With Cerebrovascular Disease; Indications for Angiography and Basis for Selecting the Type of Angiographic Study; The Natural History of Asymptomatic Carotid Ulceration; American Heart Association Consensus Committee Statement Concerning Indications for Carotid Endarterectomy in Asymptomatic Patients; American Heart Association Consensus Committee Statement Concerning Indications for Carotid Endarterectomy in Symptomatic Patients; Selective Shunting of the Carotid Artery: An Overview; The Use of Internal Carotid Artery Back Pressure to Determine Shunt Requirement; Technique of Carotid Endarterectomy; Extrathoracic Repair of the Brachiocephalic Trunks

EILEEN S. NATUZZI, M.S., M.D.
Research Fellow, University of California at San Francisco, San Francisco, California.
Accessible and Inaccessible Aneurysms of the Extracranial Carotid Artery

A. NICOLAIDES, M.S., F.R.C.S.
Professor of Vascular Surgery, St. Mary's Hospital Medical School; Honorary Consultant Vascular Surgeon, St. Mary's Hospital, London, England.
The Importance of Carotid Plaque Characteristics as Independent Variables in Predicting Stroke Risk

JOHN W. NORRIS, M.D., F.R.C.P.
Professor of Neurology, University of Toronto; Consultant Neurologist, Stroke Research Unit, Sunnybrook Medical Center, Toronto, Ontario, Canada.
The Natural History of Patients With Asymptomatic Carotid Stenosis

MARC R. NUWER, M.D., Ph.D.
Professor, Department of Neurology, University of Los Angeles School of Medicine; Department Head, Clinical Neurophysiology, University of California at Los Angeles Medical Center, Los Angeles, California.
Computed Electroencephalographic Topographic Brain Mapping; The Use of Electroencephalographic Monitoring to Determine Shunt Requirement

MARGARET O'DONOGHUE, M.D.
Assistant Professor of Neurology, Tufts University School of Medicine, St. Elizabeth's Medical Center, Boston, Massachusetts.
Medical Management of Acute Cerebral Ischemic Stroke

VICTOR PARSONNET, M.D.
Clinical Professor of Surgery, University of Medicine and Dentistry of New Jersey, New Jersey Medical School; Director of Pacemaker Center, Director, Surgical Research, Newark Beth Israel Medical Center, Newark, New Jersey.
The Management of Patients Requiring Coronary Bypass and Carotid Endarterectomy

JOHN S. PAUK, M.D., M.PH.
University of Washington Medical Center, Seattle, Washington; Department of Medicine, University of Washington Medical Center, Seattle, Washington.
A Health Policy Perspective on Carotid Endarterectomy: Cost, Effectiveness, and Cost-Effectiveness

MALCOLM O. PERRY, M.D.
Professor of Surgery and Chief of Vascular Surgery, Texas Technical University Health Sciences Center, Lubbock, Texas.
Blunt and Penetrating Injuries of the Extracranial Cerebral Vessels

TAMMY K. RAMOS, M.D.
Assistant Professor of Surgery, University of California at San Francisco; Attending Vascular Surgeon, University of California at San Francisco Medical Center, San Francisco, California.
Accessible and Inaccessible Aneurysms of the Extracranial Carotid Artery

JAMES F. REED III, Ph.D.
Director, Research and Publication Support, Lehigh Valley Hospital, Allentown, Pennsylvania.
Ocular Pneumoplethysmography

JOHN J. RICOTTA, M.D.
Professor of Surgery and Director, Division of Vascular Surgery, State University of New York at Buffalo; Chief of Surgery, Millard Fillmore Hospital, Buffalo, New York.
Immediate and Long-Term Outcome of Surgery for Asymptomatic Carotid Stenosis

THOMAS S. RILES, M.D.
Professor of Surgery, New York University Medical Center; Director, Division of Vascular Surgery, New York University Medical Center, New York, New York.
Alternatives to General Anesthesia for Carotid Endarterectomy; Surgery of the Vertebral Artery: Overview and Results; Indications for Repair of the Brachiocephalic Trunks

JAMES T. ROBERTSON, M.D.
Chief, Division of Neurological Surgery, University of Tennessee, Memphis, Tennessee.
Immediate and Long-Term Results of Carotid Endarterectomy in Reducing Stroke Risk in Patients with Hemispheric and Monocular Transient Ischemic Attack

ROBERT B. RUTHERFORD, M.D.
Professor of Surgery, University of Colorado Medical School; Vascular Surgeon, University Hospitals, Denver, Colorado.
The Importance of Percent Stenosis as an Independent Variable for Predicting Stroke Risk in Symptomatic and Asymptomatic Patients; The Importance of Establishing Uniform Reporting Standards in Evaluating the Results of Carotid Endarterectomy

R.L. SACCO, M.S., M.D.
  Assistant Professor of Neurology and Public Health
  (Epidemiology) in the Sergievsky Center, Columbia
  University; Assistant Attending in Neurology,
  Presbyterian Hospital of the City of New York, New
  York, New York.
  Morbidity and Mortality of Stroke

JAMES J. SCHULER, M.D.
  Assistant Professor of Surgery, Division of Vascular
  Surgery, University of Illinois College of Medicine,
  Chicago, Illinois.
  *Tandem Lesions of the Extracranial and Intracranial
  Carotid Artery: Management and Results*

DAVID G. SHERMAN, M.D.
  Professor and Chief, Division of Neurology, Department
  of Medicine, University of Texas Health Science Center,
  San Antonio, Texas.
  Spectrum of Pathology Responsible for Ischemic Stroke

LOUIS L. SMITH, M.D.
  Professor of Surgery, Division of Vascular Surgery,
  Loma Linda University School of Medicine; Professor of
  Surgery, Loma Linda University School of Medicine,
  Loma Linda, California.
  *Standard and Extensile Exposure of the Carotid Artery;
  Carotid Body Paragangliomas: Diagnosis, Prognosis,
  and Surgical Management*

ROBERT L. SMITH, B.S.E.E.
  President, Electro-Diagnostic Instruments, Burbank,
  California.
  Ocular Pneumoplethysmography

RONALD J. STONEY, M.D.
  Professor of Surgery, University of California at San
  Francisco; Attending Vascular Surgeon, University of
  California at San Francisco Medical Center, San
  Francisco, California.
  *Accessible and Inaccessible Aneurysms of the
  Extracranial Carotid Artery*

D. EUGENE STRANDNESS, JR., M.D.
  Professor of Surgery, University of Washington School
  of Medicine; Chief, Division of Vascular Surgery,
  University of Washington Medical Center, Seattle,
  Washington.
  Duplex Scanning and Spectral Analysis

ROY L. TAWES, JR., M.D.
  Associate Clinical Professor of Surgery, University of
  California at San Francisco; President, Peninsula
  Vascular Surgical Associates, Burlingame, California
  SPECT Scanning in Cerebrovascular Disease

D. J. THOMAS, M.A., M.D., F.R.C.P.
  Senior Lecturer, Institute of Neurology, University of
  London; Consultant Neurologist, St. Mary's Hospital,
  London, England.
  *The Effect of Risk Factor Modification and Antiplatelet
  Treatment in Reducing Stroke Risk in Patients With*

*Transient Cerebral Ischemic Attack or Prior Stroke;
Prospective Randomized Trial of Symptomatic Patients
With Carotid Artery Disease: Results of the European
Carotid Surgery Trial*

JAMES F. TOOLE, M.D.
  Teagle Professor of Neurology and Director, Stroke
  Research Center, Bowman Gray School of Medicine of
  Wake Forest University, Winston-Salem, North Carolina.
  *Transient Ischemic Attacks and Stroke in the Distribution
  of the Carotid Artery: Clinical Manifestations*

HUGH H. TROUT III, M.D.
  Clinical Professor of Surgery, George Washington
  University Medical Center, Washington, District of
  Columbia.
  *Immediate and Long-Term Results of Carotid
  Endarterectomy in Reducing Recurrent Stroke Risk in
  Patients with Prior Hemispheric Stroke; Cost-Benefit
  Analysis of Carotid Endarterectomy: A Surgical
  Perspective*

DAVID G. WEISS, Ph.D.
  Assistant Chief, Cooperative Studies Program
  Coordinating Center at Perry Point, Department of
  Veterans Affairs, VA Medical Center, Perry Point,
  Maryland.
  *Veterans Affairs Cooperative Studies Program Trial for
  Carotid Endarterectomy in Patients with Symptomatic
  Carotid Stenosis*

K. M. A. WELCH, M.D.
  Professor and Adjunct Professor, Case Western Reserve
  University, Cleveland, Ohio; Oakland University,
  Rochester, Michigan; William T. Gossett Chair, Henry
  Ford Hospital, Detroit, Michigan.
  *Magnetic Resonance Techniques in the Investigation and
  Management of Acute Ischemic Stroke*

DAVID O. WIEBERS, M.D.
  Professor and Chair, Division of Cerebrovascular
  Diseases, Mayo Clinic and Mayo Medical School;
  Consultant in Neurology and Epidemiology, Mayo Clinic
  and Mayo Medical School, Rochester, Minnesota.
  *The Importance of Symptoms in Predicting Risk for
  Subsequent Stroke Following an Initial Transient
  Ischemic Attack or Minor Stroke*

SAMUEL E. WILSON, M.D.
  Professor, Department of Surgery, University of
  California at Irvine College of Medicine, Irvine,
  California; Professor and Chair, Department of Surgery,
  University of California, Irvine Medical Center, Orange,
  California.
  *Veterans Affairs Cooperative Studies Program Trial for
  Carotid Endarterectomy in Patients with Symptomatic
  Carotid Stenosis*

ROBERT J. WITYK, M.D.
  Assistant Professor of Neurology and Medicine, The
  Johns Hopkins University School of Medicine; Co-

Director, Division of Neurology, Department of
Medicine, Sinai Hospital, Baltimore, Maryland.
*Transient Ischemic Attacks and Stroke in the Distribution
of the Vertebrobasilar System: Clinical Manifestations;
Medical Management of Vertebrobasilar Disease*

FRANK YATSU, M.D.
Professor of Neurology, Chairman Emeritus of
Neurology, University of Texas–Houston Medical
School, Houston, Texas.
*Veterans Affairs Cooperative Studies Program Trial for
Carotid Endarterectomy in Patients with Symptomatic
Carotid Stenosis*

ROBERT D. YEE, M.D., F.A.C.S.
Professor and Chairman, Department of Ophthalmology,
Indiana University School of Medicine, Indianapolis,
Indiana.
Ophthalmic Manifestations of Cerebrovascular Disease

PETER Y. YOUN, M.D.
University of Southern California County Medical
Center, Los Angeles, California.
*Computed Electroencephalographic Topographic Brain
Mapping*

CHRISTOPHER K. ZARINS, M.D.
Chidester Professor of Surgery, Stanford University;
Chief, Division of Vascular Surgery, Stanford University
Medical Center, Stanford, California.
*External Carotid Endarterectomy: Indications,
Techniques, and Results*

R. EUGENE ZIERLER, M.D.
Associate Professor of Surgery, University of
Washington School of Medicine; Attending Surgeon,
Vascular Division, University of Washington Medical
Center, Seattle, Washington.
Duplex Scanning and Spectral Analysis

Preface

Surgery for cerebrovascular disease proceeded through a rapid expansion and conceptual maturation over the past 40 years. For the last 10 years, the surgical approach to the management of patients with cerebrovascular disease, particularly carotid endarterectomy, has undergone minute investigation and has been the subject of several important prospective clinical trials. The timing of this second edition is particularly appropriate as it provides the opportunity to examine the results of these prospective randomized trials. This now brings a level of stability and maturity to our understanding of the indications and results of cerebrovascular surgery, particularly carotid endarterectomy.

Numerous scientific disciplines have contributed to the body of knowledge from which the surgeon engaged in stroke prevention can draw to better identify patients who will benefit from surgical therapy as well as to make surgical management safer for the patient. This text brings together information from a variety of disciplines, including anatomy, physiology, pathology, radiology, epidemiology, neurology, neurosurgery, and vascular surgery in order to provide a sound theoretical and practical approach to the management of patients who are at risk for stroke.

I recognize that surgeons who treat patients with cerebrovascular disorders come from several surgical specialties including general surgery, neurologic surgery, cardiac surgery, and vascular surgery. Therefore, to provide the broadest surgical perspective, recognized experts from all of these surgical specialties have been selected to contribute chapters to the book. In this manner, I hope that the text serves the needs of all surgeons treating patients with cerebrovascular disease, regardless of their surgical specialty.

The patient with cerebrovascular disease is best served by those practitioners who recognize that a comprehensive approach to the treatment will yield the best long-term results. This improved approach will include risk factor management, medical treatment, and, in appropriately selected patients, direct surgical intervention. For that reason, the text goes well beyond the technical treatise of surgical management. Chapters covering topics of natural history, diagnosis, pathogenesis, pathology, and medical management complement an extensive review of the technical aspects of surgical management as well as complications and their prevention. Finally, the immediate and long-term treatment results from various forms of therapeutic intervention are explored and reported.

In these days of cost containment and concerns of cost-effectiveness in medical management, these topics are also explored with respect to the issues of the cost of stroke as well as the cost and effectiveness in its prevention. Both the editor and the chapter contributors hope that this book will provide an integrated scientific basis to address the issues of stroke prevention and management in patients with cerebrovascular disease and present a rational and safe approach to reduce morbidity and mortality among the patients with whose care we are entrusted.

WESLEY S. MOORE, M.D.

Contents

The History of Surgery for Cerebrovascular Disease

WILEY F. BARKER

The very origin of the word *carotid* evokes a sense of humankind's early knowledge of the function of that artery. Depending on which Greek source one consults, "carotid" is said to mean "asphyxia" or "deep sleep" or "coma"—any one of which might be an appropriate derivation.

The carotid artery does have a critical role in humans as the main vascular supply to the brain. The brain is very sensitive to oxygen deprivation and responds to serious ischemia of more than a few minutes' duration with permanent deficits. Surgery of the carotid artery has, for this reason, been a most sensitive and delicate matter.

CAROTID DISEASE IN HUNTER'S TIME

Reconstructive carotid artery surgery is of recent origin, but for nearly 200 hundred years considerable knowledge that has not been fully used concerning the carotid artery and its diseases has been available. In the Hunterian Museum of the Royal College of Surgeons is a specimen of an atheromatous carotid bifurcation and an ulceration within it.[1] This lesion was found incidentally at a postmortem examination of a patient who had died of a ruptured thoracic aneurysm. What led John Hunter to identify and dissect that specimen—one that might have been so easily overlooked had he not opened the artery? In that same museum is another specimen of an aneurysm of the internal carotid artery, also dissected by John Hunter,[2] that is described in the notes in the display as follows: "An aneurysmal sac of an oval form, and about three fourths of an inch in its chief diameter, from the right internal carotid artery of a lady. It is nearly full of coagulum."

In 1800, Sir Gilbert Blane[3] reported that patient to be a 64-year-old woman who had been in good health until 5 years previously, when

[She] was suddenly seized with a fit of giddiness and dimness of sight, succeeded by acute pain in the forehead, which remained for some time. The indistinctness of vision continued for about six months.

After this she was at intervals seized with giddiness, headache, and imperfect vision. . . . [S]he continued to be subject, from time to time, to the above mentioned symptoms as long as she lived.

Without too much imagination, this could be interpreted as a description of transient ischemic episodes resulting from the clot in the carotid aneurysm.

John Hunter himself died of coronary artery disease, but the accounts of the last few months of his life suggest that he was also suffering from symptoms of intermittent cerebral ischemia; at his postmortem examination, the carotid arteries at the base of his skull were reported to be *ossified*, the term then used to describe what would soon be known as arteriosclerosis.[4, 5]

Surgical treatment of carotid artery lesions began with ligation of the carotid artery for aneurysmal disease or for trauma. Ligation was then done not to treat the distal emboli-

zation but rather to control the aneurysm itself. Sir Astley Cooper is credited with the first ligation for such an aneurysm in 1805.[6] In fact, however, a British naval surgeon, David Fleming, performed a ligation of the carotid artery in 1803, but his indication was the urgency of a bleeding carotid from a knife wound.[7] The second of Cooper's patients who underwent carotid ligation in 1808 did so well without blood flow through the ligated carotid that he finally died 13 years later from rupture of an intracranial aneurysm on the same side as the ligation. As Cooper phrased it, "The disease of which he died sufficiently attested to the freedom of the circulation as well as its force in the cerebral vessels on the side of which the carotid had been ligated."[6]

One of the early intriguing hints that more than we realize may have been known about the carotid artery is found in a description from 1835 by Barth, a French physician.[8] A report of the physical examination of one of the first patients recognized to have intermittent claudication caused by a thrombosis of the terminal aorta incidentally included the specific mention that "no murmurs were heard over the carotid arteries in the neck." Why should that particular item be noted in a physical examination at that time? One might wonder whether the early French neurologists might have had not only some inkling of the nature of occlusive diseases of the carotid artery but also some ideas as to the relationship between carotid disease and peripheral arteriosclerosis. It was only a few years earlier that it had become apparent that "senile gangrene" of the extremities was caused by proximal obstruction in the main arteries; until then, it had been thought that senile gangrene caused the vessels to become obstructed, so that there would not be excess bleeding when the gangrenous limb separated. The patient described by Barth was one of the first in whom a functional deficiency due to restriction of an arterial flow had been recognized—a blood flow that might be adequate at rest but that would not be adequate for activity. Was there also some recognition by these French physicians that a parallel phenomenon might exist between the carotid artery in the neck and the syndromes of cerebral ischemia?

An English physician exhibited a similar awareness. William Savory reported in detail in 1856[9] the case history of a 22-year-old woman with symptoms of debility, headache, episodic giddiness, and indistinct vision in the left eye. Physical examination revealed weak pulses at most stations, especially in the carotid arteries.[9] A bruit was present over the right carotid artery. After a progressive downhill course that lasted 13 months, the patient died. Postmortem examination showed diffuse lesions of the innominate, the right carotid, and the left carotid arteries. The arteries were contracted as well as thick-walled, and the right-sided vessels were completely occluded. Necrosis of the scalp and calvarium was found in the territory of the left external carotid, which was completely occluded. The other arteries were thickened and contracted; flow had been maintained only through very narrow lumina. Savory indicated in his report the probable relationship between deficient carotid blood flow and neurologic symptoms arising in the ipsilateral cerebral hemisphere.

MODERN UNDERSTANDING OF THE PATHOGENESIS OF CAROTID STROKE

Thrombi in the carotid sinus that could cause emboli were described by Chiari in 1905.[10] Given a patient at autopsy who had cerebral emboli for which no commonly recognized source could be found, Chiari opened the carotid artery along its full length and observed a thrombus on an ulcer at the bifurcation. This prompted him to examine the carotid arteries carefully in the next 400 autopsies. He observed gross thrombi on the walls of the carotid bifurcation in seven cases; in four of these patients, cerebral embolism had occurred.

Hunt[11] expressed an astute correlation in 1914 recommending that for all patients presenting with cerebral symptoms of a vascular nature, one should adopt "the same attitudes of mind toward this group of cases as toward the intermittent claudication, gangrene, and other vascular symptoms . . . ." He suggested that because the territory of the carotid in the neck seemed to fall between the jurisdiction of the neurologist and the surgeon, it was an area that was not ordinarily studied carefully during postmortem examination. Hunt also commented on the erroneous assumption that the circle of Willis is always adequate to provide collateral flow to the other side.

Fisher's thorough reports[12,13] repeated Hunt's admonitions, and he lamented the common failure of pathologists to examine the neck, for he believed that in occlusive lesions in the neck might be found the "major causes of apoplexy." While working at the Mallory Institute of Pathology, Fisher observed that in spite of the frequent clinical diagnosis of thrombosis of the middle cerebral artery, the morphologic lesion was not seen at autopsy. He reported eight cases in which occlusive disease of the arteries in the neck was diagnosed: four were proved at autopsy, two radiologically, and two on a clinical basis only. He then undertook a study that he reported 3 years later in which he had found 45 cases of total or almost total obstruction in one or both carotid arteries in a series of 432 autopsies. In 13 patients with stenoses, there were no physical findings, but there were 4 patients with cerebral emboli in whom thrombotic material was found at the bifurcation of the carotid. Fisher was astute enough to note that even the families of these asymptomatic patients had not recognized evidence of a "cerebral insult."

Based on personal experience in pathology in Boston in 1948, this author vividly remembers the sacrosanct character of the cervical carotid arteries in the postmortem examination room. They were carefully preserved and cannulated to enable the morticians to perform a more effective injection of embalming fluid for the face.

At that time, arteriography was the best way to study the carotid bifurcation, which is not so readily evaluated by external palpation as is commonly believed. It was not until Wilhelm Röntgen's findings were published in 1895 that workers began injecting material into the vessels of animals and cadavers to evaluate the anatomic relationships; by 1924, at least four investigators had injected contrast media into the blood vessels of living humans.[14–17] It was Egas Moniz of Lisbon who built on this fragmentary work and established on a firm basis the specialty of angiographic radiology,[18] which for several years focused only on the intracranial vessels.

Ten years later, Moniz and associates[19] published an account of thrombosis of the carotid artery reflecting that although this was thought to be a very unusual lesion, in fact they had found four cases of thrombosis on their first 537 angiograms. These investigators commented that had they performed arteriography on all patients with hemiplegia, they would very likely have found many more cases.

Moniz and colleagues went on to describe the clinical pattern of carotid thrombosis in these four patients. All had presented with hemiparesis or hemiplegia on the side opposite the thrombosis. In none of these patients, even those with severe aphasia, was the facial nerve more than minimally involved. Headaches occurred episodically, often long before the crisis that seemed to mark the onset of the thrombosis. There was fleeting paresthesia of the extremities, transient episodes of paresis that began in the upper extremity, occasional convulsions that were never major in nature, and aphasia when the left carotid artery was involved. In the psychological aspect of the patient there was an indifference; sometimes a euphoria toward this disease seemed characteristic. There was, however, no mention of visual disturbances in the discussion. None of the patients described the classic ipsilateral disturbances of vision as they are now understood, although one patient did have some diplopia. The authors ended their comments as follows:

In conclusion, there is a hemiplegia caused by thrombosis of the internal carotid in patients, not very old, presenting in general prodromal symptoms which we have just described. These symptoms are sufficient to suspect the etiology of a hemiplegia. Cerebral angiography will always provide a certainty of diagnosis.

The original angiographic approach of Moniz required direct puncture of the carotid artery. The final words of his first paper indicated a great need for improvement in the technical aspects of radiography. One of the great advances that was to improve the radiologic diagnosis was the technique used by Seldinger,[20] which permitted selective injection of the arteries in the region of the bifurcation as well as full pictures of the aortic arch. Digital subtraction angiography carried radiologic diagnosis one leap further.[21] Further refinements in diagnostic methods will be discussed later in this chapter.

Attempts to understand the natural history of cerebrovascular disease continue. Many important advances have been made in the neuromedical aspects, which have a direct bearing on the surgical considerations. Important inter-relationships have been found between the observations at and after surgical operation and the results of that operation and the medical course of the patient.

In a two-part presentation, Millikan and Siekert[22, 23] defined the syndromes of carotid and of vertebrobasilar insufficiency. The report to the National Research Council (London) by Yates and Hutchinson[24] indicated that (1) there was a very high degree of error in the diagnosis of cerebral ischemia, even in a sophisticated neurology service; and (2) almost all the patients who did suffer from cerebral ischemia were found at autopsy to have extracranial occlusions of their carotid or vertebral vessels. There were 74 separate infarcts distributed among 35 patients, and major stenoses or complete occlusions of the extracranial arteries were found in 32 of 35 patients with infarcts. Only 22 of the total 74 cerebral infarcts were related to intracranial arterial stenoses.

Many investigators have contributed to the knowledge of the epidemiology, the natural history, and the patterns of intermittent cerebral ischemia, thus defining the neurologic syndrome that Hunt had likened to intermittent claudication caused by peripheral arterial occlusive disease.[25-28]

Hollenhorst's report[27] on the significance of bright plaques in the retinal arterioles gave rise to recognition of a common clinical sign and an important eponym. The joint studies of extracranial disease were especially helpful in all their formats.[30, 31]

Anticoagulant and antiplatelet treatment based on the observations described in the previous paragraph at one point seemed to offer a hopeful form of therapy, but a series of prospective studies[32-36] presented some conflicting and questionable evidence for the value of these antiplatelet agents.

The relative roles played by ischemia in the specific territory of one major artery as opposed to the role played by recurrent small, even microscopic, emboli from a diseased carotid bulb were not defined clearly until well into the era of surgical intervention. Although the previously mentioned atheromatous carotid bifurcation displayed by John Hunter contained an ulcer, and although Chiari and others had noted specific instances of embolism large enough to be clearly related to the lesion in the neck, the first real clarification of the role of emboli in the common clinical picture of cerebral ischemia was clarified by Julian and his group[37] and then restated by Moore and Hall.[38]

Further understanding of the role of hemorrhage within the plaque came from Imparato and colleagues in 1979.[39] Hemorrhage within the plaque had been assumed as a rule to result from dissection behind the plaque, but Imparato and associates demonstrated that a sudden increase in the size of the plaque could arise spontaneously. Lusby and associates[40] carried the understanding of plaque one step further, noting that when such hemorrhage broke through the plaque, and the material was discharged, an atheromatous ulcer was the end result; that discharge of the material within the plaque could be one embolic episode; and that further accretion of platelets and clots could perpetuate the process of embolization.

SURGICAL THERAPY

The first considerations of therapeutic endeavors other than ligation of the carotid artery came at the end of the 19th century, when Alexis Carrel, having accomplished successful anastomoses of the carotid artery to the jugular vein in the dog[41] (an experimental model chosen because of its potential for high rates of flow), gave in to flights of fancy that suggested that such an operation might accomplish an increase of blood flow to the brain and therefore could be used to treat a variety of diseases, including microcephaly and other disturbances more clearly related to diminished blood supply. This consideration of the use of carotid-jugular shunts persisted until the 1950s, when several such opera-

tions were performed for ischemic brain syndromes at the instigation of the neurology service at Wadsworth Veterans Administration Hospital. In 1953, De Sousa Pereira[42] discussed the several modalities available at the time for the treatment of internal carotid thrombosis. These approaches included resection of the vessel, attempted thrombectomy, and attempted graft. In addition, three patients received carotid-jugular shunts, two of which had to be taken down promptly because of exacerbation of the symptoms; the third patient showed no improvement, and De Sousa Pereira was convinced that this method diminished carotid flow.

Lack of consensus for one definitive surgical approach led to the continued application of these many possible procedures, which were well outlined by Gurdjian and coworkers[43] as late as 1965, with a summary of results that was most discouraging. Their conclusions that patients did as well without surgery as with it did little to make carotid surgery popular with neurologists. Gurdjian and associates still listed as therapeutic possibilities cervical sympathectomy and the resection of the bifurcation, as well as endarterectomy.

The first hopeful surgical approach consistent with the concept of direct surgical intervention was that of Carrea and coworkers.[44] In 1951 they performed an anastomosis between the internal and external carotid arteries for a spontaneous thrombosis of the common carotid artery with moderately good results. They had observed seven patients with this problem during the preceding 4 years; in all seven cases, the bifurcation of the artery had been excised, and in five cases cervical sympathectomy had been accomplished, in deference to the concept taught by Leriche concerning arteriectomy and sympathectomy. Carrea and coworkers performed the carotid-carotideal anastomosis in one patient on the basis of a suggestion by Fisher.[12]

Better justification for the operation by Carrea and associates is in the French literature. A report by a French surgeon, LeFèvre,[45] describes an identical procedure for an acute injury of the carotid bulb. Recognizing a risk of cerebrovascular accident in his experience of four of five cases in which ligation of the three carotid arteries had been performed, and citing also that, in his experience, only 1 of 15 patients with late ligations suffered cerebrovascular accidents, he reasoned that restoration of flow through the external carotid system into the internal carotid would more than likely behave like the delayed ligation, even if thrombosis supervened later. LeFèvre chose to carry out this anastomosis instead of interposing a vein graft because it involved one suture line instead of two and because of the risk of instability of the vein graft in the presence of contamination. His patient did well.

The next important step was the publication of a case reported by Eastcott and associates.[46] Their patient had suffered a series of transient ischemic episodes, for which she had undergone resection of the carotid bulb, where there was an atheromatous lesion with nearly complete obstruction of flow to the internal carotid artery. The internal carotid artery was anastomosed to the distal end of the common carotid artery; full flow was restored, and recovery followed.

Following Eastcott's lead, Denman and associates[47] excised a completely thrombosed carotid bifurcation and replaced it with a lyophilized arterial homograft in the summer of 1954. Six months later they repeated the operation on the patient's other side.

In fact, DeBakey and associates had done a carotid endarterectomy on August 7, 1953, but it was not reported until much later.[48] Strully and colleagues[49] had attempted an endarterectomy in 1953 but could not obtain retrograde flow from the cranial end of the vessel. In the fall of 1955, Rowe[50] performed the second successful carotid endarterectomy, and in March of 1956, Cooley, Al-Namaan, and Carton[51] performed the third. It should be recognized that the intent of these three operations was as much as to extend and explore the possibilities of endarterectomy to new anatomic areas as it was to seriously embark on the treatment of stroke, although the report from Cooley's group did appear in the *Journal of Neurosurgery*.

The choice of whether to perform an endarterectomy or a grafting procedure was not a clear one. In 1957, Lyons and Galbraith[52] reported on six patients, five of whom had undergone exploration of the carotid bifurcation and the placement of a nylon shunt into the internal carotid artery from the common carotid or the subclavian artery.

The techniques of carotid artery operations became standardized during the 1960s, with Thompson and Austin,[53] Movius and associates,[54] Wylie and Ehrenfeld,[55] and Julian and associates[37] providing the basic patterns. There are still several areas of disagreement.

The use of a shunt, for instance, remains controversial; some surgeons almost always use a shunt,[56–58] some almost never,[59] and some only on a selective basis.[60–62] A common indicator in the decision of whether to use a shunt is the measurement of the pressure in the cranial side of the occluded internal carotid artery, as described by Moore and Hall.[60]

Other investigators, such as Connolly,[62] depend on the patient's ability to respond while under local anesthesia.

The choice of anesthesia remains a controversial area. A general anesthetic agent is preferred by many surgeons because of the belief that the agents used may protect the brain against hypoxia and because of the premise that the anesthesiologist has better physical and physiologic control of the patient.[63] At the same time, many surgeons who do use a general anesthetic fall back on some procedure to assure themselves that there is adequate cerebral perfusion, such as the use of an indwelling shunt as decided by preliminary stump pressures,[60] specific jugular oxygen tension,[64] and electroencephalographic (EEG) monitoring.[65] Many choose local anesthesia because it allows the surgeon a better appraisal of the cerebral responses of the patient when the carotid artery is cross-clamped.

Despite the original belief that the primary problem in carotid atherosclerosis was hydrodynamic, which had given way to the conclusion that multiple small emboli were the source of the cerebral symptoms, the surgeon who uses local anesthesia and patient responses relies on hydrodynamic factors to prove the absence of a need for a shunt.

In the natural history of any area such as cerebrovascular disease, the surgeon originally gets to treat only the most difficult category of patients, namely, those who seem doomed according to the criteria of any other therapy. So it was that some of the first patients who underwent carotid reconstruction had complete occlusions of the carotid bifurcation. Another group with a poor prognosis included those

patients who had just suffered a completed stroke. It was soon recognized that there was not great benefit in operating on those patients with a complete occlusion of the carotid instead of being able to make the diagnosis early enough to operate during the stage of stenosis.[66] Furthermore, with time, the poor results of surgery in patients with acute strokes led Thompson and associates[67] and Wylie and associates[68] to recommend against surgery at the time of complete occlusion. A consensus has developed, well stated by Javid,[58] that carotid surgery should be performed in an attempt to forestall strokes, and that usually those patients with transient ischemic episodes had declared themselves the best candidates for surgery.

More in dispute, however, became the entire issue of whether surgical therapy was of benefit to any patients. The issue seems to have been resolved with regard to symptomatic patients on the basis of the North American Symptomatic Study[69] and the European Carotid Group,[70] whose reports indicate clear benefit in clearly defined sets of patients, which are those most commonly seen. Further studies are needed to delineate the value of surgical treatment in subgroups of patients with and without symptoms.

The next step in this progression of thinking was the identification of patients who might be at risk, even though they had not yet shown transient neurologic deficits, because not in every instance is a frank stroke preceded by such warning signals. Thompson and colleagues[71] remain the strongest advocates for this approach to operation for the asymptomatic patient in whose neck a bruit can be heard, although the identification of a bruit is not as accurate a measure as some of the noninvasive testing described in the following paragraphs.

The combined presence of extracranial arterial obstruction and serious obstructive arterial disease in other areas was recognized 150 years ago. The most critical factor affecting mortality after successful cerebrovascular reconstructions remains the status of the coronary arterial tree. This poses several problems: When does one operate on the carotid arteries first and then proceed to the coronary arteries (or the abdominal aneurysm or other site), and when does one perform the coronary or aneurysm operation first? In what situations should both operations be accomplished at the same time? Bernhard and associates[72] were among the first to approach this problem in an aggressive manner. In a series of 15 patients who needed both coronary and carotid operations and who underwent surgery to the carotid artery first, 3 patients suffered fatal myocardial infarction before they could have their coronary operation. The next 16 patients with combined disease were operated on for both lesions simultaneously. These patients suffered minimal morbidity and no mortality. Since then, a large body of experience on this topic has developed.

Fibromuscular hyperplasia first became known as a lesion of an important obstructing nature in the renal arteries, but in 1965 Connett and Lansche[73] described this lesion in the carotid artery, and in 1967 Ehrenfeld and associates[74] made their first report on the surgical treatment of this important process.

Another form of obstruction to flow through the internal carotid artery is caused by elongation and kinking of the artery, so that flow is shut off just as it is when one kinks a garden hose. Elongation and coiling alone do not cause significant problems. Najafi and coworkers[75] identified this lesion and called attention to the several ways in which the vessel can be straightened; one can divide the tethering external carotid and shorten the common carotid artery by resection and end-to-end anastomosis, or one can shorten the internal carotid artery itself. The latter technique is perhaps more difficult because of the small size of the vessel and its relative inaccessibility, but there is often a small ulceration at the apex of the kink that may justify that approach.

Major problems still faced the surgeon who was dealing with a completely obstructed internal carotid artery. The distal end of the obstruction often lay in the carotid siphon area, and removal from that area was exceedingly difficult. Blaisdell and associates[76] attempted to solve this problem by injecting saline between the clot and the artery wall to loosen the clot, an approach that met with some success. Attempts to use the Fogarty catheter to displace a clot at the level of the siphon were met with near-catastrophe when the manipulation produced carotid–cavernous sinus fistulas; this occurred at two widely separated centers, which led them to combine their failures into one warning report.[77]

With the advent of microvascular techniques, which were introduced to peripheral vascular surgeons by Yasargil and coworkers,[78] a more direct reconstruction has become practicable between the major branches of the external carotid artery, such as the superficial temporal branch, by means of direct anastomosis or even the use of a vein graft to turn the flow into a cerebral vessel exposed through a small craniotomy. Chater and Popp[79] reported on 100 such cases; the best results were in those patients who were experiencing transient ischemic episodes or reversible ischemic neurologic deficits, and the worst were in those with completed strokes.

VERTEBROBASILAR DISEASE

Extracranial vascular disease of surgical significance usually is found in the carotid artery, but the other major arteries of the brachiocephalic system are also involved. In March 1954, Davis and coworkers[80] performed the first innominate endarterectomy in a 51-year-old man who had a constellation of symptoms of a more global nature: dizziness, blurring of vision, and diplopia; syncope on assumption of the erect posture; transient slight weakness of the arms and legs of several years' duration; numbness of the right hand for 2 years; intermittent claudication; and memory loss. It is hard to separate some of the peripheral arterial symptoms from the central neurologic effects of the occlusion of the innominate artery. Adequate and safe endarterectomy of the innominate and subclavian vessels was a difficult procedure. Even simple ligation of the left subclavian was a feat that had successfully evaded surgeons until William Stewart Halsted performed it in 1921.[81] It was another year and a half after Davis and associates' innominate endarterectomy before Warren and Treiman[82] performed another successful operation on the innominate artery. DeBakey's group in Houston soon carried out the first of a series of bypasses—the first one from the innominate artery to a distal implantation on the carotid and subclavian arteries[83]—and went on to demonstrate the versatility of the use of prosthetic grafts as bypasses to almost any site in the neck and brachial regions.[84]

The first more direct approach to any lesion of the vertebral artery other than an aneurysm, such as Matas had done in 1888,[85] was achieved by Cate and Scott,[86] who used endarterectomy to disobstruct the left subclavian and left vertebral arteries.

In similar clinical situations involving vertebrobasilar insufficiency, it has been noted that the combination of arterial inflow obstructions in the anterior and posterior parts of the brain is often completely relieved by an adequate restoration of flow through no more than the stenotic carotid system, given an adequate connection through the circle of Willis.[87] The hazards of the completely obstructed carotid artery take two forms. In the first there is the possibility of further thrombosis extending into the cerebral circulation; this risk currently seems uncontrollable except by means of anticoagulants. Second, further spillage of thrombi into the external carotid system from a cul-de-sac at the cervical orifice of the internal carotid has been managed, as reported by Hertzer,[88] by the division of the termination of the internal carotid artery flush with the remaining external channel to eliminate the pocket.

At the same time, an external carotid endarterectomy may be performed as well, because the external carotid artery can serve as an important source of collateral blood supply to the brain through its many collateral anastomoses with the most distal parts of the internal carotid through temporal, occipital, supraorbital, and other anastomotic networks. This justifies the attempts to restore flow through the external carotid artery by endarterectomy in the presence of symptomatic internal carotid occlusion.[89]

An intriguing hemodynamic principle was identified by Reivich and associates,[90] the subclavian "steal." An obstruction of the subclavian artery proximal to the origin of the vertebral vessels causes a reversal of blood flow down the vertebral artery and out of the total reservoir of intracranial arterial blood. In such a situation, blood flow to the posterior part of the brain can be reduced during exercise of the arm or by pharmacologic means that reduce the peripheral resistance in the affected arm. Although this phenomenon is commonly seen radiologically, it is an uncommon source of symptoms without the presence of other important obstructions to the inflow of the total cranial system. The cogent words of Jesse Thompson, one of the most distinguished carotid surgeons, seem very well to sum up this discussion[91]:

The eventual definition of the precise role of surgery in the management of cerebrovascular insufficiency must await the outcome of further studies, but it may be safely said at this time that surgical measures have already demonstrated their effectiveness in many patients with stroke syndromes.

NONINVASIVE METHODS OF DIAGNOSIS

A final chapter needs to be added to the history of noninvasive diagnosis, which began with the use of the stethoscope, as was indicated regarding Barth's patient.[8] The next major noninvasive method was ophthalmodynamometry, introduced by Baillart in 1917.[92] This method involved attempts to determine the amount of pressure on the ocular globe that would be necessary to obliterate retinal arteries—in other words, a measurement of the retinal arterial pressure. It was introduced for reasons relating to ophthalmology rather than neurology, but the method became important when it was realized that the ophthalmic artery is the last main branch of the internal carotid artery. It was an important concept, but the test was not easily performed and was highly operator-sensitive.

The use of the ultrasonic Doppler signal and measurement of the Doppler shift as occasioned by reflections from the blood cells in a vessel was introduced by Strandness and associates[93] and was soon modified by Brockenbrough[94] to evaluate reversal of flow in the supraorbital artery, a phenomenon that occurs when there is a major obstruction to the flow to the distal internal carotid artery. Under these circumstances, the rich collateralization by way of the superficial temporal artery and its anastomoses with the supraorbital artery, as well as many others, results in flow from the superficial temporal branch actually refilling the ophthalmic system and even the cerebral system on the side of the obstruction. Machleder and Barker[95] used this test to signal the frequency with which the diagnosis of internal carotid artery obstruction was being overlooked. The investigators commented on the reluctance to recognize that anomalous symptoms from the ipsilateral cortex in relation to a unilateral carotid bruit might only mean that the other carotid artery was completely obstructed, hence the title, "Stroke on the Wrong Side." This test has also turned out to be so highly operator-sensitive that it has come to have little value except in the hands of those who are very skillful and careful with it.

The use of the Doppler phenomenon in a different manner was introduced by Thomas and associates in 1974.[96] A scanning device was attached to a Doppler probe, and the subsequent images were displayed in a permanent form. The initial form of this device has been modified and improved, but there is still considerable operator sensitivity. Combining the usual ultrasonic B-mode scanning with a Doppler sensor that can read signals from a spot marked on the imaging screen permits evaluation of the quality of the content of the Doppler signal by various methods and has allowed the determination of the nature of the turbulence at an exact spot within the lumen of a vessel.[97]

These methods of evaluating the circulation noninvasively are complemented by two methods of evaluating the flow in the ophthalmic-retinal artery system. The first method, ocular plethysmography, traces the pressure waves within the eye and compares the time of arrival of the peak of the wave on the two sides with the measurement from a presumably neutral sensor on the earlobe.[98] An obstruction in the arterial tree causes a delay in the arrival of the pulse wave, and the difference between the curves representing the two eyes is presented as a third tracing. The second method, ocular pneumoplethysmography,[99] measures the minute pressure changes within small suction cups applied to the optic globe, as a high degree of negative pressure within them is returned to normal. The negative pressure is sufficient to distort the globe enough to occlude the arterial flow. As the pressure is diminished in the globe, systolic pressure waves appear and are read and calibrated to give a measurement of the ophthalmic artery pressure. Both techniques are useful within their limitations, but each reads a different physiologic parameter. These methods, however, apply primarily to the

carotid system; as yet, no reliable noninvasive monitor of the vertebrobasilar system has been introduced.

These indirect methods, however useful they have been during the historical development of arterial surgery, have been largely replaced by the duplex scanning methods, which offer not only anatomic but also physiologic information concerning the carotid artery. Many surgeons have come to rely so heavily on the information provided by the duplex scan that it threatens to replace conventional arteriography as the prime diagnostic modality in carotid disease.

Contrast arteriography itself, despite improvements in subtraction techniques and the like, is also threatened by the anatomic demonstrations made possible by computerized magnetic resonance scanning. These techniques are still in their infancy, but the quality of the anatomic information provided by them in other areas of the body[100] promises similar valuable anatomic information in the carotid and vertebral systems.

REFERENCES

1. Hunterian Museum, Royal College of Surgeons (England). Specimen P. 1171.
2. Hunterian Museum, Royal College of Surgeons (England). Specimen P. 282.
3. Blane Sir G: (No title given). *Transactions of a Society for the Improvement of Medical and Chirurgical Knowledge.* London. 1800;2:192.
4. Dobson J: *John Hunter.* Edinburgh: E & S Livingstone Ltd; 1969.
5. Gray EA: *Portrait of a surgeon. A biography of John Hunter.* London: Robert Hale Ltd; 1952.
6. Lord Brock: Astley Cooper and carotid artery ligation. *Guy's Hospital Reports (Special Number).* 1968;117:219–224.
7. Keevil JJ: David Fleming and the operation for ligation of the carotid artery. *Br J Surg.* 1949;37:92–95.
8. Barth (no initial given): Observations d'une oblitération complèt de l'aorte abdominale, recuillie dans le service de Monsieur Louis, suivie de réelections. *Archiv Gén Méd,* Second Series. 1835; VIII:26–52.
9. Savory WS: Case of a young woman in whom the main arteries of both upper extremities and of the left side of the neck were throughout completely obliterated. *Med-Chir Tr, London,* 1856;39:205–219.
10. Chiari H: Ueber Verhalten der Teilungswinkels der Carotis communis bei der Endarteritis chronica deformans. *Verh Dtsch Path Ges.* 1905;9:326–330.
11. Hunt JR: The role of the carotid arteries in the causation of vascular lesions of the brain with remarks on certain special features of the symptomatology. *Am J Med Sci.* 1914;147:704–713.
12. Fisher M: Occlusion of the internal carotid artery. *Arch Neurol Psychiatry.* 1951;65:346–377.
13. Fisher M: Occlusion of the carotid arteries. *Arch Neurol Psychiatry.* 1954;72:187–204.
14. Heuser C: Pieloradiografía con ioduro potásico y las injecionnes intravenosas en radiografía. *Sem Med (Buenos Aires).* 1919;26:424–430.
15. Berberich J, Hirsch S: Die röntgenographische Darstellung der Arterien und Venen am lebenden Menschen. *Klin Wochenschr.* 1923;2:2226–2228.
16. Sicard J, Forestier G: Iodized oil in diagnosis and therapeutics. *Bull Mém Soc Méd Hôp Paris.* 1923;47:309–314.
17. Brooks B: Intra-arterial injection of sodium iodide. *JAMA.* 1924;82:1016–1019.
18. Moniz E: L'encéphalographie artérielle, son importance dans la localization des tumeurs cérébrales. *Rev Neurol (Paris).* 1927;2:272–290.
19. Moniz E, Lima A, de Lacerda R: Hémiplegies par thrombose de la carotide interne. *Presse Mèd.* 1937;45:977–980.
20. Seldinger SI: Catheter replacement of the needle in percutaneous angiography. *Acta Radiol.* 1953;39:368–376.
21. Kruger RA, Mistretta CA, Crummy AB, et al.: Digital K-Edge subtraction radiography. *Radiology.* 1977;125:243–245.
22. Millikan CH, Siekert RG: Studies in cerebrovascular disease. I. The syndrome of intermittent insufficiency of the basilar artery system. *Proc Staff Meet Mayo Clin.* 1955;30:61–68.
23. Millikan CH, Siekert RG: Studies in cerebrovascular disease. II. The syndrome of intermittent insufficiency of the carotid artery system. *Proc Staff Meet Mayo Clin.* 1955;30:186–191.
24. Yates PO, Hutchinson EC: Cerebral infarction: the role of stenosis of the extracranial arteries. *Med Res Counc Spec Rep (London).* 1961;300:1–95.
25. Marshall J, Meadows S. The natural history of amaurosis fugax. *Brain.* 1968;91:419–434.
26. Acheson J, Hutchinson EC: Observations on the natural history of transient cerebral ischaemia. *Lancet.* 1964; ii:871–874.
27. Marshall J: The natural history of transient ischaemic cerebrovascular attacks. *Quart J Med.* 1964;33:309–324.
28. Whisnant JP, Matsumoto N, Eiveback LR: Transient cerebral ischemic attacks

in a community: Rochester, Minnesota, 1955–1969. *Mayo Clin Proc.* 1973; 48:194–198.

29. Hollenhorst RW: Significance of bright plaques in the retinal arterioles. *JAMA.* 1961;178:23–29.

30. Lyons C: Progress report of the joint study of extracranial artery occlusion of the internal carotid artery. In Millikan CH, Siekert RG, Whisnant JP, eds. *Cerebrovascular Diseases.* New York: Grune & Stratton; 1965;266.

31. Fields WS: Surgery for occlusive cerebrovascular disease: Progress report of the joint study of extracranial artery occlusion of the internal carotid artery. In Millikan CH, Siekert RG, Whisnant JP, eds. *Cerebrovascular Diseases.* New York: Grune & Stratton; 1966;245.

32. Baker RN, Broward JA, Fang HC, et al: Anticoagulant therapy in cerebral infarction: Report on cooperative study. *Neurology.* 1962;12:823–825.

33. Millikan CH: Therapeutic agents—current status: Anticoagulant therapy in cerebrovascular disease. In Millikan CH, Siekert RG, Whisnant JP, eds. *Cerebral Vascular Diseases.* New York: Grune and Stratton, 1965;181–184.

34. The Canadian Cooperative Study Group: A randomized trial of aspirin and sulfinpyrazone in threatened stroke. *N Engl J Med.* 1978;299:53–59.

35. Fields WS, Lemak NA, Frankowski RF, Hardy RJ: Controlled study of aspirin in cerebral ischemia. *Circulation.* 1980;62(V):V-90.

36. Fields WS, Lemak NA, Frankowski RF, et al: Controlled study of aspirin in cerebral ischemia. Part II: Surgical group. *Stroke.* 1978;9:309–318.

37. Julian OC, Dye WS, Javid H, Hunter JA: Ulcerative lesions of the carotid artery. *Arch Surg.* 1963;86:803–809.

38. Moore WS, Hall AJ: Ulcerated atheroma of the carotid artery: A cause of transient cerebral ischemia. *Am J Surg.* 1969;116:237–242.

39. Imparato AM, Riles TJ, Gorstein F: The carotid bifurcation plaque: pathologic findings associated with cerebral ischemia. *Stroke.* 1979;10:238–245.

40. Lusby RJ, Ferrell LD, Ehrenfeld WE, et al: Carotid plaque hemorrhage: Its role in production of cerebral ischemia. *Arch Surg.* 1982;117:1479–1488.

41. Carrel A: Les anastomoses vasculaires et leur technique operatoire. *Union Méd Can.* 1904–05;8:29–32.

42. De Sousa Pereira A: Surgical treatment of internal carotid thrombosis. *Ann Surg.* 1955;141:218–233.

43. Gurdjian ES, Darmody WR, Lindner DW, Thomas LM: Fate of patients with carotid and vertebral artery surgery for stenosis or obstruction. *Surg Gynecol Obstet.* 1965;121:326–330.

44. Carrea R, Molins M, Murphy G: Surgical treatment of spontaneous thrombosis of the internal carotid artery in the neck. Carotid-carotideal anastomosis. Report of a case. *Acta Neurol Latinoamer.* 1955;1:71–78.

45. LeFévre H: Sur un cas de plaie du bulbe carotidien per balle, traitée par la ligature de la carotid primitive, et l'anastomose bout à bout de la carotid externe avec la carotid interne. *Bull Mém Soc Chir.* 1918;44:923–928.

46. Eastcott HHG, Pickering GW, Rob C: Reconstruction of internal carotid artery in a patient with intermittent attacks of hemiplegia. *Lancet.* 1954; ii:994–996.

47. Denman FR, Ehni G, Duty WS: Insidious thrombotic occlusion of cervical carotid arteries, treated by arterial graft, a case report. *Surgery.* 1955;38:569–577.

48. DeBakey ME: Successful carotid endarterectomy for cerebrovascular insufficiency: Nineteen year follow-up. *JAMA.* 1975;233:1083–1085.

49. Strully KJ, Hurwitt ES, Blankenberg H: Thromboendarterectomy for thrombosis of the internal carotid artery in the neck. *J Neurosurg.* 1953;10:474–482.

50. Rowe WF: An early successful carotid endarterectomy, not previously reported. Presented at the Annual meeting of the Southern California Vascular Surgical Society; September 18, 1993; Coronado, CA.

51. Cooley DA, Al-Naaman YD, Carton CA: Surgical treatment of arteriosclerotic occlusion of the common carotid artery. *J Neurosurg.* 1956;13:500–506.

52. Lyons C, Galbraith G: Surgical treatment of atherosclerotic occlusion of the internal carotid artery. *Ann Surg.* 1957;146:487–498.

53. Thompson JE, Austin DJ: Surgical treatment of arteriosclerotic occlusions in the neck. *Surgery.* 1954;51:74–83.

54. Movius HJ, Zuber WF, Gaspar MR: Carotid thromboendarterectomy. *Arch Surg.* 1967;94:585–591.

55. Wylie EJ Jr, Ehrenfeld WK: *Extracranial Occlusive Cerebrovascular Disease: Diagnosis and Management.* Philadelphia: WB Saunders; 1970.

56. Thompson JE: Cerebrovascular insufficiency. In Barker WF, ed. *Peripheral Arterial Disease,* 2nd ed. Philadelphia: WB Saunders, 1975;254–302.

57. Movius HJ: Cerebrovascular insufficiency. In Gaspar MR, Barker WF, eds. *Peripheral Arterial Disease,* 3rd ed. Philadelphia: WB Saunders; 1981;330–382.

58. Javid H: Can surgery prevent stroke? *Surgery.* 1966;59:1147–1153.

59. Whitney DJ, Kahn EM, Estes JW, Jones CE: Carotid artery surgery without a temporary indwelling shunt. *Arch Surg.* 1980;115:1393–1399.

60. Moore WS, Hall AD: Carotid artery back pressure: a test of cerebral tolerance to temporary carotid occlusion. *Arch Surg.* 1969;99:702–710.

61. Moore WS, Quiñones-Baldrich WJ. In Moore WS, ed, *Vascular Surgery: A Comprehensive Review,* 2nd ed. New York: Grune & Stratton; 1966;881.

62. Connolly JE: Carotid endarterectomy in the awake patient. *Am J Surg.* 1985;150:159–165.

63. Wells BA, Keats AS, Cooley DA: Increased tolerance to cerebral ischemia produced by general anesthesia during temporary carotid occlusion. *Surgery.* 1963;54:216–223.

64. Larson CP, Ehrenfeld WK, Wade JG, Wylie EJ: Jugular venous saturation as an index of adequacy of cerebral oxygenation. *Surgery.* 1967;62:31–39.

65. Baker JD, Gluecklick B, Watson CW, et al: An evaluation of electroencephalographic monitoring for carotid surgery. *Surgery.* 1975;78:787–794.

66. Rob C: The surgery at the stage of arterial stenosis. *J Cardiovasc Surg.* 1961;2:95–96.

67. Thompson JE, Austin DJ, Patman RD: Endarterectomy of the completely occluded carotid artery for stroke. *Arch Surg.* 1962;95:791–801.

68. Wylie EJ, Hein MF, Adams JE. Intracranial hemorrhage following surgical revascularization for the treatment of acute strokes. *J Neurosurg.* 1963;21:212–215.

69. North American Symptomatic Carotid Endarterectomy Trial Collaborators: Beneficial effect of carotid endarterectomy in symptomatic patients with high-grade carotid stenosis. *N Engl J Med.* 1991;325:445–523.

70. European Carotid Surgery Trialists' Collaborative Group: MRS European Carotid Surgery Trial: interim results for symptomatic patients with severe (70–90%) or with mild (0–29%) carotid stenosis. *Lancet.* 1991;337:1235–1243.

71. Thompson JE, Patman RD, Talkington CM: Asymptomatic carotid bruit. *Ann Surg.* 1978;188:308–316.

72. Bernhard VM, Johnson WD, Peterson JJ: Carotid artery stenosis: Association with surgery for coronary artery disease. *Arch Surg.* 1972;105:837–840.

73. Connett MC, Lansche JM: Fibromuscular hyperplasia of the internal carotid artery. Report of a case. *Ann Surg.* 1965;162:59–62.

74. Ehrenfeld WK, Stoney RJ, Wylie EJ: Fibromuscular hyperplasia of the internal carotid artery. *Arch Surg.* 1967;95:284–287.

75. Najafi H, Javid H, Dye WS, et al: Kinked internal carotid artery: Clinical evaluation and surgical correction. *Arch Surg.* 1964;89:134–143.

76. Blaisdell FW, Hall AD, Thomas AN: Surgical treatment of chronic internal carotid artery occlusion by saline endarterectomy. *Ann Surg.* 1968;163:103–111.

77. Barker WF, Stern WE, Krayenbuhl H, Senning A: Carotid endarterectomy complicated by carotid cavernous sinus fistula. *Ann Surg.* 1968;167:567–572.

78. Yasargil MG, Krayenbuhl H, Jacobson JH: Microneurosurgical arterial reconstruction. *Surgery.* 1970;67:221–233.

79. Chater N, Popp J: Microsurgical vascular bypass for occlusive cerebrovascular disease: Review of 100 cases. *Surg Neurol.* 1976;6:115–118.

80. Davis JB, Grove WJ, Julian OC: Thrombotic occlusion of the branches of the aortic arch. Martorell's syndrome: Report of a case treated surgically. *Ann Surg.* 1956;144:124–126.

81. Halsted WS: Ligations of the left subclavian artery in its first portion. *Johns Hopkins Hosp Bull.* 1921;21:1–96.

82. Warren R, Treiman LJ: Pulseless disease and carotid-artery thrombosis. *N Engl J Med.* 1957;257:685–690.

83. DeBakey ME, Morris GC Jr, Jordan GL Jr, Cooley DA: Segmental thromboobliterative disease of the branches of the aortic arch. *JAMA.* 1958;166:998–1002.

84. DeBakey ME, Crawford ES, Cooley DA, Morris GC Jr: Surgical considerations of occlusive disease of the innominate, carotid and subclavian arteries. *Ann Surg.* 1959;149:690–710.

85. Cohn I: *Rudolph Matas.* Garden City, NY: Doubleday and Co; 1960.

86. Cate WR Jr, Scott HW Jr: Cerebral ischemia of central origin: Relief by subclavian-vertebral artery thromboendarterectomy. *Surgery.* 1959;45:19–31.

87. Rosenthal D, Cossman D, Ledig C, Callow AD: Results of carotid endarterectomy for vertebrobasilar insufficiency. *Arch Surg.* 1978;113:1361–1364.

88. Hertzer NR: External carotid endarterectomy. *Surg Gynec Obstet.* 1981;153:186–190.

89. Connolly JE, Stemmer EA: Endarterectomy of the external carotid artery. *Arch Surg.* 1973;106:799–802.

90. Reivich MH, Holling HE, Roberts B, Toole JF: Reversal of blood flow through the vertebral artery and its effect on the cerebral circulation. *N Engl J Med.* 1961;265:878–885.

91. Thompson JE: *Surgery for Cerebrovascular Insufficiency (Stroke).* Springfield, IL: Charles C Thomas; 1968.

92. Baillart P: Circulation artérielle rétinienne: Essais de détermination de la tension artérielle dans les branches de l'artère centrale de la rétine. *Ann d'Occul (Paris).* 1917;257–271.

93. Strandness DE, Schults RD, Sumner DS, Rushmer DF: Ultrasonic flow detection: A useful technique in the evaluation of peripheral vascular disease. *Arch Surg.* 1967;113:311–320.

94. Brockenbrough EC: Screening for prevention of stroke: Use of a Doppler flowmeter. Washington/Alaska Regional Medical Program, Information and Resource Unit, 1969.

95. Machleder HI, Barker WF: Stroke on the wrong side: Use of the Doppler ophthalmic test in cerebrovascular screening. *Arch Surg.* 1972;105:943–947.

96. Thomas GI, Spencer MD, Jones TW, et al: Noninvasive carotid bifurcation mapping: Its relation to carotid surgery. *Am J Surg.* 1974;128:164–174.

97. Barber FE, Baker DW, Nation AWC, et al: Ultrasonic duplex echo-Doppler scanner. *IEEE Trans Biomed Eng.* 1974;21:109–113.

98. Kartchner MM, McRae LP, Morrison FD: Oculoplethysmography in the diagnosis of extracranial carotid occlusive disease. *Arch Surg.* 1973;106:528–535.

99. Gee W, Mehigan JI, Wylie EJ: Measurement of collateral hemispheric blood pressure by ocular pneumoplethysmography. *Am J Surg.* 1975;130:121–127.

100. Rubin GD, Walker PJ, Dake MD, et al: Three-dimensional spiral computed tomographic angiography: An alternative imaging modality for the abdominal aorta and its branches. *J Vasc Surg.* 1993;18:656–665.

I

Epidemiology and Population at Risk

Morbidity and Mortality of Stroke

J. P. MOHR and R. L. SACCO

Stroke remains the third most common cause of death in the United States and is the leader in causes of disability.[1] Worldwide, its incidence approaches 180 cases per 100,000 deaths per year and its prevalence is roughly 500 to 600 per 100,000. All forms of stroke included, 8 to 20 percent of patients die in the first 30 days. Among survivors, early recurrence adds to the neurologic deficit and lengthens hospital stay. Late recurrence affects 4 to 14 percent of patients per year. Overall, the 5-year survival rate averages only 56 percent for men and 64 percent for women.[2] The disability occasioned by both initial and recurrent stroke causes extended stays in hospitals and leads to chronic care in institutions, with the resultant heavy strain on human and economic resources. In the United States alone, the nearly half a million people who suffer stroke annually and the current stroke survivors, numbering over 3 million, account for $29 billion in health care costs and lost productivity.

Sweeping summaries such as the foregoing give some crude idea of the magnitude of the problem. The gross facts have proved helpful for public health officials grappling with decisions on allocations of funding. However, they have proved too general to be useful to modern clinicians, who face single patients with certain clinically identifiable forms of stroke, one or more risk factors, and sometimes many different treatment options.

This chapter is directed toward those clinicians. Information is clustered according to stroke type, demographics, modifiable and non-modifiable risk factors, time from stroke, and expected course with general or no specific (placebo) therapies. The source material is drawn from hospital-based and population studies, from longitudinal analyses of the impact of attempts at modification of risk factors, and from the placebo arm of several recent clinical trials. Special attention has been given to those sources that include an effort to diagnose stroke by subtype.

STROKE SUBTYPE

From the evidence obtained in the initial hospital-based studies of stroke in the 1930s, it has been widely taught that atherothrombosis is the leading cause of stroke. This viewpoint, stemming in part from the autopsy-based studies conducted at the Boston City Hospital, defined embolism as brain infarction attributable to atrial fibrillation and valvular heart disease, and thrombosis as the remainder of cases of brain infarction.[3] These initially unchallenged definitions,

stringent for embolism and generous for thrombosis, resulted in a very small recognized incidence of embolism (3%) and a rather large estimate of thrombosis due to atherosclerosis (70%); the balance of cases were attributed to some form of hemorrhage. Some physicians may have been relieved to accept atherosclerotic thrombosis as a leading cause of stroke, since atherosclerosis as a disease is not deemed easily treatable. This attitude could lead to a view of stroke as a disease process rather like trauma, ie, mainly completed at the time of onset, with treatment options limited to dealing with the complications.

A readiness to use a generous definition for atherosclerosis as a cause of stroke persisted well into the 1960s and 1970s. (Table 2–1). Such an algorithm was used for research into stroke in the well-executed, population-based Framingham Study, a 40-year prospective study of 5070 men and women from a single community. In this population, a diagnosis of *atherothrombotic brain infarction,* diagnosed largely on the basis of risk factors, was made in 44 percent of the 693 cases of stroke and transient ischemic attacks. (Of the remainder, transient ischemic attacks accounted for 21 percent, cerebral embolism for 21 percent, intracranial hemorrhage for 12 percent, and all other causes for 2 percent).[4] This was a considerably lower frequency than that found by Aring and Merritt.

The Harvard Cooperative Stroke Registry, a prospective hospital-based study of 694 patients with stroke whose results were published in 1978, used a revised set of definitions for stroke subtype and a higher frequency of angiograms than had been applied to prior studies; it also relied in part on the then-new imaging techniques such as computed tomographic scanning.[5] These investigators found 233 cases (34%) attributed to *large artery stenosis* or *thrombosis due to atherosclerosis,* which was at that time a low frequency for arteriosclerotic stroke. The remainder of the cases included 215 (31%) explained by *embolism* (a new high for this diagnosis), 131 (19%) defined as *lacunar syndromes* (a newly introduced definition for a subtype of ischemic stroke), 70 (10%) from *intracerebral hematoma,* and 45 (6%) from *subarachnoid hemorrhage.* In this cohort, among the 138 patients who had thrombotic strokes in the carotid territory, 102 underwent angiography; all showed carotid stenosis or occlusion. Atheromatous changes of the ipsilateral carotid artery were seen in a further 33 of the 88 patients with embolic stroke who underwent complete angiography.

Growing awareness of the difficulty in uncovering an exact cause for some cases of brain infarction and dissatis-

TABLE 2–1. Evolution of Identification of Stroke Subtype

Study	Year	Cases, n	Thrombosis, %			Embolism, %		Hemorrhage, %	
			Lacune	Athero-sclerosis†	Tandem Arterial Pathology	Crypto-genic Stroke‡	Cardio-genic§	Parenchym-atous Intracerebral	Sub-arachnoid
Boston City Hospital	1935	407		81		3		15	
Framingham MA	1961	90		63		15		4	18
Rochester MN	1969	993		71		3		10	5
Harvard Registry	1978	802	17	36		20		11	7
NINDS Data Bank	1988	1802	19	6	4	28	14	13	13

*Ischemic stroke only.
†Large artery severe stenosis or occlusion attributed to atherosclerosis.
‡Infarct of undetermined cause.
§Atrial fibrillation, valvular disease, or other cause.

faction with the wide differences in estimates of the frequency of infarct subtypes prompted an even more demanding diagnostic algorithm in the NINCDS Stroke Data Bank project.[6] In this cohort of 1805 patients, based on hospital admissions for stroke seen by the investigators, additional categories for infarction were created, including *infarct with normal angiogram, tandem arterial pathology,* and *infarct of undetermined cause.* The issues of arriving at these various diagnostic categories have recently been reviewed in detail.[7] Suffice to say that the creation of these additional categories further tightened the criteria for the diagnosis of infarction attributable to large artery arteriosclerosis, and its percentage of the total plunged almost into single numbers.

Infarct of undetermined cause, later rechristened *cryptogenic stroke,*[8] was soon recognized as a major problem in diagnosis.[9] This category was and is currently used when conventional studies such as brain imaging suffice to diagnose an infarct but when Doppler or angiography does not disclose extracranial or intracranial stenoses, cardiac evaluation does not reveal a cardiac source, and the search for systemic disease yields no signs of prothrombotic states. Far from being uncommon, a negative outcome for conventional testing proved rather common, and cryptogenic stroke was diagnosed in 40 percent. Of the 508 cases in the Stroke Data Bank so labeled, 138 (27%) had been evaluated with both computed tomography and angiography. The clinical syndrome and computed tomographic and angiographic findings in 91 (65.9%) of these 138 cases of infarct of undetermined cause were clearly not attributable to large-artery thrombosis and could permit reclassification of the infarct as due to some form of embolism. It was the failure to define a source of embolus that kept them in the category of infarct of undetermined cause.

This worrisomely large number of unexplained infarcts prompted a number of studies seeking an explanation. Studies of prothrombotic states initially provided hopes that protein S deficiency would prove an important factor, but these were dashed when case-control studies suggested that protein S deficiency was not as important a factor as had initially been thought.[10] The introduction of Doppler insonations has opened a new field of detecting occlusive disease in vessels heretofore requiring angiography for their study, but such studies have not shown a high frequency of intracranial disease to explain these strokes.[11–13] A special application of Doppler studies has led to the discovery that patent cardiac

foramen ovale, formerly considered something of a medical curiosity, may actually account for just under half of these otherwise unexplained cases.[14]

These more modern efforts have all but eliminated the past practice of assigned stroke cause based on assessment of risk factors. They have also contributed to better definition of clinical cohorts for further study. Determination of stroke subtype is yielding benefits in better assessments of outcome and better insights into the clinical syndromes. One example is the better 1-year mortality prognosis for strokes labeled lacunar infarction than for other forms of stroke.[15] Ischemic stroke from embolism from a presumed carotid source seems more mild than embolism from a presumed cardiac source.[16] In the Stroke Data Bank, the probability of a carotid-brain tandem lesion was increased by the computed tomographic finding of a superficial infarct alone (odds ratio [OR] = 4.6; 95% CI = 1.5–13.7) or by a higher hematocrit level on admission. The probability of cardiac embolism was greater in patients with an initial decreased consciousness (OR = 39.2; 95% CI = 4.0–381.3) or with an abnormal first computed tomographic scan (OR = 3.2; 95% CI = 1.2–8.6).

Even the clinical course seems influenced by the stroke subtype. During the 7- to 10-day study interval from first clinical contact with patients in the Stroke Data Bank, those suffering presumed lacunar pure motor stroke worsened and improved more frequently than did those suffering from stroke of a different mechanism; the worsening symptoms of the latter group were more likely to be persistent.[17]

Overall, the findings from these inquiries have added beneficial pressure to the growing trend to create a diagnosis of stroke subtype in hopes that a treatment would be found to arrest the development of stroke in the acute stage, prevent worsening, and prevent recurrence. The goal has been to substitute the former willingness to consider stroke a single-entity condition, as was the case at one time with cancer, and see it instead as a family of disorders like the various subtypes of neoplasms and infectious diseases.

STROKE INCIDENCE

Incidence Worldwide

Although an incidence rate of 180 strokes per 100,000 deaths is the generally accepted figure worldwide, the incidence rate values vary considerably in different regions around the world. A low of 43.8 per 100,000 has been reported for Saudi Arabia in a study of 500 consecutive first-ever stroke patients whose diagnosis was pursued by computed tomographic scanning and clinical analysis.[18] In this cohort, ischemic strokes accounted for 76.2 percent, compared to those in Western populations, and the mean age was 63 ± 17 years, a bit younger than in many other countries. No ready explanation has been put forward. Annual rates as low as 120 per 100,000 for males and 56 per 100,000 for females have been reported from Perth, Australia, compared to those in Western countries.[19] Much higher rates have been reported from the Far East. Thus far, insights into the basis for the differences in these rates have not led to firm conclusions, but it is hoped that studies will lead to a better delineation of controllable risk factors.

Demographic Factors

As expected, in all studies, age plays a major role. Brain infarction has its highest incidence in the sixth to eighth decades of life, with a 2-year incidence of 4.8 per 1000 in men and 4.1 per 1000 in women. Similar risk data apply to atherothrombotic brain infarction and coronary heart disease.[20]

Race appears to influence crude incidence. In studies in the United States, the age-adjusted rates for initial stroke in south Alabama approach 208 per 100,000 for blacks and 109 per 100,000 for whites, with age-specific rates higher in blacks than in whites.[21] Rates for subarachnoid hemorrhage are highest in young black women; the reason for this difference is not known. In a study of the Northern Manhattan population,[22] the stroke incidence increased with age in both men and women in white, black, and Hispanic ethnic groups, as expected. The age-adjusted stroke incidence for men over 40 years of age was 567 per 100,000 for blacks, 351 for whites, and 306 for Hispanics. The incidence in women in the same age range was 716 per 100,000 in blacks, 361 in Hispanics, and 326 in whites. Hypertension and diabetes were more prevalent in blacks and Hispanics with stroke, whereas whites had more ischemic cardiac disease. Crude in-hospital mortality was greater in younger blacks and Hispanics compared with whites, whereas 2-year readmission rates, overall and for stroke, were similar in the three groups. This and most other studies substantiate that the greatest incidence of stroke is in black patients.

Modifiable Risk Factors

Among modifiable risk factors, hypertension overshadows the rest. Although the effect of hypertension decreases with age, it remains significant throughout life. Systolic hypertension is a greater risk factor than is diastolic, but both are independently significant for increased risk of stroke and for the occurrence of carotid stenosis. From the Framingham study, hypertension has been found to confer a relative risk of stroke of 4.0 for men and 4.4 for women. The stroke risk associated with borderline hypertension is lower (2.0), but even isolated systolic hypertension, previously thought to be benign, carries a relative risk of stroke of 2.4.[23] One overview of 14 randomized drug trials showed a 40 percent reduction in stroke risk in patients able to lower their diastolic blood pressures an average of 6 mm Hg.[24]

Cardiac disease must be considered from two viewpoints: first, the effect on the occurrence of cardiogenic embolism, itself a subtype of ischemic stroke; second, its effect on risk for stroke in general. The best-known effects apply to atrial fibrillation in the setting of rheumatic valvular disease, which confers a risk 17 times greater than that faced by people who have normal sinus rhythm. There is even a 5-fold risk for nonvalvular atrial fibrillation.[25]

Coronary artery disease is thought to confer a relative risk of 2.0, similar to that for recent myocardial infarction and congestive heart failure.[26, 27] Left ventricular hypertrophy occurs with advancing age and hypertension. The relative risk of stroke of 4.0 associated with the condition could in part be attributed to the hypertension which causes the hypertrophy.

Patent foramen ovale is also an independent risk factor for stroke.

Diabetes mellitus confers a relative risk of stroke of 1.5 to 3.0, probably secondary to microvascular disease and a greater tendency to atherosclerosis. Roughly speaking, diabetic patients have double the risk of thrombotic stroke compared with nondiabetics. The deleterious effect is less than that associated with hypertension and smoking. Glucose intolerance alone is a significant independent risk factor only in older women.[28]

Smoking is another major risk factor for thrombotic stroke.[29] Its effect is independently significant in all ages and both sexes. Some reports have associated it with a 50 percent increased risk for stroke, compared with the risk in nonsmokers.[30] The risk of stroke increases with the number of cigarettes smoked per day; the relative risk of stroke in heavy smokers (more than 45 cigarettes per day) is twice that of light smokers (fewer than 10 cigarettes per day). It appears possible to reduce the risk by cessation of smoking. Five years after the cessation of smoking, the risk for stroke in an ex-smoker approaches the risk in the general population.[25, 31]

Alcohol intake has two types of effects depending on the amount of consumption. Mild to moderate alcohol intake appears to confer something of a protective effect, at least for ischemic stroke, with a relative risk of 0.3 to 0.5 percent, which was recently confirmed in a large study. Heavy drinking carries an increased risk for stroke, especially of the hemorrhagic type. Some studies have not found an effect of ethanol after adjusting for confounding factors such as cigarette smoking and hypertension. The "J-shaped" effect (less for mild, more for heavy intake) has been observed mainly in white populations. Selection of the population for study could be a factor in these findings: in the Northern Manhattan cohort, prior heavy ethanol use was a factor in stroke recurrence, after controlling for hypertension and admission glucose, and was independent of smoking. Its effect was evident for more than 2 years. The effect was primarily observed in black and Hispanic patients, but the cohort was too small to detect a clear statistical interaction between ethanol use and the race-ethnicity factor.

A variety of blood laboratory abnormalities have some association with higher stroke incidence.[32] Hematocrit levels, both elevated[33] and decreased,[34] are thought to have a role in stroke occurrence; elevated levels are also associated with a higher frequency of worsening of ischemic stroke. The importance of lupus anticoagulant/anticardiolipin antibodies remains unsettled,[35–37] and some studies suggest that they may be only an acute-phase reactant.[38] Prothrombotic states exist after brain infarction, but their importance has been difficult to determine.[39] The association between elevated lipids and atherosclerosis in both coronary and carotid artery disease is too well known to require documentation here. Suffice to mention that a comprehensive review of 26 studies reports an association between plasma lipids and atherosclerosis, stronger in older than in younger individuals.[40] However, the Framingham Study did not support an association between total serum cholesterol and thrombotic brain infarction. Other studies have shown an association between serum lipids and extracranial carotid artery atherosclerosis that was detected by ultrasonography.[41, 42]

The evidence is unclear whether modification of risk factors prevents stroke.[43]

Observations from Clinical Trials

Clinical studies are of a slightly different cohort than population studies and studies of hospitalized patients. However, they serve to provide yet another type of insight into the risk for stroke, at least for those patients whose clinical status qualified them for participation. It is of interest to describe the fate of those in the treatment arm used to evaluate the effect of a given therapy.

For asymptomatic carotid disease, the recently concluded Asymptomatic Carotid Artery Stenosis Study (ACASS),[44] a large multicenter trial of patients with asymptomatic, high-grade internal carotid stenosis, observed a stroke rate of 10.6 percent projected over the 5 years of the study for patients treated without surgery.

Long-term oral anticoagulation therapy has been undertaken in various populations, usually compared with placebo or with aspirin. An overall risk of stroke in patients with chronic atrial fibrillation was estimated to be at least 5 percent per year, but three large prospective, double-blind trials indicate somewhat different values. In the Copenhagen Atrial Fibrillation, Aspirin, Anticoagulation Study (AFA-SAK), 1007 patients were entered over a 2-year period.[45] The incidence of transient ischemic attack, stroke, or systemic thromboembolism was 5.5 percent in the aspirin and placebo arms. In the Stroke Prevention in Atrial Fibrillation study (SPAF), 1330 patients were randomly assigned to treatment arms, and at a mean follow-up period of 1.3 years the incidence of stroke or systemic embolism was 7.4 percent in the placebo group.[46] In the Boston Area Anticoagulation Trial for Atrial Fibrillation (BAATAF), of the 420 patients randomly assigned and followed for an average of 2.2 years, ischemic stroke occurred in the control group at 2.98 percent per year.[47]

STROKE RECURRENCE

Much of the data on stroke is on the incidence of first stroke. Only with the increase in clinical trials has information on the incidence of recurrent stroke become a subject of intense concern.

Recurrence after cerebral infarction has varied widely in different studies; rates for stroke attributed to atherosclerosis have been from as low as 4 percent to as high as 12 percent per year, with aggregate rates of 6.1 percent after minor stroke and 9.0 percent after major stroke.[48]

Using a life table analysis, the Stroke Data Bank, in the largest cohort to address the frequency of recurrence by stroke subtype, found that the 30-day cumulative $\pm$ SE risk of early recurrence for all infarctions was 3.3 ± 0.4 percent.[49] In this study, the risk of early recurrence was greatest for atherothrombotic infarction ($7.9 \pm 2.2\%$, 8 of 113 patients) and least for lacunar infarction ($2.2 \pm 1.2\%$, 8 of 337 patients). Both cardioembolic infarction ($4.3 \pm 0.9\%$, 10 of 246 patients) and infarction of undetermined cause ($3.0 \pm 0.5\%$, 14 of 508 patients) had intermediate risks. History of hypertension and diabetes mellitus, as well as diastolic hypertension and elevated blood glucose concentration at admission, were associated with early recurrence. Logistic regression analysis estimated the risk of early recurrence to be 8.56 percent in those patients with coexisting hypertension and a glucose concentration of 300 mg/dL, versus 0.77 percent in the absence of these two abnormalities. Early recurrence was associated with longer median duration of initial hospital stay (27 vs 14 days) and a higher 30-day case-fatality rate (20% vs 7.4%) Increased weakness scores were associated with early recurrent stroke.

In the recent Northern Manhattan project, stroke recurrence was frequent, with 25.8 percent of patients suffering a recurrent stroke by 5 years.[50] Moreover, mortality after a recurrent stroke was greater than after the index ischemic stroke. The greatest risk of stroke recurrence or death occurred in the period immediately after the index ischemic stroke. Stroke recurred in 38 (6%) within the first 30 days, the risk decreasing and remaining relatively stable thereafter. Recurrence was not significantly different for patients with the incident ischemic strokes compared with those with prior stroke. Among the events within the first year, nearly one half of the recurrences and 37 percent of the deaths occurred in the first 30 days.

Predictors of Stroke Recurrence

The role of modifiable risk factors has been studied only recently. In Framingham, the 5-year stroke recurrence was less in those free of hypertension. In a case-control study in the Lehigh Valley, Pennsylvania, hypertension accounted for an odds ratio of 4.5 for stroke recurrence. History of hypertension and diastolic blood pressure were predictors of early recurrence and 2-year recurrence, respectively, in the NINDS Stroke Data Bank. In Rochester, Minnesota, neither level of blood pressure prior to the first stroke nor management of hypertension had any effect on stroke recurrence rates.[51]

The Stroke Data Bank found that hypertension, glucose level, and stroke subtype predicted 30-day recurrence, and only hypertension predicted 2-year recurrence.[52] The 30-day recurrence rate of stroke varied from 2.2 percent for lacunar syndromes, to 7.9 percent for large artery atherosclerotic disease, to up to 14 percent in the first 2 weeks for atrial fibrillation. In the Lehigh Valley study, the relative risk for recurrence was 41.4 for transient ischemic attack, 8.0 for myocardial infarction or other coronary artery disease, 5.6 for diabetes mellitus, and 4.5 for hypertension.[53]

For the Northern Manhattan study, recurrence was slightly more frequent among patients younger than 65, women, and black and Hispanic patients, but these differences failed to reach statistical significance.[50] Subtype of stroke showed considerable differences: those with lacunar infarcts had a significantly decreased stroke recurrence risk compared with those with atherosclerotic, cardioembolic, or cryptogenic infarcts. Recurrence was higher for those with risk factors of hypertension and was significantly increased among those with an admission glucose level of more than 140 or with a history of heavy ethanol use. In this last group, nearly half had a recurrent stroke within 5 years, compared with 22 percent with no known heavy ethanol use. No significant differences were found between heavy ethanol users and non-heavy users in the initial infarct subtype who were treated with aspirin or coumadin. Congestive heart failure, prior stroke, cigarette smoking, and diabetes were not univariate predictors of stroke recurrence.

Observations from Clinical Trials

More than 10 randomized placebo-controlled trials of platelet antiaggregants have been used to study the rate of stroke following transient ischemic attack or recurrent stroke following minor stroke.[54] Most have shown a significant risk reduction with aspirin and a higher rate with placebo. The Canadian-American Ticlopidine Study (CATS) randomly assigned 1053 patients with recent noncardioembolic stroke to receive either ticlopidine 250 mg twice daily or placebo.[55] The study excluded patients who had significant comorbidity and those with transient ischemic attack alone. The incidence of primary endpoints (ischemic stroke, myocardial infarction, and vascular death) was 15.3 percent in the placebo group.

The best known of the surgical trials is the North American Symptomatic Carotid Endarterectomy Trial (NASCET).[56] The patients were stratified to 30 to 69 percent stenosis or 70 to 99 percent stenosis as documented by angiography. After 659 patients had been randomly assigned to the high-grade stenosis group—half the number projected to be needed to prove a 10 percent risk reduction—the study was terminated because of a finding of a dramatic therapeutic benefit of surgery. In the medical group, in which almost all were treated with at least some dosing scheme of aspirin, ranging from a high of 1300 mg a day to a low of 325 mg a day, the cumulative risk of ipsilateral stroke at 2 years was found to be 26 percent, and that for major or fatal ipsilateral stroke 13.1 percent. The risk of all strokes was 27.6 percent, and the risk of death or major stroke was 18.1 percent.

The Veterans Administration study randomly assigned 189 patients with a greater than 50 percent internal carotid artery stenosis to surgical plus medical therapy (aspirin, 325 mg) versus medical therapy alone and found similar results.[57] At a mean follow-up of 11.9 months, crescendo transient ischemic attacks and stroke were found in 19.4 percent of the medical group.

WORSENING IN ISCHEMIC STROKE

The course of a given ischemic stroke has proved difficult to predict. Many patients remain stable from onset and some actually improve,[58] in some cases dramatically,[59] whereas for others, progression of disease is the outcome.

Much attention has been given to the subject of pro-

gressing stroke, since the persistent hope has been harbored that what could become a devastating deficit could be recognized and headed off in its early stages. Evidence supporting the notion of progressing stroke and of an 'ischemic penumbra' has been sought for years but has proved both an elusive and a disappointingly small or narrow zone, as can be best gleaned by the image studies carried out in recent years.[60] Neuropathologic studies have regularly indicated a very sharp border between the healthy and infarcted tissue where quantitative studies of infarction have been done in a wide variety of stroke types.[61] Whether the very high resolution image technology of the future can achieve what has eluded present technology awaits demonstration. For now, we must remain frustrated by our uncertainty about what happens when the neurologic deficit increases.

The incidence of neurologic worsening varies considerably according to the various subtypes of stroke, being least often encountered in strokes that seem to be of embolic mechanism and most often among those that appear to be caused by thrombosis, whether affecting a large or small artery.[17] The higher frequency in cases that seem to be thrombotic in nature raises the old point that the infarction may be caused by perfusion failure. But trying to settle the issue of perfusion failure by studying the clinical features of the progressing or worsening ischemic strokes has brought out two types of worsening.[6, 62] In the first, qualitative worsening, the formula of the deficit changes to involve parts not initially affected, the type of change that should correlate with spreading lesion topography and presumably reflect perfusion failure.

The second, quantitative worsening, represents intensification of the initial deficit with no change in the formula, an effect that would suggest the conversion of ischemia to infarction, an effect different from failing perfusion. Evidence to support these two types of failure has been as difficult to come by as that showing an ischemic penumbra. Few studies have been specifically directed toward this point to try to differentiate the possible separate mechanisms that could account for worsening, and even fewer of the clinical trials have been organized to pursue one or the other formula for clinical worsening.[63] Instead, most clinical trials have been directed at the goal of rounding up as many patients as will agree to the trial, a worthy goal not often achieved in itself.[64] By our calculations, the numbers needed to show an effect of any therapy are manageable but large.[65] Adding in the disappointing observation that few patients would qualify in any given institution, such a trial might prove all but unworkable.[66]

MORTALITY

Lumping together all types of cerebral infarction, the reported 30-day case fatality rates range from 15 percent to 33 percent. Estimates have been made that, within 1 year of stroke, between 30 and 52 percent of ischemic stroke patients will be dead, many because of myocardial infarction. Stroke is the cause of death only in some of the cases.[67]

Although the overall rates for ischemic stroke lumped together provide a rough guide to outcome, they mask differences in the mortality rate by ischemic stroke subtypes. In the NINCDS Stroke Data Bank, overall mortality rates approached 8 percent, with those strokes attributed to large artery atherosclerosis at the highest value of 18.8 percent. Those with lacunar infarcts had a mortality approaching 1 percent. The Framingham study obtained similar data, showing the case fatality rate from atherothrombotic infarction at 15 percent.

The mortality rate does not appear to be a function of the major territory involved. In the NINCDS Stroke Data Bank project, there was very little difference in mortality between supratentorial (12.2%) and infratentorial (13.5%) infarction.

A Cox proportional hazards model was used to analyze the recently reported cohort from the Northern Manhattan Stroke Study.[50] The independent predictors of overall mortality were: major hemispheric or basilar syndrome (RR = 2.0), congestive heart failure (RR = 2.6), admission glucose level of more than 140 (RR = 1.7), and age (RR = 1.4 for a 10-year increment in age). Patients with an index lacunar syndrome had a lower rate of mortality (RR = 0.56).

The independent predictors of 30-day mortality were major hemispheric or basilar syndrome, depressed consciousness, admission glucose level of more than 140, and congestive heart failure. When the model was restricted to 30-day survivors, depressed consciousness was not significant, indicating its relative importance for early mortality. Lacunar syndrome and age now became significant determinants of mortality.

After the first week, most stroke deaths are non-neurologic in nature. Cardiac complications are encountered very often in conjunction with stroke and occur throughout the 30-day period after stroke. Other complications include congestive heart failure, hypertension, diabetes mellitus, and older age. Relative immobilization because of the depressed level of consciousness and motor deficits is reflected in the high frequency of pneumonia, urinary tract infection, sepsis, and pulmonary thromboembolism occurring between the second and fourth weeks.

DECLINE

As recently as 1950, strokes constituted approximately 20 percent of all cardiovascular deaths, a level that has been roughly maintained since that time. A striking decline in age-specific stroke morbidity and mortality has been noted over the last 15 years in both women and men, with mortality rates falling in industrialized countries by 4.1 to 7.1 percent.[68]

While it is tempting to attribute such reports to the beneficial effects of therapy, such benefits have been difficult to demonstrate.[69] In some studies, the incidence has remained unchanged although the fatality rate has fallen[70] or the strokes have been clinically less severe.[71]

A study in Taiwan reported 31,078 deaths from cerebral infarction and 77,773 deaths from cerebral hemorrhage for groups of subjects aged 40 to 79 years during the period of 1974 to 1988.[72] The decline in age-specific mortality for this period was much more striking for cerebral hemorrhage than for cerebral infarction.

Population-based studies in Rochester, Minnesota, indicated that the mortality rates from stroke declined 76 percent during the period of 1950 to 1975.[73] The National Center for Health Statistics also showed some decline in mortality,

but not to this degree.[74] A more recent report from the same Rochester population showed an end to the decline since 1975, with a rise in event rates, especially for those patients in the older age groups. Worldwide, no study has addressed this subject in detail.

The Framingham Study showed no overall decline in incidence of stroke, but some decline in the severity of the strokes documented in men (mainly because of the dilution effect of a higher frequency of reporting of transient ischemic attacks) and in the incidence of completed stroke in women.[75] The effects seemed quite modest. The initial hope that a decline could be attributable to better management of risk factors has not yet been justified.

REFERENCES

1. Sacco RL: Ischemic stroke. In Gorelick PB, Alter M, eds. *Handbook of Neuroepidemiology*. New York: Marcel Dekker, 1994;77.
2. Sacco RL, Wolf PA, Kannel WB, et al: Survival and recurrence: The Framingham Study. *Stroke*. 1982;13:290.
3. Aring CD, Merritt HH: Differential diagnosis between cerebral hemorrhage and cerebral thrombosis. *Arch Intern Med*. 1935;56:435.
4. Wolf PA, Cobb JL, D'Agostino RB: Epidemiology of stroke. In Barnett HMJ, Mohr JP, Stein BM, Yatsu FM, eds. *Stroke: Pathophysiology, Diagnosis, and Management*, 2nd ed. New York: Churchill Livingstone, 1992;3.
5. Mohr JP, Caplan LR, Melski JW, et al: The Harvard Cooperative Stroke Registry: A prospective registry of cases hospitalized with stroke. *Neurology*. 1978;28:754.
6. Foulkes MA, Wolf PA, Price TR, et al: The Stroke Data Bank: Design, methods, and baseline characteristics. *Stroke*. 1988;19:547.
7. Brainin M: Overview of stroke data banks. *Neuroepidemiol*. 1994;13:250.
8. Mohr JP: Cryptogenic stroke. *N Engl J Med*. 1988;318:1197. Editorial.
9. Sacco RL, Ellenberg JH, Mohr JP, et al: Infarcts of undetermined cause: The NINCDS Stroke Data Bank. *Ann Neurol*. 1989;25:382.
10. Mayer SA, Sacco RL, Hurlett-Jensen A, et al: Free protein S deficiency and acute ischemic stroke. A case-control study. *Stroke*. 1993;24:224.
11. Grolimund P, Seiler RW, Aaslid R, et al: Evaluation of cerebrovascular disease by combined extracranial and transcranial Doppler sonography: Experience in 1,039 patients. *Stroke*. 1987;18:1018.
12. Caplan LR, Brass LM, Dewitt LD, et al: Transcranial Doppler ultrasound: Present status. *Neurology*. 1990;40:696.
13. Hoffmann M, Sacco RL, Chan S, Mohr JP: Noninvasive detection of vertebral artery dissection. *Stroke*. 1993;24:815.
14. DiTullio MR, Sacco RL, Gopal A, Mohr JP: Patent foramen ovale as a risk factor for cryptogenic stroke. *Ann Intern Med*. 1992;117:461.
15. Brainin M, Seiser A, Czvitkovits B, Pauly E: Stroke subtype is an age-independent predictor of first-year survival. *Neuroepidemiology*. 1992;11:190.
16. Timsit SG, Sacco RL, Mohr JP, et al: Brain infarction severity differs according to cardiac or arterial embolic source. *Neurology*. 1993;43:728.
17. Libman RB, Sacco RL, Shi T, et al: Neurologic improvement in pure motor hemiparesis: Implications for clinical trials. *Neurology*. 1992;42:1713.
18. al Rajeh S, Awada A, Niazi G, Larbi E: Stroke in a Saudi Arabian National Guard community. Analysis of 500 consecutive cases from a population-based hospital. *Stroke*. 1993;24:1635.
19. Ward G, Jamrozik K, Stewart-Wynne E: Incidence and outcome of cerebrovascular disease in Perth, Western Australia. *Stroke*. 1988;19:1501.
20. Kannel WB, Wolf PA, Verter J: Manifestations of coronary disease predisposing to stroke: The Framingham Study. *JAMA*. 1983;250:2942.
21. Gross CR, Kase CS, Mohr JP, et al: Stroke in south Alabama: Incidence and diagnostic features. A population-based study. *Stroke*. 1984;15:249.
22. Sacco RL, Hauser WA, Mohr JP: Hospitalized stroke in blacks and Hispanics in northern Manhattan. *Stroke*. 1991;22:1491.
23. Davis HD, Hachinski V: Epidemiology of cerebrovascular disease. In Anderson D, ed. *Neuroepidemiology: A Tribute to Bruce Schoenberg*. Boca Raton, FL: CRC Press, 1991:27.
24. Collins R, Peto R, MacMahon S, et al: Blood pressure, stroke and coronary heart disease: Part II. Effects of short-term reductions in blood pressure: An overview of the unconfounded randomised drug trials in an epidemiological context. *Lancet*. 1990;335:827.
25. Wolf PA, Dawber TR, Thomas HE, et al: Epidemiologic assessment of chronic atrial fibrillation and risk of stroke: The Framingham study. *Neurology*. 1978;28:973.
26. Gillum RF, Fabsitz RR, Feinleib M, et al: Community surveillance for cerebrovascular disease: The Framingham cardiovascular disease survey. *Pub Health Rep*. 1978;93:438.
27. Davis PH, Dambrosia JM, Schoenberg BS, et al: Risk factors for ischemic stroke: A prospective study in Rochester, Minnesota. *Ann Neurol*. 1987;22:319.
28. Kannel WB, McGee DL: Diabetes and cardiovascular disease: The Framingham Study. *JAMA*. 1979;241:2035.

29. Wolf PA, D'Agostino RB, Kannel WB, et al: Cigarette smoking as a risk factor for stroke: The Framingham Study. *JAMA.* 1988;259:1025.
30. Shinton R, Beevers G: Meta-analysis of relation between cigarette smoking and stroke. *Br Med J.* 1989;298:789.
31. Abbott RD, Yin Y, Reed DM, et al: Risk of stroke in male cigarette smokers. *N Engl J Med.* 1986;315:717.
32. Hart RG, Kanter MC: Hematologic disorders and ischemic stroke: A selective review. *Stroke.* 1990;21:1111.
33. Culicchia F, Tatemichi TK, Mohr JP, et al: Hematocrit and acute stroke: The NINCDS Stroke Data Bank. *Neurology.* 1986;36(suppl):139.
34. Kiyohara Y, Ueda K, Hasuo Y, et al: Hematocrit as a risk factor of cerebral infarction: Long-term prospective population survey in a Japanese rural community. *Stroke.* 1986;17:687.
35. Briley DP, Coull BM, Goodnight SH: Neurological disease associated with antiphospholipid antibodies. *Ann Neurol.* 1989;25:221.
36. Nencini P, Baruffi MC, Abbate R, et al: Lupus anticoagulant and anticardiolipin antibodies in young adults with cerebral ischemia. *Stroke.* 1992;23:189.
37. Hess DC, Krauss J, Adams RJ, et al: Anticardiolipin antibodies: A study of frequency in TIA and stroke. *Neurology.* 1991;41:1181.
38. Stern BJ, Brey RL, and the APASS Group: Anticardiolipin antibodies are associated with an increased risk of stroke recurrence. *Neurology.* 1994;44(Suppl 2):A327.
39. Takano K, Yamaguchi T, Uchida K: Markers of a hypercoagulable state following acute ischemic stroke. *Stroke.* 1992;23:194.
40. Tell GS, Crouse JR, Furberg CD: Relation between blood lipids, lipoproteins, and cerebrovascular atherosclerosis: A review. *Stroke.* 1988;19:423.
41. O'Leary DH, Anderson KM, Wolf PA, et al: Cholesterol and carotid atherosclerosis in older persons: The Framingham Study. *Ann Epidemiol.* 1992;2:147.
42. Salonen R, Seppanen K, Rauramaa R, Salonen JT: Prevalence of carotid atherosclerosis and serum cholesterol levels in eastern Finland. *Atherosclerosis.* 1988;8:788.
43. Dunbabin DW, Sandercock PAG: Preventing stroke by the modification of risk factors. *Stroke.* 1990(suppl);21:IV36.
44. The Asymptomatic Carotid Atherosclerosis Study Group: Study design for randomized prospective trial of carotid endarterectomy for asymptomatic atherosclerosis. *Stroke.* 1989;20:844.
45. Petersen P, Godtfredsen J, Boysen G, et al: Placebo-controlled, randomized trial of warfarin and aspirin for prevention of thromboembolic complications in chronic atrial fibrillation: The Copenhagen AFASAK study. *Lancet.* 1989;1:175.
46. The Stroke Prevention in Atrial Fibrillation Investigators: The stroke prevention in atrial fibrillation study: Final results. *Circulation.* 1991;84:527.
47. The Boston Area Anticoagulation Trial for Atrial Fibrillation Investigators: The effect of low-dose warfarin on the risk of stroke in patients with nonrheumatic atrial fibrillation. *N Engl J Med.* 1990;323:1505.
48. Wilterdink JL, Easton JD: Vascular event rates in patients with atherosclerotic cerebrovascular disease. *Arch Neurol.* 1992;49:857.
49. Sacco RL, Foulkes MA, Mohr JP, et al: Determinants of early recurrence of cerebral infarction. The Stroke Data Bank. *Stroke.* 1989;20:983.
50. Sacco RL, Shi T, Zamanillo MC, Kargman D: Predictors of mortality and recurrence after hospitalized cerebral infarction in an urban community: The Northern Manhattan Stroke Study. *Neurology.* 1994;44:626.
51. Meissner I, Whisnant JP, Garraway WM: Hypertension management and stroke recurrence in a community (Rochester, Minnesota, 1950-1979). *Stroke.* 1988; 19:459.
52. Hier DB, Foulkes MA, Swiontoniowski M, et al: Stroke recurrence within 2 years after ischemic infarction. *Stroke.* 1991;22:155.
53. Alter M, Friday G, Sobel E, Lai SM: The Lehigh Valley Recurrent Stroke Study: Description of design and methods. *Neuroepidemiology.* 1993;12:241.
54. Barnett HJM: 35 years of stroke prevention: Challenges, disappointments and successes. *Cerebrovasc Dis.* 1991;1:61.
55. Gent M, Blakeley JA, Easton JD, et al: The Canadian American Ticlopidine Study (CATS) in thromboembolic stroke. *Lancet.* 1989;1:1215.
56. North American Symptomatic Carotid Endarterectomy Trial Collaborators: Beneficial effect of carotid endarterectormy in symptomatic patients with high-grade carotid stenosis. *N Engl J Med.* 1991;325:445.
57. Mayberg MR, Wilson SE, Yatsu F, et al: Carotid endarterectomy and prevention of cerebral ischemia in symptomatic carotid stenosis. *JAMA.* 1991;266:3289.
58. Biller J, Love BB, Marsh EE, et al: Spontaneous improvement after acute ischemic stroke: A pilot study. *Stroke.* 1990;21:1008.
59. Minematsu K, Yamaguchi T, Omae T: Spectacular shrinking deficit: Rapid recovery from a full hemispheral syndrome by migration of an embolus. *Neurology.* 1992;42:157.
60. Powers WJ: Cerebral hemodynamics in ischemic cerebrovascular disease. *Ann Neurol.* 1991;23:231.
61. Nedergaard M, Vorstrup S, Astrup J: Cell density in the border zone around old small human brain infarcts. *Stroke.* 1986;17:1129.
62. Mohr JP: Natural history and pathophysiology of cerebral vascular disease. *Circulation.* 1991;83:172.
63. Duke RJ, Bloch RF, Turpie AGG, et al: Intravenous heparin for the prevention of stroke progression in acute partial stable stroke: a randomized controlled trial. *Ann Intern Med.* 1986;105:825.
64. Fieschi C, Argentino C, Lenzi GL, et al: Clinical and instrumental evaluation of patients with ischemic stroke within the first six hours. *J Neurol Sci.* 1989;91:311.
65. Mohr JP, Orgogozo JM, Harrison MJG, et al: Meta-analysis of oral nimodipine trials in acute ischemic stroke. *Cerebrovasc Dis.* 1994;4:197.
66. Mohr JP: Problems in formulating clinical trials. In Hacke W, delZoppo GJ, Hirschberg M, eds. *Thrombolytic Therapy in Acute Ischemic Stroke.* Berlin: Springer-Verlag, 1991.
67. Wolf PA, Kannel WB, McGee DL: Prevention of ischemic stroke: Risk factors. In Barnett HJM, Mohr JP, Stein BM, Yatsu FM, eds. *Stroke: Pathophysiology, Diagnosis, and Management.* New York: Churchill Livingstone, 1986.
68. Bonita R, Syewart A, Beaglehole R: International trends in stroke mortality: 1970–1985. *Stroke.* 1990;21:989.
69. Hypertension-Stroke Cooperative Study Group: Effect of antihypertensive treatment on stroke recurrence. *JAMA.* 1974;229:409.
70. Harmsen P, Tsipogianni A, Wilhelmsen L: Stroke incidence rates were unchanged, while fatality rates declined, during 1971–1987 in Goteborg, Sweden. *Stroke.* 1992;23:1410.
71. Stegmayr B, Asplund K, Wester PO: Trends in incidence, case-fatality rate, and severity of stroke in Northern Sweden, 1985–1991. *Stroke.* 1994;25:1738.
72. Chang CC, Chen CJ: Secular trend of mortality from cerebral infarction and cerebral hemorrhage in Taiwan, 1974–1988. *Stroke.* 1993;24:212.
73. Matsumoto N, Whisnant JP, Kurland LT, Okazaki H: Natural history of stroke in Rochester, Minnesota: An extension of a previous study, 1955 through 1969. *Stroke.* 1973;4:20.
74. Howard G, Craven TE, Sanders L, Evans GW: Relationship of hospitalized stroke rate and in-hospital mortality to the decline in US stroke mortality. *Neuroepidemiology.* 1991;10:251.
75. Wolf PA, D'Agostino RB, O'Neal MA, et al: Secular trends in stroke incidence and mortality: The Framingham Study. *Stroke.* 1992;23:1551.

The Importance of Symptoms in Predicting Risk for Subsequent Stroke Following an Initial Transient Ischemic Attack or Minor Stroke

BRUCE A. EVANS, DAVID O. WIEBERS, and H.J.M. BARNETT

Population-based studies estimate that the risk of ischemic stroke in a patient suffering a first transient ischemic attack (TIA) is approximately 12 to 13 percent for the first year and 6 percent per year over the first 5 years following the initial TIA.[1, 2] A number of studies have attempted to identify those characteristics of patients and of initial TIAs that are associated with enhanced stroke risk, to identify persons in whom special intervention may be warranted. Studies have included various referral-based series[3–10] and population-based series.[2, 11–16] Similar studies, including referral-based,[17–23] hospital population–based,[24, 25] and community population–based[26, 27] have examined patients presenting with stroke, minor stroke, or a mixture of TIA and stroke. Some of these studies used multivariate analysis to identify independent predictors of risk,[7, 8, 17, 18, 20, 21, 23, 25] but none were based on population, and thus all were prone to selection bias. To date there has been little agreement on which patient characteristics represent important predictors of increased stroke risk, which reflects the wide variety of populations studied and statistical methods used.

A further problem in using information from the aforementioned studies to help make clinical decisions in individual patients is the lack of information regarding specific stroke mechanisms. Beyond the antiplatelet agents of proven value, for which there are clinical clues identifying high-risk patients who are most likely to benefit from intervention, most interventions are mechanism-specific, such as carotid endarterectomy for carotid occlusive disease. Some information on stroke mechanism has been forthcoming from the medical arm of the North American Symptomatic Carotid Endarterectomy Trial (NASCET), which analyzed patients with severe carotid stenosis.[28, 29]

The aim of this chapter is to suggest a number of patient and clinical characteristics that previous studies and recent population-based and mechanism-specific information support as predictors of increased stroke risk in patients presenting with TIA or minor stroke. The discussion will be limited to demographic patient characteristics and symptoms specifically related to the presenting neurologic event. The issue of comorbidity as a predictor of increased stroke risk is discussed in Chapter 2.

NATURE OF THE ISCHEMIC EVENT

Ischemic stroke risk following an initial TIA has been estimated from population-based studies to be approximately 12 to 13 percent for the first year, with much of that risk occurring in the first month, and about 6 percent per year for 5 years overall.[1, 2] Our evaluation of the prognosis following an initial reversible ischemic neurologic deficit

(RIND)—a minor stroke with complete resolution—in the Rochester, Minnesota, population revealed subsequent stroke risk not significantly different from the risk found in patients with an initial ischemic stroke with persistent deficit (5.5% per year for 5 years).[30] The same study demonstrated that patients presenting with initial RIND in this population had a significantly lower risk of subsequent stroke than patients who presented with an initial TIA. The subgroup of RIND patients characterized by early resolution of symptoms (≤ 7 days) resembled the TIA group in that they had a higher overall subsequent risk of stroke and showed a tendency for the recurrent events to take place within a year of the initial event. A study of the Oxfordshire community by Dennis and associates[26] found no significant difference between the subsequent stroke risks of patients with an initial TIA (excluding patients with amaurosis only) and those with minor strokes. Minor stroke was defined in a way that allows persistent neurologic deficit of minimal functional significance.

Little information is available on the relative risk of TIA and stroke with reference to specific stroke mechanisms. Among NASCET patients with 70 percent or greater carotid stenosis randomly assigned to medical treatments, there was no significant difference between the subsequent stroke rate in patients whose qualifying event was a TIA and in those in whom it was an ischemic stroke, although the trend was toward a higher rate in the latter group (Barnett and colleagues, unpublished information). This trend may be due in part to the number of TIA patients with amaurosis fugax alone, which appears to carry a more benign prognosis.[29]

In summary, judging from population-based studies, more rapid resolution of symptoms may be associated with a slightly increased overall risk of subsequent stroke over 5 years and a somewhat more substantial increase in risk in the year following the initial event. The effect on long-term stroke risk is, however, minor, and the main role that persistent deficit plays in an intervention decision is in the determination of how much function remains at risk in the threatened cerebral circulation territory.

CLINICAL RISK FACTORS

Clinical risk factors were evaluated as predictors of subsequent stroke rate following TIA in the Rochester, Minnesota population.[30] The residents of Rochester and the surrounding area receive medical care from a limited number of providers, primarily the Mayo Clinic and its associated hospitals and one smaller group practice and its affiliated hospital. Diagnoses are coded and entered into a central index. Through the use of this system, 330 patients presenting with a first TIA between 1955 and 1979 were identified (Evans and colleagues, unpublished information). The definition of TIA used was an episode of focal neurologic symptoms with abrupt onset and rapid resolution, lasting less than 24 hours and resulting from altered circulation to a limited region of the brain.[16] The analysis was also restricted to patients whose first medical attention was within 120 days of the first TIA. In this study of outcomes following TIA, two endpoints were considered: recurrent stroke and death. Because of a recent discovery that the TIA case ascertainment with the use of this linkage system was not complete,[31] analysis was restricted to patients who had not had an outcome event (stroke) prior to first medical attention following the presenting TIA.

Rates of stroke occurrence and survival in the patients with TIA were compared with those of a population matched for age and sex with the use of Kaplan-Meier plots and the log-rank test. The variables investigated included demographics and those related to diagnostic and clinical features of the ischemic episodes. Using a Cox proportional hazards model, we plotted the time from the first medical attention after the first TIA until death or until stroke, censoring at death not due to stroke. In both cases, follow-up was limited to 10 years after first medical attention. Cox proportional hazards models were utilized first in a univariate fashion, incorporating each of the variables (Table 3–1). Subsequently, demographic, clinical, and therapeutic variables were included in a stepwise procedure to arrive at a main effects model. Two-level interactions were then included at a 0.01 significance level. Similar Cox models for the rate of survival free from stroke were constructed as a secondary analysis on the basis of follow-ups performed 30 days and 5 years after the first medical attention.

Several similar factors were also evaluated for predictive power in the patients with severe carotid stenosis from the medical arm of the NASCET study (Barnett and colleagues, unpublished information).[2, 29, 30]

TABLE 3–1. Variables Used in the Cox Model for Evaluating Risk Factors for Ischemic Stroke*

Type	Name	Description
Demographic	age	Age at TIA in years
	age 70	Dichotomous age greater than 70 years
	calyr	Continuous version of calendar year of FMA
	calyr 70	Dichotomous calendar year later than 1970
	male	Gender
	tia.fma	Days from TIA to FMA (maximum 120)
Clinical	sensory	TIAs with somatic sensory symptoms only
	hemispheric	Unilateral carotid hemispheric TIA
	vert-basilar	Vertebrobasilar TIA
	retinal	Retinal TIA only
	tia.ct	Number of TIAs before FMA (1 = 1, 2 = 2–4, 3 = ≥5)
	ntia5	> 5 TIAs before FMA (dichotomous)
Drug Use	acoag	Anticoagulant (heparin or warfarin) begun within 7 days of FMA
	ahbp	On antihypertensive drug at FMA or within 2 months

*Applied to patients in Rochester, Minnesota, with a first transient ischemic stroke. The "density" of the TIA was evaluated by examining the significance of tia.ct and ntia5 as predictors using subsets of patients whose initial TIA was within 1, 2, 4, and 12 weeks of first medical attention.

KEY: FMA = first medical attention; TIA = transient ischemic attack.

Demographic Variables

Age

Referral-based studies have provided contradictory results on the role of age as a predictor of subsequent stroke in a patient with initial TIA. Some suggest increased risk with higher age,[4, 7, 23] and others found no such relationship.[17, 18] In the Rochester population, age was a significant predictor of subsequent stroke following TIA, with a 10-year increase in age resulting in a subsequent stroke hazard ratio of 1.5 (95% confidence interval, limits, 1.2–1.8).

Gender

Although some previous referral-based and population-based studies suggest that male sex is a significant predictor of increased subsequent stroke risk after TIA or stroke,[4, 20, 32] others do not.[17, 21, 25] Although we identified a significant age-gender interaction affecting survival rate after TIA, with younger women having the best rate of survival and older women the worst, we found gender to have no significant independent effect on the risk of recurrent stroke.

Clinical Features of Transient Ischemic Attacks

Retinal versus Hemispheric

An Oxfordshire population-based study comparing the prognosis of patients with TIA and those with minor stroke showed a significantly increased risk of subsequent stroke for patients with minor stroke.[26] This significant risk increase disappeared when the 17 percent of the TIA patients who had amaurosis alone were excluded from the comparison, which implies that retinal events carry a smaller risk of subsequent brain infarction than hemispheric TIAs do. In the Rochester population, we were unable to demonstrate a significant predictive effect on subsequent stroke risk of the occurrence of amaurosis fugax alone, although a trend toward lower stroke rate was evident for those patients as compared with patients with unilateral hemispheric TIAs and vertebrobasilar TIAs. The failure to demonstrate a definite risk reduction may have been due to the low number of patients in the group with amaurosis fugax alone (18 of 330, 5.4%) or to a proportionately higher percentage of patients who had amaurosis fugax due to ipsilateral high-grade carotid stenosis.

In the NASCET patients with severe carotid stenosis who were randomly assigned to medical treatment, a subgroup with first-ever TIA showed less than half the risk of subsequent stroke than the group with hemispheric TIAs: 12% versus 28% at 2 years (Barnett and colleagues, unpublished data). A prior study, based on 119 TIA patients from the medical arm of NASCET with a 70 percent or greater ipsilateral carotid stenosis, which involved a proportional hazards analysis, showed that the risk associated with both the retinal and hemispheric TIA groups increased with increasing degree of stenosis.[29]

Posterior Circulation versus Anterior Circulation

Previous referral-based[17, 21] and population-based studies[11, 2] have demonstrated no significant difference in rates of stroke occurrence following TIA or minor stroke based on the distribution of the initial event in the anterior or posterior circulation. The Rochester population study confirms those findings.

Sensory Symptoms Only versus Other Symptoms

Only one recent study of variables affecting the stroke risk after TIA or minor stroke has evaluated the prognosis of spells consisting of sensory symptoms alone,[20] and this study found no prognostic value in the distinction. In the Rochester population studies, a sensory spell was not regarded as a TIA unless its distribution involved the face, arm and leg, or face and arm, and then only if the time-course of the symptoms and the clinical setting did not suggest a migraine-related event or focal seizure as a more appropriate diagnosis. In the current study, 56 of the 330 TIA patients had sensory symptoms alone. The presence of purely sensory symptoms had no significant effect on the risk of subsequent stroke. Similar results were seen among NASCET patients in the medical treatment arm of the study (Barnett and colleagues, unpublished information).

Recency, Number, and Frequency

At least one referral-based study of TIA identified recency of occurrence of a TIA as a risk factor for subsequent stroke.[7] Population-based studies of TIA have indicated that the subsequent stroke rate is higher in the first year, and particularly in the first month, after the initial event than it is at later times.[1, 2] This suggests that a patient whose initial TIA was relatively recent is at a higher (short-term) risk of subsequent stroke than a patient whose initial TIA was more distant (ie, 1 month or more previously).

Data from the NASCET study on patients with a 70 percent or greater carotid stenosis who were randomly assigned to medical treatment indicate a significant increased risk of subsequent stroke within 2 years in patients whose qualifying ischemic event was within 30 days of the randomization, as compared with those with a longer interval between randomization and ischemic event (30.8% versus

19.9%, P = 0.02) (Barnett and colleagues, unpublished information). Furthermore, subsequent analysis shows that the risk of stroke declines as the interval from randomization lengthens if the patient remains free of TIAs, but the risk remains high if TIAs continue to occur. In the analysis of retinal versus hemispheric events in this group of patients,[29] 60% of the subsequent 2-year risk of stroke in the retinal (risk, 17%) and hemispheric (risk, 42%) patients occurred in the first 2 months after randomization. In summary, it appears that, especially in the setting of high-grade stenosis, patients with recent TIAs are at increased risk of stroke.

Occurrence of multiple TIAs has also been reported as a predictor of increased risk of subsequent stroke in referral-based studies.[18, 20] In the Rochester patients, we found that the occurrence of five or more TIAs prior to the patient's first medical attention was a significant predictor of increased risk of subsequent stroke in the 5-year Cox model (risk ratio, 2.39, P = 0.002), with a similar trend that does not reach statistical significance in the 30-day model. A Kaplan-Meier plot shows similar results (Fig. 3–1). When the analysis is restricted to patients seen within 14 days of their initial TIA, those having experienced five or more TIAs prior to the first medical attention have a significantly increased risk of stroke compared with those with four or fewer TIAs within that time period (P = 0.02; Fig. 3–2). This difference is not seen between the groups when patients are selected who were seen for first medical attention any time after 14 days (although predictive power is limited). This suggests that a high "density" of TIAs—that is, five or more TIAs in a short period of time (1 or 2 weeks) following the initial event—signals a significantly increased risk for stroke.

CONCLUSION

The population-based studies reviewed and presented in this chapter all deal with TIA or minor stroke in general, without reference to specific mechanisms that produce cerebral ischemia. The NASCET data, although mechanism-specific, are referral-based and are also prone to distortion because of the delay of up to 120 days after the qualifying event, which biases the data toward showing a higher rate

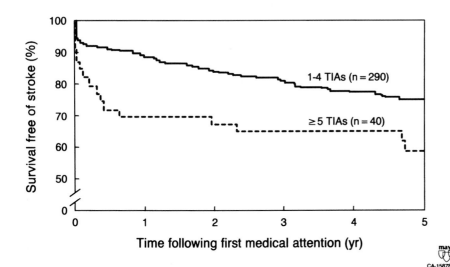

FIGURE 3–1. Rate of survival free from stroke plotted against time following the first medical attention, for two groups, one made up of patients who had experienced one to four transient ischemic attacks (TIAs) before first medical attention, and one made up of those who had experienced five or more TIAs. The difference in risk between the two groups was significant at 30 days and 5 years.

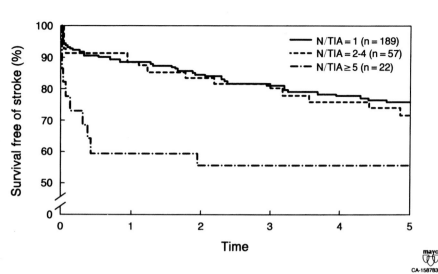

FIGURE 3–2. Rate of survival free from stroke plotted against time following the first medical attention, restricted to patients presenting within 14 days of the initial ischemic event. The patients who experienced five or more transient ischemic attacks (TIAs) within the 2-week interval (*broken line*) had a significantly worse rate of survival free from stroke than those who experienced one TIA (*solid line*) or those who experienced two to four TIAs (*dotted line*). N/TIA, number of TIAs.

of survival free from major stroke. Although the NASCET data cannot be compared directly with population-based data, they constitute the best available data for making clinical judgments regarding prognostic clinical indicators among TIA and ischemic stroke patients with severe carotid stenosis. No population-based data exist in this area. Drawing on information from population-based studies of TIA and minor stroke, supplemented by information from the control arm of this large, mechanism-specific treatment trial of patients with severe carotid stenosis, it is possible to identify a few probable demographic and clinical factors that signal an increased risk of subsequent stroke in patients presenting with TIA or minor stroke. Initial ischemic episodes with resolution of the symptoms within 1 week probably carry an increased risk of subsequent stroke, at least in the first month or two following their occurrence. Increased age correlates with an increased risk of subsequent stroke. Retinal episodes carry a better prognosis than hemispheric ischemic episodes, especially in the setting of severe ipsilateral carotid stenosis. Recent TIAs carry more risk than remote TIAs. Multiple TIAs, especially when occurring in a relatively brief interval following the initial TIA, also signal an increased risk of subsequent ischemic stroke.

REFERENCES

1. Dennis M, Bamford J, Sandercock DM, Warlow C: Prognosis of transient ischemic attacks in the Oxfordshire Community Stroke Project. *Stroke.* 1990; 21:848–853.
2. Whisnant JP, Wiebers DO: Clinical epidemiology of transient cerebral ischemic attacks (TIA) in the anterior and posterior circulation. In Sundt TMJ, ed. *Occlusive Cerebrovascular Disease: Diagnosis and Surgical Management.* New York: WB Saunders;1987;60–65.
3. Baker RN, Ramseyer JC, Schwartz WS: Prognosis in patients with transient cerebral ischemic attacks. *Neurology.* 1968;18:1157–1165.
4. Conneally PM, Dyken ML, Futty DE, et al: Cooperative study of hospital frequency and character of transient ischemic attacks. VIII. Risk factors. *JAMA.* 1978;240:742–746.
5. Evans GW, Howard G, Murros KE, et al: Cerebral infarction verified by cranial computed tomography and prognosis for survival following transient ischemic attack. *Stroke.* 1991;22:431–436.
6. Goldner JC, Whisnant JP, Taylor WF: Long-term prognosis of transient cerebral ischemic attacks. *Stroke.* 1971;2:160–167.
7. Hankey GJ, Slattery JM, Warlow CP: Transient ischaemic attacks: Which patients are at high (and low) risk of serious vascular events? *J Neurol Neurosurg Psychiatry.* 1992;55:640–652.
8. Howard G, Toole JF, Frey-Pierson J, Hinshelwood LC: Factors influencing the survival of 451 transient ischemic attack patients. *Stroke.* 1987;18:552–557.
9. Muuronen A, Kaste M: Outcome of 314 patients with transient ischemic attacks. *Stroke.* 1982;13:24–31.
10. Toole JF, Janeway R, Choi K, et al: Transient ischemic attacks due to atherosclerosis: A prospective study of 160 patients. *Arch Neurol.* 1975;32:5–12.
11. Cartlidge NEF, Whisnant JP, Elveback LR: Carotid and vertebral-basilar transient cerebral ischemic attacks: A community study, Rochester, Minnesota. *Mayo Clin Proc.* 1977;52:117–120.
12. Friedman GD, Wilson WS, Mosier JM, et al: Transient ischemic attacks in a community. *JAMA.* 1969;210:1428–1434.
13. Whisnant JP: Epidemiology of stroke: Emphasis on transient cerebral ischemic attacks and hypertension. *Stroke.* 1974;5:68–70.
14. Whisnant JP, Cartlidge NEF, Elveback LR: Carotid and vertebral-basilar transient ischemic attacks: Effect of anticoagulants, hypertension, and cardiac disorders on survival and stroke occurrence—a population study. *Ann Neurol.* 1978;3:107–115.
15. Whisnant JP, Matsumoto N, Elveback LR: The effect of anticoagulant therapy on the prognosis of patients with transient cerebral ischemic attacks in a community: Rochester, Minnesota, 1955 through 1969. *Mayo Clin Proc.* 1973;48:791–797.
16. Whisnant JP, Matsumoto N, Elveback LR: Transient cerebral ischemic attacks in a community. *Mayo Clin Proc.* 1973;48:194–198.
17. Calandre L, Bermejo F, Balseiro J: Long-term outcome of TIAs, RINDs and infarctions with minimum residuum: A prospective study in Madrid. *Acta Neurol Scand.* 1990;82:104–108.
18. Candlise L, Vegotti M, Fieschi C, et al: Italian multicenter study on reversible cerebral ischemic attacks. VI. Prognostic factors and follow-up results. *Stroke.* 1986;17:842–848.
19. Chambers BR, Norris JW, Shurvell BL, Hachinski VC: Prognosis of acute stroke. *Neurology.* 1987;37:221–225.
20. Dutch TIA Trial Study Group: Predictors of major vascular events in patients with a transient ischemic attack or nondisabling stroke. *Stroke.* 1993;24:527–531.
21. Hier DB, Foulkes MA, Swiontoniowski M, et al: Stroke recurrence within 2 years after ischemic infarction. *Stroke.* 1991;22:155–161.
22. Humphrey PRD, Marshall J: Transient ischemic attacks and strokes with recovery prognosis and investigation. *Stroke.* 1981;12:765–769.
23. Kernan WN, Brass LM: Prediction of stroke or death following a carotid territory TIA or minor stroke. *J Stroke Cerebrovasc Dis.* 1992;2(1):S67.
24. Alter M, Sobel E, McCoy RL, et al: Stroke in the Lehigh Valley: Risk factors for recurrent stroke. *Neurology.* 1987;37:503–507.
25. Sobel E, Alter M, Davanipour Z, et al: Stroke in the Lehigh Valley: Combined risk factors for recurrent ischemic stroke. *Neurology.* 1989;39:669–672.
26. Dennis MS, Bamford JM, Sandercock DM, Warlow CP: A comparison of risk factors and prognosis for transient ischemic attacks and minor ischemic stroke. The Oxfordshire Community Stroke Project. *Stroke.* 1989;20:333–339.
27. Matsumoto N, Whisnant JP, Kurland LT, Okazaki H: Natural history of stroke in Rochester, Minnesota, 1955–1969: An extension of a previous study, 1945 through 1954. *Stroke.* 1973;4:20–29.
28. NASCET Collaborators: Beneficial effect of carotid endarterectomy in symptomatic patients with high-grade carotid stenosis. *N Engl J Med.* 1991;325:445–453.
29. Streifler J, Benavente O, Harbison M, et al: Prognostic implications of retinal versus hemispheric TIA in patients with high grade carotid stenosis: Observations from NASCET. *J Stroke Cerebrovasc Dis.* 1992;2(1).
30. Wiebers DO, Whisnant JP, O'Fallon WM: Reversible ischemic neurologic deficit (RIND) in a community: Rochester, Minnesota, 1955–1974. *Neurology.* 1982;32:459–465.
31. Whisnant JP, Melton LJ 3rd, Davis PH, et al: Comparison of case ascertainment by medical record linkage and cohort follow-up to determine incidence rates for transient ischemic attacks and stroke. *J Clin Epidemiol.* 1990;43:791–797.
32. Sacco RL, Wolf PA, Kannel WB, McNamara PM: Survival and recurrence following stroke: The Framingham study. *Stroke.* 1982;13:290–295.

The Importance of Percent Stenosis as an Independent Variable for Predicting Stroke Risk in Symptomatic and Asymptomatic Patients

ROBERT B. RUTHERFORD and MAX B. MITCHELL

It seems almost axiomatic that the more severe the degree of carotid stenosis, the greater the likelihood that it will produce stroke. Occlusive disease of the carotid artery is common, in the western world at least, and it is a, if not the, major cause of stroke. Decades of study of the natural history of the relationship between carotid atherosclerosis and stroke, and the modification of the atherosclerotic process by antithrombotic drugs or by carotid endarterectomy, should have produced sufficient data to answer the question of the importance of percent stenosis as an independent predictor of stroke risk for both symptomatic and asymptomatic patients. While this relationship can be demonstrated (see later discussion), gathering proof is not easy, primarily because of a lack of uniform clinical protocols and standardized reporting practices. More difficult still is attempting to assign a specific stroke risk to a particular percent stenosis. Finally, a natural extension of such efforts would be an attempt to characterize the dimensions and shape of a line that plots stroke risk against percent stenosis, that is, to demonstrate whether the relationship is linear or whether it changes slope as a point of "critical stenosis" is approached and passed. This chapter analyzes the recent English-language literature on the subject.

SOURCES OF DATA

Although data related to this issue appear in a large number of reports in the literature, percent carotid stenosis as a predictor of stroke risk has not, to our knowledge, been the primary focus of any major clinical study. Information on this relationship must be gleaned from studies that were carried out for other purposes. The control groups of treatment trials are an obvious source of information on the natural history of carotid stenosis. Literally thousands of patients have been entered in the many randomized prospective trials of the efficacy of aspirin or other antiplatelet agents in preventing stroke. Unfortunately, the degree of carotid stenosis was not objectively determined as a routine part of the protocols of these trials. Fortunately, in the more recent trials of carotid endarterectomy at least, arteriography has been included in most protocols.

Another major source of data are studies of the natural history of an asymptomatic carotid stenosis. In a number of early studies, the carotid stenoses being followed were located contralateral to a symptomatic lesion that was treated by carotid endarterectomy.[1, 2] However, it is generally held that contralateral carotid endarterectomy probably changes the natural history of carotid stenoses, at least in terms of risk for stroke and stroke severity. A few other studies followed patients with carotid stenosis when surgery was

not performed because of reticence on the part of the patient or referring physician, but these studies did not supply adequate data for our analysis on the degree of stenosis.[3] Finally, the advent of Doppler ultrasonography and, ultimately, duplex scanning allowed serial follow-up examination of patients with asymptomatic carotid stenoses graded by degree of narrowing. These examinations are the major source of data on the outcome of asymptomatic carotid stenosis used in our analysis.

Understandably, most available data on the subject relate to asymptomatic carotid stenosis. A large randomized multicenter study of cerebrovascular arterial disease, reported in several articles in the early 1970s, provided some excellent data on symptomatic carotid stenosis, but because stroke risk appears to have changed over the last two decades, these data were not included in our analysis. In the 1980s, the effectiveness of carotid endarterectomy was again challenged,[4] primarily as a reaction to two dismal reports of community-wide experiences with that operation[5, 6] that appeared at a time when a paradoxic increase in the frequency with which carotid endarterectomy was performed in the United States was observed to occur in the face of a decreasing risk of stroke. As a result, patients with symptomatic as well as asymptomatic carotid stenoses were subjected to prospective randomized trials of carotid endarterectomy. If nothing else, the control groups of these trials have provided, or will provide, valuable data on the natural history of carotid stenosis and stroke risk. Thus, the two main sources of information examined in this chapter are data from the control groups from recent carotid endarterectomy trials and natural history studies based on Doppler ultrasonography.

PROBLEMS WITH CURRENT NATURAL HISTORY DATA RELATIVE TO THE DEGREE OF CAROTID STENOSIS AND STROKE RISK

A large number of generic problems presented difficulties when the literature was analyzed. These problems will be described, and a few of the better known studies cited as examples.

- In a great many studies, the actual degree of carotid stenosis was either not objectively measured[7] or was assessed only by indirect methods[8, 9] (eg, ocular plethysmography), which, at best, would only identify "hemodynamically significant" carotid stenosis, dividing the patient population into two broad categories based on whether the patient tested positive or negative and thus was presumed to have greater than or less than 50 percent carotid stenosis, respectively.

- In many, if not most, studies in which carotid stenosis was objectively measured, the data were arbitrarily grouped by degree of stenosis into broad categories to achieve statistical significance, again typically greater or less than a certain degree of stenosis (eg, 50% or 80%) but with no indication of the distribution of stenoses within these wide ranges.
- In general, the manner in which the degree of carotid stenosis was estimated is not uniform in the literature. In fact, sometimes the method is not even clearly described. Currently accepted practice now estimates the degree of carotid stenosis by comparing the smallest diameter in the stenosis to the normal diameter of the internal carotid artery above the stenosis. This practice was apparently not followed in some major studies that used duplex scan serial surveillance.[10] In other reports, "percent stenosis" refers to cross sectional area rather than diameter.[11, 12]
- In several studies, the duration of follow-up is given as a range with a mean figure for the entire group but is not delineated for specific subgroups of carotid stenosis.
- In some studies, stroke, transient ischemic attack (TIA), amaurosis fugax, and even asymptomatic occlusion were combined and presented as a neurologic event rate, but the risk of stroke was not separately reported for each subgroup of carotid stenosis. It might be argued, with some reason, that "stroke" should include TIAs because the temporal separation between those patients who recover completely within 24 hours and those who recover completely later (reversible ischemic neurologic deficit) is arbitrary, and a significant number of patients with TIA can be shown on computed tomography (CT) scan or magnetic resonance imaging (MRI) to have had cerebral infarct, and many cerebral infarcts are not detected clinically, occurring in patients otherwise classified as asymptomatic. In fact, a clinical classification recently proposed by vascular surgeons renames TIAs and reversible ischemic neurologic deficits *brief* and *temporary* stroke, respectively.[13, 14] This classification would of course make it easier to demonstrate increasing stroke risk with increasing stenosis and would shift the plot line upward very significantly. However, it would not be in concert with the thinking of most neurologists and most of the literature we analyzed, which focuses on lasting, if not permanent, neurologic deficit.
- In many studies (especially in trials of antiplatelet therapy or trials comparing carotid endarterectomy with antiplatelet therapy), stroke in any arterial territory was used as the endpoint and, even though an overall ratio of ipsilateral to total stroke was given in some reports, it was not supplied for subgroups with different degrees of carotid stenosis.
- A few studies focused only on the rate of unheralded stroke,[15] and although it has been and is still being argued that this is a most appropriate endpoint, we did not think it appropriate to include data from these studies in estimating stroke risk in this particular analysis.
- Similarly, in some studies, a significant number of patients were removed from the serial follow-up because

those patients underwent carotid endarterectomy, either because of the onset of TIA or amaurosis fugax or prophylactically in asymptomatic cases because of documented progression.[10, 16, 17] It is suspected that the practice of dropping patients from follow-up without their having suffered recurrent stroke may be more widespread than realized and is simply not reported.

- A significant number of otherwise excellent studies focused only on a single range of carotid stenosis (eg, over 80%), ostensibly because they wished to study the natural history of "critical stenosis" in asymptomatic patients.[15] Unfortunately, these studies did not provide a second level of carotid stenosis necessary for the type of comparative analysis carried out here.

Subtler issues, such as the definition of stroke used (often not described), the inherent variability and inaccuracy in measuring percent carotid stenosis by arteriography, the questionable validity of extrapolating duplex scan velocity data to percent stenosis based on earlier published correlations with arteriography or of using criteria developed by other investigators without internal quality control, obviously affect the reliability of data found in the literature. Clearly, many of the above limitations to analyzing the literature could be overcome by adopting standardized reporting practices (discussed in Chapter 58). Furthermore, it is apparent that more precise and sufficient information to resolve this issue still exists for (and thus could be retrieved from) many of the recent trials cited in this chapter. By necessity, for statistical strength, stroke risk reported from these trials is grouped into broad ranges of carotid stenosis. Finally, while some of the problems listed prevented our using data from many of the studies in the literature for the purpose of estimating current stroke risk relative to the degree of carotid stenosis, in other studies there was sufficient data for two or more ranges of carotid stenosis, in spite of minor flaws, to allow us to extrapolate an annual ipsilateral stroke risk with reasonable confidence.

ANALYSIS OF DATA FOR ASYMPTOMATIC STENOSES

Two studies that add significant perspective to this subject but were not included in our projections for one reason or another deserve comment.

A series of studies from the University of Washington, best represented by the report of Roederer and associates,[10] used serial surveillance by duplex scanning to document disease progression and development of symptoms in the carotid arteries of 162 asymptomatic patients referred to the vascular diagnostic laboratory. Although the study has been criticized for relying on previous correlations between duplex scan and arteriography and for measuring normal internal carotid diameter at the bulb rather than higher up, these reports nevertheless provide important information about lesion progression and establish that most symptoms develop either in patients with carotid stenosis greater than 80 percent diameter (as measured by their methods) or in those in whom the stenosis progresses to or beyond that level. Unfortunately, their data did not help in our analysis of stroke risk for different degrees of carotid stenosis because 70 of the 162 patients ultimately underwent carotid endarterectomy, mostly for progression of stenosis or the development of TIAs before the onset of stroke. In all fairness, in this study the decision to intervene rested with the referring physician and not the investigators.

Also worthy of comment are the studies performed at the University of Southern Illinois of stroke risk in patients who did not undergo surgery.[15, 18] The patients were studied by a Hokanson pulsed Doppler "arteriograph" and were grouped into three categories: group I, no stenosis; group II, less than 50 percent stenosis; group III, greater than 50 percent stenosis. The Life Table method was used to predict stroke risk. In one report,[19] the authors showed an increasing risk of localizing neurologic events (group I = 13.1%; II = 18.1%; III = 24.8%) and a less dramatic increase in stroke risk (group I = 9.8%; II = 11.1%; III = 19.3%). Unfortunately, these estimates were derived from a mixed group of patients whose initial symptoms were none (19%), nonhemispheric (45%), amaurosis fugax (5%), TIA (15%), and stroke (15%). During follow-up there were 9 strokes in 59 asymptomatic patients but no significant difference between the stroke rate for lesser than and greater than 50 percent stenosis (16.7% versus 17.6%). Subsequently, the same group reported a larger number of asymptomatic patients (n = 104) combined with a large group with nonhemispheric symptoms (n = 190).[18] Following the same protocol, the 5-year stroke risk for the combined groups showed a definite increase for increasing degrees of stenosis (group I = 9%; II = 12%; III = 18%), but the data for asymptomatic patients showed a significant trend only if TIAs were included (group I = 14%; II = 14%; III = 24%). While the data from both these reports clearly indicate greater stroke risk for patients with increasing degrees of stenosis, particularly for those with stenoses greater than 50 percent (group III) compared with lesser degrees of stenosis (group II), and estimate a 15 percent 2-year stroke risk for patients with stenoses greater than 50 percent, their data were excluded from our final analysis because patients were assigned to groups according to the side with the greatest degree of carotid stenosis and a significant number of strokes were contralateral to the side with the greatest degree of stenosis. Thus, it was not possible to obtain specific data for the ipsilateral stroke risk for certain degrees of carotid stenosis.

Another study should be mentioned primarily because it has been touted as the first completed prospective randomized trial of carotid endarterectomy versus medical therapy for asymptomatic carotid stenosis.[17] We had hoped to use data from the control (medical therapy) group because the carotid stenoses were grouped in four ranges (<50%, 50–70%, 70–90%, and >90%). However, 27 percent of the patients had undergone unilateral carotid endarterectomy *before* randomization, and the investigators operated on patients with asymptomatic stenoses that progressed beyond 90 percent, and on a significant number of patients for TIA. Altogether, 118 of 204 patients (58%) in the "nonoperated" group had had carotid endarterectomy. This method of selection, and our inability to extract the incidence of stroke for different levels of stenosis, precluded the use of this data. Considering numerous exclusions and crossovers, this trial only showed that the investigators' very selective approach to applying surgery for asymptomatic carotid stenosis did not yield statistically significantly inferior results compared with a routine policy of prophylactic carotid endarterectomy.

We narrowed our final analysis to the data from seven recent studies that related percent carotid stenosis to ipsilateral stroke risk in asymptomatic patients studied by objective means and that provided data for at least two different ranges of carotid stenosis.[11, 12, 16, 20–23] These data are summarized in Table 4–1. Two of the studies gauged the degree of stenosis arteriographically,[20, 23] on entry at least, and the other five used some form of Doppler ultrasound insonation or imaging or both. A number of extrapolations were required to convert the data to an annual ipsilateral stroke risk for percent carotid stenosis by diameter. Basically, data on carotid stenosis were either reported as percent diameter reduction or were converted to this standard from estimates based on cross sectional area. An annual ipsilateral stroke rate was derived from the cumulative numbers of strokes occurring ipsilateral to each carotid stenosis that was followed, and the mean duration of follow-up in months was divided by 12.

It can be seen from Table 4–1 that in six of the seven studies, the stroke risk increases with increasing degrees of stenosis. Only in the recent Veterans' Administration (VA) Cooperative trial of carotid endarterectomy for patients with asymptomatic stenosis was there no significant difference in the stroke risk for nonoperated control subjects between those with an initial stenosis of 50 to 75 percent versus those whose stenosis was 75 to 99 percent.[23] Unfortunately, the findings of later arteriograms, if they were performed at the time of stroke, were not included in the report, and there was no noninvasive evaluation of the degree of stenosis over time to indicate the degree of stenosis at the time of stroke. However, this criticism can be leveled at a number of other studies in the literature. In the six studies that did show a trend, the ranges of annual stroke risk varied for similar degrees of stenosis, particularly at higher levels of stenosis. With this reservation, the annual ipsilateral stroke risk for asymptomatic stenoses of less than 50 percent diameter reduction can be placed at 1 percent or less (average 0.7% per year). For the levels of stenosis over 50 percent that are represented in these six studies, the average annual ipsilateral stroke risk is just over 3 percent (mean, 3.1% per year; range, 1.7–4.8%). Thus, there would appear to be a roughly fourfold greater annual ipsilateral stroke risk for stenoses greater than 50 percent than for stenoses less than 50 percent.

These same data are graphically presented in Figure 4–1A, where data points assigned to each group are placed at the middle of their stated range of stenosis. The trend of increasing stroke risk for increasing degrees of stenosis is more readily appreciated in this graphic representation. Roughly, the slope of a straight line representing these data would cross the point representing 1 percent per year ipsilateral stroke risk at the point representing 40 percent stenosis, the 2 percent point at 60 percent stenosis, and the 3 percent point at 80 percent stenosis. Again, this attempt to put the data in their simplest terms acknowledges considerable variability, especially in estimates of the risk of ipsilateral stroke in connection with higher degrees of stenosis. In general, most reports that focus on higher grade stenosis, not included here because they lacked comparable data for lower grades of stenosis, would place the risk of stroke even higher than our analysis found. For example, data from the ongoing University of Washington surveillance of asymptomatic stenosis indicated an overall neurologic event rate of 46 percent, with a 19 percent stroke rate, in 2 years.[24]

TABLE 4–1. Asymptomatic Carotid Stenosis: Degree versus Annual Ipsilateral Stroke Rate*

Study (by Author)†	Design	Follow-Up (Mean), mo	Method	Incidence of Antiplatelet Therapy, %	Degree of Stenosis, % / Annual Stroke Rate, %					
Chambers[12]	P n = 500	23	D‡	35	0–15 / 0.7	16–49 / 1.0		50–100 / 2.8		
Hertzer[20]§	R n = 195	35	A	53			50–69 / 0.6	70–89 / 4.8		≥90 / 5.2
Hennerici[21]	P n = 235	29	D‡	35		30–55 / 0.8		>55 / 3.4		
Autret[11]	P n = 242	29	D‡	NA	1–30 / 0	30–50 / 0.8		50–99 / 1.7		
O'Holleran[22]¶	P n = 296	46	D‡	0		<50 / 0.8		≥50 / 4.2		
Norris[16]**	P n = 696	41	D‡	42	<30 / 1.0	30–50 / 0.5		>50 / 2.5		
Hobson[23]#	PR n = 218	48	D/A	84				50–75 / 2.4		>75 / 2.3

*Calculated as cumulative stroke rate divided by mean follow-up in years.
†See reference list for full bibliographic information.
‡Degree of stenosis was converted from percent reduction of vessel cross sectional area to percent reduction of vessel diameter.
§Stenosis data calculated from Fig. 6, p. 169.
¶Study number is total number of stenotic carotid arteries evaluated. The actual number of patients was 293. Strokes were not specifically identified as ipsilateral.
**Of all strokes, 75% were reported to be ipsilateral. Annual ipsilateral stroke rates calculated as 75% of total stroke rate in each category. Risk of stroke was highest during the first 2 years of follow-up. A total of 26 patients who developed ischemic symptoms underwent carotid endarterectomy. All symptomatic patients had carotid stenosis of ≥60% of the cross sectional area (47% diameter reduction).
#Only data for the medically treated group of this study was considered. Of all patients, 16% stopped antiplatelet therapy because of intolerance. There were a total of 32 strokes in the medical treatment group, of which 26 occurred within the first 2 years of follow-up.
A, angiography; D, Doppler or duplex; NA, data not available; P, prospective; PR, prospective and randomized; R, retrospective.

FIGURE 4–1 *A,* The data from the seven studies listed in Table 4–1 are plotted graphically, with group values assigned to a point midway in the given range of stenosis. *B,* The data points are submitted to curve-fitting projections for both linear and exponential functions.

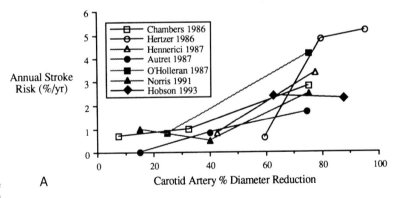

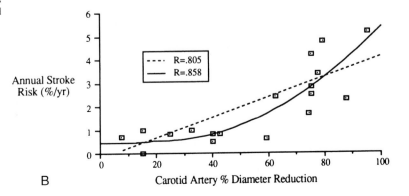

The risk of stroke as reported in this study is high early in the period following the onset of symptoms and then drops off, so that a 5-year projection of stroke risk might be closer to 5 percent per year. The authors point out that estimates of a lower stroke risk in previous reports may have been produced by the use of older continuous wave Doppler estimates of stenosis, some of which are represented in the data in Table 4–1.[1, 12, 15, 21] Modern duplex instrumentation is more accurate (sensitive) in identifying high-grade (80%) stenosis. O'Holleran and colleagues,[22] who also used Duplex scanning, also reported a high stroke risk (4.2% per year) for stenosis over 50 percent, and Hertzer and coworkers,[20] in the only study employing arteriography, reported an 8.2 percent per year stroke risk for stenoses of 70 to 89 percent. Thus, the levels of annual ipsilateral stroke risk derived from the data represented in Table 4–1 may well represent a minimal stroke risk estimate, to the extent that a number of the reports included used older Doppler techniques that are now thought to identify higher degrees of stenosis with less reliability, ie, to overestimate stenosis and thus underestimate stroke risk relative to degree of stenosis.

Furthermore, estimates of the risk of stroke with increasing degrees of carotid stenosis may be reduced by excluding patients from natural history studies or therapeutic trials because of progression of disease or transient symptoms.[10, 16, 17] The risk of carotid stenosis is shown to be very much higher when TIAs and carotid occlusions are included in the data and reported in terms of a neurologic event rate. To illustrate this approach, data for the total neurologic event rate, which were available for the seven studies represented in Figure 4–1A, are listed in Table 4–2 and plotted in Figure 4–2. The risk of any neurologic event appears to be two to three times higher than the risk of incurring a lasting neurologic deficit. Thus, to the extent that patients with TIAs and higher degrees of stenosis who have a higher stroke risk (see later discussion) have been removed from the studies used in our analysis, our estimates of stroke risk are low. Such exclusion is common clinical practice but was not even addressed in the protocols of many studies. Studies in which the practice was reported to have occurred to a significant degree were excluded from our analysis.[10, 18, 25] Nevertheless, it would appear that, for the reasons cited, the true risk of stroke for increasing degrees of carotid stenosis may have been generally underestimated.

The final question relates to the slope of the curve. Is it straight, or does it rise exponentially as a point of critical stenosis is reached and does it plateau at this point or drop down beyond it, as suggested by some (Fig. 4–3)[15, 25] These questions cannot be answered with finality from available data, although it is our impression that there is an exponential rise as a critical point of stenosis is reached, with either plateauing or possibly even a slight drop as complete occlusion is approached. An attempt to compare curve-fitting projections to the data presented in Figure 4–1A is shown in Figure 4–1B. The r value for an exponential curve is higher than that for a linear fit (0.859 versus 0.805).

It is hoped that the control group of the current Asymptomatic Carotid Atherosclerosis Study Group (ACAS) trial[26]

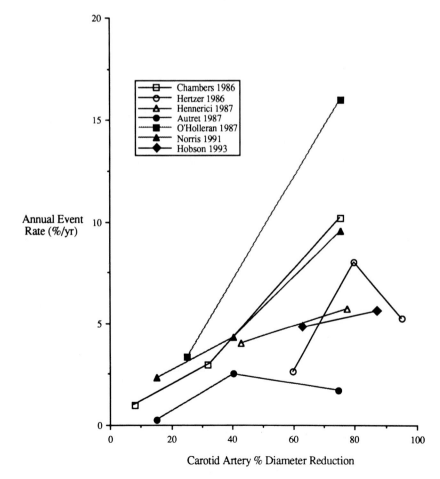

FIGURE 4–2. Data for the neurologic event rate taken from the same studies listed in Table 4–1 are plotted in the same manner as for stroke rate in Figure 4–1A. Comparison with Figure 4–1A indicates that the predicted neurologic event rate is close to three times higher than the stroke rate for patients with asymptomatic stenoses.

TABLE 4–2. Asymptomatic Carotid Stenosis: Degree versus Annual Ipsilateral Ischemic Neurologic Event Rate*

Study (by Author)†	Design	Follow-Up (Mean), mo	Method	Incidence of Antiplatelet Therapy, %	Degree of Stenosis, % / Annual Stroke Rate, %				
Chambers[12]	P n=500	23	D‡	35	0–15 / 1.0	16–49 / 3.0	50–100 / 10.2		
Hertzer[20]§	R n=195	35	A	53			50–69 / 2.6	70–89 / 8.0	≥90 / 5.2
Hennerici[21]	P n=235	29	D‡	35		30–55 / 4.0	>55 / 5.7		
Autret[11]	P n=242	29	D‡	NA	1–30 / 0.23	30–50 / 2.5	50–99 / 1.7		
O'Holleran[22]¶	P n=296	46	D‡	0		<50 / 3.3	≥50 / 16		
Norris[16]**	P n=696	41	D‡	42	<30 / 2.3	30–50 / 4.3	>50 / 9.5		
Hobson[23]#	PR n=218	48	D/A	84			50–75 / 4.8	>75 / 5.6	

*Defined as cumulative combined rate of transient ischemic attack and stroke ipsilateral to the stenotic carotid artery divided by mean follow-up in years. In cases where death not due to stroke was included as an event, such deaths were excluded from the event rate calculations in this table.

†See reference list for full bibliographic information.

‡Degree of stenosis was converted from percent reduction of vessel cross sectional area to percent reduction of vessel diameter.

§Stenosis data calculated from Hertzer et al,[20] Figure 6.

¶Study number is total number of stenotic carotid arteries evaluated. The actual number of patients was 293. Strokes were not specifically identified as ipsilateral.

**Of all events, 75% were reported to be ipsilateral. Annual ipsilateral event rates calculated as 75% of the total event rate reported in each category. For stenoses ≥50% diameter reduction, the event rate in the first year was 18%.

#Only data for the medically treated group of this study were considered. Of all patients, 16% stopped antiplatelet therapy because of intolerance or noncompliance.

A, angiography; D, Doppler or duplex; NA, data not available; P, prospective; PR, prospective and randomized; R, retrospective.

will provide sufficient additional data so that these final details can be answered. If not, data from the many recent trials could be pooled. Most data from these trials have been grouped into broad ranges for statistical analysis to achieve significance, but reanalyzing the data for percent stenosis versus stroke risk should readily answer the remaining questions, ie, as to the dimensions and shape of the line that predicts stroke risk with increasing degrees of carotid stenosis in asymptomatic patients.

ANALYSIS OF DATA FOR SYMPTOMATIC STENOSES

As one would expect, there is less usable data on patients with symptomatic stenoses. Since the prospective random-

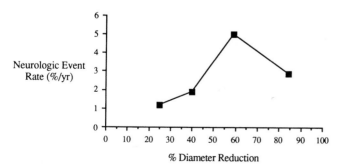

FIGURE 4–3. A commonly accepted view of the shape of the curve created by plotting stroke risk against degree of stenosis, popularized by a study by Norris and Zhu.[25]

ized multicentered trial on extracranial arterial disease, published in a number of reports in the late 1960s and early 1970s, established that carotid endarterectomy was superior to medical therapy for patients with TIAs ipsilateral to an appropriate carotid lesion,[27] symptomatic patients have been treated surgically, for the most part. There were no major studies of the natural history of symptomatic carotid stenosis until the recent challenge to the efficacy of carotid endarterectomy, which focused on both symptomatic and asymptomatic stenoses. There are three recent trials of symptomatic carotid stenosis, two of which are still in progress: the North American Symptomatic Carotid Endarterectomy Trial (NASCET),[28] the European Carotid Surgical Trialists' Collaborative Study (ECST),[29] and the brief VA Cooperative trial of carotid endarterectomy for symptomatic stenosis, reported by Mayberg and associates.[30] The data from these trials are summarized in Table 4–3. In the latter two trials, two groups separated by level of stenosis were reported in the data, and both studies show a much greater risk of ipsilateral stroke in the group with the greater degree of stenosis. The NASCET trial reported an annual ipsilateral stroke rate of 13 percent for stenosis greater than 70 percent, which falls midway between the 5 percent rate reported by the ECST trial and the 25.6 percent rate reported by the VA trial. In addition, the NASCET trial reported a definite trend toward increased risk for stroke for each of the three deciles represented in the over–70 percent stenosis group. The NASCET and ECST trials continue to gather data for the very important levels of carotid stenosis between 30 percent and 70 percent, and until these data are reported, nothing

TABLE 4–3. Symptomatic Carotid Stenosis: Degree versus Annual Ipsilateral Stroke Rate*

Study (by Author)†	Design	Follow-Up (Mean), mo	Degree of Stenosis, % / Annual Stroke Rate, %		
NASCET[28]‡	PR n = 331	24			$\frac{70-99}{13.0}$
ECST[29]§	PR n = 478	32	$\frac{0-29}{0.5}$		$\frac{70-99}{5.0}$
Mayberg[30]¶	PR n = 98	12		$\frac{50-69}{6.7}$	$\frac{>70}{25.6}$

*Calculated as the cumulative ipsilateral stroke rate divided by the mean follow-up in years. All studies included patients randomized to carotid endarterectomy plus aspirin versus aspirin alone. Data reflect only the medical treatment alone groups.

†See reference list for full bibliographic information.

‡Of the medical treatment alone group, 5% crossed over to carotid endarterectomy for reasons other than stroke. Evaluation of outcome for patients with stenosis less than 70% continues.

§Of the medical treatment alone group, 4% crossed over to carotid endarterectomy. Evaluation of outcome for patients with 30–69% stenosis continues.

¶Endpoints include stroke, crescendo transient ischemic attacks, and death. Of the medical therapy alone group, 3% crossed over to carotid endarterectomy.

PR, prospective and randomized.

definitive can be said about the slope and dimensions of a plot of the stroke risk against the degree of stenosis for symptomatic patients. However, it might be predicted that, because the risk of stroke is highest immediately after the onset of TIAs or other symptoms, the slope of a plot of stroke risk against time would have an early peak. Therefore, the predicted rate of stroke risk versus degree of stenosis for symptomatic patients may be higher when derived from short-term studies and lower from long-term studies. This is implied from a comparison of the VA[30] and ECST[10] trials. All that can be concluded at the moment is that symptomatic patients are also exposed to an increasing risk for stroke with increasing degrees of stenosis, and that this risk is very much higher for them than for asymptomatic patients, possibly as much as four times higher, at least in the early period after the onset of symptoms.

SUMMARY

- The risk of ipsilateral stroke increases with increasing degrees of carotid stenosis in both asymptomatic and symptomatic patients.
- Variability in estimates of the actual stroke risk in the current literature precludes confident prediction of the actual dimensions and shape of a line that plots annual ipsilateral stroke risk against the degree of stenosis, although a qualified attempt is made for asymptomatic patients in this report.
- Final reports from current trials still in progress on asymptomatic (ACAS) and symptomatic patients (NASCET, ECST) may provide sufficient data to allow more definitive estimates of stroke risk to be made. If not, more detailed data retrieved from recent trials should be combined and analyzed for this specific purpose.
- Our attempt to analyze the recent literature to determine the importance of percent stenosis as an independent variable in determining stroke risk highlights a significant number of major problems that result from the lack of standardized study protocols and reporting practices in the field.

REFERENCES

1. Johnson N, Burnham SJ, Flanigan DF, et al: Carotid endarterectomy: A follow-up study of the contralateral nonoperated carotid artery. Ann Surg. 1978;188:748–752.
2. Roederer GO, Langlois YE, Lusiani L, et al: Natural history of carotid artery disease on the side contralateral to endarterectomy. J Vasc Surg. 1984;1:62–72.
3. Thompson JE, Patman RD, Talkington CM: Asymptomatic carotid bruit: Long-term outcome of patients having endarterectomy compared with unoperated controls. Ann Surg. 1978;188:308–316.
4. Chambers BR, Norris JW: The case against surgery for asymptomatic carotid stenosis. Stroke. 1984;15:964–967.
5. Easton JD, Sherman DG: Stroke and mortality rate in carotid endarterectomy: 228 consecutive operations. Stroke. 1977;8:565–568.
6. Brott T, Thalinger K: Carotid endarterectomy in Cincinnati, 1980: Indications and morbidity in 431 cases. Neurology. 1983;33(suppl 2):93.
7. Wolf PA, Kannel WB, Sorlie P, McNamara P: Asymptomatic carotid bruit and the risk of stroke. JAMA. 1981;245:1442–1445.
8. Busuttil RW, Baker JD, Davidson RK, Machleder HI: Carotid artery stenosis: Hemodynamic significance and clinical course. JAMA. 1981;245:1438–1441.
9. Meissner I, Wiebers DO, Whisnant JP, O'Fallon M: The natural history of asymptomatic carotid artery occlusive disease. JAMA. 1987;258:2704–2707.
10. Roederer GO, Langlois YE, Jager KA, et al: The natural history of carotid arterial disease in asymptomatic patients with cervical bruits. Stroke. 1984;15:605.
11. Autret A, Saudeau D, Bertrand P, et al: Stroke risk in patients with carotid stenosis. Lancet. 1987;1:888–890.
12. Chambers BR, Norris JW: Outcome in patients with asymptomatic carotid stenosis. N Engl J Med. 1986;315:860–865.
13. Hye RJ, Dilley RB, Browse NL, Bernstein EF: Evaluation of a new classification of cerebrovascular disease (CHAT). Am J Surg. 1987;154:104–110.
14. Baker JD, Rutherford RB, Bernstein EF, et al: Suggested standards for reports dealing with cerebrovascular disease. J Vasc Surg. 1988;8:721–729.
15. Bogousslavsky J, Despland P, Regli F: Asymptomatic tight stenosis of the carotid artery: Long-term prognosis. Neurology. 1986;36:861–863.
16. Norris JW, Zhu CZ, Bornstein NM, Chambers BR: Vascular risks of asymptomatic carotid stenosis. Stroke. 1991;22:1485–1490.
17. CASANOVA Study Group: Carotid surgery versus medical therapy in asymptomatic carotid stenosis. Stroke. 1991;22:1229–1235.
18. Moore DJ, Miles RD, Gooley NA, Sumner DS: Noninvasive assessment of stroke risk in asymptomatic and nonhemispheric patients with suspected carotid disease. Ann Surg. 1985;202:491–505.
19. Moore DJ, Sheehan P, Kolm P, et al: Are strokes predictable with noninvasive methods: A five-year follow up of 303 unoperated patients. J Vasc Surg. 1985;2:654–660.
20. Hertzer NR, Flannigan RA, O'Hara PJ, Beven EG: Surgical versus nonoperative treatment of asymptomatic carotid stenosis. Ann Surg. 1986;204:163–171.
21. Hennerici M, Hulsbomer HB, Hefter H, et al: Natural history of asymptomatic extracranial arterial disease: Results of a long term prospective study. Brain. 1987;110:777–791.
22. O'Holleran LW, Kennely MM, McClurken M, Johnson JM: Natural history of asymptomatic carotid plaque: Five year follow up study. Am J Surg. 1987;154:659–662.
23. Hobson IRW, Weiss DG, Fields WB, et al: Efficacy of carotid endarterectomy for asymptomatic carotid stenosis. N Engl J Med. 1993;328:221–227.
24. Moneta GL, Taylor DC, Nicholls SC, et al: Operative versus nonoperative management of asymptomatic high grade internal carotid artery stenosis: Improved results with endarterectomy. Stroke. 1987;18:1005–1010.

25. Norris JW, Zhu CZ: Stroke risk and critical carotid stenosis. *J Neurol Neurosurg Psychiatry*. 1990;53:235–237.

26. The Asymptomatic Carotid Atherosclerosis Study Group: Study design for randomized prospective trial of carotid endarterectomy for asymptomatic atherosclerosis. *Stroke*. 1989;20:844–849.

27. Fields WS, Maslenikiv V, Meyer JS, et al. Joint study of extracranial arterial occlusion. *JAMA*. 1970;211(12):1993–2003.

28. NASCET: Beneficial effect of carotid endarterectomy in symptomatic patients with high-grade stenosis. *N Engl J Med*. 1991;325:445–453.

29. ECSTCG: MRC European carotid surgery trial: Interim results for symptomatic patients with severe (70–99%) or with mild (0–29%) carotid stenosis. *Lancet*. 1991;337:1235–1243.

30. Mayberg MR, Wilson ES, Yatsu F, et al: Carotid endarterectomy and prevention of cerebral ischemia in symptomatic carotid stenosis. *JAMA*. 1991;266:3289–3294.

CHAPTER 5

The Importance of Carotid Plaque Characteristics as Independent Variables in Predicting Stroke Risk

G. GEROULAKOS and A. NICOLAIDES

The European and the North American Symptomatic Carotid Endarterectomy Trial investigators reported a conclusive benefit for carotid endarterectomy for patients with symptomatic 70 to 99 percent internal carotid artery (ICA) stenosis.[1, 2] In these studies, the degree of stenosis of the ICA was the only criterion for selection of symptomatic patients at high risk for stroke. It has been suggested, however, that plaque characterization is another important factor associated with an increased risk for stroke. The purpose of this chapter is to review the literature on carotid plaque characterization, with particular emphasis on its clinical importance. The morphologic variables that will be considered can be grouped in two categories: (1) plaque surface configuration (smooth, ulcerated) and (2) plaque internal structure as determined by ultrasonography.

PLAQUE SURFACE CONFIGURATION

Definitions

There is no uniform agreement as to the definition of ulceration; however, a definition is important, lest a falsely high incidence be reported by inclusion of lumen surface irregularities. Inclusion of such findings is one of the reasons for the great diversity in the reported incidence of carotid plaque ulceration in various studies. Another factor is the use of magnifying loops in the examination of the endarterectomy specimen, so that smaller ulcers are included in the data.[3]

While in some studies no definition of plaque ulceration has been reported,[4] in others several definitions of ulceration have been proposed. According to an ultrasonic definition of plaque ulceration reported by Yao and associates,[5] an ulcerated plaque is a complex (mixed) plaque of variable echogenicity. Other investigators suggested that the surface ultrasonic characteristics of carotid plaque should be classified as smooth or irregular. A plaque is smooth when the blood-lesion interface is unbroken, and irregular when a break in the echoreflective surface of the lesion is observed, or the surface is uneven.[6] Some authors defined carotid plaque ulceration according to the gross pathologic findings of the endarterectomy specimen, such as (1) a crater at least 1 mm wide and 1 mm deep,[3] and (2) a definite surface irregularity with a punched-out characteristic.[7] Definitions based on histologic findings of the endarterectomy specimen have also been used, such as (1) microscopic foci to areas of diffuse loss of surface endothelium over most of the plaque surface,[8] and (2) deep depressions in the plaque where the endothelial lining is interrupted.[9]

Although an attempt has been made in a few studies to exclude ulceration caused by operative manipulation of the specimen, most studies fail to specify how such an exclusion was made. Standardization of a definition and of the method-

ology used to define carotid plaque ulceration appears to be an important step in comparative studies.

Ultrasonic Detection of Ulcerated Plaque

The preoperative diagnosis of the ulcerated carotid atheroma has attracted the interest of many investigators attempting to identify a group at high risk for stroke. O'Donnell and colleagues[7] compared B-mode ultrasonography and selective four-vessel arteriography findings with pathologic specimens obtained from 89 carotid endarterectomies. Whereas arteriography detected only 16 of 27 ulcerations (sensitivity, 59%), B-mode ultrasonography had a greater sensitivity (24 of 27, 89%). Both imaging techniques had comparable specificities (arteriography, 73%; B-mode ultrasonography 87%). Subsequently, two multicenter validation studies found poor agreement between preoperative imaging and pathologic specimens.[10, 11] In one of these studies, the repeatability of diagnosis of carotid ulceration by the same observer was moderate ($\kappa = 0.64$). When the interpretations of two observers were compared, the value of κ fell to 0.11. Comparable degrees of reproducibility were seen with the use of angiographic techniques; intraobserver repeatability was 0.67, and interobserver repeatability was 0.41.[12] Thus it appears that the ultrasound criteria for the diagnosis of ulcerated carotid atheroma are subjective and not easily transferable from one center or interpreter to another.

The studies investigating the ability of B-mode carotid imaging to detect ulceration failed to address the quantitative aspect of carotid plaque. A recent study[3] showed that the degree of stenosis significantly affected diagnostic sensitivities. B-mode sensitivity was 77 percent (10/13) in plaques of 50 percent or less stenosis and only 41 percent (26/63) for plaques of more than 50 percent stenosis ($P = 0.03$).

Lusby[13] stated that duplex scanning has the ability to detect the degree of stenosis based on spectral analysis and the morphologic appearance of the plaque in terms of echolucent and echodense areas. To expect this modality to detect surface ulceration goes beyond its capabilities. The recent introduction of a new generation of duplex scanners with edge-enhancing facilities, however, may considerably improve accuracy in the identification of carotid plaque ulceration.

Clinical Significance

In 1963, Julian and associates[14] were the first to discuss the issue of carotid plaque ulceration. They reported 17 cases of ulcerative carotid lesions in 231 symptomatic patients who had undergone carotid endarterectomy. Thrombi were found lying in the ulcer crater in all the cases. The authors suggested that carotid plaque ulceration is associated with an increased risk for cerebral embolization. Similar findings were reported by Moore and Hall[15] and others,[16, 17] who stressed the importance of plaque ulceration in the development of symptoms. However, this pattern has not been consistent. Imperato and coworkers,[18] in a series of 275 plaque specimens symptomatic patients and 101 plaque specimens from asymptomatic patients, all obtained from carotid endarterectomies, showed no significant difference in the incidence of ulceration and intraluminal thrombus between the symptomatic and asymptomatic plaques. More recently in a clinicopathologic study, Fisher and coworkers[19] found that the occurrence of transient ischemic attacks (TIAs) and amaurosis fugax did not correlate with the presence of plaque ulceration.

One of the reasons for these conflicting reports may be the time interval between the occurrence of the symptoms and the operation, which has not been recorded in any of the studies cited. It may be that some of these ulcers heal following a single attack of TIA or amaurosis fugax. Lusby and colleagues[20] reported re-endothelialization in a number of plaque lesions in patients for whom the interval between symptom onset and surgery was longer than 3 weeks. We believe that this point should be addressed in all future studies.

In an early study from our unit,[4] carotid endarterectomy specimens were examined for macroscopic ulceration, and the findings were correlated with the prevalence of cerebral infarction on the computed tomographic (CT) scan in 65 patients. Of those patients, 55 were symptomatic and 13 asymptomatic. A macroscopic ulcer seen with the naked eye was found in 42 specimens (three bilateral operations). Twenty-six (62%) of the patients with ulceration had one or more ipsilateral infarcts. In contrast, only 2 (8%) of the 26 patients without ulceration had infarcts. These data showed a strong association between internal carotid plaque ulceration and infarction detected on CT scans. Further evidence for the clinical importance of ulcerative carotid lesions is provided by the North American Symptomatic Carotid Surgery Trial.[21] Review of 593 angiograms showing severe stenosis led to recognition of ulceration with reasonable certainty in 34 percent of patients assigned to the medical therapy group and in 36 percent of those assigned to the surgery group. At 2 years, a nonfatal stroke or any death due to a vascular event had occurred in 30 percent of the group with ulcer that was assigned to medical care alone, and in 17 percent of the group without an ulcer (log rank test: $P = 0.0054$).

It appears from these studies that the presence of carotid plaque ulceration has a clinical relevance, which is likely to help in the identification of groups at high risk for stroke.

CONSISTENCY OF THE PLAQUE

Background

High-resolution ultrasonography has the major advantage over arteriography in that it can be used to characterize atherosclerotic plaques.

A classification that allows a closer study of the character and behavior of atherosclerotic plaque was first introduced

by Reilly and associates[22] in 1982. Two distinct echo patterns were recognized. The first pattern was termed *homogeneous*. Homogeneous lesions were characterized by uniformly high- or medium-level echoes. There was a close correlation between a homogeneous ultrasound pattern and a fibrous lesion. The second ultrasonographic plaque pattern was termed *heterogeneous*. Heterogeneous lesions demonstrated high-, medium-, and low-level echoes. There was a close association between the heterogeneous ultrasound pattern and the presence of intraplaque hemorrhage, lipids, cholesterol, and a loose stroma. A refinement of this classification was introduced by Steffen and coworkers in 1988.[23] Four plaque types were defined, based on the degree of echolucency seen on B-mode scan:

Type I: Dominantly echolucent lesions with a thin echogenic cap (Fig. 5–1).
Type II: Substantially echolucent lesions with small areas of echogenicity (Fig. 5–2).
Type III: Dominantly echogenic lesions with small areas of echolucency (Fig. 5–3).
Type IV: Uniformly echogenic lesions (equivalent to homogeneous) (Fig. 5–4).

Geroulakos and colleagues[24] have added the type V plaques, which could not be classified because of acoustic shadowing artifact (Fig. 5–5). They also reported a good interobserver agreement for this classification ($\kappa = 0.79$).

In another classification system, carotid plaques were distinguished as calcified, dense, or soft.[25]

Studies correlating histologic characteristics with B-mode ultrasound imaging of carotid plaques show that fibrous plaques are highly echogenic, increased lipid content causes the plaque to become more echolucent, and calcium could cause extensive shadowing.[7, 26, 27] It has been proposed that increased lipid concentration could make carotid plaques

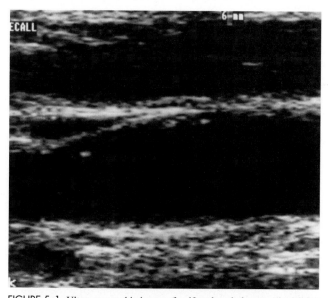

FIGURE 5–1. Ultrasonographic image of uniformly echolucent, "invisible" (type I) plaque causing a 75 percent stenosis in a patient who presented with transient ischemic attacks. (From Geroulakos G, Domjan J, Nicolaides A, et al.: Characterisation of symptomatic and asymptomatic carotid plaques using high resolution real time ultrasound. *Br J Surg.* 1993;80:1274–1277; Oxford: Blackwell Science Ltd.)

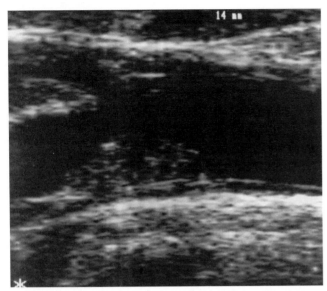

FIGURE 5–2. Ultrasonographic image of predominatly echolucent (type II) plaque. (From Geroulakos G, Domjan J, Nicolaides A, et al.: Characterisation of symptomatic and asymptomatic carotid plaques using high resolution real time ultrasound. *Br J Surg.* 1993;80:1274–1277; Oxford: Blackwell Science, Ltd.)

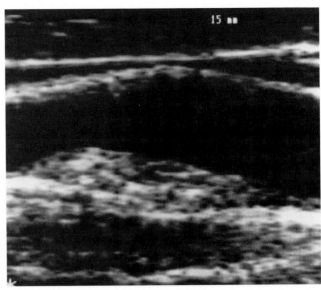

FIGURE 5–4. Ultrasonographic image of uniformly echogenic (type IV) plaque. (From Geroulakos G, Domjan J, Nicolaides A, et al.: Characterisation of symptomatic and asymptomatic carotid plaques using high resolution real time ultrasound. *Br J Surg.* 1993;80:1274–1277; Oxford: Blackwell Science, Ltd.)

unstable and prone to embolization.[28, 29] Similar findings have been reported for aortic plaques. In a cadaveric study, ulceration and thrombosis were shown to be characteristic of aortic plaques in which a high proportion of the volume was occupied by extracellular lipid.[30]

Decreased echogenicity could indicate either lipid deposits or intraplaque hemorrhage. In 1982, Lusby and coworkers[20] reported a close association between hemorrhage within the plaque and ipsilateral symptoms, a finding that has been confirmed by a number of other investigators.[8, 18] However, there is no uniform agreement on the extent of intraplaque hemorrhage and its clinical significance in the pathogenesis of cerebrovascular events. A study focusing on the microana-

tomic and chemical features of symptomatic and asymptomatic plaques concluded that hemorrhage is a feature commonly seen in carotid plaques; the study did not distinguish between symptomatic and asymptomatic plaques.[31] Feeley and associates[28] reported that hemorrhage occurred in only 2 percent and 1 percent of asymptomatic and symptomatic carotid plaques, respectively. However, the need to distinguish between intraplaque hemorrhage and lipid may not be so critical, as both types of material render the plaque potentially unstable.[13]

This echographic assessment of plaque structure is based on a subjective, qualitative evaluation of the carotid plaques. Most recently, two techniques were introduced for a quanti-

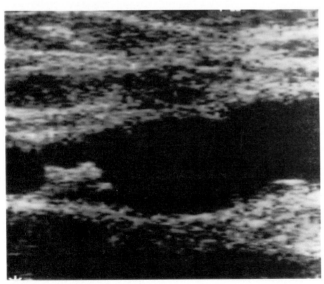

FIGURE 5–3. Ultrasonographic image of predominantly echogenic (type III) plaque. (From Geroulakos G, Domjan J, Nicolaides A, et al.: Characterisation of symptomatic and asymptomatic carotid plaques using high resolution real time ultrasound. *Br J Surg.* 1993;80:1274–1277; Oxford: Blackwell Science, Ltd.)

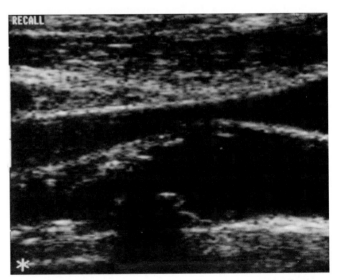

FIGURE 5–5. Typical example of type V plaque. As a result of a dense acoustic shadow produced by a calcified plaque on the proximal wall of the carotid bulb, the plaque on the distal wall cannot be classified to any of the other groups.

tative, objective assessment of the ultrasonic characterization of atherosclerotic plaque.

Videodensitometric analysis of B-mode ultrasound images of arteries has shown significant differences in gray-level intensities between fibrous plaques and plaques with increased concentrations of cholesterol and necrotic material.[32] Under standardized conditions, videodensitometry may be a valid method for detecting differences in the morphology of atherosclerotic plaques.

In vivo, radiofrequency-based, ultrasonic tissue characterization has been found to be effective in distinguishing lipidic, fibrotic, and calcific components in human atherosclerotic plaques.[33] This relatively simple, quantitatively displayed information may represent an important improvement for future studies of carotid plaque characterization.

Clinical Significance

Steffen and colleagues[22] reported that in patients with symptomatic lesions, for all degrees of stenosis, echolucent type I and type II lesions were more common (67%), whereas in patients without symptoms the more common lesions were echogenic type III and type IV (86%). Geroulakos and coworkers[24] confirmed that these findings hold for patients with stenoses greater than 70 percent. In addition, the same authors demonstrated that echolucent plaques in patients with stenosis greater than 70 percent are associated with an increased number of cerebral infarctions.[34]

Several natural history studies have shown that echolucent plaques are associated with an increased rate of TIA and stroke.

The first prospective study relating ultrasonic plaque morphology to the development of cerebrovascular symptoms was reported by Johnson and associates in 1985.[25] Asymptomatic plaques were classified according to ultrasonographic characteristics as calcified, dense, or soft. At the end of a 3-year follow-up, a large proportion of patients with no symptoms and soft plaques had become symptomatic, whereas only a small proportion of those with calcified plaques developed symptoms. These findings were confirmed by Sterpetti and coworkers,[35] who performed follow-up examinations on 135 asymptomatic and 79 symptomatic patients with a total of 238 carotid plaques. During a mean follow-up period of 34 months, 27 new focal neurologic deficits occurred. Multivariate analysis showed that the ultrasonographic pattern (heterogeneous plaques) and the severity of stenosis were independent variables.

Most recently, in a prospective series of 242 patients, Bock and associates[36] found that vessels with echolucent carotid plaques were associated with a 5.7 percent annual rate of TIA and stroke, significantly greater than the 2.4 percent rate found among patients with vessels with echogenic plaques.

These reports provide sufficient evidence to suggest that the ultrasonic internal structure of the carotid plaques is a contributing factor to the development of cerebrovascular events.

CONCLUSIONS

The European Symptomatic Carotid Surgery Trial[1] has shown that only a small number (21%) of symptomatic patients with severe carotid stenosis will experience a stroke within 3 years of the onset of symptoms. In this study, the degree of stenosis was the only selection criterion. Similar results were shown by the North American Symptomatic Carotid Endarterectomy Trial.[2] The indications for carotid endarterectomy must be better defined, and to achieve this, stratification of patients into risk-of-stroke categories is essential. The identification of a high-risk subgroup will lead to the refinement of the selection criteria in patients with severe symptomatic stenosis and will increase the therapeutic benefit from surgery by reducing the number of unnecessary operations.

There is now strong evidence to suggest that the surface characteristics and ultrasonic internal structure of carotid plaque are factors that contribute to the development of cerebrovascular events; however, various studies have shown the significance of individual factors. No prospective studies at present are assessing the combined effect of the degree of stenosis, surface ulceration, ultrasonic plaque characterization, and the status of the collateral cerebral reserve on the incidence of ipsilateral stroke. There is no doubt that such a natural history study is urgently needed and should be performed in asymptomatic subjects with severe carotid stenosis, since ethical considerations preclude further natural history studies in symptomatic patients with critical carotid stenosis.

REFERENCES

1. Medical Research Council European Carotid Surgery Trial: Interim results for symptomatic patients with severe (70–99%) or with mild (0–29%) carotid stenosis. *Lancet.* 1991;337:1235–1243.
2. North American Symptomatic Carotid Endarterectomy Trial Collaborators: Beneficial effect of carotid endarterectomy in symptomatic patients with high grade carotid stenosis. *N Engl J Med.* 1991;325:445–453.
3. Comerota AJ, Katz ML, White JV, Grosh JD: The preoperative diagnosis of the ulcerated carotid atheroma. *J Vasc Surg.* 1990;11:505–510.
4. Zukowski AJ, Nicolaides AN, Lewis RT, et al: The correlation between carotid plaque ulceration and cerebral infarction seen on CT scan. *J Vasc Surg.* 1984;1:782–786.
5. Yao JST, Francfort J, Flinn WR, Bergan JJ: Sonic characterization of carotid artery plaque and its surgical significance. In Bergan JJ, Yao JST, eds. *Arterial Surgery:* New Diagnostic and Operative Techniques. Orlando: Grune and Stratton; 1988:161–170.
6. Fitzgerald DE, O'Farrell CM: Prognostic value of ultrasound morphology in carotid atherosclerosis. *Int Angiol.* 1993;12:337–341.
7. O'Donnell TF, Erodes L, Mackey WC, et al: Correlation of B-mode ultrasound imaging and arteriography with pathologic findings at carotid endarterectomy. *Arch Surg.* 1985;120:443–449.
8. Fryer JA, Myers PC, Appleberg M: Carotid intraplaque hemorrhage: The significance of neovascularity. *J Vasc Surg.* 1987;6:341–349.
9. Van Damme H, Vivario M: Pathologic aspects of carotid plaques: surgical and clinical significance. *Int Angiol.* 1993;12:299–311.
10. Katz ML, Johnson M, Pomajzl MJ, et al: The sensitivity of real-time B-mode carotid imaging in the detection of ulcerated plaques. *Bruit.* 1983;8:13–16.
11. Ricotta JJ, Bryan FA, Bond MG, et al: Multicenter validation study of real time (B-mode) ultrasound, arteriography and pathologic examination. *J Vasc Surg.* 1987;6:512–520.
12. O'Leary DH, Bryan FA, Goodison MW, et al: Measurement variability of carotid atherosclerosis: Real-time (B-mode) ultrasonography and angiography. *Stroke.* 1987;18:1011–1017.
13. Lusby RJ: Plaque characterisation: Does it identify high risk groups? In Bernstein EF, Callow AD, Nicolaides AN, Shifrin EG, eds. *Cerebral Revascularisation.* London: Med-Orion Publishing Co, 1993:93–107.
14. Julian OC, Dye WS, Javid H, Hunter JA: Ulcerative lesions of the carotid artery bifurcation. *Arch Surg.* 1963;86:803–809.
15. Moore WS, Hall AD: Ulcerated atheroma of the carotid artery: A cause of transient cerebral ischemia. *Am J Surg.* 1968;116:237–242.
16. Bartynski WS, Darbouze P, Nemir P: Significance of ulcerated plaque in transient cerebral ischemia. *Am J Surg.* 1981;141:353–357.
17. Hertzer NR, Beven EG, Benjamin SP: Ultramicroscopic ulcerations and thrombi of carotid bifurcation. *Arch Surg.* 1977;112:1394–1402.
18. Imperato AM, Riles TS, Mintzer R, Baumann G: The importance of hemorrhage

in the relationship between gross morphologic characteristics and cerebral symptoms in 376 carotid artery plaques. *Ann Surg.* 1983;197:195–203.

19. Fisher CM, Ojemann RG: A clinico-pathological study of carotid endarterectomy plaques. *Rev Neurol.* 1986;142:573–589.

20. Lusby RJ, Ferrell LD, Ehrenfeld WK, et al: Carotid plaque hemorrhage. Its role in production of cerebral ischaemia. *Arch Surg.* 1982;117:1479–1488.

21. Streifler JY, Fox AJ, Hachinski VC, Barnett HJM: The importance of plaque ulceration in symptomatic patients with high grade stenosis: Observations from the NASCET. *Stroke.* 1992;23:160.

22. Reilly LM, Lusby RJ, et al: Carotid plaque histology using real-time ultrasonography. *Am J Surg.* 1983;146:188–193.

23. Steffen CM, Gray-Weale AC, Byrne KE, et al: Carotid atheroma: Ultrasound appearance in symptomatic and asymptomatic vessels. *Aust N Z J Surg.* 1989;59(7):529–534.

24. Geroulakos G, Ramaswami G, Nicolaides A, et al: Characterization of symptomatic and asymptomatic carotid plaques using high resolution real time ultrasound. *Br J Surg.* 1993;80:1274–1277.

25. Johnson JM, Kennelly MM, Decesare D: Natural history of asymptomatic carotid plaque. *Arch Surg.* 1985;120:1010–1012.

26. Goes E, Janssens W, Maillet B, et al: Tissue characterization of atheromatous plaques: Correlation between ultrasound image and histological findings. *J Clin Ultrasound.* 1990;18:611–617.

27. Wolverson MK, Bashiti HM, Peterson GJ: Ultrasonic tissue characterization of atheromatous plaques using a high resolution real time scanner. *Ultrasound Med Biol.* 1983;9:599–609.

28. Feeley TM, Leen EJ, Colgan MP, et al: Histologic characteristics of carotid artery plaque. *J Vasc Surg.* 1991;13:719–724.

29. Seeger J, Kligman N: The relationship between carotid plaque composition and neurological symptoms. *J Surg Res.* 1987;43:78–85.

30. Davies MJ, Richardson PD, Woolf N, et al: Risk of thrombosis of human atherosclerotic plaques: Role of extracellular lipid, macrophage, and smooth muscle cell content. *Br Heart J.* 1993;69:377–381.

31. Bassiouny HS, Davis H, Massawa N, et al: Critical carotid stenosis: morphologic and chemical similarity between symptomatic and asymptomatic plaques. *J Vasc Surg.* 1989;9:202–212.

32. Mercuri M, Bond MG: B-mode ultrasound characterisation of atherosclerosis. *J Cardiovasc Tech.* 1992;10:277–291.

33. Urbani MP, Picano E, Prenti G, et al: In vivo radiofrequency-based ultrasonic tissue characterization of the atherosclerotic plaque. *Stroke.* 1993;24:1507–1512.

34. Geroulakos G, Domjan J, Nicolaides A, et al: Ultrasonic carotid plaque characterization and the risk of cerebral infarction on computed tomography. *J Vasc Surg.* 1994;20:263–266.

35. Sterpetti AV, Schultz RD, Feldhaus RJ, et al: Ultrasonographic features of carotid plaque and the risk of subsequent neurologic deficits. *Surgery.* 1988;104:652–660.

36. Bock RW, Gray-Weal AC, Mock PA, et al: The natural history of asymptomatic ulcerative lesions of the carotid artery. *J Vasc Surg.* 1993;113:1352.

CHAPTER 6

Risk Factors Predisposing to Stroke

MARK L. DYKEN

Stroke mortality trends reported in western nations, including the United States, have shown an impressive decrease.[1-13] This decline is real and cannot be accounted for by changes in, or inaccuracies of, diagnoses on death certificates.[14, 15] Until the early 1970s, stroke mortality in the United States declined at a rate of around 1 percent per year. Since then, the decline has been approximately 5 percent per year.[8] Although in some geographic areas, this decrease has lessened,[16-18] in the entire United States, stroke-related deaths have decreased consistently and geographic variations have narrowed.[9, 12, 19] These changes are much greater than those for cardiovascular disease in general. A number of erudite reviews suggest that the effective treatment of hypertension may be the major factor in lowering the rate of stroke mortality,[20-28] but other factors may also contribute.[12, 29] Although better treatment for stroke once it has occurred may have added somewhat to the decline in incidence, the evidence is overwhelming that the major changes are related to prevention.[30] Prevention, in turn, is most likely related to the improved recognition and treatment of risk factors. It is therefore imperative to the prevention and understanding of stroke and to the development of rational therapy that these factors and their relative degrees of risk be clearly identified.

Estimates of the prevalence of clinical varieties of cerebrovascular disease vary widely depending on where the studies were performed and whether the data are from hospital records or from epidemiologic population surveys. Because the prevention of stroke depends on identification of the risk factors in the general population, population studies are used whenever possible in this report. The population studies[4, 31, 32] indicate that atherothrombotic ischemic infarction is the most common variety of cerebrovascular disease, accounting for nearly two thirds of all incidents of stroke. Cerebral embolization from a recognized embolic source and causing infarction is reported to occur in 5 to 14 percent of all stroke events, but as hospital-based diagnoses become more sophisticated, an increased percentage of infarctions previously diagnosed as atherothrombotic are now being attributed to emboli. Hemorrhage, including intraparenchymal and subarachnoid, is present in about 14 to 20 percent of all stroke events. If transient ischemic attacks were included, the total incidence of cerebrovascular disorders would be increased by 10 to 25 percent.

The medical and social impact of cerebrovascular disease in the United States is discussed in Section XV. Although the death rate continues to drop, stroke is still the third leading cause of death in the United States, following heart disease and cancer, and is the leading cause of major disability.[32-34] Reliable estimates indicate that the annual direct cost of health care for stroke victims in 1976 was $3.3 billion and that the total costs were between $6.6 and $8.5 billion.[35] Thus, if stroke could be prevented, or the decrease continued, the economic benefits to the nation would be extremely large and the decrease in human suffering incalculable.

To prevent stroke, it is necessary to identify and correct the predisposing factors in persons at high risk. The frequency and relative impact of these factors have been and are being identified in free-living populations through means of epidemiologic studies such as those performed in Framingham, Massachusetts,[32] and by the Mayo Clinic Study of the population of Rochester, Minnesota.[4] There is a high likelihood that a concerted effort to reduce and treat risk factors will continue to decrease the incidence of stroke.

RISK FACTORS

Risk factors must be considered individually and in combination. Some appear to be major risks for stroke by themselves, others become more important when in combination, and some are important only when in combination with others. For this reason, a format similar to that of the American Heart Association Subcommittee on Risk Factors will be followed.[36] First, factors will be considered alone and then in combination. As the major purpose in identifying risk factors is to treat them, so that cerebrovascular disease can be prevented, the factors will also be categorized by the strength of their established relationship to stroke and by the proven or theoretic effectiveness of treatment. These points are summarized in Table 6–1, which outlines the factors by category.

Single and Well-Documented Risk Factors

This section reviews those risk factors whose individual association with increased risk for stroke has been established. The following sections consider those factors that are not as well established and those that appear to make a special contribution when in combination with others.

Treatment Effective

The most important risk factors are, of course, those that not only have a strong predictive relationship to stroke but also are treatable, and for which the treatment has been shown to decrease the incidence of later stroke. For this reason, these factors are discussed first.

Hypertension. Of all the risk factors for stroke, hypertension is considered the most important. It is strongly related to both atherothrombotic brain infarction and intraparenchymal hemorrhage. Hypertension is also very common and has an adverse impact on a large portion of the population.[21, 37-40] The risk of stroke is directly related to the elevation of blood pressure.[41] Women with hypertension are at as great a risk for stroke as men, and the risk persists in the elderly, in whom most strokes occur. The Framingham study indicates that control of hypertension is as important for stroke prevention in the eighth and ninth decades of life as it is at younger ages.[32] In this population, when all the components of blood pressure are studied in relation to the incidence of brain infarction, systolic pressure is most closely linked to stroke. The results of the biennial clinical examination performed as part of the Radiation Effects Research Foundation in Japan[42] indicate that in this Japanese population, a

TABLE 6–1. Risk Factors for Stroke

Single Risk Factor
Well documented
    Treatment effective
        HYPERTENSION!
        Cardiac disease
        Cigarette smoking
        Transient ischemic attacks
        Alcohol consumption
        Increasing hematocrit (?)
    Value of treatment not established
        Diabetes mellitus
        Prior stroke
        Increasing blood fibrinogen level
        Sickle cell disease
        Asymptomatic bruits
        Lupus anticoagulant
    Treatment not feasible
        Age
        Gender
        Heredofamilial factors
        Race
Less well documented
    Treatable
        High cholesterol and lipid levels
        Use of oral contraceptives
        Sedentary physical activity
        Obesity
        Migraine and migraine equivalents
    Treatment not feasible
        Geographic location
        Season and climate
        Socioeconomic factors
Multiple Risk Factors as Found in:*
Framingham risk profile[33, 190]
Paffenberger and Williams study[135]
Women of childbearing age
Gothenburg, Sweden trial[192]
Lehigh Valley trial[195]

*See text for details on the referenced studies.
Modified from Dyken ML, Wolf PA, Barnett HJM, et al: Risk factors in stroke: A statement for physicians by the Subcommittee on Risk Factors and Stroke of the Stroke Council. *Stroke*, 1984;15:1105. Used with permission. Copyright © 1984 American Heart Association.

single blood pressure measurement is not sufficient to predict risk. An accumulated value or an average over time was more reliable. In addition, an increase in blood pressure with time was a particular risk factor for cerebral hemorrhage. Cerebral hemorrhage was more strongly related to diastolic than to systolic blood pressure, whereas cerebral infarction appeared to be more strongly related to systolic than to diastolic blood pressure. The Framingham study also suggests that antecedent blood pressure elevation is a significant risk factor for subarachnoid hemorrhage.[43]

For infarction, the increased risk of stroke associated with systolic hypertension is probably a direct result of elevated pressure rather than a reflection of underlying arterial rigidity. As hypertension becomes more effectively controlled, the accelerated decline in stroke mortality is not unexpected.[9] It is interesting that the Framingham study indicated a declining incidence of stroke only for women who underwent more intensive treatment and achieved more effective control of blood pressure than did men.[18, 44] Effective treatment of hypertension cannot be accepted unequivocally as the only reason for the decline, because stroke mortality was already declining before effective antihypertensive therapy became available. Nevertheless, all evidence in balance overwhelm-

ingly supports the conclusion that efforts to control hypertension have been a major contributor to the recent decline in the death rate from stroke. A number of clinical studies have demonstrated a reduction in stroke incidence and mortality when hypertension is treated.[21–26, 45, 46] Observations from the Hypertension Detection and Follow-Up Program[22] indicate that elderly hypertensive persons, compared with younger ones, demonstrate as great or greater a reduction in stroke morbidity and mortality when blood pressure is well controlled. In the United States from 1972 to 1977, age-adjusted death rates for hypertension-related cardiovascular disease declined 20 percent, whereas for cardiovascular disease unrelated to hypertension, the decline was only 9 percent.

Cardiac Disease. Although hypertension at any level is the most potent of all treatable risk factors, other factors also influence the risk of stroke. Following hypertension, the most important risk factor for stroke is heart disease. Persons with cardiac impairment of any sort, whether symptomatic or not, independent of blood pressure, carry more than twice the risk for stroke than do persons with normal cardiac function. This is true whether cardiac impairment is determined by the presence of overt diseases such as coronary heart disease and congestive heart failure, evidence of left ventricular hypertrophy by ECG and x-ray readings, or arrhythmias.[47] Coronary heart disease is also the major cause of death among stroke survivors as well as among patients with transient ischemic attacks or carotid bruits. Atrial fibrillation, even in the absence of rheumatic heart disease, is strongly correlated with stroke, specifically embolic stroke.[39, 48–50] In the Framingham study,[51, 52] even after adjustment for increased age and blood pressure, patients with chronic nonrheumatic atrial fibrillation developed strokes more than five times as often as those without fibrillation, which suggests a direct association. Atrial fibrillation in conjunction with rheumatic heart disease was associated with a 17-fold increase. Stroke occurrence increased as the duration of the atrial fibrillation increased, with no evidence of a particularly vulnerable period.

Since the publication of the first edition of this book in 1987, four randomized studies have been performed that demonstrate a marked reduction in the rate of stroke for patients on low-intensity anticoagulation therapy with warfarin.[53–57] Although the studies were not double-blinded, in each the design was rigid and the differences were great and unlikely to be related to chance. In the Stroke Prevention in Atrial Fibrillation studies (SPAF),[56, 57] 325 mg of aspirin a day was associated with significant relative risk reduction in stroke. In the Copenhagen[55] and the Boston trials[53] no aspirin effect was demonstrated. In the Boston study, aspirin was not randomly assigned but was taken at the discretion of the patient, and in the Copenhagen study, the dose was only 75 mg a day and the patients were much older than those in SPAF. Therefore these studies are not comparable.

Cigarette Smoking. At the time of the first edition of this book, the relationship of cigarette smoking to atherothrombotic brain infarction was not clear. During the interval between the two editions, a number of studies have established cigarette smoking to be a major treatable risk factor. After a 26-year follow-up, the Framingham study[58] established that cigarette smoking was a significant independent risk factor for stroke. The risk increases with the number of cigarettes and decreases significantly in 2 years after cessation of smoking, reverting to that of nonsmokers at 5 years. Other large epidemiologic studies have reported similar results, including a study of young and middle-aged women,[59] middle-aged men,[60] residents of Copenhagen,[61] and men of Japanese ancestry,[62] among others.[63] The Nurses' Health Study[64] also reported that excess risks among former smokers largely disappeared 2 to 4 years after cessation.[64]

Transient Ischemic Attacks. Transient ischemic attacks (TIAs) are episodes of focal ischemic neurologic deficit in the blood flow of an arterial vessel to the brain that last less than 24 hours. Although the occurrence of TIAs appears to be a highly significant risk factor for stroke,[65] the Framingham study included patients who had had TIAs who also exhibited other significant risk factors, such as hypertension and cardiac disease, coronary heart disease, left ventricular hypertrophy as shown by ECG examination, and congestive heart failure, more frequently than other persons of the same age and sex. Also, diabetes was present more frequently among the women in this study. Therefore, TIA as a risk factor is greatly influenced by other stroke risk factors,[32] which suggests that the risk for impending stroke associated with TIA might be greatly reduced if co-occurring conditions are treated. Although it is clear that TIAs are strong predictors of stroke, they may not make a large contribution to the total problem of stroke because only about 10 percent of all strokes are preceded by TIAs.[50, 66, 67] In addition, it is estimated that atherothrombotic disease in a surgically accessible lesion accounts for less than 15 percent of strokes. Further, atherothrombotic disease of the large extracranial arteries, including the carotid arteries, is associated with no more than one third of all strokes.[66]

Nevertheless, there is increasing evidence that the risk for stroke can be appreciably decreased in individuals who experience TIAs. One of the most promising approaches to therapy is related to what is assumed to be the platelet-antiaggregating effect of aspirin.

Aspirin has been known to be effective for some time. At least nine studies of the effects of aspirin for treating patients with TIAs or minor stroke were reported before 1990.[68–79] In all but two, a statistical benefit was established.[70, 77] Since then, the Swedish Aspirin Low-dose Trial (SALT)[80] reported that 75 mg of aspirin a day results in a statistically significant 18% reduction in stroke and death. This suggests that low-dose aspirin is effective but gives no information concerning whether it is as effective as doses of 975 mg a day or higher. Although the value of aspirin in secondary stroke prevention has been established, the most appropriate dose is still under question.[81]

Ticlopidine, another platelet-antiaggregant, also effectively reduces recurrent stroke and death in patients who have experienced TIA, mild stroke, or moderate stroke. In the Ticlopidine Aspirin Stroke Study (TASS),[82] patients receiving ticlopidine compared with those receiving aspirin showed a 21 percent decrease in all types of stroke at 3 years, and a 47 percent risk reduction at 1 year. The Canadian American Ticlopidine Study (CATS) demonstrated the drug's superiority over placebo in patients with moderate to severe stroke.[83] In these studies, almost 1 percent of the patients experienced serious neutropenia but, in every case, it occurred within 3 months and recovery occurred rapidly when drug administration was stopped.

In 1991, two large prospective randomized studies, the North American Symptomatic Carotid Endarterectomy Trial (NASCET)[84] and the European Carotid Surgery Trial (ECST),[85] established that symptomatic patients with severe (70–99%) stenosis who underwent endarterectomy experienced markedly fewer strokes in the territory of the symptomatic artery. The ECST study also conclusively demonstrated that endarterectomy on arteries with less than 30 percent stenosis was not beneficial. In each study, operative morbidity and mortality were acceptably low. A third well-designed prospective study, a Veterans' Affairs multicenter study, was terminated early because of these results.[86] Despite early termination, final analysis in the Veterans' Affairs study revealed a statistical difference in outcome similar to that of the NASCET study. Therefore, endarterectomy performed by a surgeon who has a low complication rate and on a patient with a 70 to 99 percent stenosis of a carotid artery that is symptomatic is effective. It is of no benefit when the stenosis is 30 percent or less.

The value of the operation for symptomatic patients with 30 to 70 percent stenosis and for any asymptomatic patient should be determined by ongoing studies now in progress.

Alcohol Consumption. Studies in recent years have better clarified the relationship of alcohol consumption to various types of stroke. The positive association between hemorrhagic stroke and alcohol intake observed and reported by the Honolulu Heart study and the Hisayama study in Japan[87, 88] has been reinforced.[89–91] In more recent reports, alcohol intake was associated with two to three times the risk for hemorrhagic stroke, particularly subarachnoid hemorrhage, but was not related independently to ischemic stroke.[89] Studies in Scandinavia have implicated alcohol intoxication as a precipitating factor for both infarction and subarachnoid hemorrhage.[92] The Framingham study suggested an association of alcohol intake with the incidence of stroke in general as well as with brain infarction in men.[47] Recent reports have offered possible explanations for the different results from the various studies. A number of studies[93–97] reported that low levels of alcohol intake were associated with a decreased risk for stroke, and moderate to high levels of intake with an increased risk. Gorelick and associates[98] reported that the apparent effects of acute alcohol consumption were not independent of those of cigarette smoking. Alcohol consumption and cigarette smoking have been shown to increase blood viscosity,[99] and cigarette smoking is more frequent among heavy drinkers, as is hemoconcentration with increased hematocrit. Rebound thrombocytosis during abstinence from alcohol has been suggested as a mechanism predisposing to stroke. Cardiac rhythm disorders also have been associated with acute alcohol intoxication.[100]

Other Drugs. In addition to alcohol and cigarettes, other drug abuse has become an increasing problem in the United States and in other countries.[101] Common drugs known to be associated with stroke include opiates (heroin), amphetamines and related drugs, cocaine, and phencyclidine hydrochloride. Stroke can be produced either by the direct effect of the drug or by complications of its method of administration, for example, infection or emboli from intravenous injection. Heroin use may be associated with either ischemic or hemorrhagic stroke. Amphetamines, amphetamine-related drugs (phenylpropanolamine hydrochloride), cocaine, and phencyclidine hydrochloride are more likely to be associated with hemorrhage because of elevated blood pressure or vasculitis or both. Recent studies suggest that stroke related to cocaine use is increasing, occurs primarily in the young, follows any route of administration of the drug, is frequently associated with intracranial aneurysms and malformations, and involves hemorrhage more commonly than infarction.[102]

Elevated Hematocrit. Not only did the Framingham study[103] call attention to a relationship between high hemoglobin (or high hematocrit) levels and increased incidence of cerebral infarction, it also indicated that within the normal range, the risk was directly proportional to the hemoglobin concentration. This finding was true for both sexes. However, when the study results were adjusted for blood pressure and smoking, the hemoglobin level, as a separate risk factor, was not statistically significant.[103] Nevertheless, a Japanese autopsy study[104] and several clinical and radiologic studies of patients with stroke[105, 106] support these observations. In patients with elevated hematocrit values, the associated decreased cerebral blood flow was increased by 50 percent following venisection.[107] Harrison and coworkers[108] found a direct correlation between hemoglobin levels and the size of brain infarcts and suggested that this was caused by decreased collateral flow secondary to increased viscosity.

Value of Treatment Not Established

A number of factors have been established as significant risks for cerebrovascular disease, but unfortunately there is no convincing evidence that treatment of them will decrease the likelihood that a stroke will occur. Nevertheless, they need to be identified, as in most cases treatment should be initiated for other reasons and might have some beneficial effect on the risk for stroke. Also, it is likely that when the reasons for the association between these factors and an increased risk for stroke are better understood, other therapeutic possibilities will become evident.

Diabetes Mellitus. Diabetes is a major risk factor for the development of stroke, along with hypertension and heart disease. Much of the risk is because of coexistent hypertension,[6, 65] but there is a significant independent impact, which is greater for women than for men. The risk persists with advancing age in both sexes. Although diabetes should be treated, to date there is no evidence that treatment will reduce the risk for stroke.[10, 109, 110]

Previous Stroke. Once a stroke has occurred, the risk of recurrent stroke increases 10 to 20 times.[111, 112] Although it might at first appear to be too late, the knowledge of this increased risk offers the opportunity to institute vigorous therapy for associated diseases and other risk factors, which might decrease the likelihood of a repeat insult and more severe dysfunction or death.

Fibrinogen. Two prospective long-term studies recently reported that an increased blood fibrinogen level is an independent risk factor for stroke. The results of the two studies, one performed in Sweden[113] and the other as part of the Framingham study,[114] were similar. Although fibrinogen levels were related to other risk factors, such as blood pressure, serum cholesterol, and cigarette smoking, fibrinogen levels still made an independent contribution to risk. Although cause and effect cannot be assumed, a number of therapeutic interventions may be possible if there is such a relationship,

as the theoretic adverse effects of increased fibrinogen levels may manifest in several different ways.

Sickle Cell Disease. The occurrence of stroke associated with homozygous sickle cell anemia varies from as low as 2.4 percent to as high as 17 percent. When the diagnoses are substantiated by hemoglobin electrophoresis, hemiplegia is reported in 13 to 17 percent of cases.[115] Other neurologic signs are much more common. Treatment of the neurologic complications once they occur does not have a beneficial effect. The effectiveness of prophylactic therapy in preventing stroke has not been established.

Asymptomatic Carotid Bruits. Two prospective epidemiologic studies indicate that individuals with an asymptomatic bruit have a much greater risk for stroke than those without,[116, 117] but there is considerable controversy concerning whether the source of the bruit should be treated. Because of this controversy, this chapter details reasons for categorizing bruits with those factors for which a treatment has not been established.

The Framingham study[117] reported that 21 (12.3%) of 171 patients with bruits who were prospectively followed developed permanent stroke during up to 8 years of follow-up. Although it was not possible to calculate the annual incidence from the data reported, Wolf personally analyzed the Framingham data at this author's request and noted that the rate was about 1.25 percent per year for men and 1.5 percent per year for women (Wolf P.A., personal communications). Although the stroke rate in patients with bruits was 2.6 times that in patients without bruits, in only six patients was there an atherothrombotic infarction in the arterial distribution of the artery exhibiting the bruit. In eight, the infarction was not ipsilateral. In four it was due to a cerebral embolus, and in three it was caused by a subarachnoid hemorrhage. Therefore, only six strokes could possibly have been prevented if a lesion on the side of the asymptomatic bruit had been removed. Of the 43 patients who died, the cause of death was cardiovascular in 34.

A second major epidemiologic prospective study, performed in Evans County, Georgia, obtained similar data from a different population.[116] In contrast with Framingham, a northern middle-class white community, Evans County is in the South and the population is more than 40 percent black. From 1620 patients surveyed, 72 patients with bruits were identified. During a 6-year follow-up, 10, or 13.9 percent, of the 72 individuals with bruits experienced a stroke, compared with 52, or 3.4 percent, of the 1548 without bruits. The calculated annual incidence rate was 2.4 percent. Of those with bruits, three had a spontaneous stroke on the same side as the bruit. In one, stroke occurred as a complication of endarterectomy, in two stroke resulted from multiple causes, in two a death certificate did not establish the side of stroke, and in two stroke was a result of intracranial hemorrhage. Therefore, although each study concluded that an asymptomatic bruit was a major risk factor for stroke, because the stroke occurred randomly, it is unlikely that removal of the atherosclerotic lesion producing the bruit would have affected the outcome in terms of stroke occurrence. In a hospital-based frequency study of TIAs, neither carotid bruit nor the degree of stenosis added any additional risk for stroke or death over the TIA alone.[118]

Some investigators recommend that because a bruit usually reflects atherosclerosis of the artery at the site, individuals with a bruit should undergo a thorough examination for a surgically accessible lesion. They reason that this lesion may be part of the increased risk and therefore should be removed. No prospective random studies exist to indicate the benefit or lack of benefit of endarterectomy for asymptomatic bruit.

The Carotid Artery Stenosis with Asymptomatic Narrowing: Operation Versus Aspirin (CASANOVA) trial, a multicenter randomized trial, involved 410 patients with asymptomatic stenosis (50–90%) of the internal carotid artery.[119] There were no significant differences in the number of neurologic deficits and deaths between patients receiving medical therapy and patients undergoing surgery. Unfortunately from a statistical standpoint, all patients with greater than 90 percent stenosis received surgery. If the stenosis progressed to greater than 90 percent during the study, surgery was performed.

The Mayo Asymptomatic Carotid Endarterectomy Study Group terminated their study after only 71 patients had been randomized because a significantly higher number of primary and secondary endpoints had been reached in the surgical group.[120] This outcome, however, does not reflect the lack of effectiveness of endarterectomy. In this study, only the medical group received aspirin. The investigators concluded that the results were likely related to the absence of aspirin therapy in the surgical group.

A Veterans' Administration Cooperative Study[121] reported a significantly decreased number of ipsilateral events in patients who underwent surgery. Unfortunately, these were primarily transient events, and the results could have been influenced by bias. The numbers of the primary, hard, nonsubjective endpoints of stroke and death were not significantly different.

The Asymptomatic Carotid Atherosclerosis Study (ACAS) has now enrolled more than 1200 of its planned 1500 patients.[122] When this study is completed, the value of endarterectomy for asymptomatic patients may be known.

The evidence indicates that the asymptomatic bruit is a potent risk factor for stroke or death, but it does not yet support the value of surgical intervention. Still, it is very important to identify the patient with an asymptomatic bruit; then an aggressive approach can identify other risk factors so that they can be treated.

Lupus Anticoagulant and Anticardiolipin Antibodies. A number of reports have noted an association between lupus anticoagulant or abnormal anticardiolipin antibodies and an increased risk for stroke in patients with no overt evidence of collagen-vascular disease.[123–127] To date, no studies have shown any treatment to be effective in decreasing this risk.

Treatment Not Feasible

In this section, a number of factors are considered that have an established known risk for stroke but unfortunately, or in some cases fortunately (as for age and sex), are not correctable by therapeutic intervention.

Age. In our society, an increasing number of persons are able to survive for a relatively long time. As age is the single most important risk factor for stroke, the percentage of the population at high risk is also rising proportionately. For each successive 10 years after 55 years of age, the stroke rate in that age group more than doubles.[31, 111] Although the

prevention of stroke is even more critical as the numbers of elderly persons increase, age is not treatable. It must be noted, however, that despite the strong relationship between stroke and increasing age, the National Survey of Stroke reports that 29.6 percent of strokes occur before 65 years of age and that youth does not necessarily preclude the occurrence of stroke.[50]

Gender. For all patients, independent of other risk factors, the incidence of stroke is generally about 30 percent higher in men than in women.[31, 32] Although the difference varies, it is present at all ages. The National Survey of Stroke[111] reported that in short-term general hospitals, for each 10-year period between 35 and 65 years of age, the average annual initial stroke incidence rate in each age group was always higher for men than for women.

Although some experimental and clinical studies suggested that the administration of female sex hormones to men retarded the progression of atherosclerosis and reduced the mortality from coronary and cerebrovascular disease,[128–132] long-term cooperative studies comparing estrogens with placebo failed to demonstrate any beneficial effect on men with cerebral infarction.[133] Not only did estrogens (Premarin, 1.25 mg and 2.5 mg) fail to reduce the incidence of cerebral infarction, transient ischemia, or death, but they were associated with an overall high death rate, largely due to cancer and various other diseases.

Heredofamilial. A number of studies have reported a marked excess of stroke deaths among the parents and male and female relatives of patients with cerebrovascular disease.[134–137] Although there was an increased incidence of other familial diseases, such as hypertension and diabetes mellitus, among the groups studied, all the excess stroke deaths could not be accounted for by co-incidence of other risk factors.

Race. Studies indicate, consistently, that black persons in the United States have higher death rates from stroke than white persons. This finding has been related to a finding of increased hypertension.[138–143] In southeastern United States, black persons have an especially high rate of death from stroke at all ages and in both sexes. Studies conducted in Japan and Hawaii strongly suggest, however, that racial variation is environmentally and not genetically determined. In Japan, the incidence and mortality rates for stroke have been very high for most of this century and exceed those for heart disease.[104, 144–148] In Hawaii, stroke incidence rates for Japanese residents appear similar to those for white Americans.[87, 149, 150] Thus, if the death rates truly reflect stroke incidence in Japan, then environmental factors would be the most likely explanation for the difference. Some evidence suggested that a high-sodium diet is related to the higher incidence of hypertension and that this might be a potent environmental factor,[151, 152] but a recent 10-year update of a study of dietary and other stroke risk factors in Hawaiian Japanese men did not demonstrate any relation between salt intake and the incidence of stroke.[149] In this cohort of Japanese ancestry, the risk factors were remarkably consistent with other American studies. For thromboembolic infarction, the independent risk factors included elevated blood pressure, glucose intolerance, older age, electrocardiographic evidence of left ventricular hypertrophy or strain, cigarette smoking, and proteinuria. For intracranial hemorrhage, the independent risk factors included older age, elevated blood pressure, cigarette smoking, increased serum uric acid, and decreased serum cholesterol level. Electrocardiographic evidence of left ventricular hypertrophy or strain significantly increased the risk of cerebral hemorrhage but was not associated with subarachnoid hemorrhage. Pathologic studies do show that Japanese persons in Japan have more intracranial than extracranial occlusive disease compared with non-Japanese or Hawaiian Japanese persons.[153-155]

Single and Not Well-Documented Factors

A number of factors considered to be risk factors for cerebrovascular disease are either controversial or unestablished as such. Future studies may better define the degree, or the lack, of importance.

Treatable, But Effect on Stroke Unknown

Although there are a number of factors that are not well documented to be risks for stroke, they may be quite important for a number of reasons. Many are risk factors for other serious conditions, such as heart and peripheral vascular disease, and indeed may have some relation to stroke. Regardless, the patient's general health could be appreciably improved if each factor were recognized and treated, and in the process at least, risk for stroke would not be unfavorably affected.

Elevated Blood Cholesterol and Lipids. Reports of the relationship of stroke to elevated blood cholesterol and lipid levels are conflicting.[6, 156-160] In the Framingham study,[6] an increased risk was present only in those patients under the age of 50.

Oral Contraceptives. Retrospective case control studies report that oral contraceptive use is associated with fourfold to 13-fold increase in the relative risk of cerebral infarction.[161-163] However, when smoking was controlled as a risk factor, Petitti and associates[164] found no independent effect related to the use of birth control pills except for subarachnoid hemorrhage. It is suggested that the risk of stroke is further enhanced by coexistent hypertension, a history of migraine, age exceeding 35 years, prolonged use of oral contraceptives, presence of diabetes or hyperlipidemia, and, in particular, cigarette smoking. This is discussed further in the section on multiple risk factors. The risk seems to be greatest for women taking oral contraceptives that are rich in estrogen.[162]

A number of reviews suggest that the evidence for an association of oral contraceptives with stroke is inconclusive.[165-168] In fact, the incidence of stroke in the 15- to 45-year-old age group is the same in men and women; furthermore, no substantial increase in stroke mortality has been noted in these age groups since oral contraceptives became available.[169] The Subcommittee on Risk Factors of the Stroke Council of the American Heart Association did not reach an agreement concerning the risk of oral contraceptive use and advised readers to review the referenced studies to draw an independent conclusion.[36]

Physical Inactivity. Studies of the incidence of stroke in persons involved in a variety of sedentary, as opposed to physically active, occupations have shown no significant differences.[104, 170-172] Although the Framingham study suggested a relationship between sedentary work and stroke, this was not statistically significant. In a study of longshoremen, men with sedentary jobs had coronary death rates one third higher than those of cargo handlers, but the rates for stroke were similar in both groups.

Obesity. Obesity has not been established as a separate risk factor, independent of hypertension and diabetes, for stroke.[32] Obesity can be related to hypertension, and an increase in weight is often associated with an increase in severity of hypertension. This direct relationship between weight change and change in blood pressure is independent of basal weight level.[173] Obesity also contributes to impaired glucose tolerance. Therefore, although obesity is not a direct risk factor for stroke, it must be considered to be a very potent risk factor for hypertension and glucose intolerance, which in turn increase the likelihood of stroke.

Migraine and Migraine Equivalents. A relationship between migraine headaches and stroke is commonly reported. Persistence of ischemic deficit following an attack is defined as ''complicated migraine'' and appears to be one of the recognized causes of stroke, particularly in young people.[174-177] Although a number of reports suggest that those with migraine cephalgia are at increased risk for stroke, migraines are also associated with a number of other factors that are established risks for stroke.[178-180] In a thorough review, Henrich[44] concluded that the contribution of migraine to other known risk factors for thromboembolic stroke needs to be examined further by controlled studies.

Treatment Not Feasible

In this section, some factors are described that may or may not have a relationship to stroke, but even if they do, treatment is not practicable.

Geographic Location. Cerebrovascular disease is more common in the southeastern United States than in the northern Midwest, regardless of sex or race.[181-183] Despite these rather definite regional differences, few well-documented environmental factors have been identified that contribute substantially to the occurrence of stroke.

Season and Climate. A general relationship has been reported between the frequency of stroke deaths and extremes in temperature.[184-187] Unconvincing attempts have been made to correlate these observations with conditions as diverse as atmospheric pollution and increased respiratory infections.

Socioeconomic Factors. Studies relating stroke to socioeconomic status are conflicting. For example, in England a weak but direct correlation between cerebrovascular disease and high socioeconomic status was reported,[188] and in the United States it was observed that men who died because of strokes were poorer than those in the control group.[189]

Multiple Risk Factors

Analyses of data from the Framingham study have described a general cerebrovascular risk profile that can be used to identify that 10 percent of the population that will have at least one third of the strokes.[32, 190] The risk profile consists of five factors: elevated systolic blood pressure, elevated serum cholesterol, glucose intolerance, cigarette smoking, and left ventricular hypertrophy as shown by electrocardiography. The probability of a person's experiencing a stroke within the next 2 to 10 years of his or her life is determined by adding up the points assigned on the basis of the risk factors of age, gender, history of cigarette smoking, systolic blood pressure, antihypertension treatment, diabetes, prior cardiovascular disease, atrial fibrillation, and left ventricular hypertrophy as shown by electrocardiography.

Various other combinations of risk factors have been described. Paffenbarger and Williams[136] reported that combinations of smoking, elevated systolic blood pressure, and a low ponderal index (height in inches divided by cube root of weight in pounds) are associated with an increasing stroke mortality rate. When all three factors were present, risk was increased eightfold. Combinations of three other factors in a patient of college age (body height, one parent dead, and not a varsity athlete) resulted in a fourfold increase in the mortality rate secondary to stroke. The most important single factor of the six was elevated blood pressure.

Longstreth and Swanson,[191] in an in-depth review, noted that much of the controversy concerning the relationship between oral contraceptives and stroke might be because most studies were of young populations with a lower incidence of stroke. Because of this, a multiple-factor effect might be lost, particularly if an important component was older age. From their analysis, they observed that most women who had strokes and were on oral contraceptives had other risk factors, such as hypertension. They concluded that use of oral contraceptives, cigarette smoking, and age above 35 years are particularly potent in combination.

Increasing blood pressure, abdominal obesity, increased plasma fibrinogen level, and maternal death from stroke in Gothenburg, Sweden, were, in combination, significant for stroke risk.[192]

Transient ischemic attacks, myocardial infarction, and other heart disease in the Lehigh Valley study constituted a significantly greater risk than other combinations studied.[193]

SUMMARY

The evidence reviewed indicates that stroke can be decreased significantly by treating certain major risk factors. Foremost among these are the independent factors of hypertension, clinical evidence of cardiac disease, TIAs, cigarette smoking, use of street drugs, and possibly a high hematocrit value. Treatment of these conditions will reduce the incidence of stroke morbidity and mortality. Active programs need to be initiated and continued so that risk factors can be identified in the population at large. Upon identification, effective therapy should be initiated and maintained, particularly for hypertension.

There are other definite major risk factors for which there is no compelling evidence that specific treatment now available will result in a decrease in stroke rate. These include diabetes mellitus, increased blood fibrinogen, previous stroke, and asymptomatic carotid artery bruits. On the other hand, a number of other factors are not as strongly correlated with increased risk of stroke but can be effectively treated. These include high-fat diet, elevated blood lipids, cigarette smoking, excessive alcohol intake, sedentary activity, and obesity. Although not convincingly related to stroke, they are definite risk factors for other factors that are, in turn, related to stroke, eg, hypertension and heart disease. There-

fore, it would appear that these, too, should be identified and treated if possible. When treatment is not possible, observation of the patient should be continued for the purpose of identifying other treatable factors and of implementing new treatment modalities when they are identified.

It is becoming more apparent that a number of factors, of very low or no risk at all by themselves, may be important factors in combination with other characteristics. These combinations also make risk-factor identification and treatment more practicable. For example, some individual risk factors are so prevalent that to recognize and adequately treat them might completely occupy all of the currently available medical personnel. It is assumed that as much as 40 percent of the adult population of the United States has some degree of hypertension. General health programs such as those initiated by the American Heart Association recommending weight reduction, modification of diet, and exercise regimens might be effective.

For intensive medical survey and treatment programs, a smaller number of individuals at extremely high risk need to be identified. The Framingham study concluded that a general cerebrovascular risk profile including five factors could identify the 10 percent of the population who would have one third to one half of all strokes. These factors were elevated levels of blood pressure, elevated serum cholesterol levels, abnormal glucose tolerance, cigarette smoking, and left ventricular hypertrophy as determined by electrocardiogram. Other data reviewed suggest that two sets of three factors in a single individual indicate a risk for increasing stroke mortality. One group was smoking, elevated systolic blood pressure, and low ponderal index. The other, for college students, was body height, a parent dead, and not a varsity athlete. For women of childbearing age, the combination of oral contraceptive medication, cigarette smoking, and age above 35 years is particularly dangerous.

Although one cannot assume a cause-and-effect relationship for each of these multiple factors, it is quite important to identify them. When each is treated, the probability greatly increases that at least one treatment will be effective in reducing stroke incidence and mortality.

REFERENCES

1. Acheson RM: Mortality from cerebrovascular accidents and hypertension in the Republic of Ireland. *Br J Prev Soc Med.* 1960;14:139.
2. Borhani NO: Changes and geographic distribution of mortality from cerebrovascular disease. *Am J Public Health.* 1965;55:673.
3. Dyken ML, Calhoun RA: Changes in stroke mortality: Effects on evaluating and predicting outcome for therapeutic studies. In Reivich M, Hurtig HI, eds. *Cerebrovascular Diseases.* New York: Raven Press; 1983;51.
4. Garraway WM, Whisnant JP, Furlan AJ, et al: The declining incidence of stroke. *N Engl J Med.* 1979;300:449.
5. Haberman S, Capildeo R, Rose FC: The changing mortality of cerebrovascular disease. *Q J Med.* 1978;47:71.
6. Kannel WB: Epidemiology of cerebrovascular disease. In Russell RWR, ed. *Cerebral Arterial Disease.* Edinburgh: Churchill Livingstone; 1976;1.
7. Kannell WB, Thom TJ: Implications of the recent decline in cardiovascular mortality. *Cardiovasc Med.* 1979;4:983.
8. Levy RI: Declining mortality in coronary heart disease. *Arteriosclerosis.* 1982;1:312.
9. Levy RI: Stroke decline: Implications and prospects. *N Engl J Med.* 1979;300:490. Editorial.
10. Metropolitan Life Insurance Company: Recent trends in mortality from heart disease. *Stat Bul Metropol Life Ins Co.* 1975;56:2.
11. Prineas RJ: Cerebrovascular disease occurrence in Australia. *Med J Aust.* 1971;2:509.
12. Soltero I, Liu K, Cooper R, et al: Trends in mortality from cerebrovascular diseases in the United States, 1960 to 1975. *Stroke.* 1978;9:549.

13. Wylie CM: Cerebrovascular accident deaths in the United States and in England and Wales. *J Chronic Dis.* 1962;15:85.

14. Florey CD, Du V, Senter MG, Acheson RM: A study of the validity of the diagnosis of stroke in mortality data. I. Certificate analysis. *Yale J Biol Med.* 1967;40:148.

15. Israel RA, Klebba AJ: A preliminary report on the effect of eighth revision ICDA on cause of death statistics. *Am J Public Health.* 1969;59:1651.

16. Broderick JP, Phillips SJ, Whisnant JP, et al: Incidence rates of stroke in the eighties: The end of the decline of stroke? *Stroke.* 1989;20:577.

17. Howard G: Decline in stroke mortality in North Carolina: description, predictions, and a possible underlying cause. *Ann Epidemiol.* 1993;3:488.

18. McGovern PG, Burke GL, Sprafka JM, et al: Trends in mortality, morbidity, and risk factor levels for stroke from 1960 through 1990: The Minnesota Heart Survey. *JAMA.* 1992;268:753.

19. Feinleib M, Ingster L, Rosenberg H: Time trends, cohort effects, and geographic patterns in stroke mortality: United States. *Ann Epidemiol.* 1993;3:458.

20. Wolf PA: Lewis A. Conner Lecture: Contributions of epidemiology to the prevention of stroke. *Circulation.* 1993;88:2471.

21. Carter AB: Hypotensive therapy in stroke survivors. *Lancet.* 1970;1:185.

22. Hypertension Detection and Follow-up Program Cooperative Group: Five year findings of the hypertension detection and follow-up program. III. Reduction in stroke incidence among persons with high blood pressure. *JAMA.* 1982;247:633.

23. Management Committee: The Australian therapeutic trial in mild hypertension. *Lancet.* 1980;1:1261.

24. Taguchi J, Freis ED: Partial reduction of blood pressure and prevention of complications in hypertension. *N Engl J Med.* 1978;291:329.

25. Veterans Administration Cooperative Study Group on Antihypertensive Agents: Effects of treatment on morbidity in hypertension. I. Results in patients with diastolic blood pressures averaging 115 through 129 mm Hg. *JAMA.* 1967; 202:1028.

26. Veterans Administration Cooperative Study Group on Antihypertensive Agents: Effects of treatment on morbidity in hypertension. II. Results in patients with diastolic blood pressures averaging 90 through 114 mm Hg. *JAMA.* 1970; 213:1143.

27. Whisnant JP: The decline of stroke. *Stroke.* 1984;15:160.

28. Wolf PA: Risk factors for stroke. *Stroke.* 1985;16:359.

29. Hachinski V: Decreased incidence and mortality of stroke. *Stroke.* 1984;15:376.

30. Anderson GL, Whisnant JP: A comparison of trends in mortality from stroke in the United States and Rochester, Minnesota. *Stroke.* 1982;13:804.

31. Kurtzke JF: Epidemiology of cerebrovascular disease. In National Institute of Neurological and Communicative Disorders and Stroke and National Heart and Lung Institute: *Cerebrovascular Survey Report for Joint Council Subcommittee on Cerebrovascular Disease* (revised). Rochester, MN: Whiting Press, 1980;135.

32. Wolf PA, Kannel WB, Verter J: Current status of risk factors for stroke. In Barnett HJM, ed. *Neurologic Clinics.* Vol. 1:1. Philadelphia: WB Saunders Company; 1983;317.

33. American Heart Association: *Heart Facts 1984.* Dallas: American Heart Association; 1982.

34. Kurtzke JF: Epidemiology and risk factors in thrombotic brain infarction. In Harrison MJG, Dyken ML, eds. *Cerebrovascular Disease.* London: Butterworth & Co., Ltd. 1983;27.

35. Adelman SM: The National Survey of Stroke: Economic impact. *Stroke.* 1981; 12(suppl I):I-69.

36. Dyken ML, Wolf PA, Barnett HJM, et al: Risk factors in stroke. *Stroke.* 1984;15:1105.

37. Kannel WB, Wolf PA, McGee DL, et al: Systolic blood pressure, arterial rigidity, and risk of stroke. The Framingham study. *JAMA.* 1981;245:1225.

38. Paffenberger RS Jr, Wing AL: Characteristics in youth predisposing to fatal stroke in later years. *Lancet.* 1967;1:753.

39. Sacco RL, Wolf PA, Kannel WB, McNamara PM: Survival and recurrence following stroke. The Framingham study. *Stroke.* 1982;13:290.

40. Wolf PA: Hypertension as a risk factor for stroke. In Whisnant JP, Sandok B, eds. *Cerebral Vascular Diseases.* New York: Grune & Stratton; 1975;105.

41. Kannel WB, Wolf PA, Verter J, McNamara PM: Epidemiologic assessment of the role of blood pressure in stroke: The Framingham study. *JAMA.* 1970; 214:301.

42. Shimizu Y, Kato H, Lin CH, et al: Relationship between longitudinal changes in blood pressure and stroke incidence. *Stroke.* 1984;15:839.

43. Sacco RL, Wolf PA, Bharucha NE, et al: Subarachnoid and intracerebral hemorrhage: Natural history, prognosis, and precursive factors in the Framingham study. *Neurology.* 1984;34:847.

44. Henrich JB: The association between migraine and cerebral vascular events: An analytical review. *J Chronic Dis.* 1987;40:329.

45. Collins R, Peto R, MacMahon S, et al: Blood pressure, stroke, and coronary heart disease, part 2: short-term reductions in blood pressure; overview of randomised drug trials in their epidemiological context. *Lancet.* 1990;335:827.

46. MacMahon S, Peto R, Cutler J, et al: Blood pressure, stroke, and coronary heart disease, part 1: Prolonged differences in blood pressure: Prospective observational studies corrected for the regression dilution bias. *Lancet.* 1990;335:765.

47. Wolf PA, Kannel WB, Verter J: Current status of risk factors for stroke. In Barnett HJM, ed. *Neurologic Clinics.* Vol 1: Philadelphia: WB Saunders Company; 1983;317.

48. Friedman GD, Loveland DB, Ehrlich SP Jr: Relationship of stroke to other cardiovascular disease. *Circulation.* 1968;38:533.

49. Kannel WB, Abbott RD, Savage DD, McNamara PM: Epidemiologic features of chronic atrial fibrillation: The Framingham study. *N Engl J Med.* 1982;306:1018.

50. Weinfeld FD, ed: The National Survey of Stroke. (National Institute of Neurological and Communicative Disorders and Stroke.) *Stroke.* 1981;12(suppl I):I-1.

51. Wolf PA, Dawber TR, Thomas HE Jr, Kannel WB: Epidemiologic assessment of chronic atrial fibrillation and risk of stroke: The Framingham study. *Neurology.* 1978;28:973.

52. Wolf PA, Abbott RD, Kannel WB: Atrial fibrillation as an independent risk factor for stroke: The Framingham Study. *Stroke.* 1991;23:1242.

53. The Boston Area Anticoagulation Trial for Atrial Fibrillation Investigators: The effect of low-dose warfarin on the risk of stroke in patients with nonrheumatic atrial fibrillation. *N Engl J Med.* 1990;323:1505.

54. Ezekowitz MD, Bridgers SL, James KE, et al, for the Veterans Affairs Stroke Prevention in Nonrheumatic Atrial Fibrillation Investigators: Warfarin in the prevention of stroke associated with non-rheumatic atrial fibrillation. *N Engl J Med.* 1992;327:1406.

55. Petersen P, Boysen G, Godtfredsen J, et al: Placebo-controlled randomized trial of warfarin and aspirin for prevention of thromboembolic complications in chronic atrial fibrillation. The Copenhagen AFASAK Study. *Lancet.* 1989;1:175.

56. Stroke Prevention in Atrial Fibrillation Investigators: Preliminary report of the Stroke Prevention in Atrial Fibrillation Study. *N Engl J Med.* 1990;322:863.

57. Stroke Prevention in Atrial Fibrillation Investigators: Stroke Prevention in Atrial Fibrillation Study: Final results. *Circulation.* 1991;84:527.

58. Wolf PA, D'Agostino RB, Kannel WB, et al: Cigarette smoking as a risk factor for stroke: The Framingham study. *JAMA.* 1988;259:1025.

59. Colditz GA, Bonita R, Stampfer MJ, et al: Cigarette smoking and risk of stroke in middle-aged women. *N Engl J Med.* 1988;318:937.

60. Menotti A, Mariotti S, Seccareccia S, Giampaoli S: The 25 year estimated probability of death from some specific causes as a function of twelve risk factors in middle aged men. *Eur J Epidemiol.* 1988;4:60.

61. Boysen G, Nyboe J, Appleyard M, et al: Stroke incidence and risk factors for stroke in Copenhagen, Denmark. *Stroke.* 1988;19:1345.

62. Abbott RD, Yin Y, Reed DM, Yano K: Risk of stroke in male cigarette smokers. *N Engl J Med.* 1986;315:717.

63. Shinton R, Beevers G: Meta-analysis of relation between cigarette smoking and stroke. *Br Med J.* 1989;298:789.

64. Kawachi I, Colditz GA, Stampfer MJ, et al: Smoking cessation and decreased risk of stroke in women. *JAMA.* 1993;269:232.

65. Schoenberg BS, Schoenberg DG, Pritchard DA, et al: Differential risk factors for complete stroke and transient ischemic attacks (TIA): Study of vascular diseases (hypertension, cardiac disease, peripheral vascular disease) and diabetes mellitus. In Duvoisin RC, ed. *Transactions of the American Neurological Association.* Vol. 105. New York: Springer Publishing Company; 1980;165.

66. Mohr JP, Caplan LR, Melski JW, et al: The Harvard Cooperative Stroke Registry: A prospective registry. *Neurology.* 1978;28:754.

67. Whisnant JP: Epidemiology of stroke: Emphasis on transient cerebral ischemia attacks and hypertension. *Stroke.* 1974;5:68.

68. Bousser MG, Eschwege E, Haguenau M, et al: Essai cooperatif controle "AICLA." Prevention secondaire des accidents ischemiquers cerebraux lies a l'atherosclerose par l'aspirine et le dipyridamole. *Rev Neurol (Paris).* 1981;5:333.

69. Bousser MG, Eschwege E, Haguenau M, et al: "A.I.C.L.A." controlled trial of aspirin and dipyridamole in the secondary prevention of atherothrombotic cerebral ischemia. *Stroke.* 1983;14:5.

70. Britton M, Helmers C, Samuelsson K: High dose acetylsalicylic acid after cerebral infarction: A Swedish co-operative study. *Stroke.* 1987;18:325.

71. Canadian Cooperative Study Group: A randomized trial of aspirin and sulfinpyrazone in threatened stroke. *N Engl J Med.* 1978;299:53.

72. European Stroke Prevention Study Group: ESPS: Principal end points. *Lancet.* 1987;ii:1351.

73. Fields WS, Lemak NA, Frankowski RF, Hardy RJ: Controlled trial of aspirin in cerebral ischemia. *Stroke.* 1977;8:301.

74. Fields WS, Lemak NA, Frankowski RF, Hardy RJ: Controlled trial of aspirin in cerebral ischemia. Part II: Surgical group. *Stroke.* 1978;9:309.

75. Guiraud-Chaumeil B, Rascol A, David J, et al: Prevention des recidives des accidents vasculaires cerebraux ischemiques par les anti-aggregants plaquettaires. *Rev Neurol (Paris).* 1982;138:367.

76. Ruether R, Dorndorf W: Aspirin in patients with cerebral ischemia and normal angiograms or non-surgical lesions: The results of a double-blind trial. In Breddin K, Dorndorf W, Loew D, et al, eds. *Acetylsalicylic Acid in Cerebral Ischemia and Coronary Heart Disease.* Stuttgart: Schattauer; 1978;97.

77. Sorenson PS, Pedersen H, Marquardsen J, et al: Acetylsalicylic acid in the prevention of stroke in patients with reversible cerebral ischemic attacks. A Danish Cooperative Study. *Stroke.* 1982;13:15.

78. UK-TIA Study Group: United Kingdom Transient Ischaemic Attack (UK-TIA) aspirin trial: Interim results. *Br Med J.* 1988;296:315.

79. UK-TIA Study Group: The United Kingdom Transient Ischaemic Attack (UK-TIA) aspirin trial: Final results. *J Neurol Neurosurg Psychiatry.* 1991;54:1044.

80. The SALT Collaborative Group: Swedish Aspirin Low-Dose Trial (SALT) of 75 mg aspirin as secondary prophylaxis after cerebrovascular ischaemic events. *Lancet.* 1991;338:1345.

81. Dyken ML, Barnett HJM, Easton JD, et al: Low-dose aspirin and stroke: "It ain't necessarily so." *Stroke.* 1992;23:1395. Editorial.

82. Hass WK, Easton JD, Adams HP Jr, et al: A randomized trial comparing ticlopidine hydrochloride with aspirin for the prevention of stroke in high-risk patients. *N Engl J Med.* 1989;321:501.

83. Gent M, Blakely JA, Easton JD, et al: The Canadian American Ticlopidine Study (CATS) in thromboembolic stroke. *Lancet.* 1989;1:1215.

84. NASCET Collaborators: Beneficial effect of carotid endarterectomy in symptomatic patients with high-grade carotid stenosis. *N Engl J Med.* 1991;325:445.

85. European Carotid Surgery Trialists' Collaborative Group: MRC European Surgery Trial: Interim results for symptomatic patients with severe (70–99%) or with mild (0–29%) carotid stenosis. *Lancet.* 1991;337:1235.

86. Mayberg MR, Wilson SE, Yatsu F, et al, for the Veterans Affairs Cooperative Studies Program 309 Trialist Group: Carotid endarterectomy and prevention of cerebral ischemia in symptomatic carotid stenosis. *JAMA.* 1991;266:3289.

87. Kagan A, Popper JS, Rhoads GG, et al: Epidemiologic studies of coronary heart disease and stroke in Japanese men living in Japan, Hawaii and California: Prevalence of stroke. In Scheinberg P, ed. *Cerebrovascular Diseases.* New York: Raven Press; 1976;267.

88. Kagan A, Harris BR, Winkelstein W Jr, et al: Epidemiologic studies of coronary heart disease and stroke in Japanese men living in Japan, Hawaii and California: Demographic, physical, dietary and biochemical characteristics. *J Chronic Dis.* 1974;27:345.

89. Donahue RF, Abbott RD, Reed DM, Yano K: Alcohol and hemorrhagic stroke. The Honolulu Heart Program. *JAMA.* 1986;255:2311.

90. Klatsky AL, Armstrong MA, Friedman GD: Alcohol use and subsequent cerebrovascular disease hospitalizations. *Stroke.* 1989;20:741.

91. Stampfer MJ, Colditz GA, Willett WC, et al: A prospective study of moderate alcohol consumption and the risk of coronary disease and stroke in women. *N Engl J Med.* 1988;319:267.

92. Lee K: Alcoholism and cerebrovascular thrombosis in the young. *Acta Neurol Scand.* 1979;59:270.

93. Camargo CA: Moderate alcohol consumption and stroke: The epidemiological evidence. *Stroke.* 1989;20:1611.

94. Gill JS, Shipley MJ, Hornby RH, et al: A community case-control study of alcohol consumption in stroke. *Int J Epidemiol.* 1988;17:542.

95. Gill JS, Zezulka AV, Shipley MJ, et al: Stroke and alcohol consumption. *N Engl J Med.* 1986;315:1041.

96. Palomaki H, Kaste M: Regular light-to-moderate intake of alcohol and the risk of ischemic stroke: Is there a beneficial effect? *Stroke.* 1993;24:1828.

97. Rodgers H, Aitken PD, French JM, et al: Alcohol and stroke: A case-control study of drinking habits past and present. *Stroke.* 1993;24:1473.

98. Gorelick PB, Rodin MB, Langenberg, et al: Is acute alcohol ingestion a risk factor for ischemic stroke? Results of a controlled study in middle-aged and elderly stroke patients at three urban medical centers. *Stroke.* 1987;18:359.

99. Dintenfass L: Elevation of blood viscosity, aggregation of red cells, haematocrit values and fibrinogen levels with cigarette smokers. *Med J Aust.* 1975;1:617.

100. Ettinger PO, Wu CF, De La Cruz C Jr, et al: Arrhythmias and the "holiday heart": Alcohol-associated cardiac rhythm disorders. *Am Heart J.* 1978;95:555.

101. Brust JCM: Stroke and substance abuse. In Barnett HJM, Mohr JP, Stein BM, Yatsu FM, eds. *Stroke: Pathophysiology, Diagnosis and Management.* Vol 2. New York: Churchill Livingstone; 1986;903.

102. Klonoff DC, Andrews BT, Obana WG: Stroke associated with cocaine use. *Arch Neurol.* 1989;46:989.

103. Kannel WB, Gordon T, Wolf PA, McNamara P: Hemoglobin and the risk of cerebral infarction: The Framingham study. *Stroke.* 1972;3:409.

104. Katsuki S, Omae T, Hirota Y: Epidemiological and clinicopathological studies on cerebrovascular disease. *Kyushu J Med Sci.* 1964;15:127.

105. Pearson TC, Thomas DJ: Physiological and pharmacological factors influencing blood viscosity and cerebral blood flow. In Tognoni G, Garattini S, eds. *Drug Treatment and Prevention in Cerebrovascular Disorders.* Amsterdam: Elsevier North Holland; 1979;33.

106. Tohgi J, Yamanouchi H, Murakami M, Kameyama M: Importance of the hematocrit as a risk factor in cerebral infarction. *Stroke.* 1978;9:369.

107. Thomas DJ, Marshall J, Russell RWR, et al: Effect of haematocrit on cerebral blood-flow in man. *Lancet.* 1977;ii:941.

108. Harrison MJG, Pollock S, Kendall BE, Marshall J: Effect of haematocrit on carotid stenosis and cerebral infarction. *Lancet.* 1981;ii:114.

109. Olivares L, Castaneda E, Grife A, Alter M: Risk factors in stroke: A clinical study in Mexican patients. *Stroke.* 1973;4:773.

110. Paffenberger RS Jr, Wing AL: Chronic disease in former college students. XI. Early precursors of nonfatal stroke. *Am J Epidemiol.* 1971;94:524.

111. Robins M, Baum HM: The National Survey of Stroke: Incidence. *Stroke.* 1981;12(suppl I):I-45.

112. Toole JF, Janeway R, Choi K, et al: Transient ischemic attacks due to atherosclerosis: A prospective study of 160 patients. *Arch Neurol.* 1975;32:5.

113. Wilhelmsen L, Svardsudd K, Korsan-Bengtsen K, et al: Fibrinogen as a risk factor for stroke and myocardial infarction. *N Engl J Med.* 1984;311:501.

114. Wolf PA, Kannel WB, Meeks SL, et al: Fibrinogen as a risk factor for stroke: The Framingham study. *Stroke.* 1985;16:139.

115. Portnoy BA, Herion JC: Neurological manifestations in sickle-cell disease, with a review of the literature and emphasis on the prevalence of hemiplegia. *Ann Intern Med.* 1972;76:643.

116. Heyman A, Wilkinson WE, Heyden S, et al: Risk of stroke in asymptomatic persons with cervical arterial bruits: A population study in Evans County, Georgia. *N Engl J Med.* 1980;302:838.

117. Wolf PA, Kannel WB, Sorlie P, McNamara P: Asymptomatic carotid bruit and risk of stroke: The Framingham study. *JAMA.* 1981;245:1442.

118. Conneally PM, Dyken ML, Futty DE, et al: Cooperative study of hospital frequency and character of transient ischemic attacks. VIII. Risk factors. *JAMA.* 1978;240:742.

119. CASANOVA Study Group: Carotid surgery versus medical therapy in asymptomatic carotid stenosis. *Stroke.* 1991;22:1229.

120. Mayo Asymptomatic Carotid Endarterectomy Study Group: Results of a randomized controlled trial of carotid endarterectomy for asymptomatic carotid stenosis. *Mayo Clin Proc.* 1992;67:513.

121. Hobson RW II, Weiss DG, Fields WS, et al, and The Veterans' Affairs Cooperative Study Group: Efficacy of carotid endarterectomy for asymptomatic carotid stenosis. *N Engl J Med.* 1993;328:221.

122. Toole JF, Hobson RW, Howard VJ, Chambless LE: Nearing the finish line? The Asymptomatic Carotid Atherosclerosis Study. *Stroke.* 1992;23:1054.

123. Coull BM, Bourdette DN, Goodnight SH, et al: Multiple cerebral infarctions and dementia associated with anticardiolipin antibodies. *Stroke.* 1987;18:1107.

124. Hart RG, Miller VT, Coull BM, Bril V: Cerebral infarction associated with lupus anticoagulants: preliminary report. *Stroke.* 1984;15:114.

125. Levine SR, Kim S, Deegan MJ, Welch KMA: Ischemic stroke associated with anticardiolipin antibodies. *Stroke.* 1987;18:1101.

126. Levine SR, Welch KM: Cerebrovascular ischemia associated with lupus anticoagulant. *Stroke.* 1987;18:257.

127. Young SM, Fisher M, Sigsbee A, Errichetti A: Cardiogenic brain embolism and lupus anticoagulant. *Ann Neurol.* 1989;26:390.

128. London WT, Rosenberg SE, Draper JF, et al: The effect of estrogens on atherosclerosis: A postmortem study. *Ann Intern Med.* 1961;55:63.

129. Marmorston J: Effect of estrogen treatment in cerebrovascular disease. In Millikan CH, Siekert RG, Whisnant JP, eds. *Cerebral Vascular Diseases.* New York: Grune & Stratton; 1965;214.

130. Rivin AV, Dimitroff SP: The incidence and severity of atherosclerosis in estrogen-treated males and in females with a hypoestrogenic or hyperestrogenic state. *Circulation.* 1954;9:533.

131. Stamler J, Pick R, Katz LN: Experiences in assessing estrogen antiatherogenesis in the chick, the rabbit, and man. *Ann N Y Acad Sci.* 1956;64:596.

132. Stamler J, Pick R, Katz LN, et al: Effectiveness of estrogens for therapy of myocardial infarction in middle-aged men. *JAMA.* 1963;183:632.

133. Veterans Administration Cooperative Study Group: Estrogenic therapy in men with ischemic cerebrovascular disease: Effect on recurrent cerebral infarction and survival. Final report of the Veterans Administration cooperative study of atherosclerosis, Neurology Section. *Stroke.* 1972;3:427.

134. Gifford AJ: An epidemiological study of cerebrovascular disease. *Am J Public Health.* 1966;56:452.

135. Heyden S, Heyman A, Camplong L: Mortality patterns among parents of patients with atherosclerotic cerebrovascular disease. *J Chronic Dis.* 1969;22:105.

136. Paffenbarger RS Jr, Williams JL: Chronic disease in former college students. V. Early precursors of fatal stroke. *Am J Public Health.* 1967;57:1290.

137. Kiely DK, Wolf PA, Cupples A, et al: Familial aggregation of stroke: The Framingham Study. *Stroke.* 1993;24:1366.

138. Eckstrom PT, Brand FR, Edlavitch SA, Parrish HM: Epidemiology of stroke in a rural area. *Public Health Rep.* 1969;84:878.

139. Heyman A, Karp HR, Heyden S, et al: Cerebrovascular disease in the biracial population of Evans County, Georgia. *Arch Intern Med.* 1971;128:949.

140. Nichaman MZ, Boyle E Jr, Lesene TP, Sauer HI: Cardiovascular disease mortality by race, based on a statistical study in Charleston, South Carolina. *Geriatrics.* 1962;17:724.

141. Ostfeld AM, Shekelle RB, Klawans H, Tufo HM: Epidemiology of stroke in an elderly welfare population. *Am J Public Health.* 1974;64:450.

142. Parrish HM, Payne GH, Allen WC, et al: Mid-Missouri stroke survey: A preliminary report. *Mo Med.* 1966;63:816.

143. Peacock PB, Riley CP, Lampton TD, et al: The Birmingham stroke, epidemiology and rehabilitation study. In Stewart GT, ed. *Trends in Epidemiology: Application to Health Service Research and Training.* Springfield, IL: Charles C. Thomas; 1972;231.

144. Fusa K, Fusa K, trans: An epidemiological study of hypertension: A prospective study of incidence of cerebrovascular disease and myocardial infarction in an area in Tohoku District of Japan. *J Jap Soc Intern Med.* 1974;63:630.

145. Hatano S: Experience from a multicentre stroke register: A preliminary report. *Bull WHO.* 1976;54:541.

146. Katsuki S, Hirota Y, Akazome T, et al: Epidemiological studies in Hisayama, Kyushu Island, Japan. I. With particular reference to cardiovascular status. *Jpn Heart J.* 1964;5:12.

147. Tanaka H, Ueda Y, Hayashi M, et al: Risk factors for cerebral hemorrhage and cerebral infarction in a Japanese rural community. *Stroke.* 1982;13:62.

148. Ueda K, Omae T, Hirota Y, et al: Decreasing trend in incidence and mortality from stroke in Hisayama residents, Japan. *Stroke.* 1981;12:154.

149. Kagan A, Popper JS, Rhoads GG, Yano K: Dietary and other risk factors for stroke in Hawaiian Japanese men. *Stroke.* 1985;16:390.

150. Worth RM, Kato H, Rhoads GG: Epidemiologic studies of coronary heart disease and stroke in Japanese men living in Japan, Hawaii and California: Mortality. *Am J Epidemiol.* 1975;102:481.

151. Sasaki N: The salt factor in apoplexy and hypertension: Epidemiological studies in Japan. In Yamori Y, Lovinberg W, Freis E, eds. *Perspectives in Cardiovascular Research.* New York: Raven Press; 1978;467.

152. Takahashi E, Sasaki N, Takeda J, Ito H: The geographic distribution of cerebral hemorrhage and hypertension in Japan. *Human Biol.* 1957;29:139.

153. Mitsuyama Y, Thompson LR, Hayashi T, et al: Autopsy study of cerebrovascular disease in Japanese men who lived in Hiroshima, Japan and Honolulu, Hawaii. *Stroke.* 1979;10:389.

154. Resch JA, Okabe N, Loewenson RB, et al: Pattern of vessel involvement in cerebral atherosclerosis: A comparative study between a Japanese and Minnesota population. *J Atheroscler Res.* 1969;9:2339.

155. Takeya Y, Popper JS, Shimizu Y, et al: Epidemiologic studies of coronary heart disease and stroke in Japanese living in Japan, Hawaii and California: Incidence of stroke in Japan and Hawaii. *Stroke.* 1984;15:15.

156. Dyer AR, Stamler J, Paul O, et al: Serum cholesterol and risk of death from cancer and other causes in three Chicago epidemiological studies. *J Chronic Dis.* 1981;34:249.

157. Farid NR, Anderson J: Cerebrovascular disease and hyperlipoproteinemia. *Lancet.* 1972;i:1398.

158. High-density lipoprotein. *Lancet.* 1981;i:478. Editorial.

159. Ladurner G, Cornauer U, Ott E, et al: Gefassbund and Lipide bei ischämischer Hirnerkrankung. *Psychiatria et Neurologia (Thessalonika)* 1978;1:1.

160. Mathew NT, Davis D, Meyer JS, Chander K: Hyperlipoproteinemia in occlusive cerebrovascular disease. *JAMA.* 1975;232:262.

161. Collaborative Group for the Study of Stroke in Young Women: Oral contraception and increased risk of cerebral ischemia or thrombosis. *N Engl J Med.* 1973;288:871.

162. Handin R: Thromboembolic complications of pregnancy and oral contraceptives. *Prog Cardiovasc Dis.* 1974;16:395.

163. Layde PM, Beral V, Kay CR: Further analyses of mortality in oral contraceptive users. (Royal College of General Practitioners' Oral Contraception Study). *Lancet.* 1981;i:541.

164. Pettiti DB, Wingerd J, Pellegrin F, Ramcharan S: Risk of vascular disease in women. Smoking, oral contraceptives, noncontraceptive estrogens, and other factors. *JAMA.* 1979;242:1150.

165. Comer TP, Tuerck DG, Bilas RA, et al: Comparison of strokes in women of childbearing age in Rochester, Minnesota and Bakersfield, California. *Angiology.* 1975;26:351.

166. Schoenberg BS, Whisnant JP, Taylor WF, Kempers KD: Strokes in women of childbearing age: A population study. *Neurology.* 1970;20:181.

167. Shearman RP: Oral contraceptives: Where are the excess deaths? *Med J Aust.* 1981;1:698.

168. Stadel BV: Oral contraceptives and cardiovascular disease. *N Engl J Med.* 1981;305:612.

169. Wiseman RA, MacRae KD: Oral contraceptives and the decline in mortality from circulatory disease. *Fertil Steril.* 1981;35:277.

170. Johnson KG, Yano K, Kato H: Cerebral vascular disease in Hiroshima, Japan. *Jpn J Chronic Dis.* 1967;20:545.

171. Marquardsen J: The natural history of acute cerebrovascular disease: A retrospective study of 769 patients. *Acta Neurol Scand.* 1969;45(suppl 38):11.

172. Paffenbarger RS Jr, Laughlin ME, Gima AS, Black RA: Work activity of longshoremen as related to death from coronary heart disease and stroke. *N Engl J Med.* 1970;282:1109.

173. Messerli FH: Cardiovascular effects of obesity and hypertension. *Lancet.* 1982 i:1165.

174. Bogousslavsky J, Regli F, VanMelle G, et al: Migraine stroke. *Neurology.* 1988;38:223.

175. Bogousslavsky J, Regli F: Ischemic stroke in adults younger than 30 years of age: Cause and prognosis. *Arch Neurol.* 1987;44:479.

176. Hilton-Jones D, Warlow CP: The causes of stroke in the young. *J Neurol.* 1985;232:137.

177. Rothrock JF, Walicke P, Swenson MR, et al: Migrainous stroke. *Arch Neurol.* 1988;45:63.

178. Chen TC, Leviton A, Edelstein S, Ellenberg JH: Migraine and other diseases in women of reproductive age: The influence of smoking on observed associations. *Arch Neurol.* 1987;44:1024.

179. Hogan MJ, Brunet DG, Ford PM, Lillicrap D: Lupus anticoagulant, antiphospholipid antibodies and migraine. *Can J Neurol Sci.* 1988;15:420.

180. Pfaffenrath V, Pollmann W, Autenrieth G, Rosmanith U: Mitral valve prolapse and platelet aggregation in patients with hemiplegic and non-hemiplegic migraine. *Acta Neurol Scand.* 1987;75:253.

181. Kuller L, Anderson H, Peterson D, et al: Nationwide cerebrovascular disease morbidity study. *Stroke.* 1970;1:86.

182. Nefzger MD, Acheson RM, Heyman A: Mortality from stroke among U.S. veterans in Georgia and five western states. I. Study plan and death rates. *J Chronic Dis.* 1973;26:393.

183. Nefzger MD, Heyman A, Acheson RM: Stroke, geography and blood pressure. *J Chronic Dis.* 1973;26:389. Editorial.

184. Bull GM: Meterological correlates with myocardial and cerebral infarction and respiratory disease. *Br J Prev Soc Med.* 1973;27:108.

185. Haberman S, Capildeo R, Rose FC: The seasonal variation in mortality from cerebrovascular disease. *J Neurol Sci.* 1981;52:25.

186. Knox EG: Meterological associations of cerebrovascular disease mortality in England and Wales. *J Epidemiol Community Health* 1981;35:220.

187. Rogot E, Padgett SJ: Associations of coronary and stroke mortality with temperature and snowfall in selected areas of the United States, 1962–1966. *Am J Epidemiol.* 1976;103:365.

188. Acheson RM, Fairbairn AS: Record linkage in studies of cerebrovascular disease in Oxford, England. *Stroke.* 1971;2:48.

189. Acheson RM, Heyman A, Nefzger MD: Mortality from stroke among U.S. veterans in Georgia and five western states. III. Hypertension and demographic characteristics. *J Chronic Dis.* 1973;26:417.

190. Wolf PA, D'Agostino RB, Belanger AJ, Kannel WB: Probability of stroke: A risk profile from the Framingham Study. *Stroke.* 1991;22:312.

191. Longstreth WT Jr, Swanson PD: Oral contraceptives and stroke. *Stroke.* 1984;15:747.

192. Welin L, Svardsudd K, Wilhelmsen L, et al: Analysis of risk factors for stroke in a cohort of men born in 1913. *N Engl J Med.* 1987;317:521.

193. Sobel E, Alter M, Davanipour Z, et al: Stroke in the Lehigh valley: Combined risk factors for recurrent ischemic stroke. *Neurology.* 1989;39:669.

II

Pathology

CHAPTER

7

Spectrum of Pathology Responsible for Ischemic Stroke

DAVID G. SHERMAN, J. DONALD EASTON, and KATHLEEN S. KAGAN-HALLET

Brain infarction or transient ischemia is the end result of a number of underlying disorders that may impair blood flow to the brain. Arterial disease may produce ischemia by a flow-impeding stenosis, thrombotic occlusion, or embolization of thrombotic material. Venous thrombosis, through a number of mechanisms, may produce brain infarction in the brain region drained by the involved vein or sinus. Valvular and other cardiac disorders promote intracardiac thrombi, with the potential for embolization to the brain. The reason for a given episode of brain ischemia may be either obvious and singular or occult and multifactorial. Many patients have both arterial and cardiac disease with superimposed systemic disorders that may either promote intravascular coagulation or impede blood flow.

ATHEROSCLEROSIS

Atherosclerosis of the cerebral vessels is the most common disorder producing brain ischemia. The production of atherosclerotic lesions appears to be multifactorial. The concentration and nature of circulating lipids and lipid transporting proteins appear to be major factors in the pathogenesis of atherosclerosis. Elevated serum cholesterol, low-density lipoproteins, and reduced circulating concentrations of high-density lipoproteins promote the development of atherosclerotic plaques. Both dietary and hereditary factors influence the levels of these circulating lipid compounds.[1–3] Endothelial injury also promotes the development of atherosclerotic plaque. Injury to the vascular endothelium exposes the subendothelial connective tissue to which circulating platelets adhere, covering the damaged intravascular surface. These adherent platelets promote the proliferation of smooth muscle cells through the production of platelet-derived growth factor. This smooth muscle cell proliferation leads to expansion of the endothelium and forms the substrate for the development of the atheromatous plaque.[4, 5] The known risk factors for atherosclerosis, such as hypertension, diabetes mellitus, familial hyperlipidemia, and diet, presumably promote the development of atherosclerosis by either altering lipid metabolism or damaging the vascular endothelium.

Cerebral atherosclerosis produces a characteristic gross appearance during life. Changes can be visualized on the cerebral angiogram or by noninvasive studies of the cerebral vessels. Pathologically, yellow streaks can be seen on the endothelial surface, along with firm yellow and white plaques that may either narrow or occlude the vascular lumen. These plaques may remain smooth on their surface or contain pitted, irregular ulcerations with or without attached thrombus. The vessels become rigid and elongated, sometimes with dilatations and fusiform aneurysm formation. Cross sections of plaque may or may not contain underlying hemorrhage.

Microscopically, atherosclerotic plaques contain increased interstitial collagen and elastic substance, along with foam cells filled with lipid and cholesterol crystals.

LIPOHYALINOSIS AND FIBRINOID NECROSIS

Lipohyalinosis and fibrinoid necrosis are pathologic changes that may occur in the small penetrating vessels supplying the basal ganglia and internal capsule. Lipohyalinosis is characterized by thinning of the connective tissue in the vessel wall, surrounding oil red O-positive lipid material and, frequently, hemosiderin-filled macrophages. These changes occur predominantly in vessels with a diameter of less than 200 μm.[6, 7] Fibrinoid necrosis resembles lipohyalinosis but stains more intensely eosinophilic and stains strongly for phosphotungstic acid hematoxylin, whereas lipohyalinosis does not. Both lipohyalinosis and fibrinoid necrosis of the arterioles are thought to be small vessel changes produced by hypertension. Fibrinoid necrosis is more commonly seen with severe acute hypertension, whereas lipohyalinosis occurs with chronic hypertension. These small artery pathologic changes cause the small infarcts responsible for the formation of lacunae commonly seen in the internal capsule, basal ganglia, and thalamus of chronically hypertensive patients. Lacunae also occur as a result of atheromatous occlusion of the larger penetrating arterioles measuring 400 to 900 μm in diameter. The lacunae produced by occlusion of these larger, more laterally placed penetrating vessels tend to be of larger diameter, often measuring 1.5 cm or more.[8, 9]

FIBROMUSCULAR DYSPLASIA

Fibromuscular dysplasia is characterized by segmental proliferation of fibrous tissue and degenerative changes in the cerebral arteries. The pathologic changes most commonly affect the arterial media, less commonly the adventitia or the intima. The proliferation of fibrous tissue produces ringlike narrowing of the arterial lumen. This ringlike narrowing alternates with regions of medial thinning and elastic disruption; this leads to dilatation and aneurysm formation. Fibromuscular dysplasia may lead to dissections of the cerebral vessels and is associated with an increased frequency of intracranial aneurysms that are not necessarily in the distribution typically associated with berry aneurysms.

Fibromuscular dysplasia affects the renal arteries in 90 percent of cases and in only 10 percent of cases demonstrates cerebral involvement. Thirty percent of patients with fibromuscular dysplasia of a cerebral artery have coexistent renal artery involvement. The internal carotid artery is the most frequent cerebral artery involved; rarely the vertebral, posterior cerebral, occipital, and middle cerebral arteries may be affected.[10-12] Seventy-five to 85 percent of patients have bilateral cerebral artery involvement. The internal carotid artery has a characteristic gross and radiographic appearance. Alternating bands of constriction and dilatation produce the string-of-beads appearance, usually beginning 2 to 2.5 cm distal to the carotid bifurcation, and typically sparing the region of the carotid bifurcation.[13, 14] Cerebral symptoms may be produced by hemodynamic mechanisms through progressive stenosis of the cerebral vessels or by the formation of thrombus and thromboembolic occlusion. In addition, dissection of the involved artery may occur and carotid-cavernous fistulas and intracranial aneurysms may develop (see Chapter 51).

SUBACUTE ARTERIOSCLEROTIC ENCEPHALOPATHY

Subacute arteriosclerotic encephalopathy (Binswanger disease) is an uncommon cause of cerebral ischemia.[15-18] Areas of gliosis in the subcortical white matter and degeneration of axons and myelin with some cystic areas of infarction are the characteristic features of this disorder. The gray matter and subcortical association fibers are generally spared. Microscopic examination shows the small arteries and arterioles to be affected, with narrowing or occlusion of the lumen by hyalinization of the wall and intimal fibrosis, medial hypertrophy, and splitting of the internal elastic lamina. Small cystic lacunar infarcts are often also present in the basal ganglia. The computed tomography scan may reflect the changes in the subcortical white matter by showing symmetric areas of diminished white matter density with dilated cerebral ventricles. The clinical picture is that of progressive dementia in a chronically hypertensive patient, with features resembling multi-infarct dementia. The pathogenesis of Binswanger disease is not entirely clear but is commonly attributed to the small artery changes produced from sustained hypertension that either impairs flow to the white matter, particularly in the most distal territories of the penetrating vessels, or produces intermittent focal edema resulting from poorly controlled hypertension.

AMYLOID ANGIOPATHY

Amyloid or congophilic angiopathy is a degenerative vasculopathy of the elderly. The prevalence of this disease

increases progressively after the seventh decade. The pathologic characteristics are deposition of Congo red–positive amyloid in the media and adventitia of small and medium-sized cortical and leptomeningeal arteries. The amyloid is birefringent under polarized light. This amyloid deposition produces narrowing or occlusion of the arterial lumen intramural clefts producing a characteristic ''double barrel'' appearance, thickening of the basement membrane, fragmentation of the internal elastic laminae, and loss of endothelial cells. Electron microscopy shows the amyloid material to be composed of 9 to 11 nm diameter β-amyloid fibrils.

Amyloid angiopathy is the presumed cause for a number of subcortical or lobar intracerebral hemorrhages occurring in all lobes of the brain, with some preference for the parietal and occipital regions.[19-21] The weakened vessel wall leads to miliary aneurysm formation and intracerebral hemorrhage, which may be recurrent. Amyloid angiopathy may occasionally be familial but is not associated with systemic amyloidosis. Hypertension may or may not be present, and the brain often contains the amyloid-containing senile plaques and neurofibrillary tangles of Alzheimer's disease.

VASCULITIS

A number of different forms of cerebral arteritis or vasculitis have been described. In most forms of vasculitis the precise pathophysiology is unclear, although many have a presumed immunologic basis. The classification of these disorders is based on their microscopic appearance, the size of the vessel involved, associated involvement of other organ systems, and the presence or absence of other laboratory and radiologic features.[22, 23]

POLYARTERITIS NODOSA

Polyarteritis nodosa is a vasculitis that may affect the central or peripheral nervous system through involvement of small and medium-sized arteries. The involved vessels typically show bifurcational lesions characterized by infiltrates of polymorphonuclear leukocytes, intimal proliferation, degeneration of the vascular wall with fibrinoid necrosis, and occasional luminal thrombosis. More than half of affected patients are hypertensive. Twenty to 40 percent have central nervous system involvement with ischemic infarction, and about 50 percent have ischemic peripheral neuropathies. Polyarteritis nodosa, like many other forms of noninfectious vasculitis, has a presumed immunologic basis and develops when circulating immune complexes are filtered and deposited in the walls of arteries and venules, promoting inflammatory infiltration of the vessel wall with subsequent destructive changes.

ALLERGIC ANGIITIS

Allergic angiitis and granulomatosis are forms of vasculitis that occur in patients with a history of allergy and frequent lung involvement with peripheral eosinophilia.[24] Small and medium-size arteries and capillaries are infiltrated with granulomas and eosinophils, with associated fibrinoid necrosis. Similar vascular changes are seen in patients with hypersensitivity vasculitis, which develops following a drug-induced allergy, infection, or serum sickness or is associated with Schönlein-Henoch purpura. Skin involvement is frequent in these forms of hypersensitivity vasculitis due to inflammatory changes in the superficial veins, often producing palpable purpuric nodules.

WEGENER GRANULOMATOSIS

Wegener granulomatosis produces a cytologically atypical granulomatous infiltration of the small arteries and veins, with associated fibrinoid necrosis and eventual fibrosis with luminal narrowing and occlusion.[25] Involvement of the lung, skin, and kidneys is common. Cranial nerves II, III, IV, and VI are the most frequent intracranial structures affected. Ischemic peripheral neuropathies may also develop.

LYMPHOMA

Lymphomatoid granulomatosis is a vasculitis resulting from the infiltration of neoplastic lymphocytoid and plasmacytoid cells into the vessel wall. Peripheral leukocytosis is common in these patients.[26]

ISOLATED CEREBRAL GRANULOMATOUS ANGIITIS

Isolated granulomatous angiitis of the central nervous system is typically not accompanied by non–central nervous system arteritis.[27] This disorder is rare, occurs in all ages, and is characterized by segmental involvement of small arteries and venules, especially in the leptomeninges. Microscopically, lymphocytes and plasma cells infiltrate the vessel wall and are accompanied by granulomas with giant cells. Aneurysmal dilatation and rupture may occur, producing subarachnoid or intracerebral hemorrhages. Diffuse small areas of infarction, with or without associated petechiae, are also produced in the brain. Angiography may demonstrate beading of the small arteries, or it may be completely normal.

GIANT CELL ARTERITIS

Giant cell arteritis takes the form of either temporal arteritis or the much less frequent Takayasu arteritis, or pulseless disease. Temporal arteritis is characterized pathologically by segmental panarteritis with mononuclear cell infiltrates and multinucleated giant cells involving the temporal arteries, other branches of the external carotid artery, and rarely the vertebral or other intracranial vessels.[26, 29] Ninety-five percent of patients with temporal arteritis are over 50 years of age; visual changes from ischemia of the optic nerve, or occasionally the retina, occur in 36 to 58 percent of patients.[30] A moderate to marked elevation of the erythrocyte sedimentation rate is common in patients with temporal arteritis. Takayasu arteritis is a rare form of giant cell arteri-

tis involving the aortic arch and its major branches. This disorder is most frequent in young Asian females and may be associated with symptoms of carotid distribution ischemia, hypertension, headache, and carotid sinus sensitivity.[31]

HERPES ZOSTER ARTERITIS

Granulomatous arteritis may develop in the intracranial vessels of patients following herpes zoster ophthalmicus. In affected persons, a carotid distribution infarction develops 4 to 6 weeks following ophthalmic herpes zoster. The characteristic angiographic changes consist of single or multiple smooth, tapered segmental narrowings in either the A2 segment of the proximal pericallosal artery or the M1 segment of the middle cerebral artery, or both. Segmental narrowing has also been identified in the perisellar carotid siphon. Occasionally lesions have also been demonstrated in the basilar artery. Microscopically, there is a granulomatous angiitis of the affected arteries with infiltration of the vessel wall by lymphocytes, histiocytes, and plasma cells. There is necrosis of the arterial wall, and occasionally multinucleated histiocytes are seen.[32–34]

AMPHETAMINE-ASSOCIATED ARTERITIS

Amphetamine abuse has been associated with brain ischemia and infarction as well as intracerebral hemorrhage. Angiography has demonstrated segmental arterial narrowing with a characteristic beaded appearance of involved intracranial vessels. Inflammatory infiltration of the vessel wall with luminal narrowing has been demonstrated pathologically in some patients. Intracerebral hemorrhage may occur after either oral or intravenous amphetamine use; however, some of these patients do not have angiographic or pathologic evidence of arteritis.[35–37] Some of the hemorrhages may be caused by sudden, severe arterial hypertension.

INFECTIOUS ARTERITIS

A number of infectious disorders involving the meninges may produce focal arteritis. These include syphilis, tuberculosis, cat scratch fever, and other bacterial and fungal infections.[22]

ARTERIAL DISSECTION

Arterial wall dissection is an uncommon cause of brain ischemia. The extracranial carotid artery is most frequently involved; however, the major intracranial vessels and the vertebral arteries may be affected. The dissection may begin as an intimal tear with extravasation of blood into the vascular wall or possibly as hemorrhage within the vessel wall, narrowing the vessel lumen. If a second intimal tear distal to the dissection develops, a double lumen may be noted by angiography or pathologic examination. Pseudoaneurysms sometimes develop, but the most frequent finding is an irregular narrowing of the internal carotid artery distal to the carotid sinus extending to the base of the skull. Dissections may occur spontaneously in either normal vessels or diseased arteries, or they may be associated with trauma. Cystic medial degeneration, fibromuscular hyperplasia, Marfan syndrome, and arteriosclerotic degeneration have all been associated with vascular dissections. Traumatic injuries range from severe blunt or direct trauma to rotational and extension injuries occurring with chiropractic neck manipulations or less obvious forms of head movement and trauma.[38]

MOYAMOYA DISEASE

Moyamoya disease is a rare vascular disorder named for the characteristic angiographic appearance of occlusion of the carotid siphon with filling of the so-called rete mirabile collateral vessels, yielding a hazy puff-of-smoke appearance. This disorder was first and is most frequently described as occurring in Asian children. It produces symptoms of recurrent cerebral ischemia. Adults with moyamoya disease more commonly experience subarachnoid or intracerebral hemorrhage.[39–40] The etiology of most cases of moyamoya disease is unclear. It may represent a pattern of collateral development resulting from many causes of distal internal carotid artery occlusion. Pathologically there is no evidence of arteritis. There is generally hypoplasia of the media, with subintimal proliferation. The walls of the small anastomotic vessels are thin and are the presumed fragile substrate of the intracranial hemorrhages occurring in these patients.

VENOUS AND DURAL SINUS THROMBOSIS

Venous thrombosis may produce either brain infarction or hemorrhage. Many disorders may produce venous sinus or cortical vein thrombosis, including disorders that affect blood coagulation, cause changes in the venous wall, and lead to reduced blood flow through the venous channels. The common underlying conditions include pregnancy, malignancy (especially leukemia), and infectious and inflammatory disorders of the sinuses and middle ear. Pathologically the venous sinuses appear distended, and there is often infarction of adjacent brain, with edema and petechial or even gross parenchymal hemorrhage. Surviving patients may have recanalization of the thrombosed vessel. The walls of the veins may either be normal or contain malignant or inflammatory cells, depending on the underlying disorder predisposing to thrombosis.[41]

CARDIOGENIC BRAIN EMBOLISM

Cardiogenic emboli account for approximately 15 percent of all ischemic brain infarctions. The emboli arise from diseased valves or from thrombi within the left ventricle or the left atrium. Degenerative changes in the mitral and aortic valves and in prosthetic valves provide a surface for thrombus formation, leading to brain or systemic embolization. In addition, calcific or other degenerative material from the valve may embolize into the arterial circulation. Emboliza-

tion of infected material produces an ischemic stroke in about 20 percent of patients with infectious endocarditis. Approximately 1 in 6000 patients with mitral valve prolapse experiences transient or permanent brain ischemia, presumably caused by embolized platelet-fibrin material originating on the functionally abnormal valve leaflets. In nonbacterial thrombotic endocarditis, platelet-fibrin thrombi form on the atrial surface of the mitral valve and the ventricular surface of the aortic valve along the lines of valve closure. Nonbacterial (marasmic) thrombotic endocarditis is seen in patients with malignant neoplasms or chronic wasting illnesses, and about 30 percent of these patients experience embolic brain ischemic events.

Mural thrombus within the left ventricle may embolize to the brain. Following myocardial infarction, an area of dyskinetic ventricular wall or a ventricular aneurysm may be the site of thrombus formation and subsequent embolization. Cardiomyopathies are also associated with intraventricular thrombus formation and systemic embolism.

Atrial fibrillation is the most common cardiac condition associated with an embolic stroke. The fibrillating, poorly contracting atrium forms thrombi within its appendage or on its wall. Although atrial fibrillation associated with mitral stenosis leads to the greatest risk of embolization, atrial fibrillation without valvular disease is also accompanied by increased risk of ischemic stroke. Other less common causes of cardiogenic embolism include paradoxic embolism with persistent atrial septal defects and intracardiac tumors.[42]

CONCLUSION

The spectrum of pathology producing brain ischemia is extremely broad. Disease of the arteries, especially atherosclerosis, is the presumed basis for ischemia in most patients. Degenerative disorders of the arteries, inflammatory vasculopathies, and trauma are causative in others. Emboli may arise from diseased heart valves or from thrombi formed within the left ventricle or left atrium that embolize to the brain. Venous sinus or cortical vein thrombosis associated with a predisposing systemic illness may also produce brain infarction or hemorrhage. Emboli may arise from diseased valves or from thrombi formed within the left ventricle or left atrium.

REFERENCES

1. Mancini M, Pauciullo P: Clinical relevance of hyperlipidemia [review]. *Cardiovasc Drug Ther.* 1990;4:1385–1388.
2. Benditt EP: Origins of human atherosclerotic plaques: The role of altered gene expression. *Arch Pathol Lab Med.* 1988;112:997–1001.
3. Raines EW, Ross R: Smooth muscle cells and the pathogenesis of the lesions of atherosclerosis [review]. *Br Heart J.* 1993;69:530–537.
4. Tennant M, McGeachie JK: Platelet-derived growth factor and its role in atherogenesis: A brief review. *Aust N Z J Surg.* 1991;61:482–488.
5. Fisher M: Atherosclerosis: Cellular aspects and potential intervention [review]. *Cerebrovasc Brain Metab Rev.* 1991;3:114–133.
6. Boiten J, Lodder J: Large striatocapsular infarcts: Clinical presentation and pathogenesis in comparison with lacunar and cortical infarcts. *Acta Neurol Scand.* 1992;86:298–303.
7. Mohr JP: Lacunes. In Barnett HMJ, Mohr JP, Stein BM, Yatsu FM, eds. *Stroke, Pathophysiology, Diagnosis and Management,* 2nd ed. New York: Churchill Livingstone; 1992:539–544.
8. Besson G, Hommel M: Historical aspects of lacunes and the "lacunar controversy." *Adv Neurol.* 1993;62:1–10.
9. Besson G, Hommel M: Lacunar syndromes. *Adv Neurol.* 1993;62:141–160. Review.

10. Bellot J, Gherardi R, Poirier J, et al: Fibromuscular dysplasia of cervico-cephalic arteries with multiple dissections and a carotid-cavernous fistula: A pathological study. *Stroke*. 1985;16:255–261.

11. Saygi S, Bolay H, Tekkok H, et al: Fibromuscular dysplasia of the basilar artery: A case of brainstem stroke [review]. *Angiology*. 1990;41:658–661.

12. Morgenlander JC, Goldstein LB: Recurrent transient ischemic attacks and stroke in association with an internal carotid artery web. *Stroke*. 1991;22:94–98.

13. Furie DM, Tien RD: Fibromuscular dysplasia of arteries of the head and neck: Imaging findings. *AJR Am J Roentgenol*. 1994;162:1205–1209.

14. Pappada G, Parzarasa G, Sani R, Formaggio G: Intracranial fibromuscular dysplasia: Report of two cases and review of the literature. *J Neurol Sci*. 1987;31:13–8.

15. Bibikian V, Ropper AH: Binswanger's disease: A review. *Stroke*. 1987;18:1–12.

16. Bennett DA, Wilson RS, Gilley DW, Fox JH: Clinical diagnosis of Binswanger's disease. *J Neurol Neurosurg Psychiatry*. 1990;53:961–965.

17. Kinkel WR, Jacobs L, Polachini I, et al: Subcortical arteriosclerotic encephalopathy (Binswanger's disease). *Arch Neurol*. 1985;42:951–959.

18. Bogousslavsky J: Binswanger's disease. In Barnett HMJ, Mohr JP, Stein BM, Yatsu FM, eds. *Stroke, Pathophysiology, Diagnosis and Management*, 2nd ed. New York: Churchill Livingstone; 1992:805–819.

19. Vonsattel JPG, Myers RH, Hedley-White ET, et al: Cerebral amyloid angiopathy without and with cerebral hemorrhages: A comparative histological study. *Ann Neurol*. 1991;30:637–649.

20. Mandybur TI: Cerebral amyloid angiopathy: The vascular pathology and complications. *J Neuropathol Exp Neurol*. 1986;45:79–90.

21. Greenberg SM, Vonsattel JPG, Stakes JW, et al: The clinical spectrum of cerebral amyloid angiopathy. *Neurology*. 1993;43:2073–2079.

22. Jennette JC, Falk RJ, Andrassy K, et al: Nomenclature of systemic vasculitides: Proposal of an international consensus conference. *Arthritis Rheumatol*. 1994;37:187–193.

23. Greenan TJ, Grossman RI, Goldberg HI: Cerebral vasculitis: MR imaging and angiographic correlation. *Radiology*. 1992;182:65–72.

24. Sigal LH: The neurologic presentation of vasculitic and rheumatologic syndromes. *Medicine*. 1987;66:157–180.

25. Schwartz RA, Churg J: Churg-Strauss syndrome [review]. *Br J Dermatol*. 1992;127:199–204.

26. Capone PM, Mechtler LL, Bates VE, et al: Multiple giant intracranial aneurysms associated with lymphomatous granulomatosis. *J Neuroimaging*. 1994;4:109–111.

27. Lie JT: Primary (granulomatous) angiitis of the central nervous system: A clinico-pathologic analysis of 15 new cases and a review of the literature. *Hum Pathol*. 1992;23:164–171.

28. Caselli RJ, Hunder GG: Neurologic aspects of giant cell (temporal) arteritis. *Rheum Dis Clin North Am*. 1993;19:941–953.

29. Hunder GG, Lie JT, Garonzy JJ, Weyland CM: The pathogenesis of giant cell arteritis. *Arthritis Rheum*. 1993;36:757–761.

30. Hamed CM, Guy JR, Moster ML, Bosley T: Giant cell arteritis in the ocular ischemic syndrome. *Am J Ophthalmol*. 1992;113:702–705.

31. Bengtsson BA, Andersson R: Giant cell and Takayasu's arteritis [review]. *Curr Opin Rheumatol*. 1991;3:15–22.

32. Herkes GK, Storey CE, Joffe R, MacKenzie RA: Herpes zoster arteritis: Clinical and angiographic features. *Clin Exp Neurol*. 1987;24:169–174.

33. Lexa FJ, Galetta SL, Yousem DM, et al: Herpes zoster ophthalmicus with orbital pseudotumor syndrome complicated by optic nerve infarction and cerebral granulomatous angiitis: MR-pathologic correlation. *AJNR Am J Neuroradiol*. 1993;14:185–190.

34. MacKenzie RA, Ryan P, Karnes WE, Okazaki H: Herpes zoster arteritis: Pathologic findings. *Clin Exp Neurol*. 1987;23:219–224.

35. Bostwick DG: Amphetamine induced cerebral vasculitis. *Hum Pathol*. 1981;12:1031–1033.

36. Stoessl AJ, Young GB, Feasby TE: Inracerebral hemorrhage and angiographic beading following ingestion of catecholaminergics. *Stroke*. 1985;16:734–736.

37. Fredericks RK, Lefkowitz DS, Challa VR, Troost BT: Cerebral vasculitis associated with cocaine abuse. *Stroke*. 1991;22:1437–1439.

38. Caplan LR, Baquis GD, Pessin MS, D'Alton J: Dissection of the intracranial vertebral artery. *Neurology*. 1988;38:868–877.

39. Kaufman M, Little BW, Berkowitz BW: Recurrent intracranial hemorrhage in an adult with moya moya disease: Case report, radiologic studies and pathology. *Can J Neurol Sci*. 1988;15:430–434.

40. Yonekawa Y, Goto T, Nobuyoski O: Moyamoya disease: Diagnosis, treatment and recent achievement. In Barnett HJM, Mohr JP, Stein BM, Yatsu FM, eds. *Stroke, Pathophysiology, Diagnosis and Management*, 2nd ed. New York: Churchill Livingstone; 1992:721–747.

41. Bousser M-G, Barnett HJM: Cerebral venous thrombosis. In Barnett HJM, Mohr JP, Stein BM, Yatsu FM, eds. *Stroke, Pathophysiology, Diagnosis and Management*, 2nd ed. New York: Churchill Livingstone; 1992:517–537.

42. Caplan LR: Brain embolism, revisited. *Neurology*. 1993;43:1281–1287.

CHAPTER 8

Lesions, Dynamics, and Pathogenetic Mechanisms Responsible for Ischemic Events in the Brain

RICHARD W. BOCK and ROBERT J. LUSBY

Full appreciation of the the dominant role of extracranial atherosclerosis as the primary cause of cerebral ischemia was reached only in the latter half of the 20th century. Until then, the carotid arteries were removed at autopsy only rarely, and their importance in the pathogenesis of stroke remained hidden. In the early 1950s, clinical observations and subsequent pathologic studies by Fisher[1, 2] and Hutchinson and Yates[3] demonstrated the significance of both carotid and vertebral artery disease. It is now recognized that cerebral infarction arising from these vessels accounts for almost three fourths of the strokes in the community.[4] The Framingham study revealed a thromboembolic cause for 78 percent of strokes, of which only 2 percent were associated with a known cardiac source of emboli.[5] Other major causes of stroke included subarachnoid hemorrhage (8–12%) and primary intracerebral hemorrhage (5–10%).[4, 5]

Stroke can result from other, less common causes. Emboli may arise from the heart in association with old and recent myocardial infarction, rheumatic heart disease, myocarditis, congestive cardiomyopathy, thrombotic endocarditis, infective myocarditis, and, rarely, atrial myxoma. Other causes include inherited and acquired hypercoagulable states, giant cell arteritis, polyarteritis nodosa, and tuberculous meningitis. Trauma, fibromuscular dysplasia, and spontaneous dissection of the extracranial and intracranial vessels may also cause cerebral ischemia.

In all these conditions, flow through the cerebral arteries may be compromised partially (stenosis) or completely (occlusion); the resulting ischemia may be either temporary or permanent. The affected vessels may be large or small, and the distal tissues may be supplied by well-developed collateral vessels or by none at all. Ischemic events in the brain follow a reduction in blood flow to a level below that required to maintain normal physiologic function, but the interplay of some of these factors determines the severity of brain damage. The ischemic event is transient if blood flow is quickly restored. Prolonged reduction in flow causes loss of viable tissue, leading to infarction. Infarction is the dominant cause of completed stroke.

THE LESIONS OF CEREBRAL INFARCTION

Infarction of brain tissue may vary in size from a massive lesion in the territory of a single major vessel, such as the middle cerebral artery, to small peripheral areas of the cerebral cortex or underlying white matter supplied by smaller branches or arterioles. Sudden occlusion of a vessel may induce ischemia to an extent that, even in the presence of potential collaterals, there is insufficient blood flow to maintain cell metabolism.

Cerebral ischemia causes ischemia, cell death, and necro-

sis of nerve cells and fibers; similar changes in the glial cells soon follow. Necrosis of small blood vessels occurs as part of the ischemic process, with the extravasation of red blood cells. When extravasation of erythrocytes is minimal, a pale infarct occurs. More extensive perivascular extravasation produces hemorrhagic infarcts, particularly in the cortical area. The finding of hemorrhagic infarction suggests an embolic etiology.[6] One mechanism of postinfarction extravasation of blood involves fragmentation of the embolus, dislodgement, and subsequent revascularization of damaged vessels. In the region of cerebral infarction there are zones of underperfusion and overperfusion. Clinically, areas of enhanced blood flow may be seen on computed tomographic (CT) scans in the days following the development of an infarct; however, old infarcts are devoid of such activity.

Soon after infarction, degradation and liquefaction of lipid in and around the myelin sheaths occurs. Interstitial fluid accumulates and early acute swelling follows. Phagocytic cells infiltrate the area and begin removal of fatty and necrotic tissues. The degree of cerebral edema depends on infarct size, and it generally peaks at 4 to 5 days. Interstitial fluid, lipid, and engorged microglial phagocytes account for much of the swelling. The healing phase is heralded by resolution of edema, development of new vessels, and formation of granulation tissue composed of astrocytes and a few fibroblasts. Eventually, a dense neuroglial scar is formed with shrinkage, cavitation, and scarring in the surrounding tissue.[7, 8]

Death from acute stroke generally results from the rapid swelling of the brain in association with extensive cerebral ischemia and tissue breakdown. Transtentorial herniation and resulting increased brain-stem pressure, along with rupture of small arteries to the midbrain and pons, lead to further extension of the ischemic process and the arrest of brain-stem function.[9]

LACUNAR INFARCTS

Lacunae are small, cavitary ischemic infarcts. They are located deep to the cortex, characteristically in the internal capsule and basal ganglia. Lacunar infarcts arise from occlusions of the small penetrating vessels of the lenticulostriate and thalamoperforate arteries. Because of their small size, they are generally associated with pure motor or pure sensory symptoms.[10] Lacunae are rare in the cerebral cortex, the major white matter of the cerebral hemispheres, the visual radiations, the corpus callosum, the medulla, and the spinal cord, despite the presence of similar small vessels in these areas.[11] The lack of collateral supply for these small penetrating vessels causes wedge-shaped infarctions, the apex arising from the site of occlusion. Capsular infarcts arising from distal penetrating branch arteries 200 to 400 μm in size produce infarcts 2 to 3 mm^3 or smaller, which are often difficult to detect on CT scanning.[12] More proximal occlusions at the mouth of a penetrating vessel will produce greater areas of infarction up to 15 mm³. These "superlacunae" can produce large defects that are detectable at several levels of a CT scan.

Until recently, lacunar strokes were routinely ascribed to small vessel disease at the site of occlusion and were felt to be secondary to hypertension and its effects on the small intracranial perforating vessels. Embolism from larger, more proximal vessels was not thought to be involved in lacunar stroke, and investigations in search of such disease were not generally performed. More recently, experimental[13] and clinical[14, 15] proof of large-vessel embolism in cases of classic lacunar stroke has emerged, leading to a fundamental reassessment of the disorder. Millikan and Futrell[16] emphasized that the "lacune hypothesis" of small-vessel disease is a fallacy, that large vessel embolism is likely a common etiology, and that the term "lacunar stroke" should be used simply to signify a small stroke. Patients suffering lacunar strokes should therefore receive the same investigations as other ischemic stroke patients, as they have a similar prospect for identification of a treatable (extracranial) etiology.

ATHEROSCLEROSIS AND CEREBRAL ISCHEMIA

Atheroma is the most common arterial lesion giving rise to the development of cerebral ischemia. The term was first applied to arterial pathology by von Haller in 1735, when he described a lesion of the artery that, on sectioning, exuded "a yellow, pultaceous gruel-like material." Flory[17] recognized the pathologic significance of atheromatous embolization and described the occlusion of small- and medium-sized vessels of the kidney and spleen distal to the erosion of atheromatous plaques. In 1904, Marchand[18] introduced the term "atherosclerosis" to describe lesions of the arteries

showing both fatty degeneration and connective tissue proliferation.

In its earliest form, this disease is seen as a fatty streak containing large amounts of lipid within macrophages and smooth muscle cells. Later, as the lesion grows and thickens, it becomes a fibrous plaque, which involves the inner layers of the vessel wall and protrudes into the lumen. It is composed of smooth muscle cells and connective tissue with a high percentage of collagen. At this stage, the microscopic appearance of the lesion is still monotonous, and on gross examination it appears smooth and homogeneous. As these smooth, fibrous plaques continue to grow, they may increasingly encroach on the vessel lumen. The artery may enlarge in response to plaque growth,[19] which in turn allows for further plaque enlargement.

A few plaques remain smooth and fibrous as they grow beyond moderate degrees of stenosis. However, with such growth usually comes a new stage in plaque development: plaque degeneration. These complex plaques (Fig. 8–1) contain areas of surface ulceration, intraplaque hemorrhage, lipid (cholesterol) vacuolization, and calcification. As plaques enlarge, portions may undergo softening, often as a result of relative ischemia in the center of the plaque.[20] Mechanical stress applied to these complex lesions may result in the breakdown of the overlying intimal surface. It is uncommon for such breakdowns to occur without evidence of intraplaque hemorrhage.[21, 22] Plaque calcification is often a marker for development of complex plaque but is probably not an independent risk factor for embolization.[23] The remaining lesions are unstable and friable and are linked to the development of cerebrovascular ischemia through embolization (Fig. 8–2).[24–26] They are discussed individually in the following sections.

Ulceration

Ulceration of carotid artery plaques is commonly found in complex lesions and is closely linked to the development

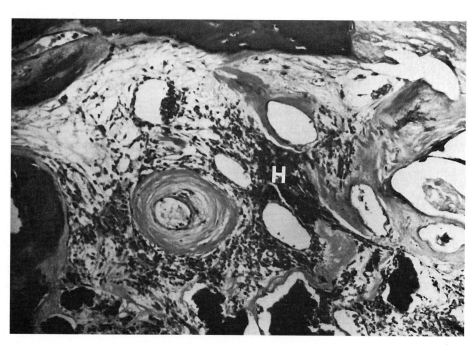

FIGURE 8–1. Micrograph from a complex plaque showing areas of focal hemorrhage (H) and new vessels. In the center is one hyalinized vessel and throughout the field are numerous thin-walled capillaries. (Original magnification × 125.)

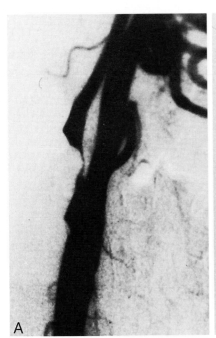
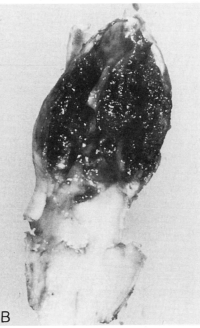

FIGURE 8–2. *A* and *B,* Angiogram demonstrating a high-grade stenosis of the origin of the internal carotid artery. The specimen was removed at operation and contained a large intraplaque hemorrhage that occupies most of the stenotic lesion.

of transient ischemic attack (TIA) and stroke.[23, 24, 27, 28] The term "ulcer" denotes a pit or recess in an atherosclerotic plaque rather than any loss of the intimal layer (most ulcers have an intact endothelial covering). Breakdown of the fibrous cap over a complex plaque is a frequent cause of ulceration. These lesions vary from shallow superficial erosions (Fig. 8–3), often over calcific deposits, to deep ulcers that penetrate into plaques and commonly contain recent intraplaque hemorrhage or complex lipid, cholesterol, and calcium elements (Fig. 8–4).[29] Ulcers may cause cerebrovascular symptoms at the time of formation through embolization of the overlying cap. More commonly, they serve as a nidus for clot formation; embolization or propagation of thrombus beyond the ulcer's borders may follow.

Retrospective studies of carotid plaque ulceration have demonstrated annual stroke rates between 4.5 and 12.5 percent.[24, 27] The randomized, prospective North American Symptomatic Carotid Endarterectomy Trial (NASCET) included a study of carotid plaque ulceration in patients with symptomatic stenoses exceeding 75 percent. In patients with angiographically demonstrated ulcers who were randomly assigned to the medical (aspirin) group, the 2-year risk of stroke ranged from 26 to 73 percent as the degree of stenosis increased from 75 to 95 percent. Patients with similar stenosis but no ulcer showed no increasing risk of stroke with higher degrees of stenosis, and all groups benefited significantly from carotid endarterectomy.

Intraplaque Hemorrhage

Intraplaque hemorrhage at the carotid bifurcation is a dominant factor in the pathogenesis of carotid stroke.[21, 23, 30, 31] Up to 85 percent of symptomatic patients exhibit intraplaque hemorrhage in association with intimal disruption (Fig. 8–5).[22, 32–34] Intraplaque hemorrhage is the most common pathologic finding in plaques removed from symptomatic patients. By contrast, plaques removed from asymptomatic patients show little evidence of intraplaque

hemorrhage, and ulceration is rarely seen (Fig. 8–6).[21] Intraplaque hemorrhage becomes more frequent as carotid stenosis increases,[35, 36] leading some investigators to suggest that the diagnosis of intraplaque hemorrhage may be at least as important as the determination of percentage stenosis in identifying patients at risk for stroke.[37] The fact that most strokes are associated with sudden, major changes in the degree of stenosis[30] provides further indirect evidence for a dominant role of intraplaque hemorrhage in the pathogenesis of stroke.

Two mechanisms have been proposed for the development of hemorrhage within the plaque. Dissection and tracking of blood into the softened central portion of a complex plaque may follow plaque fracture and intimal disruption (Figs. 8–7 and 8–8). Alternatively, the vasa vasorum growing into the plaque may be disrupted, leading to a contained intraplaque hemorrhage without direct communication with the lumen (Fig. 8–9). It is probable that both mechanisms contribute to the clinical findings. Determination of the age of the hemorrhage has given further weight to the argument that intraplaque hemorrhage occurs in association with symptoms. The plaques removed from symptomatic patients exhibit an acute or recent inflammatory response adjacent to the hemorrhage in which polymorphonuclear cells and macrophages are seen. Healing and repair processes are found in which macrophage engulfment of hemosiderin, giant cell formation, and the development of new vessels occur (Fig. 8–10). This inflammatory reaction was noted in more than 92 percent of plaques removed from patients with symptoms of cerebral ischemia, in contrast to a low incidence of 27 percent in plaques removed from asymptomatic patients.[21] Up to 75 percent of patients undergoing carotid endarterectomy within 1 week of the onset of symptoms had evidence of an acute hemorrhage. Recent hemorrhage was seen in 75 percent of patients whose symptoms developed from 1 to 6 weeks after operation. Evidence of multiple hemorrhages based on pathologic criteria was seen in 81 percent of symptomatic patients, many of whom experienced several attacks of cerebral ischemia.[21] The inflammatory reaction that follows acute intraplaque hemorrhage appears to be a response to injury within the vessel wall, which results in a spectrum of endpoints.

Plaques containing intraplaque hemorrhage (as well as those with ulceration) may evolve over time, either healing or degenerating further (Fig. 8–11). The well-documented reduction in stroke incidence after 1 year following the onset of cerebral ischemic attacks may correlate with the development of a well-healed lesion. When progression to stroke occurs, it may be a result of further hemorrhage within the friable vascular plaque or degenerative breakdown and embolization.

Lipid Sequestration

Complex atherosclerotic plaques may also contain large sequestrations of lipid, in the form of cholesterol crystals (Fig. 8–12) or as discrete collections of pure lipid (Fig. 8–13). Symptoms of cerebral ischemia are correlated with increased content of both substances.[26] In addition, increasing degrees of carotid stenosis also correlate with cholesterol content, as do ulceration and intraplaque hemorrhage. Conversely, increased content of collagen (the predominant component of smooth, fibrous plaques) is associated with a low risk of ischemic symptoms.[26]

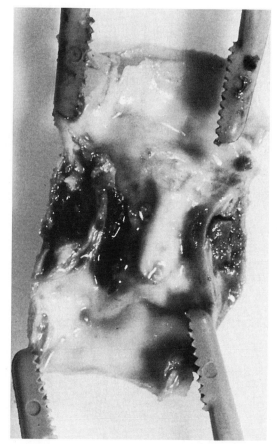

FIGURE 8–4. Deep ulcer overlying an area of intraplaque hemorrhage. Note the luminal thrombus on the surface adjacent to the ulcer.

Distribution of Lesions

Among the vessels supplying the brain, formation of complex, unstable lesions is probably more common in the extracranial carotid arteries than elsewhere. For reasons detailed below, the carotid bifurcation and the proximal internal carotid artery are particularly susceptible to plaque formation and subsequent degeneration. While stenotic lesions of the vertebral arteries are common, they are usually less heterogeneous and hemorrhagic than carotid bifurcation plaques.[20, 29] Most vertebral plaques are smooth, fibrous, and proximal, rarely extending beyond 2 to 3 mm from the ostia (Fig. 8–14).[21] The innominate and subclavian arteries may develop either fibrous or complex plaques, and hemorrhagic lesions are commonly found (Figs. 8–15 and 8–16). Symptoms may arise from these lesions as a result of progressive narrowing leading to decreased distal flow, or from emboli arising from the degeneration and breakdown of the plaques. Finally, the intracranial vessels may develop atherosclerotic lesions. While it is generally assumed that these lesions are more fibrous and less likely to produce embolization, few investigations of intracranial plaque morphology have been performed.

HEMODYNAMICS OF PLAQUE FORMATION

The location of clinically important atheromatous plaques at points of arterial bifurcation or branching has led investi-

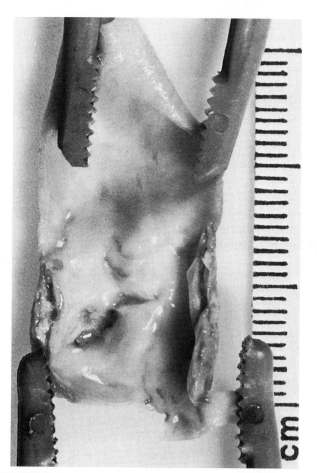

FIGURE 8–3. Shallow ulcer seen in an endarterectomy specimen. A calcific plate was present at the base of the ulcer.

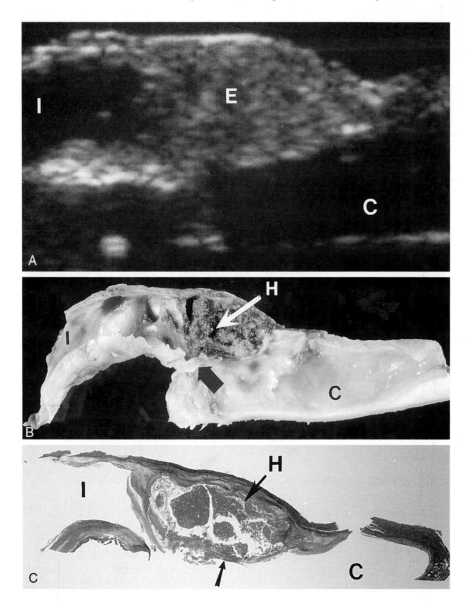

FIGURE 8–5. Symptomatic carotid bifurcation plaque exhibiting intraplaque hemorrhage and high-grade stenosis. *A,* Ultrasonographic image demonstrating the echolucent lesion *(E),* interposed between the common *(C)* and internal *(I)* carotid arteries. *B,* Gross photograph of the same plaque with intraplaque hemorrhage *(H).* *Heavy arrow* depicts the small residual lumen. *C,* Special stain shows the intraplaque hemorrhage *(H)* and clearly demonstrates resultant overlying ulceration *(small arrow).*

gators to seek a hemodynamic basis for their development. Common sites of atherogenesis in the cerebrovascular system include the carotid artery bifurcation, the origins of the vertebral artery at the subclavian arteries, the origins of the carotid and innominate arteries, the carotid siphon, and origins of the anterior cerebral arteries.[38-40] Sites of direct branching from the basilar artery may also be involved.[10, 12] Approximately two thirds of cerebrovascular lesions are in the surgically accessible extracranial vessels. Most of these occur at the carotid bifurcation (57%), with the origin of the vertebral artery (30%) and origin of great vessels (13%) accounting for the remainder.[41, 42]

Investigation into the specific hemodynamic factors that trigger carotid plaque development began more than 30 years ago. Many researchers assumed that endothelial injury in areas of high shear stress was responsible for atherogenesis. However, in 1971 Caro and associates[43] reported an elegant series of experiments using glass models of the carotid bifurcation. They demonstrated that the regions along the carotid bifurcation and bulb long known to have a predilection for plaque formation actually experience *low* shear stress. Conversely, regions of high shear stress seemed to correlate with known regions of relative resistance to atherogenesis. These studies were confirmed a decade later by Bharadvaj and coworkers,[44] who found that oscillatory as well as low shear stress correlated with known patterns of plaque development. These areas of low and oscillatory shear stress corresponded to the lateral wall of the carotid bulb, opposite and lateral to the flow divider, whereas regions of high shear stress and presumed resistance to atherogenesis included the medial internal carotid artery and the flow divider itself. Nazemi and associates[45] demonstrated similar findings with pulsatile flow, and Zarins and associates[46] added studies of autopsy specimens to data obtained from the glass models and confirmed the conclusions of previous investigators. Other studies documented an acceleration in atherogenesis with increased heart rate[47] and demonstrated the role of arterial wall compliance in modulating the oscillations of shear stress.[48]

Although these studies provide strong evidence for the role of low and oscillatory shear stress in the development of mild and perhaps moderate degrees of carotid stenosis,

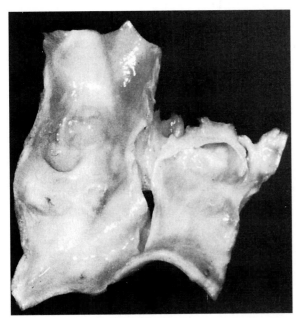

FIGURE 8–6. Carotid endarterectomy specimen removed from an asymptomatic patient. Although irregular, the plaque is predominantly fibrous without evidence of hemorrhage or ulceration.

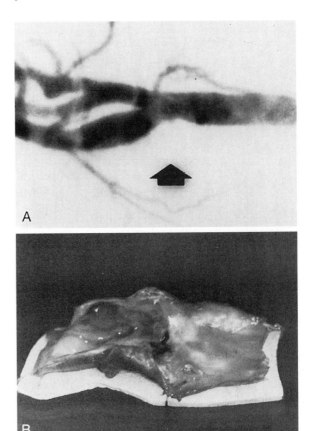

FIGURE 8–7. A, Angiogram showing a stenotic lesion at the carotid bifurcation. B, Operative specimen shows plaque fracture on the surface of the mound.

they do not explain the progression of lesions to tight stenosis or the development of complex plaques with ulceration, hemorrhage, and macroscopic lipid sequestration. With the development of a focal atheroma, the medial thickness of the carotid bulb changes in relation to the less affected (proximal and distal) regions of the vessel.[49] Segmental changes in vessel distensibility that result from the uneven distribution of plaque can produce sudden alterations in compliance[50] and in the presence of asymmetric plaque may also be important in the development of plaque hemorrhage.[51] Abrupt changes in vessel compliance have been associated with disruptive stresses in the wall, leading to dilation.[52] Further alterations in local shear stress ensue, producing either low stress and a predisposition to further atherogenesis, or sharply higher shear stress, which may lead to acute plaque fracture and intraplaque hemorrhage.

The composition and thickness of the wall also influence the tangential tension (force per unit area), a factor distinct from shear stress. With the development of nondistensible, often asymmetric atheroma, changes in wall structure and topography occur, producing imbalances in tangential ten-

sions (Fig. 8–17). Alterations in these forces, possibly associated with exacerbations in systemic blood pressure, may contribute not only to the gradual development of atheroma but also to the sudden development of plaque fracture and intraplaque hemorrhage.[51] Vibration may also play a role: carotid artery bruits, often heard in the presence of atheroma, result from vessel wall movement at high frequencies within the audible range.[53] There is evidence that particular frequencies cause changes in the structural components or the vessel walls, particularly in the integrity of elastin and collagen.[54, 55]

Another hemodynamic force may predispose to sudden changes in plaque structure. The Bernoulli principle states that the product of pressure and velocity remains constant.

FIGURE 8–8. Low-power longitudinal section of the lesion shown in Figure 8–7. A large intraplaque hemorrhage is seen within the plaque along with an ulcerative defect on the luminal surface.

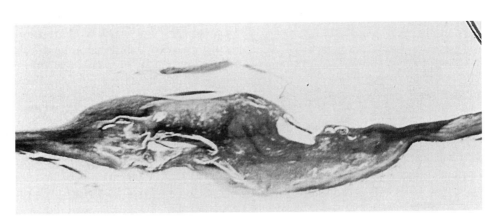

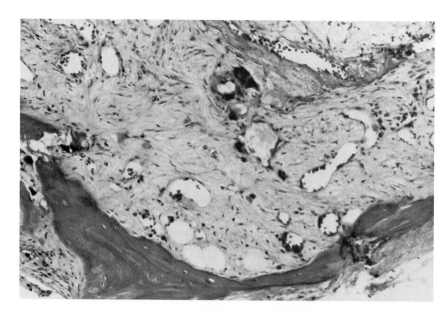

FIGURE 8–9. High-power micrograph of plaque from a carotid artery showing multiple new vessels arising from the vasa vasorum. Disruption of these new vessels gives rise to intraplaque hemorrhage.

As blood flows through a stenosis, its velocity increases, while pressure decreases. Thus a pressure gradient exists across the plaque and produces an "unroofing" force (Fig. 8–18). This force, when applied across a complex plaque, may result in plaque fracture and intraplaque hemorrhage with accompanying embolization, progression to critical stenosis, or occlusion. This sudden change in plaque shape and size correlates well with the clinical finding that strokes are usually associated with abrupt, unpredictable changes in degree of stenosis.[30]

ANEURYSMAL DISEASE

Whereas stenosing lesions of the extracranial vessels are frequent, aneurysms are distinctly uncommon. When they do occur, the commmon and internal carotid arteries are generally involved, but even in that case the incidence is low: only 8 cervical carotid aneurysms were noted in a review of 5000 carotid angiograms.[56] In addition to atherosclerosis (Figs. 8–19 and 8–20), trauma, fibromuscular dysplasia, cystic medial necrosis, and infection (syphilitic, bac-

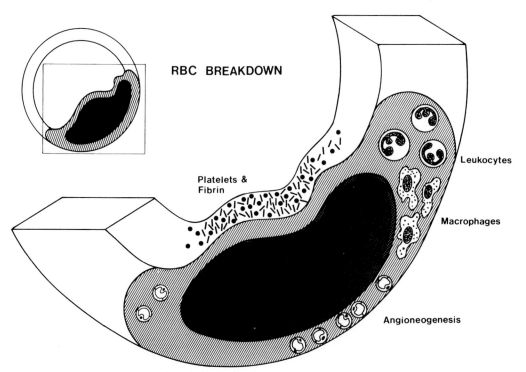

RBC BREAKDOWN

Leukocytes

Platelets & Fibrin

Macrophages

Angioneogenesis

FIGURE 8–10. Diagrammatic representation of inflammatory elements involved in response to development of intraplaque hemorrhage. (From Lusby RJ, Ferrell LD, Wylie EJ: The significance of intraplaque haemorrhage in the pathogenesis of carotid atherosclerosis. In Bergan, JJ, Yao ST, eds. *Cerebrovascular Insufficiency,* 2nd ed. New York: Grune & Stratton, 1983:41.)

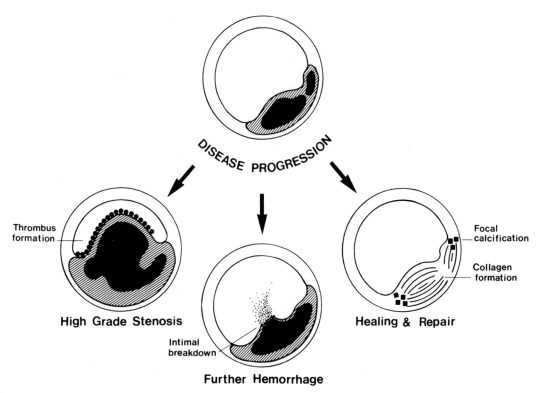

FIGURE 8–11. Diagram illustrating possible sequence of events in carotid artery following the development of an intraplaque hemorrhage. (From Lusby RJ, Ferrell LD, Wylie EJ: The significance of intraplaque haemorrhage in the pathogenesis of carotid atherosclerosis. In Bergan, JJ, Yao ST, eds. *Cerebrovascular Insufficiency,* 2nd ed. New York: Grune & Stratton, 1983:41.)

terial, and fungal) may cause aneurysm formation. De facto carotid artery aneurysms may be produced by improperly wide patch closure applied at carotid endarterectomy (see Chapter 47). False aneurysms may also occur following vein patch closure of the vessel (Fig. 8–21), but overall rates of pseudoaneurysm formation probably do not differ among patients receiving patch versus primary closure.[57] Thrombus formation within the wall of the aneurysm is often a source of emboli, but many aneurysms appear as asymptomatic bulges in the neck.[58]

ARTERIAL ELONGATION, TORTUOSITY, AND KINKING

Elongation of the carotid artery may be a manifestation of atherosclerosis or a result of abnormal development. The carotid artery is formed from the third aortic arch and the dorsal aorta. It is normally redundant and kinked in the early stages of development, but this condition is corrected as the heart descends into the thorax. Some residual length may remain until later development, as noted in the high inci-

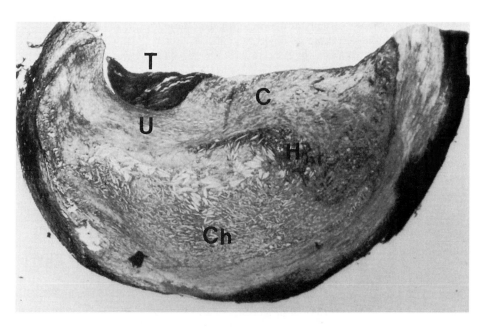

FIGURE 8–12. Low-power cross section of atheromatous plaque with dense fibrous cap *(C)* overlying a large deposit of cholesterol crystals *(Ch).* A luminal thrombus *(T)* lies in a small ulcer crater *(U)* on the plaque surface, and a small intraplaque hemorrhage is present *(H).*

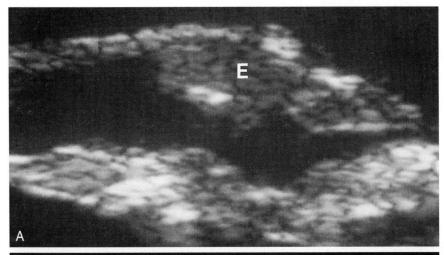

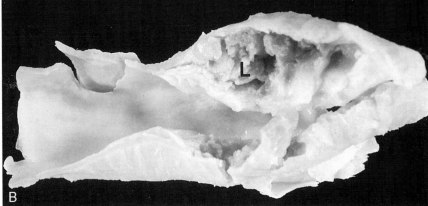

FIGURE 8–13. *A,* Ultrasonographic image of a symptomatic carotid plaque demonstrating an echolucent lesion *(E). B,* Surgical specimen reveals that a lipid collection *(L)* within the complex plaque is responsible for the echolucent appearance on the ultrasonogram.

dence of redundancy seen in infant angiograms.[59] Up to 21 percent of adult carotid angiograms demonstrate elongation, varying from minimal changes to kinks and 360-degree loops. Excessive lengthening or redundancy may result in kinking capable of producing such hemodynamic changes as turbulent flow and pressure-reducing lesions. Carotid artery kinks may become symptomatic with turning of the head.[60] Up to 70 percent of coils and kinks are associated with atherosclerotic lesions,[61] usually at the origin of the internal carotid artery (Fig. 8–22). Carotid kinks and coils have also been associated with spontaneous dissection.[62, 63]

FIBROMUSCULAR DYSPLASIA

Fibromuscular dysplasia was first recognized as a cause of cerebral ischemia in 1965.[64] It is now known to involve both the carotid and vertebral arteries as well as the intracranial vessels. Hyperplasia of the media is the most common feature, although three other lesions—intimal fibroplasia, medial fibroplasia, and premedial dysplasia—may occur. Fibromuscular dysplasia is segmental, affecting long conducting arteries with few primary branches. The lesions occur more frequently in females and are often bilateral. They tend to occur in a young population and may present with acute dissections, complete occlusions, or abnormal kinks as well as the classic beaded-vessel appearance.[16, 63] This subject is covered more fully in Chapter 51.

TRAUMATIC VASCULAR LESIONS

Sudden extension of the head or a direct blow to the neck can cause an intimal tear in the carotid or vertebral arteries, with subsequent formation of thrombotic emboli or complete occlusion. The initial event may be asymptomatic; however, with the formation of thrombus on the exposed medial surface, late sequelae may occur because of altered flow states associated with the retraction and curling up of the intima (Figs. 8–23 and 8–24).[65, 66] The vertebral arteries are also susceptible to injury from hyperextension and rotational strain.[67–71] Intimal disruption and dissection with secondary thrombosis may follow stretching of the vertebral arteries over cervical bony prominences. Chiropractic manipulation may cause brain-stem stroke,[69, 70, 72] and the posterior inferior cerebellar artery syndrome has been associated with neck traction following fracture of the cervical vertebrae.[73] Penetrating trauma of the carotid vessels may lead to death by hemorrhage, stroke, or airway compromise, but such injuries sometimes remain occult until weeks or months later, when intimal defects may produce temporary or permanent symptoms of cerebral ischemia.

CAROTID ARTERY DISSECTION

Spontaneous dissection of the carotid artery has become recognized more frequently with the increased use of angiog-

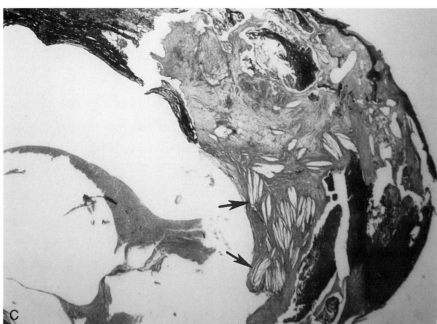

FIGURE 8-13 *Continued. C,* Modified elasto-chrome demonstrating the same lipid collection. *D,* Higher magnification view of another section, demonstrating cholesterol clefts. (From Bock RW, Lusby RJ: Carotid plaque morphology and interpretation of the echolucent lesion. In Labs KH, ed. *Diagnostic Vascular Ultrasound.* Kent, England: Edward Arnold, Ltd., 1992:256.)

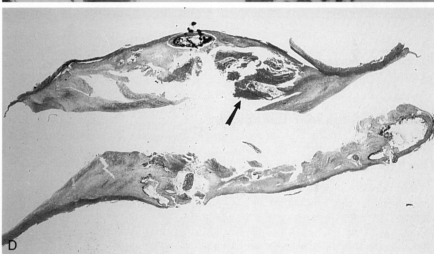

raphy[74–77] and magnetic resonance imaging[78] in the diagnosis of cerebral ischemia. Its clinical incidence has been estimated at 2.6 per 100,000 population.[79] Dissection generally occurs in the absence of atherosclerosis and follows an intimal tear. The dissection occurs in the outer layers of the media, causing stenosis of the lumen, which may progress to total occlusion or undergo spontaneous resolution.[76] The nonoperative treatment of these lesions has limited the availability of tissue for examination, but altered vessel wall structure with diminished smooth muscle fibers, degenerative internal elastic laminae, and increased ground substance have been found on microscopic examination.[80] Cystic medial necrosis, fibromuscular dysplasia, and carotid elongation and kinking have been associated with the disease.[62, 63] Symptoms of transient or permanent ischemia may occur, with emboli arising from thrombus formed at the entry site or as a result of thrombotic occlusion. The fact that resolution occurs in some patients with restoration of a normal-caliber vessel probably indicates a healing and repair response within the vessel wall, leading to closure of the false lumen (Fig. 8–25).

RADIATION-INDUCED INJURY

Exposure to radiation has long been linked with atherogenesis in patients who have a history of exposure and absence of other risk factors. Recent evidence confirms that radiation accelerates atherogenesis in humans.[81] Patients typically present with atherosclerotic lesions limited to that segment of the vessel exposed to irradiation.[82–84] There appears to be a time-related pattern of disease.[85] Within the first 5 years, the dominant pathology involves intimal damage with mural thrombus formation. During the subsequent 5-year period, fibrotic occlusions tend to occur. Elongated, stenotic, atheromatous lesions are common, and periarterial fibrosis may be severe. They often appear quite similar to spontaneously occurring atherosclerotic lesions, but their

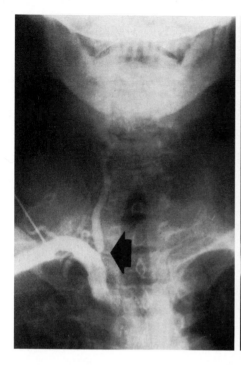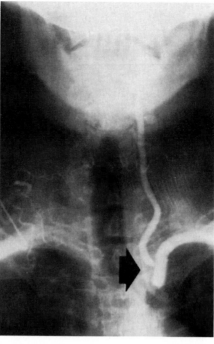

FIGURE 8-14. Angiogram showing bilateral tight stenotic lesions involving the origins of the vertebral arteries in a patient with vertebrobasilar insufficiency.

distribution is different, with many radiation-induced lesions occurring proximal to the bifurcation.[85]

EARLY THEORIES OF CEREBRAL ISCHEMIA

The Vasospastic Theory

Until the latter half of this century, transient and permanent ischemia was thought to be caused by vasospasm. Raynaud in 1862 postulated that transient loss of vision was the result of intermittent cerebral spasms, likening the phenomenon seen in the fingers to ischemic events in the brain.[86] Peabody in 1891[87] suggested spasmodic contraction of the muscular coat of the middle cerebral artery as a cause of transient ischemia and stroke. This explanation of the pathophysiology provided a rationale for the use of cervical sympathetic ganglionectomy and for treatment with vasodilators in an effort to overcome the angiospastic response.[88–90] Eastcott and associates[91] argued against this theory on the basis that selective involvement of just a few vessels was unlikely in the absence of any local stimulus. Millikan[92] pointed out that nitrous oxide studies of blood flow following stellate ganglion block showed no significant change in flow. Furthermore, he noted that stellate blockade did not influence attacks of intermittent carotid or vertebrobasilar insufficiency. The evidence against this theory was overwhelming by the early 1960s, and by then the hemodynamic mechanical flow reduction theory was taking shape.

The Flow-Reduction Theory

Despite the recognition early in this century by Chiari[93] and Hunt[94] that carotid artery stenosis was related to stroke, routine visualization of the neck vessels awaited development of angiography.[95] In 1951 Denny-Brown,[96] while questioning the vasospastic theory, put forward the suggestion that circulatory insufficiency due to carotid or basilar stenosis was related to defects in collateral circulation. Subsequently, Rothenberg and Corday[97] demonstrated experimentally that ligation of carotid arteries in monkeys resulted in electroencephalographic (EEG) changes and restoration to normal when the blood flow resumed. Although this theory of stenosis and flow reduction gained increasing acceptance, doubt persisted as to the precise nature of the development of symptoms. In 1956, Meyer and coworkers[98] used a tilt-table apparatus in an effort to induce symptoms. Patients with symptomatic carotid and basilar disease generally displayed EEG changes with tilting, but only 10 percent developed symptoms. The case for carotid artery stenosis was strengthened by the demonstration that surgery to remove the lesion resulted in reversal of symptoms. Although this theory dominated the approach to surgical therapy, several aspects failed to stand up to critical analysis.

Early in the development of the hemodynamic theory, it was noted that carotid ligation was not associated with increasing attacks of cerebral ischemia and could in fact result in the cessation of attacks. It was also difficult to reconcile the intermittent nature of ischemic attacks with the presence of constant stenosis. Adams and colleagues in 1963[99] studied cerebral blood flow in patients with carotid and vertebral artery stenosis; total cerebral blood flow prior to surgery was normal in these symptomatic patients, and endarterectomy did not result in any increase. Nonetheless, the incidence of ischemic attacks was sharply reduced. While an explanation for the inconsistencies could lie in intermittent attacks of systemic hypotension, in most patients with stenotic or occlusive disease this seemed unlikely. Kendall and Marshall[100] studied 37 patients with frequent ischemic attacks and were unable to reproduce those symptoms with the deliberate induction of systemic hypotension. Millikan[92] pointed out that many patients develop symptoms at rest, often while recumbent or sitting. Evidence from oculo-

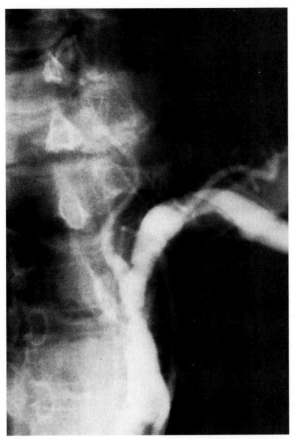

FIGURE 8–15. Angiogram of left subclavian artery showing a stenotic lesion proximal to the origin of the vertebral artery.

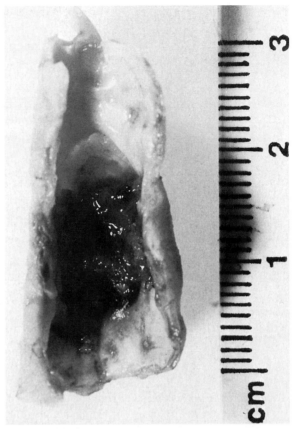

FIGURE 8–16. Plaque removed from subclavian artery stenosis (see Fig. 18–5). Fresh thrombus overlying an ulcerative hemorrhagic lesion was found. The patient suffered intermittent vertebrobasilar symptoms and emboli to his left index finger.

plethysmographic studies suggested that up to 84 percent of patients with high-grade lesions do not progress to stroke and that 60 percent do not have recurrent ischemic episodes.[101] Furthermore, transient cerebral symptoms generally disappear following occlusion of the vessel that supplies the relevant hemisphere. These factors led to further doubt regarding the role of stenosis alone in producing symptoms of transient ischemia.

The international randomized trial of extracranial-intra-

cranial arterial bypass has failed to confirm the hypothesis that increased blood flow is effective in preventing cerebral ischemia in patients with atherosclerotic disease in the carotid and middle cerebral arteries. The difficulty in distinguishing between cerebral ischemic events of hemodynamic origin resulting from poor circulatory perfusion and those events caused by arterial emboli was recognized in this study. Advocates of the bypass operation postulated that it

FIGURE 8–17. Angiogram of carotid bifurcation showing the increased radius (r) at the site of division. The disparity in segmental tangential tension associated with posterior wall plaque is illustrated. P, pressure; d, wall thickness; H, hemorrhage. (From Lusby RJ, Ferrell LD, Wylie EJ: The significance of intraplaque haemorrhage in the pathogenesis of carotid atherosclerosis. In Bergan, JJ, Yao ST, eds. *Cerebrovascular Insufficiency,* 2nd ed. New York: Grune & Stratton, 1983:41.)

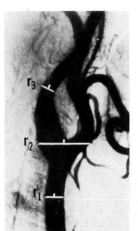

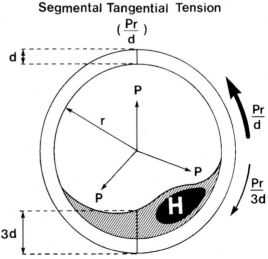

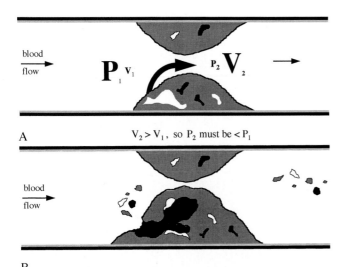

FIGURE 8-18. *A*, The Bernoulli principle applied to a complex carotid plaque. The product of pressure *(P)* and velocity *(V)* remains constant. Pressure decreases inside and distal to the stenosis as velocity increases. *B*, Unroofing forces across the plaque *(arrow)*, caused by the pressure differential across the plaque, have resulted in plaque fracture and intraplaque hemorrhage.

might benefit patients with ischemia from either cause by improving cerebral perfusion and providing additional collateral circulation or, in patients with ischemia of embolic origin, providing a sufficient increase in perfusion to promote early passage and disintegration of an embolus. The results indicated with strong statistical power that fatal and nonfatal strokes were not prevented by increasing cerebral perfusion with anastomosis of the superficial temporal artery to the middle cerebral artery.[102]

PATHOGENESIS OF CEREBRAL ISCHEMIA: CURRENT CONCEPTS

Overwhelming evidence now supports the central role of large-vessel embolism and thrombosis in the pathogenesis of both transient ischemia and stroke. Emboli from diseased but patent extracranial carotid arteries are the most common cause. Thrombosis and occlusion of the carotid arteries may also result in stroke, often via secondary, embolic phenomena rather than by reduction in blood flow to the affected hemisphere. Hemodynamic factors are important, but through an indirect mechanism: blood flow and collateral circulation determine what damage, if any, is caused by thromboembolic events in vessels supplying the brain.

The Thromboembolic Theory

The concept that an embolism of thrombus and other particles may cause cerebral ischemia is not new,[92, 103, 104] and a continuing accumulation of evidence supports the notion that degenerative events at the carotid artery bifurcation are closely related to the onset of symptoms.[22, 32–34] Hollenhorst first described the presence of plaques in the retinal arteries of patients with transient blindness.[104] The plaques were composed of birefringent cholesterol crystals,

which clearly had embolized from a more proximal vessel. Following the appearance of symptoms and initial detection, some of these emboli disappeared, whereas others remained stationary or moved more distally, occasionally leading to arterial occlusion. Evidence for embolization of platelet thrombi to the retinal vessels came from clinical observations of Russel[105] and pathologic studies of McBrien and colleagues.[106] The latter workers performed histologic examinations on the retinal vessels of a patient who had episodic transient monocular blindness; emboli were found consisting of platelets, leukocytes, and small quantities of lipid material. Ehrenfeld and associates[107] recognized that these emboli originated in the carotid artery. These investigators showed that the intermittent monocular blindness and episodes of cerebral ischemia ceased on removal of the ulcerated carotid lesions.

Events in the retinal vessels, although difficult to document because of the timing of events and availability of equipment, provided irrefutable evidence of cerebrovascular embolism and its relationship to ischemic symptoms. Evidence linking cerebral ischemic events to the development of ulceration in the carotid vessels awaited the development of CT scanning. Eastcott and associates[91] demonstrated macroscopic carotid plaque ulceration in 72 percent of patients with TIAs, of whom 88 percent had ipsilateral cerebral infarcts on CT scanning. In contrast to these findings, carotid plaque ulceration and CT evidence of brain infarcts were

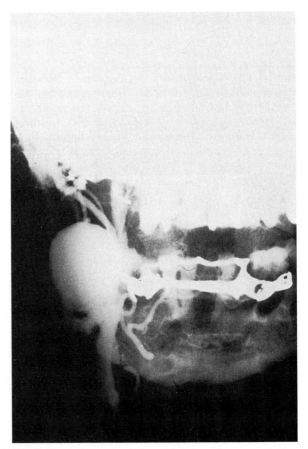

FIGURE 8-19. Angiogram showing an aneurysm of the extracranial internal carotid artery.

infrequent in asymptomatic patients in their study (Figs. 8–26 through 8–28). Other studies have confirmed a close correlation between carotid plaque ulceration, ischemic symptoms, and CT evidence of cerebral infarction.[34]

Emboli may consist of loosely aggregated or tightly bound platelets, thrombotic particles, cholesterol crystals, semiliquid lipids, breakdown products of intraplaque hemorrhages, or atherosclerotic plaque itself, including calcific and even bony material. It is understandable that a wide range of clinical outcomes may follow embolism of these varied materials to cerebral vessels of varying size and collateral supply. Relief of symptoms after embolism may follow (1) the dissolution of platelet emboli by lytic action, (2) fragmentation of emboli at a downstream bifurcation, with particles traveling to more distal branches and disappearing or no longer obstructing flow, or (3) the effective rerouting of blood through collateral channels, rendering the embolus clinically insignificant (Fig. 8–29).[92]

The carotid bifurcation plaque appears to be the most important source of embolism associated with monocular and hemisphere ischemic symptoms, even in the absence of tight or critical stenosis. Several studies have shown that fewer than half of patients with documented hemisphere and monocular ischemic attacks have hemodynamically significant lesions.[21, 30, 51, 108–110] Ulceration of the luminal surface is a common finding in these lesions, either alone or in conjunction with intraplaque hemorrhage (Figs. 8–30 and 8–5C). Luminal ulceration can give rise to a variety of

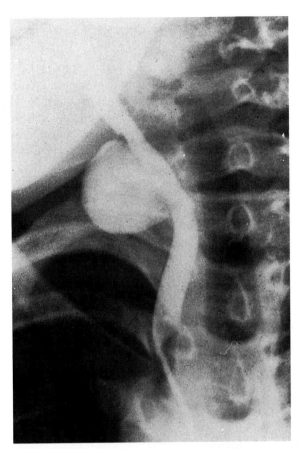

FIGURE 8–21. False aneurysm of common carotid artery. This 12-year-old patient had previously undergone resection and patch of a true aneurysm of the carotid artery associated with a collagen deficiency of the vessels.

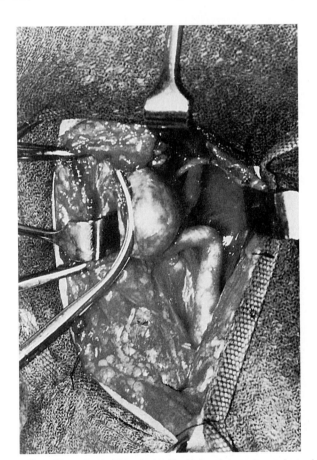

FIGURE 8–20. Operative photograph displaying the aneurysm shown in Figure 8–19. Note the elongation and kinking of the internal carotid artery associated with this lesion.

emboli, including the fibrous cap dislodged from the surface of the plaque, luminal thrombus formed over the ulcerated surface, platelet emboli loosely attached to the luminal surface over an ulcer, subintimal contents of a plaque including the breakdown products of an intraplaque hemorrhage, cholesterol crystals, and fibrous, calcific, and bony fragments (Fig. 8–31). Larger clumps of degenerative plaque may be less inclined to disaggregate and thus cause permanent occlusion of cerebral vessels, resulting in stroke (Figs. 8–32 and 8–12). Clinicopathologic correlations have shown that patients recovering from stroke have a higher incidence of plaque ulceration than patients with transient ischemic symptoms,[111] suggesting that embolization of plaque fragments may be more likely to produce permanent symptoms. Finally, plaque degeneration may be followed by healing rather than progression to stroke; this repair process is associated with additional formation of collagen and with focal calcification (see Fig. 8–11).

Intraplaque hemorrhage is the most common pathologic finding seen in symptomatic patients, and it is closely linked to embolic cerebral ischemic events. It is not always associated with macroscopic ulceration,[21, 33] but it may nonetheless cause embolism. Luminal thrombus formation can occur over the surface of an intraplaque hemorrhage and may be a source of platelet and thrombotic emboli (Figs. 8–33 and 8–34).[21] Acute intraplaque hemorrhage may cause minute intimal disruption or splaying of endothelial cells, exposing underlying collagen; platelet adhesion and thrombus forma-

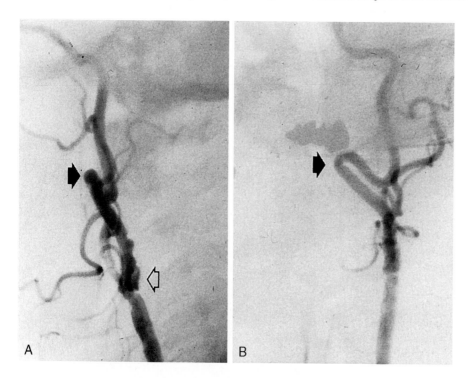

FIGURE 8–22. *A* and *B,* Angiogram in two planes demonstrating an elongated internal carotid artery with an associated kink *(dark arrow).* A coincidental atheromatous plaque is seen at the carotid bifurcation *(light arrow).*

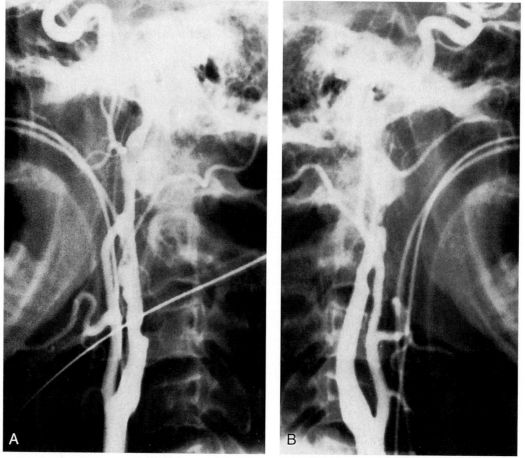

FIGURE 8–23. *A* and *B,* Bilateral intimal tears with local dissection and thrombus deposition found post mortem in this patient, who suffered a hyperextension injury in a high-speed vehicular accident.

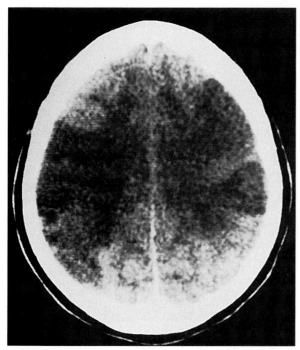

FIGURE 8–24. Premortem computed tomographic scan of the patient with bilateral cerebral infarction shown in Figure 8–23. Cerebral symptoms related to embolic occlusion of intracerebral vessels in the presence of patent though narrowed internal carotid arteries developed 12 hours after admission.

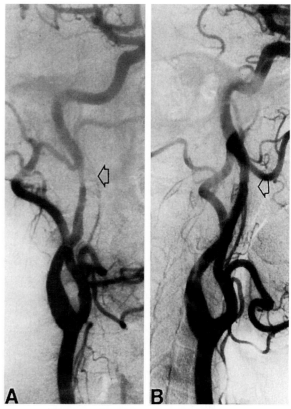

FIGURE 8–25. *A,* Angiogram showing stenosis associated with an acute dissection of the internal carotid artery *(arrow). B,* The artery has undergone spontaneous repair with resolution of the stenosis.

tion may then follow. Another site for platelet deposition is within the fully endothelialized pit formed by an ulcer (Fig. 8–35).

It is postulated that platelet emboli arising from these lesions, in which the lumen is essentially intact, are most likely to produce the fleeting ischemic attack; the pure platelet emboli undergo rapid dissolution with corresponding resolution of symptoms.[51] Platelet emboli arising in such circumstances would appear most likely to respond to aspirin therapy for control of transient ischemic attacks.[112] The failure of aspirin to prevent major strokes in many instances

may be due to its inability to prevent embolization resulting from plaque degeneration, intraplaque hemorrhage, and acute plaque fracture.[51]

Mechanisms of Ischemic Stroke

It seems clear that stroke does not occur as a result of slow, steady, predictable growth of smooth, homogeneous

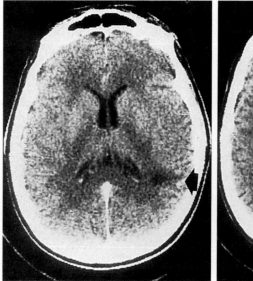
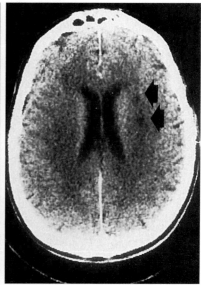

FIGURE 8–26. Computed tomographic scan showing multiple small infarcts obtained from a patient experiencing transient ischemic attacks.

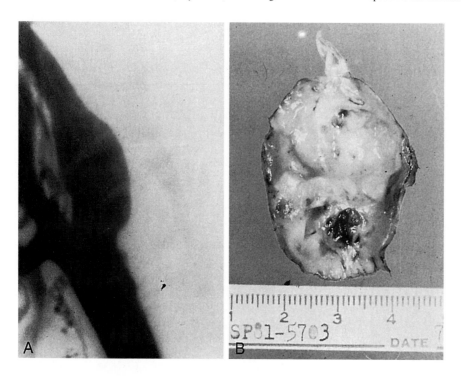

FIGURE 8–27. Angiogram *(A)* and operative specimen *(B)* obtained from the patient shown in Figure 8–26. A small ulcer is seen at the base of the plaque.

plaque. Clinically significant carotid lesions do not grow like rings on a tree (Fig. 8–36). Thromboembolic stroke is unpredictable and sudden, and it occurs in conjunction with intraplaque hemorrhage, plaque degeneration, ulceration, fracture, rupture, and other abrupt changes in plaque morphology. It is theorized that these pathologic processes cause cerebral ischemia by at least four distinct mechanisms.

Large Artery Embolism. The most common pathway for development of ischemic stroke is via embolism from the large, extracranial arteries, generally the carotid bifurcation. Embolization occurs via the processes described earlier, and embolic fragments enter the bloodstream, are carried distally, and lodge in intracerebral vessels downstream. Depending on the size of the embolus, this may occur in the intracranial internal carotid artery, the middle or anterior cerebral arteries, or in their more distal branches downstream. Collateral flow around these arteries is commonly inadequate to protect against cerebral ischemia and cell death, and a cerebral infarction results in the corresponding vascular territory served by the occluded vessel. The collateral blood supply and the location of the embolus determine the size of the infarct. Disaggregation of the embolus may follow soon after the acute event. If this occurs before cell death, a transient ischemic attack results; otherwise ischemic stroke ensues.

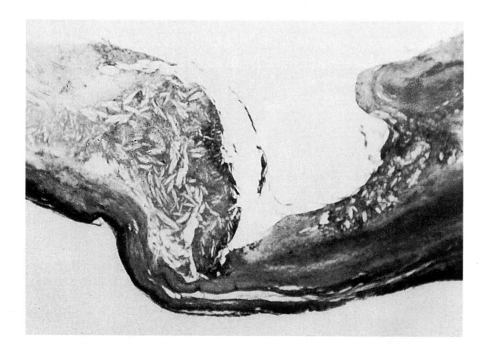

FIGURE 8–28. Photomicrograph of the ulcer displayed in Figure 8–27 showing cholesterol crystals and atheromatous debris in the ulcer cavity.

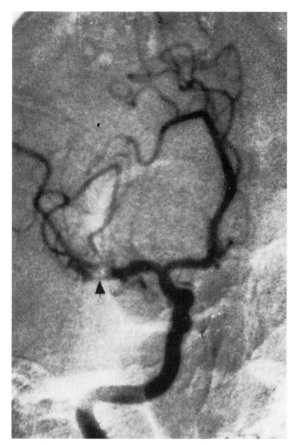

FIGURE 8–29. Embolus lodged in the middle cerebral artery *(arrow).*

Most ischemic strokes occur in the absence of acute carotid occlusion, and most occur in association with only moderate hemodynamic compromise. Diagnostic investigations performed following a stroke occurring in this setting often fail to demonstrate "critical" carotid stenosis. Ulceration may elude noninvasive and angiographic diagnosis. Intracranial angiography may or may not demonstrate a filling defect in an intracranial vessel. Usually the patient is left with a patent, moderately diseased carotid artery, no other obvious source of embolus, and a classic ischemic stroke.

Large Artery Occlusion and Pure "Hemodynamic" Stroke. Less commonly, acute changes in plaque structure (general plaque fracture or intraplaque hemorrhage or both) will cause sudden occlusion of the carotid artery. Flow to the ipsilateral hemisphere is thus compromised in the absence of embolism. In this scenario, the fate of brain tissue downstream rests with the collateral circulation. Many patients with adequate collateral circulation (either from the contralateral hemisphere, the ipsilateral posterior circulation, smaller collateral routes, or some combination) suffer either transient ischemia or no symptoms at all, but some develop acute stroke. Because total and regional cerebral blood flow is usually preserved after simple carotid occlusion, because many patients are found with old occlusions and no clinical history or findings of stroke, and because most strokes occur in the absence of extracranial arterial occlusion, this mechanism is thought to be less common than embolic stroke.

Occlusion with Clot Propagation and Secondary Embolization. Carotid artery occlusion can cause stroke via another mechanism: secondary embolization. In this scenario, occlusion is followed by clot propagation distally along the internal carotid artery. When the propagating thrombus reaches the first branch able to provide enough retrograde flow to keep the vessel open (usually the ophthalmic artery), further extension of the clot ceases. However, the fresh, fragile tail of the thrombus (see Fig. 8–33*B*) remains in an open flow channel and remains a nidus for further clot formation. Secondary, vessel-to-vessel embolization of the tip of this fresh clot can then occur with devastating results downstream: the involved brain tissue is already at risk because

FIGURE 8–30. *A,* Digital subtraction angiogram of the carotid artery showing an ulcerative lesion in the bulbous origin of the internal carotid artery. *B,* The operative specimen shows the central defect in the plaque.

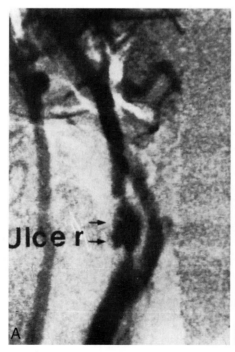

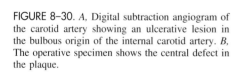

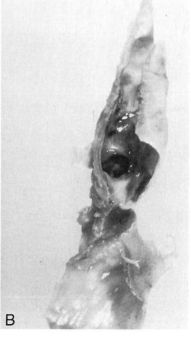

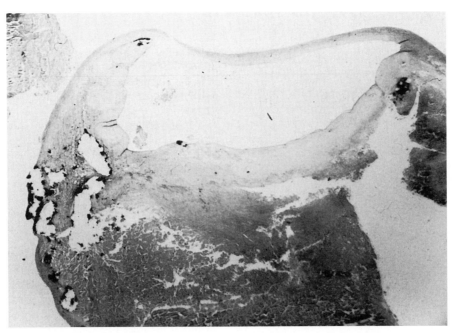

FIGURE 8–31. Cross section of carotid artery with small residual lumen. Focal calcification has developed at the edge of a large intraplaque hemorrhage. The contents of this complex plaque are potential emboli.

of compromised flow, and collateral, compensatory mechanisms are already maximized. Stroke, often extensive, follows this secondary embolic process. This mechanism may explain why patients with carotid occlusion and only minimal initial symptoms remain at risk for ipsilateral stroke long after the occlusive event, why aspirin and coumarin may sometimes prevent stroke after carotid occlusion, and why devastating stroke may follow carotid occlusion even in patients with an open circle of Willis and good collateral flow.

PREDICTION OF STROKE

There are no reliable clinical predictors of stroke. Bruits correlate poorly with outcome, and only 10 to 15 percent of strokes are preceded by TIA.[113] Angiography, the first diagnostic modality employed in evaluating the cerebral vasculature, is invasive and relatively risky: data from a recent randomized prospective multicenter study have shown that the angiographic stroke rate is 1.2 percent.[114] Although it provides acceptable evaluation of percentage stenosis, two-plane angiography can still significantly underestimate stenotic lesions. Angiography provides almost no information regarding other characteristics of atherosclerotic lesions; it is largely useless in the diagnosis of intraplaque hemorrhage and lipid sequestration. Retrospective studies have shown that angiography is also unreliable in the diagnosis of plaque ulceration,[115] and the prospective NASCET trial confirmed little agreement between gross and angiographic diagnoses of ulcers.[116] Often, angiograms that are purported to show

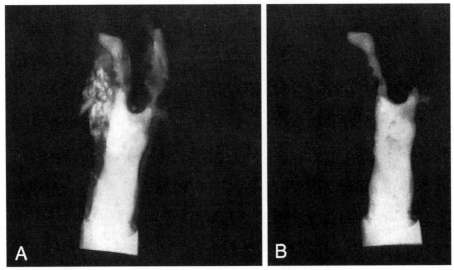

FIGURE 8–32. Radiograph of carotid artery with opaque cast of lumen. A large calcified lesion at the origin of the internal carotid artery is shown *(A)*, not present when the cast alone is radiographed *(B)*.

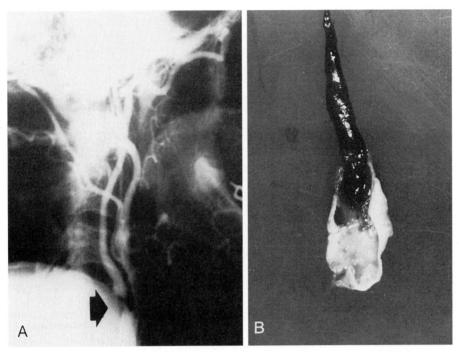

FIGURE 8–33. *A,* Angiogram showing high-grade stenosis that had progressed to total occlusion by the time of operation *(arrow). B,* Specimen shows thrombotic occlusion developing over site of recent intraplaque hemorrhage.

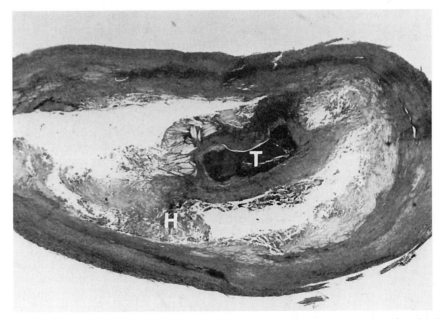

FIGURE 8–34. Cross section of carotid artery with occlusion of the residual lumen *(T)* secondary to extensive circumferential plaque formation and recent intraplaque hemorrhage *(H).*

ulceration may in fact demonstrate two foci of intraplaque hemorrhage with intervening uninvolved plaque.[117]

Carotid arteriography may be flawed in another more fundamental way: its use in determining the degree of stenosis may be clinically irrelevant. Critical analysis of the literature demonstrates that the oft-cited link between increasing degrees of stenosis and clinical stroke is tenuous at best, particularly when the analysis excludes "100% stenotic" (occluded) vessels. These vessels, commonly included in the literature on carotid stenosis, are inoperable and are physiologically completely different from high-grade stenoses.[30] Recent data from the randomized prospective ACAS report[114] confirm this assertion: absolutely no tendency toward increasing stroke rates was seen with increasing levels of stenosis between 90 and 99 per cent in an asymptomatic population. Percentage of stenosis, it seems, may simply be an overexact determination of the presence or absence of a significant carotid plaque burden.

The Doppler function of duplex ultrasonography is frequently used in an effort to identify individuals at risk for stroke. Doppler information regarding flow velocity through the carotid bifurcation is extrapolated to provide an estimation of the degree of stenosis. When interpretation is restricted to broad categories of stenosis, these data are fairly reproducible. Unfortunately, up to 93 percent of strokes in asymptomatic individuals occur in the absence of pre-existing critical (> 80%) stenosis.[30] High-grade stenosis is clearly a risk factor for cerebral ischemia, but epidemiologically, such lesions cause the minority of ischemic strokes.

B-mode ultrasonography is an excellent tool for the diagnosis of intraplaque hemorrhage and lipid sequestration. Ultrasonographic studies of symptomatic patients may demonstrate predominantly echolucent areas, which correlate with the pathologic finding of intraplaque hemorrhage.[22, 118, 119] These lesions correlate with the development of symptoms at least as well as measurement of the degree of stenosis.[118, 120-123] The few cases of false-positive diagnosis of intraplaque hemorrhage are generally associated with lipid collections.[118] Since both intraplaque hemorrhage and lipid collections are associated with symptoms of cerebral ischemia, it may be argued that the ultrasonographic diagnosis of echolucency is more important than the pathologic differentiation between hemorrhage and lipid within the plaque. Such a change in reporting and interpretation would lead to even better accuracy of B-mode ultrasonography as well as enhanced clinical relevance.

Unfortunately, ultrasonography is ineffective in the diagnosis of plaque ulceration,[121, 124] although one study suggests that ultrasonographic (as well as angiographic) detection of plaque ulceration improves somewhat at lesser degrees of stenosis.[125] Another recent report of computer-assisted assessment of three-dimensional plaque ultrastructure shows more promise in the search for an ideal diagnostic and predictive modality.[126]

The use of each of these modalities in an effort to predict stroke implies one assumption: that the plaque will harbor some identifiable characteristic that will correlate with the occurrence of future stroke. Unfortunately, almost all available data concerning characteristics of cerebrovascular atherosclerotic lesions involve the retrospective correlation between ischemia and lesion appearance or percentage stenosis observed *after* the ischemic event. It may be that plaques destined to produce stroke harbor absolutely no definable characteristic until the moment that plaque fracture, intraplaque hemorrhage, acute occlusion, or other complication occurs, or that such characteristics (eg, moderate degree of stenosis) are so common that little useful predictive value exists.

One new means of predicting stroke involves the measurement of cerebral vasoregulatory reserve. Normal subjects exhibit cerebrovascular autoregulation over a wide range of variation in flow. Several tests employ the measurement of cerebral flow, either by transcranial Doppler[127] or xenon-enhanced computed tomography.[128, 129] Baseline flow studies are compared with results obtained after the production of cerebral vasodilation with either inspired carbon dioxide or acetazolamide. Patients with impaired collateral reserve are identified by a drop in cerebral blood flow; by retrospective analysis they are at increased risk for subsequent stroke. These data are compatible with the thromboembolic theory of cerebral ischemia, as the collateral circulation appears important in determining the clinical effect of embolic events.

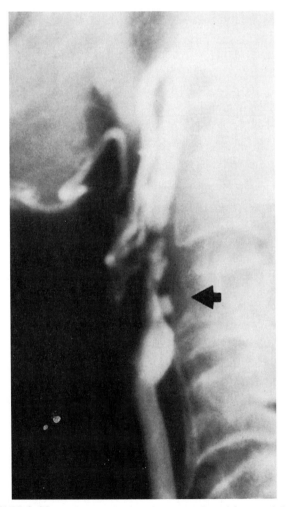

FIGURE 8–35. Angiogram showing pit *(arrow)* formed by re-endothelialized ulcer. This is a potential site at which platelet emboli might form.

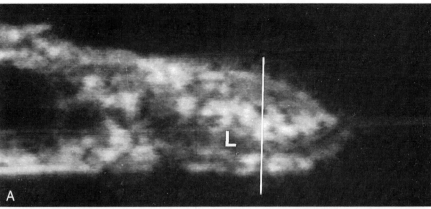

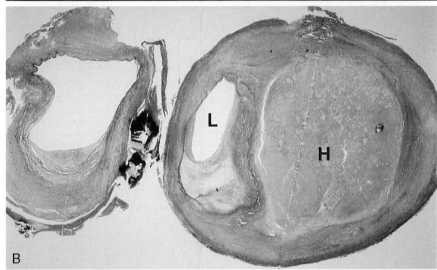

FIGURE 8–36. Ultrasonographic image *(A)* and gross specimen *(B)* of a highly stenotic plaque of the carotid bifurcation. The external carotid artery is relatively free of disease. The *white line* on part *A* marks the level of the transverse section taken through the specimen. Note the intraplaque hemorrhage *(H)*, the development of which has almost certainly caused abrupt, marked change in the residual lumen *(L)*.

REFERENCES

1. Fisher M: Transient monocular blindness associated with hemiplegia. *Arch Ophthalmol.* 1952;47:167.
2. Fisher M: Occlusion of the carotid arteries: Further experience. *Arch Neurol Psychol.* 1954;72:187.
3. Hutchinson EC, Yates PO: Carotid-vertebral stenosis. *Lancet.* 1957;2:722.
4. Whisnant JP, Fitzgibbon JP, Kurland LT, et al: Natural history of stroke in Rochester, Minnesota, 1945 through 1954. *Stroke.* 1971;2:11.
5. Kannel MB, Wolf PA, Verter JL, et al: Epidemiologic assessment of the role of blood pressure and stroke: The Framingham Study. *JAMA.* 1970;214:301.
6. Adams JH: Patterns of cerebral infarction. *Scott Med J.* 1967;12:335.
7. Adams RD: Mechanisms of apoplexy as determined by clinical and pathological correlation. *J Neuropathol Exp Neurol.* 1954;13:1.
8. Fisher CM, Adams RD: Observations on brain embolism with special reference to the mechanisms of hemorrhagic infarcts. *J Neuropathol Exp Neurol.* 1951;10:92.
9. Millder D, Adams JH: Pathophysiology and management of increased intracranial pressure. In Critchley M, O'Leary JL, Jennett B, eds. *Scientific Foundations of Neurology.* London: William Heineman; 1972.
10. Fisher CM: The arterial lesions underlying lacunes. *Acta Neuropathol (Berl).* 1969;12:1.
11. Mohr JP: Lacunes. *Stroke.* 1982;13:3.
12. Fisher CM: Capsular infarcts. *Arch Neurol.* 1979;36:65.
13. Futrell N, Watson B, Dietrich W, et al: A new model of embolic stroke produced by photochemical injury to the carotid artery of the rat. *Ann Neurol.* 1988;23:251.
14. Horowitz DR, Tuhrim S, Weinberger JM, Rudolph SH: Mechanisms in lacunar infarction. *Stroke.* 1992;23:325.
15. Cacciatore A, Russo L, Jr.: Lacunar infarction as an embolic complication of cardiac and arch angiography. *Stroke.* 1991;22:1603. See comments.
16. Millikan C, Futrell N: The fallacy of the lacune hypothesis. *Stroke.* 1990;21:1251. See comments.
17. Flory CM: Arterial occlusions produced by emboli from eroded aortic atheromatous plaques. *Am J Pathol.* 1945;21:549.
18. Marchand F: Über Arteriosclerose. *Verh Dtsch K Inn Med.* 1904;21:23.
19. Masawa N, Glagov S, Zarins CK: Quantitative morphologic study of intimal thickening at the human carotid bifurcation: I. Axial and circumferential distribution of maximum intimal thickening in asymptomatic, uncomplicated plaques. *Atherosclerosis.* 1994;107:137.
20. Ross R, Glomset JA: The pathogenesis of atherosclerosis. *N Engl J Med.* 1976;295:369.
21. Lusby RJ, Ferrell LD, Ehrenfeld WK, et al: Carotid plaque hemorrhage: Its role in the production of cerebral ischaemia. *Arch Surg.* 1982;117:1479.
22. O'Donnell TF, Erdoes L, Mackey WC, et al: Correlation of B-mode ultrasound imaging and arteriography with pathological findings at carotid endarterectomy. *Arch Surg.* 1984;120:443.
23. Avril G, Batt M, Guidoin R, et al.: Carotid endarterectomy plaques: Correlations of clinical and anatomic findings. *Ann Vasc Surg.* 1991;5:50.
24. Moore WS, Boren C, Malone JM, et al.: Natural history of nonstenotic, asymptomatic ulcerative lesions of the carotid artery. *Arch Surg.* 1978;113:1352.
25. Van Damme H, Vivario M: Pathologic aspects of carotid plaques: Surgical and clinical significance. *Int Angiol.* 1993;12:299.
26. Seeger JM, Barratt E, Lawson GA, Klingman N: The relationship between carotid plaque composition, plaque morphology, and neurologic symptoms. *J Surg Res.* 1995;58:330.
27. Dixon S, Pais SO, Raviola C, et al: Natural history of nonstenotic, asymptomatic ulcerative lesions of the carotid artery: A further analysis. *Arch Surg.* 1982;117:1493.
28. Eliasziw M, Streifler JY, Fox AJ, et al: Significance of plaque ulceration in symptomatic patients with high-grade carotid stenosis: North American Symptomatic Carotid Endarterectomy Trial. *Stroke.* 1994;25:304.
29. Virchow R: Phlogose und Thrombose im Gefässsystem. In *Gesammelte Abhandlungen zur Wissenschlaftlichen Medizin.* Frankfurt: Meidinger Sohn; 1856.
30. Bock RW, Gray-Weale AC, Mock PA, et al: The natural history of asymptomatic carotid artery disease. *J Vasc Surg.* 1993;17:160; Discussion, 170.
31. Imparato AM, Riles TS, Mintzer R, et al: The importance of haemorrhage in the relationship between gross morphologic characteristics and cerebral symptoms in 376 carotid artery plaques. *Ann Surg.* 1983;197:197.
32. Persson AV, Robichaux WT, Silverman M: The natural history of the significant events in carotid plaque developments. *Arch Surg.* 1983;118:1948.
33. Edwards JH, Kricheff I, Gorstein F, et al: Atherosclerotic subintimal haematoma of the carotid artery. *Radiology.* 1979;133:123.
34. Zukowski AJ, Nicolaides AN, Lewis RT, et al: The correlation between carotid plaque ulceration and cerebral infarction on CT scan. *J Vasc Surg.* 1984;1:782.

35. Beach KW, Hatsukami T, Detmer PR, et al: Carotid artery intraplaque hemorrhage and stenotic velocity. *Stroke.* 1993;24:314.

36. Sterpetti AV, Hunter WJ, Schultz RD: Importance of ulceration of carotid plaque in determining symptoms of cerebral ischemia. *J Cardiovasc Surg.* 1991;32:154.

37. Leahy AL, McCollum PT, Feeley TM, et al: Duplex ultrasonography and selection of patients for carotid endarterectomy: Plaque morphology or luminal narrowing? *J Vasc Surg.* 1988;8:558.

38. Hutchinson EC, Yates PO: The cervical portion of the vertebral artery: A clinico-pathological study. *Brain.* 1956;79:319.

39. Fisher CM, Gore I, Okabe N, et al: Atherosclerosis of the carotid and vertebral arteries: Extracranial and intracranial. *J Neuropathol Exp Neurol.* 1965;24:455.

40. Imparato AM, Lin JPT: Vertebral arterial reconstruction internal plication and vein patch angioplasty. *Ann Surg.* 1967;166:213.

41. Blaisdell FW, Hall AD, Thomas AN, et al: Cerebrovascular occlusive disease: Experience with panarteriography in 300 consecutive cases. *Cal Med.* 1965;103:321.

42. Hass WK, et al: Joint study of extracranial arterial occlusion. II. Arteriography techniques sites and complications. *JAMA.* 1968;203:961.

43. Caro CG, Fitzgerald JM, Schroter RC: Atheroma and arterial wall shear: Observation, correlation and proposal of a shear dependent mass transfer mechanism for atherosclerosis. *Proc R Soc Lond B Biol Sci.* 1971;117:109.

44. Bharadvaj BK, Mabon RF, Giddens DP: Steady flow in a model of the human carotid bifurcation. Part I. Flow visualization. *J Biomech.* 1982;15:349.

45. Nazemi M, Kleinstreuer C, Archie J, Jr: Pulsatile two-dimensional flow and plaque formation in a carotid artery bifurcation. *J Biomech.* 1990;23:1031.

46. Zarins CK, Giddens DP, Bharadvaj BK, et al: Carotid bifurcation atherosclerosis. Quantitative correlation of plaque localization with flow velocity profiles and wall shear stress. *Circ Res.* 1983;53:502.

47. Beere PA, Glagov S, Zarins CK: Experimental atherosclerosis at the carotid bifurcation of the cynomolgus monkey. Localization, compensatory enlargement, and the sparing effect of lowered heart rate. *Arterioscler Thromb.* 1992;12:1245.

48. Anayiotos AS, Jones SA, Giddens DP, Glagov S, Zarins CK: Shear stress at a compliant model of the human carotid bifurcation. *J Biomech Eng.* 1994;116:98.

49. Heath D, Smith P, Harris P, et al: The atherosclerotic human carotid sinus. *J Pathol.* 1973;110:49.

50. Lusby RJ, Woodcock JP, Machleder HI, et al: Transient ischaemic attacks. The static and dynamic morphology of the carotid bifurcation. *Br J Surg.* 1982;69(Suppl):S41.

51. Lusby RJ, Ferrell LD, Wylie EJ: The significance of intraplaque haemorrhage in the pathogenesis of carotid atherosclerosis. In Bergan JJ, Yao ST, eds. *Cerebrovascular Insufficiency.* New York: Grune & Stratton; 1983:41.

52. Gonza ER, Mason WF, Marble AE, et al: Necessity for elastic properties in synthetic arterial grafts. *Can J Surg.* 1974;17:1.

53. McDonald DA: *Blood Flow in Arteries,* 2nd ed. Baltimore; Williams & Wilkins; 1974.

54. Bougner DR, Roach MR: Effect of low frequency vibration on arterial wall. *Circ Res.* 1973;29:136.

55. Gersten JW: Relation of ultrasound effects to orientation of tendon in ultrasound field. *Arch Phys Med Rehabil.* 1956;37:201.

56. Trippel OH, Haid SP, Kornmesser TW, et al: Extracranial carotid aneurysms. In Bergan J, Yao JS, eds. Aneurysm: Diagnosis and Treatment. New York: Grune & Stratton; 1982:493.

57. Branch C Jr, Davis C Jr: False aneurysm complicating carotid endarterectomy. *Neurosurgery.* 1986;19:421.

58. Weber RC, Barker WF: Aneurysms of the extracranial internal carotid artery. *Arch Surg.* 1969;99:501.

59. Moore WS: Pathology in extracranial cerebrovascular disease. In Rutherford RB, ed. *Vascular Surgery.* Philadelphia: WB Saunders; 1977:1057.

60. Poindexter J Jr, Patel KR, Clauss RH: Management of kinked extracranial cerebral arteries. *J Vasc Surg.* 1987;6:127.

61. Koskas F, Bahnini A, Walden R, Kieffer E: Stenotic coiling and kinking of the internal carotid artery. *Ann Vasc Surg.* 1993;7:530.

62. Barbour PJ, Castaldo JE, Rae-Grant AD, et al: Internal carotid artery redundancy is significantly associated with dissection. *Stroke.* 1994;25:1201.

63. Pozzati E, Giuliani G, Acciarri N, Nuzzo G: Long-term follow-up of occlusive cervical carotid dissection. *Stroke.* 1990;21:528.

64. Palubinskas AJ, Ripley HR: Fibromuscular hyperplasia in extrarenal arteries. *Radiology.* 1964;82:451.

65. Clarke PR, Dickson J, Smith BJ: Traumatic thrombosis of the internal carotid artery following a nonpenetrating injury and leading to infarction of the brain. *Br J Surg.* 1955;43:215.

66. Kauffman HH, Lind TA, Clark DS: Nonpenetrating trauma to the carotid artery with secondary thrombosis and embolism treatment by thrombolysin. *Acta Neurochir.* 1977;37:219.

67. Carpenter S: Injury of neck as cause of vertebral artery thrombosis. *J Neurosurg.* 1961;18:849.

68. Simeone FA, Goldberg HI: Thrombosis of the vertebral artery from hyperextension injury of the neck. *J Neurosurg.* 1968;29:540.

69. Sherman DG, Hart RG, Easton JD: Abrupt change in head position and cerebral infarction. *Stroke.* 1981;12:2.

70. Kruger BR, Okazaki H: Vertebral-basilar distribution infarction following chiropractic cervical manipulation. *Mayo Clin Proc.* 1980;55:322.

71. Toole JF, Tucker SH: Influence of head position upon cerebral circulation. Studies on blood flow in cadavers. *Arch Neurol.* 1960;2:616.

72. Hamann GF, Felber S, Schimrigk K: Cervicocephalic artery dissections and chiropractic manipulations. *Lancet.* 1993;342:114. Letter.

73. Suechting RL, French LA: Posterior inferior cerebellar artery syndrome following a fracture of the cervical vertebrae. *J Neurosurg.* 1955;12:187.

74. Anderson R, Schechter M: A case of spontaneous dissecting aneurysm of the internal carotid artery. *J Neurol Neurosurg Psychiatry.* 1959;22:195.

75. Brice JG, Cromptom MR: Spontaneous dissecting aneurysms of the cervical internal carotid artery. *Br Med J.* 1964;27:90.

76. Ehrenfeld WK, Wylie EJ: Spontaneous dissection of the internal carotid artery. *Arch Surg.* 1976;111:1294.

77. Gee W, Kaupp HA, McDonald KM, et al: Spontaneous dissection of internal carotid arteries: Spontaneous resolution documented by serial ocular pneumoplethysmography and angiography. *Arch Surg.* 1980;115:944.

78. Ast G, Woimant F, Georges B, et al: Spontaneous dissection of the internal carotid artery in 68 patients. *Eur J Med.* 1993;2:466.

79. Schievink WI, Mokri B, Whisnant JP: Internal carotid artery dissection in a community. Rochester, Minnesota, 1987–1992. *Stroke.* 1993;24:1678.

80. Roome NS Jr, Aberfeld DC: Spontaneous dissecting aneurysm of the internal carotid artery. *Arch Neurol.* 1977;34:251.

81. Feehs RS, McGuirt WF, Bond MG, et al: Irradiation: A significant risk factor for carotid atherosclerosis. *Arch Otolaryngol Head Neck Surg.* 1991;117:1135.

82. Silverberg GD, Britt RH, Goffinet DR: Radiation induced carotid artery disease. *Cancer.* 1978;41:130.

83. Glick B: Bilateral carotid occlusive disease following irradiation for carcinoma of the vocal cords. *Arch Pathol Lab Med.* 1972;93:352.

84. McCready RA, Hyde GL, Bivins BA, et al: Radiation induced arterial injuries. *Surgery.* 1983;93:306.

85. Butler MJ, Lane RHS, Webster JHH: Irradiation injury to large arteries. *Br J Surg.* 1980;67:341.

86. Raynaud A (1862). Quoted by Loeb C: Protracted transient ischemic attacks. *Eur Neurol* 1980;19:1.

87. Peabody GL: Relations between arterial disease and visceral changes. *Trans Am Physicians.* 1891;6:154.

88. Risteen WA, Volpitto PP: Role of stellate ganglion block in certain neurologic disorders. *South Med J.* 1946;39:431.

89. Gilbert NC, DeTakats C: Emergency treatment of apoplexy. *JAMA.* 1948;136:659.

90. Johnson HC, Walker AE: The angiographic diagnosis of spontaneous thrombosis of internal and common carotid arteries. *J Neurosurg.* 1951;8:631.

91. Eastcott HHG, Pickering GR, Rob CG: Reconstruction of internal carotid artery in a patient with intermittent attacks of hemiplegia. *Lancet.* 1954;2:994.

92. Millikan CH: The pathogenesis of transient focal cerebral ischaemia. *Circulation.* 1965;32:438.

93. Chiari H: Über das Verhalten des Teilungs Winkels der Carotis Communis bei der endarterutig Chronica Deformans. *Verh Dtsch Ges Pathol.* 1905;9:326.

94. Hunt JR: The role of the carotid arteries in the causation of vascular lesions of the brain with certain features of symptomatology. *Am J Med Sci.* 1914;147:704.

95. Moniz E, Lima A, del'Acerda R: Hemiplegies par thrombose de la carotide interne. *Presse Med.* 1937;45:977.

96. Denny-Brown D: Symposium on specific methods of treatment: Treatment of recurrent cerebrovascular symptoms and the question of vasospasm. *Med Clin North Am.* 1951;35:1457.

97. Rothenberg SF, Corday E: Etiology of transient cerebral stroke. *JAMA.* 1957;164:2005.

98. Meyer JS, Leiderman H, Denny-Brown D: Electroencephalographic study of insufficiency of the basilar and carotid arteries in man. *Neurology.* 1956;6:455.

99. Adams JE, Smith MC, Wylie EJ: Cerebral blood flow and hemodynamics in extracranial vascular disease: Effect of endarterectomy. *Surgery.* 1963;53:449.

100. Kendall RE, Marshall J: Role of hypertension in the genesis of transient focal cerebral ischaemic attacks. *Br Med J.* 1963;2:344.

101. Busuttil RW, Baker JD, Davidson RK, et al: Carotid artery stenosis: Hemodynamic significance and clinical course. *JAMA.* 1981;245:1438.

102. Barnett HJM and the EC/IC Bypass Study Group: Failure of extracranial-intracranial arterial bypass to reduce the risk of ischaemic stroke: Results of an international randomized trial. *N Engl J Med.* 1985;313:1191.

103. Gunning AJ, Pickering GW, Robb-Smith AHT, et al: Mural thrombosis of the internal carotid artery and subsequent embolization. *Q J Med.* 1964;33:155.

104. Hollenhorst RW: Significance of bright plaques in the retinal arterioles. *JAMA.* 1961;175:23.

105. Russel RW: Observations on the retinal blood vessels in monocular blindness. *Lancet.* 1961;2:1422.

106. McBrien DJ, Bradley RD, Ashton N: The nature of retinal emboli in stenosis of the internal carotid artery. *Lancet.* 1963;1:691.

107. Ehrenfeld WK, Hoyt WF, Wylie EJ: Embolization and transient blindness from carotid atheroma: Surgical considerations. *Arch Surg.* 1966;93:181.

108. Eisenberg RL, Nemzek WR, Moore WS, et al: Relationship of transient ischaemic attacks and angiographically demonstrable lesions of the carotid artery. *Stroke.* 1977;8:483.

109. Pessin MS, Duncan GW, Mohr JP, et al: Clinical and angiographic features of carotid transient ischaemic attacks. *N Engl J Med.* 1977;296:358.

110. Thiele BL, Young JV, Chikos PM, et al: Correlation of arteriographic findings and symptoms in cerebrovascular disease. *Neurology.* 1980;30:1041.

111. Lusby RJ, Ferrell LD, Reilly LM, et al: Stroke: The significance of carotid plaque haemorrhage with ulceration. *Stroke.* 1983;14:133.

112. Barnett HJM, et al: Canadian Cooperative Study Group: A randomized trial of aspirin and sulfinpyrazone in threatened stroke. *N Engl J Med.* 1978;299:53.

113. Whisnant J, Matsumoto N, Elvebeak L: Transient ischemic attacks in a community: Rochester, Minnesota, 1955–69. *Mayo Clin Proc.* 1973;48:194.

114. Executive Committee for the Asymptomatic Carotid Atherosclerosis Study (ACAS): Endarterectomy for asymptomatic carotid stenosis. *JAMA* 1995;273:1421.

115. Estol C, Claasen D, Hirsch W, et al: Correlative angiographic and pathologic findings in the diagnosis of ulcerated plaques in the carotid artery. *Arch Neurol.* 1991;48:692.

116. Streifler JY, Eliasziw M, Fox AJ, et al: Angiographic detection of carotid plaque ulceration: Comparison with surgical observations in a multicenter study. North American Symptomatic Carotid Endarterectomy Trial. *Stroke.* 1994;25:1130.

117. Bock R, Lusby R: Carotid plaque morphology and interpretation of the echolucent lesion. In Labs, KH, ed. *Diagnostic Vascular Ultrasound.* Kent, England: E Arnold, Ltd, 1992:256.

118. Reilly LM, Lusby RJ, Hughes L, et al: Carotid plaque histology using real-time ultrasonography: Clinical and therapeutic considerations. *Am J Surg.* 1983;188:193.

119. Steffen CM, Gray-Weale AC, Byrne KE, et al: Carotid artery disease: Plaque ultrasound characteristics in symptomatic and asymptomatic vessels. *Stroke.* 1986;17.

120. Feeley TM, Leen EJ, Colgan MP, et al: Histologic characteristics of carotid artery plaque. *J Vasc Surg.* 1991;13:719.

121. Widder B, Paulat K, Hackspacher J, et al: Morphological characterization of carotid artery stenoses by ultrasound duplex scanning. *Ultrasound Med Biol.* 1990;16:349.

122. Geroulakos G, Ramaswami G, Nicolaides A, et al: Characterization of symptomatic and asymptomatic carotid plaques using high-resolution real-time ultrasonography. *Br J Surg.* 1993;80:1274.

123. Goes E, Janssens W, Maillet B, et al: Tissue characterization of atheromatous plaques: Correlation between ultrasound image and histological findings. *J Clin Ultrasound.* 1990;18:611.

124. Barry R, Pienaar C, Nel CJ: Accuracy of B-mode ultrasonography in detecting carotid plaque hemorrhage and ulceration. *Ann Vasc Surg.* 1990;4:466.

125. Comerota AJ, Katz ML, White JV, Grosh JD: The preoperative diagnosis of the ulcerated carotid atheroma. *J Vasc Surg.* 1990;11:505.

126. Hatsukami TS, Thackray BD, Primozich JF, et al: Echolucent regions in carotid plaque: Preliminary analysis comparing three-dimensional histologic reconstructions to sonographic findings. *Ultrasound Med Biol.* 1994;20:743.

127. Kleiser B, Widder B: Course of carotid artery occlusions with impaired cerebrovascular reactivity. *Stroke.* 1992;23:171.

128. Yonas H, Smith HA, Durham SR, et al: Increased stroke risk predicted by compromised cerebral blood flow reactivity. *J Neurosurg.* 1993;79:483.

129. Webster MW, Makaroun MS, Steed DL, et al: Compromised cerebral blood flow reactivity is a predictor of stroke in patients with symptomatic carotid artery occlusive disease. *J Vasc Surg.* 1995;21:338; Discussion, 344.

III

Clinical Considerations

Transient Ischemic Attacks and Stroke in the Distribution of the Carotid Artery: Clinical Manifestations

JAMES F. TOOLE, STEVEN W. DIBERT, and GARY J. HARPOLD

Stroke and its complications are the third leading cause of death in the western world and many Asiatic nations. Stroke is the most frequently encountered entity in the field of neurology and often involves a wide range of medical specialties.[1] It behooves practitioners caring for the at-risk population to become familiar with the warning signs and clinical presentations of cerebrovascular disease. This chapter deals with the entities of transient ischemic attacks (TIAs), reversible ischemic neurologic deficits, and stroke. The clinical manifestations of cerebral ischemia in the carotid territory, including the ophthalmic artery, are discussed.

References to cerebrovascular disease date back to antiquity. By the middle of the nineteenth century, the premonitory symptoms of cerebral infarction were recognized. In his 1893 edition of *A Manual of Diseases of the Nervous System*, Gowers reported the following about what we now call TIAs[2, 3]:

In thrombosis from atheroma . . . the premonitory symptoms are frequent. They depend on the interference with the supply of blood due to the disease of the vessels. They may exist for months before the onset or only for a few hours. The most common are dull headache, giddiness, tingling, numbness, slight weakness in one-half of the body, sometimes limited to a single limb and often but not always corresponding in seat to the subsequent paralysis; less commonly, there is defective articulation or some mental change, failure of memory or irritability due to the general malnutrition of the brain that is produced by widespread arterial disease. In all cases, their presence is far more significant than their absence.

This description is just as applicable today as it was in 1893.

Since that time, much has been written regarding cerebrovascular disease and the warning signs that often precede a permanent stroke. During the 1950s, Fisher[4] described numerous patients who suffered recurrent transient neurologic deficits before succumbing to an internal carotid artery occlusion on the ipsilateral side. In 1955, Millikan and Siekert[5, 6] described the more common carotid and vertebral artery territories involved in TIAs. Fisher,[7] in 1958, reviewed a large series of patients with cerebral thrombosis and found that 50 percent had a history of transient ischemic events before a persistent stroke. The incidence of TIAs preceding a major stroke may vary from as low as 5 to as high as 75

percent.[3] The 1971 Evans County, Georgia, study reported by Heyman and coworkers[8] revealed that approximately 13.8 patients out of 1000 at all ages had a history of TIAs and that this frequency rose to 18 per 1000 for individuals over the age of 65. The 1973 Seal Beach, California, study reported by Stallones and associates[9] showed a TIA frequency of 1 per 1000 in the over-65 age group. A cumulative summary of several studies demonstrated that the risk of stroke in TIA patients at 1 year is about 12 percent, for an estimated relative risk of about 14; the absolute risk of stroke at 5 years is about 30 percent, and the relative risk per year over 5 years is 7. Sixty percent of these strokes are ipsilateral.[10]

In 1975, the Ad hoc Committee of the National Institutes of Neurologic Communicable Diseases and Stroke (NINCDS) defined TIAs as focal neurologic deficits of sudden onset that resolve completely within 24 hours.[11] Indeed, most TIAs strike suddenly without warning, with the neurologic deficit usually developed to its full extent within a few seconds, and certainly by 1 to 2 minutes.[12, 13] Even though the classification of TIA requires that the deficit resolve within 24 hours, clinical experience shows that most patients recover within 15 to 20 minutes of its onset. Although, by definition, recovery is complete, recent data by Frank Wood (personal communication, 1993) demonstrated detectable neuropsychologic changes, presumably caused by permanently disrupted circulation, in patients having repeated TIAs. But on clinical grounds, bedside examination should show no evidence of localized neurologic deficits after 24 hours have elapsed.

Embolism and perfusion failure are the two major causes of TIA symptoms. In embolic TIAs, the size and composition of the embolic particle, along with the availability of a collateral circulation, determine the location, symptoms, and time until resolution. Most emboli proceeding up the carotid arteries travel to the middle cerebral artery and lodge at its bifurcations in the sylvian fissure area. There is little evidence that embolic infarcts have much of an ischemic penumbra. Studies have demonstrated a sharp demarcation between infarcted tissue and normal brain tissue, indicating that collaterals are either completely effective or useless.[14]

Hypoperfusion ischemia commonly affects watershed areas lying between the major cerebral vessels. The TIA symptoms commonly resolve once sufficient cerebral perfusion pressure has been acquired. Flow-related TIAs are typically short in duration and have stereotypical symptoms; they often come in clusters. Embolic TIAs tend to last longer than hypoperfusion TIAs and may affect multiple locations.[15, 16] Repeated episodes in a carotid distribution suggest the carotid bifurcation as the source. Multiple vascular territories suggest a cardiac origin.

A number of TIAs occurring over a short period of time are known as crescendo TIAs. Patients having crescendo TIAs require emergency treatment, often including intravenous anticoagulation therapy. Crescendo TIAs correlate strongly with atherosclerotic carotid disease in 85 percent of cases.[17]

The distinction between TIAs and minor strokes is partly artificial, since recent studies have shown that approximately 24 percent of patients with TIAs have residual infarction on cerebral computed tomography (CCT).[18] The question is whether a patient with these findings should be classified as having a TIA or an infarction. A term gaining acceptance is cerebral infarction with transient symptoms (CITS). The prognosis of CITS differs from that of TIAs (unpublished observation), and CITS should be a consideration in the selection of medical or surgical management. For example, TIA patients seem to be at minimum risk from endarterectomy or anticoagulation treatment because of a normal neurologic examination, but the underlying silent infarction in patients with CITS may convert from ischemic to hemorrhagic if either treatment is used.[19] The Oxfordshire community stroke project found no major epidemiologic factors that could help distinguish TIAs from minor ischemic strokes. Patients with TIAs appeared to have a lower risk of dying or having major strokes than those who had minor ischemic events. The apparent difference was due to the good prognosis in patients with amaurosis fugax.[20]

Reversible ischemic neurologic deficits are defined as focal neurologic deficits of sudden onset that are similar to TIAs but of longer duration. By definition, the deficit must last longer than 24 hours but resolve completely by the end of 7 days. Debate still continues as to whether a reversible ischemic neurologic deficit represents a long TIA or a completed stroke with a rapid recovery.[11, 21, 22] The definition of infarction then becomes a neurologic deficit lasting longer than 7 days from which varying degrees of recovery may be made.[11]

As in most areas of medicine, the history from the patient or the family is all-important in the evaluation and classification of patients with transient neurologic deficits. Overall, 90 percent of carotid episodes last less than 6 hours, and 90 percent of vertebrobasilar episodes last less than 2 hours.[23] Half of all TIAs resolve within 30 minutes, so the symptoms have resolved in a majority of patients by the time they receive medical attention. TIAs may also occur during sleep and go completely unnoticed. Few physicians have witnessed a TIA and studied its clinical manifestations. Many patients have been known to ignore minor TIAs or to resist seeking medical attention until a major deficit is encountered. Table 9–1 lists neurologic defects that may go ignored by patients and those defects that bring patients to medical attention. Careful history taking is essential to assess prior events and the vascular territories affected. Some events that at first sound like TIAs may later prove to be physiologic events

TABLE 9–1. Patient Reaction to Possible Symptoms of Transient Ischemic Attacks

Defect	Seldom Ignored		Often Ignored or Misinterpreted
Vision			
Diplopia	X		
Field cut			
Dominant	X		
Nondominant			X
Amaurosis fugax	X		
Sensory loss			
Dominant hemisphere	X	or	X
Nondominant hemisphere			X
Motor defect			
Dominant hemisphere	X		
Nondominant hemisphere			X
Intellectual disturbance			X
Amnesia	X	or	X
Mild memory defect			X
Aphasia	X		
Reading difficulty			X

unrelated to localized cerebral hypoperfusion or embolization.

Important aspects of the physical examination include a full neurologic examination, blood pressure measurement, palpation of the carotid arteries and peripheral pulses, cardiac and carotid auscultation, and a thorough funduscopic exam. Patients who develop carotid artery stenosis are at increased risk for cerebral infarction, but they are more likely to die of coronary atherosclerosis. Therefore, patients with carotid artery stenosis must be thoroughly evaluated for both cardiac and cerebrovascular disease.[19]

Before discussing the clinical manifestations related to compromised perfusion in various carotid territories, discussion should first be directed toward differentiating what is and is not a TIA. Table 9–2 provides a list of episodic disturbances that are not characteristic of TIAs in either the posterior or anterior circulatory territory. Episodic alterations in consciousness, including syncope, are often misdiagnosed as TIAs and often prove, after extensive and costly diagnostic workups, to be secondary to either cardiac abnormalities or seizure disorders. Likewise, tonic or clonic activity (especially generalized), marching of the sensory deficits, and bowel and bladder incontinence all point toward epilepsy and not cerebrovascular insufficiency. Exceptions to this

TABLE 9–2. Signs and Symptoms Not Characteristic of Transient Ischemic Attacks

Unconsciousness, including syncope
Tonic and/or clonic activity
March of a sensory deficit
Vertigo alone
Dysphagia alone
Dysarthria alone
Bowel or bladder incontinence
Loss of vision, with alteration of consciousness
Focal symptoms associated with migraine
Scintillating scotomata
Confusion alone
Amnesia alone

include focal motor seizures, which are discussed later in this chapter. Isolated episodes of vertigo, dysphagia, or dysarthria alone are not typical of TIAs. Confusion or amnesia likewise should not be considered a manifestation of TIAs. They are more likely due to global cerebral dysfunction secondary to metabolic or iatrogenic causes or systemic hypoperfusion. Visual loss with alternations of consciousness also point toward a cardiac abnormality as the likely cause. However, these events are still referred on a regular basis to neurologists and vascular surgeons under the diagnosis of TIAs. Migraine accompaniments, which include a variety of motor, somatic, and special sensory manifestations, are frequently misdiagnosed as TIAs.[24, 25] Likewise, episodic nocturnal hypoglycemia, as described by Silas and colleagues,[26] may masquerade as TIAs. In their patient, a right hemiparesis present upon awakening resolved after the infusion of intravenous glucose.

Intracranial mass lesions may produce transient focal deficits that can be confused with TIAs. In 1983, Ross described four patients with TIA-like symptoms and signs resulting from intracranial neoplasms.[27] Debate still remains as to the pathophysiology of these events. Theories regarding transient cerebrovascular steal phenomena, sudden changes in hydrostatic pressures within the tumor, spreading zones of neural depression, and rapid changes in mass effect due to intratumor necrosis and hemorrhage have all been proposed. Welsh and coworkers[28] and later Master and coworkers[29] reported patients with chronic subdural hematomas presenting with transient focal neurologic dysfunction. Again, the causative pathophysiology for these occurrences is unclear. Vascular compromise due to pressure on cortical vessels, neuronal dysfunction due to cerebral edema, postictal paralysis, and spreading cortical depression have all been postulated. CCT is of great value in the evaluation of TIA patients and in ruling out a mass lesion as the cause of the clinical picture.

Cerebral aneurysms may produce TIA symptoms. Fisher and associates[30] described a series of patients found to have cerebral aneurysms during evaluation for TIAs. The vascular lesions were in the correct distributions for the observed deficits, and it is postulated that there was embolization from the aneurysmal sac.

Table 9–3 completes the picture with a list of the common manifestations of transient ischemic events involving the

TABLE 9–4. Manifestations of Carotid Artery Transient Ischemic Attacks

Syndrome	Description
Motor defect	Weakness, poor use, or paralysis: contralateral side
Sensory defect	Numbness, loss of sensation, or paresthesia: contralateral side
Speech and/or language defect	Dysarthria or dysphasia
Visual defect	Unilateral blindness, ipsilateral side (amaurosis fugax), or contralateral field defect
Mental change	Associated with other signs
Headache	In association with other symptoms or signs
Lightheadedness	
Visual hallucinations	
Seizure activity, often focal	
Combination of above	

vertebrobasilar system.[31, 32] These syndromes are discussed in detail in Chapter 10. When a patient presents with a history of crossed motor and sensory findings, bilateral or shifting sensory defects, or episodes of multiple cranial nerve dysfunction, the suspicion of vertebrobasilar insufficiency must be raised. Episodic visual loss involving complete or partial defects in both homonymous fields may point to occipital lobe ischemia in the distribution of the posterior cerebral artery. Episodic ataxia, imbalance, unsteadiness, or disequilibrium not typically vertiginous, if combined with dysarthria, should point the examiner toward the vertebrobasilar system involving the brain stem structures. Drop attacks, classically a sign of vertebrobasilar insufficiency, are episodic losses of tone without alteration of consciousness, resulting in embarrassing and often injurious falls without warning.

Table 9–4 lists common signs and symptoms related to carotid distribution TIAs.[24] The time course and symptoms of TIAs in the anterior circulation have been shown to be related to the severity of atherosclerotic disease in the carotids. TIAs in the distribution of the internal carotid artery lasting longer than 1 hour are associated with a widely patent internal carotid artery and are often due to cardiogenic embolism. Patients with both hemispheric and retinal TIAs tend to have severe carotid disease.[15, 33] Perhaps the most common and easily understood manifestations of carotid territory TIAs are contralateral motor deficits ranging from mild paresis to complete paralysis involving the face, arm, and leg. The motor deficits may be accompanied by varying degrees of sensory deficits, resulting in numbness and paresthesias on the contralateral side. Speech and language function may be affected alone or in conjunction with motor and sensory deficits. The extent of the language dysfunction may range from mild dysarthria to a severe combined expressive and receptive loss. Localized hemispheric events resulting in defects of higher cortical function are discussed later in this chapter.

OPHTHALMIC ARTERY ISCHEMIA

Transient visual defects frequently bring a patient to medical attention. As the first intracranial branch of the internal carotid artery, the ophthalmic artery is often the target for

TABLE 9–3. Signs and Symptoms of Vertebrobasilar Ischemia

Syndrome	Description
Motor defect	Weakness, clumsiness, or paralysis; bilateral or shifting
Sensory defect	Numbness, including loss of sensation or paresthesias; bilateral or shifting
Visual defect	Loss of vision, complete or partial in both homonymous fields
Ataxia	Imbalance, unsteadiness, or disequilibrium, not associated with vertigo
Speech defect	Dysarthria with other brain stem signs
Drop attacks	Episodic loss of muscle tone without alteration in consciousness
Any combination of the above	

artery-to-artery embolization, resulting in transient visual loss. Classically, the term *amaurosis fugax* has been given to fleeting attacks of visual loss that may occur in up to 40 percent of patients with TIAs of the carotid distribution.[34, 35] The visual loss is painless and monocular, occurring on the side of the offending carotid artery lesion. The visual loss may be complete and is often described by the patient as a window shade coming down across the visual field. The visual loss may affect only part of the visual field, depending on the size of the embolus and the extent of travel through the retinal vessels before lodging and occluding flow. On examination, the clinician may see a bright yellow, highly refractile body in a retinal vessel, usually at a branch bifurcation. These refractile bodies as described by Hollenhorst[36] represent cholesterol crystals embolized from degenerating plaques in the carotid system. Retinal emboli, which are white in appearance, may represent calcified emboli from cardiac valvular disease or platelet emboli from atherosclerotic plaques in the carotid vessels. The visual loss in amaurosis fugax lasts for minutes to hours and slowly resolves in the reverse order in which it came. This resolution most likely represents the fragmentation of the embolus and its migration farther distally.

It should be noted that a slow constriction of the visual field progressing to total or near-total blindness, followed by central resolution and clearing to the periphery, is suggestive of a diffuse ocular hypoperfusion that is more likely caused by disturbed cardiac output and systemic hypotension than cerebrovascular disease. Since amaurosis fugax is usually the result of embolized material from the carotid bifurcation, these attacks are ipsilateral to the side of the disease. Interestingly, one case report by Pejic[37] in 1982 described a case of simultaneous bilateral amaurosis fugax in a patient with bilateral symptomatic carotid lesions. Following bilateral carotid endarterectomy, this patient suffered no further visual episodes.

An important entity in the differential diagnosis of amaurosis fugax is ischemic optic neuropathy.[38] This may occur in two forms: the atherosclerotic form occurs most frequently between the ages of 50 and 70, secondary to atherosclerotic disease of the vessels supplying the optic nerve; and the arteritic form often occurs in conjunction with giant cell arteritis affecting other cranial vessels. Regardless of the cause, visual loss may occur over hours to days. Visual acuity is almost always decreased, and field testing frequently demonstrates an inferior nasal defect. Funduscopic examination reveals blurring of the disc margins, with adjacent flame-shaped hemorrhages. These findings are in striking contrast to those in the amaurosis fugax patient, in whom vision has usually returned by the time the patient reaches medical attention, when funduscopic examination may or may not show retinal emboli.

Two cases of unilateral angle-closure glaucoma following ipsilateral carotid distribution TIAs were reported by Coppeta and Monteiro.[39] The cause is unknown. It remains to be seen whether the acute glaucoma was secondary to mydriasis induced by the ischemic attacks or whether the angle-closure glaucoma produced vasovagal symptoms and hypotension, which in turn caused transient cerebral ischemia.

ANTERIOR CEREBRAL ARTERY ISCHEMIA

The paired anterior cerebral arteries supply the anterior two thirds to three fourths of the medial surface and, to some extent, the parasagittal surface of the cerebral hemisphere. Branches of the anterior cerebral artery also perfuse the majority of the corpus callosum, the frontal poles, and the medial orbital surfaces of the frontal lobe. Deep branches penetrate the anterior limb of the internal capsule to supply the head of the caudate nucleus.

Occlusion of the proximal anterior cerebral artery prior to the connection with the anterior communicating artery may produce no significant problems. Collateral flow from the contralateral side may be adequate to perfuse both anterior cerebral artery distributions. Occlusion of one anterior cerebral artery distal to the connection of the anterior communicating artery usually results in a contralateral monoparesis of the lower extremity as well as a sensory defect. Depending on the vascular distribution, sensory and motor defects in the contralateral arm may be encountered, but the face is spared. Urinary incontinence may be present in varying degrees, and frontal lobe signs such as paratonia (gegenhalten) and pathologic reflexes such as grasping and sucking responses may be present. Frontal lobe ischemia may result in disorders of behavior, slowness of response, easy distractability, poor power of concentration, and a soft whispering voice. Bilateral occlusions of the anterior cerebral arteries result in paraplegia, incontinence, abulia, and aphasia. Occlusion of Heubner's branch of the left anterior cerebral artery may result in a diminution or arrest of spontaneous speech, agraphia, and varying degrees of anomia, but the ability to repeat spoken or written sentences is preserved. This has been called a transcortical motor aphasia.

MIDDLE CEREBRAL ARTERY ISCHEMIA

The middle cerebral artery territory is composed of the lateral portions of the cerebral hemispheres and, to varying extents, the deep gray nuclei. Specifically, this territory encompasses the lateral and anterior surfaces of the frontal lobe, motor and sensory speech areas, major and minor motor control areas, and sensory cortex. Superior aspects of the temporal lobe and insular cortex are also supplied by middle cerebral branches. Deeper penetrating branches perfuse the corona radiata, posterior limbs of the internal capsule, putamen, globus pallidum, and posterior portion of the caudate nucleus.

The middle cerebral artery may become occluded at its major trunk or at any one of its distal branches, each producing different neurologic deficits. Occlusion of the middle cerebral artery trunk results in a contralateral hemiplegia, hemianesthesia, and homonymous hemianopia. If the dominant hemisphere is involved, aphasia results, whereas a nondominant hemispheric lesion produces abnormalities of praxis and spatial orientation. Total occlusions of the middle cerebral artery trunk are not frequent occurrences. Most middle cerebral artery occlusions are the result of embolic phenomena to distal branches.

The middle cerebral artery has two main divisions: the superior and inferior branches. Superior branch occlusion results in contralateral face, arm, and leg paralysis, similar to that associated with a middle cerebral artery trunk occlusion. However, there may be less deterioration in alertness with a branch occlusion. Acutely, in dominant hemisphere ischemia, there may be a global aphasia that gradually improves to a primary motor aphasia with hesitant and dis-melodic speech. Because of the contribution to the leg cortex by the anterior cerebral artery, contralateral leg weakness can be quite variable. Ischemia of the rolandic branches, sparing Broca's area, may result in a sensory motor paralysis with dysarthria rather than aphasia. Likewise, branch occlusions may result in very little sensory motor deficit but a severe motor aphasia.

The inferior division of the middle cerebral artery is affected less often than the superior one. Lesions in this territory frequently result in a receptive aphasia if the dominant hemisphere is involved, amorphosynthesis if the nondominant hemisphere is involved, and a homonymous visual field defect.

One study demonstrated that the location of TIAs in areas perfused by the middle cerebral artery had an effect on resolution time. TIAs in the inferior division were longer (median 45 minutes) compared with those in the superior division (median 20 minutes). TIAs in the inferior division of the middle cerebral artery were also more likely to arise from an embolic source.[40]

ANTERIOR CHOROIDAL ARTERY ISCHEMIA

Occlusion of the anterior choroidal artery alone is a rare event. Foix and coworkers[41] reported the classic clinical syndrome of an anterior choroidal artery infarct as contralateral hemiplegia, hemihypesthesia, and homonymous hemianopia. The ischemic territory in their case involved the posterior internal capsule and other adjacent white matter tracts. Other cases have been reported in which infarction in the right internal capsule produced visual neglect, constructional apraxia, alexia, and motor impersistence. To add to the clinical spectrum, other anterior choroidal artery infarcts have produced symptoms of pure sensory loss, pure motor loss, hemiataxia with hemisensory loss, and acute pseudobulbarism. Bilateral infarcts are uncommon but can produce acute pseudobulbar palsy, with sparing of the limbs; bilateral hemisensory and hemimotor deficit, with bilateral upper quadrantanopia; or bilateral pure motor hemiparesis, with facial-buccal-lingual palsy.

The most likely pathogenesis is a vasculopathy caused by long-standing hypertension or diabetes. Embolism is possible, since the anterior choroidal artery has a larger diameter (0.7–2.0 mm at the origin) than most deep penetrating vessels and thus could receive an emboli. Further studies are needed to establish the etiology.

The prognosis of an anterior choroidal artery territory stroke is poor when it occurs bilaterally; however, unilateral infarcts usually have a good prognosis, with only mild impairment noted after several months of convalescence. Visual and sensory impairments have been reported to improve while motor deficits improved little.[42] The optimal treatment is unknown. Controlling the patient's hypertension is the main therapy. There is probably no role for the use of anticoagulants due to the risks of hemorrhagic conversion in advanced small vessel disease.

LACUNAR SYNDROMES

Lacunar infarcts are small infarcts that occur primarily in the basal ganglia, internal capsule, and brain stem, resulting

TABLE 9–5. Lacunar Syndromes

Syndrome	Location of Infarction	Deficit
Pure motor hemiparesis	Contralateral internal capsule or basis pontis	Paresis of face, arm, and leg
Pure sensory stroke	Contralateral thalamus	Paresthesia of arm, face, and leg
Dysarthria-clumsy hand	Contralateral internal capsule or basis pontis	Dysarthria, hemiataxia
Ataxic hemiparesis	Contralateral internal capsule or basis pontis	Hemiparesis, ipsilateral ataxia

from occlusion of small penetrating branches. The residual of the infarct is a cavity known as a lacuna that ranges in size from 3 mm (very small) to 2 cm (large). The larger lacunae result primarily from atheroma occlusion, and the smaller ones from lipohyalinosis. The most common sites of lacunar infarcts, in descending frequency, are putamen, caudate, thalamus, pons, internal capsule, and convolutional white matter.[43] In over 90 percent of cases, the patient is hypertensive (blood pressure greater than 140/90 mm Hg).

Fisher[43] and Mohr[44] described four lacunar syndromes, which account for the majority of lacunar infarcts (Table 9–5). The pure sensory stroke or TIA is the most common lacunar manifestation. The infarct is usually the result of lipohyalinosis. In a pure sensory ischemic event, there are paresthesias involving one side of the body (but no weakness), homonymous hemianopia, aphasia, and apractagnosia.[45] These signs and symptoms may be related to ischemia in the internal capsule, adjacent to white matter tracts. A sensory defect may also occur with involvement of the contralateral thalamus, with ischemia in the territory of the posterior cerebral artery. However, Dibert examined a patient with a pure sensory stroke involving only the vibration and proprioceptive modalities; this was caused by a pontine lacuna involving the medial lemniscus. Thus, if individual long tracts are involved, consideration of a brain stem lacuna must be entertained. Pure motor hemiparesis is the second most frequent lacunar syndrome. In contrast to the pure sensory syndrome, the pure motor syndrome is mainly the result of atherosclerosis. Pure motor hemiparesis may be the result of ischemia in the contralateral internal capsule, basis pontis, or medullary pyramid. Both capsular and pontine lesions may produce identical pictures, and the differentiation between vertebral artery ischemia and carotid territory pathology must be made.

The majority of lacunar syndromes are believed to result from atheroma, except for the pure sensory syndrome, which results from lipohyalinosis. This is important in management, since anticoagulation in the presence of lipohyalinosis has a higher probability of causing hemorrhage. Because of their location, lacunar syndromes are rarely associated with certain neurologic signs and symptoms as described in Table 9–6.

OTHER MANIFESTATIONS OF TRANSIENT CEREBRAL ISCHEMIA

Focal seizure activity is important in the differential diagnosis of TIAs. However, it is known that transient embolic

TABLE 9–6. Signs and Symptoms Not Characteristic
of Lacunar Infarctions

Aphasia
Apractagnosia of the minor hemisphere
Sensorimotor stroke
Homonymous hemianopia
Isolated severe memory impairment
Coma
Stupor
Seizures
Monoplegia
Loss of consciousness

events may be accompanied by focal seizure activity without alterations in consciousness. This often takes the form of the sudden onset of involuntary movements of an extremity followed by paresthesia, which must be differentiated from postictal paralysis.

Another interesting manifestation of transient cerebral ischemia was reported in 1982 by Margolin and Marsden.[46] They described four patients who had episodic dyskinetic movements that ceased after carotid artery disease was diagnosed and treated either medically or with carotid endarterectomy. These case reports indicate that ischemia in the deep nuclei of the hemispheres may produce involuntary movement disorders as a result of embolic phenomena. Another case report described a patient who exhibited prosopagnosia as the only manifestation of transient cerebral ischemia.[47] This patient later manifested a more classic TIA involving right arm and leg paresthesias, with a sensory defect.

It is worth emphasizing that whether dealing with a TIA or stroke from embolic causes, the clinical signs and symptoms may be secondary to a single embolus producing finite and easily localizable deficits or to a shower of emboli producing deficits attributable to multiple vascular territories. As discussed in Chapter 8, the evaluation with regard to the site of emboli and a history differentiating single and bilateral hemispheric events are critical.

REFERENCES

1. Wolf PA, Dawber TR, Thomas HE, et al: Epidemiology of stroke. In Thompson RA, Green JR, eds. *Advances in Neurology,* Vol 16. New York: Raven Press; 1977:5.
2. Gowers WR: *A Manual of Diseases of the Nervous System.* Philadelphia: Blakiston; 1893.
3. McDowell F: Transient cerebral ischemia: Diagnostic considerations. *Prog Cardiovasc Dis.* 1980;22:309.
4. Fisher CM: Occlusion of the internal carotid artery. *Arch Neurol Psych* 1951;65:346.
5. Millikan CH, Siekert RC: Studies in cerebrovascular disease. I. The syndrome of intermittent insufficiency of the carotid arterial system. *Mayo Clin Proc.* 1955;30:186.
6. Siekert RC, Millikan CH: Studies in cerebrovascular disease. II. Some clinical aspects of thrombosis of the basilar artery. *Mayo Clin Proc.* 1955;30:93.
7. Fisher CM: Intermittent cerebral ischemia. In Wright IS, Millikan CH, eds. *Transactions of the Second Conference on Cerebral Vascular Disease.* New York: Grune & Stratton; 1958:8.
8. Heyman A, Karp HR, Heyden S, et al: Cerebrovascular disease in the biracial population of Evans County, Georgia. *Stroke.* 1971;2:509.
9. Stallones RA, Dyken ML, Fang HLH, et al: Epidemiology for stroke facilities planning. *Stroke.* 1972;3:360.
10. Crouse JR: Assessment and management of carotid disease. *Annu Rev Med.* 1992;43:301.
11. Ad hoc Committee NINCDS: A classification and outline of cerebrovascular diseases. II. *Stroke.* 1975;6:564.
12. Dyken M, Jones F: Transient ischemic attacks. *Compr Ther.* 1981;7:6.
13. Millikan CH, McDowell FH: Treatment of transient ischemic attacks. *Stroke.* 1978;9:299.
14. Nedergaard M, Vorstrup S, Astrup J: Cell density in the border zone around old small human brain infarcts. *Stroke.* 1986;17:1129.
15. Pessin MS, Duncan GW, Mohr JP, Poskanzer DC: Clinical and angiographic features of carotid transient ischemic attacks. *N Engl J Med.* 1977;296:358.
16. Caplan LR, Stein RW: *Stroke: A Clinical Approach.* Boston: Butterworths; 1986.
17. Rothrock JF, Lyden PD, Yee J, Wiederhort WC: ''Crescendo'' transient ischemic attacks: Clinical and angiographic correlations. *Neurology.* 1988;38:198.
18. Murros KE, Evans GW, Toole JF, et al: Cerebral infarction in patients with transient ischemic attacks. *J Neurol.* 1989;236:182.
19. Toole JF: The Willis lecture: Transient ischemic attacks, scientific method, and new realities. *Stroke.* 1991;22:99.
20. Dennis MS, Bamford JM, Sandercock PAG, Warlow CP: A comparison of risk factors and prognosis for transient ischemic attacks and minor strokes: The Oxfordshire community stroke project. *Stroke.* 1989;20:1494.
21. Loeb C: Transient ischemic attack, protracted transient ischemic attack and completed stroke. *Eur Neurol.* 1983;22(1):68.
22. Gratzl O, Schmiedek P: Microneurosurgical arterial anastomoses in patients with prolonged reversible ischemic neurological deficit (PRIND). In Fein J, Reichman H, eds. *International Symposium on Microvascular Anastomoses for Cerebral Ischemia, Chicago 1974.* Heidelberg: Springer-Verlag; 1978.
23. Hachinski V, Norris JW: *Diagnosis of Transient Ischemic Attacks: The Acute Stroke.* Philadelphia: FA Davis; 1985:65.
24. Wiley R: The scintillating scotoma without headache. *Ann Ophthalmol.* 1979;11:581.
25. Fisher C: Late-life migraine accompaniments as a course of unexplained transient ischemic attacks. *J Can Sci Neurol.* 1980;7:9.
26. Silas J, Grant D, Maddocks J: Transient hemiparetic attacks due to unrecognized nocturnal hypoglycemia. *Br Med J.* 1981;1282:132.
27. Ross RT: Transient tumor attacks. *Arch Neurol.* 1983;40:633.
28. Welsh JE, Tyson GW, Winn HR, et al: Chronic subdural hematoma presenting as transient neurologic deficits. *Stroke.* 1979;10:564.
29. Master ML, Johnston DE, Reinmuth OM: Chronic subdural hematoma with transient neurological deficits: A review of 15 cases. *Ann Neurol.* 1983;14:539.
30. Fisher M, Davidson R, Marcus E: Transient focal cerebral ischemia as a presenting manifestation of unruptured cerebral aneurysm. *Ann Neurol.* 1980;8:367.
31. Jones HR: Disease of the vertebral basilar system. *Prim Care.* 1979;6:733.
32. Ueda K, Toole JF, McHenry LC: Carotid and vertebrobasilar transient ischemic attacks: Clinical and angiographic correlation. *Neurology (NY).* 1979;27:1094.
33. Toole JF, Yuson CP: Transient ischemic attacks with normal arteriograms: Serious or benign prognosis? *Ann Neurol.* 1977;1:100.
34. Carlow TJ, Bicknell JM: Stroke and the eye: Diagnostic clues and treatment approaches. *Geriatrics.* 1981;36:28.
35. Diener HC, Ruprecht KW: Ocular key symptoms of extracranial cerebrovascular disease. *Arch Psychiatry Nervenk.* 1981;230:129.
36. Hollenhorst RW: Significance of bright plaques in retinal arteries. *JAMA.* 1961;178:23.
37. Pejic R: Bilateral and simultaneous amaurosis fugax. *J Ind State Med Assoc.* 1982;75:396.
38. Bender M, Rudolph S, Stacy C: The neurology of the visual and oculomotor systems. In Baker A, Baker L, eds. *Clinical Neurology,* Vol 1. Hagerstown, MD: Harper & Row; 1983:6.
39. Coppeta J, Monteiro M: Angle-closure glaucoma and transient ischemic attacks. *Am J Ophthalmol.* 1985;99:493.
40. Bogousslavsky J, Van Melle G, Regli, F: Middle cerebral artery pial territory infarcts: A study of the Lausanne stroke registry. *Ann Neurol.* 1989;25:555.
41. Foix C, Chavany J, Hillemand P, et al: Obliteration of the anterior choroidal artery. *Bull Soc Ophtalmol Fr.* 1982;37:221.
42. Helgason CM: A new view of anterior choroidal artery territory infarction. *J Neurol.* 1988;235:387–391.
43. Fisher CM: Lacunar strokes and infarcts: A review. *Neurology (NY).* 1982;32:871.
44. Mohr JP: Lacunes. *Stroke.* 1982;13:3.
45. Fisher CM: Pure sensory stroke and allied conditions. *Stroke.* 1982;13:434.
46. Margolin D, Marsden L: Episodic dyskinesias and transient cerebral ischemia. *Neurology (NY).* 1982;32:1379.
47. Marti-Vilatta J, Dalmau J, Santola M: Prosopagnosia, a transient ischemic attack. *Stroke.* 1981;12:702.

SUGGESTED READING

Toole JF: *Cerebrovascular Disorders.* 4th ed. New York: Raven Press; 1990.

CHAPTER 10

Transient Ischemic Attacks and Stroke in the Distribution of the Vertebrobasilar System: Clinical Manifestations

LOUIS R. CAPLAN and ROBERT J. WITYK

HISTORICAL BACKGROUND

Five decades ago, Kubik and Adams[1] described the clinical and necropsy findings in 18 patients who died of brainstem infarction caused by occlusion of the basilar artery. Their report was one of the first careful and detailed clinicopathologic analyses of any stroke syndrome. The authors emphasized that knowledge of the clinical findings in patients with brain-stem infarction might permit diagnosis during life of what they considered to be an invariably fatal disease. Kubik and Adams noted that the symptoms and signs of basilar artery occlusion begin abruptly, usually without premonitory warning. They did not mention preceding transient ischemic attacks (TIAs), a phenomenon brought to the attention of the medical community somewhat later (1951) by Fisher.[2] Describing the symptoms in a series of patients with occlusion of the internal carotid artery (ICA), Fisher emphasized the frequency of transient attacks of ocular or cerebral ischemia that he called TIAs. Fisher also noted that occlusive disease in the anterior circulation is not always, as traditionally believed, in the intracranial middle cerebral artery, but instead is found in the ICA in the neck, a location potentially surgically accessible. Shortly after Fisher's report, Hutchinson and Yates[3, 4] examined the vertebrobasilar arterial systems of cadavers in whom the vertebral arteries were removed with the cervical vertebrae. These workers found a high incidence of occlusive disease of the vertebral arteries in the neck and described the associated clinical findings.

Also in the 1950s, a number of senior neurologic clinicians on both sides of the Atlantic Ocean, armed with Fisher's[2] concept of warning TIAs and the symptoms described by Kubik and Adams,[1] reported several series of patients with transient episodes of ischemia that they localized to the posterior circulation. Denny-Brown,[5] Fang and Palmer,[6] Williams,[7] Williams and Wilson,[8] and Millikan and Siekert[9] all described transient ischemic attacks in the posterior circulation, a syndrome they labeled vertebrobasilar insufficiency (VBI). They recognized these attacks as likely precursors to potentially fatal brain-stem infarction. In that era, it was fashionable to use warfarin as a treatment for coronary disease and for venous thrombosis with pulmonary embolism. As a result of uncontrolled observations in series of patients with VBI, enthusiasm for the use of warfarin for this condition grew, and the drug was widely used in the medical community in the United States during the 1960s and 1970s. During the 1950s and early 1960s, attention was also redirected toward the neck vessels, especially the proximal subclavian and vertebral arteries after the subclavian steal syndrome was recognized and described.[10–14]

The past two decades have witnessed remarkable advances in technology and an awakening of interest in stroke. More detailed information about stroke syndromes and subtypes has become available with the advent of safer angiography, noninvasive vascular studies (duplex ultrasonography, transcranial Doppler, and magnetic resonance angiography), and better brain imaging with computed tomography and magnetic resonance imaging. The general term *carotid insufficiency* is no longer used to characterize the large heterogeneous group of patients with ischemia of the anterior circulation. Instead, subgroups of more homogeneous patients with ICA occlusion, ICA stenosis, lacunar disease, middle cerebral artery occlusion, or embolization are widely recognized. Similarly, disease of the posterior circulation is not homogeneous but also consists of various different patterns that depend on the location, severity, and type of vascular pathology, the location and extent of the brain ischemia, and the make-up of the blood itself.[15, 16] The general designation VBI, useful when we had no definitive information, has outgrown its utility. Treatment should not simply be geared toward the presence of posterior circulation symptoms or whether the patient has TIAs, progressing stroke, or a fixed deficit, since these terms only describe the tempo of the illness and say nothing about the nature of the vascular lesion.[17]

This chapter first reviews the important anatomic features and the pathology of the vertebrobasilar arterial system. A discussion of general signs and symptoms of disease of the posterior circulation and its differential diagnosis is followed by a description of subgroups of patients who are clinically recognizable by their constellation of symptoms and signs. Treatment is discussed in Chapters 77, 78, and 79.

KEY ANATOMIC FEATURES

The vertebral arteries arise at a rather acute angle as the first branches of the subclavian arteries. Their course is traditionally divided into four segments. In the first segment, the artery is directed cephalad until it enters the transverse foramen of C6 or C5. In its second segment, the artery is entirely within the transverse foramina of the cervical vertebral column from C6 to C2. The distal extracranial vertebral artery, the third segment, is that portion of the vessel after its exit from C2, until it pierces the dura to enter the cranium. This segment is very tortuous. The artery courses posterolaterally, circles the posterior arch of C1, and passes between the atlas and occiput within the suboccipital triangle. Covered by muscle, ligaments, and the atlanto-occipital membrane, the distal extracranial segment is pressed against bone. The vertebral artery is relatively fixed at its origin and in its second and intracranial segments. The other segments, especially the third, are more loosely anchored and are especially vulnerable to trauma or injury during neck motion. The extracranial vertebral artery gives off a number of muscle branches; rich collateral circulation is available from the ascending cervical and transverse cervical branches of the thyrocervical trunk, the occipital branches of the external carotid arteries, and other branches of the parent subclavian and external carotid arteries and from the contralateral vertebral artery. The fourth segment of the vertebral artery is its intracranial segment until the two vertebral arteries merge to form the basilar artery at the pontomedullary junction.

The intracranial vertebral artery supplies primarily the medulla and the inferior surfaces of the cerebellum. The two most important branches of the intracranial vertebral arteries are the posterior inferior cerebellar arteries (PICAs), which usually emerge laterally from approximately the midportion of the vessel, and the anterior spinal arteries, which branch medially from the more distal vertebral artery to merge with the contralateral anterior spinal artery to descend along the medulla and cervical spinal cord as a midline anterior vessel. The basilar artery runs along the base of the pons on the clivus and is somewhat wider at its origin, tapering as it courses toward its termination at the pontomesencephalic junction. The basilar artery supplies the pons and has two major circumferential branches: The anterior inferior cerebellar artery (AICA) supplies the lateral pontine tegmentum and the inferior rostral cerebellum; and the superior cerebellar artery (SCA) emerges laterally from the distal basilar artery to supply the pontine and caudal mesencephalic tegmentum and the superior surface of the cerebellum. Smaller but constant branches penetrate the brain stem and supply the medial and paramedial basal and tegmental regions (Fig. 10–1).

Small penetrating arteries arise from the distal basilar artery and course through the posterior penetrating substance to supply the paramedian rostral midbrain, thalamus, and hypothalamus. The initial portion of the posterior cerebral arteries, the tributaries of the basilar artery, is called the basilar communicating artery. After receiving the posterior communicating branch from the internal carotid artery, the posterior cerebral artery (PCA) courses around the brain stem, giving off thalomogeniculate branches to the lateral thalami. The major branches of the posterior cerebral artery supply the posterior and medial temporal lobes and the medial occipital lobes, including the striate visual cortex on the banks of the calcarine fissure. The vertebral, basilar, and posterior cerebral arteries are illustrated in Figure 10–2.

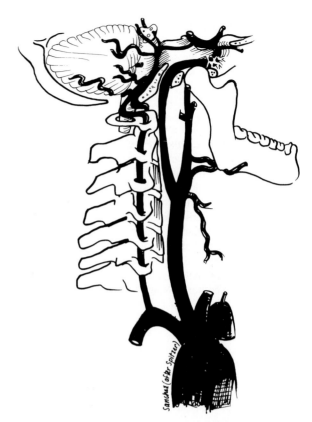

FIGURE 10–2. Diagrammatic representation of vertebrobasilar arterial tree. (Drawn by Dr. Juan Sanchez-Ramos; used with permission.)

VASCULAR PATHOLOGY

Congenital Variations

Congenital variations are very common. In about 8 percent of individuals, the left vertebral artery originates directly from the aortic arch,[18] as can be seen when the left vertebral artery does not fill with dye after a left brachial dye injection. Rarely, the right vertebral artery arises from the innominate artery directly and not from the subclavian artery. The distal segment of the vertebral artery may be hypoplastic or nonexistent; the vertebral artery is then said to end in PICA. The vertebral arteries are frequently asymmetric; in 45 percent of patients the left is larger, in 21 percent the right is larger, and in 34 percent the arteries are approximately equal.[18] One vertebral artery may be quite hypoplastic, in which case the corresponding transverse foramina are small. The PICA and AICA arteries are often reciprocally related in size. For example, a large PICA may supply nearly the entire inferior surface of the cerebellum, while the ipsilateral AICA is quite small and has little cerebellar supply. Sometimes the AICA is dominant and the PICA small. The distal basilar segments are also variably formed. During early fetal life, the ICA supplies the posterior cerebral hemispheres and brain stem through the posterior communicating posterior cerebral arteries. In one third of patients, this primitive vascular pattern persists, and the connecting segment from the basilar artery to the PCA, variously called the basilar communicating or mesencephalic artery, remains vestigial.[19] In these cases, the PCA fills from carotid injection but not after vertebral artery opacification. In 2 percent of patients, this primitive circula-

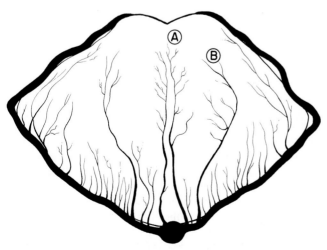

FIGURE 10–1. Pontine penetrating arteries. *A*, Median; *B*, Paramedian.

tory pattern is bilateral; even more rarely, the distal basilar segment is hypoplastic and ends in the SCAs.

Occasionally, primitive connections from the ICA to the vessels of the posterior circulation persist into adult life. The most common case (1–2% of adults) involves the trigeminal artery, which arises from the ICA at the entrance to the cavernous sinus and joins the basilar artery between the AICA and SCA branches after penetrating the sella turcica and the dura along the clivus. The next most common pattern involves the hypoglossal artery, which originates from the ICA in the neck, usually between T3 and C1, and enters the hypoglossal canal to join the lower basilar artery. Much more rarely persisting are the otic artery, which branches from the ICA within the petrosal bone to the midbasilar artery, and the proatlantal intersegmental artery, which branches from the nuchal ICA or external carotid artery to the suboccipital vertebral artery. In patients with persisting fetal communicating channels, the vertebral and basilar arteries proximal to the channel may be hypoplastic.

Atherosclerosis

Atherosclerosis is by far the most frequent vascular pathology in patients with posterior circulation ischemia. Fatty streaks, fibrous plaques, calcified lesions, and complicated lesions consisting of plaques with superimposed hemorrhage, ulceration, or thrombus have all been identified within the larger arteries of the vertebrobasilar system and do not differ qualitatively from the findings of anterior circulation atherosclerosis.[22, 25] The most common site of atherosclerotic stenosis is at the origin of the vertebral arteries. Plaque sometimes extends from the subclavian artery to encircle the proximal vertebral artery like a ring. Proximal vertebral artery lesions are common in white patients but are rare in black patients.[26] The intracranial artery just after it pierces the dura and the more distal vertebral artery are other sites of atherosclerotic predilection. In the second portion of the vertebral artery, a ladderlike arrangement of fibrous plaques is found related to adjacent cervical spine bars or osteophytes, but stenosis of the artery in this segment is rare.[25] Clots in the extracranial vertebral artery usually develop at sites of atherosclerotic stenosis and seldom form long anterograde or retrograde extensions.[23, 24]

Within the basilar artery, stenosis or occlusion is commonly thought to be most frequent in the proximal 2 cm of the vessel. A review of the angiographic literature suggests that basilar thrombosis is just as common in the middle and distal segments.[26] Distal basilar artery stenosis is more common in black patients.[27] When thrombosis occurs within the basilar artery, the thrombus usually has limited propagation,[1, 23] generally extending only to the orifice of the next long circumferential branch, AICA or SCA. The proximal posterior cerebral arteries also are sites of atherosclerosis, especially in black patients, but occlusion of posterior cerebral artery branches is usually embolic.[23] Black persons also have a higher incidence of narrowing of the orifices of the long circumferential branches, PICA, AICA, and SCA.[27] Larger paramedian basilar artery branches can become occluded when plaque within the vessel or artery blocks or extends into the orifice of the branch, or when a microatheroma begins within the branch.[28, 29]

Lipohyalinosis

The pathology of atherosclerosis of penetrating arteries less than 200 μm in size is qualitatively distinct from that of larger vessels. A hyalin material that stains positively with fat stains accumulates subintimally in these vessels, and fibrinoid necrosis or degeneration affects the vascular walls. Weakening of the walls leads to aneurysmal bulges and to disruption of the lumen. This process, variously called lipohyalinosis or fibrinoid degeneration,[30] is most common in hypertensive patients and is identical to the vascular lesion found in the kidneys in hypertensive nephrosclerosis. Obliteration of the lumina of small penetrating vessels leads to distal ischemia and small infarcts (lacunae), usually within the basis pontis.

Embolism

Embolic occlusion within the posterior circulation most often affects the intracranial vertebral artery, the distal basilar bifurcation, or the posterior cerebral artery or its branches. Emboli that are large enough to traverse the vertebral artery usually pass through the larger basilar artery but become trapped distally within the basilar apex or its tributaries.[31] The most frequent loci of infarction are in the cerebellum and occipital lobes. In the Michael Reese Stroke Registry, approximately 20 percent of emboli affected the posterior circulation[32]; the posterior circulation accounts for about one fifth of the blood flow to the cranial contents. Emboli may arise from the heart or from occlusive disease more proximally within the vertebrobasilar system—so-called artery-to-artery emboli. In a series of 30 pathologically verified PCA occlusions studied by Castaigne and colleagues,[23] 15 represented artery-to-artery emboli in the form of atheromatous debris or clot originating in the proximal vertebral or basilar arteries. Embolization of clot from a stenosed or occluded vertebral artery has been well documented.[33–38]

Trauma and Dissection

The vertebral artery can be injured during sudden neck rotation or movement or after direct neck injury.[39–44] Chiropractic manipulation has caused pathologically and radiographically documented vertebral artery injury.[42] The most common location for injury is the third segment of the vertebral artery near C2 and C1 before the artery pierces the dura. Injury to the vascular intima of the vertebral artery activates clotting mechanisms, and thrombus forms in the distal vertebral artery. Clot may propagate or embolize to the distal basilar tree. Dissection of blood flow between the intima and media, formation of aneurysm,[45] and even perforation of the artery[43] have been noted. In most patients with traumatic dissection of the distal extracranial vertebral artery, the syndrome is unilateral, and ischemia is limited to the lateral medulla, pons, and ipsilateral cerebellum. When initial findings indicate bilateral brain stem ischemia, the course is often progressive and fatal.[41] In about one third of patients, ischemic symptoms develop at the time of neck motion or injury; in another third, symptoms develop minutes or days later; and in the last third, symptoms progress after onset.[43] Spontaneous dissections of the extracranial vertebral artery are unusual but have been reported.[46–56] The lesion is usually bilateral; the distal extracranial vertebral arteries are irregularly narrowed, especially in the horizontal segments that circle around C1. Long segmental narrowing (string sign) and aneurysmal pouches are common angiographic findings within the third segment of the vertebral artery. Occasionally, spontaneous or traumatic dissection can affect the first portion of the vertebral artery.[49]

Encroachment by osteophytes in the cervical spine on the extracranial vertebral artery is a common angiographic finding, particularly in elderly patients.[50] These lesions rarely cause vertebrobasilar symptoms in patients except in cases in which the contralateral vertebral artery is occluded or hypoplastic, and symptoms of brain-stem ischemia can be reproduced with particular head positions.[51] Some cases of postoperative cerebellar infarction may be related to prolonged, unusual head positions, resulting in transient stasis of blood flow in the vertebral artery.[52] After surgery, mobilization of the neck could allow embolization of the clot, resulting in posterior circulation infarction. Spontaneous dissection of the intracranial vertebral and basilar arteries has also been described.[57–61] Headache, neck pain, and subarachnoid hemorrhage are typical presentations, but patients with chronic dissecting aneurysms may develop symptoms from thrombosis and brain-stem ischemia.

MISCELLANEOUS VASCULAR PATHOLOGIES

Fibromuscular Dysplasia

Fibromuscular dysplasia of the vertebral arteries is less common than involvement of the ICA.[62] Vertebral artery dysplasia, when present, usually affects the distal vertebral artery between C3 and the posterior arch of the atlas. Angiographically, typical string-of-beads appearance with alternating zones of narrowing and dilatation are observed. Occasionally smooth concentric long regions of tubular stenosis or a diverticulum-like smooth or corregated outpouching of the vessels is seen. Osborn and Anderson[63] reviewed 25 of their own cases of fibromuscular dysplasia and found 6 with vertebral artery involvement, all bilateral and all accompanied by ICA disease. Rarely, the AICA[63] or PCA has fibromuscular dysplasia. Patients with extracranial or intracranial fibromuscular dysplasia have a predilection for accompanying intracranial aneurysms.[64–66]

Migraine

The basilar and posterior cerebral arteries seem to have a propensity for vasospasm. Classic migraine, with its somatosensory and visual symptoms and diminished blood flow to the posterior hemispheres, is a disorder of the PCAs. Basilar migraine has been described in young women.[67] I have seen a number of adults with intermittent symptoms related to the posterior circulation, generally lasting 30 to 90 minutes and usually unaccompanied by headache, with widely patent vertebral and basilar arteries. Spells in these adults have not been affected by heparin, warfarin, or antiplatelet agglutinating agents but have improved with administration of methysergide (Sansert) or phenytoin (Dilantin).[68] Some ischemic episodes that are difficult to explain may be migraine. In nine personally examined patients with migraine and posterior circulation ischemia, two had narrowing of the basilar artery and four had occlusion of the basilar artery.[69] In one patient with basilar artery occlusion, the vessel later reopened, as discovered on repeat studies.

Arteritis

Temporal arteritis[70, 71] and use of oral birth control pills[72] have been associated with stenosis or occlusion of the distal extracranial vertebral artery before dural penetration. Subclavian artery involvement in temporal arteritis is also well described[70, 73–75] and can cause subclavian steal syndrome.[75]

Sickle cell disease can cause occlusion of small and large vessels in the posterior circulation, usually with extensive intimal proliferation and fibrodysplasia.[76] Fungal and tuberculous meningitic basal exudates can lead to a reaction within the vessel that is usually called Huebner arteritis. Arteries within the interpeduncular fossa that supply the midbrain and thalamus are most often involved. Syphilis and polyarteritis nodosa can also affect posterior circulation vessels, but the loci of predilection have not been carefully studied because of the rarity of documented necropsy and angiographically studied cases.

Saccular Aneurysms

Saccular aneurysms are not especially common in the posterior circulation but accounted for 3.6 percent (64 of 1769) of aneurysms in a large series analyzed by Bull.[77] The most common posterior circulation sites for aneurysm are the basilar apex (about 60%), the vertebral-PICA junction (20%), and the basilar-SCA junction (11%). Aneurysms of the basilar apex may grow quite large, splaying the cerebral peduncles and producing considerable mass effect.

Basilar Artery Ectasia

Basilar artery ectasia is perhaps more common than saccular aneurysms and has distinctive radiographic and clinical features. Fusiform ectatic basilar arteries are visualized on computed tomography scan as focal bands of increased attenuation, with prominent enhancement after infusion of contrast agent. The enhancing band is usually curvilinear and occupies or crosses the cerebellar pontine angle.[78–80] MRI also identifies vertebrobasilar dolichoectasia and is superior at anatomic definition of brain stem or cranial nerve involvement.[80] These elongated dilated vessels produce symptoms by pressure and traction on cranial nerves and the brain stem. The orifices of branching vessels are also sometimes blocked by plaque or clot within the arteries, leading to TIA or stroke.[81–83] Occipital or neck ache, trigeminal distribution pain, hemifacial spasm, facial weakness, and tinnitus are frequent findings.[82] The larger fusiform ectatic basilar aneurysms may also compress the basis pontis or cerebral peduncles or present as cerebellopontile angle masses. Occasionally these lesions block the flow of cerebrospinal fluid, usually at the level of the third ventricle, and hydrocephalus develops.[81, 84] Vertebral artery giant aneurysms have also been reported; mass effect is usually lateral to the medulla and may be spinal.[85–87]

MAJOR DIFFERENCES BETWEEN THE ANTERIOR AND POSTERIOR CIRCULATIONS AND THEIR PATHOLOGY

The vertebral arteries form a paired system of vessels that unite to form a larger vessel. Such a configuration is very rare in the human body; one of the only other loci is also within the posterior circulation, where two small anterior spinal branches merge to form a larger single anterior spinal artery. By contrast, each ICA supplies one anterior cerebral hemisphere. Occlusion or hypoplasia of one vertebral artery is often tolerated well because of compensatory flow from the opposite side. If a distal vertebral artery becomes occluded, however, and the contralateral vertebral artery is hypoplastic or previously occluded, there may be serious problems because of the lack of reserve flow. When there are two arteries, the patient is usually safe when the first one fails but is seriously endangered when the second one fails.

The posterior circulation is blessed with very rich collaterals. In the neck, the frequent small vertebral branches and nearby external carotid and thyrocervical branches are ready to help reconstitute the vertebral artery if it blocks proximally. Occlusions usually occur over a short portion of the artery. By contrast, the ICA has no neck branches; when the ICA occludes at its orifice, clot frequently propagates up to its next branch, the intracranial ophthalmic artery. Collateral supply to the medullary, pontine, and mesencephalic tegmentam is rich, with supply coming from many small tributaries of various penetrating and circumferential branches. The tegmentum is often spared from ischemia even after basilar artery occlusion.

There is a higher frequency of congenital variations and retained fetal patterns in the posterior circulation. This can lead to vascular occlusive disease at an atypically young age. A congenital deficiency in some vessels also helps explain the extent of symptoms in some patients with seemingly minor occlusive disease.

In the posterior circulation, a much higher proportion of tissue is fed by small penetrating arteries. In the cerebral hemispheres, the cortex, because of its many convolutions, or gyri, far outmeasures in volume the gray matter and internal capsule of the basal nuclei, and receives blood flow from the large, external arteries. The deeper structures are fed by penetrating arteries. In the posterior circulation, however, the cerebellar cortex has a proportionately smaller volume, and so a higher proportion of the brain stem and cerebellar tissues is fed by penetrating vessels from the vertebral, basilar, and circumferential arteries. For this reason, lacunae are relatively more common in the posterior circulation, perhaps accounting for the fact that in many patients with posterior circulation infarcts, the disease follows a relatively benign course.[88]

Emboli less commonly go to the posterior circulation than to the anterior circulation. The posterior circulation receives only about 20 percent of the intracranial flow and probably receives approximately 20 percent of the emboli.[32] Emboli in the anterior circulation must often end up in branches of the middle cerebral artery. Similarly, in the posterior circulation, emboli go to the circumferential and PCA branches.

The geometry of the vertebral artery origin is quite different from that of the ICA. The common carotid artery leads directly (at about a 180-degree angle) to the ICA, a vessel of nearly the same caliber. By contrast, the vertebral arteries are much smaller than their parent subclavian arteries and arise at nearly a 90-degree angle. Less is known about the morphology and pathology of the origin of the vertebral artery, since direct endarterectomy is seldom performed and there are few surgical specimens. The differences in geometry should not lead to an assumption that the same morphology will be found in the ICA and vertebral arteries. More work must be done in this area before the pathology of proximal vertebral artery lesions is clarified. Does the proximal vertebral artery serve as a nidus for fibrin and platelet emboli?

SIGNS AND SYSTEMS OF POSTERIOR CIRCULATION ISCHEMIA

To understand and recall the signs and symptoms of posterior circulation ischemia, it is best to visualize the major anatomic structures and systems and their functions and to consider manifestations by anatomic and physiologic systems. There are few independent pathognomonic symptoms. Once a particular symptom is reported, the clinician should seek confirmation of location by searching for objective signs that can verify the system involved. We shall consider signs and symptoms in the same section because they should be thought of together by the physician attempting to localize the neurologic lesion.

Vestibulocerebellar System

The paired vestibular nuclei are located in the lateral medullary and pontine tegmenta. They have intimate connections with the flocculonodular lobes of the cerebellum. Ischemia of these structures causes vertigo or feelings of disequilibrium in the patient. Some patients complain of frank whirling dizziness or rotational turning, but others speak of swaying, falling, or being off balance. Dysfunction of the vestibular nuclei causes nystagmus, often rotatory. Usually the nystagmus is coarse and of larger amplitude when the patient looks toward the side of the lesion and of smaller amplitude and quicker when he or she looks toward the opposite side. Vertical nystagmus also results from lesions in the pontine tegmentum in the vicinity of the vestibular nuclei. The nystagmus can cause a sensation of objects moving in space.

Cerebellar ischemia causes a feeling of being off balance as well as difficulty with coordinated limb movement and walking. On examination, the most important abnormalities include leaning or veering when the patient is sitting or standing, gait ataxia and titubation, and difficulty in the performance of fine alternating movements of the limbs. A particularly useful diagnostic sign of cerebellar disease is to ask the patient to elevate both arms together rapidly, brake them quickly, and then drop the arms together again, stopping short of hitting the knees or a table. The arm ipsilateral to the cerebellar lesion usually lags behind the other arm but overshoots and rebounds as it reaches the target.

Extraocular Movements

The nucleus of the sixth cranial, or abducens, nerve lies near the midline in the pontine tegmentum, whereas the nuclei of the third and fourth cranial nerves lie more rostrally in the paramedian midbrain tegmentum. These nuclei and their corresponding cranial nerves are responsible for motor control of individual eye muscles. The medial longitudinal fasciculi coordinate lateral gaze and contain connections between the sixth nerve nucleus on one side and the contralateral third nerve nucleus; they also lie in the paramedian tegmentum from the medulla to the rostral midbrain. The paramedian pontine reticular formation, often called the pontine lateral gaze center, lies slightly more lateral in the pontine tegmentum. Connections with the abducens nucleus help generate conjugate gaze to the ipsilateral side. In the rostral midbrain tegmentum are various nuclei, including the rostral interstitial nucleus of the medial longitudinal fasciculi, that help coordinate upward and downward gaze. The most common symptom of ischemia to these eye control regions is diplopia. Less often, patients report tilting of the environment, moving of objects (oscillopsia), or difficulty in looking to the side.

Ischemia to the paramedian pontine reticular formation leads to a conjugate gaze palsy toward the side of the lesion. In a lesion of the left cerebral hemisphere, a patient with right hemiplegia might have eyes that deviate to the left and might be unable to look voluntarily to the right. In the pons, a patient with a paramedian left tegmental basal lesion might also have a right hemiplegia but would be unable to look left. Involvement of the medial longitudinal fasciculi leads to dysconjugate gaze paralysis; that is, the third and sixth nerves do not work in coordination on lateral gaze. A lesion of the left medial longitudinal fasciculus would cause a failure of adduction of the left eye when the patient looks right; nystagmus of the right abducting eye would also be present. Sometimes the medial longitudinal fasciculus and paramedian pontine reticular formation on the same side are involved together. The resulting eye movement is limited to abduction of the contralateral eye and has been called the one-and-a-half syndrome;[89] if each lateral gaze is scored as one, only one-half gaze is left. Lesions within the rostral vertical gaze centers would cause a failure of up or down gaze, sometimes with one or both eyes down, down and in, or overconverged. Lesions of the individual cranial nerves or their nuclei cause paralysis only of the muscles innervated by that nerve. Ocular skew, a condition in which there is constant vertical displacement of the two eyes in all gaze directions, can also be the result of tegmental brain-stem ischemia.

Vestibular and extraocular deficits are very important to recognize and understand, since they are invariably localized to the posterior circulation. Moreover, they are tegmental functions, analysis of which can pinpoint the rostrocaudal level of the lesion, that is, medulla versus pons or midbrain. Since the brain stem at its various levels has different vascular supplies, the location of the diseased vessel can often be predicted on the basis of knowledge of the region of ischemia.

Pupillary Abnormalities

The size of the pupils depends on the balance between sympathetic and parasympathetic innervation. The sympa-thetic system begins in the hypothalamus, from which fibers descend bilaterally in the lateral reticular formation of the brain stem. Parasympathetic pupilloconstricter fibers are located in the Edinger-Westphal nucleus of the oculomotor nerve in the region of the midbrain, just basal and lateral to the cerebral aqueduct. The pupillary reflex arc is located in the rostral brain stem; visual fibers from the optic tract go to the superior colliculus and then synapse in the third nerve. Abnormalities of the pupils are rarely noted by patients. Sympathetic dysfunction (usually resulting from lateral tegmental lesions) leads to small pupils. Lesions of the nuclei of the third nerve cause dilated fixed pupils with poor light reaction. When sympathetic and parasympathetic lesions are combined, the pupils are at midposition and fixed. In lesions of the rostral brain stem that interrupt the pupillary reflex arc, the pupils are unreactive. In more caudal lesions below the reflex arc, the pupils react normally.

Motor Deficits

The descending corticospinal tracts lie alongside one another in the base of the brain stem. A unilateral lesion of the base at any level, cerebral peduncle, basis pontis, or medullary pyramid causes paralysis of the opposite limbs, a hemiparesis. The face is affected if the lesion is high enough to include corticobulbar fibers to the facial nuclei in the pons. A bilateral lesion of the base will produce quadriparesis. Patients with vertebrobasilar ischemia may complain of unilateral or bilateral limb weakness or, less often, of alternating weakness, first of one side and then the other.

The seventh nerve nucleus in the lateral pontine tegmentum contains motor fibers that control motion of the ipsilateral face. The ambiguous nucleus just caudal, in the same tegmental location, controls the pharynx, palate, and larynx. The hypoglossal nucleus is a midline structure in the caudal medullary tegmentum. Lesions of these respective nuclei, or their cranial nerves, produce paralysis of the bulbar muscles that they control. Lesions of the facial nerve or its nucleus cause paralysis of the face that is often noted by the patient as difficulty in handling fluids in the mouth or inability to shut the eye. A particularly diagnostic finding is paralysis of one side of the face and motor paralysis of the opposite limbs, so-called crossed motor signs. Lesions of the ambiguous nucleus or of the ninth and tenth cranial nerves can cause hoarseness and dysphagia, with observable weakness of the pharynx, palate, or larynx. Lesions of the twelfth nerve cause slurred speech and paralysis of the ipsilateral tongue. Weakness of the bulbar muscles can result from dysfunction of either the individual motor nuclei described or of the descending corticobulbar fibers to these nuclei. Bilateral lesions of the corticofugal pyramidal system cause pseudobulbar paralysis, manifested by dysarthria, dysphagia, and weakness of the face, pharynx, palate, larynx, and tongue. Jaw, facial, and gag reflexes are often exaggerated, and emotional stimuli cause an overreaction of laughing or crying.

Sensory Abnormalities

The brain stem contains three sensory tracts of clinical importance, the spinal tract of V and spinal nucleus of V, the spinothalamic tract, and the medial lemniscus. The spinal tract and spinal nucleus of V are located in the lateral tegmentum of the medulla and pons. Ischemia in this region is sometimes associated with jabbing pain or heat in the ipsilateral eye or face, loss of the ipsilateral corneal reflex, and decreased pain and temperature perception in the ipsilateral face. Patients sometimes report numbness or lack of feeling in the face.

The spinothalamic tract also courses through the lateral tegmentum just lateral to the spinal tract and spinal nucleus of V. The effects of lesions of this tract are not usually recognized by the patient, but a loss of pin-prick and temperature sensibility in the contralateral limbs and trunk is detectable on examination. The leg fibers are most lateral in the spinothalamic tract and are adjacent to trunk fibers so a small lateral lesion might produce pain and temperature loss only in the opposite leg and lower trunk, with a sensory level on the trunk. Because of their proximity, the spinal tract of V and the spinothalamic tract share the effects of lesions of the lateral pontine and medullary tegmenta. A pathognomonic crossed sensory loss results, with diminished pain and temperature sensation in the face on one side and in the opposite limbs and trunk. Touch perception and position sense are spared in lateral tegmental lesions.

The medial lemniscus is a paramedian structure that courses through the brain stem just dorsal to the corticospinal fibers near the tegmentobasal junction. Lesions of the medial lemniscus are invariably combined with corticospinal tract dysfunction in cerebrovascular disease. Limb weakness and numbness are reported by the patient. Unlike in the cerebral cortex of higher animals like humans, where the more sophisticated sensory and motor regions (sometimes referred to as the homunculus) lie just behind one another in the precentral and postcentral gyri, motor and sensory control regions in the brain stem do not run parallel. Therefore, weakness of the left arm and leg might be accompanied by tingling of only the left arm. Dysfunction of the medial lemniscus is reported by the patient as tingling, prickling, or numbness of the body or limbs. Because the two medial lemnisci are adjacent to each other, bilateral numbness is frequent, which differentiates it from unilateral hemispheral disease. The medial lemnisci and spinothalamic tracts join in the upper brain stem on their way to the posterior ventral nuclei of the thalamus. Involvement of this sensory lemniscus or of the lateral thalamus causes decrease in all types of sensory function in the contralateral face, limbs, and trunk. Numbness or paresthesias of the affected parts results, with detectable decrease in the appreciation of touch, pain, temperature, and position-sense. Despite severe lesions of the lateral thalamus, sensory loss may be slight because of the diversion of sensory fibers to other systems, including the reticular formation.

Auditory Dysfunction

The auditory nuclei are located in the tegmentum of the lateral recess of the fourth ventricle near the pontomedullary junction. Auditory pathways, including the trapezoid body and the medial geniculate body, are also located within the brain stem. Occasionally patients with lateral tegmental pontine lesions (in the AICA territory) develop ipsilateral deafness. Bilateral tinnitus and hearing loss can occur with basilar artery occlusion, presumably because of ischemia involving the internal auditory arteries.[90]

Abnormalities of Visual Perception

The primary striate visual cortex is located on the banks of the calcarine fissure and is fed by the PCAs, the end tributaries of the basilar artery. When both PCAs are affected, as would happen if an embolus blocked both orifices, bilateral abnormalities of visual perception result. If only one PCA is affected, the symptoms and signs relate only to the contralateral visual field. Patients with unilateral striate infarcts usually report difficulty seeing to the opposite side; darkness, a shadow, grayness, and missing one half or part of objects are other descriptions used. The patient is usually aware of the visual loss. When the entire PCA territory on one side is infarcted, patients usually develop visual neglect and do not pay attention to objects in the contralateral visual field, a phenomenon not present in purely calcarine infarcts. As the visual-field defect develops, or as it starts to clear, visual hallucinations or scintillations can develop in the blind field.[91] Also, visual perservations in the blind field may develop.[31, 92] When the left posterior cerebral artery territory is involved, the patient may be unable to read but retains the ability to write or spell.[93–95] Examination of the patient with a unilateral PCA lesion reveals a homonymous hemianopia, sometimes with sparing of the macular region. When the left PCA territory is involved, the patient may be unable to name colors correctly or read words or phrases, although writing and letter- and number-naming are most often preserved.[93–95] Some patients with right PCA lesions cannot revisualize in their own minds what objects or people look like. When the visual-cortical ischemia is bilateral, cortical blindness and bilateral visual-field defects are observed.

Amnesia

The major cortical and subcortical structures subserving memory are supplied with blood by the basilar artery and PCAs. The Papez circuit, the traditional memory zone, includes the mammillary bodies, the mammillothalamic tract, the fornices, and the hippocampi. A bilateral lesion within this region usually causes permanent amnesia; that is, the patient cannot make new memories and has no recall for events after the stroke.[96, 97] Unilateral lesions within the dominant medial temporal lobe can also cause amnesia that lasts at least 6 months.[94, 95, 98] Usually the patient does not complain of the amnesia; it is generally noted by the spouse, friends, or associates. Amnesia is almost always accompanied by other findings, most often a hemianopia.

Headache

Headache is a prominent symptom in many patients with occlusive cerebrovascular disease and may precede other symptoms of ischemia.[99] Richard Bright in 1836 first called attention to posterior headache in patients with vascular disease.[68, 100] He described a patient with ''neck pain in the back of the head, like a rheumatic pain, generally at the same spot on the right side of the back part of the head.''[68] Steady or pulsatile headache is often located in the occiput and is unilateral in most patients with vertebral artery occlusion. The headache associated with vertebral occlusion is usually centered just below the external occipital protruberance and extends into the suboccipital neck regions close to the midline.[100] Headache can extend to the frontal region. In basilar occlusion, the headache is more often generalized but can also favor the occiput or top of the head. Patients with PCA occlusion frequently have pain in or just above the eyes. Table 10–1 lists the most prominent symptoms and signs of posterior circulation ischemia.

DIFFERENTIAL DIAGNOSIS

The symptoms and signs described relate generally to the brain stem, cerebellum, and posterior hemispheres, anatomic regions supplied by the vertebrobasilar arteries and their tributaries. Although these findings do suggest a pathologic anatomy, they are not disease-specific. Any illness that involves these structures could produce similar signs and symptoms. Dizziness is commonly caused by peripheral vestibular and labyrinthine disease. Multiple sclerosis can cause nystagmus, dysarthria, and gait ataxia. Posterior fossa tumors can cause prominent cranial-nerve and brain-stem symptoms. A posterior circulation vascular etiology is suggested (1) when the ecologic background is appropriate, for example, in an older patient with pre-existing diabetes, hypertension, or coronary or peripheral vascular disease; (2) when there is a characteristic tempo of illness, that is, onset after awakening, TIAs, or sudden, gradual, or stepwise accumulation of a deficit during a period of minutes, hours, or a few days (tumors and multiple sclerosis develop more gradually over weeks or months); and (3) on the basis of confirmatory laboratory features, especially computed tomography, magnetic resonance imaging, and angiography, with an infarct or hemorrhage visible on computed tomography scan verifying the vascular nature of the lesion (whereas a visualizable tumor would make a vascular etiology improbable).

Sometimes the symptoms of posterior circulation disease are not anatomically specific. Bilateral disease of the cerebral hemispheres, for example, resulting from near syncope or bilateral ICA occlusive disease, can produce dizziness, dim vision, or bilateral weakness or numbness. Objective signs are more important. Nystagmus, extraocular muscle palsy,

intranuclear ophthalmoplegia, and cerebellar signs cannot be mimicked by anterior circulation lesions. The constellation of symptoms may be more important than any single individual symptom. For example, dizziness unaccompanied by other central nervous system symptoms or signs that last for 6 weeks or more is rarely, if ever, the result of vertebrobasilar disease.[101] If, however, the dizziness were accompanied by diplopia and limb clumsiness occurring in spells, the diagnosis of posterior circulation ischemia would be clear cut. Dizziness is a particularly confounding symptom, since it can be caused by disease of many different regions.[102] Some investigators have emphasized the importance of so-called drop attacks, characterized by sudden loss of postural tone in the legs with the patient's dropping to the floor without loss of consciousness. Unfortunately, sudden falling can be caused by many pathophysiologic mechanisms and is a common reflex in the elderly. We have not found it particularly helpful as a localizing symptom. We do not know of a patient with definite vertebrobasilar occlusive disease in whom drop attacks were the only symptom.

PATTERNS OF POSTERIOR CIRCULATION DISEASE

Different portions of the vertebrobasilar arterial system supply specific anatomic loci (as emphasized in the section on anatomy). Lesions at different loci within the vascular system cause different symptoms and signs and different patterns of ischemia. The remainder of the chapter describes the most common clinical patterns. Further details of these syndromes have been described elsewhere.[68]

Occlusive Disease of the Subclavian and Proximal Extracranial Vertebral Arteries

In occlusive disease of the proximal vertebral artery system, the usual neurologic symptoms are transient spells of dizziness, altered vision, or diplopia. The lesions are relatively benign; TIAs are common but strokes are rare, probably because of the great potential for collateral circulation.

Disease of the subclavian artery proximal to the vertebral artery branch may cause posterior circulation ischemia. When both vertebral arteries are patent, blood sometimes courses from the opposite vertebral artery to the vertebral artery on the affected side and then travels retrograde down the vertebral artery to supply the ischemic arm. Fisher[11] called the siphonage of blood from the vertebral system to the arm the subclavian "steal" syndrome, a name that stuck. The most frequent symptoms associated with subclavian occlusive disease relate to the arm. Fatigue, claudication on exercise, paresthesia, sensitivity to cold, and heaviness or coolness of the arm are often reported. Severe ischemia of the arm is rare, probably because of the usually slow development of the lesion and because of the presence of rich collaterals. Headache is also a common symptom. Recurrent throbbing pain in the mastoid region radiating to the parietal and occipital areas was the most severe symptom of the first patient reported, that of Reivich and colleagues.[10] The most frequent neurologic symptom is dizziness or frank vertigo, usually described as a turning feeling or sensation

TABLE 10–1. Ischemia of the Posterior Circulation

Symptoms	Signs
Dizziness or vertigo	Nystagmus
Gait ataxia	Vertical gaze palsy
Inability to stand	Dysconjugate gaze
Bilateral limb weakness	Internuclear ophthalmoplegia
Alternating weakness on both sides of body	Ocular skew
	Bilateral limb weakness
Bilateral numbness	Crossed motor weakness (ipsilateral palsy of nerves VI, VII, XII and contralateral hemiparesis)
Crossed weakness	
Diplopia	
Crossed paresthesia or numbness	Crossed sensory loss (ipsilateral face and contralateral body)
Bilateral loss of vision	Unilateral gaze palsy (contralateral hemiparesis)
Poor memory	
Tinnitus or deafness	Palsy of nerve VI or VII
Difficulty seeing to one side	Hemianopia, bilateral hemianopia
Occipital or neck ache	Amnesia

of light-headedness, rocking, swaying, or tilting. Visual blurring often accompanies vertigo and is characterized by the sensation of objects moving or the inability to focus, probably because of vestibular dysfunction and nystagmus. Occasionally, bilateral dim vision is described. Diplopia was noted in about 15 percent of patients with subclavian steal syndrome in a combined series.[68] Perioral or limb numbness and unilateral or bilateral weakness occur, but infrequently. Hemiparesis and hemisensory loss are very rare.

On examination, the most important abnormalities relate to the ischemic arm. The blood pressure is generally at least 20 mm Hg lower on the involved side. The pulse is invariably small, absent, or difficult to palpate in the arm on the involved side, compared with the opposite arm. The arm or hand may feel cool or appear more cyanotic than the opposite arm when both are held above heart level. A bruit is sometimes audible over the supraclavicular area. Sometimes the bruit radiates to the ipsilateral mastoid process; vertebral bruits can be bilateral because of the increased flow in the opposite vertebral artery. Another helpful sign is production of arm or cerebral ischemia by exercising of the arm with the diminished pulse.

Diagnosis is usually possible by noninvasive means. In fact, subclavian steal patients are now commonly discovered when they are referred to laboratories performing noninvasive studies for peripheral vascular disease, bruit, or extracranial vascular disease, and the ischemia to the arm is discovered incidental to the major complaint.[103] Forearm blood flow measurements by oscillography, venous occlusive arm plethysmography, and Doppler techniques are all usually diagnostic. Liljequist and associates[104] documented abnormalities of directional Doppler ultrasonography at the level of the transverse process of the atlas in 22 patients with angiographically verified subclavian steal syndrome. The relative velocity of pulse-wave propagation in the two arms is another useful test; a delay in propagation correlates well with angiographically confirmed subclavian stenosis or occlusion.[105] Digital angiography or standard arterial angiography remains the definitive diagnostic technique.

The left subclavian artery is involved three times more frequently than the right innominate or subclavian arteries in occlusive disease. Subclavian occlusive disease is not always associated with retrograde vertebral flow. Only 10 of 20 patients studied by Berguer and coworkers[105] showed evidence of reversal of vertebral artery flow. Left subclavian steal syndrome is relatively benign; although TIAs are common, brain stem infarcts are exceedingly rare. However, patients with subclavian steal syndrome usually have severe atherosclerosis and may have severe accompanying disease of the ICAs in the neck.[103, 106] In all cases of hemiplegia in patients with subclavian steal syndrome appropriate ICA lesions have been present, or the ICA contralateral to the hemiparesis has not been visualized angiographically. In a review of 53 patients with verified subclavian steal syndrome, 15 had unilateral motor or sensory attacks or deficits; of these, 10 had severe disease of the contralateral ICA. In the other 5, insufficient angiographic details were available about the appropriate ICA-MCA system.[106]

Disease of the right subclavian artery, although less common, is more serious because of occasional involvement of the right ICA. The right innominate artery usually rises higher in the supraclavicular fossa than its left counterpart

does. A clot in the right subclavian or axillary artery may propagate into the innominate artery and embolize to the right ICA or intracranial anterior circulation, causing a left hemiplegia. Cervical rib syndrome,[107, 108] ununited arm fracture with chronic pain,[109] the use of crutches, and trauma can all cause the initial right subclavian artery lesion. Baseball pitchers, perhaps because of the repetitive throwing motion that their arms perform, are particularly susceptible to subclavian disease.

The most common cause of subclavian occlusive disease is atherosclerosis. Congenital lesions such as preductal coarctation of the aorta associated with patent ductus arteriosus, atresia of the left subclavian artery, or pseudocoarctation of the aorta with a kinked left subclavian artery[110] occasionally cause this syndrome. Sometimes subclavian steal syndrome develops following surgical manipulation of the subclavian artery, as in the Blalock-Taussig operation for repair of the tetralogy of Fallot. Takayasu disease and temporal arteritis[75] have also been implicated.

The neurologic symptoms in patients with stenosis or occlusion of the vertebral artery at its origin are virtually identical to those reported by patients with subclavian steal syndrome. TIAs are common, but frank strokes are much rarer. Surgeons have performed ligation of the vertebral artery to treat subclavian steal syndrome without causing important posterior circulation ischemia. Fisher reported five patients with bilateral occlusions at the origin of the vertebral artery.[111] All patients had TIAs, but only one patient had persistent neurologic signs, and that patient also had occlusion of the ICA at the siphon on the appropriate side to explain the symptoms.[111]

Intracranial embolism had been documented in a number of patients with occlusion or severe stenosis of the vertebral artery origin.[23, 37, 38, 68, 112] The comparable situation in the anterior circulation is well known, that is, a patient who presents with the sudden onset of symptoms referable to middle cerebral artery branch occlusion. At angiography, the ICA on the same side is shown to be occluded, the clot presumably arising from the fresh occlusion and embolizing intracranially. Undoubtedly, a fresh clot at the vertebral artery orifice can also embolize. The most common recipient sites of emboli from the vertebral artery origin are the intracranial vertebral artery (commonly involving the PICA), the distal basilar artery, the SCA, and the PCA.[112] Traumatic occlusion of the proximal or second segment of the vertebral artery is less benign, presumably because of the rapid onset that allows little time for collaterals to develop and because of the frequency of intimal injury and clot formation.

The morphology of vertebral artery atherosclerosis has not been studied in as much detail as ICA disease has because of the rarity of vertebral endarterectomy. Proximal vertebral artery disease is known to be rare in black persons.[27] It is unknown whether ulceration of the proximal vertebral artery with fibrin-platelet emboli occur.[113] Digital subtraction angiography is usually adequate to visualize severe disease of the origin of the vertebral artery. A diagnostic digital subtraction angiogram is pictured in Figure 10–3. Real-time B-mode ultrasonography and color-coded Doppler imaging allow noninvasive assessment of the extracranial vertebral arteries in a manner similar to that used in carotid noninvasive studies.[114, 115] Ultrasonography of the vertebral

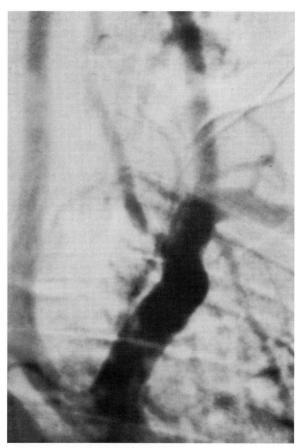

FIGURE 10–3. Digital subtraction angiogram showing stenosis of the proximal vertebral artery at its origin.

artery origin is technically more difficult but may be a useful diagnostic tool.

Occlusive Disease of the Distal Extracranial and Intracranial Vertebral Arteries

Occlusive disease of the distal vertebral arteries most often causes ischemic symptoms referrable to the lateral medulla and cerebellum. Knowledge of the findings in patients with lateral medullary and cerebellar infarction should allow the clinician to recognize distal vertebral artery disease.

Knowledge of the anatomy of the lateral medulla will help the physician understand the symptoms and signs of ischemia. Currier and coworkers[116] analyzed the most frequently involved regions of the lateral medulla; their report includes a diagrammatic section of the medulla demonstrating the lesion. The structures affected as well as their signs and symptoms are as follows:

Spinal tract and nucleus of V. Ischemia to this nucleus causes, on the side of the lesion, sharp pain or a burning sensation in the face, facial numbness, decreased corneal reflex, and loss of pin-prick and temperature sensibility on the face.

Vestibular nuclei. Ischemia to this region causes vertigo and nystagmus that are usually coarse and rotational to the side of the lesion.

Descending sympathetic fibers. In ischemia of the lateral reticular formation, there is ipsilateral ptosis and meiosis.

Spinothalamic tract. Patients do not usually report abnormal sensation or loss of sensation, but diminished pin-prick and temperature perception are present in the opposite trunk and limbs on testing. If the lesion extends medially, it may also involve the quintothalamic fibers that have crossed from the opposite side. In that case, the entire contralateral body and face are affected. The patients can, however, differentiate between the sensory loss related to the descending trigeminal complex and that related to the quintothalamic tract.

Ambiguous nucleus. This structure is also rather medially placed in the tegmentum and is often spared in superficial lesions. This motor nucleus controls pharangeal, laryngeal, and palatal movement; dysfunction usually produces dysphagia and hoarseness. Food or secretions become caught in the piriform recess, and often a high-pitched crowing cough is used to extricate the material. The ipsilateral pharynx does not elevate well, and ipsilateral vocal cord paralysis can be detected by laryngoscopy.

Restiform body. Also called the inferior cerebellar peduncle, this structure contains fibers from the vestibular nuclei and spinocerebellar tracts going into the cerebellum. Lesions of this tract cause clumsiness of the ipsilateral limbs and poor sitting and standing balance. The patient leans, veers, or lurches toward the side of the lesion.

Dorsal motor nucleus of the vagus nerve. Involvement of this parasympathetic nucleus or of the descending sympathetic fibers causes prominent autonomic signs and symptoms.

Tachycardia, labile blood pressure, and postural hypotension are noted in lateral medullary ischemia. Vomiting is another common accompaniment, probably because of involvement of the vomiting center in the floor of the fourth ventricle or in relationship to the vertigo and vestibular dysfunction. Ondine's curse, a failure of automatic breathing when the patient is asleep, is usually the result of bilateral lateral pontine or medullary lesions but has been reported after unilateral lateral medullary infarction.[117]

Lateral medullary ischemia is sometimes combined with infarction of the cerebellum, in which case there is a higher fatality risk. The swollen cerebellum may compress the fourth ventricle and cause fatal brain stem compression and hydrocephalus. Headache, head tilt, and decreased alertness are clues that the cerebellum as well as the lateral medulla is ischemic.

Often infarction is limited to the cerebellum, and the brain stem remains unscathed. Cerebellar infarction is difficult to diagnose clinically. Some patients complain of occipital and neck ache or of neck stiffness. When the cerebellum is quite swollen, patients may resist head movement and hold their necks stiffly and, often, tilted. Gait ataxia is a most important abnormality. Most often, the patients cannot walk well and at times are unable to sit or stand without help. Classic cerebellar signs, such as finger-to-nose ataxia, intention tremor, and toe-to-object ataxia, are often not present. Arm rebound on rapid elevation or depression of the outstretched arms is probably the result of hypotonia and is common. Sometimes the lower extremity deep tendon reflexes are exaggerated and pendular, despite flexor plantar responses. Vomiting is also common.

Cerebellar infarction is a potentially mortal lesion when the infarct is large and edematous. When cerebellar swelling occurs, patients usually develop some decrease in the level of alertness and an increase in the incidence of headache. Bilateral extensor plantar reflexes, horizontal conjugate gaze palsy to the side of the lesion, and ipsilateral or bilateral sixth nerve palsies are other signs of brain-stem compression and are indications for urgent treatment. The computed tomography scan can be very helpful diagnostically but, in our experience, may not show the infarct immediately or even during the first 24 hours. Figure 10–4 shows a computed tomography scan and the brain of a patient who died of a hemorrhagic cerebellar infarction after the development of pressure. Key features on a computed tomography scan indicative of pressure are obliteration or shift of the fourth ventricle and obliteration of the cerebellopontile and ambient cisterns, in addition to hypodensity in the cerebellum. On computed tomography or magnetic resonance imaging scans, it is very important to identify the fourth ventricle and observe the cisternal structures.

The most common underlying vascular lesion in patients with lateral medullary or cerebellar infarction or both is occlusive disease of the distal extracranial or intracranial vertebral artery before the PICA branch. The extracranial vertebral artery is most often injured during neck turning or chiropractic manipulation. The timing of symptoms has been described in the section on vascular pathology under the heading Trauma and Dissection. Headache and neck pain are common and are usually posteriorly located. Angiography shows dissection or occlusion of the vertebral arteries near C1. Spontaneous dissection produces a syndrome indistinguishable from trauma, is usually bilateral, and demonstrates similar angiographic findings.[49] In fact, the only distinction may be that the causative trauma was minor or considered too inconsequential to report. In traumatic spontaneous dissection, the risk of infarction is greatest at or shortly after the dissection. Fresh thrombus propagates or embolizes from the point of injury. With time, dissections heal, and the lumen usually returns to normal. Sometimes a telltale aneurysmal pouch remains as a marker of the injury.

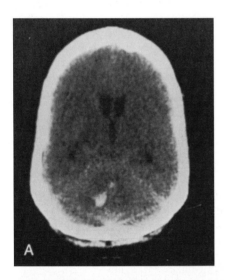

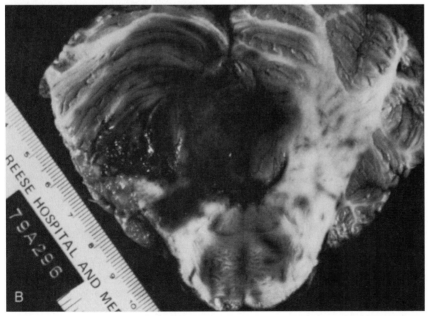

FIGURE 10–4. *A,* Computed tomography scan showing hemorrhagic infarct in the left cerebellum. Note obliteration of cisterns. *B,* Brain at postmortem examination.

Figure 10–5 is an angiogram from a patient with bilateral spontaneous vertebral dissections.

The intracranial vertebral artery lesion most often results from atherosclerosis, which can produce severe stenosis just after the artery pierces the dura (Fig. 10–6). Fisher et al. and associates[33] showed that the most frequent vascular lesion studied at necropsy in patients with lateral medullary infarction is occlusion of the intracranial vertebral artery before the PICA branch. Sypert and Alvord[118] showed that a similar vascular lesion was responsible for cerebellar infarction in a necropsy study. Others have confirmed the preponderance of PICA territory cerebellar infarction.[119, 120] In black patients, occlusion of the PICA branch is probably more common than occlusion of the parent artery.[27] Black patients and Asian patients have similar patterns of occlusion that are different from those in white patients. At times the distal vertebral artery lesion blocks flow into the anterior spinal artery branch of the vertebral artery. A medial medullary infarct results, which is characterized by contralateral hemiparesis, usually sparing the face, and paralysis of the ispilateral tongue. Numbness or tingling of the contralateral limbs is due to ischemia to the medial lemniscus, which is located medially just dorsal to the medullary pyramid and ventral to the twelfth nerve nucleus. Medial and lateral ischemia can be combined in patients with vertebral occlusion, a contralateral hemiparesis being added to symptoms and signs of lateral medullary ischemia.[33, 121, 122] The occluded thrombosed vertebral artery can also serve as the nidus of embolization to the more distal basilar artery tree. Vertebral artery occlusion and cerebellar infarction can also be caused by embolism from the heart or proximal subclavian-vertebral system.

Although unilateral intracranial vertebral artery lesions are sometimes relatively well tolerated, bilateral lesions almost always cause severe ischemia.[123] Unilateral severe vertebral artery stenosis or occlusion can have bilateral manifestations if the opposite vertebral artery is hypoplastic or had been previously occluded. Patients with bilateral occlusion of the intracranial vertebral artery are often hypertensive or diabetic or both. Symptoms or signs evolve very gradually, sometimes taking up to 2 months.[124] Posturally related symptoms are common.[124, 125] When the patient sits or stands erect, collateral flow is decreased sufficiently to cause an attack or increase the pre-existing deficit. In nine personally studied cases of bilateral distal vertebral artery occlusions, the patients' conditions worsened despite anticoagulation therapy. Other investigators have treated patients surgically by creating an occipital-to-PICA shunt,[126–129] and stabilization or improvement resulted. Ischemic symptoms are usually referable to the medulla and cerebellum. Bilateral pyramidal and cerebellar dysfunction are present. Failure of automatic respiration is also more common after bilateral lateral medullary lesions[124] and can be the cause of death. Respiratory monitoring of these patients is very important.

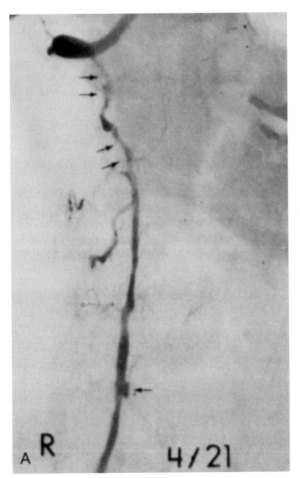
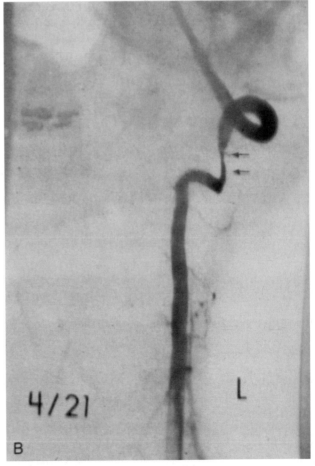

FIGURE 10–5. Bilateral "spontaneous" vertebral artery dissections. *A*, Right vertebral artery, lateral view. *B*, Left vertebral artery, lateral view.

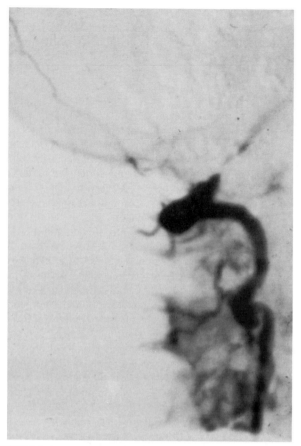

FIGURE 10–6. Lateral view of severe stenosis of the vertebral artery just after piercing the dura to begin its intracranial course.

Occlusion of the Proximal or Midbasilar Artery

Kubik and Adams[1] considered basilar occlusion a mortal disease. We now know that there is a wide spectrum of deficit, from TIA to severe quadriplegia and death. The basilar artery supplies the pons; the most vulnerable region in the pons is the pontine base bilaterally. The tegmentum and lateral regions of the brain stem and cerebellar hemispheres are usually protected because of collateral circulation. Collateral circulation usually flows from the vertebral arteries to the PICAs and then around the cerebellum to AICA or SCA branches. Blood also travels through the ICAs into the posterior communicating arteries to supply the rostral basilar segments. Occlusion of the basilar artery is most often caused by thrombosis superimposed on atherosclerotic narrowing.

Basilar artery occlusion is often heralded by TIAs characterized by dizziness and by alternating or bilateral numbness or weakness. The stroke usually develops in the morning or when the patient rises from a nap and may fluctuate or progress over 24 to 96 hours.[37, 130] Progression after 4 days is unusual.[130, 131] A posturally related increase in symptoms is common during the initial week.[125] Conjugate horizontal gaze palsies, one-and-a-half syndrome, and ocular bobbing[132] are ocular motor signs indicating tegmental pontine damage. The arms and legs are often weak bilaterally and extensor toe signs are bilateral. The locked-in syndrome is a term used to describe patients with severe bulbar and limb paralysis who are unable to communicate because of paralysis but are awake and alert.[133, 134] Patients with bilateral medial tegmental ischemia are usually comatose.[135] Survival depends on the development of collateral circulation. The diagnosis of basilar artery occlusion can only be made with certainty by angiography. Occasionally, occlusion of basilar artery branches bilaterally can cause bilateral infarction of the basis pontis and can mimic occlusion of the basilar artery.[29]

Occlusive Disease of Penetrating Basilar Branches and Lacunae

Differentiation of small-vessel disease from occlusive disease of larger vessels (vertebral or basilar arteries) is crucial for prognosis and choice of therapy. Branch occlusion in the posterior circulation is usually caused by a plaque within the basilar artery obliterating a branch or by a microatheroma obstructing the orifice of the branch.[28, 136] Lacunar infarcts are usually caused by fibrinoid degeneration and obliteration of the wall of a branch.[30] The most common lacunar syndromes in the posterior circulation are pure motor hemiparesis caused by a lacune in the basis pontis,[137] ataxic hemiparesis caused by a lacune in the pons or midbrain,[138] dysarthria-clumsy hand syndrome caused by a small lesion in the medial pons,[139] and pure sensory stroke caused by a thalamic lacune.[140, 141]

The two most commonly occluded branches are the median pontine penetrating artery and the thalamogeniculate artery. Occlusion of the former leads to contralateral hemiparesis, sometimes accompanied by contralateral paresthesia, or an ipsilateral intranuclear ophthalmoplegia or conjugate gaze paresis. The lesion causing this syndrome would have to be limited to the territory of one penetrating branch. Occlusion of the thalamogeniculate artery causes contralateral hemisensory symptoms and clumsiness and ataxia of the contralateral limbs.[142, 143] In the lateral thalamus are located the ventral posterior medial and lateral nuclei, which are way stations for somatosensory input, and the ventral anterior and ventral lateral nuclei, which are way stations for basal ganglia and cerebellar connections. Disruption of these motor pathways causes hemichorea and hemiataxia on the same side as the sensory symptoms. Computed tomography occasionally documents a small infarct in the lateral thalamus. Although other branch disease might be predicted, there has been no pathologic confirmation except for the reports of Fisher and Caplan[28] and Fisher.[29] Figure 10–7 is a diagrammatic representation of the mechanism and common loci of branch disease.

Disease of Long Circumferential Cerebellar Arteries

The PICA, AICA, and SCA course around the brain stem at medullary, pontine, and mesencephalic levels, respectively. Ischemia within the territory of these arteries is most often the result of occlusion of the parent arteries. MRI of the posterior fossa reveals characteristic lesions in cerebellar stroke that allow identification of the vessel involved.[144] PICA territory infarcts are mostly caused by vertebral artery occlusion. SCA territory infarcts are most often due to distal

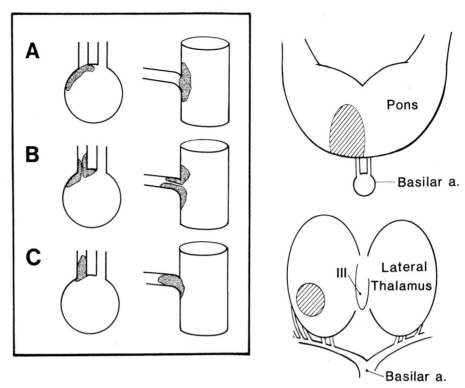

FIGURE 10–7. Diagram of mechanism of branch disease and its most frequent sites in the thalamus and pons. *A,* Basilar artery plaque. *B,* Junctional plaque in basilar artery extending into a branch. *C,* Branch atheroma with clot. (Drawn by Harriet Greenfield; used with permission.)

basilar artery embolism with blockage of the orifice of this branch. Only AICA territory infarction is most often due to occlusion of this branch. Occlusive disease of branches, so-called microatheroma, is more common in black persons than in white persons.[27]

The signs and symptoms of PICA infarction have already been described under lateral medullary and cerebellar infarction. The AICA supplies an identical area more rostral in the pons at the level of the facial nucleus. The core territory involves the middle cerebellar peduncle,[145] which can be easily seen by magnetic resonance imaging. Also, the internal auditory artery usually branches from the AICA, so that vertigo and unilateral hearing loss may rarely represent TIAs in the AICA territory.[146] Ipsilateral facial palsy and ipsilateral deafness are clues that the lesion is lateral pontine and not medullary.[147, 148] Other common findings include dizziness, ipsilateral facial numbness, and hemiataxia.

Isolated SCA infarcts are rare, and the clinical findings associated with SCA infarction are often overshadowed by associated lesions involving the PICA and the rostral basilar territory.[149–152] Most SCA infarcts are caused by cardiogenic or artery-to-artery embolism, which accounts for the frequent association with other areas of infarction, particularly in the rostral basilar territory. Because the lesion is above the spinal tract of V, the ipsilateral facial pain and loss of facial sensibility found in PICA territory lesions are not seen. Instead, there is contralateral hemisensory loss usually affecting pain and temperature sensations. In more rostral lesions, touch and position sense are also affected because of involvement of the medial lemniscus after merger of the spinothalamic tracts. Ipsilateral cerebellar limb dysfunction with spontaneous slow involuntary arm movements and dysmetria are also found. Dysarthria is a common finding and a Horner syndrome or ipsilateral sixth nerve palsy can be

seen with involvement of the pontine tegmentum. Deafness can also occur because of the involvement of fibers afferent to the medial geniculate body. The lesion is above the seventh, eighth, and tenth nerve nuclei; thus, weakness related to these nerves is not found in SCA territory infarcts.

Distal Basilar Artery Occlusion

Blockage of the basilar apex is most often embolic but can be due to intrinsic occlusive disease, especially in black patients.[27] The resulting clinical syndrome has been described as the top of the basilar syndrome.[31, 153, 154] Infarction is usually in the midbrain and thalamus in the distribution of penetrating vessels and in PCA territory unilaterally or bilaterally. When ischemia is limited to the brain stem, the principal findings relate to abnormalities of eye movement, level of alertness and consciousness, and behavior. Eye signs include limited upward or downward gaze,[155] hyperconvergence of the eyes sometimes accompanied by spasms,[156] failure of eye abduction (pseudo-sixth-nerve palsy),[31] retraction of the upper eyelids, skew deviation of the eyes, and small poorly reacting pupils. Bilateral third nerve palsies can also occur.[157, 158]

The rostral reticular formation is in the medial thalamus adjacent to the third ventricle and is supplied by rostral basilar artery penetrating branches. Tatemichi and colleagues[154] described the clinical findings in 11 patients with infarcts limited to this vascular distribution, which they termed "paramedian thalamopeduncular infarction." Four patients presented with stupor and coma at onset due to bilateral thalamic infarction, and one developed severe persistent amnesia. A number of the other patients had a combination of change in mental status and oculomotor dysfunction.

Persistent memory loss[159] and peduncular hallucinations[160] can also occur from infarctions in the thalamus and rostral brain stem.

Posterior Cerebral Artery Occlusive Disease

The PCA territory includes the occipital lobe and the inferior and medial portions of the temporal lobe. Various branches of the PCA supply specific regions and are usually identifiable by computed tomography.[161] Occlusion of PCA branches is most often embolic,[23, 162] but intrinsic disease of the PCA does occur,[163] especially in black persons.[27] Angiography is necessary to make this distinction. The most important abnormalities in patients with PCA infarcts relate to vision, memory, sensation, higher cortical function, and behavior.

Vision

Infarction of the striate cortex or the geniculocalcarine tract causes a homonymous hemianopia in the contralateral visual field. The patient is usually aware of the deficit and describes it as darkness or as a void to one side. Sparing of the macular zone is common. At times, the visual defect is partial; for example, it affects only color recognition, in which case the deficit is called a hemiachromatopsia. This defect is discovered by testing of the visual fields with confrontation using a colored pin. Scintillations can herald the visual field defect or may occur as the lesion is receding.[91, 164] Visual perseverations may develop as well after partial clearing of the visual deficit.[31] When the lateral occipital lobe or entire PCA territory is infarcted, the patient neglects the opposite side of visual space, especially in the case of right PCA infarcts. Optokinetic nystagmus is preserved in infarcts limited to striate cortex but is lost in large lesions extending into the parietal lobe.[31, 165] Memory defects have been described in the section on amnesia.

Higher Cortical Function Abnormalities

Left PCA lesions can cause Gerstmann syndrome (agraphia, left-right confusion, finger agnosia, and dyscalculia) by undercutting the angular gyrus.[95, 166] Alexia without agraphia is a striking syndrome that has been extensively described in the literature.[93–95] Anomic aphasia,[95] transcortical sensory aphasia,[167] and associative visual agnosia[95, 168] are other findings associated with left PCA infarction. In right PCA infarction, defective revisualization of objects and dreams devoid of visual imagery have been described. Hemisensory loss is also common and is caused by ischemia to the ventrolateral thalamus or to sensory fibers traveling in the temporal and parietal lobes toward the primary and secondary somatosensory cortex.[31] Figure 10–8 is a representative computed tomography scan of a patient with unilateral PCA territory infarction.

Bilateral infarcts are almost always caused by thrombosis or embolism of the basilar artery distally. The clinical setting of their development and the behavioral aspects of this syndrome make diagnosis difficult. Bilateral ischemia of the limbic cortex results in an agitated delirium in which patients are very hyperactive and restless.[169, 170] Agitation and com-

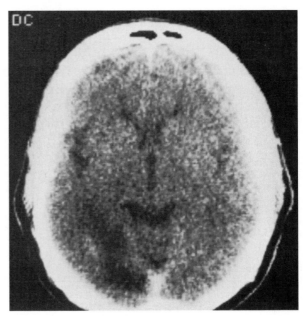

FIGURE 10–8. Computed tomography scan showing left posterior cerebral artery territory infarct.

plete lack of ability to make new memories (amnesia) leads to the patients' being completely unable to give any account of their problems. We have seen several such patients suddenly go berserk on a medical ward, most having been admitted for cardiac complaints. A psychiatrist is usually called, and sometimes an acute psychosis is diagnosed. When the patient is carefully examined, the presence of cortical blindness and amnesia clarifies the nature of the lesion. Cortical blindness is due to bilateral infarction of the calcarine cortex.[171] Often patients with this affliction deny that they are blind or are unaware of it (Anton syndrome). When the lower banks of the calcarine cortex are infarcted, bilateral upper quadrant visual-field defects, prosopagnosia[172] (difficulty matching or recognizing faces), and defects of color vision result.[173, 174]

An important constellation of signs in bilateral PCA disease is called Balint syndrome.[175] Knowledge of its features is very helpful in diagnosis of posterior hemispheral disease. Findings include simultanagnosia, optical ataxia, and apraxia of gaze.

Simultanagnosia

Patients see things piecemeal; they may see part of a letter or picture or object. If several objects are held before them, they will notice only one, belatedly seeing another if they change the direction of their gaze. They are unable to read, as they omit words and phrases. The patient can be tested for simultanagnosia by being made to read a paragraph, look at a picture, or enumerate the number of objects or numbers on a piece of paper while the physician watches.

Optical Ataxia

The patient cannot direct the arm in coordination with vision and reaches past things.[176] This defect can be tested by the physician's asking the patient to point to an object in

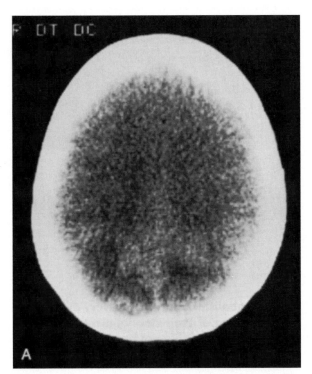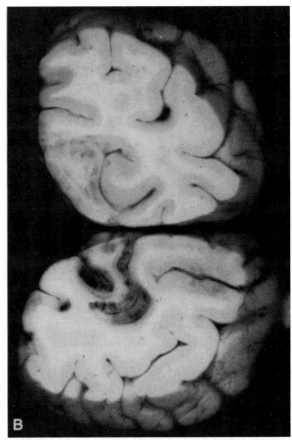

FIGURE 10–9. *A,* Computed tomography scan showing bilateral posterior cerebral artery territory lucency. *B,* Brain at postmortem examination, showing bilateral posterior cerebral artery hemorrhagic infarction.

the room or on a picture or to trace with a pencil over a line drawing.

Apraxia of Gaze

These patients cannot look where they want to or where the physician has asked them to direct their gaze. The patient should be asked to look first at the extended right thumb, then at the left thumb as the physician observes the patient's gaze.

Detection of PCA disease relies heavily on tests of visual function. The human brain is highly developed visually. To omit testing of the visual fields and visual behavior in a patient with central nervous system disease would be like failing to examine the heart or lungs of a medical patient. Computed tomography can often verify the bilateral PCA territory hypodensity (Fig. 10–9).

Motor Weakness

Infarcts resulting from proximal PCA occlusion can clinically mimic middle cerebral artery territory infarction.[177] Since penetrating branches from the proximal PCA supply the cerebral peduncle and the lateral thalamus, occlusion at this level can cause hemiplegia (cerebral peduncle), sensory loss (thalamus), and hemianopia (occipital lobe).

REFERENCES

1. Kubik C, Adams R: Occlusion of the basilar artery: A clinical and pathologic study. *Brain.* 1946;69:73.
2. Fisher CM: Occlusion of the internal carotid artery. *Arch Neurol Psychiatr.* 1951;65:345.
3. Hutchinson E, Yates P: The cervical portion of the vertebral artery. A clinico-pathological study. *Brain.* 1956;79:319.
4. Hutchinson E, Yates P: Caratico-vertebral stenosis. *Lancet.* 1957;i:2.
5. Denny-Brown D: Basilar artery syndromes. *Bull N Engl Med Cent.* 1953;15:53.
6. Fang H, Palmer J: Vascular phenomena involving brainstem structures. *Neurology (NY).* 1956;6:402.
7. Williams D: The syndromes of basilar insufficiency. In Garland H, ed. *Scientific Aspects of Neurology.* Baltimore: Williams & Wilkins; 1961;202.
8. Williams D, Wilson T: The diagnosis of the major and minor syndromes of basilar insufficiency. *Brain.* 1962;85:741.
9. Millikan C, Siekert R: Studies in cerebrovascular disease. The syndrome of intermittent insufficiency of the basilar arterial system. *Mayo Clin Proc.* 1955;30:61.
10. Reivich M, Holling E, Roberts B, et al: Reversal of blood flow through the vertebral artery and its effect on cerebral circulation. *N Engl J Med.* 1961;265:878.
11. Fisher CM: A new vascular syndrome: ''The subclavian steal.'' *N Engl J Med.* 1961;265:912. Editorial.
12. North R, Fields W, DeBakey M, et al: Brachial-basilar insufficiency syndrome. *Neurology (NY).* 1962;12:810.
13. Patel A, Toole J: Subclavian steal syndrome: Reversal of cephalic blood flow. *Medicine (Baltimore).* 1965;44:289.
14. Siekert R, Millikan C, Whisnant J: Reversal of blood flow in the vertebral arteries. *Ann Intern Med.* 1964;61:64.
15. Caplan L: Vertebrobasilar disease: Time for a new strategy. Modern Concepts in Cerebrovascular Disease. XV(3): 1980. *Stroke.* 1981;12:111.
16. Caplan L: Treatment of cerebral ischemia: Where are we headed? *Stroke.* 1984;15:571.
17. Caplan L: Are terms such as completed stroke or RIND of continued usefulness? *Stroke.* 1983;14:431.
18. Fields WS: Collateral circulation in cerebrovascular disease. In Vinken P, Bruyn

G, eds. *Handbook of Clinical Neurology,* Vol 11. Amsterdam: North-Holland; 1972;168.

19. Gillilan L: Anatomy and embryology of the arterial system of the brainstem and cerebellum. In Vinken P, Bruyn G, eds. *Handbook of Clinical Neurology,* Vol 11. Amsterdam: North-Holland; 1972;24.

20. Szdzuy D, Lehman R: Hypoplastic distal part of the basilar artery. *Neuroradiology.* 1972;4:118.

21. Lie T: Congenital malformations of the carotid and vertebral arterial systems, including the persistent anastamoses. In Vinken P, Bruyn G, eds. *Handbook of Clinical Neurology,* Vol 12. Amsterdam: North-Holland; 1972;289.

22. Baker A, Iannone A: Cerebrovascular disease. I. The large arteries of the circle of Willis. *Neurology (NY).* 1959;9:321.

23. Castaigne P, Lhermitte F, Gautier J, et al: Arterial occlusions in the vertebral-basilar system. *Brain.* 1973;96:133.

24. Fisher C, Gore I, Okabe N, et al: Atherosclerosis of the carotid and vertebral arteries: Extracranial and intracranial. *J Neuropathol Exp Neurol.* 1965;24:455.

25. Moosy J: Morphology, sites and epidemiology of cerebral atherosclerosis. *Proc Assoc Res Nerv Men Dis.* 1966;51:1.

26. Pessin MS, Gorelick PB, Kwan ES, Caplan LR: Basilar artery stenosis: Middle and distal segments. *Neurology.* 1987;37:1742.

27. Gorelick P, Caplan L, Hier D, et al: Racial differences in the distribution of posterior circulation occlusive disease. *Stroke.* 1985;16:785.

28. Fisher CM, Caplan L: Basilar artery branch occlusion: A cause of pontine infarction. *Neurology (NY).* 1971;21:900.

29. Fisher CM: Bilateral occlusion of basilar artery branches. *J Neurol Neurosurg Psychiatr.* 1977;40:1182.

30. Fisher CM: The arterial lesions underlying lacunes. *Acta Neuropathol.* 1967;12:1.

31. Caplan L: "Top of the basilar" syndrome: Selected clinical aspects. *Neurology (NY).* 1980;30:72.

32. Caplan L, Hier D, D'Cruz I: Cerebral embolism in the Michael Reese Stroke Registry. *Stroke.* 1983;14:530.

33. Fisher CM, Karnes W, Kubik C: Lateral medullary infarction: The pattern of vascular occlusion. *J Neuropathol Exp Neurol.* 1961;20:323.

34. McCusker E, Rudick R, Honch G, et al: Recovery from the locked-in syndrome. *Arch Neurol.* 1982;39:145.

35. Fisher CM, Karnes WE: Local embolism. *J Neuropathol Exp Neurol.* 1965;24:174.

36. George B, Laurian C: Vertebro-basilar ischemia with thrombosis of the vertebral artery: Report of two cases with embolism. *J Neurol Neurosurg Psychiatr.* 1982;45:91.

37. Caplan L: Occlusion of the vertebral or basilar artery. *Stroke.* 1979;10:277.

38. Caplan L, Rosenbaum A: Role of cerebral angiography in vertebrobasilar occlusive disease. *J Neurol Neurosurg Psychiatr.* 1975;38:601.

39. Ford F, Clark D: Thrombosis of the basilar artery with softenings in the cerebellum and brainstem due to manipulation of the neck. *Bull Johns Hopkins Hosp.* 1956;98:37.

40. Heros R: Cerebellar infarction resulting from traumatic occlusion of a vertebral artery. *J Neurosurg.* 1979;51:111.

41. Kreuger B, Okazaki H: Vertebral-basilar distribution infarction following chiropractic cervical manipulation. *Mayo Clin Proc.* 1980;55:322.

42. Robertson J: Neck manipulation as a cause of stroke. *Stroke.* 1981;12: 1.

43. Sherman D, Hart R, Easton JD: Abrupt change in head position and cerebral infarction. *Stroke.* 1981;12:2.

44. Katirji M, Reinmuth O, Latchaw R: Stroke due to vertebral artery injury. *Arch Neurol.* 1985;43:242.

45. Pawl G, Shaw C, Wray L: True traumatic aneurysm of the vertebral artery. *J Neurosurg.* 1980;53:101.

46. Fisher CM, Ojemann R, Roberson G: Spontaneous dissection of cervico-cerebral arteries. *J Can Sci Neurol.* 1978;5:9.

47. Ringel S, Harrison S, Norenberg M, et al: Fibromuscular dysplasia: Multiple "spontaneous" dissecting aneurysms of the major cranial arteries. *Ann Neurol.* 1977;1:301.

48. Goldstein S: Dissecting hematoma of the cervical vertebral artery. *J Neurosurg.* 1982;56:451.

49. Caplan L, Zarins C, Hermatti H: Spontaneous dissection of the extracranial vertebral artery. *Stroke.* 1985;16:1030.

50. Meyer JS, Sheehan S, Bauer RB: An arteriographic study of cerebrovascular disease in man. *Arch Neurol.* 1960;2:27.

51. Rosengart A, Hedges T, Teal PA, et al: Intermittent downbeat nystagmus due to vertebral artery compression. *Neurology.* 1993;43:216.

52. Tettenborn B, Caplan LR, Sloan MA, et al: Postoperative brainstem and cerebellar infarcts. *Neurology.* 1993;43:471.

53. Bladin P: Long segment stenotic lesions of cervical arteries in cerebrovascular disease. *Proc Aust Assoc Neurol.* 1974;11:13.

54. Bradac G, Kaernbach A, Bolk-Weischedel D, et al: Spontaneous dissecting aneurysm of cervical cerebral arteries. *Neuroradiology.* 1981;21:149.

55. Mas J, Goeau C, Bousser M, et al: Spontaneous dissecting aneurysm of the internal carotid and vertebral arteries: Two case reports. *Stroke.* 1985;16:125.

56. Mokri B, Houser DW, Sandok BA, Piepgras DG: Spontaneous dissections of the vertebral arteries. *Neurology.* 1988;38:880.

57. Allen G, Cohen R, Preziosi T: Microsurgical endarterectomy of the intracranial vertebral artery for vertebrobasilar transient ischemic attacks. *Neurosurgery.* 1981;81:56.

58. Watson AJ: Dissecting aneurysm of arteries other than the aorta. *J Pathol Bacteriol.* 1956;72:439.

59. Wolman L: Cerebral dissecting aneurysms. *Brain.* 1959;82:276.

60. Escourolle R, Gautier J, Rosa A, et al: Aneurysme dissequant vertebro-basilaire. *Rev Neurol.* 1972;128:95.

61. Caplan LR, Baquis GD, Pessin MS, et al: Dissection of the intracranial vertebral artery. *Neurology.* 1988;38:868.

62. Houser OW, Baker H, Sandok B, et al: Cephalic arterial fibromuscular dysplasia. *Radiology.* 1971;101:605.

63. Osborn A, Anderson R: Angiography spectrum of cervical and intracranial fibromuscular dysplasia. *Stroke.* 1977;8:617.

64. Frens D, Petajan J, Anderson R, et al: Fibromuscular dysplasia of the posterior cerebral artery: Reports of a case and review of the literature. *Stroke.* 1974;5:161.

65. Handa J, Kamijo Y, Handa H: Intracranial aneurysms associated with fibromuscular hyperplasia of the renal and internal carotid arteries. *Br J Radiol.* 1970;43:483.

66. Mettinger K: Fibromuscular dysplasia and the brain. II. Current concepts of the disease. *Stroke.* 1982;13:53.

67. Bickerstaff E: Basilar artery migraine. *Lancet.* 1961,i:15.

68. Caplan L: Vertebrobasilar occlusive disease. In Barnett H, Mohr J, Stein B, Yatsu F, eds. *Stroke: Pathophysiology, Diagnosis and Management.* New York: Churchill Livingstone; 1986;549.

69. Caplan LR: Migraine and vertebrobasilar ischemia. *Neurology.* 1991;41:55.

70. Goodwin J: Temporal arteritis. In Vinken P, Bruyn G, eds. *Handbook of Clinical Neurology,* Vol. 39. Amsterdam: North-Holland; 1980;313.

71. Wilkinson I, Russel R: Arteries of the head and neck in giant cell arteritis. *Arch Neurol.* 1972;27:378.

72. Bickerstaff E: *Neurological Complications of Oral Contraceptives.* Oxford: Clarendon Press; 1975.

73. Hamrin B: Polymyalgia arteritica with morphological changes in the large arteries. *Acta Med Scand.* 1972;533(suppl):4.

74. Klein R, Hunder G, Stanson A, et al: Large artery involvement in giant cell (temporal) arteritis. *Ann Intern Med.* 1975;83:806.

75. Pollock M, Blennerhassett J, Clarke A: Giant cell arteritis and the subclavian steal syndrome. *Neurology (NY).* 1973;23:653.

76. Merkel K, Grinsberg P, Parker J, et al: Cerebrovascular disease in sickle cell anemia: A clinical, pathological, and radiological correlation. *Stroke.* 1978;9:45.

77. Bull J: Contribution of radiology to the study of intracranial aneurysms. *Br Med J.* 1962;2:1701.

78. Deeb Z, Janetta P, Rosenbaum A, et al: Tortuous vertebrobasilar arteries causing cranial nerve syndromes: Screening by computed tomography. *J Comput Tomogr.* 1965;3:774.

79. Moseley I, Holland I: Ectasia of the basilar artery; the breadth of the clinical spectrum and the diagnostic value of computed tomography. *Neuroradiology.* 1979;18:83.

80. Giang DW, Perlin SJ, Monajati A, et al: Vertebrobasilar dolichoectasia: Assessment using MR. *Neurology.* 1988;30:518.

81. Hirsh L, Gonzalez C: Fusiform basilar aneurysm simulating carotid transient ischemic attacks. *Stroke.* 1979;10:598.

82. Denny-Brown D, Foley J: The syndrome of basilar aneurysm. *Trans Am Neurol Assoc.* 1952;77:30.

83. Pessin MS, Chimowitz MI, Levine SR, et al: Stroke in patients with fusiform vertebrobasilar aneurysms. *Neurology.* 1989;39:16.

84. Ekbom K, Greitz T, Kugelberg E: Hydrocephalus due to ectasia of the basilar artery. *J Neurol Sci.* 1969;8:465.

85. Ashbury A: Case records of the Massachusetts General Hospital (case 27–1969). *N Engl J Med.* 1969;281:34.

86. Barrows L, Kubik C, Richardson E: Aneurysms of the basilar and vertebral arteries. A clinico-pathologic study. *Trans Am Neurol Assoc.* 1956;81:181.

87. Sundt T, Piepgras D, Houser O, et al: Interposition saphenous vein grafts for advanced occlusive disease and large aneurysms in the posterior circulation. *J Neurosurg.* 1982;56:205.

88. Chambers BR, Norris J, Hackinski V, et al: Favorable influences in stroke survival. *Neurology (NY).* 1983;33(suppl 2):163.

89. Fisher C: Some neuro-opthalmological observations. *J Neurol Neurosurg Psychiatr.* 1967;30:383.

90. Huang MH, Huang CC, Ryu SJ, Chu NS: Sudden bilateral hearing impairment in vertebrobasilar occlusive disease. *Stroke.* 1993;24:132.

91. Kolmel H: Complex visual hallucinations in the hemianopic field. *J Neurol Neurosurg Psychiatr.* 1985;48:29.

92. Critchley M: Perseveration in the domain of vision. In Locke S, ed. *Modern Neurology.* Boston: Little Brown; 1969;347.

93. Dejerine J: Contribution à l'étude anatomo-pathologique et clinique des différentes variétés de cecite verbale. *CR Soc Biol (Paris).* 1892;4:61.

94. Geschwind N, Fusillo M: Color naming deficits in association with alexia. *Arch Neurol.* 1965;18:137.

95. Caplan L, Hedley-White T: Cueing and memory dysfunction in alexia without agraphia. *Brain.* 1974;97:251.

96. Victor M, Angevine J, Mancall E, et al: Memory loss with lesions of hippocampal formation. *Arch Neurol.* 1961;5:244.

97. Symonds C: Disorders of memory. *Brain.* 1966;89:624.

98. Mohr J, Leicester J, Stoddard L, et al: Right hemianopia with memory and color deficits in circumscribed left posterior cerebral artery territory infarction. *Neurology (NY).* 1971;21:1104.

99. Mohr J, Caplan L, Melski J, et al: The Harvard Cooperative Stroke Registry: A prospective registry. *Neurology (NY).* 1978;28:754.

100. Fisher CM: Headache in cerebrovascular disease. In Vinken P, Bruyn G, eds. *Handbook of Clinical Neurology.* Vol. 5. Amsterdam: North-Holland; 1968;124.

101. Fisher CM: Vertigo in cerebrovascular disease. *Arch Otolaryngol.* 1967;85:529.
102. Caplan L: Treatment of the dizzy patient. *Drug Ther.* 1983;8:40.
103. Hennerici M, Klemm C, Rautenberg W: The subclavian steal phenomenon: A common vascular disorder with rare neurologic deficits. *Neurology.* 1988;38:669.
104. Liljequist L, Ekerstrom S, Nordhus O: Monitoring direction of vertebral artery blood flow by Doppler shift ultrasound in patients with suspected subclavian steal. *Acta Chir Scand.* 1981;147:421.
105. Berguer R, Higgins R, Nelson R: Non-invasive diagnosis of reversal of vertebral artery blood flow. *N Engl J Med.* 1980;302:1349.
106. Baker R, Rosenbaum A, Caplan L: Subclavian steal syndrome. *Contemp Surg.* 1974;4:96.
107. Symonds C: Two cases of thrombosis of subclavian artery with contralateral hemiplegia of sudden onset, probably embolic. *Brain.* 1927;50:259.
108. Hoobler S: The syndrome of cervical rib with subclavian lateral thrombosis and hemiplegia due to cerebral embolism. *N Engl J Med.* 1942;226:942.
109. Yates A, Guest D: Cerebral embolism due to an ununited fracture of the clavicle and subclavian thrombosis. *Lancet.* 1928;ii:225.
110. Lochaya S, Kaplan B, Shaffer AB: Pseudocoarctation of the aorta will bicuspid aortic valve and kinked left subclavian artery, a possible cause of subclavian steal. *Am Heart J.* 1967;73:369.
111. Fisher CM: Occlusion of the vertebral arteries. *Arch Neurol.* 1970;22:13.
112. Caplan LR, Amarenco P, Rosengart A, et al: Embolism from vertebral artery origin occlusive disease. *Neurology.* 1992;42:1505.
113. Caplan L: Extracranial vertebral artery: Progress in cerebrovascular disease. *Stroke.* 1984;19:25.
114. Weinberger J: Non-invasive imaging of the cervical vertebral artery in the diagnosis of vertebrobasilar insufficiency. *J Stroke Cerebrovasc Dis.* 1991;1:21.
115. Trattnig S, Hübsch P, Schuster H, Pölzleitner D: Color-coded Doppler imaging of normal vertebral arteries. *Stroke.* 1990;21:1222.
116. Currier R, Giles C, DeJong R: Some comments on Wallenberg's lateral medullary syndrome. *Neurology (NY).* 1962;12:778.
117. Levin B, Margolis G: Acute failure of automatic respirations secondary to a unilateral brainstem infarct. *Ann Neurol.* 1977;1:583.
118. Sypert G, Alvord E: Cerebellar infarction: A clinicopathological study. *Arch Neurol.* 1975;32:357.
119. Duncan G, Parker S, Fisher CM: Acute cerebellar infarction in the PICA territory. *Arch Neurol.* 1975;32:364.
120. Lehrich J, Winkler G, Ojemann R: Cerebellar infarction with brainstem compression: Diagnosis and surgical treatment. *Arch Neurol.* 1970;22:490.
121. Duffy P, Jacobs G: Clinical and pathologic findings in vertebral artery thrombosis. *Neurology (NY).* 1958;8:862.
122. Hauw J, Der Agopian P, Trelles L, et al: Les infarctus bulbaires. *J Neurol Sci.* 1976;28:83.
123. Caplan LR, Pessin MS, Scott RM, et al: Poor outcome after lateral medullary infarcts. *Neurology.* 1986;36:1510.
124. Caplan L: Bilateral distal vertebral artery occlusion. *Neurology (NY).* 1983;33:552.
125. Caplan L, Sergay S: Positional cerebral ischemia. *J Neurol Neurosurg Psychiatr.* 1976;39:385.
126. Sundt T, Whisnant J, Piepgras D, et al: Intracranial bypass grafts for vertebral basilar ischemia. *Mayo Clin Proc.* 1978;53:12.
127. Roski R, Spetzler R, Hopkins L: Occipital artery to posterior inferior cerebellar artery bypass for vertebrobasilar ischemia. *Neurosurgery.* 1982;10:44.
128. Hopkins L, Budney J, Spetzler R: Revascularization of the rostral brainstem. *Neurosurgery.* 1982;10:364.
129. Ausman J, Nicoloff D, Chou S: Posterior fossa revascularization anastamosis of vertebral artery to PICA with interposed radial artery graft. *Surg Neurol.* 1978;9:281.
130. Jones HE, Millikan C, Sandok B: Temporal profile (clinical course) of acute vertebrobasilar system cerebral infarction. *Stroke.* 1980;11:173.
131. Patrick B, Ramirez-Lassepas M, Snyder B: Temporal profile of vertebrobasilar territory infarction. *Stroke.* 1980;11:643.
132. Fisher CM: Some neuro-opthalmical observations. *J Neurol Neurosurg Psychiatr.* 1967;30:383.
133. Kemper T, Romanul F: State resembling akinetic mutism in basilar artery occlusion. *Neurology (NY).* 1967;17:74.
134. Plum F, Posner J: *The Diagnosis of Stupor and Coma,* 3rd ed. Philadelphia: FA Davis; 1980.
135. Chase T, Moretti L, Prensky A: Clinical and electroencephalographic manifestations of vascular lesions of the pons. *Neurology (NY).* 1968;18:357.
136. Caplan LR: Intracranial branch atheromatous disease: A neglected, understudied, and underused concept. *Neurology.* 1989;39:1246.
137. Fisher CM: Pure motor hemiplegia of vascular origin. *Arch Neurol.* 1965;13:30.
138. Fisher CM: Ataxic hemiparesis: A pathologic study. *Arch Neurol.* 1978;35:126.
139. Fisher CM: A lacunar stroke: The dysarthria-clumsy hand syndrome. *Neurology (NY).* 1967;17:614.
140. Fisher CM: Thalamic pure sensory stroke: A pathologic study. *Neurology (NY).* 1978;28:1141.
141. Fisher CM: Pure sensory stroke and allied conditions. *Stroke.* 1982;13:434.
142. Dejerine J, Roussy G: Le syndrome thalamique. *Rev Neurol.* 1906;14:521.
143. Caplan LR, DeWitt D, Pessin MS, et al: Lateral thalamic infarcts. *Arch Neurol.* 1988;45:959.
144. Amarenco P: The spectrum of cerebellar infarctions. *Neurology.* 1991;41:973.
145. Amarenco P, Hauw JJ: Cerebellar infarction in the territory of the anterior and inferior cerebellar artery. *Brain.* 1990;113:139.
146. Oas JG, Baloh RW: Vertigo and the anterior inferior cerebellar artery syndrome. *Neurology.* 1992;42:2274.
147. Adams R: Occlusion of the anterior inferior cerebellar artery. *Arch Neurol Psychiatr.* 1943;49:765.
148. Atkinson WJ: The anterior inferior cerebellar artery. *J Neurol Neurosurg Psychiatr.* 1949;12:137.
149. Amarenco P, Hauw JJ: Cerebellar infarction in the territory of the superior cerebellar artery. *Neurology.* 1990;40:1383.
150. Kase CS, Norrving B, Levine SR, et al: Cerebellar infarction: Clinical and anatomic observations in 66 cases. *Stroke.* 1993;24:76.
151. Davison C, Goodhart S, Savitsky N: The syndrome of the superior cerebellar artery and its branches. *Arch Neurol Psychiatr.* 1935;33:1143.
152. Mills CK: Hemianesthesia to pain and temperature and loss of emotional expression on the right side with ataxia of the upper limb on the left. *J Nerv Ment Dis.* 1908;35:331.
153. Mehler MF: The rostral basilar artery syndrome: Diagnosis, etiology, prognosis. *Neurology.* 1989;39:9.
154. Tatemichi TK, Steinke W, Duncan C, et al: Paramedian thalamopeduncular infarction: Clinical syndromes and magnetic resonance imaging. *Ann Neurol.* 1992;32:162.
155. Christoff N: A clinicopathological study of vertical eye movements. *Arch Neurol.* 1974;31:1.
156. Gay A, Brodkey J, Miller J: Convergence retraction nystagmus. *Arch Ophthalmol.* 1963;70:456.
157. Facon E, Steriade M, Werthein N: Hypersomnie prolongée engendrée per des lésions bilatérales du systéme activateur medial: Le syndrome thrombotique de la bifurcation du tronc basilaire. *Rev Neurol.* 1958;98:117.
158. Segarra J: Cerebral vascular disease and behavior. I. The syndrome of the mesencephalic artery. *Arch Neurol.* 1970;22:408.
159. Malamut BL, Graff-Radford N, Chawluk J, et al: Memory in a case of bilateral thalamic infarction. *Neurology.* 1992;42:163.
160. McKee AC, Levine DN, Kowall NW, et al: Peduncular hallucinosis associated with isolated infarction of the substantia nigra pars reticularis. *Ann Neurol.* 1990;27:500.
161. Kinkle W, Newman R, Jacobs L: Posterior cerebral artery branch occlusions: CT and anatomic considerations. In Berguer R, Bauer R, eds. *Vertebrobasilar Arterial Occlusive Disease.* New York: Raven Press; 1984;117.
162. Pessin MS, Lathi ES, Cohen MB, et al: Clinical features and mechanism of occipital infarction. *Ann Neurol.* 1987;21:290.
163. Pessin MS, Kwan ES, DeWitt LD, et al: Posterior cerebral artery stenosis. *Ann Neurol.* 1987;21:85.
164. Brust J, Behrens M: Release hallucinations: As the major symptom of posterior cerebral artery occlusion. A report of 2 cases. *Ann Neurol.* 1977;2:432.
165. Smith JL: *Optokinetic Nystagmus.* Springfield, IL: Charles C Thomas; 1963;69.
166. Critchley M: *The Parietal Lobes.* London: WA Arnold; 1953.
167. Kertesz A: Association of visual agnosia and trancortical sensory aphasia. *Ann Neurol.* 1982;12:96.
168. Rubens A, Benson D: Associative visual agnosia. *Arch Neurol.* 1971;24:305.
169. Horenstein S, Chamberlin W, Conomy J: Infarction of the fusiform and calcarine regions: Agitated delerium and hemianopia. *Trans Am Neurol Assoc.* 1962;92:357.
170. Medina J, Rubino F, Ross E: Agitated delirium caused by infarction of the hippocampal formation and fusiform and lingual gyri. *Neurology (NY).* 1974;24:1181.
171. Symonds C, MacKenzie I: Bilateral loss of vision from cerebral infarction. *Brain.* 1957;80:415.
172. Damasio A, Damasio H, Van Hoesen G: Prospagnosia: Anatomic basis and behavioral mechanisms. *Neurology (NY).* 1982;32:331.
173. Damasio A, Yamada T, Damasio H, et al: Central achromatopsia: Behavioral, anatomic and physiologic aspects. *Neurology (NY).* 1980;30:1064.
174. Pearlman A, Birch J, Meadows J: Cerebral color blindness: An acquired defect in hue discrimination. *Ann Neurol.* 1979;5:253.
175. Hecaen H, DeAjuriaguerra J: Balint's syndrome (psychic paralysis of visual fixation) and its minor forms. *Brain.* 1954;77:373.
176. Damasio A, Benton A: Impairment of hand movements under visual guidance. *Neurology (NY).* 1979;27:170.
177. Chambers BR, Brooder RJ, Donnan GA: Proximal posterior cerebral artery occlusion simulating middle cerebral artery occlusion. *Neurology.* 1991;41:385.

Ophthalmic Manifestations of Cerebrovascular Disease

11

ROBERT S. HEPLER and ROBERT D. YEE

Recognition of the carotid arteries as the major source of stroke is a surprisingly recent event. In 1951, Fisher published an article in which he stated that "recent clinical and pathological studies have led me to the conclusion that thrombosis of the internal carotid artery . . . may well prove to be one of the major causes of apoplexy."[1] Prior to his observations, intrinsic middle cerebral occlusion was considered the major cause of stroke. Fisher emphasized the great significance of amaurosis fugax, particularly when combined with contralateral weakness or sensory change, as an indicator of carotid disease.

Another milestone was the publication in 1961 of Hollenhorst's article on bright plaques in retinal arterioles.[2] Hollenhorst noted a nearly 10 percent incidence of visible plaques in the retinal arterioles of 235 patients with proven occlusive carotid disease. He concluded that the physician should look for such plaques and, upon finding them, should refer the patient for an evaluation of the cardiovascular system.[2] A Hollenhorst plaque is shown at the bifurcation of a retinal arteriole in Figure 11–1. Small plaques such as this one might be found in patients without visual symptoms but are of the same diagnostic importance as plaques found in patients with symptoms.

Another important aspect of the relationship between the eye and the carotid artery was identified by Kearns and Hollenhorst in 1963.[3] Their article and others since 1963 describing other ocular manifestations of poor blood flow to the eye have increased the awareness of visual symptoms and ophthalmic signs as important clues to the existence of carotid and vertebrobasilar disease.

VASCULAR SUPPLY OF THE EYE AND VISUAL PATHWAYS

The arterial blood supply of the eyeball and the optic nerve within the orbit is derived from the ophthalmic artery, which is the first branch of the internal carotid artery after it exits the cavernous sinus. Details of the vascular supply to the retina and optic disk are highly relevant to our topic. The ophthalmic artery enters the orbit through the optic canal and gives off a branch called the central retinal artery. This artery penetrates the sheaths of the intraorbital portion of the optic nerve about 10 mm behind the globe and runs forward to the eye within the center of the nerve. The central retinal artery is shown within the optic nerve and at the optic nerve head in Figure 11–2. The central retinal artery usually divides into superior and inferior branches, which can be seen within the cup (the physiologic excavation) of the disk. A second division occurs at or near the disk, creating nasal and temporal retinal arteries. The vessels lose their muscular coats after the second branching and are then arterioles in size and anatomy.

The retinal arterioles continue to branch dichotomously and do not have anastomoses. The capillary beds then supply the inner half of the retina, including the bipolar cells, the retinal ganglion cells, and their axons within the nerve fiber layer. There is little overlap between the capillary beds of adjacent arteriolar branches. Occlusion of the superior branch of the central retinal artery results in loss of the lower visual field (inferior altitudinal hemianopia). The visual-field defect will have a border precisely at the horizontal meridian, and pale swelling of the inner layers of the retina due to ischemia of the ganglion cells and their axons will end at the horizontal meridian. The capillary beds of the superior and inferior artery branches meet at this meridian and do not overlap. Most episodes of monocular amaurosis fugax are caused by transient obstruction of the central retinal artery or its branches by emboli. When emboli are detected on funduscopy, they are within retinal arteries or arterioles.

The short posterior ciliary arteries arise from the ophthalmic artery and further divide into many small branches that penetrate the eye at the insertion of the optic nerve and adjacent areas in the back of the globe. The short posterior ciliary arteries provide the main source of arterial flow to the capillary plexus of the optic nerve head. The central retinal artery and the arterial pial plexus of the retrobulbar optic nerve also contribute to the capillary plexus of the nerve head (see Fig. 11–2).[4, 5] Occlusion of the short posterior ciliary arteries causes the pale swelling of the optic disk seen in anterior ischemic optic neuropathy.

A cilioretinal artery has been observed in 14 to 50 percent of humans. This vessel probably originates from a branch of a short posterior ciliary artery, is located at the temporal margin of the optic disk, and supplies part of the central area of the retina called the macula (see Fig. 11–2). Central vision can be spared in some patients with obstruction of the central retinal artery, since the cilioretinal artery is not a branch of the central retinal artery.

The orbital portion of the optic nerve is supplied by ophthalmic artery branches that form a capillary plexus within the pia mater of the nerve. Anastomoses are common between branches of the ophthalmic artery and branches of the middle meningeal artery (external carotid artery) within the orbit. Therefore, the external carotid artery can be the major or sole source of arterial blood flow to the eye and intraorbital optic nerve in the presence of obstruction of the internal carotid artery.

The retrobulbar and intracanalicular segments of the optic nerve are supplied by branches from the internal carotid artery. Branches from the internal carotid artery, anterior cerebral artery, and anterior communicating artery provide arterial perfusion to the intracranial optic nerve. The optic chiasm has a large collateral arterial blood supply, fed by branches from the internal carotid, anterior cerebral, anterior communicating, basilar, posterior communicating, and posterior cerebral arteries. Infarction of the chiasm is unusual because of its rich collateral supply. The anterior choroidal artery and other branches of the internal carotid artery perfuse the optic tract. The lateral geniculate body is supplied by the anterior and posterior choroidal arteries. Branches of the middle cerebral artery and of the posterior cerebral artery

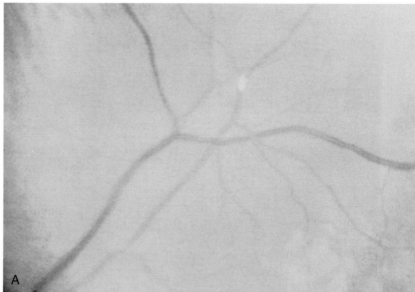

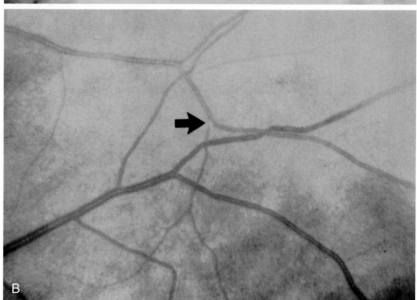

FIGURE 11-1. Bright plaques of Hollenhorst are sometimes easy to visualize (A) but sometimes require meticulous search of the fundi (B).

serve the superior and inferior optic radiations, respectively. The visual cortex of the occipital lobe is perfused primarily by branches of the posterior cerebral artery. However, the middle cerebral artery contributes to an extensive system of collateral vessels at the pole of the occipital lobe. This collateral blood flow accounts for the sparing of central vision in some patients with ischemia of the occipital lobes.

The choroid and the outer retinal layers in the back of the eye are supplied by branches of the short posterior ciliary arteries. The remainder of the choroid, outer retinal layers, and anterior segment of the eye (ciliary body, iris, and cornea) are supplied by the long posterior ciliary arteries and anterior ciliary arteries, which are also branches of the ophthalmic artery. Obstruction of flow within the ophthalmic artery can result in ischemia of the entire globe. The venous flow from the eye (central retinal vein, anterior and posterior ciliary veins, and vortex veins) and orbit enters the cavernous sinus via the superior and inferior ophthalmic veins. Arteriovenous communications in carotid-cavernous fistulas cause distention and arterialization of veins of the eye and orbit.

SYMPTOMS

Ophthalmic symptoms of cerebrovascular disease can be divided into amaurosis fugax and the vertebrobasilar equivalent of transient homonymous visual disturbance; fixed visual reduction due to infarction of the retina or optic nerve or both; fixed peripheral field loss due to temporal, parietal, or occipital lobe infarction; low-pressure glaucoma; and symptoms of the ocular ischemia syndrome.

Amaurosis fugax (transient monocular loss of vision) is often the first symptom of vascular obstructive disease. In the overwhelming majority of cases, amaurosis fugax is not associated with symptoms of ischemia of the contralateral hemisphere. Therefore, although clinicians should ask the patient about such symptoms, they should not be led astray by a response that the patient has not experienced contralateral weakness, sensory change, or clumsiness during amaurosis fugax. Amaurosis fugax typically lasts only a few seconds to a very few minutes—less than five. It may be perceived as a graying out or even a blacking out of vision

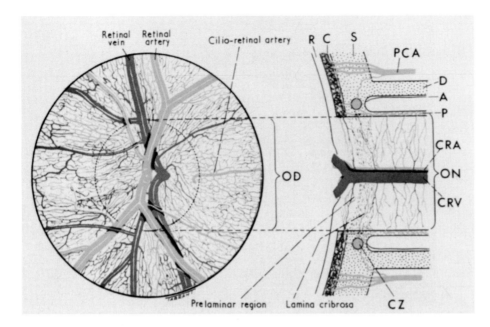

FIGURE 11–2. Diagram of the vascular supply of the optic nerve head and the retina. A, arachnoid; C, choroid; CRA, central retinal artery; CRV, central retinal vein; CZ, circle of Zinn and Haller; D, dura; OD, optic disk; ON, optic nerve; P, pia; PCA, posterior ciliary arteries; R, retina; S, sclera. (From Hayreh SS: Blood supply of the optic nerve and its role in optic neuropathy, glaucoma, and oedema of the optic disk. *Br J Ophthalmol* 1969;53:721. Published by BMJ Publishing Group.)

in one eye. Usually the occurrences are spontaneous, without identifiable postural associations or other predisposing factors. When it is caused by marginal perfusion past a major carotid obstructive lesion, amaurosis fugax is likely to be a repetitive constriction of the field from the periphery to the center of vision of the involved eye. On the other hand, when amaurosis fugax is caused by showers of soft emboli, the attacks are extremely abrupt and the area of visual impairment varies from episode to episode, depending on which retinal and optic nerve arterioles are transiently occluded. Although the perception of flashing lights or shooting stars in the area of impaired vision is commonly encountered with occipital disturbances (migraine), occasionally such subjective disturbances are part of retinal or optic nerve ischemia. Unless the patient is a poor observer, it should be possible to differentiate between amaurosis fugax and cerebral visual disturbances on the basis of duration and frequency of attacks, age of the patient at onset, monocularity versus binocularity, and associated symptoms.

Transient bilateral blurring of vision is an important warning sign of vascular insufficiency in the brain, particularly in the occipital lobes. While such blurring is often due to thromboembolic disease arising within surgically inaccessible parts of the vertebrobasilar system, this is not always the case. Sometimes the recurrent bilateral visual loss comes from surgically accessible areas of the vertebral system, sometimes the cause is cardiac (reduced cardiac output, emboli from aortic valve or mural thrombi), and sometimes the visual symptoms are indirectly related to poor perfusion pressure from the carotid system. For instance, a patient with congenital or acquired low perfusion from the basilar artery with longstanding dependence on the carotid system may develop symptoms of occipital ischemia from acquired obstructions in the carotid system. Therefore, transient bilateral blurring of vision provides a good reason to investigate both the anterior and the posterior cerebral circulation.[6]

Transient episodes of bilateral visual disturbance due to ischemia are not nearly as stereotyped as the recurrent episodes of migrainous individuals. The episodes may even be

hard for the patient to describe, beyond an overall impairment of vision lasting a few seconds to a few minutes and requiring interruption of activity or occupation. The typical patient may not identify any homonymous character of the visual disturbance. The visual impairment may be described as a sensation of looking through haze or fog, and there may be flashes of light in the involved field of vision. If more generalized posterior fossa ischemia is involved, the visual episodes may be associated with diplopia, ataxia, dysphagia, and perioral paresthesias.

Transient visual loss can be caused by eye diseases other than vascular insufficiency. Examples of such disorders include glaucoma (particularly subacute angle closure glaucoma), uveitis, subluxation of the lens, and corneal edema. These nonvascular causes are readily ruled out by an ophthalmologist's evaluation. The subluxated lens in a patient with Marfan's syndrome is shown in Figure 11–3. The lens has moved downward and medially in the right eye.

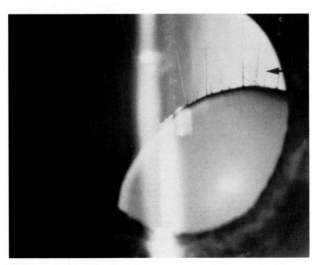

FIGURE 11–3. Subluxated lens in a patient with Marfan's syndrome. *Arrow* indicates zonules of the lens.

The lens is not centered within the pupil. Its edge and several lens zonules can be seen within the pupil after it has been dilated with mydriatic drops. Refractive errors and blurred vision occur when the visual axis does not pass through the center of the lens.

The optic disks of a patient with subacute angle closure glaucoma are shown in Figure 11–4. The 61-year-old woman had experienced several episodes of blurred vision in her right eye over a period of 3 years. She reported that the entire field of vision in that eye was blurred for several hours at a time, particularly when she was dining in a darkened restaurant. She did not have pain, redness of the eye, and tearing, the expected symptoms of acute angle closure glaucoma. The intraocular pressure was normal in the left eye but was abnormally high in the right eye. The anterior chamber angle, through which the aqueous humor normally is drained from the eye, was partially obstructed by the peripheral portions of the iris. The left optic disk is normal in appearance (see Fig. 11–4B). The optic cup can be seen as the pale, excavated area in the center of the disk and is about 20 percent of the horizontal and vertical diameters of the disk. The cup of the right disk is abnormally enlarged to about 70 percent of the horizontal diameter of the disk and to 90 percent of its vertical diameter (see Fig. 11–4A). A computerized study of the central 30 degrees of the right visual field (Octopus perimetry) is shown in Figure

11–4C. Areas that normally have a high sensitivity to light are lighter in shading; areas of low sensitivity in the visual-field defect are darker. A dense arcuate scotoma in the inferior visual field extends from the blind spot below gaze fixation. A dense sector-like scotoma is present in the nasal field. The visual field of the left eye is normal.

Migraine is the most common cause of transient visual disturbance.[7] Symptoms typically begin in adolescence or young adulthood and consist of transient visual loss preceded by a warning aura that is difficult for the patient to describe and may or may not be followed by headache. The frequency of episodes is extremely variable, from several per month to one per 5 to 10 years. The visual symptoms are usually homonymous and consist of an expanding partial scotoma in which there may be flashing lights or a picket-fence phenomenon. Patients often describe the loss of part of what they are looking at (eg, not seeing half of someone's face) during the episode. Duration of the visual disturbance is highly characteristic, in the range of 20 minutes. Age of onset, time of duration of the visual disturbance, and stereotyped behavior are characteristics that help identify migraine and distinguish it from other causes of transient visual loss.

A particularly important cause of transient visual loss is chronic papilledema. Unlike the typical visual loss of amaurosis fugax or transient ischemia of the occipital cortex, the visual loss in papilledema is often postural.[8] It is most likely

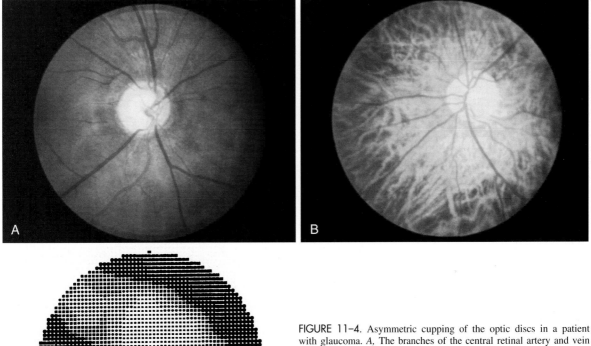

FIGURE 11–4. Asymmetric cupping of the optic discs in a patient with glaucoma. A, The branches of the central retinal artery and vein at the cup are displaced nasally, and the cup is enlarged in the right eye (to the left in the figure). B, Note the smaller cup (central excavation) in the left eye (to the right in the figure). C, Computerized perimetric study (Octopus) of central 30 degrees of the right eye. Note the dense (black) inferior arcuate scotoma.

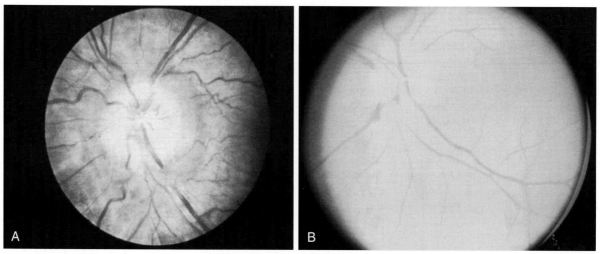

FIGURE 11–5. *A,* Left optic disk of a patient with chronic papilledema. Note the dilation and tortuosity of the retinal veins, hyperemia of the disk, obscuration of the disk margins, and elevation of the disk tissue. *B,* Pale swollen disk of the left eye in a patient with anterior ischemic optic neuropathy. Note the splinter-shaped hemorrhages in the retina at the nasal margins of the disk.

to occur as the patient gets up from the bed or chair. It may occur bilaterally, since severe papilledema is usually bilateral but not necessarily in both eyes at the same time. Transient visual loss is not necessarily an indication that permanent visual loss will occur.[9] The swollen disk of papilledema is hyperemic and markedly elevated, compared with the pale swollen disc of anterior ischemic optic neuropathy, with which it might otherwise be confused.[10] The left optic disk of a patient with chronic papilledema is shown in Figure 11–5*A.* The margins of the disk are obscured by the opaque swollen tissue of the optic disk. Dilation of capillaries and venules at the surface of and within the optic disk produces a reddish discoloration of the disk. Deviation of the retinal blood vessels anteriorly (toward the observer) and then posteriorly as they leave the optic cup is caused by marked elevation of the disk. Normally, the retinal blood vessels are slightly obscured by axons of the retinal ganglion cells that overlie them in the nerve fiber layer. In Figure 11–5, the blood vessels are distinctly seen owing to atrophy of axons within the nerve fiber layer, which distinguishes chronic from acute papilledema. Visual loss in papilledema usually lasts only a few to several seconds but can persist up to a minute or more. Between episodes of visual impairment, central vision of the patient with papilledema is usually normal, unlike that in the patient with acute ischemic optic neuropathy or optic nerve papillitis.

The same obstructive or embolizing processes that cause amaurosis fugax or transient impairment of occipital circulation can lead to permanent anoxic sequelae of optic nerve, retina, or cerebral hemisphere. There may or may not be antecedent warning symptoms before permanent loss of vision. When the optic nerve is involved, there is acute loss of either central or peripheral vision—in one eye only. Obstruction of blood flow to the optic nerve head in the short posterior ciliary arteries causes anterior ischemic optic neuropathy, with pallor and swelling of the optic disk. In Figure 11–5*B,* the left optic disk in a patient with anterior ischemic optic neuropathy has a whitish discoloration resulting from lack of blood flow in small blood vessels of the disk and swelling of axons. The disk tissue is elevated, and

the disk margins are obscured. Small splinter and flame-shaped hemorrhages and cotton wool spots are often found on or near the disk. The visual loss is generally major as well as sudden. Almost any part of the visual field may be affected, but a particularly common pattern is loss of either the upper or lower half of the field in one eye. This so-called altitudinal pattern of field loss derives from the nature of the posterior ciliary arterial circulation, which is divided into upper and lower divisions of supply to the optic nerve.[5]

Computerized visual fields of a 52-year-old man with ischemic optic neuropathy are presented in Figure 11–6. The patient awakened one morning with impairment of the lower field of vision of the left eye. Examination of the disk showed subtle pale swelling primarily in the upper half of the disk, and the visual field demonstrates a patchy defect in the bottom half of the field of the left eye. Demarcation

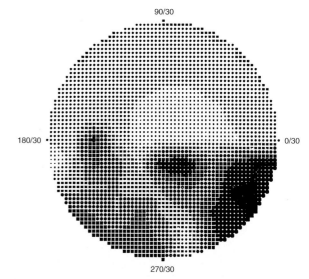

FIGURE 11–6. Computerized perimetric study (Octopus) of the central 30 degrees in a patient with anterior ischemic optic neuropathy of the left eye. Note the inferior altitudinal defect whose border is aligned with the horizontal meridian. The visual field of the right eye is normal.

of the normal and abnormal visual field along the horizontal meridian is characteristic of ischemic optic neuropathy. The patient was evaluated for temporal arteritis, hypertension, diabetes mellitus, clotting disorders, and carotid obstructive disease, but no cause was found. The abnormality in such causes is presumed to involve the intrinsic microvasculature of the anterior aspect of the optic nerve. In this case, as in most, the course was stable, the visual-field defect persisted unchanged with time, and the patient was advised of an approximate 30 percent chance of occurrence of a similar process in the second eye. Curiously, additional episodes very seldom occur in an eye that has previously experienced acute anterior ischemic optic neuropathy.[11]

Altitudinal field loss can also result from occlusion of the upper and lower divisions of the central retinal artery. Occlusion of either branch or the central retinal artery is a reason for urgent referral and treatment. Although at one time it was stated erroneously that all potential function of the retina or optic nerve was lost permanently within minutes of obstructed blood flow, such is not always the case. If the patient is seen within a few hours of onset of occlusion, the ophthalmologist treats such cases with intermittent digital compression of the eye through closed lids (20 seconds on, 10 seconds off), with intraocular pressure–reducing agents (acetazolamide 500 mg orally or intravenously), and with carbon dioxide-enriched air administered by having the patient rebreathe into a paper bag or breathe carbogen gas. The goal of such urgent treatment is mechanical dissolution of soft emboli and increase in arteriolar flow by reduction in intraocular pressure. Once the urgent treatment phase is past, diagnostic evaluation of the underlying cause is in order.

It is important to emphasize that anterior ischemic optic neuropathy is a very common disorder that is seldom the result of carotid obstructive disease. While it is appropriate for the physician to review the history and ophthalmologic findings carefully in consideration of possible carotid occlusive disease, the overwhelming majority of cases of typical anterior ischemic optic neuropathy appear to be caused by intrinsic optic nerve vascular disease.[11–13] Contrast studies of the carotid circulation are not indicated in typical cases. Hypertension and diabetes mellitus are common precursors. Giant cell arteritis is an occasional but very important cause to consider in any elderly patient with sudden visual loss because of the opportunity to prevent loss of vision in the other eye.[14] Without treatment with systemic corticosteroids, approximately 30 to 50 percent of patients will suffer from ischemic optic neuropathy in the other eye. The second eye is usually affected within a few weeks after the first eye. For this reason, every patient with acute ischemic optic neuropathy should have a Westergren sedimentation rate measurement immediately. The sedimentation rate is markedly elevated in most patients with active giant cell arteritis. Typically the patient is 70 years of age or older, and the Westergren sedimentation rate is at least equal in number to the chronologic age. The loss of vision is major. Unlike most patients with nonarteritic ischemic optic neuropathy, the patient with giant cell arteritis is likely to be blind or nearly blind in the involved eye. Vigorous immediate treatment with systemic corticosteroids significantly reduces the risk of infarction of the patient's other optic nerve or retina.[15] Prednisone is given orally at a dosage of 1 mg/kg body weight daily. However, some experts treat with 250 mg of methylprednisolone intravenously every 6 hours initially, since visual loss in the second eye can occur within a few days even after oral prednisone is administered. Corticosteroids usually do not improve vision in the initially affected eye in giant cell arteritis. They are also probably not effective in improving vision in an eye with nonarteritic ischemic optic neuropathy. Recently, fenestration of the optic nerve sheath immediately behind the eye has been reported to improve vision in nonarteritic ischemic optic neuropathy.[16] However, the efficacy of this treatment is still controversial.[17]

A multicenter, prospective, randomized study compared visual outcomes in patients who underwent optic nerve sheath fenestration and patients who did not have surgery.[18] Both groups had individuals in whom vision improved, but the frequency of worsened vision was higher in the surgical group. The study's authors did not recommend optic nerve sheath fenestration for nonarteritic ischemic optic neuropathy.

A history of systemic symptoms and signs associated with giant cell arteritis should be sought. The optic disks of a patient with giant cell arteritis are shown in Figure 11–7. The 84-year-old woman shown lost all vision in her right eye 3 weeks before seeing an ophthalmologist, but she thought there was just something wrong with her glasses and she sought no medical attention until she awakened with no vision in either eye. She had also ignored a 25-pound weight loss over the prior 3 months, systemic malaise, anorexia, pain in her muscles, and tender spots in both temples. All of these symptoms she attributed to her old age. The right optic disk is atrophic (see Fig. 11–7A). The disk is pale, the retinal arterioles are narrow, and the retinal nerve fiber layer is markedly thinned. The fundus of the left eye shows pale swelling of the retinal nerve fiber layer and a cherry red spot at the fovea caused by occlusion of the central retinal artery (see Fig. 11–7B). The retinal arterioles are narrow, and the disk tissue is pale and swollen. The Westergren sedimentation rate was 90 mm/hour. A temporal artery biopsy showed infiltration of the walls by chronic inflammatory cells, including epithelioid cells and giant cells, establishing the diagnosis of giant cell arteritis (see Fig. 11–7D). Despite corticosteroid therapy, the patient died 6 months later of coronary artery occlusion, which may have been arteritic.

Retinal emboli may not necessarily cause permanent visual defects. Many cases of visually asymptomatic bright Hollenhorst plaques are seen without associated retinal infarction. The symptoms of retinal infarction are areas of blindness in the visual fields which may be central, producing a very noticeable loss of vision, or may be peripheral in areas of the field not very apparent to the patient.

The patient whose fundi are depicted in Figure 11–8 presented to her opthalmologist with acute visual loss in the left eye. She was only 58 years old but had a 90-pack-per-year history of cigarette smoking, was hypertensive and diabetic, and had emphysema. Vision in the right eye was lost suddenly several years before. The right disk is severely atrophic with neovascular shunt vessels at the margins above and below. The left fundus shows a variety of hard (above, at arteriolar bifurcation) and soft emboli. Unfortunately, none of the emboli was dislodged by ocular massage, intravenous acetazolamide (Diamox), or inhalation of carbogen.

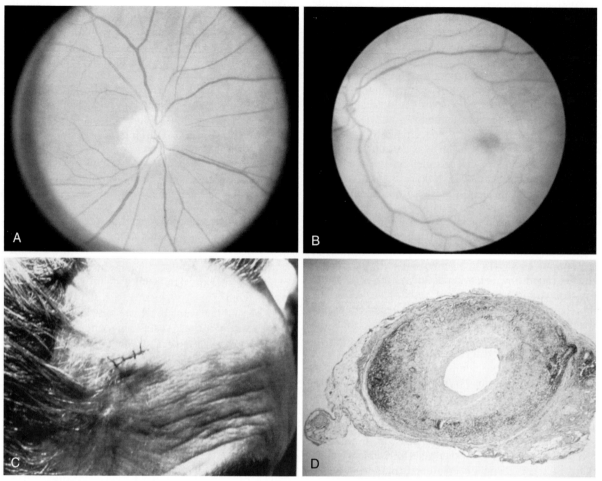

FIGURE 11-7. *A,* Atrophic right optic disk in a patient with giant cell arteritis. *B,* Acutely infarcted left optic disk and retina in the same patient. *C,* Right temporal artery biopsy site. *D,* Histopathologic specimen from the biopsy. Note the inflammation of the vessel walls, including epithelioid and giant cells.

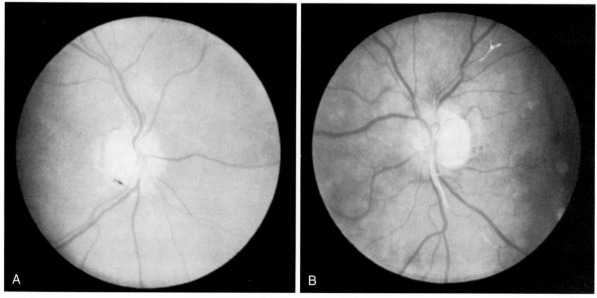

FIGURE 11-8. Fundi of a patient with bilateral internal carotid atheromas, 100 percent obstruction in the right carotid artery and 70 percent obstruction in the left carotid artery. *A,* The right disk shows optic atrophy, resulting from previous anterior ischemic optic neuropathy or occlusion of the central retinal artery. Neovascular shunt vessels are present on the disk. *B,* The left fundus shows multiple hard and soft emboli.

The patient had patchy visual loss in her left eye corresponding to the location of her emboli.

Loss of vision resulting from infarction behind the optic nerves is extremely variable in pattern and dependent on the area of localization. Because of an extremely abundant blood supply, the optic chiasm and optic tract are seldom involved by ischemia. Unless both cerebral hemispheres are involved, the one common feature of all disturbances of vision arising behind the chiasm is their homonymous character, but this information may not be readily volunteered by the patient. Many patients who have even a complete right or left homonymous hemanopia fail to realize what it is that is wrong with their vision. They may report that they bump into objects on their right or their left. If they are aware of a visual problem to the right or left, they often incorrectly state that the problem is in the right or left eye. Particularly in the elderly, it is often difficult to characterize their visual symptoms accurately in this regard. Localization can be suspected clinically by the associated neurologic features. For instance, occipital strokes are often asymptomatic except for the visual field defects. On the other hand, temporal and parietal lobe lesions produce moderate to severe neurologic disturbances of speech, paralysis, sensory abnormality, or agnosia, depending on the area of involvement—in addition to homonymous hemianopia.

Glaucoma is a common disorder causing progressive visual loss and usually caused by increased intraocular pressure. Occasionally, patients with peripheral visual loss and optic nerve appearance typical of glaucoma present to the ophthalmologist without any documentable increase in intraocular pressure. In these patients, carotid occlusion is occasionally found to be the cause of their optic nerve degeneration. Therefore, the ophthalmologist may seek the assistance of the vascular surgeon in assessing such cases, although unfortunately most of the time so-called low-pressure glaucoma proves to be idiopathic.

Pain or inflammation of the eye or both may be a symptom of carotid obstructive disease. Chronic ocular ischemia may produce several ocular abnormalities, characterized by gradual reduction in vision, irritation, light sensitivity, and pain. The pain is sometimes characteristic in that it may be relieved by placing the head in a dependent position.[16]

NEURO-OPHTHALMOLOGIC EVALUATION IN CEREBROVASCULAR DISEASE

Before discussing ophthalmic signs, it is appropriate to stress the importance of symptoms in assessing the patient who may have cerebrovascular disease. The character of the visual loss, bilaterality versus unilaterality, the episodic nature of events, any progressive component, relationship of events to exertion (such as in subclavian steal syndrome), postural associations, and the presence of systemic disease must be reviewed in detail before physical signs are addressed. Many of the patients in question show no abnormalities on clinical examination; hence the need for proper assessment of the symptoms.

In evaluating the patient who may have cerebrovascular disease, the ophthalmologist will first determine the best potential vision, with refractive errors corrected by glasses, reported in terms of Snellen test type acuity (eg, 20/20, 20/40, 20/200). A general ophthalmologic examination will include observations of the external ocular structures, pupillary reactions, and integrity of eye movements, and slit-lamp biomicroscopy of the anterior chambers, measurement of intraocular pressures, assessment of the visual fields, and funduscopic examination.

The patient experiencing amaurosis fugax most often has no demonstrable abnormalities on neuro-ophthalmologic examination. However, careful assessment may show reduced visual acuity (from emboli or reduced flow affecting the optic nerve or retina), abnormal visual fields on the involved side, or changes in intraocular pressure compared with the normal side. Intraocular pressure may be reduced because of poor perfusion of the ciliary body, which reduces production of aqueous humor, or may be high because of neovascular glaucoma. Neovascular glaucoma is a dreaded complication. Untreated, it promptly leads to a fibrovascular occlusion of the anterior chamber angle through which aqueous humor is normally drained from the eye. The effect is a severe elevation of intraocular pressure, with pain and blindness.

An afferent pupillary defect on the involved side is apparent if there is any substantial reduction in optic nerve or retinal function compared with the normal opposite side. The afferent pupillary defect is a particularly important sign of significant reduction in optic nerve or retinal function and is a sign for which any trained physician can look, not just an ophthalmologist. Examination requires a flashlight with fresh batteries; the patient is asked to look steadily at a distant object, preferably a target at least 10 feet away. The examiner holds the flashlight 6 inches away from the right eye, then the left eye, as shown in Figure 11–9. Each eye is stimulated by the light for about 3 seconds; the light is then moved quickly to the other eye. If acute ischemic optic neuropathy is present in the right eye, for example, both pupils will constrict faster and more extensively when the left eye is stimulated. This effect is best seen by noting that the left pupil constricts briskly when the left eye is stimulated, and of course the right pupil will dilate when the light returns to the right side. The visual fields are usually normal between episodes of amaurosis fugax unless there has been permanent ischemic damage to the retina or optic nerve.

Funduscopy is particularly important in patients who complain of either amaurosis fugax or bilateral visual disturbance due to hemispheric ischemia. The pupils should be dilated to facilitate detailed examination of the optic nerve heads and retinal peripheral vascular structures. In examining the optic nerve head, the physician should look carefully for differences in color, vascularity, and any signs of asymmetric glaucomatous cupping or atrophy of the disk (see Fig. 11–4). In comparing the two disks, it must be remembered that the multifocal nature of vascular disease may have produced changes in the presumed normal side, and these changes may limit absolute comparisons.

Intraretinal embolic material is either hard or soft. Bright Hollenhorst plaques are examples of the former. They are cholesterol chips that tend to lodge at bifurcations of arterioles. They are highly refractile and may glisten brightly only when the ophthalmoscope is oriented at a specific angle. Otherwise they may be nearly invisible. Bright plaques may be single or multiple and tend to be permanent once they are lodged in position. The plaques frequently appear to be

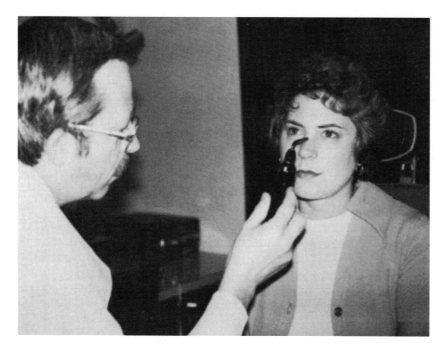

FIGURE 11–9. Swinging flashlight test.

larger than the lumen of the vessel containing them, although this is only an optical artifact that occurs because the column of visible red blood cells is smaller than the surrounding zone of plasma in the vessel. Bright plaques usually originate from the depths of an atheromatous ulcer but may arise from aortic valve calcifications.

Soft emboli are composed of atheromatous material or platelet aggregations, presumably arising from areas of thrombus formation on the surface of atheromatous ulcerations. They are usually white and conform to the shape of the arteriole. Because of their nature, soft emboli may move through the circulation rapidly and thus be visible only transiently. They tend to occur in showers during a time of subjective visual disturbance and break up as they are pushed by the column of arterial blood into the peripheral retinal circulation. Within a few minutes they may move through the circulation and disappear from funduscopic view, leaving no permanent effect on the vision. A small, white soft embolus is located at a bifurcation of the inferior temporal arteriole in Figure 11–10A. The fundus of the right eye is normal. Slight pallor and swelling of the retinal nerve fiber layer along the inferotemporal vessels was seen. A fluorescein angiogram was obtained by injecting fluorescein dye into an arm vein. A fundus camera was used to photograph the transit of dye within the retinal blood vessels. In Figure 11–10B, arteriolar and venous vessels in which blood is flowing are filled with dye and are white; vessels with poor blood flow are dark. The embolus has obstructed flow at the bifurcation of the inferotemporal arteriole. A branch of the inferotemporal vein that drains the retinal area perfused by the obstructed arteriole is dark because of the poor arteriolar flow.

The ocular ischemia syndrome occurs as a result of impaired perfusion of the entire eye.[19–21] Signs include poor

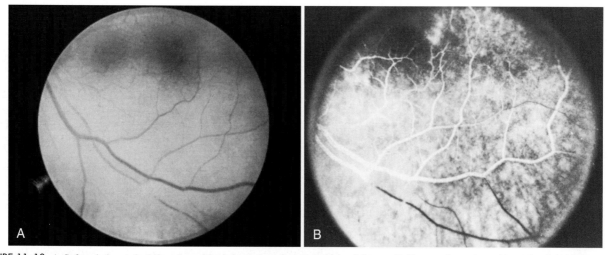

FIGURE 11–10. A, Soft embolus at the bifurcation of the inferotemporal arteriole in the right eye. B, Fluorescein angiographic study of the right eye. Note filling of all of the retinal vessels with dye (white), except branches of the inferotemporal arteriole and vein.

vision resulting from cataract formation, uveitis, abnormally low intraocular pressure (impaired blood flow to the ciliary body), or abnormally high pressure (due to neovascular obliteration of the anterior chamber angle). The external examination clue to these internal changes lies in engorgement of the conjunctival and episcleral blood vessels, which gives the eye an inflamed appearance. The characteristic internal abnormalities are confirmed on slit-lamp biomicroscopic examination of the anterior segment of the eye and with tonometry. The right eye of a 42-year-old man with ocular ischemia is shown in Figure 11–11. The cause of ocular ischemia in this striking case was iatrogenic. Six months previously the patient had undergone a trapping procedure of the right carotid artery to eliminate the noise of a traumatic carotid-cavernous sinus fistula. He had normal visual function in the right eye prior to surgery. Balloon embolization to directly close the fistula is less likely than a trapping operation to produce this disastrous complication. Dilation and tortuousness of the conjunctival blood vessels are marked. Edema and irregularities of the surface of the cornea produce an irregular light reflex. The pupil is dilated and nonreactive, and a dense cataract is present. This patient has neovascular glaucoma. The right eye of a 62-year-old woman with less severe ocular ischemia is shown in Figure 11–12A. Changes in the conjunctival vessels are slight. A mild cataract was present, allowing the fundus to be seen. Figure 11–12B shows the retinal veins to be dilated and tortuous. Many flame-shaped hemorrhages are seen.

Testing for visual field abnormalities is modified according to the suspected abnormality and the condition of the patient. For instance, the alert, observant young patient with amaurosis fugax can be tested with sensitive quantitative perimetry using equipment such as the Octopus (Fig. 11–13). By contrast, an elderly, confused patient who has just had major impairment of the middle cerebral artery of the dominant hemisphere will probably have a gross defect of visual field on the contralateral side. This gross defect can best be confirmed by placing fingers or hands into the right and left halves of the field and observing to which side the patient looks. This kind of testing can give valid information about the nature of the field defect, even in the presence of a severe aphasia that prevent speech. Simple confrontation tests can be effective in alert, cooperative patients. A hand comparison test is shown in Figure 11–14A. The patient covers an eye and fixates the physician's nose with the other eye. The patient is asked to compare the clarity of hands held equidistant from fixation in the right and left hemifields. A patient with an incomplete hemianopia will usually report that the hand in the defective hemifield is blurred. A finger-counting test is shown in Figure 11–14B. While fixating the physician's nose the patient is asked to count the fingers that are held up in one hand or in both hands simultaneously. The fingers in a hemianopic field are usually missed.

Occipital lobe visual-field defects are otherwise neurologically silent. The patient walks into the examination suite speaking and moving all extremities normally, as long as the defect is purely occipital. Occipital defects typically produce highly congruous field defects, which are likely to be multiple and irregular in contour but perfectly superimposable, one eye upon the other. They have been likened to cookie-cutter fields because of the superimposable defects. A partial left homonymous hemianopia is shown in Figure 11–15. The 25-year-old man shown had undergone resection of a right occipital arteriovenous malformation. The computerized visual fields of each eye show defects, the borders of which line up along the vertical meridian and whose density and shape are extremely symmetric.

Parietal lobe visual-field defects are homonymous and tend to involve the lower field more than the upper—corresponding to impaired function in the upper fibers of the visual pathway, which tend to travel in the parietal lobe. Because the corresponding retinal fibers from the two retinas are not grouped as closely in the parietal lobe as in the occipital lobe, the defects are not nearly so congruous. A partial left homonymous hemianopia is shown in Figure 11–16. Note the differences in density and shape of the defects in the two eyes in this patient with a right parietal lobe infarction. In general, the asymmetry or incongruity of hemianopic defects increases the more anteriorly located the lesions are in the visual pathways. The most asymmetric homonymous hemianopic defects are produced by lesions of the optic tracts. Congruity cannot be used to localize lesions if the hemianopias are complete. Patients with parietal lobe lesions can show a host of neurologic signs and symptoms

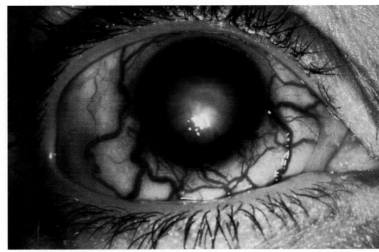

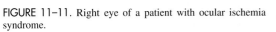

FIGURE 11–11. Right eye of a patient with ocular ischemia syndrome.

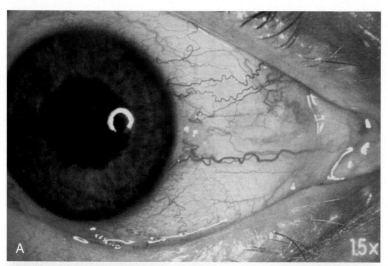

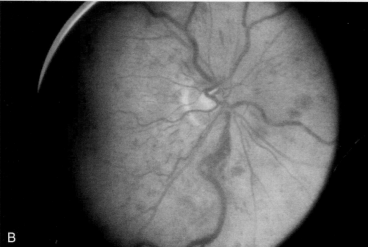

FIGURE 11-12. *A,* Right eye of another patient with ocular ischemia syndrome. *B,* Fundus of the right eye. Note the dilation and tortuousness of the retinal veins and the retinal hemorrhages caused by ocular ischemia syndrome. The fundus view is partially obscured by a developing cataract.

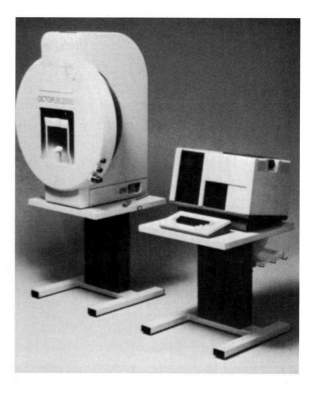

FIGURE 11-13. The Octopus quantitative perimeter is one example of several commercially available instruments that detect and record visual-field defects.

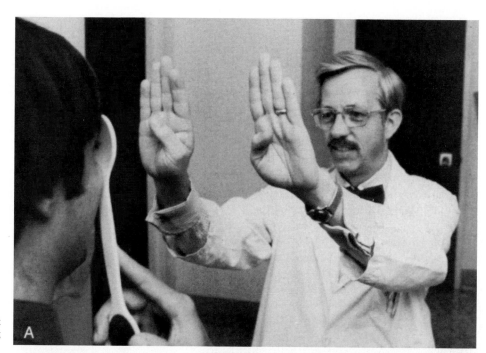

FIGURE 11–14. *A*, Hand-comparison test of the visual fields. *B*, Finger-counting test.

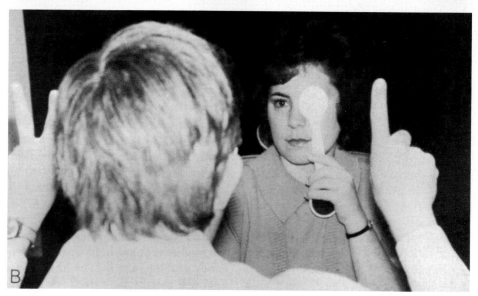

related to their parietal lobe dysfunction; these will help identify the area of brain abnormality.

Temporal lobe visual-field defects result from impairment of the lower fibers of the visual pathways, which sweep laterally around the lateral ventricle (Meyer's loop) before passing back to the occiput. Interruption of these lower fibers, which are not well sorted yet, produces an upper homonymous defect that has been termed "pie-in-the-sky" because it is in the upper region and wedge-shaped. Figure 11–17 shows a homonymous right superior quadrant defect in a young woman who had undergone left temporal lobectomy for intractable seizures. As in parietal lobe lesions, associated neurologic signs and symptoms assist in the localization of the defect.

Precise quantitation of neuro-ophthalmologic findings can assist in following the course of cerebrovascular disease. In addition to recording the results of intraocular pressure and

visual-field tests, the examiner should consider taking fundus photographs of optic nerve abnormalities and intraretinal emboli to aid in determining later whether changes have taken place. Such photographs can be obtained in many ophthalmologists' offices. Neuro-ophthalmologic assessment may include comparative palpation and auscultation in the area of the carotid bifurcation. However, it is not unusual for the patients in whom vascular assessment is being made to have severe obstruction on one side or the other side, or both. Prolonged or overly energetic manipulation of the carotid artery should be avoided, particularly in the elderly.

No discussion of this topic would be complete without reference to ophthalmodynamometry, which is limited in usefulness by so many false negative results as to make interpretation difficult.[22, 23] Congenital variations in arterial circulation, variables in collateral circulation around areas of obstruction, and failure to demonstrate nonobstructive but

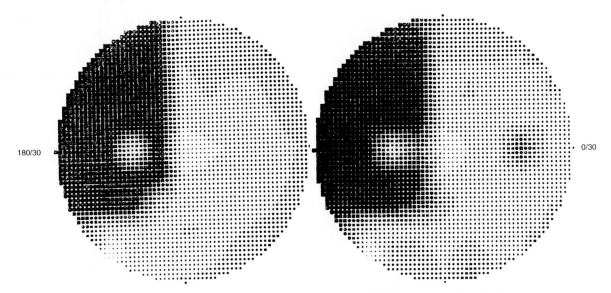

FIGURE 11-15. Congruous left homonymous hemianopia resulting from a right occipital lesion.

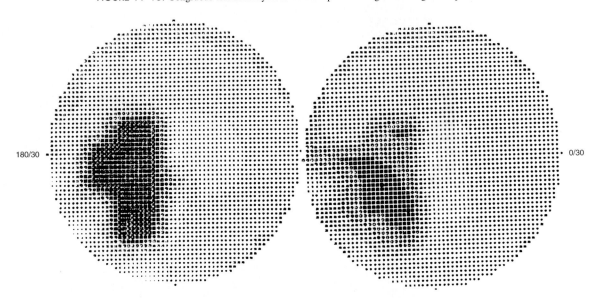

FIGURE 11-16. Incongruous left homonymous hemianopia resulting from a right parietal lesion.

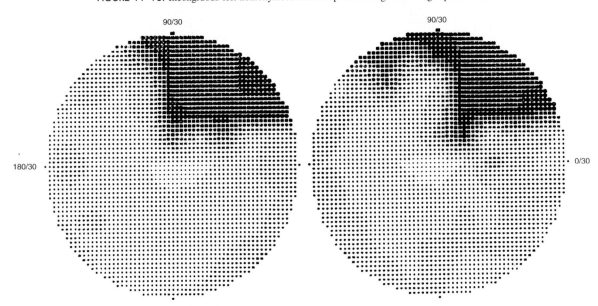

FIGURE 11-17. Incongruous right homonymous, superior quadrant defect "pie-in-the-sky" after left temporal lobectomy.

dangerous embolizing lesions lead to a false sense of security when an ophthalmodynamometric reading is reported to be normal. Much more useful noninvasive flow studies will be discussed in later chapters of this book.

In summary, symptoms and signs of visual dysfunction provide many useful clues in the assessment of the patient who may have cerebrovascular disease. The vascular surgeon should be acquainted with many of these and should consult with ophthalmologic colleagues for thorough assessment of patients with visual symptoms. Careful, informed review of the details of episodic visual loss is particularly important in patients with cerebrovascular disease, since the symptoms may be highly significant even in the absence of any demonstrable visual signs between occurrences. If there is any question about the interpretation of symptoms of visual disturbance, prompt ophthalmologic consultation is recommended.

REFERENCES

1. Fisher MF: Occlusion of the internal carotid artery. *Arch Neurol Psychiatry.* 1951;65:346.
2. Hollenhorst RW: Significance of bright plaques in the retinal arterioles. *Trans Am Ophthalmol Soc.* 1961;59:252.
3. Kearns TP, Hollenhorst RW: Venous-stasis retinopathy of occlusive disease of the carotid artery. *Mayo Clin Proc.* 1963;38:304.
4. Hayreh SS: Blood supply of the optic nerve head and its role in optic neuropathy, glaucoma, and oedema of the optic disc. *Br J Ophthalmol.* 1969;53:721.
5. Risco JM, Grimson BS, Johnson PT: Angioarchitecture of the ciliary artery circulation of the posterior pole. *Arch Ophthalmol.* 1981;99:864.
6. Hoyt WF: Transient bilateral blurring of vision. *Arch Ophthalmol.* 1963;70:746.
7. Duke-Elder S, Scott GI: *System of Ophthalmology.* Vol. 12. St. Louis: CV Mosby;1971.
8. Cogan DG: Blackouts not obviously due to carotid occlusion. *Arch Ophthalmol.* 1961;66:180.
9. Rush JA: Pseudotumor cerebri. *Mayo Clin Proc.* 1980;55:541.
10. Hoyt WF, Beeston D: *The Ocular Fundus in Neurologic Disease.* St. Louis: CV Mosby;1966.
11. Boghen DR, Glaser JS: Ischemic optic neuropathy. *Brain.* 1975;98:689.
12. Hayreh SS, Podhajsky P: Visual field defects in anterior ischemic optic neuropathy. *Doc Ophthalmol.* 1979;19:53.
13. Miller NR: Anterior ischemic optic neuropathy: Diagnosis and management. *Bull NY Acad Med.* 1980;56:643.
14. Keltner JL: Giant-cell arteritis, signs and symptoms. *Ophthalmology.* 1982;89:1101.
15. Glaser JS: Neuro-ophthalmology. In *Topical Diagnosis: Prechiasmal Visual Pathways.* Hagerstown, MD: Harper & Row, 1978:61.
16. Sergott RC, Cohen MS, Bosley TM, Savino PJ: Optic nerve decompression may improve the progressive form of nonapteritic ischemic optic neuropathy. *Arch Ophthalmol.* 1989;107:1734.
17. Yee RD, Selky AK, Purvin VA: Outcomes of optic nerve sheath decompression for nonarteritic ischemic optic neuropathy. *J Neuro-ophthalmol.* 1994;14:70.
18. The Ischemic Optic Neuropathy Decompression Trial Research Group: Optic nerve decompression surgery for nonarteritic anterior ischemic optic neuropathy (NAION) is not effective and may be harmful. *JAMA* 1995;273:625.
19. Knox DL: Ischemic ocular inflammation. *Am J Ophthalmol.* 1965;60:995.
20. Young LH, Appen RE: Ischemic oculopathy. A manifestation of carotid artery disease. *Arch Neurol.* 1981;38:358.
21. Countee RW, Gnanadev A, Chavis P: Dilated episcleral arteries: A significant physical finding in assessment of patients with cerebrovascular insufficiency. *Stroke.* 1978;9:42.
22. Batko KA, Appen RE: Ophthalmodynamometry. A reappraisal. *Ann Ophthalmol.* 1979;11:1499.
23. Sanborn GE, Miller NR, Maguire M, Kumar AJ: Clinical-angiographic correlation of ophthalmodynamometry in suspected carotid artery disease. Prospective study. *Arch Ophthalmol.* 1981;99:1811.

CHAPTER 12

Clinical Evaluation and Differential Diagnosis of Patients with Cerebrovascular Disease

SHELDON E. JORDAN

In the evaluation of a patient with possible cerebrovascular disease, the initial strategy is to determine three things: whether a vascular event occurred, which vessel was occluded, and what mechanism caused the occlusion. If these points cannot be determined, it will be difficult to select appropriate tests or therapy. As an example, consider a patient who presents with a transient hemiparesis. An angiogram may be performed in this case without a consideration of possible underlying mechanisms. If a small plaque is seen at the carotid bifurcation, endarterectomy may be performed. If the actual mechanism in this particular case was cardiac embolization to the brain, however, the endarterectomy may not improve the patient's overall prognosis.

The patient's main presenting neurologic sign or symptom sometimes enables the examiner to determine which area of the brain is involved. Once localization is determined, the particular vessel at fault is identified by looking at vascular distribution patterns. The temporal profile or the presence of prodromal events may help in determining the underlying mechanisms. The occurrence of systemic signs and symptoms may also be of some value; for example, if a patient presents with a transient neurologic event but also has intermittent atrial fibrillation, the possibility of cardiac embolization might come to mind. Certain demographic characteristics may also be helpful; for example, stroke in young adults is often due to cardiac embolization or coagulopathy, whereas stroke in older persons tends to be attributable to atherosclerosis or arteriolosclerosis of cerebral vessels. Once the most likely underlying mechanism is determined, the appropriate tests can be selected to confirm or reject the working hypothesis.

This chapter aims to improve clinicians' ability to interpret signs and symptoms. If clinicians are willing to formulate opinions of underlying mechanisms as the examination proceeds, confirmatory tests and therapy can be ordered in a more efficient way.

THE PATIENT INTERVIEW

General Considerations

Patients may present with undiagnosed problems, or they may arrive with angiograms in hand and working diagnoses. In the initial evaluation, it is wise to take an approach that is unbiased by test results or the opinions of others. Set aside the angiograms and scans and listen to the patient describe the problem and tell you what is wrong. It is also important to speak with the patient's family. Eyewitness reports can be critical in confirming the patient's account and filling in missing details. Seasoned clinicians often say that history is 90 percent of the diagnosis; examination plays only a confirmatory role, and any test that requires electricity to perform should be viewed with skepticism. Many mistakes are made by relying too heavily on apparently abnormal test results while forgetting to obtain an adequate history.

If a compelling history cannot be obtained, it may be appropriate to perform bedside provocative tests in order to jog the patient's memory. For example, with a young patient experiencing dizziness, a battery of bedside provocative maneuvers might include hyperventilation, head positioning maneuvers and tilt table testing. When the patient's dizziness is reproduced, the mechanism of the spontaneous steps may be elucidated.[1-3]

As the patient is describing his or her complaints, the examiner may begin to form opinions about the patient on the basis of observation. The patient's level of alertness and ability to concentrate on a task should be observed. An opinion about the patient's memory and language function can be formed as the patient tries to recollect specific facts from the history.

Visual Complaints

Visual symptoms associated with transient ischemia are generally of three types: diplopia, obscuration of vision, and the occurrence of certain positive experiences such as shimmering effects or hallucinations.

Transient diplopia alone is a relatively nonspecific symptom that may or may not be an indication of an ischemic event. However, diplopia in association with certain additional neurologic signs or symptoms may indicate vertebrobasilar cerebrovascular disease. A brainstem ischemic event should be considered when diplopia occurs in association with unilateral or bilateral sensory or motor complaints, vertigo, ataxia, or dysarthria.

As a result of ischemia, vision may be obscured wholly or partly in one or both eyes. A patient may have difficulty deciding whether a previous event affected just one eye or both eyes. An astute patient may have tried alternately covering and uncovering each eye; if covering one eye alleviated the visual obscuration, a monocular event is likely. Likewise, the movement of a scotoma or scintillating image with manipulation of the globe, as in "rubbing the eye," suggests a monocular event.

Monocular ischemic events are generally localized to circulatory disturbances in the central retinal artery distribution or in the posterior ciliary vascular network, that is, in the retina or optic nerve or both. By contrast, binocular events suggest pathology affecting the optic chiasm, optic tracks, visual radiations, or calcarine cortex. These areas are subserved by the middle cerebral and posterior cerebral arteries. If a patient has not performed a cover-uncover test, a binocular event can still be suspected if the patient reports seeing only the right or left half of a room or a face. Note that each eye views both halves of the visual field, so a monocular event should not produce an inability to see half of an object.

The actual detailed description of a monocular event in terms of its onset and progression may help in determining the underlying mechanism. With transient embolic occlusion of retinal arterioles, the patient may describe a shade falling from above or rising from below and rapidly obscuring all vision in one eye or blacking out vision in the upper or lower half. Visual obscuration progresses over seconds and typically lasts 5 minutes or less; the recovery process often occurs as a shade drawing up or down until vision is restored. This type of event can be contrasted with the development of obscured vision that spreads inward from the periphery, leaving a rapidly diminishing area of retained central vision. This "iris-diaphragm type" of visual loss can be simulated by gently pressing on the globe and is not characteristic of transient monocular blindness due to an embolism.[4, 5] The "iris-diaphragm type" of monocular loss occurs with increased intraocular pressure and systemic hypotension and might be expected when there are other causes of diminished ocular perfusion, such as aortic arch syndrome, arteritis, anomalous ophthalmic artery, and ophthalmic artery stenosis.[6–8] On occasion, transient monocular blindness can also be caused by a variety of local and systemic conditions, including optic nerve compression, papilledema, optic nerve hyaline bodies, anemia, polycythemia, and thrombocytosis.[9–11]

The descending or ascending shade type of monocular blindness could conceivably occur with transient ischemia related to the posterior ciliary circulation, but conditions that result in disturbed ciliary circulation tend to present as a permanent loss of vision or with brief periods of fluctuation followed by a rapidly progressive visual loss. The latter type of visual loss is seen with acute ischemic optic neuropathy and temporal arteritis.[10]

A slow progression of transient monocular blindness over a course of 15 to 20 minutes suggests a migraine phenomenon.[12, 13] Headache may or may not be an accompaniment of migraine.[14] By contrast, headache is rarely, if ever, reported with embolic transient monocular blindness. The occurrence of additional neurologic signs or symptoms in patients with amaurosis fugax can sometimes help elucidate the underlying mechanism. For example, in patients presenting with amaurosis fugax and separate episodes of contralateral hemiparesis, subsequent angiography frequently demonstrates carotid bifurcation atherosclerosis or carotid artery dissection.[15, 16] Patients presenting with amaurosis fugax but without a history of additional transient focal signs referable to the ipsilateral carotid may or may not have angiographic abnormalities. Caution is advised, however, when trying to compare clinical studies that purport to evaluate patients with amaurosis fugax.[16–19] The variable frequency of abnormal carotid angiograms in such patients may relate to the inclusion of cases without regard to the precise characteristics of the onset and progression of transient monocular visual obscurations.

Homonymous hemianopsia that gradually grows in size over the course of 5 to 20 minutes, with or without an associated headache, suggests a migraine.[12] Hemianopia associated with ischemia of the middle cerebral or posterior cerebral artery distributions tends to have an abrupt onset.[20] To make matters confusing, migraine accompaniments occasionally have an abrupt onset and evolution, mimicking the more ominous transient ischemic attack (TIA). In these cases, the diagnostician may be rescued by a prior history of more typical migraines or the weight of evidence obtained after imaging tests.

In patients with persistent hemianopic defects, the history may be helpful in differentiating posterior cerebral artery distribution ischemia from middle cerebral artery distribution ischemia. Patients with posterior cerebral lesions are often aware and complain of a blackness or void to one side; patients with middle cerebral artery occlusions are often unaware of their deficits, bumping into objects on one side of the room without realizing why. The persistence of afterimages and the presence of sparkling scintillations at the edge of a hemianopic field defect is more characteristic of posterior cerebral ischemia than middle cerebral artery disease.[21]

Simultaneous bilateral visual obscuration, or so-called cortical blindness, that results from an ischemic mechanism is usually due to involvement of the posterior cerebral artery. However, bilateral fluctuating blurring can be experienced with a variety of neurologic and systemic problems. In these circumstances, a consideration of the clinical context should help clarify the diagnosis. For example, darkening or blurring of vision can occur as a prodrome to syncope; the diagnosis may be apparent if there are accompanying signs such as pallor, sweating, or palpitations. Fluctuating blurred vision, mimicking a TIA, can be seen in medication toxicity; side effects from anticonvulsants, carbamazepine, and phenytoin are examples of this problem. Neurologic conditions such as intracranial hypertension and multiple sclerosis can cause brief bilateral blurring; again, the clinical context may come to the diagnostician's rescue.

Hemiplegia with simultaneous hemianopia occurs most often with large infarctions in the middle cerebral artery distribution; however, hemiplegia and hemianopia can also be seen with occlusion in the proximal portion of the posterior cerebral artery and, on rare occasion, with occlusion of the anterior choroidal artery.[22]

To complicate the analysis of hemianopia further, ischemia in the posterior cerebral distribution may result from embolization through the anterior circulation, since in a small percentage of the population the posterior cerebral artery derives its major blood supply through the posterior communicating artery and not from the vertebrobasilar circulation.

Scintillations and other positive phenomena can occur with lesions of the retina as well as with lesions affecting the central visual pathways. Hoyt[4] described bright sparks arising from the blind spot in one eye that then dart off toward the periphery; these phenomena suggest the passage of microemboli through branches of the retinal arterioles. Scintillating scotomata associated with migraine were discussed above, but it should be noted that similar scintillating scotomata that have an abrupt onset may be seen with posterior circulation TIAs. Sterotyped, repetitive, formed or unformed hallucinations, particularly within a hemianopic field, can be seen with occipital lobe infarction. Brief, episodic hallucinations in this setting can be due to a seizure focus resulting from brain infarction; obviously, seizure foci can also result from other structural etiologies such as tumors. Visual perseverations, disordered visual recognition (agnosia), and complex visual hallucinations (peduncular hallucinosis) can be observed with ischemia in the vertebrobasilar and posterior cerebral artery distribution.

Sensory and Motor Complaints

Sensory and motor symptoms are frequent manifestations of anterior and posterior circulation ischemia; however, transient or persistent motor and sensory symptoms may also occur with a variety of intracranial structural pathologies, including tumors and hemorrhages; with functional disturbances such as migraines and seizures; and during hypoglycemic episodes in insulin-treated diabetics.

The initial task is to decide whether the event is related to an ischemic or nonischemic event. Sometimes this distinction can be made with attention to the history. For example, migraines and seizures may have prominent "positive" features such as paresthesias. In the case of focal motor seizures, stereotyped, rhythmic clonic activity can be seen. By contrast, TIAs usually have little in the way of "positive" symptoms; typically they feature diminished function, such as hypesthesia or paralysis. A potential source of confusion may be an occasional patient with focal motor seizures that cause only an arrest of movement, or a patient with brief clonic activity followed by prominent postictal paralysis. The next task is to decide whether the anterior or posterior circulation is involved. A final objective is to guess whether extracranial large vessel atherosclerosis, intracranial small vessel arteriolosclerosis, or cardiac embolization is a likely mechanism for the ischemic event.

In sorting out the history, it is frequently noted that patients have a hard time deciding whether a transient event was purely motor, purely sensory, or a combination of both. When using the word "numbness," patients may mean either weakness or an alteration of sensation. Weakness is apparent if the patient had trouble elevating the arm. If the patient was unable to feel a touch sensation applied to the affected limb with the opposite hand, sensory loss was probably present at the time of the event. Note, however, that difficulties with coordination—for example, when a patient reports trouble buttoning a shirt—may result from either a motor impairment or a loss of sensory input.

With a persistent ischemic focal neurologic deficit, the pattern of involvement may have some value in localizing the lesion and determining the stroke mechanism. For example, infarction characterized by sensory loss on one half of the body is frequently attributable to a thalamic lesion caused by small vessel disease in the distribution of the posterior circulation.[23–25] Pure motor syndromes involving the face, arm, and leg are often caused by infarctions of the internal capsule, frequently as a result of small vessel occlusive disease.[26–30] When weakness affects only one limb or the face is spared, a mechanism based on intrinsic small vessel disease becomes less likely; embolic mechanisms need to be considered in these cases.[31–33] Branch vessel occlusion in the pons due to small vessel disease in the posterior circulation may also present with a pure motor syndrome.[28]

A combination of sensory and motor complaints referable to the same distribution in a patient who has sustained a TIA or infarction suggests a lesion in the contralateral cerebral cortex.[22] The most likely cause is a larger vessel embolization or thrombosis. In unusual cases, sensorimotor strokes

occur with smaller vessel occlusions in the posterior limb of the internal capsule.[34] Transient or persistent ischemic events alternately or simultaneously affecting both sides of the body most likely represent thromboembolism in the vertebrobasilar circulation.[22, 35]

The association of certain signs and symptoms also helps with localization and potentially with the determination of the underlying mechanism. Unilateral or bilateral sensorimotor signs along with cranial nerve disturbances such as diplopia suggest vertebrobasilar disease.[35] The simultaneous or sequential occurrence of transient monocular blindness and contralateral hemisensory loss or hemiparesis strongly suggests thromboembolism due to carotid bifurcation atherosclerosis or carotid dissection.[15, 16] The association of aphasia with sensory and motor complaints usually indicates embolization or thrombosis affecting the middle cerebral distribution.[36] The occurrence of headache may suggest intracerebral hemorrhage, although headaches occasionally occur with transient or persistent ischemic attacks affecting large vessels, particularly with vascular dissection, but not with events related to penetrating vessel ischemia (lacunes).[37] Nausea and vomiting associated with headache are more likely associated with intracerebral hematoma or subarachnoid hemorrhage than with a bland infarction. Note, however, that headache associated with nausea and vomiting may be seen with brain stem ischemia or with cerebellar swelling associated with infarction. Migraine can also be associated with headache, nausea, and vomiting, with or without the concurrence of sensory and motor focal signs. Therefore, it is especially important to rule out the possibility of intracranial hemorrhage with an appropriate imaging study in patients who present with motor or sensory deficits along with headache, nausea, or vomiting.

Focal motor or sensory seizures are rarely, if ever, seen with lacunar infarction alone.[37] Focal seizures are occasionally seen with large vessel thrombosis in the anterior circulation distribution.[38] Seizures are also seen with embolization to cerebral vessels as well as with a variety of structural lesions that may irritate or compress cerebral cortical structures, including intracerebral hematoma, subarachnoid hemorrhage, tumor abscess, or encephalitis. Brief nonrhythmic jerking that is not a typical seizure may also be seen with cortical ischemic events.[39]

The historical profile of a transient deficit may also help determine the mechanism. A series of stereotyped TIAs may occur with carotid bifurcation atherosclerosis, intracerebral small vessel disease, or migraine accompaniments.[14, 24, 40] Cardiac embolization is likely to distribute randomly in either hemisphere; it does not tend to cause multiple stereotyped events.

The onset of a transient sensory or motor event may also be of some help in determining mechanism. With TIAs due to large artery thromboembolism, the onset is abrupt; if the arm and face are involved, both areas are affected almost simultaneously from the onset. By contrast, with focal accompaniments of migraine, there is often a slow spread of involvement from one body part to another over 5 to 20 minutes.[14] For example, a patient may complain of paresthesia of a hand that gradually, over 10 minutes, begins to affect the face; after an additional 5 minutes, the patient may start to complain of dysphasia.

The overall duration of a transient event may also have

some diagnostic significance.[41] TIAs associated with stenotic lesions of the carotid artery tend to be brief, lasting 5 to 10 minutes. By comparison, patients with TIAs due to embolization from a cardiac source tend to experience events that last an hour or longer. In contrast to TIAs, focal seizures tend to be brief, lasting seconds to a couple of minutes, but postictal paralysis can last many minutes or hours. An initiating focal clonic event belies a seizure mechanism, but unfortunately for the diagnostician, clonic activity can be unapparent or absent.

The temporal profile for the onset and progression of a persistent deficit may be of some help in the determination of stroke mechanism.[37] A history of stereotyped TIAs with normal periods in between may be seen as a prodrome of a stroke due to carotid atherosclerosis or intracranial small vessel disease. Sometimes, patients with orthostatic hypotension and a mild or severe intracranial stenosis present with stereotyped TIAs; diabetics with autonomic dysfunction, for example, occasionally present in this manner. It is rare for patients with cardiac embolization to experience repeated stereotyped prodromal events. A slow onset over the course of days or weeks can be seen with carotid thrombosis; however, other structural pathologies such as cerebral tumors or subdural hematomas should be considered. A stepwise or fluctuating onset suggests large artery thrombosis or lacunar infarction. The latter onset would be unusual for embolization, hematoma, or ruptured aneurysm; an abrupt onset is more typical in these cases. It is important to note that these rules are general and have many exceptions; for example, large artery thrombosis may have an abrupt onset and may also occur without any preceding TIAs in up to 50 percent of cases.[37]

There is an important warning in the analysis of historical profiles: patients with completed strokes may demonstrate spontaneous fluctuations in their deficits that are not related to recurrent embolization or to new ischemic injury. Each fluctuation should not be treated as a new ischemic event, nor should it prompt a new round of diagnostics or a change in therapy. Motor deficits temporarily worsened by fever or fatigue are examples of relatively harmless fluctuations. Certain types of deficits, by their nature, tend to wax and wane: dizziness and aphasia fall into this category and are discussed later.

Dizziness

Dizziness is a common presenting complaint of patients with vertebrobasilar ischemia; in most patients presenting with dizziness alone, however, a nonvascular cause is eventually identified.[1, 35, 42–44] In evaluating dizziness, a variety of neurologic and systemic problems need to be considered in the differential diagnosis, including imbalance in the elderly, syncope and presyncopal spells, hyperventilation attacks, transient confusional states, transient global amnesia, and seizures. An analysis of triggering factors gleaned from the history can often narrow down diagnostic possibilities. If recollections and eyewitness reports are not helpful, it may be possible to reproduce the experience at the bedside; this provocative approach is discussed in a separate section of this chapter. It may be quite a challenge to decide which patients' dizziness has a cerebrovascular basis and which patients' complaints are nonvascular in nature.

The examiner should attempt to clarify the nature of the subject's experience.[42] Descriptions that include a sensation of movement or spinning, perhaps associated with nausea, suggests a disturbance of the inner ear or brain stem vestibular pathways. Vestibular disorders may produce feelings of light-headedness without a clear-cut expression of vertigo; however, dizziness without a feeling of movement or spinning may be related to a wider variety of causes, including cardiac arrhythmias, orthostatic hypotension, vasovagal attacks, hypoglycemia, and transient global ischemia.

The next step in evaluating the cause of dizziness is to collect historical facts that may differentiate peripheral dysfunction from a central disturbance. Note that most cases of peripheral vestibulopathy are probably not due to large vessel vertebrobasilar atherosclerosis but may be due to either small vessel disease or a variety of intrinsic inner ear disorders. In cases of a purely peripheral vestibulopathy, the future occurrence of a major brain stem stroke is relatively unlikely. By contrast, many cases of a central vestibulopathy in the appropriate clinical setting may be associated with vertebrobasilar ischemia and with a higher risk for major infarction of the posterior circulation.

The occurrence of certain associated signs and symptoms may help differentiate peripheral from central vestibulopathies. When dizziness is accompanied by only tinnitus or hearing loss, a peripheral lesion is most likely. When hearing is disturbed in the setting of vertebrobasilar ischemia, many other brain stem–related complaints are usually encountered simultaneously.[43]

The patient should be questioned carefully for other signs of brain stem involvement that would help in establishing a central localization. These signs and symptoms include dysarthria, facial numbness, hemiparesis, headache, diplopia, binocular visual disturbance, and unilateral or bilateral weakness or numbness. These additional signs of brain stem dysfunction may accompany the complaint of dizziness or occur as independent events. In either circumstance, the association of vertigo with other manifestations of brain stem dysfunction makes a central lesion more likely than a purely peripheral vestibulopathy.[45]

Speech and Language Disturbance

Dysarthria, a pure speech disturbance, needs to be distinguished from aphasia or dysphasia, a language disorder.[46, 47] The former is a relatively nonlocalizing complaint and may be seen with ischemia in the anterior or posterior circulation. Aphasia suggests a disturbance in the anterior circulation of the dominant hemisphere. (The dominant hemisphere for language is the left side in right-handed individuals and in more than 50 percent of left-handed individuals.) From history alone it is difficult to differentiate a transient language disturbance from a transient speech disturbance. If articulation is relatively spared but word substitutions or neologisms are being produced, a language disturbance is likely. If speech production is severely affected so that the patient is mute or severely dysarthric, a concurrent language deficit might be difficult to ascertain retrospectively unless there was an associated comprehension, reading, or writing difficulty. Further discussion about the bedside evaluation of aphasic patients can be found in the section dealing with the mental status examination.

PHYSICAL EXAMINATION

General Strategy and Tactics

The physical examination actually begins during the interview session. Much is learned about the functioning of the central nervous system by observing the patient's level of alertness, memory, ability to communicate, and ability to move and perceive the environment. The formal physical examination should be tailored to confirm those initial impressions.

On the basis of the history, the examiner should have formulated an opinion about localization and underlying mechanism. The examination should be planned to evaluate specifically the main areas of concern suggested by the history; less pertinent portions of the examination are performed for screening purposes only.

As an example, a patient who is entirely asymptomatic but who presents with a bruit should have a careful examination, including palpation and auscultation of peripheral pulses; the remainder of the neurologic examination would be performed as a screening maneuver to evaluate for possible subclinical ischemic events. The following sections describe ways in which the basic examination can be tailored to evaluate specific problems.

Vascular Examination

The brachial blood pressures should be taken in both arms. A 20 mm Hg difference between the two arms may indicate subclavian artery stenosis; the latter would also be suspected if there was a significant pulse delay or unilateral pulse absence when simultaneously palpating over both radial arteries. As the radial pulses are being palpated, it is worthwhile to inspect the fingernail beds and hands for evidence of embolic phenomena.

Auscultation with a stethoscope should proceed in a logical sequence, starting with the heart and working rostrally to the neck and cranium. First listen along the apex and left sternal border and possibly into the axilla for murmurs that might indicate mitral valve disease. Next listen at the base of the heart for aortic murmurs that could radiate upward to the carotid vessels. With the bell of the stethoscope, listen over the carotid arteries in the low neck and in the mid cervical region, and also at the angle of the jaw in sequence along the anterior border of the sternocleidomastoid muscle. Bruits may also arise from the supraclavicular region due to subclavian artery or vertebral artery disease. For detecting orbital bruits, the bell may be applied over one closed eye while the contralateral eye is fixating on a distant object. Sometimes intracranial bruits are also heard well over the mastoid.

To determine the significance of a cervical bruit, several features should be considered: location, overall loudness, duration and timing with respect to systole, pitch, and response to compression maneuvers.[48, 49] Bruits due to internal carotid artery stenosis are loudest in the mid and upper cervical regions up the angle of the jaw. By contrast, radiated cardiac murmurs are often heard in the precordium, at the base of the neck, in the supraclavicular regions, and over the carotid vessels along the anterior portion of the sternocleidomastoid muscle. Internal carotid artery bruits due to cervical bifurcation stenoses radiate poorly to the orbits, but a bruit in the latter location may suggest distal internal carotid stenosis or increased collateral flow due to contralateral internal carotid artery occlusion. Cervical bruits due to increased flow can also be heard contralateral to an internal carotid artery occlusion or high-grade stenosis.

Simultaneous compression of the superficial temporal and facial arteries may diminish the intensity of an external carotid artery bruit, but it will not substantially change bruits associated with internal carotid stenosis.

Several additional features may be helpful in determining the degree of carotid stenosis: loudness, duration, timing, and pitch. It is important to note, however, that these features are difficult to quantify without the aid of carotid phonangiography instrumentation.[50–52] With less than 50 percent carotid stenosis, bruits are soft; the loudness increases for greater degrees of arterial narrowing up to 85 to 90 percent stenosis. With even greater degrees of stenosis, the bruits again become soft and may actually become inaudible, possibly due to diminished flow or a diminished pressure gradient associated with the development of distal collaterals. Provided there has been no systemic change such as correction of fever, onset of anemia, or decrease in systemic pressure or cardiac output, the loss of a previously noted carotid bruit may indicate a sudden increase in arterial narrowing or occlusion of a previously patent vessel.

With increased arterial narrowing, carotid bruits increase in duration and may be heard throughout systole or even past the second heart sound into diastole. Pitch is also correlated with the residual diameter of the vessel lumen. The predominant sound frequency for a bruit due to low-grade stenosis is often less than or equal to 175 Hz. For residual arterial lumina less than or equal to 3 mm, the predominant frequency is greater than 175 Hz and is often in the 300 Hz range.[50] For the nonmusically inclined clinician, it is difficult to learn about pitch for the purpose of bedside examinations. Furthermore, bruits typically encompass a wide frequency band, making bedside bruit analysis difficult even for a trained ear. To help with bruit description, one readily available teaching device is the tuning fork. The lowest-frequency tuning fork commonly available resonates at 128 Hz; a bruit with a similar pitch may not be associated with marked stenosis. The 256 and 512 Hz tuning fork may demonstrate the range of pitch associated with higher-grade stenoses.

After listening for cervical bruits, the examiner should place the stethoscope over the abdomen and groin to search for bruits in these locations. The abdomen should also be palpated for pulsatile masses, and the femoral, popliteal, and pedal pulses should be examined. The feet should be evaluated for evidence of embolization and for trophic changes. Age may be an important factor in the interpretation of distal pulse deficits. The unilateral absence of a pedal pulse in a young patient may suggest cardiac embolization, whereas the loss of distal pulses in an elderly patient may be more suggestive of atherosclerotic peripheral vascular disease.

To summarize, it is important to fully characterize a bruit. Location and response to compression maneuvers are two features that are helpful in localizing the source of a bruit. The degree of stenosis may be roughly estimated when several features are considered, including loudness, duration and timing with respect to the cardiac cycle, and pitch.

Systemic influences should be considered, including hypertension, hypotension, anemia, fever, and cardiac output. Caution is advised when trying to compare clinical studies regarding cervical bruits; different methods of characterization make it difficult to compare studies.[53–56]

Neuro-Ophthalmologic Examination

Examination of the visual system begins with a test of visual acuity. The development of hyperopia within a short time span may be a result of ischemic shortening of the long axis of the eye or hardening of the lens, which may occur ipsilateral to carotid stenosis or occlusion. This abrupt change in visual acuity may be seen with multiple-arch vessel stenosis, as in Takayasu disease.[57]

Simple bedside tests are available to help distinguish retinal disease from optic nerve disease.[10] These tests include photostress testing, color and light brightness perception, and the swinging flashlight test.

The inability of visual acuity to recover quickly after a photostress test can be a sign of retinal disease. To perform this test, best corrected visual acuity is determined individually in each eye. With the defective eye covered, the normal eye is subjected to a strong light for 10 seconds; the light is removed and the patient is instructed to read the next larger line on the eye chart as soon as possible. For example, if the baseline vision were 20/20, the next larger line would be 20/25. This recovery process is timed and recorded in seconds. The same process is repeated for the defective eye, and the recovery times are compared. Abnormalities in recovery time reflect a delay in regeneration of visual pigments following exposure to bright light. An asymmetry in recovery times may occur with ischemia to the retina.[58] By contrast, in a lesion confined to the optic nerve, recovery times will be more comparable between the defective and normal eyes.

With monocular visual loss due to retinal disease, color perception and light perception are relatively preserved. By contrast, with optic nerve disease, colors look washed out and bright lights appear dim. To test these phenomena, a brightly colored object or a bright light is shown to each eye alternately, and the subject is asked to compare the color or light intensity.

The swinging flashlight test is a key maneuver in distinguishing retinal disease and optic nerve disease from more central problems. The subject should be placed in a room with dim ambient lighting. A bright flashlight is shone in one eye as the patient is asked to fixate on a distant object. The light is then moved to the opposite eye. Normally no overall dilation should be seen when the light is switched over; significant dilation of the pupil when the light is swung over to it suggests an afferent pupillary defect. With mild or moderate visual loss, an afferent pupillary defect usually indicates a lesion of the optic nerve or chiasm. Note that with the swinging flashlight test, only the pupil being illuminated is observed. By contrast, if both pupils are observed simultaneously under the illumination of the ambient light or when a bright light is shone into both eyes, the pupils should be of equal size with an afferent pupillary defect. A unilateral visual defect in acuity or visual field does not cause unequal pupils when viewing the pupils simultaneously unless there is a concomitant disease of the iris or a defect in pupillary motor innervation.

It is interesting to note that patients who present with amaurosis fugax may have abnormalities in retinal function or during optic nerve testing even at times remote from a spell of transient monocular blindness.[58]

For screening of visual field defects, several bedside techniques are available.[10] A small brightly colored object, such as the colored top of an eyedrop bottle, can be used to test for loss of color sensitivity when shown to each visual field quadrant of each eye. Fading of the color in a hemifield or quadrant may suggest an early field defect. Confrontation tests include showing both of the examiner's hands in front of each eye on either side of the vertical meridian. If the patient perceives a diminution or distortion of one hand, a subtle field defect may have been discovered. Counting fingers held simultaneously in two quadrants is another way of screening for field defects. To screen for smaller scotomata, an Amsler grid may be used. If the grid is unavailable, a newspaper may be shown to each eye separately. A small cross drawn in the middle of the newspaper will help the patient fixate. With one hand the patient can then point out which areas of the printed page disappear.

The type of field defect can be helpful in determining the site of a possible ischemic process. Purely monocular defects indicate retinal or optic nerve infarction. If a defect is due to a retinal vascular lesion, the apex of the scotoma is often at the blind spot.[10] The latter phenomenon is a consequence of the distribution of retinal vessels coming off the disc. By contrast, optic nerve lesions produce monocular defects with the apex of the scotoma at the central fixation point. Binocular field defects may affect homologous parts of the field; the latter usually indicates optic tract, optic radiation, or occipital lobe disease. Lesions beyond the optic chiasm and up to the occipital lobe tend to produce field defects that are sharpest at the vertical meridian. Homonymous field defects that involve exactly the same parts of the visual field are called congruous defects. Congruous homonymous hemianopia can occur with occipital lobe or optic radiation defects. Incongruous hemianopia is most often seen with optic tract or optic radiation localizations.

Homonymous hemianopia caused by lesions of the occipital lobe secondary to posterior cerebral artery ischemia can sometimes be differentiated from a similar defect caused by involvement of the visual radiations deep to the parietal and temporal lobes and in the distribution of the middle cerebral artery.[21] Patients with posterior cerebral artery lesions often complain of a void or blackness to one side; patients with ischemia of the middle cerebral artery often neglect their field defects. Patients with occipital lobe lesions often experience poorly formed scintillations in the hemianopic field; this phenomenon is rarely experienced with lesions in the optic radiations due to middle cerebral artery distribution ischemia. Perseveration of an afterimage is occasionally seen with posterior cerebral artery disease, but rarely with middle cerebral artery lesions. Motor paralysis is uncommon in patients with occlusion of the posterior cerebral artery unless the proximal part of the artery is also occluded, with ischemia affecting the cerebral peduncle.[59] By contrast, with middle cerebral artery distribution strokes, motor involvement is a frequent concomitant. Optokinetic nystagmus is often preserved with occipital lobe lesions but is typically lost with lesions deep to the parietal lobe and in the distribution of the middle cerebral artery.

After testing for visual acuity, pupillary responsiveness, and visual fields, the eye itself is inspected. Dilated episcleral vascular networks are seen with severe ipsilateral carotid artery stenosis and may be an indication of anastomotic connections between the internal and external carotid circulation. In aortic arch disease associated with Takayasu syndrome, this hyperemia may be present in up to 80 percent of cases.[57, 60–62] Ipsilateral to severe carotid stenosis, rubeosis iridis may be seen; this consists of a web of small interweaving blood vessels growing on the outer surface of the iris.[62] Frank hyphema or haziness of the anterior chamber may result from cellular debris from the neovascular network.

Examination of the fundus in patients with chronic ocular ischemia demonstrates scattered cotton wool patches; these are produced by focal ischemia of the nerve fiber layer of the retina. Microaneurysms, hemorrhages, and venous dilation may be seen with prolonged ischemia. Anastomotic arteriovenous connections may occur in the midperiphery or encircle the optic disc.[60, 62]

An asymmetric hypertensive retinopathy may occur with unilateral carotid stenosis or occlusion. The eye ipsilateral to the carotid lesion may be relatively protected from systemic hypertension so that the hypertensive retinopathy is less in comparison with the contralateral eye.

During funduscopic examination, the retinal vessels should be carefully scanned for the presence of emboli. Bright yellow or orange refractile emboli that temporarily lodge at arteriolar bifurcations apparently represent cholesterol crystals, which have been associated with atheromas at carotid bifurcations.[63–67] However, cholesterol emboli may arise from locations other than the carotid bifurcation, such as the aortic arch. It follows that some patients with cholesterol emboli may have normal-appearing carotid angiograms.[19] Often patients with cholesterol emboli are free of visual symptoms at the time of the examination. By contrast, patients in the midst of a spell of amaurosis fugax may have dull gray-white emboli moving through a segment of an arteriole; these are apparently due to platelet-fibrin aggregates.[68, 69] Fixed, dull-white calcific or fibrin emboli may also be seen.[62] With the latter type of emboli, a pale portion of retina may be seen downstream from the occluded arteriole; often a visual field scotoma correlates with the area of ischemic retina. Calcific emboli may arise from calcified cardiac valves; it is unknown how often they arise from carotid atheromatous plaques.

With fixed retinal branch occlusions, the retina distal to the affected vessel appears opaque and pale. The arterioles are small, and the veins are normal or slightly enlarged in diameter. The blood may appear to segment in the veins. With time, the pale portion of the retina may seem less apparent, but the arterioles remain relatively narrowed.

With acute optic nerve ischemia, the underlying pathology is usually that of a small vessel disease affecting the posterior ciliary circulation. The disc appears pale and swollen, later replaced by a pale atrophic disc. In rare instances, optic disc infarction or optic atrophy may be seen in patients with amaurosis fugax and in association with carotid bifurcation atherosclerosis or with embolization from a proximal source.[70, 71] In patients with unilateral ischemic optic neuropathy, efforts should be made to exclude the diagnosis of temporal arteritis so that appropriate steroid therapy may be instituted to save vision in the contralateral eye. A history of headache, generalized muscle aches, jaw claudication with chewing, and an elevated sedimentation rate might suggest a diagnosis of temporal arteritis, particularly in an elderly individual.

Sensory and Motor Examination

Provided that hemorrhage can be excluded,[72] a pure motor hemiplegia is often attributable to lacunar infarction of the internal capsule or, on occasion, pontine infarction; in either case, intrinsic small vessel disease seems to be the underlying mechanism.[33, 73] However, from motor signs alone it may be difficult to localize a lesion to a particular level of the corticospinal tract and to a particular vascular distribution. In these cases, associated focal findings may help the diagnostician. For example, with brain stem ischemia, the patient may have dysconjugate eye movement or may have difficulty looking away from the side of paralysis. With paralysis due to cortical injury and in the distribution of the middle cerebral artery, dysconjugate gaze is not typically found. Furthermore, with cortical lesions, the patient has most difficulty looking to the same side of the paralysis, in contrast to lesions affecting the brain stem. It is useful to remember that hemispheric function is concerned with the environment of the contralateral side of the body. With involvement of the cortical eye fields of the ipsilateral frontal lobe, the eyes are unable to gaze toward the contralateral side of the body; they tend to deviate toward the affected hemisphere.

The pattern of sensory disturbance may be helpful in localizing the lesion. A hemisensory loss involving all modalities indicates a lesion in the upper brain stem, thalamus, or deep parietal white matter. When position sense, two-point discrimination, tactile localization, and graphesthesia are affected relatively more than pain, temperature, and light touch sensation, a cerebral lesion is suggested. The converse suggests a brain stem localization. Bilateral sensory or motor signs suggest brain stem involvement.

When hemiparesis and sensory loss affect the same parts of the body, a thalamic, hemispheric white matter, or cortical lesion is probable. When sensory and motor deficits are coextensive, a lesion affecting the sensorimotor cortex or adjacent white matter is suggested; the affected vessel would typically be the middle cerebral artery or middle cerebral artery branch. Rarely, combined sensorimotor syndromes are seen with small vessel occlusions in the area of the contralateral capsule and thalamus.[34]

A pure hemisensory stroke is often caused by lacunar infarction associated with small vessel disease affecting branches of the posterior cerebral artery, with resultant thalamic infarction. Rarely, a pure sensory stroke occurs with cortical branch vessel disease.[74]

BEDSIDE EVALUATION OF THE DIZZY PATIENT

To help the patient characterize the type of dizziness experienced, a variety of bedside maneuvers can be performed in an attempt to reproduce the experience.[44] Check blood pressure change both lying and standing for 3 minutes to rule out orthostatic hypotension as a cause of dizziness. The patient's description of light-headedness during this evaluation is a starting point. Note that occasionally a patient has dizziness when standing up with only a minimum diminution of blood pressure; some of these patients may have multiple vessel occlusive disease.[75] Prolonged upright positioning, as in tilt table testing, can be used to evaluate patients with syncope of unknown cause. Although this test lacks diagnostic specificity for the evaluation of fainting, the prodromal sensations of presyncope may help the diagnostician if the sensations engendered reproduce those occurring in spontaneous episodes.

Turning the head to extreme lateral position while sitting or standing may also reproduce dizziness due to a mechanical compression of the vertebral artery from cervical spondylosis and cervical bands, as well as other anomalies at the cervical portion of the vertebral artery.[76]

The head and body positioning maneuvers are variously named Nylen-Barany or Hallpike maneuvers. The patient is seated with his or her back to the end of the examining table. The head and entire body are then brought backwards rapidly, with the head hanging over the edge 45 degrees and rotated initially to the left; then, in an additional trial, it is rotated to the right. The patient is observed during the head-turned position for at least 1 minute during each trial; the patient's report of vertigo and the examiner's observation of nystagmus are noted. Vertigo and nystagmus due to benign peripheral vestibular disease commonly develop after several seconds in a particular position; they gradually diminish after several more seconds and then become more difficult to elicit after repeated trials in the same head position.[44] Vertigo and nystagmus due to peripheral vestibulopathy are often best seen only in one head-turned position, and the nystagmus has a typical rotatory character. By contrast, vertigo due to a central brain ischemic lesion may be associated with nystagmus of sudden onset that persists in a given trial and fails to extinguish after repeated trials in a given head position.[44, 45, 77, 78] The nystagmus may change its direction and be elicitable in a variety of head positions.

The presence of other brain stem findings on examination would also confirm a central vestibular lesion.[43, 45] One should look carefully for ocular dysconjugacy during the evaluation of eye movements, dysarthria, incoordination, and visual field defects.

Other maneuvers applied at the bedside include hyperventilation for 3 minutes, gentle carotid sinus massage for 10 seconds, a Valsalva maneuver, and sudden turning while walking. If the history suggests a subclavian steal syndrome, repetitive arm exercises may produce limb claudication, perhaps followed by dizziness.

Occasionally a patient presents in the midst of a vertiginous attack with nystagmus. Sometimes the character of the nystagmus helps distinguish a peripheral vestibular process from a central vestibulopathy, for example, due to an ischemic lesion. Acute peripheral vestibulopathy usually causes unidirectional nystagmus, with a fast phase away from the side of the lesion; nystagmus increases in amplitude when gaze is toward the side of the fast phase. With vertebrobasilar ischemic lesions, as in cerebellar infarction, nystagmus may change directions, depending on the direction of gaze.[45] Ipsilateral cerebellar signs are also frequently present.

To summarize, efforts at the bedside should be directed toward a reproduction of the patient's experience of dizziness. These maneuvers may help decide what mechanism produced dizziness in a particular case. It is possible, by bedside examination, to distinguish a peripheral vestibulopathy from a central vestibulopathy that might be due to an ischemic process.

EVALUATION OF ALTERED MENTAL STATUS

Much of the mental status examination proceeds as the history is being taken and general physical exam is being performed. Observations at the time of the examination should be characterized in terms of important components of mental functioning. Alertness, attention, and distractibility are considered first. Drowsiness or stupor is often seen with subarachnoid hemorrhage, large supratentorial infarctions or bleeds, or infratentorial lesions compressing and distorting the brain stem. Direct ischemia to the reticular formation of the brain stem tegmentum can also produce drowsiness or stupor. Drowsiness in a patient with a presentation of vertigo and nystagmus along with ataxia and nausea should raise the possibility of acute cerebellar bleed or infarction; this may require emergency neurosurgical intervention before the brain stem structures are critically compressed. Lacunar infarctions due to smaller supratentorial branch vessel occlusions do not typically produce drowsiness.

An alert patient who is easily distracted by extraneous stimuli and without other localizing signs may have a diffuse impairment of the central nervous system, as might be seen with metabolic encephalopathy. Inattention to one side of the body or to one side of a room, otherwise known as unilateral neglect, indicates focal damage to the contralateral parietal lobe. Observations may include a patient lying in bed with a leg hanging off the side in an awkward position or a patient ignoring objects or people off to one side. Unilateral neglect may be so profound that the patient may fail to shave on one side of the face or may forget to place one arm in the sleeve of a robe.

Language is initially tested during the history taking; several categories of function should be considered during this period of observation. Spontaneous or conversational verbalizations are analyzed. Slow, hesitant output with poor articulation and short phrase lengths characterize nonfluent aphasias.[46, 47] The words produced are mostly nouns, with a striking lack of the usual grammatical sentence structure; there is a lack of the usual connectives such as prepositions, articles, adverbs, adjectives, and verbs. A patient with a profound nonfluent aphasia may be able to produce only stereotyped verbal outputs such as a single word or syllable that is repeated. Nonfluent output is generally seen with involvement of the anterior portion of the left hemisphere in right-handed individuals; it can also occur in those left-handed individuals (more than 50%) in whom the left hemisphere is dominant.

Conversational speech of a patient with dysarthria alone should be differentiated from the speech of a patient with nonfluent asphasia. The former has problems with articulation and with the normal rhythm and melody of speech, but there is no problem with phrase length, word finding, or grammatical sentence structure.

Fluent asphasia is characterized by relatively effortless output and normal articulation. The speed of word production is relatively preserved. Phrase length is normal, as is melodic quality. Pauses, however, may be noted when the patient is trying to find a word. Frequently the pauses are filled in with circumlocutions when the patient is trying to find a word. Frequently the pauses are filled in with circumlocutions when the patient cannot generate the correct word; for example, instead of saying "watch," the patient may say "the thing on my arm to tell time." In spite of abundant output, little meaning may be conveyed. Word substitutions, paraphasias, or nonsensical words (neologisms) are produced. When most of the words are substituted or nonsensical, the verbalization becomes incomprehensible. The term *jargon aphasia* may be used to describe this type of verbal output. Fluent aphasia is generally associated with lesions in the temporoparietal areas of the dominant hemisphere.

During the formal part of the bedside examination, the examiner should ask the patient to repeat words and short phrases. An inability to repeat suggests damage to the perisylvian region.

Comprehension is tested when the patient is asked to perform various tasks on verbal command during the physical examination. If a patient has difficulty following commands, a distinction needs to be made between poor comprehension of the task and apraxia, which is the inability to formulate an appropriate motor response. To facilitate this distinction and to test more specifically for comprehension, the patient should be asked to respond with a limited activity, such as finger pointing or a yes or no answer, to increasingly complicated questions. For example, the examiner may begin by asking the patient to point to the ceiling. If the patient points appropriately, that shows evidence of comprehension as well as the ability to perform the motor act associated with pointing. A more complicated question then helps determine the limits of the patient's comprehension; for example, the patient may be asked to point to a receptacle for something that has burned. If the patient points correctly to an ashtray, comprehension for more complicated phrases is relatively intact.

Writing should be tested by asking the patient to write words and sentences. Alexia (the inability to read) without agraphia (the inability to write) is often seen with a lesion in the occipital area. Agraphia, particularly with severe difficulty in the basic mechanics of writing but relative preservation of reading or comprehension, is seen with frontal lobe damage. A combined disturbance in both reading and writing is frequently seen with lesions of the dominant temporoparietal region.

Short-term memory is tested by asking the patient to remember three unrelated words for 5 minutes and by asking the patient to identify the present location, the date, and the time. An abrupt but transient loss of short-term memory associated with relative retention of remote memory in the absence of other localizing features is called transient global amnesia; this condition has a relatively benign prognosis. However, memory loss with associated focal findings such as hemianopia is more likely to be a manifestation of ischemia of the posterior circulation.

The ability to add and subtract as well as to name individual fingers of the right and left hand should be formally tested. Dyscalculia and right-left finger confusion or finger agnosia are associated with lesions in the dominant inferior parietal region.

As a final task in the mental status examination, the patient should be asked to copy a cube and a complex figure. For example, a clock face should be drawn to verbal command, with instructions to place all the numbers and designate a specific time on the clock. Nondominant parietal lobe injury may be associated with an inability to copy figures. A patient with nondominant parietal lobe disease may also manifest neglect; the left half of the clock may not be drawn, or the left side of the copied figure may be omitted.

INITIAL AND ROUTINE LABORATORY TESTS

A complete blood count and differential and platelet count are obtained on all patients. Polycythemia and thrombocytosis can be contributing factors to ischemic cerebrovascular disease. The basic laboratory tests should also include electrolytes, glucose, blood urea nitrogen, creatinine, and urinalysis. These studies should be examined before contrast imaging studies are performed because the risk of exacerbating renal failure is high in patients with pre-existing renal disease, particularly in the setting of diabetes or dehydration. A sedimentation rate may be helpful in evaluating elderly patients with possible cranial arteritis. In younger patients, a sedimentation rate and antinuclear antigen may be valuable to screen for collagen vascular disease, which occasionally presents with transient focal signs and symptoms. A fluorescent treponemal antibody absorption test is reasonable to screen for neurosyphilis. Note that the Veneral Disease Research Laboratory (VDRL) test is occasionally negative in late neurosyphilis. A prothrombin time and partial thromboplastin time should be obtained in all cases. Additional tests for coagulopathy are often indicated: in the absence of typical atherosclerotic risk factors, in patients with prior venous or arterial occlusions, and in young patients with unapparent causes for stroke. Testing may include antithrombin III, protein C, protein S, and plasminogen assays and antiphospholipid antibody titers. The latter antibody test is important in cases with the above historical features and in patients with a history of spontaneous abortions and false-positive VDRL test results, with or without evidence of systemic lupus. A chest radiograph and an electroencephalogram baseline are also helpful. The electrocardiogram (ECG) should be scanned for signs of acute myocardial ischemia and for arrhythmias, including atrial fibrillation. Patients with cerebrovascular disease often have concomitant ischemic heart disease.

Patients with nonischemic pathology may have a presentation similar to that of a stroke. Aneurysms, arteriovenous malformations, tumors, subdural hematomas, and other focal lesions all have to be excluded with an appropriate brain imaging study. Initially, a noncontrast computed tomography (CT) scan of the brain is probably adequate for most patients; this study can rule out most large mass lesions and most intracranial hemorrhages. If clinically warranted, a contrast CT scan can be obtained later, perhaps after an angiogram; this sequence spares the patient additional exposure to contrast dye. Presently, compared with CT, magnetic resonance imaging is not an acceptable alternative because the magnetic field is a relatively hostile environment for monitoring devices and other supportive equipment that may be needed for acute stroke patients. After the acute phase, if necessary, a magnetic resonance image can be obtained to further clarify stroke mechanisms or to visualize vascular structures. CT, however, has sufficient sensitivity and specificity for acute hemorrhage; this feature is critical in the evaluation of patients presenting with acute focal neurologic deficits.

In many cases, an imaging study of the carotid bifurcation will be ordered. The indications, advantages, and drawbacks to ultrasonic imaging or angiography are discussed in other chapters of this book.

CARDIOLOGIC TESTS

Beyond the initial chest radiograph and ECG, additional cardiac evaluation may be needed for three reasons: (1) to evaluate for potential sources of embolization to the brain, (2) to identify patients at high risk of coronary artery disease with subsequent myocardial infarction and death due to ischemic heart disease, and (3) to monitor the secondary effects of cerebral infarction on cardiac function.

Cardiac disease is thought to produce signs of focal ischemia, usually on the basis of embolization to the brain. Only rarely is a drop in cardiac output associated with the production of focal cerebral dysfunction.

Potential sources of embolization include a variety of valvular diseases, such as rheumatic heart disease, congenital heart disease, mitral annulus calcification, endocarditis, and mitral valve prolapse.[79–87] Certain dysrhythmias may be associated with the development of intracardiac clot and secondary embolization; these conditions include atrial fibrillation with and without valvular disease, sick sinus syndrome, and bradycardia-tachycardia syndrome.[88, 89] Intracardiac clot can also develop in areas of myocardial dyskinesia due to myocardial infarction or cardiomyopathy. Other rare conditions such as atrial myxoma may predispose to systemic and cerebral embolization. Conditions such as mitral valve prolapse and mitral annulus calcification can occur in otherwise normal individuals, so the relevance of these valvular anomalies to a given case of cerebral ischemia may be difficult to prove.

Patients with histories of cardiac disease, abnormal cardiologic examinations, or abnormal routine ECGs frequently have potential cardiac sources for embolization. These can be detected by noninvasive tests such as standard transthoracic echocardiography techniques. In unselected stroke patients who lack clinical evidence of cardiac disease by routine examination, however, transthoracic echocardiography rarely demonstrates an abnormality with the potential to produce systemic or cerebral embolization.[89–91]

Contrast effects can be used to detect embolization associated with clinically inapparent right-to-left shunts due to small atrial septal defects and patent foramen ovale. Ultrasound contrast effects caused by microbubbles in agitated saline and other agents can be used to detect right-to-left shunts with provocative maneuvers such as Valsalva or cough, using transthoracic echocardiography or transcranial Doppler. Transesophageal echocardiography can be quite sensitive in detecting right-to-left shunts because of the probe's proximity to the atrial structures, as compared with transthoracic techniques. Transesophageal techniques can also be used to visualize potential sources of embolization from aortic arch atheromas.[92–97]

Even without a specific history or examination suggesting cardiac disease, certain patients might be expected to have a higher incidence of abnormalities on echocardiography and Holter monitoring examination, including patients less than 45 years of age and patients with CT scans or magnetic resonance imaging scans that show evidence of multiple areas of nervous system involvement. By contrast, other patients probably have a low incidence of echocardiographic abnormalities, suggesting an identifiable course of embolization; such cases include patients presenting with typical lacunar syndromes, since these are usually due to small vessel disease. Older patients with typical hemispheric ischemic events and appropriate lesions demonstrated at the carotid bifurcation would be expected to have a lower incidence of abnormalities on echocardiography compared with similar patients without lesions detectable by angiography or ultrasonography.

To summarize, echocardiography and Holter monitoring are not necessarily routine tests for all stroke patients; however, if the clinical presentation suggests embolization or if the cardiac history or examination is abnormal, echocardiography or Holter monitoring should be performed. Patients with a negative cardiac history and examination, and those with appropriate lesions demonstrable by angiography at the carotid bifurcation, all tend to have a lower yield of abnormal test results by echocardiography or Holter monitoring techniques.

Certain clinical presentations of ischemic stroke are thought to be commonly associated with embolic mechanisms; these cases include patients with Wernicke aphasia,[37] Broca aphasia,[98] global aphasia without hemiparesis,[99] the angular gyrus syndrome,[100] and other branch vessel syndromes.[36] If patients with these conditions do not demonstrate an obvious source of embolization from the carotid bifurcation on the angiogram, and if the CT scan does not show a tumor or bleed, the possibility of cardiac embolization should be considered. Some patients with amaurosis fugax may have an identifiable carotid source for embolization. Others with amaurosis fugax and negative carotid angiograms may have cardiac sources for embolization. In patients with no apparent vertebrobasilar atherosclerosis, certain events referable to the posterior circulation may suggest embolization, including homonymous hemianopia and various forms of the ''top of the basilar syndrome.'' Patients with branch vessel occlusions on angiography but negative angiograms at the carotid bifurcation may have cardiac sources for embolization.

In patients presenting with TIA or carotid bruit, the risk of myocardial infarction or cardiac death is higher than the risk of stroke.[101] If we are to have a substantial impact on the morbidity and mortality in patients with cerebrovascular disease, these patients should be screened for coronary artery disease. Any patient with an obvious history of angina should be evaluated according to the institutional routine for symptomatic coronary disease. Further epidemiologic evaluation needs to be performed for patients with TIAs in whom an obvious history of angina is lacking. It has been suggested that these patients should be evaluated for subclinical coronary disease.[102]

After an acute stroke, cardiac function should be monitored for dysrhythmia, such as ventricular tachycardia or heart block, and for evidence of myocardial ischemia. These cardiac sequelae are not infrequent after a cerebral infarct and may relate to stroke-induced increases in sympathetic tone.

In summary, there are three major concerns that may indicate the need for additional cardiologic testing: (1) a search for potential sources of emboli in certain high-risk patients, (2) evaluation for coronary artery disease in an attempt to improve long-term survival, and (3) observation for cardiac sequelae of acute stroke, including the development of dysrhythmias and evidence of myocardial ischemia.

CONCLUSION

In evaluating patients with transient or permanent ischemic events, the initial goal is to identify which part of the brain is involved. Based on knowledge of vascular distribution patterns, the vessel at fault can often be suggested from the initial evaluation. Then a best guess about the underlying mechanism evolves. Correctly identifying the underlying mechanism in a given case helps in choosing appropriate tests and therapy. Our best guesses are often sketchy and phrased in terms of probabilities. However, if we fail to consider the probabilities and begin to treat all patients in a routine manner, we are likely to be inefficient and perhaps misled in our efforts to provide appropriate therapy.

REFERENCES

1. Drachman DA, Hart CW: An approach to the dizzy patient. *Neurology.* 1972;22:323.
2. Glick TA: *Neurologic Skills.* Boston: Blackwell Scientific, 1993.
3. Harper AF: *The Neurologic Examination.* Philadelphia: JB Lippincott, 1992.
4. Hoyt WF: Ocular symptoms and signs. In Ehrenfeld WK, ed. *Extracranial Occlusive Cerebral Vascular Disease.* Philadelphia: WB Saunders; 1970:64.
5. Ewing CC: Recurrent monocular blindness. *Lancet.* 1968;1:1035.
6. Wikes WN, Adams G, Cullen JP: Temporal arteritis and visual loss associated with position. *Neuro-ophthalmology.* 1984;4:107.
7. Weinberger J, Bender A, Young W: Amaurosis fugax associated with ophthalmic artery stenosis. *Stroke.* 1980;11:290.
8. Weinberg PE, Patronas NI, Kim KS, Melin O: Anomalous origin of the ophthalmic artery in patients with amaurosis fugax. *Arch Neurol.* 1981;38:315.
9. Walsh TJ: *Neuro-ophthalmology: Clinical Signs and Symptoms.* Philadelphia: Lea & Febiger; 1978.
10. Glaser JS: *Neuro-ophthalmology.* Hagerstown, MD: Harper & Row; 1978.
11. Cogan DG: Blackouts not obviously due to carotid occlusion. *Arch Ophthalmol.* 1961;66:180.
12. Selby G: *Migraine and Its Vanants.* Sydney: Adis Health Science Press; 1983.
13. Hedges T, Lackman R: Isolated ophthalmic migraine in the differential diagnosis of cerebral-ocular ischemia. *Stroke.* 1976;7:379.
14. Fisher CM: Late-life migraine accompaniments as a cause of unexplained transient ischemic attacks. *Can J Neurol Sci.* 1980;7:9.
15. Harrison, MJG, Marshall J: Indications for angiography and surgery in carotid artery disease. *Br Med J.* 1975;1:616.
16. Wilson L, Russell RWR: Amaurosis fugax in carotid artery disease—indications for angiography. *Br Med J.* 1977;2:435.
17. Sorenson PN: Amaurosis fugax. *Acta Ophthalmol (Copenh).* 1983;61:583.
18. Adams H, Putman S, Corbett J, et al: Amaurosis fugax, the results of arteriography in 59 patients. *Stroke.* 1983;14:742.
19. Mungas GE, Baker WH: Amaurosis fugax. *Stroke.* 1977;8:232.
20. Hoyt WF: Transient bilateral blurring of vision: Considerations of specific ischemic symptoms of vertebral basilar insufficiency. *Arch Ophthalmol.* 1963;70:476.
21. Caplan LR: ''Top of the basilar'' syndrome. *Neurology (NY).* 1980;30:72.
22. Adams R, Victor M: *Principles of Neurology*, 3rd ed. New York: McGraw-Hill; 1985.
23. Fisher CM: Pure sensory stroke involving face, arm and leg. *Neurology (NY).* 1965;15:76.
24. Fisher CM: Pure sensory stroke and allied conditions. *Stroke.* 1982;13:434.
25. Rosenberg N, Koller R: Computerized tomography in pure sensory stroke. *Neurology (NY).* 1981;31:217.
26. Fisher CM: Lacunes: Small, deep cerebral infarcts. *Neurology (NY).* 1965;15:774.
27. Fisher CM: Capsular infarcts. *Arch Neurol.* 1979;36:65.
28. Rascol A, Clanet M, Manelfe C, et al: Pure motor hemiplegia: Computed tomography study of 30 cases. *Stroke.* 1982;13:11.
29. Mohr JP: Lacunes. *Stroke.* 1982;13:3.
30. Weisber L: Computed tomography in pure motor hemiparesis. *Neurology (NY).* 1979;29:490.
31. Aleksic S, George A: Pure motor hemiplegia with occlusion of the extracranial carotid artery. *J Neurol Sci.* 1973;19:331.
32. Pullicino P, Nelson RC, Kendall BE, et al: Small deep infarcts diagnosed by computed tomography. *Neurology (NY).* 1980;30:1090.
33. Melo TP, Bogousslavsky J, van Melle G, et al: Pure motor stroke: A reappraisal. *Neurology (NY).* 1992;42:789.
34. Mohr JP, Kase CS, Meckler RJ, Fisher CM: Sensorimotor stroke due to thalamocapsular ischemia. *Arch Neurol.* 1977;34:739.
35. Williams D, Wilson TG: The diagnosis of the major and minor syndromes of basilar insufficiency. *Brain.* 1964;85:741.
36. Waddington MM, Ring BA: Syndromes of occlusion of the middle cerebral artery branches. *Brain.* 1968;91:685.
37. Mohr JP, Caplan LR, Melski JW, et al: The Harvard cooperative stroke registry—a prospective registry. *Neurology (NY).* 1978;28:754.
38. Cocito L, Favale E, Reni L: Epileptic seizures in cerebral arterial occlusive disease. *Stroke.* 1982;13:189.
39. Baquis GD, Pessin M, Scott M: Limb shaking—a carotid TIA. *Stroke.* 1985;16:444.
40. Fisher CM: Concerning recurrent transient cerebral ischemic attacks. *Can Med Assoc J.* 1962;86:1091.
41. Harrison MJG, Marshall J, Thomas DJ: Relevance of duration of TIAs in carotid territory. *Br Med J.* 1978;1:1578.
42. Baloh R: *Dizziness, Hearing Loss and Tinnitus—Essentials of Neuro-otology.* Philadelphia: FA Davis; 1984.
43. Fisher CM: Vertigo in cerebral vascular disease. *Arch Otolaryngol.* 1967;85:529.
44. Troost BT: Dizziness and vertigo in vertebrobasilar disease. Part I. Peripheral and systemic causes of dizziness. *Stroke.* 1980;11:301.
45. Troost BT: Dizziness and vertigo in vertebrobasilar disease. Part II. Central causes and vertebral basilar disease. *Stroke.* 1980;11:413.
46. Strub R, Black FW: *The Mental Status Examination in Neurology.* Philadelphia: FA Davis; 1977.
47. Benson DF: *Aphasia, Alexia and Agraphia.* New York: Churchill Livingstone; 1979.
48. Toole JF: *Cerebrovascular Diseases*, 3rd ed. New York: Raven Press; 1984.
49. Kartchener MM, McRae LP: Auscultation for carotid bruits in cerebrovascular insufficiency. *JAMA.* 1969;210:494.
50. Duncan GW, Gruber JO, Dewey F, et al: Evaluation of carotid stenosis by phonoangiography. *N Engl J Med.* 1979;293:1124.
51. Kartchener MM, McRae LP: Noninvasive evaluation and management of the ''asymptomatic'' carotid bruit. *Surgery.* 1977;82:840.
52. Kartchener MM, McRae LP, Morrison FD: Noninvasive detection and evaluation of carotid occlusion disease. *Arch Surg.* 1973;106:528.
53. Heyman A, Wilkenson WE, et al: Risk of stroke in asymptomatic persons with cervical bruits. *N Engl J Med.* 1980;302:838.
54. Riles T, Liekerman A, Kopelman I, Imparato A: Symptoms, stenosis, and bruit. *Arch Surg.* 1981;116:218.
55. Henerici M, Aulich A, Sandermann W, Freund HJ: The incidence of asymptomatic extracranial arterial disease. *Stroke.* 1981;12:750.
56. Ziegler DK, Ziteli T, Dick A, Sebaugh J: Correlation of bruits over the carotid artery with angiographically demonstrated lesions. *Neurology (NY).* 1971;21:860.
57. Bonventre MV: Takayasu's disease revisited. *NY State J Med.* 1960, 1974.
58. Heckenlively JR, Yee RD, Krauss HR, et al: Visual physiologic and ocular evaluation in carotid occlusive disease. *Doc Ophthalmol.* 1981;27:131.
59. Benson DF, Tomlinson EB: Hemiplegic syndrome of the posterior cerebral artery. *Stroke.* 1971;2:559.
60. Shimizu K, Sano K: Pulseless disease. *J Neuropathy Clin Neurol.* 1951;1:37.
61. Ishikawa K: Natural history and classification of occlusive thromboaortopathy (Takayasu's disease). *Circulation.* 1978;57:27.
62. Parker JP: Neuro-ophthalmological aspects of cerebral vascular disease. In Smith RR, ed. *Stroke in the Extracranial Vessels.* New York: Raven Press; 1984:69.
63. Hollenhorst RW: Ocular manifestations of insufficiency for thrombosis of the internal carotid artery. *Trans Am Ophthalmol Soc.* 1958;56:474.
64. Hollenhorst RW: Ocular manifestations of carotid arterial thrombosis. *Med Clin North Am.* 1960;44:897.
65. Pfaffenbach D, Hollenhorst RW: The significance of bright plaques in the retinal arterial tree. *Trans Am Ophthalmol Soc.* 1972;70:337.
66. Ehrenfeld WK, Hoyt W, Wylie E: Embolization and transient blindness from carotid atheroma. *Arch Surg.* 1966;93:787.
67. Hollenhorst RW: Significance of bright plaques in retinal arterioles. *JAMA.* 1961;178:23.
68. Fisher CM: Observations of the fundus oculi with transient monocular blindness. *Neurology (NY).*
69. Fisher CM: Transient monocular blindness associated with hemiplegia. *Trans Am Neurol Assoc.* 1951;50:154.

70. Waybright EA, Selhorst JB, Combs J: Anterior ischemic optic neuropathy with internal carotid artery occlusion. *Am J Ophthalmol.* 1982;93:42.
71. Lieberman MF, Shaki A, Green WR: Embolic ischemic optic neuropathy. *Am J Ophthalmol.* 1978;86:206.
72. Mori E, Tabuchi M, Yamadori A: Lacunar syndrome due to intracerebral hemorrhage. *Stroke.* 1985;16:454.
73. Fisher CM, Curry HB: Pure motor hemiplegia of vascular origin. *Arch Neurol.* 1965;13:30.
74. Derouesne C, Mas J, Bolgert F, Castaigne P: Pure sensory stroke caused by a small cortical infarction in the middle cerebral artery territory. *Stroke.* 1984;15:660.
75. Sundt TM, Sibert RG, Piepgras GG, et al: Bypass surgery for vascular disease of the carotid system. *Mayo Clin Proc.* 1976;51:677.
76. Bauer RB: Mechanical compression of the vertebral arteries. In Berguer R, Bauer RB, eds. *Vertebrobasilar Occlusive Disease.* New York: Raven Press; 1984;45.
77. Corvera J, Benitiz L, Lopez-Rios G, et al: Vestibular and ocular motor abnormalities in vertebral basilar insufficiency. *Ann Otol.* 1980;89:370.
78. Barber HO, Dionne J: Vestibular findings in vertebral basilar ischemia. *Ann Otol.* 1971;80:805.
79. Nishide M, Irino T, Gotch M, et al: Cardiac abnormalities in ischemic cerebral vascular disease: Studies by two dimensional echocardiography. *Stroke.* 1983;14:541.
80. Barnett HJM, Jones MW, Boughner DR, Kostuk WJ: Cerebral ischemic events associated with prolapsing mitral valve. *Arch Neurol.* 1976;33:777.
81. Rolak L, Robey R, Vereni M, Haruti Y: Coronary artery disease in patients with cerebrovascular disease: A prospective study. *Ann Neurol.* 1983;14:132.
82. Barnett HJM, Boughner DR, Taylor DW, et al: Further evidence relating mitral valve prolapse to cerebral ischemic events. *N Engl J Med.* 1980;302:139.
83. Watson R: TIA stroke and mitral valve prolapse. *Neurology (NY).* 1979;29:886.
84. De Bono DP, Warlon CP: Mitral annulus calcification and cerebral or retinal ischemia. *Lancet.* 1979;2:383.
85. Abernathy WS, Willis PW: Thromboembolic complications of rheumatic heart disease. *Cardiovasc Clin.* 1973;5:131.
86. Biller J, Challa V, Toole JF, Howard V: Nonbacterial thrombotic endocarditis: Clinicopathologic correlations of 99 patients—a neurological perspective. *Arch Neurol.* 1982;39:95.
87. Barletta GA, Gegliardi R, Benvenuti L, Fantini F: Cerebral ischemic attacks as a complication of aortic and mitral valve prolapse. *Stroke.* 1985;16:219.
88. Britton M, Gustafsson C: Nonrheumatic atrial fibrillation as a risk factor for stroke. *Stroke.* 1985;16:182.
89. Abdon NJ, Zettervall O, Carlson J, et al: Is occult atrial disorder a frequent cause of nonhemorrhagic stroke? Long term EKG in 86 patients. *Stroke.* 1982;13:832.
90. Come PC, Riley MF, Bivis NK: Roles of echocardiography and arrhythmia monitoring in the evaluation of patients with suspected systemic embolization. *Ann Neurol.* 1983;13:527.
91. Robbins JA, Sagar KB, French M, Smith PJ: Influence of echocardiography on management of patients with systemic emboli. *Stroke.* 1983;14:546.
92. DiTullio M, Sacco RL, Mohr JP, et al: Patent foramen ovale as a risk factor for cryptogenic stroke. *Ann Intern Med.* 1992;117:461.
93. Hoffman T, Kasper W, Meinertz, et al: Echocardiographic evaluation of patients with clinically suspected arterial emboli. *Lancet.* 1990;336:1421.
94. Pearson AC, Labovitz AJ, Tatineni S, et al: Superiority of transesophageal echocardiography in detecting cardiac sources of emboli in patients with cerebral ischemia of unknown etiology. *J Am Coll Cardiol.* 1991;17:66.
95. Teague SM, Sharma MK: Detection of paradoxical cerebral echo contrast embolization by transcranial Doppler ultrasound. *Stroke.* 1991;22:740.
96. DiTullo M, Massaro A, Hoffman, et al: Transcranial Doppler with contrast injection in stroke patients with patent foramen ovale. *Circulation.* 1991;84:451.
97. Nemec JJ, Marwick TH, Lorig RJ, et al: Comparison of transcranial Doppler ultrasound and transesophageal contrast echocardiography in the detection of intraatrial right to left shunts. *Am J Cardiol.* 1991;68:1498.
98. Mohr JP, Pessin MS, Finklestein S, et al: Broca aphasia—pathological and clinical aspects. *Neurology (NY).* 1978;28:311.
99. Horn GV, Hawes A: Global aphasia without hemiparesis: A sign of embolic encephalopathy. *Neurology (NY).* 1982;32:403.
100. Marinkovic SV, Kovacevic MS, Kostic VS: The isolated occlusion of the angular gyri artery—a correlative neurological and anatomical study—case report. *Stroke.* 1984;15:366.
101. Adams HP, Kassell NF, Mazuz H: The patient with transient ischemic attacks: Is this the time for a new therapeutic approach? *Stroke.* 1984;15:371.
102. Myers MG, Norris JW, Hachinski VC, et al: Cardiac sequelae of acute stroke. *Stroke.* 1982;13:838.

IV

Hemodynamic Assessment and Imaging

CHAPTER
13

Computed Tomography of Stroke

JOHN R. BENTSON

It is generally recognized that the development of computed tomography was a major advance in imaging technology, one of the most fundamental advances since the discovery of the roentgen ray. The potentials of computed tomography (CT) in brain imaging were recognized from the beginning, and the role of CT in the imaging of a wide variety of brain disorders, including cerebrovascular diseases, can hardly be overemphasized.

HISTORY

Prior to the development of CT, no imaging method was available to demonstrate the actual structure of brain tissue. The traditional diagnostic tests relied on injection of gas into the cerebrospinal fluid spaces or injection of iodinated contrast media into blood vessels in order to gain some idea of the shape of the brain. Angiography also contributed information about the blood vessels, blood flow, and the effects of disease on these vessels. The limitations of these tests were apparent to Dr. William H. Oldendorf, who built a simple experimental gadget to demonstrate that the makeup of a complex structure could be determined by passing a beam of radiation through it at different angles.[1] The results of his experiments were published in 1961, before the computer technology required for further development had become available.

The first CT scanner was developed by Godfrey Hounsfield, an engineer at the Central Research Laboratories of EMI Ltd. in England.[2] The first clinical unit using this technology was installed in Wimbledon, England, in 1971.

Many technologic advances have been made since that time to improve the speed, resolution, and reliability of scanners. Early scanners were of a translate-rotate type, whereas modern scanners use rotation only, as well as a fanbeam, which allows the reduction of scanning time per slice from a minute or more to a few seconds. With improved and more numerous detectors and other refinements, resolution has been remarkably improved. Such additions as dynamic scanning and xenon-inhalation techniques provide further information regarding blood flow to various portions of the brain. Although the potentials of CT scanning were recognized from the time of the early, relatively crude images, refinements in the technology have made CT scanners essential equipment in all major hospitals.

PRINCIPLES

Basically, computed tomography owes its value as an imaging modality to its ability to scan selected thin sections of tissue, minimizing the effects of interference from adjacent tissue, and to its superior ability to detect slight variations in tissue density. A closely collimated beam of photons, generated by an x-ray tube, is passed through the tissue to be examined. The proportion of photon absorption by the tissue is determined by a detection apparatus, and this information is stored and processed by a computer. In order to determine the location of the tissues responsible for the absorption of photons, the photon beam must be passed through the body repeatedly at a large number of angles, so that a method of mathematic reconstruction can be applied. If the slice of anatomy examined is considered to have a grid or matrix structure, and if each element of the matrix (pixel) is assigned a shade of gray determined by its computed attenuation characteristic or absorption coefficient, an image can be produced that will faithfully reflect relative electron densities of that tissue. Reducing pixel size will result in better image resolution up to a point, whereupon the practical penalties of image graininess, prolonged scanning time, and required increased photon beam density with associated increased radiation exposure will prevent further reduction of pixel size.

Interpretation of CT scans entails the appreciation of density differences of pixels related to their different absorption values. Tissues with high absorption values appear white (eg, bone), whereas tissues and other areas with low absorption values appear dark (eg, air, fat). Density of brain tissue is nearly uniform, with gray matter being slightly more dense than white matter. Water has a lower density than brain tissue, making differentiation of cerebrospinal fluid from brain tissue relatively simple, and also making edematous tissue detectable because of its lower density. Freshly coagulated blood is relatively dense, which is of considerable importance in the computed tomography of hematomas. There may be difficulties in distinguishing blood from calcification, but such a differentiation is often possible if the appearance of the abnormality and its absorption coefficient values are examined. These values can be higher for calcification than for blood.

Accurate interpretation of CT scans demands familiarity

with a large variety of artifacts that plague CT scanning. Artifacts can be generated by motion, metal, dense bone structures, improper centering, calibration problems, and so forth. Artifacts vary with different CT scanners, producing further difficulty in distinguishing between true absorption abnormalities and artifacts. Besides the examiner's ability to distinguish between artifacts and real abnormalities, accurate interpretation of CT scans depends on the ability to assemble observations that can be linked logically to support specific diagnoses.

TRANSIENT ISCHEMIC ATTACKS

Transient ischemic attacks (TIAs) are acute neurologic dysfunctions related to brain ischemia that last less than 24 hours. These are usually caused by either emboli to brain vessels or arteriosclerotic narrowing of arteries supplying the brain, with the acute event often precipitated by transient hypotension. The passing of symptoms is presumably related to improvement in brain perfusion, either from the breaking-up of emboli or thrombus or by the restoration of blood pressure.

Computed tomography scans of patients with TIAs generally show no abnormalities. Bradac and Oberson[3] found no CT findings associated with TIAs in a series of 200 patients, most of whom were scanned during the first 4 weeks following the attacks. The few positive scans showed only atrophy or the results of previous infarctions. In the same group of patients, cerebral angiography demonstrated abnormalities in about 80 percent, showing a variety of findings such as stenosis, ulceration or occlusion of the carotid arteries in the neck, arteriosclerotic abnormalities of intracranial vessels, arteritis, and fibromuscular dysplasia.

Such has been the general experience with CT scanning of TIAs. However, CT scans are often performed in cases of TIAs for two reasons. First, it is often clinically unclear in the early stages whether one is dealing with a TIA or an early stroke. Second, other pathologic states such as tumor or cerebral inflammatory disease can clinically mimic TIAs, and these causes can be detected by CT scanning (Fig. 13–1). The possibility of other lesions, such as tumors or inflammatory conditions, may be given as a reason to support the desirability of using contrast-infused CT scans for suspected TIAs, but there is no general agreement on this point.

COMPUTED TOMOGRAPHY SCANNING IN ACUTE ISCHEMIC INFARCTION

Early CT scanning of stroke patients is generally done to distinguish ischemic or bland infarcts from intracranial hemorrhage, in order to help make therapeutic decisions, such as the possible use of anticoagulation medication. Early reports stated that CT scanning performed in the first 48 hours after ischemic strokes generally showed negative results.[4–6] The time at which first CT manifestations appear is variable, depending on such factors as size and completeness of infarction. Although the detection rates of early infarcts were disappointing with the early scanners, improved scanners permitted the detection of nearly 90 percent of infarcts within the first 24 hours.[7] The most common early CT findings are areas of decreased attenuation of the brain and subtle evidence of mass effect, such as effacement of sulci and subarachnoid cisterns. These findings are related to the accumulation of edema fluid within the affected tissue, a process that begins within the first few hours following the

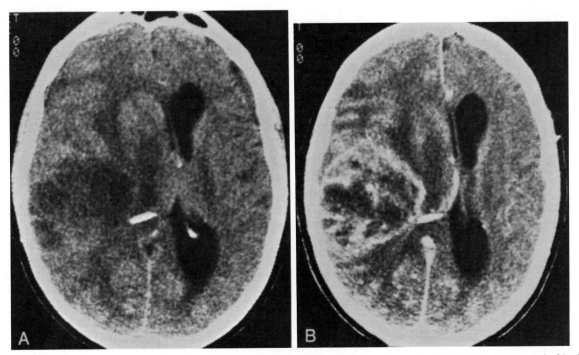

FIGURE 13–1. Surprising computed tomography (CT) scan in a 58-year-old patient with acute aphasia and mild hemiparesis, suspected of having had a transient ischemic attack (TIA). *A*, Noncontrast CT scan shows extensive hypodensity of the right cerebral hemisphere and marked mass effect, neither of which is consistent with TIA or early infarction. *B*, Contrast-enhanced scan shows irregular enhancement of a large tumor, later proved to be a glioblastoma.

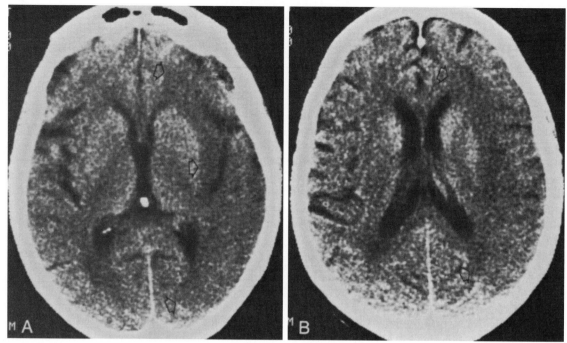

FIGURE 13–2. *A and B,* Acute infarct of the middle cerebral artery territory. This scan, performed 12 hours after the onset of stroke, shows a subtle hypodensity *(arrowheads)* of the entire middle cerebral artery territory except for the basal ganglia region, which indicates sparing of the striate arteries. Note the obliteration of the left cerebral sulci and narrowing of the left sylvian fissure, signs of early mass effect.

onset of infarction.[8] The hypodensity of the early infarct is very subtle, and its detection requires both high-resolution scanning and the absence of motion on the part of the patient. If the early scan shows no abnormalities, a scan performed later than 48 hours after the event is almost certain to show the infarct. Whether this later scan is necessary is debatable, since the clinical diagnosis of stroke can generally be made by then, other causes of acute neurologic symptoms having been ruled out by the early scan.

Another early sign associated with cerebral infarction is the hyperdense artery sign, seen most commonly in the middle cerebral artery. The hyperdensity, related to clotted blood, generally predicts a large infarction. In some cases, this may be the only sign of infarction on early CT scans.[9, 10]

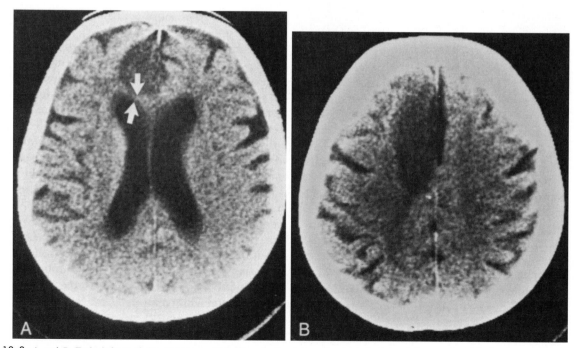

FIGURE 13–3. *A and B,* Early infarct of the anterior cerebral artery territory. Location is typical, involving a strip of brain tissue adjacent to the falx, sparing the corpus callosum *(arrows).* The most posteriorly located part of the anterior cerebral artery territory is spared, probably because of collateral flow from posterior cerebral artery branches.

Magnetic resonance imaging (MRI) is more sensitive than CT in detecting early infarcts and has been advocated for this purpose. The advantages of MRI relate to higher sensitivity for detecting brain edema, better demonstration of subtle sulcal compression, and changes within arteries indicating obstruction or slow flow.[11, 12] CT remains the imaging modality generally used when acute infarcts are suspected, however, as it may be more expedient and is equally sensitive for the detection of acute bleeding.

Since the early evidence of infarction can be subtle, some points regarding the specific appearance of infarction should be kept in mind. First, the areas of infarction tend to correspond to vascular territories, and crossover between major vessel areas is uncommon. The middle cerebral artery territory is the area most often involved, and involvement of a portion of that territory is more common than that of the entire territory. Middle cerebral artery infarcts often result in compression of the sylvian fissure as an early sign, with effacement of sulci or mass effect on the ventricles being less commonly observed.[7] A second important observation is that the low attenuation, related to the formation of edema fluid within the infarcted tissue within a few hours after onset, is found to involve both gray and white matter. This observation helps to distinguish infarcts from neoplasms, abscesses, or demyelinating disease, all of which typically have edema patterns that involve only the white matter.

Typical infarction patterns related to the middle cerebral, anterior cerebral, and posterior cerebral arteries are illustrated in Figures 13–2 to 13–4. It should be noted that most infarcts are not necessarily wedge-shaped but do extend to involve both gray and white matter. Central infarcts of the basal ganglia and adjacent white matter can occur as a result

of striate artery occlusions. Although intrinsic disease of the striate arteries is the most common cause of these deep infarcts, they may also result when the horizontal portion of the middle cerebral or anterior cerebral arteries is occluded by emboli, dissections, or other causes. In such cases, collateral flow can occur to the more distal branches of the parent arteries, sparing territories other than the basal ganglia from infarction. By paying close attention to the location of the infarct on the CT scan, the examiner can often determine which striate vessels are involved. For example, infarction of branches of the medial striate arteries results in infarction of the anterioinferior part of the corpus striatum. Lateral striate artery occlusions affect the posterolateral corpus striatum and the periventricular white matter cephalad to that region. Anterior choroidal artery occlusions will infarct the posterior limb of the internal capsule, portions of the uncus, the amygdaloid nucleus, and the hippocampus.[13]

Infarcts of the cerebellum are less common and are more often unilateral than bilateral. Less than half of these infarcts are detectable by computed tomography.[14] Again, the location of the infarct may make it apparent that it involves the superior cerebellar, posteroinferior cerebellar, or anteroinferior cerebellar artery territories.[15] Acute infarcts of the brain stem are generally difficult or impossible to see on CT scans and are better appreciated by MRI. In general, all acute infarcts are better demonstrated by MRI than by CT. However, practical matters such as the difficulty of eliminating motion in patients who are acutely disoriented or obtunded must also be considered in the choice of the examination technique.

Another pattern of infarction is that occurring in the border zones, or watershed regions, between the major vascular territories.[16-18] Such infarction is also referred to as hemodynamic infarction. These infarcts generally occur in older persons who have occlusive disease of one or more major arterial trunks. When perfusion pressure is further reduced by such factors as cardiac dysrhythmias, treatment of hypertension, or even nocturnal hypotension, infarction of border zones may occur because the perfusion pressure in the terminal vascular branches is normally lower. Those areas in which border zone infarcts are most often seen are on the cerebral convexity between the anterior and middle cerebral artery territories and the parieto-occipital region between the posterior and middle cerebral arteries. The low density of the infarcted area characteristically extends from the cortex deeply into the periventricular white matter (Fig. 13–5).

One further type of infarction that should be kept in mind is venous infarction, resulting from occlusion of either dural venous sinuses or cerebral veins, or both. A number of conditions predispose to occlusion of these venous channels, including septic causes such as meningitis, empyema, sinusitis, and mastoiditis, and aseptic causes such as severe dehydration, pregnancy, use of oral contraceptives, disseminated intravascular coagulation, leukemia, intracranial neoplasms, and arteriovenous malformations.[19] Mortality is high in cases of venous sinus occlusion, and early recognition of the condition is essential. There are several features of venous infarcts that distinguish them from arterial infarcts. Low-density regions related to venous infarcts tend to be less well defined and may not be seen unless the scan is closely scrutinized. The infarcted area may involve more than one arterial territory, with the parasagittal region being most

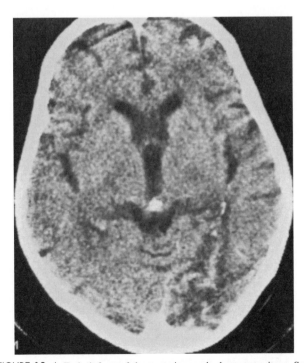

FIGURE 13–4. Early infarct of the posterior cerebral artery territory. Scan shows hypodensity of the left occipital lobe extending to the falx and extension anteriorly to the inferior surface of left temporal lobe, indicating involvement of temporal lobe branches of posterior cerebral artery also. There are irregular strands of high density in a gyral pattern, indicating cortical bleeding secondary to the infarction.

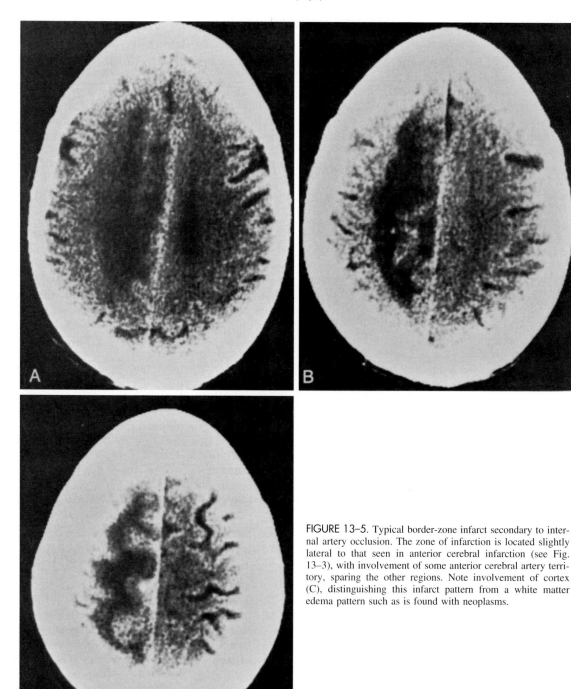

FIGURE 13–5. Typical border-zone infarct secondary to internal artery occlusion. The zone of infarction is located slightly lateral to that seen in anterior cerebral infarction (see Fig. 13–3), with involvement of some anterior cerebral artery territory, sparing the other regions. Note involvement of cortex (C), distinguishing this infarct pattern from a white matter edema pattern such as is found with neoplasms.

often involved. Nonenhanced scans often show petechial bleeding into gyri, or even frank parenchymal hemorrhage.[20] Gyral enhancement is common following contrast infusion. A characteristic sign found in more than one half of the cases is the empty delta sign, in which sections of perpendicular to the superior sagittal sinus show its walls to be contrast-enhanced but its interior, filled with clotted blood, to be of lower density.[19, 20] The falx and tentorium may show an unusual degree of enhancement attributable to enlarged collateral venous pathways. Because cases occur in which computed tomography is nonspecific or may even show normal results, angiography is recommended to confirm or rule out the presence of venous thromboses.

CHANGES IN APPEARANCE OF INFARCTS WITH TIME

When an infarct first becomes visible on CT scans, its borders may be indistinct. Over the next few days, the infarct becomes more readily visible because of greater accumulation of edema fluid, and the infarct margins then becomes sharper. At the same time, the area of the infarct may change. It may become smaller as some of the tissue at the margin of the infarct is revitalized by collateral blood flow. In other cases, the area of infarction may enlarge because of propagation of intravascular clotting or increase of edema (Fig. 13–6). Mass effect due to edema peaks between the third and fifth days.[21, 22] The degree of mass effect is generally small considering the amount of brain tissue involved, which constitutes another characteristic feature of infarction on CT. However, major infarcts, such as those involving the entire middle cerebral artery territory, not infrequently result in sufficient mass effect to cause subfalcial and transtentorial herniation (see Fig. 13–6), which in turn may result in extension of infarction to the occipital lobe secondary to compression of the posterior cerebral artery against the tentorium. Eventually, the density of an infarcted area on CT approximates that of cerebrospinal fluid. This is not surprising, since phagocytosis of necrotic brain tissue eventually results in large cystic spaces.

The progressively decreasing attenuation of the infarcted tissue may be interrupted by the "fogging" effect seen during the second and third weeks after the infarct.[23, 24] This temporary increase in attenuation of the area of infarction may be sufficient to mask the presence of an infarct on noninfused CT scans taken during that time. This effect is probably related to formation of highly vascular granulation tissue within the region of infarction at this time. Cases in which the fogging effect is prominent also tend to show strong contrast enhancement, so that diagnosis of infarct during this period is not difficult if both preinfusion and postinfusion scans are performed.

The appearance of an infarct may also be altered by the complication of bleeding into the infarcted area. The degree of bleeding varies considerably, ranging from marginal petechial bleeding to massive hemorrhage. Petechial bleeding, when extensive, can be recognized on CT scans as regions of increased attenuation involving primarily gray matter and having a gyral distribution pattern (Figs. 13–4 and 13–7).[5] When such petechial hemorrhage is extensive, the infarct is called a hemorrhagic infarct, not to be confused with a primary cerebral hemorrhage. This hemorrhagic phenomenon develops more often in infarcts caused by emboli,[25] which is probably due to the commonly occurring disintegration of the embolus, with subsequent return of perfusion pressure to infarcted tissue, causing leakage of blood through injured capillaries. Supporting this theory is the frequent observation that patients in whom hemorrhagic infarcts develop have had earlier CT scans showing no evidence of such bleeding.[26] Bleeding into infarcted tissue may also be provoked by elevation of blood pressure and by the use of heparin.[27] In contrast to the appearance of hemorrhagic infarcts, primary intracerebral hematomas are shown to be more dense and more homogeneous on CT, do not show a gyral pattern, are not limited to the gray matter, and are usually round or oval in shape (Fig. 13–8).

CONTRAST ENHANCEMENT IN INFARCTION

Intravenous infusion of an iodinated contrast medium is of great importance in the detection by CT of a wide variety of diseases but is of more limited use in the diagnosis of stroke. Enhancement of the infarcted area rarely occurs during the first 5 days, and contrast infusion may indeed obscure the hypodensity of the infarcted area at this time. However,

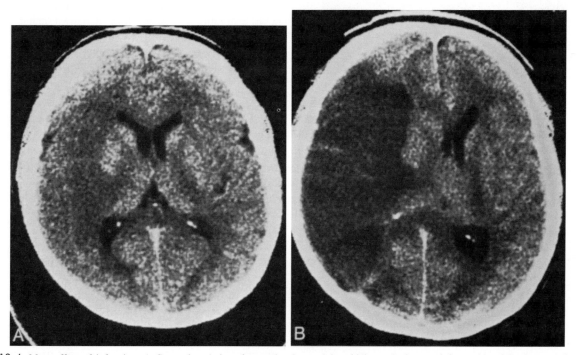

FIGURE 13–6. Mass effect of infarction. A, Scan taken 1 day after stroke shows right middle cerebral artery infarct with minimal mass effect and ill-defined borders. B, Scan taken 2 days later shows marked hypodensity and marked mass effect from edema fluid, also clear definition of borders. Edema of this degree often proves fatal.

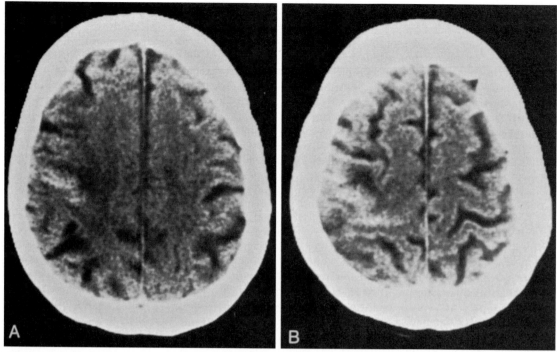

FIGURE 13–7. *A and B,* Recent infarction with cortical bleeding. The gyriform hyperdensities of the right parietal lobe are the best indication of infarction in this elderly patient, with white matter edema and sulcal effacement being less evident. It is important to recognize such bleeding, which may be subtle, because of the hazards of anticoagulating such patients.

there is great variation in the incidence of contrast enhancement during the first few days, depending on such factors as the etiology and extent of infarction and the amount of contrast material used. Few infarcts become enhanced during the first week when modest doses of contrast medium are

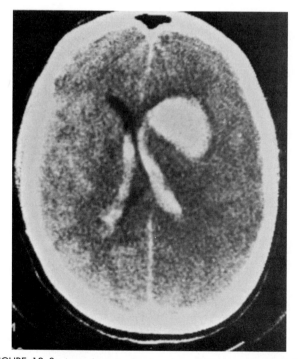

FIGURE 13–8. Acute hypertensive hematoma. This hematoma probably originated in the head of the caudate or anterior lenticular nucleus, more anterior than the typical hypertensive bleed. Note the thin ring of hypodensity around the hematoma and the rupture of the hematoma into the displaced lateral ventricles.

used.[24] Using a dose of contrast material twice that normally used (80 g iodine), Hayman and associates[28] noted enhancement in 72 percent of patients within the first 28 hours after infarction and also observed that persistent enhancement on 3-hour delayed scans correlated well with later development of hemorrhagic infarction. Embolic infarcts are more likely to show early enhancement than are those of other etiologies, which is probably related to the breakup of the embolus with restoration of blood flow. Contrast enhancement in infarcts is related mainly to the accumulation of contrast media in the extracellular space, deposited there because of damage to the capillary endothelium with resultant blood-brain barrier breakdown.[29] This breakdown develops within a few hours of the ischemic event, but there is little if any enhancement for several days, probably because of low blood flow to the infarcted area.[30] The development of new capillaries at the margins of the infarcted area, beginning several days after the infarction, also contributes to the enhancement.[31] The third possible mechanism of the development of enhancement, so-called luxury perfusion, is believed less likely to be a major factor, partly because delayed scans show increased and more diffuse staining of brain tissue by contrast, more in keeping with extravasation of contrast medium into the brain tissue.[5, 32]

Although contrast enhancement is seen only in the minority of infarcts in the first week, it occurs in the great majority (70% to 90%) during the second week.[5, 24] Thereafter, the degree of contrast enhancement begins to slowly decrease, but enhancement may be present for as long as 12 weeks after the stroke.[33]

Enhancement involves mainly the cortical and deep gray matter. The most common pattern is that of irregular strips of enhanced material that follow the gyral pattern to some degree or may be nonhomogeneous without a clear pattern. Other patterns of enhancement occur, including homogeneous and ringlike patterns. There is some tendency for the enhancement pattern to change, with the most common change being from generalized enhancement to ringlike enhancement (Fig. 13–9).[33] Ringlike enhancement is most often seen in deep cerebral infarcts, such as those of the basal ganglia. Both homogeneous and ringlike enhancement may be diagnostically troublesome, resembling the enhancement patterns of neoplasms and abscesses. Noting that there is little or no associated mass effect may help make this differentiation. If there is still a problem, it may be resolved by performance of a follow-up scan in a couple weeks, since the degree of enhancement decreases with time. Enhancement is more often seen in cases of large infarction, probably accounting for the observation that there is an association

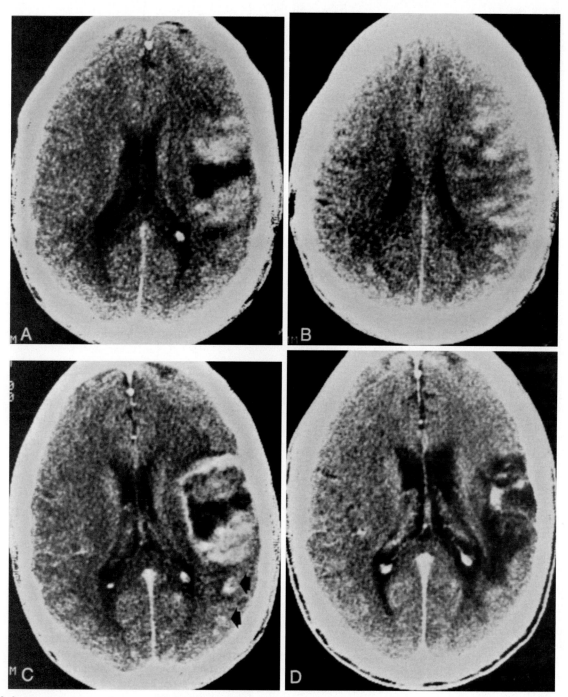

FIGURE 13–9. Changing patterns of contrast enhancement. A, Contrast-infused scan, taken approximately 2 weeks after middle cerebral territory stroke, showing areas of strong enhancement separated by a hypodense region. An earlier scan at 2 days showed only hypodensity, similar to that seen in Figure 13–2. B, Same scan, higher section. At this level, the more typical infarct pattern of gyriform enhancement is seen. C, One week later, a ring stain is seen on the infused scan, resembling neoplasm such as glioblastoma or metastasis more than infarct. However, note the separate regions of enhancement seen posteriorly (arrows), also present on higher sections, which together with lack of mass effect, should suggest infarct even if previous scans had not been available. D, Three months later, a contrast-infused scan shows contraction of the infarcted region, now hypodense except for residual central enhancement. The left lateral ventricle has enlarged due to the loss of volume of the infarcted region.

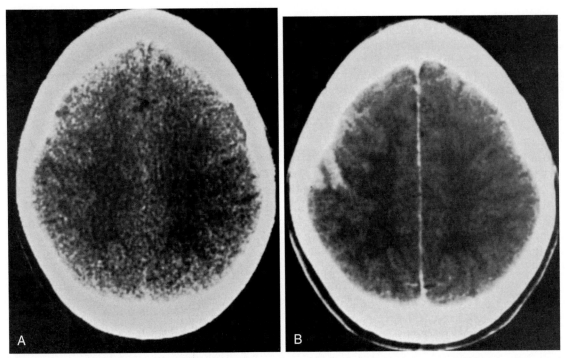

FIGURE 13–10. Small cortical infarct. *A*, No abnormalities were apparent on noninfused scan. *B*, Following contrast infusion, there is strong enhancement of two gyri in the right frontoparietal cortex. This type of infarct, without apparent white matter involvement, may be missed on magnetic resonance imaging.

between contrast enhancement of infarcts and poor prognosis.[33]

There is one type of infarction that is only visible on contrast-infused CT scans. This is a small infarct that involves only small segments of cerebral cortex (Fig. 13–10). The lack of white matter involvement apparently accounts for the lack of white matter edema, making the infarct invisible on noninfused scans. Another curious feature of such infarcts is that they may also be invisible on MRI.[34]

LACUNAR INFARCTS

Several features of lacunar infarcts set them apart from other cerebral infarcts. They involve relatively small volumes of tissue but may have profound clinical effects. These cylindrical infarcts often extend through the basal ganglia and into the paraventricular white matter. They are often very difficult or impossible to detect in the acute phase by CT and may only become visible weeks later (Fig. 13–11). The ability to become enhanced is generally not a prominent feature of lacunar infarcts. Older lacunar infarcts are easily seen on CT, even though they are relatively small, partly because the long axis of the infarct corresponds to the longest dimension of the CT boxel.

The arteries involved in lacunar infarction are mainly the striate arteries of the anterior, middle, and posterior cerebral arteries. The type of artery involved may be determined by the location of the abnormality on CT. For example, striate arteries arising from the anterior cerebral artery supply mainly the head of the caudate nucleus, part of the putamen, and the anterior limb of the internal capsule. The anterior choroidal artery supplies the globus pallidus and part of the internal capsule. The lateral striate branches of the middle

cerebral artery supply the body of the caudate, part of its head, portions of the internal capsule, and paraventricular white matter. Thalamic infarction usually involves obstruction of one or more of the posterior perforating arteries

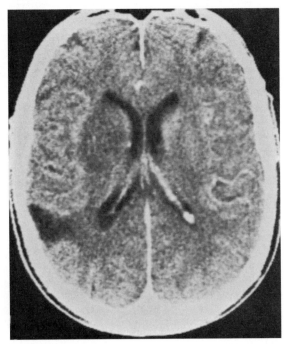

FIGURE 13–11. Early basal ganglia infarct. Scan taken 3 days after stroke showed hypodensity and mild mass effect in the right basal ganglia region but no enhancement. This infarct was visible at this early stage because of its large size; it later became a smaller, more hypodense, and typically rounded lacunar infarct. An old wedge-shaped infarct is seen in the right parietal lobe.

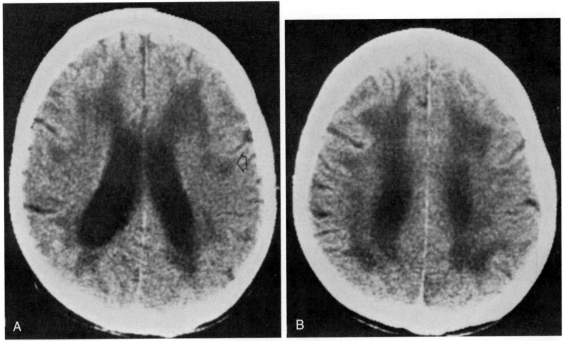

FIGURE 13–12. Binswanger disease. Typical features are the irregularity and marked extension outward from the lateral ventricles of the ischemia-related hypodensities. Hypodensities may be isolated, giving a more lacunar appearance *(arrow).*

arising from the posterior cerebral or posterior communicating arteries.[35–37]

BINSWANGER DISEASE

Computed tomography has demonstrated that Binswanger disease occurs more commonly than had been thought. In this disease, also called subcortical arteriosclerotic encephalopathy, the long penetrating arteries of the brain are affected by arteriosclerosis, mainly in elderly patients who have chronic hypertension. This results in small infarcts of the deep white matter and in regions of demyelination and incomplete infarction.[38–41] Characteristic lacunar infarcts may be found also. The typical CT finding in these cases consists of areas of decreased density of the deep white matter of the cerebrum, mainly in the paraventricular regions (Fig. 13–12). These low-density areas tend to be asymmetric and nonhomogeneous and often extend a considerable distance laterally from the lateral ventricles. The cerebral cortex is not involved, but there may be lacunar infarcts in the basal ganglia. The distinction between Binswanger disease and the common symmetric paraventricular hypodensities of old age may be blurred. Paraventricular lucencies are also prominent in normal-pressure hydrocephalus but are generally more homogeneous and less extensive in this condition, in which the lateral ventricles tend to be larger and smoother than in Binswanger disease. High cortical sulci are less prominent in normal-pressure hydrocephalus as well.

CEREBRAL HEMATOMAS

One of the great advantages of CT in the diagnosis of stroke is its ability to show clearly the presence of acute hematomas, their size and location, whether they extend into the ventricular or subarachnoid spaces, and the degree of brain displacement that has resulted. Early bleeds are better detected by CT than by MRI, whereas the opposite is true in early ischemic infarcts.

Acute hematomas have CT densities in the 50- to 90-Hounsfield unit range, are generally well circumscribed, and have smooth borders (see Fig. 13–8). Within a few hours a zone of decreased density surrounds the hematoma; this one enlarges over the next several days, often associated with some increase in mass effect. The low-density region is initially edema but later includes the periphery of the hematoma, which decreases in CT density.[42, 43] The hematoma slowly undergoes changes related to hemoglobin breakdown and becomes less dense on CT scans. The rate at which this happens varies, depending partly on the size of the hematoma, but most hematomas will be isodense relative to brain tissue at about 2 to 5 weeks.[42–44] Resorption takes place more quickly about the periphery of the hematoma, contributing to the size of the low-density zone around the hematoma and giving the CT illusion that the volume of the hematoma is decreasing faster than it really is. Eventually, the hematoma becomes lucent and may change in shape, going from being round to lenticular or even slitlike. Calcification occasionally occurs in old hematomas, as may happen in old ischemic infarcts as well.[45]

Contrast-enhanced CT scans may demonstrate an enhancing ring around a hematoma, beginning about 1 week after onset and lasting up to 6 weeks.[43] This ring is several millimeters wide and occurs within the zone of decreased density surrounding the hematoma. In its early stages, the ring may be modified by steroid administration, supporting the hypothesis that the ring enhancement is related to blood-brain barrier breakdown. In later stages, several weeks after onset, the ring stain is no longer decreased by steroids,

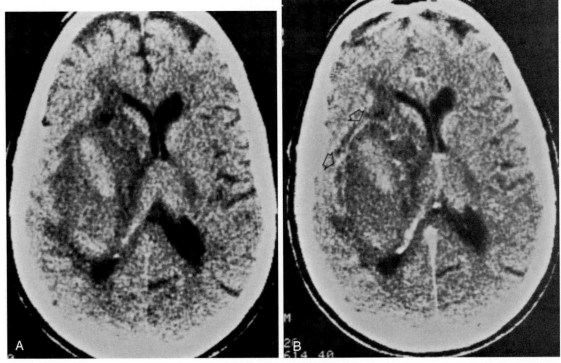

FIGURE 13–13. Subacute hematoma. *A,* Noninfused scan shows mass effect and areas of high and low density deep in the right cerebral hemisphere. This hematoma is probably a few weeks old, but the time of origin, surprisingly, was unknown. *B,* Contrast-infused scan shows a thin rim of enhancement incompletely surrounding the hematoma (arrowheads). This typical ring and the typical central high-density region help make the diagnosis of hematoma, but neoplasm may be difficult to rule out in such cases.

probably because vascular granulation tissue has formed around the hematoma and contributes to the ring stain.[44] If a contrast-infused scan, performed several weeks after a hematoma has occurred, shows a ring stain around an isodense or hypodense area, there is a good possibility that the

hematoma will mistakenly be considered a neoplasm or an abscess (Fig. 13–13). As with ring stains in cases of bland infarcts, a follow-up scan will show no enlargement of the ring and may show a decrease in its intensity.[46]

The precise localization of cerebral bleeds afforded by CT

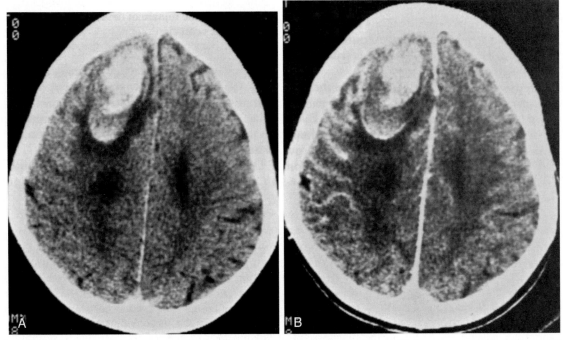

FIGURE 13–14. Proved amyloid angiopathy in an elderly patient. *A,* The anterior frontal location of this hematoma is atypical for one of hypertensive origin, and other causes must be considered more likely. Bleeding has probably occurred more than once, judging from the different densities within the hematoma. *B,* Infused scan shows a ring stain around the hematoma, but does not show arteriovenous malformation or tumor.

is of help in determining the etiology of the bleeds. After trauma, hypertension is the most common cause of cerebral bleeds. These most often begin in the putamen, sometimes in the caudate nucleus or thalamus, and rarely elsewhere. Ventricular spread occurs quite often, but subarachnoid extension is rare. The tendency of these bleeds to occur in the basal ganglia is probably related to the tendency of hypertension to produce small aneurysms on the striate arteries.[47, 48] Bleeds occurring elsewhere in the cerebrum may rarely be of hypertensive origin, but careful search should be made for other causes. Arteriovenous malformations may cause bleeding anywhere in the intercranial space. Contrast-infused CT scans usually show the characteristic enlarged vessels of the arteriovenous malformation in the vicinity of the bleed but will usually not show the small or cryptic arteriovenous malformations. Amyloid angiopathy is being recognized more often as a cause of cerebral bleeding in the elderly (Fig. 13–14).[49] Aneurysms may bleed into cerebral tissue, particularly when the aneurysm arises from the anterior communicating or pericallosal arteries or the knee of the middle cerebral artery. Some metastases bleed, especially those of malignant melanoma and choriocarcinoma. Other causes of cerebral hemorrhage include anticoagulation therapy, platelet deficiency, angiitis, and other vascular malformations, such as cavernous hemangiomas and even venous angioma.[20]

REFERENCES

1. Oldendorf W: Isolated flying-spot detection of radiodensity discontinuities displaying the internal structural pattern of a complex object. *IRE Trans Bio-Med Elect BME* 1961;8:68.
2. Hounsfield G: Computerized transverse axial scanning (tomography). I. Description of system. *Br J Radiol*. 1973;46:1016.
3. Bradac G, Oberson R: CT and angiography in cases of occlusive disease of supratentorial cerebral vessels. *Neuroradiology*. 1980;19:193.
4. Wing D, Norman D, Pollock J, Newton T: Contrast enhancement of cerebral infarcts in computed tomography. *Radiology*. 1976;121:89.
5. Inoue Y, Takemoto K, Miyamoto T, et al: Sequential computed tomography scans in acute cerebral infarction. *Radiology*. 1980;135:655.
6. Campbell J, Houser W, Stevens J, et al: Computed tomography and radionuclide imaging in the evaluation of ischemic stroke. *Radiology*. 1978;128:695.
7. Wall S, Brant-Zawadski M, Jeffrey R, Barnes B: High frequency CT findings within 24 hours after cerebral infarction. *AJR Am J Roentgenol*. 1982;138:307.
8. Schuler F, Hossman K: Experimental brain infarcts in cats. II. Ischemic brain edema. *Stroke*. 1980;11:593.
9. Pressman B, Tourje E, Thompson J: An early CT sign of ischemic infarction: Increased density in a cerebral artery. *AJNR Am J Neuroradiol*. 1987;8:645.
10. Tomsick T, Brott T, Barsan W, et al: Thrombus localization with emergency cerebral CT. *AJNR Am J Neuroradiol*. 1992;13:256.
11. Bryan R, Levy L, Whitlow W, et al: Diagnosis of acute cerebral infarction: Comparison of CT and MR imaging. *AJNR Am J Neuroradiol*. 1991;12:611.
12. Yuh W, Crain M, Loes D, et al: MR imaging of cerebral ischemia: Findings in the first 24 hours. *AJNR Am J Neuroradiol*. 1991;12:621.
13. Sterbini C, Agatiello L, Stocchi A, Solivetti F: CT of ischemic infarctions in the territory of the anterior choroidal artery: A review of 28 cases. *AJNR Am J Neuroradiol*. 1986;8:229.
14. Kingsley W, Jacobs L: Evaluation of computed tomography in vascular lesions of the vertebrobasilar territory. *J Neurol Neurosurg Psychiatr*. 1980;43:193.
15. Hinshaw D, Thompson J, Hasso A, Casselman E: Infarctions of the brainstem and cerebellum: A correlation of computed tomography and angiography. *Radiology*. 1980;137:105.
16. Denny-Brown D: Recurrent cerebrovascular episodes. *Arch Neurol*. 1960;2:194.
17. Zulch K: Uber die Entstehung und Lokalisation der Hirninfarkte. *Zentralbl Neurochir*. 1961;21:158.
18. Wodarz R: Watershed infarctions and computed tomography: A topographical study in cases with stenosis or occlusion of the carotid artery. *Neuroradiology*. 1980;19:245.
19. Buonanno F, Moody D, Ball M, Laster D: Computed cranial tomographic findings in cerebral sinovenous occlusion. *J Comput Assist Tomogr*. 1978;2:281.
20. Rao K, Knipp H, Wagner E: Computed tomographic findings in cerebral sinus and venous thrombosis. *Radiology*. 1981;140:391.
21. Wing S, Norman D, Pollock J, Newton T: Contrast enhancement of cerebral infarcts in computed tomography. *Radiology*. 1976;121:89.
22. Yock D, Marshall W: Recent ischemic brain infarcts at computed tomography: Appearances pre- and post-contrast infusion. *Radiology*. 1975;117:599.
23. Becker H, Desch H, Hacker H, Pencz A: CT fogging effect with ischemic cerebral infarcts. *Neuroradiology*. 1979;18:185.
24. Shriver E, Olsen T: Contrast enhancement of cerebral infarcts: Incidence and clinical value in different states of cerebral infarction. *Neuroradiology*. 1982;23:259.
25. Fisher C, Adams R: Observations on brain embolism with special reference to the mechanism of hemorrhagic infarction. *J Neuropathol Exp Neurol*. 1951;10:92.
26. Cronquist S, Brismar J, Kjellin K, Söderström C: Computer assisted axial tomography in cerebrovascular lesions. *Acta Radiol [Diagn]*. 1975;16:135.
27. Wood M, Wakim K, Sayre G, et al: Relationship between anticoagulants and hemorrhagic cerebral infarction in experimental animals. *Arch Neurol Psychiatr*. 1958;79:390.
28. Hayman L, Evans R, Bastion F, Hinck V: Delayed high dose contrast CT: Identifying patients at risk of massive hemorrhagic infarction. *Am J Neuroradiol*. 1981;2:139.
29. Gado M, Phelps M, Coleman R: An extravascular component of contrast enhancement in cranial computed tomography. *Radiology*. 1975;117:595.
30. O'Brien M, Jordan M, Waltz A: Ischemic cerebral edema and the blood-brain barrier. Distribution of pertechnetate, albumin, sodium, and antipyrene in brains of cats after occlusion of the middle cerebral artery. *Arch Neurol*. 1974;30:461.
31. Hayman L, Sakai F, Meyer J, et al: Iodine enhanced CT pattern after cerebral artery embolization in baboons. *Am J Neuroradiol*. 1980;1:233.
32. Soin J, Burdine J: Acute cerebral vascular accident associated with hyperperfusion. *Radiology*. 1976;118:109.
33. Pullicino P, Kendall B: Contrast enhancement in ischemic lesions: Relationship to prognosis. *Neuroradiology*. 1980;19:235.
34. Weinstein M, LaValley A, Rosenbloom S, Duchesneau P: Limitations of MRI for the detection of gray matter lesions. Reported at 1986 American Society of Neuroradiology Meeting, San Diego, CA.
35. Manelfe C, Clanet M, Gigaud M, et al: Internal capsule: Normal anatomy and ischemic changes demonstrated by computed tomography. *Am J Neuroradiol*. 1981;2:149.
36. Takahashi S, Goto K, Fukasawa H, et al: Computed tomography of cerebral infarction along the distribution of the basal perforating arteries. Part I. Striate arterial group. *Radiology*. 1985;155:107.
37. Takahashi S, Goto K, Fukawawa H, et al: Computed tomography of cerebral infarction along the distribution of the basal perforating arteries. Part II. Thalamic arterial group. *Radiology*. 1985;155:119.
38. Caplan L, Schoene W: Clinical features of subcortical arteriosclerotic encephalography (Binswanger disease). *Neurology (NY)*. 1978;28:1206.
39. Rosenberg G, Kornfeld M, Stovring J, Bicknell J: Subcortical arteriosclerotic encephalopathy (Binswanger): Computerized tomography. *Neurology (NY)*. 1979;29:1102.
40. Goto K, Ishii N, Fukasawa H: Diffuse white matter disease in the geriatric population: A clinical, neuropathological, and CT study. *Radiology*. 1981;141:687.
41. Zeumer H, Schonsky B, Sturm K: Predominant white matter involvement in subcortical arteriosclerotic encephalopathy (Binswanger disease). *J Comput Assist Tomogr*. 1980;4:14.
42. Dolinskas C, Bilaniuk L, Zimmerman R, Kuhl D: Computed tomography of intracerebral hematomas. I. Transmission CT observations on hematoma resolution. *AJR Am J Roentgen*. 1977;129:681.
43. Dolinskas C, Bilaniuk L, Zimmerman R, et al: Computed tomography of intracerebral hematomas. II. Radionuclide and transmission CT studies of the perihematoma region. *AJR Am J Roentgen*. 1977;129:689.
44. Laster D, Moody D, Ball M: Resolving intracerebral hematomas: Alternation of the "ring sign" with steroids. *AJR Am J Roentgen*. 1978;130:935.
45. Kapila A: Calcification in cerebral infarction. *Radiology*. 1984;153:685.
46. Zimmerman R, Leeds N, Naidich T: Ring blush associated with intracerebral hematomas. *Radiology*. 1977;122:707.
47. Cole F, Yates P: The occurrence and significance of intracerebral microaneurysms. *J Pathol Bacterial*. 1967;93:393.
48. Kido D, Gomez D, Santos-Buch C, et al: Microradiographic study of cerebral and ocular aneurysms in hypertensive rabbits. *Neuroradiology*. 1978;15:21.
49. Vinters H, Gilbert J: Amyloid angiopathy: Its incidence and complications in the aging brain. *Stroke*. 1981;12:118.

CHAPTER 14

Magnetic Resonance Techniques in the Investigation and Management of Acute Ischemic Stroke

K. M. A. WELCH, PETER B. BARKER, and YUE CAO

Nuclear magnetic resonance (NMR) in condensed matter was discovered more than four decades ago. Since then, NMR has proved a fundamental and invaluable tool in the fields of chemistry and physics. One application has resulted in the development of NMR for anatomic imaging, the impact of which has been compared with that of the development of radiography. The ability of NMR, or magnetic resonance imaging (MRI), to differentiate gray from white matter and diseased from normal brain, as well as its apparent lack of biologic hazard, provides an unparalleled opportunity for sequential study of the evolution of cerebral infarction and hemorrhage in vivo.

A somewhat different application of NMR is in in vivo spectroscopy. The technique first demonstrated was phosphorus 31 NMR spectroscopy. The spectrum has resonance peaks representing inorganic phosphate (P_i), phosphocreatine, and the α, β, and γ phosphate groups of adenosine-5'-triphosphate (ATP) and can be processed to measure pH and magnesium concentrations. No less important has been the development of proton (^{1}H) magnetic resonance spectroscopy (MRS), which makes available important measures for the stroke specialist, such as lactate and N-acetyl aspartate (NAA), a putative neuronal marker. In most recent years, it has become possible to produce whole brain slice images of the ^{31}P and ^{1}H spectral components. This technique is called spectroscopic imaging (SI). MR techniques also have been developed for the measurement of cerebral perfusion and cerebral blood flow (CBF), although these measures require validation. One such technique, known as functional magnetic resonance imaging (fMRI), which is sensitive to both blood flow and oxygenation, is now being used extensively in experimental studies of cortical localization. This technique may have value in determining reorganization of the brain after focal stroke.

The chapter on MR in the first edition of this book was written in the early days of MR science and thus dealt with fundamental principles that are now well known and available in teaching texts; accordingly, they are omitted here. For these same reasons, we will only briefly refer to routine diagnostic MRI in stroke as well as MR angiography. This chapter will focus on the value of established and newer MR methods that can be applied to the diagnosis and management of acute ischemic stroke, with emphasis on future applications of MR to fill previously unmet needs of the treating clinician.

THE CLINICAL PROBLEM

The clinician who treats acute stroke requires an imaging technique for the rapid and early identification of stroke. Recently developed MR techniques may be of use not only to diagnose stroke but also in the assessment of stroke prior to innovative treatments, such as with thrombolytic and cytoprotective drugs. If one imaging technique could provide

early and reliable predictions of eventual ischemic cell damage and volume of infarction, it would be of immense value for judging the effectiveness of therapy. CBF measurement, computed tomographic scanning, and metabolic imaging have limited clinical acceptability in this regard. Along the same lines, some clear marker of the state and extent of tissue viability remaining would be valuable to judge whether therapy is still worthwhile when patients are studied at later times after stroke onset. Time alone is an inadequate indicator of the therapeutic window, especially when the time of stroke onset is uncertain. Thus, there is a need to *predict the evolution* of stroke in a way that more precisely and with greater resolution identifies the progression of cellular damage at the moment of investigation. This also would be of value for treatments such as thrombolysis, in which knowledge of the degree and extent of tissue necrosis and of the consequent potential for brain hemorrhage is of utmost importance.

For the acute management of stroke, it is desirable to have one measuring device, thereby shortening the time of the early investigative process and permitting treatment at the earliest possible time. This device should be readily available, rapid, and noninvasive and should provide the maximum number of measurements, including diagnostics. Currently, however, the technology is such that hours of study would be necessary to achieve such complete information in one session. The challenge is to (1) reduce the time needed for the methods to be applied and (2) identify the most critically important measures for the diagnosis, staging, and prediction of outcome of stroke.

Another major need in the management of ischemic stroke relates to monitoring the recovery process and the inexactitude of the clinical examination as a measure of outcome. An objective measurement of irreversible cellular injury and information on the effectiveness of brain plasticity and how this can be enhanced by physical procedures and drugs are thus sorely needed. Such measures should also stimulate the rehabilitation sciences themselves. This chapter indicates that MR technology may also be of value in achieving such objectives.

High field magnets (>1.5 tesla) are now installed in general hospitals throughout the world. MR technology at these field strengths can observe anatomic structure, identify arterial occlusion, and measure CBF, metabolism, and integrity of the blood-brain barrier. It has the potential to distinguish reversible from irreversible ischemic cell damage and to identify cortical neuronal reorganization after brain injury. These methods are discussed subsequently, and strategies are proposed whereby MR measures are best applied in acute stroke investigation and management. First, however, we briefly review and critique those procedures that may already be available and have been tested for their potential to provide an early prediction of eventual tissue infarction after onset of ischemia.

EXISTING TECHNIQUES

Computed tomographic scanning is limited in value because it is unable to detect the ischemic focus acutely. Currently, single photon emission computed tomography is usually used in the clinical situation to measure CBF. The technique is predictive of neurologic deficit at the onset of ischemia,[1] and strong associations have been found between the degree and duration of CBF reduction and irreversible cell death in rigorously controlled and reproducible stroke models,[2] but this technique has limited utility in clinical patients. The time delay between stroke onset and the time of study contributes to this limitation, as does the heterogeneity of CBF in human ischemic foci caused by such factors as variable collateral vasocapacitance and reperfusion. In addition, the initial ischemic insult activates a cascade of cellular events that apparently proceed independently of the subsequent CBF levels.[3] Measures of CBF combined with blood volume and brain oxygen consumption using positron emission tomography (PET) provide information on regions of "misery perfusion," in which the fraction of the O_2 extraction is indicative of cell viability.[4] But PET scanners are not in general clinical use, and the measurements are often time consuming. Furthermore, PET, unlike MRI, cannot provide routine diagnostic measures and employs radioactive tracers.

It must be realized that to employ multiple techniques to measure essential anatomic and functional information for the diagnosis and management of acute stroke presents logistical problems that have a high chance of delaying treatment beyond the optimal time window of therapeutic opportunity. Thus, there is a need to search for new approaches to predict stroke that will have greater practical clinical application in the acutely ill patient.

MAGNETIC RESONANCE EXAMINATION OF ISCHEMIA

Magnetic resonance techniques can noninvasively measure specific parameters that are sensitive to the biophysical environment of water in tissue.[5] These include the water ^1H spin-lattice (T_1) and spin-spin (T_2) relaxation times, spin density, and the translational (apparent) diffusion coefficient of water (ADC_w). MRI readily identifies change in the ^1H NMR parameters of water that occur following ischemic stroke.[6–17] There is a progressive increase in T_2, which, however, does not maximize until approximately 24 hours after the onset of stroke. Similar results have been found for changes in T_1; proton spin density increases are observed even later,[8] although in the case of cerebral embolism they may change more rapidly.[18]

The acute increase in T_2 following ischemia forms the basis for the diagnostic utility of MRI in ischemic stroke. The increase is thought to reflect developing vasogenic edema, but the mechanisms remain to be determined. Unlike the increase in T_1 relaxation time, which reflects the accumulation of bulk water, T_2 changes are influenced by the protein content of the fluid as ischemia evolves. Decrease in bound intracellular water may be a contributing factor, possibly because of ischemic changes in the cellular environment, for example, protein breakdown.[19] Whatever the mechanisms, the clinical diagnosis of stroke uses techniques that generate T_2-weighted images, considered the "gold standard" measure because of the conformity of T_2-weighted MR images with histopathologic identification of ischemic lesions post mortem.[20, 21]

When a gray scale is used to represent signal intensity, infarction appears bright (high signal intensity) on T_2-weighted images and dark (low signal intensity) on T_1-weighted images. In hemorrhagic conditions, however, T_1 tends to shorten in the subacute phase and appears bright on T_1-weighted images. Subacute hemorrhage is easily differentiated on T_1-weighted images but is more difficult to detect in the acute phase. This is because the increased intensity seen on T_1-weighted images takes days to develop as blood elements break down and iron is deposited in the tissues. Hemorrhage also causes increased signal intensity on T_2-weighted images, owing to prolongation of T_2 initially by both clot and edema, but this is not specific because of T_2 prolongation by infarction. On T_1-weighted images, obtained early after stroke, hemorrhage may appear as an area of isosignal in white matter or as an area of decreased intensity indistinguishable from an infarct. Nevertheless, with the appropriate pulse paradigms, such as gradient echo sequences, MRI can be superior to computed tomography in detecting petechial hemorrhage in the tissues.

DIFFUSION IMAGING

Recently, MRI was adapted to generate images whose contrasts are based on the translational motion (diffusion) of water and thus may be more specific for tissue characterization.[22] Diffusion is a process whereby water molecules move in a random fashion owing to thermal energy (brownian movement). A technique utilizing intravoxel incoherent motion, based on the pulsed gradient spin echo technique developed originally by Stejskal and Tanner,[23] has been developed to generate images that can be used to calculate the ADC_w. In brain matter, the diffusion of water is impeded by cellular membranes, organelles, macromolecules, and other cellular structures. The intensity of diffusion images, therefore, depends on such factors as tortuosity of the diffusion path, cell membrane permeability, and the exchange of free water with bound water.

The diffusion imaging technique has been used to study cerebral ischemia,[6–11] which, shortly after onset, causes a decline in the ADC_w by a factor of approximately two, representing a *decrease* in the translational movement of water. This decline is rapid (within minutes), and precedes changes in any other ^1H NMR parameters of water. Moseley and colleagues[6] reported that the ADC_w declines significantly within the first 3 minutes after middle cerebral artery (MCA) occlusion in the cat, and that by 12 minutes after ischemia the ADC_w falls by 25 to 30 percent. Additionally, Mintorovitch and associates[24] demonstrated that acute decreases in the ADC_w were independent of changes in total brain water content, although increases in brain water content occurred after 60 minutes of MCA occlusion. Thus, ADC_w measurements are sensitive to changes in the environment of water independent of changes in total water content. Our studies of permanent focal ischemia in the rat have shown that after an initial fall and the lapse of 8 to 24 hours, the ADC_w values begin to recover toward the normal range and then attain values that are higher than normal over 7 days. Similar changes, although with a much protracted time-course, have been recorded in human stroke (see later discussion).[25]

There is considerable interest in the mechanisms responsible for the ischemia-induced decline in the ADC_w, but the physical basis for these changes remains to be determined. A full discussion of these mechanisms is beyond the scope of this chapter; however, in brief, proposed mechanisms include temperature effects, increased tortuosity of the extracellular diffusion paths, restriction by reduced cellular membrane permeability, shifts in water from extracellular to intracellular space, membrane depolarization, and cytotoxic edema.[10, 11, 26–38] The rapidity of the decline in the ADC_w after ischemia suggests that, at least initially, it is not a result of the gross secondary changes in ischemic tissue histopathology, such as vasogenic edema or tissue necrosis.

The decline in the ADC_w following cerebral ischemia is associated with a specific threshold level of regional CBF. With the use of bilateral common carotid artery occlusion in the gerbil,[10] it was demonstrated that the decline in the ADC_w does not begin until regional CBF (measured by H_2^- clearance) reaches a level of approximately 15 mL/100 g^{-1} per minute, a threshold similar to that associated with the loss of membrane potential. The increased signal intensity of diffusion-weighted images was also associated with breakdown of energy metabolism, acidosis, cellular ionic shifts, and decreased Na^+, K^+, and ATPase activity.[39] The mechanisms responsible for the rise in the ADC_w subsequent to the initial decrease have been less intensively studied but are probably the reverse of those responsible for its initial decline as well as impairment of those processes responsible for the physiologic restriction of brain water diffusion. The ADC_w increase may mark the disruption of cell membrane structure, necrosis, and loss of cells (ie, the breakdown of barriers to diffusion).

There have been few published studies of diffusion-weighted imaging in human stroke. Chien and coworkers[40] investigated 15 patients with focal cerebral ischemia and infarction within 24 hours (n = 3) and up to 4 years, some studied serially (n = 4). They found an increase of the "average ADC_w" in ischemic lesions compared with normal control subjects at these subacute and chronic times of study, observing further increases as time progressed. They attributed this to vasogenic edema complicating the subacute strokes and to gliosis or encephalomalacia in the 2- to 4-year-old strokes. On the other hand, Warach and colleagues[25] studied 32 ischemic stroke patients with different techniques, at times from 2 to 12 hours (n = 12) and up to 12 days, in whom the ADC_w ratio, calculated as the ADC_w in homologous brain regions divided by that in the stroke region, was low acutely, reached a nadir at 24 hours, and then remained low. There was then no change in the ADC_w at up to 2 months, but chronic infarcts were associated with a relative increase in the ADC_w, although not until 4 months. The differences in these results can probably be explained on technical grounds as well as by the use of different controls. Indeed, the control values of Warach and colleagues[25] were higher than expected, although the use of ratios adjusted for this in part. Both studies had small numbers of patients, particularly at the early time-points of the investigation. The techniques used were less advanced than are currently available so that, for example, movement artifact could not be easily corrected and only two images were available for

calculation of the ADC_w. Further, measurement of an average ADC_w value from a single locus of an ischemic focus of well-known heterogeneity may add to the variability. Nevertheless, although the interpretation of the findings is limited by the aforementioned problems, these were seminal studies in the application of diffusion-weighted imaging to human stroke. In a more recent publication, Warach and colleagues overcame many of the technical limitations of their prior studies by using the fast imaging technique of echoplanar imaging for diffusion measurements. The time-course of ADC_w change then approximated that found in the earlier studies by Chien and colleagues, which were from the same laboratory.

Our own studies are more in accord with those of Chien and coworkers.[40] In the majority of our patients, we observed an increase of ADC_w as early as 24 hours after stroke onset, but a prolonged decrease of ADC_w was found in one third. We judge that this is probably because we investigated a population of patients of whom the majority had embolism-induced ischemia, which is known to be associated with more rapid necrosis of brain tissue. Similar findings have been reported in abstract form by de Crespigny and associates.[41] Thus, although more extensive investigations are required in clinical patients at all stages of stroke evolution, it appears that the average ADC_w in human ischemic foci may be decreased at acute times of investigation and subsequently rebound to increased levels as ischemia evolves to cellular necrosis. Although the directions of ADC_w change in humans are the same as in animal models of ischemia, it remains to be determined whether the degree and duration of change are the same and to what extent heterogeneity of ADC_w change is present in an ischemic focus.

A major value of diffusion imaging is obviously the ability to detect ischemia in human stroke at least 6 hours before there is any detectable T_2 change. This is of particular importance with the advent of reperfusion therapy and potential cytoprotective therapeutic drugs. Because reperfusion therapy with thrombolytic agents can result in serious complications due to cerebral hemorrhage, a correct diagnosis becomes imperative. As we mentioned at the outset of this chapter, information on tissue histopathology is equally essential, first because reperfusion of necrotic tissue, as well as promoting hemorrhagic conversion of the tissue, may predispose to the development of massive reperfusion edema, herniation, and death. It is also important to know whether potentially reversible cellular damage is in place or whether cellular necrosis has advanced to a degree that renders the use of cytoprotective drugs unwarranted. This information would also be of immense value in the testing of these treatment strategies. We propose a strategy of identifying specific MR signatures of ischemic histopathology based on the use of T_2-weighted and diffusion-weighted imaging. The reasoning for this strategy is now outlined.

Magnetic Resonance Correlates of Ischemic Histopathology

There is evidence that diffusion-weighted imaging and quantitation of ADC_w may predict histopathologic outcome of cerebral ischemia.[10, 27, 42–47] Sevick and colleagues[46] showed that the signal intensity of diffusion-weighted images correlated with lack of lesion staining by 2,3,5-triphenyltetrazolium chloride. Minematsu and colleagues[47] showed similar findings in the rat MCA occlusion model. Conventional MR images using T_2 obtained during the stage of cerebral infarction correlate well with the histopathology of the lesion.[20, 21] This is despite the fact that T_2 essentially characterizes vasogenic edema rather than cellular change, so that it is insensitive to ischemic tissue damage before vasogenic edema develops. Further, the stroke region appears homogeneous on T_2-weighted images, and it is usually impossible to detect different regions of tissue damage in the lesion. On the other hand, ADC_w is sensitive to early ischemia and can reveal heterogeneity in regions of ischemia that are homogeneous on T_2-weighted images.[42] ADC_w alone can provide earlier and more specific information on regional ischemic histopathology, particularly when shifts in values can be observed over time.[48]

Our laboratory has expended a major experimental effort to examine the relationships of MR measures to tissue histopathology in rat models of permanent and transient focal cerebral ischemia.[9, 19, 27, 43, 44, 48–50] Ours is one of few laboratories to have successfully accomplished serial measures over prolonged time periods of up to 1 week. These studies have provided strong support that diffusion-weighted imaging combined with T_2-weighted imaging may be a powerful tool in predicting ischemic histopathology. The data obtained in these experiments indicated a reduction in ADC_w, with gradation of change in terms of time and degree from minimally to severely injured tissue. Elevation of T_2 seemed to follow a similar gradation of change, which was, however, delayed compared with that of ADC_w. It is especially interesting to note that in the most heavily injured areas, the value of ADC_w turns toward normal values, coincident with the emergence of eosinophilic neurons, which signify neuronal damage. The subsequent increase of ADC_w, therefore, probably indicates a loss of cell membrane integrity (ie, allowing the unrestricted movement of water molecules) and cell necrosis. According to our results, the ability to distinguish the return toward a normal ADC_w value that is caused by injury from the return to normal that is expected of recovery depends on T_2 changes, which, when elevated, represent the former. A major point to be made is that high ADC_w and high T_2 together represent cellular necrosis. Even when T_2 subsequently declines back

toward normal values, the ADC_w remains elevated and remains a signature of cellular necrosis. In this instance, what causes T_2 decline from previously elevated values in severely damaged tissue remains to be determined, but possibly the decline reflects a decrease in vasogenic edema or a shortening of T_2 relaxation properties because of paramagnetic elements in the tissues, such as red blood cells from the petechial hemorrhage associated with tissue necrosis. The dynamic relationships of ADC_w and T_2 are diagrammed in Figure 14–1, from which five different signatures of ischemic histopathology can be obtained.

Further studies in the rat model of MCA occlusion have shown that, after permanent occlusion for 2 hours,[44] a low ADC_w predicts to a high degree of probability cellular necrosis at 1 week, measured histopathologically. A low ADC_w at 1 hour, however, was not predictive. This study, taken together with the results obtained from the other studies described, offers important conclusions for the interpretation of human stroke data.

1. A low ADC_w alone (Fig. 14–1, signature B) in acute stroke can be associated with the potential for cellular recovery or eventual cell necrosis, or both, depending on subsequent ischemic events, and thus, if used alone, has low probability of predicting cell necrosis.

2. A low ADC_w with high T_2 (Fig. 14–1, signature C) in ischemic brain may have a better probability of predicting, but is not a marker for, eventual cell necrosis, although events leading to irreversible cell death may or may not have commenced.

3. High ADC_w with high T_2 (Fig. 14–1, signature E) is a *marker* of cell necrosis in the tissue, and the time between the transition from low to high ADC_w values (Fig. 14–1, signature D) probably marks the onset and progression of cell necrosis, although irreversible cell death may have occurred prior to this time.

Clinical Application of the Model

In clinical practice, stroke patients cannot be studied at the precise time of stroke onset or serially over prolonged time periods, with the result that moment-to-moment shifts

FIGURE 14–1. Diagram of the dynamic changes in the apparent diffusion coefficient of water (ADC_w) and the spin-spin relaxation time (T_2) in the central region of an ischemic focus, based on the experimental data obtained from the rat model of middle cerebral artery occlusion. Note that including normal, six different combinations of ADC_w and T_2 occur over time as ischemic histopathology progresses, and that consequently this provided five different signatures of histopathology from early ischemic damage to infarction. The signatures are discussed further in the text, as are ADC_w and T_2.

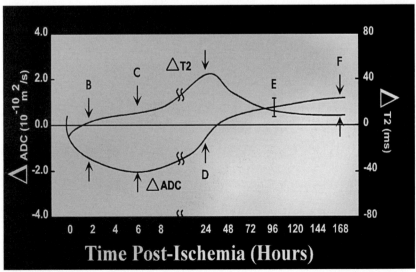

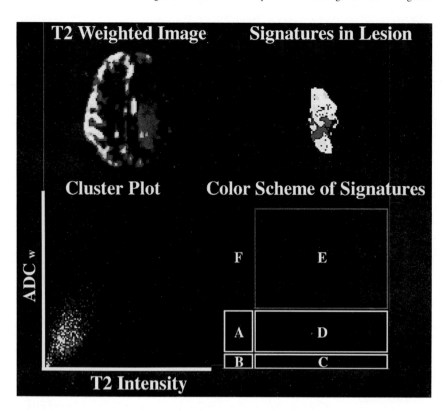

FIGURE 14-2. Demonstration of how we use cluster analysis of a scattergram of ADC_w and T_2 (T_2-weighted intensity in this example) to generate the different signatures of histopathology and their topography. The "color scheme" is shown here in shades of gray. See text for definitions of ADC_w and T_2.

in ADC_w cannot be observed. Instead, a "snapshot" of events is obtained at the earliest possible time and possibly on one or two other occasions during a stroke evaluation. Thus, based on experimental observations,[48] at these less acute time-points, the ADC_w in tissue destined for necrosis may be low, normal, or high as the ADC_w shifts from low to high values, and there will be a heterogeneous distribution of ADC_w values throughout central and peripheral regions. Furthermore, there must be some measure by which a "normal" value of ADC_w in its transition to high values in

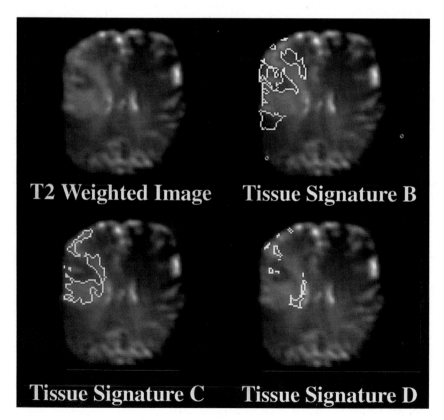

FIGURE 14-3. Illustration of how the pixel clusters generated as in Figure 14–2 are projected onto the T_2-weighted image of a 72-hour-old middle cerebral artery stroke. Note how signature B (low ADC_w) is distributed in peripheral segments of the stroke focus and around the sylvian fissure. In this case, the prominent signatures are B and C, indicating that the majority of tissue has not yet begun the progression to necrosis, although a small proportion of the tissue does show a transition to necrosis (signature D). See text for definitions of ADC_w and T_2.

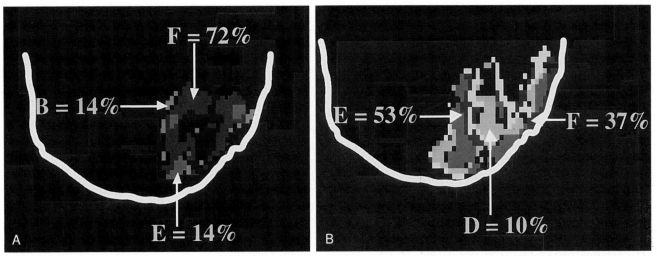

FIGURE 14–4. The progression of signatures toward necrosis over time in an embolic infarct. *A*, Cerebral infarct at day 1. *B*, Cerebral infarct at day 2. Note that signature B (low ADC_w alone) is at the margin and is taken up into the expanded lesion. The reason for the large percentage of signature F (high ADC_w/normal T_2) remains to be determined. See text for definitions of ADC_w and T_2.

regions undergoing active cellular necrosis can be distinguished from normal ADC_w values in recovering tissue. For these reasons, another complementary measure, perhaps more than one, is likely to be important to characterize the evolving ischemic histopathology. We believe that the combined measurement of ADC_w with T_2 (see Fig. 14–1) achieves these aims. The biophysical mechanisms of T_2 change are better known than those of the ADC_w.[5] The T_2 correlates of histopathology, although regionally and dynamically limited, are established.[20, 21]

Figures 14–2 through 14–5 provide examples of how we have processed cases of human stroke to generate the tissue signatures of ischemic histopathology based on our experimental model. Figure 14–2 shows how a scattergram of the ADC_w and T_2 is generated and how normal values can be defined from visually directed cluster analysis. From this, regions corresponding to the signatures can be constructed,

and the clusters of abnormal signatures projected back onto the stroke image. Figure 14–3 shows that in an image obtained 72 hours after stroke affecting the MCA territory, an area of low ADC_w (signature B) is found at the margins. These regions were not seen on the pure T_2 image and presumably were destined either for recovery or to be taken up into an expanding infarct. Figure 14–4 shows an embolic infarct with signature B present to a minor degree at 24 hours, which is then taken up in the expanding infarct at 48 hours. It is common to find signatures D, E, and F at early times in embolic stroke, compatible with the known histopathology of rapid necrosis. Finally, Figure 14–5 shows a 4-day-old stroke in which the D signature of transitional necrosis predominates, being replaced by the signatures of established necrosis, E and F, at 70 days. Note that despite the normal shrinkage of the established infarct, it is possible to track the shifts in proportions of the ischemic signatures.

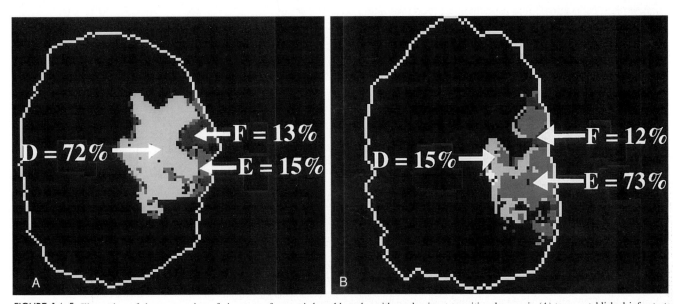

FIGURE 14–5. Illustration of the progression of signatures from a 4-day-old stroke with predominant transitional necrosis *(A)* to an established infarct at 70 days *(B)*.

We have now processed over 50 cases of acute stroke and can clearly track progression through all the signatures to established necrosis. Signature B appears to be short-lived and is only infrequently seen beyond 48 hours. The model is sensitive to rapid necrosis and can discriminate embolic from thrombotic patterns of necrosis.

At the outset, it is important to note that there are different time-courses of change between ADC_w and T_2,[48] which provides support that the ADC_w is influenced by other factors than bulk flow of water. So it is possible to observe low ADC_w in the presence of high T_2, indicating that ADC_w remains sensitive to cellular change when T_2 is influenced by vasogenic edema. In the early stage of cerebral ischemia, before the development of vasogenic edema, the ADC_w is decreased without a change in T_2.[48] Although a low ADC_w has been associated with some form of cellular change, it is uncertain what level of damage is needed to bring about ADC_w reduction. Data from reperfusion models of focal cerebral ischemia suggest that low ADC_w is sensitive not only to eventual cell death but also to a degree of cellular impairment that is compatible with cell recovery.[44] The predictive probability of ADC_w is also influenced by the degree and time-course of ADC_w reduction as well as the region of the lesion.[44, 48] In acute human stroke studied before vasogenic edema develops, that is, before T_2 elevation, the potential for cellular recovery in regions of low ADC_w would be supported if the volume of the eventual infarct were less than the volume of early ADC_w reduction. It should also be possible to identify the regionality of probable recovery, perhaps present in more peripheral zones. On the one hand, the knowledge that a low ADC_w does not rule out the potential for cell recovery is encouraging for the use of ADC_w to monitor the effects of cytoprotective drugs. On the other, however, the documentation that a low ADC_w can be caused by a spectrum of cellular change from potentially reversible metabolic deficit to destined cell necrosis[45] means that, in clinical practice, other measures may be essential to discriminate degrees of recoverability, especially at later times of study.

Experimental studies have shown, now confirmed by human stroke observations, that as ischemia progresses and T_2 becomes elevated, the ADC_w may remain low.[48] Whether the development of vasogenic edema and consequent increase of T_2 in the presence of a low ADC_w predicts that the tissue has undergone irreversible ischemic damage remains to be determined. Van Bruggen and associates[42] studied a photoactivation model of focal cerebral infarction and found that a hyperintense rim of the lesion seen on diffusion-weighted images was associated with edema without cell necrosis. Pierpaoli et al.[45] found to the contrary in the same model that this region was associated with cell necrosis identified by electronmicroscopy. The latter investigation also showed that the same MR characteristics were present in the necrotic core of the lesion in the earlier time-point of its evolution. We have shown in a more representative model of focal ischemia that, in core regions of the lesion, low ADC_w in the presence of high T_2 is a predictor of eventual ischemic necrosis.[27, 48] But in the peripheral zones of the lesion, an initial reduction of the ADC_w occurred in tissue that had minor histopathologic change but in which T_2 was minimally or not increased after the ADC_w value had recovered its normal level.

Thus, it remains to be determined whether a low ADC_w and high T_2 have histopathologic correlates in human stroke of (1) vasogenic edema in ischemic regions destined for recovery, (2) eventual cell necrosis, or (3) both (depending on stroke region). We believe that this signature represents a probable predictor of cell necrosis; if so, this would have important implications for human stroke assessment. One implication is that when brain regions are identified with this signature, although the cascade of events leading to cell necrosis may have begun, there still may be some potential benefit from cytoprotective drugs working at later points in the cascade, perhaps in more peripheral zones of the ischemic focus. Secondly, cellular necrosis has not yet occurred in these brain regions, so perhaps there will be less compliance of these tissues to hemorrhagic conversion or massive enhancement of vasogenic edema after reperfusion therapy. These hypotheses can all be investigated in clinical stroke using the combined measures of ADC_w and T_2 and the ability of ADC_w to detect cellular ischemic change in the presence of vasogenic edema.

At some time in the course of permanent ischemia, which appears to depend on the duration and degree of ischemia as well as the region of the lesion forming in the distribution of the occluded artery, the ADC_w value begins to return to the normal range and then becomes abnormally high owing to cell loss and tissue necrosis.[48] Our animal data strongly

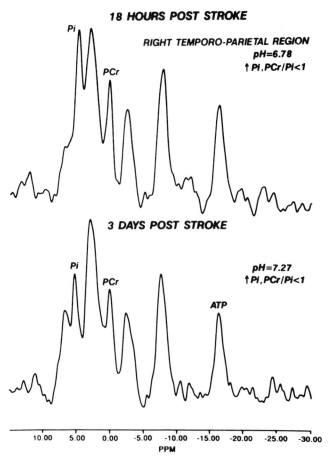

FIGURE 14–6. ''Flip-flop'' of pH from acidotic to alkalotic over time in a patient with ischemic infarction of the right middle cerebral artery territory. The phosphorus 31 spectra are obtained from the center of the infarction on two separate occasions. PPM, parts per million.

support that this "flip-flop" of ADC_w from low to high values is associated with necrosis of cells in which it occurs. Therefore, if a snapshot image is taken in later stages of clinical stroke evolution, when cellular necrosis has occurred, we can expect to find regions of high T_2 in association with ADC_w values in a normal range, in which tissue the ADC_w had previously been low. This will be a marker of active cell necrosis and also of the transition to established necrosis, which is characterized by a high ADC_w in association with a high T_2.

The significance of an available predictor and marker of cell necrosis cannot be overemphasized. T_2-weighted images have been unable to discriminate regions of necrosis from less involved tissue in a subacute ischemic focus, which is essential if MR techniques are to be used for any other purpose than diagnostics in stroke patients. In combination with diffusion-weighted imaging, however, the availability of such a cell necrosis predictor and marker opens the possibility of identifying tissue that may respond to cytoprotective therapy and perhaps extending the therapeutic window or opening it for those patients in whom the time of stroke onset cannot be determined with certainty. At the least, such tissue signatures might indicate, at subacute stages of stroke, whether the total lesion is beyond recovery. The present review indicates that diffusion-weighted imaging together with T_2-weighted imaging can identify both reversible and irreversible components of the ischemic lesion, in which the response of the reversible component to cytoprotective therapy can be revealed and monitored by the same MR measures.

MAGNETIC RESONANCE SPECTROSCOPY

Phosphorus 31

To evaluate the utility of spectroscopy in the practical management of acute ischemic stroke, we investigated early human focal ischemia with ^{31}P MR spectroscopy to characterize the temporal evolution and relationship of brain pH and phosphate energy metabolism.[51–57] Analysis of the ^{31}P spectrum enables the measurement of phosphocreatine, P_i, ATP, pH, and intracellular magnesium $[Mg^{2+}]$. Serial localized spectroscopic measurements of ischemic brain pH in clinical patients indicated a progression from acute acidosis to subacute (18 hours and beyond) and chronic alkalosis (Fig. 14–6). When acidosis was present, there was a significant elevation in the relative signal intensity of P_i and significant reductions in signal intensities of α-ATP and γ-ATP in stroke patients compared with the same signals in control subjects. Ischemic brain pH values directly correlated with the relative signal intensity of phosphocreatine and inversely correlated with the signal intensity of P_i. Furthermore, hyperglycemia worsened brain acidosis and metabolic breakdown.

Brain pMg (where $pMg = -\log[Mg^{2+}]$) was significantly lower in the ischemic focus of all stroke patients when compared with that of normal control subjects. Ischemic brain pMg was also significantly reduced when the pH of the stroke region was acidotic and when the phosphocreatine index was reduced (Fig. 14–7). Brain pMg was significantly reduced in acute stroke (0–1 days) and at days 2 to 3 (subacute) after stroke. During the temporal evolution of stroke, pH returned to normal levels by days 2 to 3, but pMg did not return to normal until days 4 to 10, at a time when ischemic brain pH had become significantly alkalotic. We found, therefore, that elevation of ischemic brain $[Mg^{2+}]$ was temporally linked to the acidotic phase of human stroke as well as to the breakdown of energy metabolism.

The data therefore suggested a link between high-energy phosphate metabolism and brain pH, especially during the period of ischemic brain acidosis. Acute stroke therapy potentially could be instituted during this period because it may mark a therapeutic window. Nevertheless, although localized ^{31}P MR spectroscopy can be performed in a reasonable time-frame (5–10 minutes), the resolution is poor (20

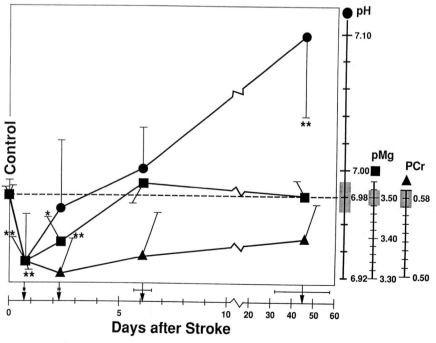

FIGURE 14–7. Evolution of human brain pMg (see text), pH, and phosphocreatine (PCr) as a function of time after stroke. *Arrows* along the time axis indicate mean time after stroke (± SEM) for the four time subgroups studied. Normal control values are plotted at time zero and are also represented across time by the horizontal *dashed* line. *Shaded bars* represent ± SEM of mean control values. Statistically significant deviations from control levels are marked by *double asterisks* ($P < .0$) or a *single asterisk* ($P = .03$).

mL at best) and the single voxel approach is inadequate to detect the metabolic heterogeneity of the evolving ischemic focus. Spectroscopic imaging of ^{31}P is now available. Although this may be a necessary approach to identify metabolic heterogeneity, the resolution is still limited and the time of data collection is too lengthy (30 minutes) to make this an option for the rapid assessment needed in acute stroke management.

Proton

Numerous proton spectroscopy studies of models of cerebral ischemia have indicated the potential of the method to detect ischemia on the basis of increased levels of lactate.[58–60] However, proton spectroscopy of the human brain was not possible on a routine basis until the pioneering work of Frahm and colleagues,[61] who demonstrated that high-resolution localized spectroscopy was possible using the STEAM sequence. This group was also the first to record a proton spectrum of a human infarct, demonstrating high lactate and a near-total depletion of NAA.[62] Following this publication, several groups studied either acute[63–65] or chronic[66, 67] ischemia in humans using single voxel localization techniques. A significant drawback of this methodology, as with ^{31}P MR spectroscopy, is that it provides no information regarding the spatial extent of the abnormalities and also requires prior knowledge of the stroke location for correct voxel placement. Therefore, there has been an effort to develop SI methods that map metabolite levels over wider regions of the brain. Early attempts used one-dimensional SI,[68, 69] which gave only limited coverage, and more recently single-slice two-dimensional SI.[70, 71] With the development of multi-slice two-dimensional SI,[72, 73] it became possible to completely map supratentorial metabolite levels in acute stroke for the first time.

Generally, there is a consensus that elevated lactate levels are observed in the acute stage of stroke and can be used to delineate ischemic tissue. Tissue that has already progressed to infarction, however, will show decreased NAA, indicative of neuronal loss, as well as possible anatomic or signal changes on conventional MR images. Thus, MR spectroscopic imaging has the potential to identify ischemic tissue and distinguish it from infarcted tissue.

Figure 14–8 shows representative data from a patient who was first scanned 3 hours after symptom onset. MRI results at this time were normal, but MR angiography showed a high-grade stenosis or complete occlusion of the right internal carotid artery (ICA) and low flow in the right MCA (Fig. 14–8A). Spectroscopic images performed at this time showed elevated lactate levels throughout much of the right MCA territory, with the highest lactate level in the right basal ganglia (Fig. 14–8B and C). Only slight reductions in NAA were apparent. Follow-up scans performed 1 week later showed that the basal ganglia region progressed to infarction, with high T_2 signal (Fig. 14–8D) and complete absence of NAA but that the previously ischemic lateral regions were spared.

The technique also has its limitations. Scan time is long (approximately 30 minutes) and the spatial resolution is coarse (approximately 1 cm^3); the technique is approaching the resolution limit (which is limited by the sensitivity of the signal-to-noise ratio). Also, animal studies have shown that the decrease in NAA following onset of ischemia is a relatively slow process (eg, 50% decrease after 6 hours in one study). Therefore, tissue that is no longer viable may still have significant NAA levels, and tissue with this characteristic (high lactate, normal NAA and T_2), while possibly representing the penumbra, cannot definitely be assumed to be salvageable by therapeutic intervention. This same issue renders the NAA metabolite unsuitable for assessment of whether enough viable tissue is available to make cytoprotection therapy worthwhile. Therefore, NAA measurement may be most suitable for assessing outcome rather than predicting ischemia.

MAGNETIC RESONANCE MEASUREMENTS OF CEREBRAL PERFUSION AND FLOW

Techniques for MR imaging of cerebral perfusion, using a bolus injection a gadolinium contrast agent, have been pioneered by the group at Massachusetts General Hospital.[74] Rapid, susceptibility-weighted MR images are sequentially recorded during bolus injection of the contrast agent. This group has shown that the area under the Δ versus time curve, where $\Delta = -\ln(S/S_0)/TE$ (S is the MR signal intensity; S_0 is the preinjection MR signal intensity), is proportional to relative cerebral blood volume (CBV). Attempts have also been made to calculate CBF using this type of methodology.[75] However, a number of assumptions are required to make such quantitative measurements, and it appears that, for the time being, the technique is best used as a qualitative measure of cerebral perfusion and that, in patients with unilateral deficits, bilateral comparisons may be used to detect perfusion abnormalities. A number of investigations have shown that bolus arrival time (BAT) may be more sensitive than CBV in detecting perfusion abnormalities. In patients with occluded vessels, BATs were significantly longer than in contralateral hemispheres with patent vessels. There are two possible reasons for increased BAT: (1) blood flow may be decreased, with increased mean transit times (MTT), since CBF = CBV/MTT,[25] or (2) the flow may be collateral or contralateral, with the result that the bolus has to traverse a longer path to reach the ischemic region. It is also possible that both mechanisms are involved.

Figure 14–9 shows representative T_2, CBV, and BAT images from one patient who had a left MCA stroke. At this early time-point, T_2 MRI results are normal; CBV images are also fairly unremarkable. However, BAT images clearly show a delayed arrival of contrast material throughout the left MCA distribution. Follow-up MR scans performed 3 and 8 days later revealed a large left MCA infarct.

A significant technical limitation of this perfusion technique is the fact that with conventional gradient-echo imaging, only one slice can be recorded with an acceptable time resolution (1 to 3 seconds). In acute stroke, the location of the lesion is often uncertain and imaging techniques that provide whole-brain coverage are therefore required. One solution to this problem is to use high-speed multi-slice echo planar imaging, as has been demonstrated by the group at Massachusetts General Hospital for bolus-tracking experiments.[76] However, echo planar imaging is a demanding technique requiring specialized gradient hardware, which is not

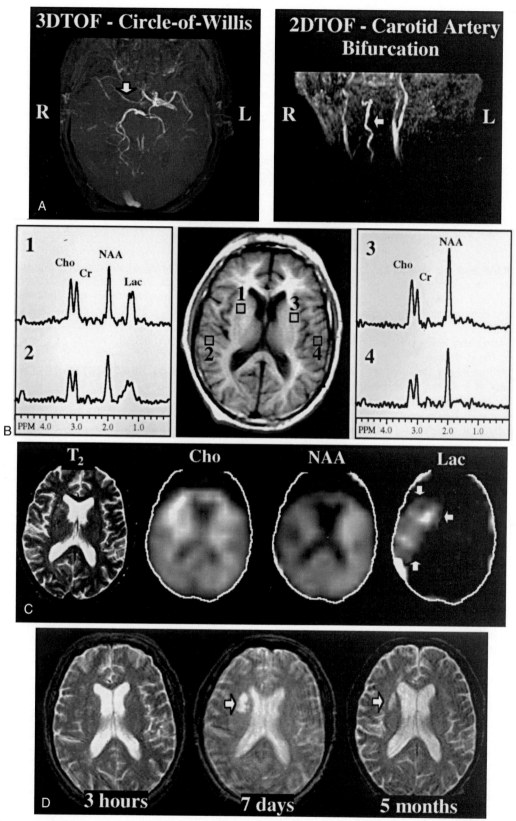

FIGURE 14–8. Representative data from one case. The patient was first scanned 3 hours after symptom onset. Magnetic resonance imaging at this time was normal, but magnetic resonance angiography showed a high-grade stenosis or complete occlusion of the right internal carotid artery (ICA) and low flow in the right middle cerebral artery (MCA) *(A)*. Spectroscopic images performed at this time showed elevated lactate throughout much of the right MCA territory, with the highest lactate in the right basal ganglia *(B* and *C)*. Only slight reductions in *N*-acetyl aspartate (NAA) were apparent. Follow-up scans performed 1 week later showed that the basal ganglia region progressed to infarction, with high T_2 (see text for definition) signal *(D)* and complete absence of NAA (not shown in this figure), but that the previously ischemic lateral regions were spared.

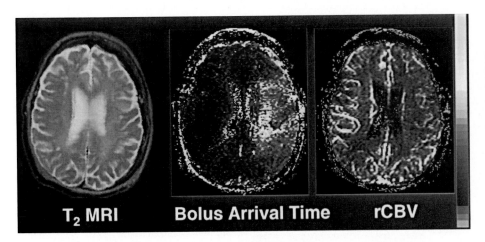

FIGURE 14–9. Representative T_2, cerebral blood volume (CBV), and bolus arrival time (BAT) images from one patient who had a left middle cerebral artery (MCA) stroke. At this early time-point, T_2-weighted magnetic resonance images were normal; CBV images are also fairly unremarkable. However, BAT images clearly show a delayed arrival of the contrast material throughout the left MCA distribution. Follow-up magnetic resonance scans performed 3 and 8 days later revealed a large left MCA infarct. See text for definition of T_2.

generally available, and the images can contain significant spatial distortions because of magnetic susceptibility effects. An alternative, based on the BURST imaging sequence,[77] has recently been demonstrated by the group at the National Institutes of Health.[78]

Perfusion imaging also has significant biologic limitations. Although tissue blood flow is a critical parameter in acute stroke, an isolated perfusion measurement may be of limited value, particularly if it is not quantitative. Stroke outcome depends strongly on the duration of the ischemic insult and on other parameters, such as arterial oxygenation and glucose supply and the extent to which these compounds are metabolized.[79] Nevertheless, brain regions with evidence of abnormal perfusion and no other abnormality (eg, T_2 hyperintensity or NAA deficit) are consistent with ischemic tissue at risk for infarction. Perfusion imaging may therefore be useful in selecting patients suitable for thrombolytic or other therapies.

Ideally, a flow technique should avoid the use of exogenous tracer agents that may either have potentially toxic properties or require an invasive procedure for administration. Also, because thresholds of flow are critical to the degrees of brain injury in occlusive cerebrovascular disease, a method for the measurement of true tissue flow is desirable. Recently, an atraumatic and quantitative steady-state indicator dilution technique for MRI of regional CBF in rats has been proposed, with promising initial results.[80, 81] In experimental MRI of regional CBF, the protons of arterial blood are inverted in the neck of a small animal, for example, a rat. In the presence of a magnetic gradient in the direction of carotid arterial inflow, an inversion of the inflowing protons in arterial blood is performed. The arterial protons thus labeled flow into the brain in a time much less than the persistence of the inversion, that is, the T_1 of blood. The persistence of the inversion label in the tissue, the T_1 of the tissue, is short on a flow time scale. Thus, this is the MRI equivalent of a CBF study using a short-lived indicator in which the steady-state concentration of the indicator, inverted protons in the tissue, is directly proportional to the flow to the tissue. Although the technique can be applied to animals in a suitably robust and reproducible form, there are problems in extending the studies to humans. Most of the systematic errors of the method lead to underestimation of flow. These errors are, however, estimable and uniform. Errors deriving from MRI temporal system instabilities, coupled with magnetization transfer effects, can lead to errors in CBF estimates, which cannot be corrected in a linear manner without improvements in imaging techniques to shorten total imaging times and thus minimize temporal systematic errors. Therefore, at this time, the measurement of true tissue blood flow in human brain by MRI must be considered experimental.

FUNCTIONAL MAGNETIC RESONANCE IMAGING

In the last 3 years, fMRI techniques[76, 82–85] have been developed to detect functional changes in the brain. The most versatile of these techniques is based on detecting local changes in blood deoxyhemoglobin concentration in active regions of the brain.[86, 87] Many PET experiments have demonstrated that during brain activation, the CBF increased about 29 to 50 percent,[88–91] and the regional oxygen consumption increased only about 5 percent,[88] which resulted in an increased regional cerebral blood oxygenation level and reduced concentrations of deoxyhemoglobin in active regions of brain. These physiologic changes during brain activity increase MRI signal intensities, which are sensitive to relative concentrations of paramagnetic deoxyhemoglobin and diamagnetic oxyhemoglobin. The fMRI signal changes detected by this technique are called blood oxygen level–dependent signals. The fMRI technique is noninvasive, and can be used routinely and repeatedly. Furthermore, MR methodology can provide both anatomic and functional information and can produce images with higher temporal and spatial resolutions than PET. The feasibility of mapping visual,[92, 93] motor,[94, 95] sensory,[96] language,[97] working memory,[98] and auditory activation[99] using fMRI techniques has been demonstrated by many investigators. Clinical applications of fMRI have been initiated to explore, for example, presurgical planning,[100] studying brain reorganization after perinatal unilateral injury,[101] and mapping epilepsy foci.[102, 103]

Evidence for recovery of function following stroke has been accumulated for many years, but the understanding of mechanisms is limited in the clinical situation. Brain plasticity can be considered as a fundamental factor in the recovery, however. This phenomenon is especially prominent in the developing nervous system, but it persists to some extent throughout the lifespan. There is little information on the nature of functional recovery and reorganization following stroke, such as time-course, spatial location, and mechanism.

Increased understanding of brain plasticity may provide useful information to enhance patient rehabilitation and may increase the number of patients who can partially or completely recover from brain injury. Furthermore, certain drugs may be useful in speeding up the process of recovery by enhancing plasticity. These mechanisms probably begin in the early stages after stroke, which justifies early studies of reorganization. Thus this topic is considered appropriate in the acute management of stroke because it is such reparative processes that cytoprotective therapy is designed to maintain.

An example to illustrate how such strategies may be appropriate is as follows. We have studied eight normal right-handed subjects and three recovering stroke patients while they performed a finger opposition task in which the thumb *sequentially* touched each of the four digits. In normal subjects, activation was found primarily in the contralateral motor cortex with slight ipsilateral activation (Fig. 14–10). We measured the volume of tissue between the anterior margin of the precentral gyrus and the posterior margin of the postcentral gyrus (rolandic area) of each hemisphere activated by movement of the *contralateral* (C) and *ipsilateral* (I) hands. The average ratios of activated volumes, I/C, of left hemisphere and right hemisphere were 0.12 ± 0.05 (mean ± standard error of mean) and 0.05 ± 0.04, respectively. These results are consistent with findings of other investigators: each hemisphere of right-handed normal subjects is primarily activated by contralateral hand movements and has little ipsilateral representation.[93, 95, 104]

In three stroke patients who had motor deficits of upper limbs after stroke but had improved their motor abilities of upper limbs at the time of the study, we found that paretic hand movement resulted in increased activation of the ipsilateral primary motor cortex and adjacent areas (in the intact hemisphere) (Fig. 14–11). The average I/C value in the intact hemisphere was 0.73 ± 0.62 (n = 3). In two of the patients, the extent of activation was found in the lateral frontal lobe with movement of either hand. The average ratio of activated

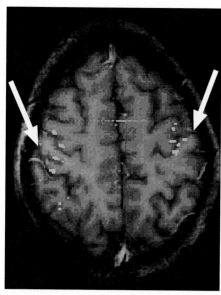

FIGURE 14–11. Cross sectional images of brain structure and function of a right-handed stroke patient during movements of the paretic (right) hand. Bilateral activation (*bright areas,* indicated by *arrows*) was observed near the central sulcus during the paretic hand movements.

brain volume in the bilateral frontal lobes to that in the contralateral primary motor cortex was 1.02 ± 0.56 (n = 3) for the unaffected hand movements. For the paretic hand movements, this ratio was 0.90 ± 0.63 (n = 3).

The results obtained from these patients are summarized in Table 14–1. These data suggest that some areas of intact cerebral cortex (ipsilateral primary motor cortex, its adjacent areas, and frontal lobe), which are traditionally not involved in the motor function in normal people, may be recruited to compensate in the function of the damaged cortex in hemiparetic stroke patients.

Clearly these studies are in their infancy as applied to stroke but constitute a major opportunity to expand the scientific basis of stroke rehabilitation, hitherto plagued with the abscence of objective measuring devices to monitor outcomes and consequent reliance on frequently unsatisfactory neurologic or behavioral measures.

RECOMMENDED STRATEGY FOR ACUTE FOCAL ISCHEMIC STROKE INVESTIGATION AND MANAGEMENT

As we stated at the outset of this chapter, for the acute management of stroke it is desirable to have one measuring

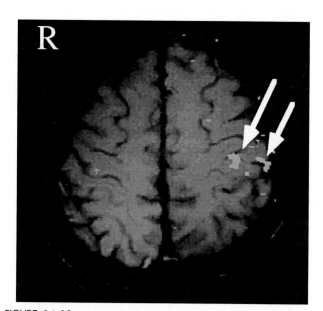

FIGURE 14–10. A typical example of cross sectional images of brain structure and function of a right-handed normal subject during movements of the right hand. Primarily, contralateral activation (*bright areas* indicated by *arrows*) was observed in the sensorimotor cortex.

TABLE 14–1. Summary of Stroke Patient Outcomes

Patient	Intact Hemisphere (I/C volume ratio)	Good Hand Movements (TF/CPMC volume ratio)	Paretic Hand Movements (TF/CPMC volume ratio)
1	2.00	1.00	0.72
2	0.00	2.00	1.86
3	0.26	0.06	0.10
mean ± sem	0.75 ± 0.63	1.02 ± 0.56	0.90 ± 0.63

C, contralateral; CPMC, contralateral primary motor cortex; I, ipsilateral; sem, standard error of mean; TF, bilateral frontal lobes.

device, thereby shortening the time of the early investigative process and permitting treatment at the earliest possible time. This device should be readily available, rapid, and noninvasive and should provide the maximum number of measurements, including diagnostics. We recommend that the measuring device be the MR spectrometer with capability for fast imaging of structure and function. The patient should be transferred to the MR suite as soon as possible after admission, and the following measures should be performed.

Standard Diagnostic Imaging

Magnetic Resonance Angiography. MR angiography provides the evidence needed to confirm arterial occlusion. For thrombolytic therapy, the site of occlusion may also prove important because it may influence the dosage regimen. For example, distal occlusive thrombus in branch arteries may be less well organized than a thrombus in the internal carotid artery. Further, evidence of clot dissolution and reperfusion may be obtained by repeat angiography during the same imaging session.

Proton Density, T_1-, and T_2-Weighted Magnetic Resonance Imaging. Although standard MRI has a low yield in the acute detection of focal ischemia, it remains essential to have standard diagnostic brain images to identify preexisting abnormalities of structure.

Advanced Diagnostic Imaging

Diffusion-Weighted Imaging. This technique is essential to detect acute ischemia within at least 6 hours of onset. Although not an imperative or a contraindication to treatment, diagnostic substantiation of acute ischemic stroke prior to potentially harmful modes of therapy provides the highest standard of care.

At this stage, we recommend postprocessing of the diffusion-weighted and T_2-weighted images to produce ADC_w and T_2 maps, which are then further processed to provide maps and quantitation of the tissue signatures of ischemic histopathology described in previous sections of the chapter. This facilitates decision-making in terms of safety of reperfusion strategies and the appropriateness of cytoprotective treatment. For clinical research into the effectiveness of such strategies and objective measurement of outcome, volumetric analysis of infarct size and knowledge of the proportions of potentially viable and salvageable tissue will be essential. The value of this approach is to replace time as the therapeutic window and extend the opportunity of treatment to those patients presenting beyond the stringent time limits employed in current investigative clinical trials. At this time, these patients constitute the large majority and will continue to do so until health and emergency care systems change to meet the imperatives of acute stroke managment. The investigative strategies we propose, including standard and advanced imaging paradigms, can be completed within 20 to 30 minutes of the patient's entering the magnet.

Research Magnetic Resonance Imaging

Spectroscopic Imaging. At this time, the role of spectroscopy in the acute evaluation of stroke remains experimental and is best focused on mechanisms. When more rapid techniques are developed, it seems possible that measures such as pH may be useful in defining the therapeutic window.

Cerebral Hemodynamics. It remains to be determined whether the addition of a further measure such as CBF to the assessment of tissue signatures will improve the early detection of cells that are injured by ischemia but remain responsive to cytoprotection. Currently, some perfusion measures require contrast material and all add time to the evaluation. Functional MRI has strong potential to assess brain reorganization but introduces time and clinical constraints in the acute setting with critically ill patients.

In conclusion, we believe that magnetic resonance provides the most comprehensive information needed for acute stroke diagnosis and management and permits treatment and early outcome monitoring in a single setting.

REFERENCES

1. Astrup J, Siesjo BK, Symon L: Thresholds in cerebral ischemia: The ischemic penumbra. *Stroke.* 1981;12:723.
2. Marcoux FW, Morawetz RB, Crowell RM, et al: Differential regional vulnerability in transient focal cerebral ischemia. *Stroke.* 1982;13:339.
3. Welch KMA, Barkley GL: Biochemistry and pharmacology of cerebral ischemia. In Barnett HJM, Mohr JP, Stein MB, Yatsu FM, (eds). *Stroke: Pathophysiology, Diagnosis and Management.* New York: Churchill Livingstone; 1986:75.
4. Baron JC, Frackowiak RSJ, Herholz K, et al: Use of PET methods for measurement of cerebral energy metabolism and hemodynamics in cerebrovascular disease. *J Cerebral Blood Flow Metab.* 1989;9:723.
5. Mansfield P, Morris PG: Water in biological systems. In Waugh, JS, ed. *NMR Imaging in Biomedicine.* London: Academic Press; 1982;15.
6. Moseley ME, Cohen Y, Mintorovitch J, et al: Early detection of regional cerebral ischemia in cats: Comparison of diffusion- and T_2-weighted MRI and spectroscopy. *Mag Reson Med.* 1990;14:330.
7. Shimizu H, Chileuitt L, Mintorovitch J, et al: Early detection of cerebral ischemia by diffusion-weighted MRI after middle cerebral artery occlusion and reperfusion in rats. *J Neurosurg.* 1990;72:36A.
8. Knight RA, Ordidge RJ, Helpern JA, et al: Temporal evolution of ischemic damage in rat brain measured by proton nuclear magnetic resonance imaging. *Stroke.* 1991;22:802.
9. Moseley ME, Mintorovitch J, Asgari H, et al: Diffusion/perfusion MR characterization of hyperacute cerebral ischemia. *Proc X Ann Mtg Soc Magn Reson Med.* 1991;1:330.
10. Busza AL, Allen KL, Gadian DG, Crockard HA: Early changes demonstrated by diffusion-weighted MR imaging in experimental cerebral ischemia. *Proc X Ann Mtg Soc Magn Reson Med.* 1991;1:328.
11. Benveniste H, Hedlund IW, Johnson GA: Mechanism of detection of acute cerebral ischemia in rats by diffusion-weighted magnetic resonance microscopy. *Stroke.* 1992;23:756.
12. Naruse S, Horikawa Y, Tanaka C, et al: Proton nuclear magnetic resonance studies of brain edema. *J Neurosurg.* 1982;56:747.
13. Buonanno FS, Pykett IL, Brady TJ, et al: Proton NMR imaging in experimental ischemic infarction. *Stroke.* 1983;14:178.
14. Mano I, Levy RM, Crooks LE, Hosobuichi Y: Proton nuclear magnetic resonance imaging of acute experimental cerebral ischemia. *Invest Radiol.* 1983;17:345.
15. Horikawa Y, Naruse S, Tanaka C, et al: Proton NMR relaxation times in ischemic brain edema. *Stroke.* 1986;17:1149.
16. Bederson JB, Bartkowski HM, Meen K, et al: Nuclear magnetic resonance imaging and spectroscopy in experimental brain edema in a rat model. *J Neurosurg.* 1986;64:795.
17. Kato H, Kogure K, Ohtomo H, et al: Characterization of experimental ischemic brain edema utilizing proton nuclear magnetic resonance imaging. *J Cereb Blood Flow Metab.* 1986;6:212.
18. Ordidge RJ, Helpern JA, Knight RA, et al: Investigation of cerebral ischemia using magnetization transfer contrast (MTC) MR imaging. *Magn Reson Imag.* 1991;9:895.
19. Shimosegawa E, Inugami A, Okudera T, et al: Embolic cerebral infarction: MR findings in the first 3 hours after onset. *AJR Am J Roentgenol* 1993;160:1077.
20. Bose B, Jones SC, Lorig R, et al: Evolving focal cerebral ischemia in cats: Spatial correlation of nuclear magnetic resonance imaging, cerebral blood flow, tetrazolium staining, and histopathology. *Stroke.* 1988;19:28.
21. Brant-Zawadzki M, Pereira B, Weinstein P, et al: MR imaging of acute experimental ischemia in cats. *AJNR Am J Neuroradiol* 1986;7:7.
22. LeBihan D, Breton E, Lallemand D, et al: MR imaging of intravoxel incoherent motions: Application to diffusion and perfusion in neurologic disorders. *Radiology.* 1986;161:401.
23. Stejskal EO, Tanner JE: Spin diffusion measurements: Spin-echoes in the presence of a time-dependent field gradient. *J Phys Chem.* 1965;42:288.

24. Mintorovitch J, Baker LL, Yang GY, et al: Diffusion-weighted hyperintensity of early cerebral ischemia: Correlation with brain water content and ATPase activity. *Proc Soc Magn Reson Med.* 1991;10:329. Abstract.

25. Warach S, Chien D, Li W, et al: Fast magnetic resonance diffusion-weighted imaging of acute human stroke. *Neurology.* 1992;42:1717.

26. Moonen CT, Pekar J, de Vleeschouwer MH, et al: Restricted and anisotropic displacement of water in healthy cat brain and in stroke studied by NMR diffusion imaging. *Magn Reson Med.* 1991;19:327.

27. Helpern JA, Dereski MO, Knight RA, et al: Histological correlations of nuclear magnetic resonance imaging parameters in experimental cerebral ischemia. *Mag Reson Imag.* 1993;11:241.

28. Lynch LJ: Water relaxation in heterogeneous and biological systems. In Cohen JS, ed, *Magnetic Resonance in Biology,* Vol. 2. New York; John Wiley & Sons; 1980:280.

29. Kuntz ID, Kauzmann W: Hydration of proteins and polypeptides. In Anfinsen CB, Edsall JT, Richards FM, eds. *Advances in Protein Chemistry.* Vol. 28. New York: Academic Press; 1995:297, 314.

30. Inuzuka T, Tamura A, Sato S, et al: Changes in the concentrations of cerebral proteins following occlusion of the middle cerebral artery in rats. *Stroke.* 1990;21:917.

31. Fung LWM, Narasimhan C, Lu HZ, Weaterman MP: Reduced water exchange in sickle cell anemia red cells: A membrane abnormality. *Biochem Biophys Acta.* 1989;982:167.

32. Benga G, Morariu VV: Membrane defect affecting water permeability in human epilepsy. *Nature.* 1977;265:636.

33. Serbu AM, Marian A, Popescu O, et al: Decreased water permeability of erythrocyte membranes in patients with duchenne muscular dystrophy. *Muscle Nerve.* 1986;9:127.

34. Fritz OG Jr, Swift TJ: The state of water in polarized and depolarized frog nerves. *Biophys J.* 1986;7:675.

35. Tanner JE: Transient diffusion in a system partitioned by permeable barriers. Application to NMR measurements with a pulsed field gradient. *J Chem Phys.* 1978;69(4):1748.

36. Tanner JE, Stejskal EO: Restricted self-diffusion of protons in colloidal systems by the pulsed-gradient, spin-echo method. *J Chem Phys.* 1978;49(4):1768.

37. Cooper RL, Chang DB, Young AC, et al: Restricted diffusion in biophysical systems. *Biophys Acta.* 1970;230:482.

38. Tanner JE: Self diffusion of water in frog muscle. *Biophys J.* 1979;28:107.

39. Moseley ME, Brant-Zawadzki M, Berry I, et al: Magnetic resonance imaging and 31-P and 1-H spectroscopy of experimental brain ischemia. *Am J Neuroradiol.* 1986;7:538.

40. Chien D, Kwong KK, Gress DR, et al: MR diffusion imaging of cerebral infarction in humans. *AJNR Am J Neuroradiol* 1992;13:1097.

41. de Crespigny A, Yenari M, Enzmann D, et al: Navigated spin-echo diffusion imaging of human stroke. *Soc Mag Reson Med.* 1994;Abstract 137.

42. van Bruggen N, Cullen BM, King MD, et al: T2- and diffusion-weighted magnetic resonance imaging of a focal ischemic lesion in rat brain. *Stroke.* 1992;23:576.

43. Dereski MO, Chopp M, Knight RA, et al: The heterogeneous temporal evolution of focal ischemic neuronal damage in the rat. *Acta Neuropathol.* 1993;85:327.

44. Jiang Q, Zhang ZG, Chopp M, et al: Temporal evolution and spatial distribution of the diffusion constant of water in rat brain after transient middle cerebral artery occlusion. *J Neurol Sci.* 1993;120:123.

45. Pierpaoli C, Righini A, Linfante I, et al: Histopathologic correlates of abnormal water diffusion in cerebral ischemia: Diffusion-weighted MR imaging and light electron microscopic study. *Radiology.* 1993;189:439.

46. Sevick RJ, Kucharczyk J, Mintorovitch J, et al: Diffusion-weighted MR imaging and T₂-weighted MR imaging in acute cerebral ischemia: Comparison and correlation with histopathology. *Acta Neurochirurgica Suppl.* 1990;51:210.

47. Minematsu K, Li L, Fisher M, et al: Diffusion-weighted magnetic resonance imaging: Rapid and quantitative detection of focal brain ischemia. *Neurology.* 1992;42:235.

48. Knight RA, Dereski MO, Helpern JA, et al: MRI assessment of evolving focal cerebral ischemia: Comparison with histopathology in rats. *Stroke.* 1994;25:1252.

49. Dereski MO, Chopp M, Knight RA, et al: Focal cerebral ischemia in the rat: Temporal profile of neutrophil responses. *Neurosci Res Commun.* 1992;11:179.

50. Garcia JH, Yoshida Y, Chen H, et al: Progression from ischemia injury to infarct following middle cerebral artery occlusion in the rat. *Am J Pathol.* 1993;142:623.

51. Levine SR, Welch KMA, Helpern JA, et al: Prolonged deterioration of ischemic brain energy metabolism and acidosis associated with hyperglycemia: Human cerebral infarction studied by serial 31P NMR spectroscopy. *Ann Neurol.* 1988;23:416.

52. Welch KMA, Levine SR, Helpern JA: Pathophysiologic correlates of cerebral ischemia. The significance of acid-base shifts. *Funct Neurol.* 1990;5:21.

53. Martin GB, Paradis NA, Helpern JA, et al: 31-Phosphorus NMR spectroscopy of human brain after cardiac arrest. *Stroke.* 1991;22:462.

54. Levine SR, Helpern JA, Welch KMA, et al: Human focal cerebral ischemia: Evaluation of brain pH and energy metabolism with P-31 NMR spectroscopy. *Radiology.* 1992;185:537.

55. Welch KMA, Levine SR, Martin G, et al: Magnetic resonance spectroscopy in cerebral ischemia. *Neurol Clin.* 1992;10:1.

56. Halvorson HR, Vande Linde AMQ, Helpern JA, Welch KMA: Assessment of magnesium concentrations by 31P NMR in vivo. *NMR Biomed.* 1992;5:53.

57. Helpern JA, Vande Linde AMQ, Welch KMA, et al: Acute elevation and recovery of intracellular [Mg²⁺] following human focal cerebral ischemia. *Neurology.* 1993;43:1577.

58. Gadian DG, Frackowiak RS, Crockard HA, et al: Acute cerebral ischaemia: Concurrent changes in cerebral blood flow, energy metabolites, pH, and lactate measured with hydrogen clearance and 31P and 1H nuclear magnetic resonance spectroscopy. I. Methodology. *J Cereb Blood Flow Metab.* 1987;7:199.

59. Monsein LH, Mathews VP, Barker PB, et al: Irreversible regional cerebral ischemia: Serial MR imaging and proton MR spectroscopy in a nonhuman primate model. *AJNR Am J Neuroradiol.* 1993;14:963.

60. Petroff OA, Prichard JW, Ogino T, Shulman RG: Proton magnetic resonance spectroscopic studies of agonal carbohydrate metabolism in rabbit brain. *Neurology.* 1988;38:1569.

61. Frahm J, Bruhn H, Gyngell ML, et al: Localized high-resolution proton NMR spectroscopy using stimulated echoes: Initial applications to human brain in vivo. *Magn Reson Med.* 1989;9:79.

62. Bruhn H, Frahm J, Gyngell ML, et al: Cerebral metabolism in man after acute stroke: New observations using localized proton NMR spectroscopy. *Magn Reson Med.* 1989;9:126.

63. Felber SR, Aichner FT, Sauter R, et al: Combined magnetic resonance imaging and proton magnetic resonance spectroscopy of patients with acute stroke. *Stroke.* 1992;23:1106.

64. Gideon P, Henriksen D, Sperling B, et al: Early time course of N-acetylaspartate, creatine and phosphocreatine, and compounds containing choline in the brain after acute stroke. *Stroke.* 1992;23:1566.

65. Henriksen O, Gideon P, Sperling B, et al: Cerebral lactate production and blood flow in acute stroke. *J Magn Reson Imag.* 1992;2:511.

66. Berkelbach van der Sprenkel JW, Luyten PR, van Rijen PC, et al: Cerebral lactate detected by regional proton magnetic resonance spectroscopy in a patient with cerebral infarction. *Stroke.* 1988;19:1556.

67. Sappey MD, Calabrese G, Hetherington HP, et al: Proton magnetic resonance spectroscopy of human brain: Applications to normal white matter, chronic infarction, and MRI white matter signal hyperintensities. *Magn Reson Med.* 1992;26:313.

68. Petroff OAC, Graham GD, Blamire AM, et al: Spectroscopic imaging of stroke in humans: Histopathology correlates of spectral changes. *Neurology.* 1992;42:1349.

69. Graham G, et al: Early temporal variation of cerebral metabolites after human stroke. *Stroke.* 1993;24:1891.

70. Hugg JW, Duijn JH, Matson GB, et al: Elevated lactate and alkalosis in chronic human brain infarction observed by 1H and 31P MR spectroscopic imaging. *J Cereb Blood Flow Metab.* 1992;12(5):734.

71. Duijn JH, Matson GB, Maudsley AA, et al: Human brain infarction: Proton MR spectroscopy. *Radiology.* 1992;183:711.

72. Duyn JH, Gillen J, Sobering G, et al: Multisection proton MR spectroscopic imaging of the brain. *Radiology.* 1993;188:277.

73. Barker PB, Gillard JH, van Zijl PCM, et al: Acute stroke: Evaluation with serial proton magnetic resonance spectroscopic imaging. *Radiology.* 1994;723:192.

74. Rosen BR, Belliveau JW, Vevea JM, et al: Perfusion imaging with NMR contrast agents. *Magn Reson Med.* 1990;14:249.

75. Rempp KA, Brix G, Wenz F, et al: Quantification of regional cerebral blood flow and volume with dynamic susceptibility contrast-enhanced MR imaging. *Radiology.* 1994;193:637.

76. Belliveau JW, Kennedy DN, McKinstry RC, et al: Functional mapping of the human visual cortex by magnetic resonance imaging. *Science.* 1991;254:716.

77. Hennig J, Hoddap M: Burst imaging, MAGMA 1993;1:39.

78. Duyn JH, van Gelderen P, Liu G, Moonan CTW: Fast volume scanning with frequency-shifted BURST MRI. *Magn Reson Med.* 1993;32:429.

79. Hossman K-A: Viability thresholds and the penumbra of focal ischemia. *Ann Neurol.* 1994;36:557.

80. Williams DS, Detre JA, Leigh JS, Koretsky AP: Magnetic resonance imaging of perfusion using spin inversion of arterial water. *Proc Natl Acad Sci U S A.* 1992;89:212.

81. Dixon WT, Du LN, Faul DD, et al: Projection angiograms of blood labeled by adiabatic fast passage. *Magn Reson Med.* 1986;3(3):454.

82. Ogawa S, Tank DW, Menon R, et al: Intrinsic signal changes accompanying sensory stimulation: Functional brain mapping using MRI. *Proc Natl Acad Sci U S A.* 1992;89:5951.

83. Kwong KK, Belliveau JW, Chesler DA, et al: Dynamic magnetic resonance imaging of human brain activity during primary sensory stimulation. *Proc Natl Acad Sci U S A.* 1992;89:5675.

84. Bandettini PA, Wong EC, Hinks PS, et al: Time course EPI of human brain function during task activation. *Magn Reson Med.* 1992;25:390.

85. Frahm J, Bruhn H, Merboldt KD, Hanicke W: Dynamic MR imaging of human brain oxygenation during rest and photic stimulation. *J Magn Res Imag.* 1992;2:501.

86. Ogawa S, Lee T, Nayak AS, Glynn P: Oxygenation-sensitive contrast in magnetic resonance image of rodent brain at high magnetic fields. *Magn Reson Med.* 1990;14:68.

87. Turner R, LeBihan DL, Moonen CTW, et al: Echo-planar time course MRI of cat brain oxygenation changes. *Magn Reson Med.* 1991;22:159.

88. Fox PT, Raichle ME: Focal physiological uncoupling cerebral blood flow and oxidative metabolism during somatosensory stimulation in human subjects. *Proc Natl Acad Sci U S A.* 1986;83:1140.

89. Fox PT, Raichle ME, Mintun MA, Dence C: Nonoxidative glucose consumption during focal physiological neural activity. *Science.* 1988;241:462.

90. Deiber MP, Passingham RE, Colebatch JG, et al: Cortical areas and the selection of movement: A study with positron emission tomography. *Exp Brain Res.* 1991;84:393.

91. Fox PT, Meizin FM, Allman JM, et al: Retinotopic organization of human visual cortex mapped with positron emission tomography. *J Neurosci.* 1987;7:913.

92. Menon RS, Ogawa S, Tank DW, Ugurbil K: 4 Tesla gradient recalled echo characteristics of photic stimulation-induced signal changes in the human primary visual cortex. *Mag Reson Med.* 1993;30:380.

93. Schneider W, Casey BJ, Noll DC: Functional MRI mapping of stimulus rate effects across visual processing stages. *Hum Brain Map.* 1994;1:117.

94. Kim SG, Ashe J, Hendrich K, et al: Functional magnetic resonance imaging of motor cortex: Hemispheric asymmetry and handedness. *Science.* 1993;261:615.

95. Rao SM, Binder JR, Bandettini PA, et al: Functional magnetic resonance imaging of complex human movements. *Neurology.* 1993;43:2311.

96. Hammeke TA, Yetkin FZ, Mueller WA, et al: Functional magnetic resonance imaging of somatosensory stimulation. *Neurosurg.* 1994;35:677.

97. Hinke R, Hu X, Stillman A, et al: Functional magnetic resonance imaging of Broca's area during internal speech. *Cog Neurosci Neuropsych.* 1993;4:675.

98. Cohen JD, Forman SD, Braver TS, et al: Activation of the prefrontal cortex in a nonspatial working memory task with functional MRI. *Human Brain Mapping.* 1994;1:293.

99. Binder JR, Rao SM, Hammeke TA, et al: Temporal characteristics of functional magnetic resonance signal change in lateral frontal and auditory cortex. *Proc Magn Reson Med.* 1993;1:5.

100. Jack CR Jr, Thompson RM, Butts RK, et al: Sensory motor cortex: Correlation of presurgical mapping with functional MR imaging and invasive cortical mapping. *Radiology.* 1994;190:85.

101. Cao Y, Vikingstad M, Huttenlocher PR, et al: Functional magnetic resonance studies of the reorganization of the human hand sensorimotor area after unilateral brain injury in the perinatal period. *Proc Natl Acad Sci U S A.* 1994;91:9612.

102. Cao Y, Towle VL, Levin DN, et al: Conventional 1.5 T functional MRI localization of human hand sensorimotor cortex with intraoperative electrophysiologic validation. *Proc Soc Magn Res Med.* 1993;3:1417.

103. Jackson GD, Connelly A, Cross JH, et al: Functional magnetic resonance imaging of focal seizures. *Neurology.* 1994;44:850.

104. Cao Y, Towle VL, Levin DN, Balter JM: Functional mapping of human motor cortical activation by conventional MRI at 1.5 T. *J Mag Res Imag.* 1993;3:869.

CHAPTER 15

Positron Emission Tomography

JOHN C. MAZZIOTTA

To understand the complex interrelationships that occur during cerebral ischemia and stroke requires examination of the relationship among blood flow, metabolism, and other physiologic variables as a function of the site of injury, the time course of the injury, and the etiology of the ischemia. Positron emission tomography (PET) has already demonstrated its ability to provide just this sort of pathophysiologic information. The great majority of clinical studies performed with PET have been aimed at the elucidation of the pathophysiology of cerebrovascular disease.

Traditional approaches to neurologic imaging in the study of cerebrovascular disease focused on structural abnormalities as tools in diagnosis. Angiography and computed tomography provided new insights into the structural processes that accompany clinical syndromes. An understanding of the mechanisms that influence the acute and chronic responses of the brain to diminished perfusion, however, requires the type of pathophysiologic information provided by PET. Knowledge of the pathophysiologic states that accompany specific stroke syndromes in individual patients over time, and of the clinical phenomena pertaining to outcome, provides the best opportunity for understanding the mechanisms underlying stroke. Most important, such data are critical to the design of specific therapies to avoid irreversible cerebral injury due to perfusion insufficiencies.

Noninvasive physiologic studies previously performed in patients with cerebrovascular disease were limited to the measurement of blood flow alone and suffered from insufficient spatial resolution due to the use of two-dimensional image-detection systems. The application of PET to cerebrovascular disease research has provided information on the temporal course of blood flow, oxygen, and glucose metabolism as well as the respective extraction fractions for these substrates. In using tracer kinetic methods to study cerebrovascular disease, one must be constantly aware of the limitations imposed by tracer kinetic principles. Stroke, as the name implies, is an acute event wherein rapid changes in biochemical pathways occur. These unstable situations, in which substrate availability is (at least initially) rate limiting, may constrain certain PET estimates.

Despite these problems, carefully executed detailed studies of cerebral ischemia performed with PET provided a first glimpse at the complex interrelationships of flow and metabolism, as well as tissue pH and substrate availability, as a function of time in these disorders. Invasive measures of animal models of stroke plus PET studies of spontaneous cerebral ischemia in humans can be performed with identical tracer kinetic techniques to obtain a more detailed understanding of these pathophysiologic mechanisms. Such comparisons can validate or refute certain stroke models and provide the necessary understanding of the abnormal cellular biochemical processes that occur in response to perfusion insufficiencies in humans.

TECHNICAL ASPECTS OF POSITRON EMISSION TOMOGRAPHY

Positron emission tomography is a complex methodology that produces brain images that depict physiologic processes (Fig. 15–1). Despite its relatively recent development, PET is already capable of providing information about local cerebral blood flow (LCBF), local cerebral metabolic rate of oxygen (LCMRO$_2$), local cerebral metabolic rate of glucose (LCMRglc), local cerebral blood volume (LCBV), and local oxygen extraction fractions (LOEF). Such information is

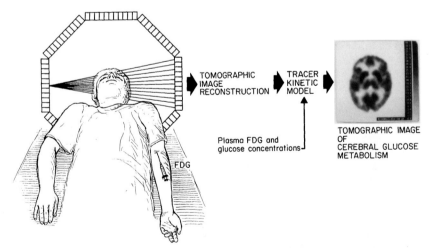

FIGURE 15–1. The sequence of events involved in the tomographic measurement of the local cerebral metabolic rate for glucose with the use of (^{18}F)2-fluoro-2-deoxy-D-glucose (*FDG*). About 40 minutes after intravenous injection of FDG, tomographic data are collected and cross-sectional images are reconstructed of the ^{18}F tissue activity distribution. Plasma FDG and glucose concentrations are entered into the computer of the tomograph, which also contains the operational equation of the FDG tracer kinetic model. Images are then converted to local cerebral metabolic rates for glucose in units of μmol/minute/g of tissue. Tomographic images are displayed on a television screen with a gray scale in proportion to local cerebral metabolic rate for glucose (black being the highest) and numerical values shown beside the scale. Lines through the head show the 180 degree emission of two photons in positron decay that are recorded by a surrounding ring of detectors. (From Phelps ME, Mazziotta JC, Schelbert HR: Studies of cerebral function and dysfunction. Positron computed tomography for studies of myocardial and cerebral functions. *Ann Intern Med.* 1983;9:339; with permission.)

possible because of PET's ability to measure—noninvasively and quantitatively—local tissue radioactivity concentrations in much the same manner as they are measured in animals by means of tissue autoradiography. Such studies require the combined efforts of nuclear physicists and chemists, neuroscientists, and technicians. They also require access to a cyclotron, since many physiologically useful positron-emitting isotopes have short (eg, seconds to minutes) half-lives. In addition, carefully designed tracer kinetic mathematical models are needed to accurately describe the process being imaged with PET. Although these requirements are extensive and expensive, the resultant three-dimensional images provide truly physiologic data (as opposed to structural data) about brain function—a capability not previously available to the clinician or neuroscientist in human studies.[1-4]

PHYSICAL PRINCIPLES

It is the special combination of physical and chemical properties of positron-labeled compounds that allows for their reliable imaging in a quantifiable manner. The positron-emitting isotopes that have acceptable radiation-dose properties and physical half-lives and that have been incorporated into tracer methods to study biologic systems include ^{15}O ($t\frac{1}{2}$ = 123 seconds), ^{11}C ($t\frac{1}{2}$ = 20 minutes), ^{13}N ($t\frac{1}{2}$ = 10 minutes), and ^{18}F ($t\frac{1}{2}$ = 110 minutes). The first three isotopes are substituted for their corresponding natural elements, and ^{18}F is used to replace hydrogen or the hydroxyl group.[2-4]

The unique physical properties of positron decay permit accurate and quantifiable imaging.[2, 3, 5] Positrons are positively charged electrons that are emitted from certain unstable nuclei as they decay to more stable nuclei. When a positron combines with an electron, they annihilate (ie, the masses of the electron and positron are converted to electromagnetic radiation) and produce a pair of high-energy (511 keV) annihilation photons. The detection of these events utilizes the fact that the annihilation photons are emitted in essentially opposite directions. PET devices use rings or multiple banks of opposed detectors (Fig. 15–2). These detectors are electronically linked in opposition to accept only those events that are recorded simultaneously (within 10–20 nanoseconds) at opposing detectors. This approach provides an electronic form of collimation and establishes the origin of the recorded radiation to well-defined regions between the opposing detectors. The system, known as coincidence detection, also rejects radiation originating above or below the tomographic plane of interest. Using these methods, only a thin (1–2 cm) slice of tissue is sampled, with relatively uniform resolution across the slice. The data from each set of detectors are collected over time at many linear positions and angles around the cross section of the brain. At this point, the collected tissue count rate profiles resemble data collected using computed tomography systems. The data are then processed in a fashion mathematically similar to that for computed tomography data to reconstruct the final two-dimensional map of the tissue radioactivity concentrations in the brain slice. Finally, the image is corrected for the attenuation of the emitted radioactivity that occurs as it passes through the cranial structures. Final image resolution is currently in the range of 5 to 10 mm. The ECAT III (CTI, Knoxville, TN) device achieves spatial resolutions as high as 5 to 6 mm. The theoretical limit of resolution is on the order of a few millimeters; however, the practical limit of resolution, dictated mainly by financial factors, is in the range of 3 to 5 mm.[6]

Physiologic Variables

Characterization of the local function of the brain requires measurement of numerous variables, depending on the problem under study. The primary variables of interest studied thus far with PET include LCBF, LCMRO$_2$, and LCMRglc, which normally form the supply-and-demand basis of local function in the brain. That is to say, under normal conditions, glucose and oxygen metabolism are related by a constant stoichiometric relationship, and blood flow is determined by metabolic demand (ie, metabolic regulation of flow or flow metabolism coupling). Although a complete discussion of the mathematical models and methods used for each of these determinations is beyond the scope of this chapter, a brief description of each is included.

Local cerebral blood flow has been measured with PET by a variety of techniques. The most commonly used methods determine LCBF by the use of ^{15}O-labeled compounds or ^{13}N-labeled ammonia. LCBF can be measured by the clearance of a single breath inhalation of $C^{15}O_2$ or bolus intravenous injection of $H_2^{15}O$, followed by redundant sampling with the PET device over a 4- to 8-minute period.[7] Alternatively, the subject can be made to inhale $C^{15}O_2$ continuously until the concentration of the radioisotope reaches a dynamic equilibrium in the brain.[8, 9] This point occurs when the radioactivity delivered from the lung equals that due to the physical decay of the isotope and the biologic clearance. Although the ^{15}O tissue concentrations obtained with the continuous inhalation method are nonlinearly related to cerebral blood flow, the effect can be corrected to provide measurements of absolute LCBF. These corrections are best at low to normal flow values.

The use of $^{13}NH_3$ also produces a nonlinear estimate of cerebral blood flow, but it has been used to examine relative perfusion in stroke and seizure patients; the results demonstrate good correlation with changes in metabolism. Krypton-

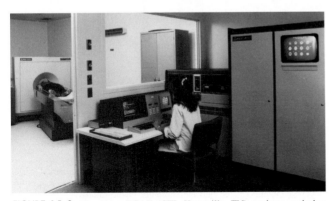

FIGURE 15–2. The NeuroECAT (CTI, Knoxville, TN) positron emission tomography system at the University of California Los Angeles. (From Phelps ME, Mazziotta JC, Schelbert HR: Studies of cerebral function and dysfunction. Positron computed tomography for studies of myocardial and cerebral functions. *Ann Intern Med.* 1983;9:339; with permission.)

77 and other diffusible agents have also been combined with PET to measure blood flow.

Cerebral glucose metabolism can be measured tomographically by the use of either ^{18}F-fluorodeoxyglucose (FDG) or ^{11}C-deoxyglucose injected intravenously.[10–12] Using an extension of the Sokoloff [13]model to determine glucose metabolic rate with deoxy analogues of natural glucose, one can obtain images that represent cerebral glucose utilization patterns approximately 30 to 40 minutes following injection. During this time, deoxyglucose is taken up by cells in proportion to their functional activity (ie, metabolic rate), and the final image represents the local integrated sum of neuronal activity during the 30- to 40-minute uptake.[1–4, 13]

Local cerebral metabolic rate for oxygen utilization can be determined by the continuous inhalation of $^{15}O_2$-labeled O_2.[8, 9] After LCBF is measured by the continuous inhalation of $C^{15}O_2$, LCMRO$_2$ can be measured by switching the inhaled gas delivered to the subject to ^{15}O-labeled O_2. The image obtained during the continuous inhalation of $^{15}O_2$ is then corrected for the blood-flow component (ie, $^{15}O_2$ is metabolized to $H^{15}O_2$, which is redelivered to the brain in proportion to cerebral blood flow). by dividing the $^{15}O_2$ image by the $C^{15}O_2$ image. This ratio image is proportional to the LOEF or to the arteriovenous oxygen difference divided by the arterial oxygen concentration. When this ratio image of LOEF is multiplied by the blood flow and the arterial oxygen concentration, LCMRO$_2$ values are obtained.

Local cerebral blood volume can be determined following a single breath inhalation of ^{11}C-labeled CO, which binds to hemoglobin in the red blood cells, thereby trapping the tracer in the vascular compartment.[14] Images obtained using these methods produce quantitative distributions of the blood volume per gram of brain substance. The images provide a clear delineation of the large intracranial arteries, veins, and venous sinuses.

Models also exist for the calculation of cell membrane–facilitated transport of glucose using ^{11}C-labeled methylglucose. Blood-brain barrier integrity can be determined using ^{68}Ga-labeled EDTA.[15] Radiopharmaceuticals and tracer kinetic models are currently being tested to study protein synthesis with ^{11}C-labeled L-leucine,[16] dopamine receptor sites, and benzodiazepine receptor sites as well as the use of inert lipophilic agents that can be used as tracers to determine the distribution and integrity of myelin in the brain.

APPLICATION OF POSITRON EMISSION TOMOGRAPHY TO CEREBROVASCULAR DISEASE

Temporal Pathophysiologic Sequence of Completed Stroke

Basic to an understanding of cerebrovascular disease is knowledge of the temporal pathophysiologic sequence of events that occurs following reduced perfusion to the brain. Table 15–1 synthesizes data derived from PET studies that depict this sequence of abnormal events following reductions in perfusion pressure to local brain regions.[17] This hypothetical sequence of events reflects initial data obtained with PET and will probably change and become more refined as additional studies are performed. It does, however, demonstrate the ability of PET to examine a complex sequence of events over time and across multiple processes to establish the natural pathophysiologic history of a complex disease process.

Blood Flow and Volume, Oxygen Utilization, and Oxygen Extraction

Initial studies using ^{15}O-labeled compounds to measure LCBF, LCMRO$_2$, and LOEF were performed at relatively late times (3 days or more) after the stroke ictus.[18–28] A number of generalizations can be made about these initial studies. First, all demonstrated a reduction in oxygen metabolism in tissue that ultimately showed complete infarction by diminished attenuation values on computed tomography. Second, perfusion was typically in excess of oxygen requirements for the tissue and resulted in a uniformly decreased oxygen extraction fraction in these late cases. Third, cerebral blood flow was typically in excess of metabolic needs and was quite variable. LCBF values could be high, low, or normal in the area of ultimate infarction. In addition, the pattern of flow abnormalities was heterogeneous within the area of ultimate infarction.[20, 22]

These studies (Fig. 15–3) suggested that oxygen utilization and extraction fraction were more reliable predictors of ultimate tissue outcome and that a threshold for tissue viability could be determined.[20, 22, 23, 29, 30] An initial threshold value of 58 µmol O_2/minute/100 g for LCMRO$_2$ was found to predict a poor clinical outcome and presumed nonviability

TABLE 15–1. Temporal Pathophysiologic Sequence of Events Following Reduced Perfusion to the Brain*

State	CMRO$_2$	CBF/CBV	OEF	CBF
Decreased hemodynamic reserve	Normal	Decreased	Normal	Normal
Decreased oxygen extraction reserve	Normal	Decreased	Increased	Decreased
Ischemia	Decreased	Decreased	Increased‡	Decreased
Early infarction†	Decreased	Variable	Decreased	Variable
Late infarction	Decreased	Variable	Normal	Decreased

*Possible pathophysiologic sequence of events that occurs in humans as cerebral perfusion pressure is progressively reduced from states of mild hypoperfusion to cerebral infarction. This scenario is the product of combining numerous positron emission tomography (PET) studies in cerebrovascular disease. As more information is obtained, this hypothetical composite will evolve and change. As discussed in the text, PET studies provide the types of physiologic data that allow for such hypotheses to be developed, tested, validated, or refuted.

†Dependent on site, duration, and severity. Threshold for infraction, CMRO$_2$ <56 µmol O_2/min/100 g (or <40% of contralateral side); CBF <20 mL/min/100 g.

‡CBF/CBV <5.5 leads to increased OEF.

CBF, cerebral blood flow; CBV, cerebral blood volume; CMRO$_2$, cerebral metabolic rate of oxygen; OEF, oxygen extraction fraction.

Adapted from Frackowiak RS, Wise RJ: Positron tomography in ischemic cerebrovascular disease. *Neurol Clin.* 1983; 1:183; with permission.

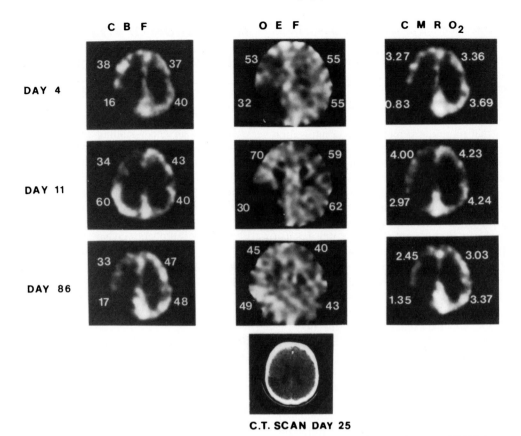

FIGURE 15-3. Cerebral blood flow *(CBF)*, oxygen extraction fraction *(OEF)*, and cerebral metabolic rate of oxygen *(CMRO₂)* measured using the ^{15}O continuous inhalation technique in a patient with cerebrovascular disease. Clinically, the patient demonstrated global aphasia, apraxia, and right homonymous hemianopia without motor or sensory deficits. Computed tomography scan showed an infarct in the left middle cerebral artery territory sparing the motor cortex, as demonstrated on day 25. An angiogram demonstrated occlusion of the left internal carotid artery. Positron emission tomography studies were obtained on days 4, 11, and 86 following the onset of symptoms. Values indicated are as follows: CBF, mL/min/100 g; OEF, percentage values; and CMRO₂, mL O₂/min/100 g. Within the core area of the infarct, blood flow was very low on day 4, but oxygen metabolism was even more depressed, as evidenced by the lower OEF value relative to that of the remainder of the brain (''luxury perfusion''). On day 11 there was focal hyperemia with continuing luxury perfusion, the OEF being at about one half of the contralateral value, and oxygen metabolism, although improved, was still reduced. On day 86, both blood flow and oxygen metabolism reached very low values in the infarcted area and were essentially coupled. Such studies can be used to grade and classify various ischemic versus infarcted cerebral regions and could be helpful in both diagnostic and therapeutic decisions, as discussed in the text. Gray scale is proportional to quantitative rates, with white indicating the highest value. (From Baron JC, Bousser MG, Lebrun K, et al.: Commissariet de l'Energie Atomique, Service Hopitalier Frederic Joliot Orsay, and the Hôpital de la Salpetrière, Paris, France; with permission.)

of damaged tissue.[30] Low oxygen utilization with severely reduced oxygen extraction is representative of cell death. The high variability in LCBF values has been attributed to derangements in vascular autoregulation, to capillary hyperplasia, and to postinfarct reperfusion by various investigators, depending on the time of its occurrence.[22, 31] This luxury perfusion was originally labeled as such by Lassen[32] during the mid-1960s, when regional cerebral blood flow studies documented its occurrence following infarction. The great variability in regional cerebral blood flow measurements obtained using ^{133}Xe was extremely difficult to interpret. In light of the combined flow-metabolism data, it is now clear that flow is a relatively unreliable predictor of ultimate tissue outcome following cerebral ischemia.[17, 20, 22, 25, 27–29, 31]

Baron and colleagues[23] made an important observation when they reported that 18 percent of their patients had increased oxygen extraction fractions following the stroke ictus. The state of increased oxygen extraction, termed ''misery'' or ''critical'' perfusion, occurred in all three of their patients who were tested early (3 days or less following the ischemic insult).

The observation that an increased oxygen extraction frac-

tion was more likely to occur soon after the onset of clinical symptoms from cerebrovascular disease led Wise and colleagues[31] to study patients at much earlier times following stroke ictus. Twenty-eight cases were studied in all. Nine patients were examined less than 3 days following the onset of their stroke symptoms. Patients were restudied at 7 days, and half of them were studied again at 3 to 6 weeks. In those patients studied less than 12 hours after the onset of symptoms, all but one had an increased oxygen extraction fraction (Fig. 15–4). The one exceptional patient had extremely low LCBF values (less than 5 mL/min/100 g) and oxygen utilization (less than 22 μmol O₂/min/100 g). Twelve of 14 patients studied at 24 hours or more after the symptoms, however, had decreased oxygen extraction fractions (see Fig. 15–4). In the follow-up studies, eight of nine patients had a decrease in oxygen extraction fractions between the first and second studies. The typical time of this transition was 12 to 24 hours after the onset of symptoms (see Table 15–1). The reason for the change in extraction fraction was commonly due to an increase in CBF, but in some cases it was attributed to the combined decrease in flow and oxygen utilization, with the reduction of the latter

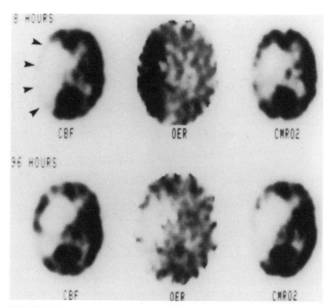

FIGURE 15–4. Critical perfusion and luxury perfusion. The transition is demonstrated from a high oxygen extraction rate *(OER)* in the lesion at an early stage (8 hours after onset of symptoms of ischemia) to a low OER accompanied by cerebral, low oxygen consumption rate *(CMRO₂)* at a later stage (96 hours) in the same patient. Note the greater severity of the changes in the subcortical structures supplied by deep penetrating end arteries. There was no clinical change between measurement. CBF, cerebral blood flow. (From Frackowiak RS, Wise RJ: Positron tomography in ischemic cerebrovascular disease. *Neurol Clin* 1983;1:183; with permission.)

process being greater. Typical values for the oxygen extraction fraction at early times (mean time 14 hours) were 0.7 ± 0.12 and at late times (4 days) 0.34 ± 0.23.[31] At these later times, Wise and coworkers[31] saw the same variability in cerebral blood flow previously reported in studies performed late after the onset of clinical symptoms.[20, 22, 25–30] These data demonstrate that (1) luxury perfusion can occur with high, low, or normal absolute values of cerebral blood flow; (2) increases in oxygen extraction fraction are transient and relatively short in duration; (3) no improvement in oxygen utilization was ever observed, indicating an irreversible disruption of oxidative metabolism; and (4) the drop in oxygen extraction fraction with time may reflect tissue reperfusion, further decreases in oxygen utilization, or both.[31]

All patients in the studies described above had persistent symptoms and completed infarction. Gibbs and colleagues,[33, 34] Frackowiak and associates,[35] and Powers and coworkers[36] examined patients with less severe cerebral ischemia to investigate the relationship among cerebral blood volume, oxygen utilization, and cerebral blood flow. In these patients, a change in the normal ratio of cerebral blood flow to cerebral blood volume occurred. Although normal persons, on average, have a value of 10.2 ± 0.9 for this ratio, patients with carotid occlusions have reductions in this relationship and a value of 6.9 ± 1.4 for the hemisphere ipsilateral to the carotid occlusion.[33, 34] Gibbs and coworkers[33, 34] observed that the oxygen extraction fraction began to increase when this ratio dropped below a value of 5.5.

Combining all these data, one arrives at the temporal sequence of flow, volume, oxygen extraction, and utilization relationships depicted in Table 15–1. Initially, when perfu-

sion pressure to the brain is reduced, the patient remains symptom free due to compensatory mechanisms (vasodilation). Oxygen extraction and utilization remain within the normal range. Further reductions in cerebral perfusion initiate an additional reserve mechanism—further desaturation of arterial blood—with a resultant increase in oxygen extraction fraction (Fig. 15–5). According to Gibbs and associates,[33, 34] this should occur when the flow-volume ratio is reduced below the threshold of 5.5. Imaging at this point would demonstrate local increases in blood volume and extraction fraction, with reduced flow and normal oxygen utilization. Further reductions in brain perfusion exceed the reserve of the system to meet metabolic demands, and oxygen utilization drops. This condition, which fulfills the criteria for ischemia, occurs in proportion to the severity and duration of the ischemia and is attended clinically by neurologic deficits.[17, 31] Imaging during this period demonstrates an increased oxygen extraction fraction and decreased oxygen utilization. If the severity and duration of the ischemia are such that irreversible tissue damage occurs, the oxygen extraction fraction will drop, typically at around 24 hours after the initial insult, and cerebral blood flow assumes the more variable pattern described above.[31] At this point, oxygen utilization and extraction are low, blood flow is variable but typically in excess of metabolic needs, and the site of these abnormalities predicts ultimate structural tissue damage that will ultimately be identifiable by computed tomography.

Although still speculative, the available PET data make this a plausible working hypothesis for the sequence of

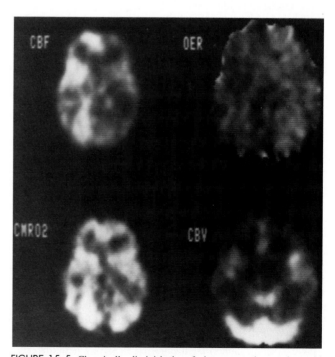

FIGURE 15–5. Chronically diminished perfusion reserve in a patient with a unilateral complete carotid occlusion. The ipsilateral (right) hemisphere shows a lower cerebral blood flow *(CBF)* (−26%) but a higher oxygen extraction rate *(OER)* (+30%) and a similar oxygen consumption rate *(CMRO₂)* (−2%) compared with the contralateral side. This is accompanied by an increase in the cerebral blood volume *(CBV)* of the affected side (±24%), indicating compensatory vasodilation. (From Frackowiak RS, Wise RJ: Positron tomography in ischemic cerebrovascular disease. *Neurol Clin* 1983;1:183; with permission.)

the pathophysiologic events that occur as a consequence of progressive cerebral perfusion reductions. Information about glucose utilization, pH, and other variables is needed to understand the temporal sequence of pathophysiologic events that occur to produce ischemic brain infarction. One should also keep in mind that cerebrovascular disease is not a single entity in terms of its nature or time course. Therefore, many different descriptions of these heterogeneous pathophysiologic events will undoubtedly emerge with further PET investigations.

Wise and coworkers[31] also reported that the distribution of these abnormal flow-metabolism relationships varies between cortical and subcortical zones. These investigators found that at a given point in time, deep areas (ie, lenticular nuclei and thalamus) had decreased oxygen extraction fractions relative to overlying cortex. For example, in nine of their patients, these subcortical zones had oxygen extraction fractions of 0.45, whereas the ipsilateral overlying cortex had a mean value of 0.67. This discrepancy was attributed to the lack of collateral circulation in the deep zones, which are fed by penetrating end arteries. This finding suggests that the time course for irreversible injury produced by leptomeningeal arterial occlusion may be more rapid for these end artery deep zones, placing them at increased jeopardy for irreversible tissue damage. Therapeutic schemes designed to save viable brain tissue may therefore have to be instituted within extremely short times after the onset of symptoms to salvage these deep structures. Finally, at extremely late times, all reports indicate that the oxygen extraction fraction slowly increases and approaches but never reaches normal values.[26, 30]

Cerebral Perfusion and Glucose Utilization

Relative cerebral perfusion, using ^{13}N-ammonia,[37] and LCMRglc were reported by Kuhl and associates[38] in 10 patients (Fig. 15–6). Two of these patients were studied soon (2 days or less) after the onset of stroke symptoms. In these patients, glucose utilization exceeded perfusion, although both were depressed, a situation analogous to the state of increased oxygen extraction in the above-described early ^{15}O studies. Three patients studied at 2 weeks following stroke ictus had perfusion values in excess of glucose utilization. In five patients studied at 2 months or longer after the onset of stroke symptoms, glucose metabolism and perfusion were matched, and a defect was seen on CT that was typically smaller than the metabolic abnormality detected with PET. This late coupling between flow and glucose metabolism was similarly reported by Celesia and colleagues[39] who used ^{18}F-fluoromethane to measure cerebral blood flow.

In no instance thus far has increased glucose utilization (above normal values) been reported in stroke patients. Hypermetabolism for glucose has been found at very short times (10–90 minutes) following occlusion of blood flow in animal models of acute stroke.[40, 41] It may be that PET measurements have been too distant from the initial event to observe these acute changes. However, most cerebrovascular disease patients have been studied with ^{15}O PET techniques, so there is limited data on LCMRglc in this disease process.

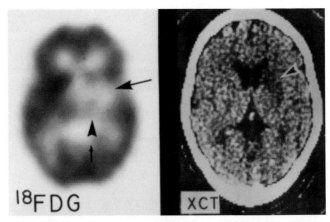

FIGURE 15–6. Cerebral glucose metabolism in a subject with an ischemic infarct. Computed tomography (X-CT) demonstrates a deep basal ganglia infarct on the right side. Positron emission tomography with (^{18}F)2-fluoro-2-deoxy-D-glucose (^{18}FDG) demonstrates a larger area of hypometabolism than the structural defect would suggest. In the metabolic image, not only is the right basal ganglia involved in its entirety but there is ipsilateral depression in the local cerebral metabolic rate of glucose of the thalamus (arrowhead) and of a zone of cortex (arrow). (From Kuhl DE, Phelps ME, Kowell AP, et al: Effects of stroke on local cerebral metabolism and perfusion: Mapping by emission computed tomography of ^{18}FDG and ^{13}NH₃. Ann Neurol. 1980;8:47; reprinted with permission.)

Blood Flow, Oxygen, and Glucose Stoichiometry in Stroke

An increasing number of studies have demonstrated that in situations in which oxygen utilization and extraction are low (completed stroke) and blood flow is variable in magnitude, glucose utilization is either normal or only mildly impaired.[17, 34, 42] In these situations, an abnormally low oxygen-to-glucose molar utilization ratio has been reported, ranging from 1.2 to 2.0 for patients with low oxygen extraction fractions.[42, 43] It remains to be seen whether this abnormal relationship is coupled in completed stroke at this abnormally low value or whether there is a temporal sequence to this relationship as well. Initial studies indicate that coupling may occur in the infarct zone with reductions in both glucose and oxygen extraction fractions.[44] Speculative causes for the relative preservation of glucose utilization despite a reduction in oxygen utilization include (1) irreversible mitochondrial damage, with cessation of oxidative energy metabolism of the tricarboxylic acid, or Krebs, cycle but preservation of the Embden-Meyerhof pathway activity; (2) anaerobic glycolysis of macrophages that have infiltrated the infarcted zone; and (3) artifactual overestimations produced by the use of the deoxyglucose method in pathologic tissues.[43, 45, 46] Nevertheless, in chronic stroke patients, no indication for changes in the lumped constant was found. Changes in the rate constants produced underestimations of LCMRglc when low metabolic rate states were examined.[47] The complex temporal sequence of these pathologic stoichiometric relationships will undoubtedly be the focus of future PET studies on stroke.

Tissue pH and Blood-Brain Barrier Integrity

Techniques for the measurement of tissue pH using a weak acid such as ^{11}C-dimethyloxazolidine-dione have been reported.[48, 49] Syrota and coworkers[49] described such studies in nine patients examined at 10 to 24 days after the onset of stroke symptoms. Tissue acidosis at the site of the infarction was never observed. Normal or slightly elevated tissue pH was found in five patients, and a marked increase in pH (>20% higher than the contralateral hemisphere) was noted in four patients. The increase in tissue pH was linearly coupled with a decrease in oxygen extraction fraction and found to be independent of blood flow. Although the cause of this tissue alkylosis is unknown, possible explanations considered by these investigators included decreased production of acidotic tissue metabolites in necrotic stroke sites, increases in the extracellular fluid space, or combinations of both.

Blood-brain barrier integrity has been examined using ^{68}Ga-EDTA and PET in patients with cerebrovascular disease and compared with computed tomography images performed with and without intravenous administration of iodinated contrast material.[15] The results demonstrate that PET evidence of barrier disruption occurred between 6 and 60 days after the stroke onset (mean time 22.9 days), and 6 of 14 patients without contrast enhancement on computed tomography were found to have blood-brain barrier disruption using PET and ^{68}Ga-EDTA. The different results obtained with the two methods were attributed to the differences in size and chemical properties of the two agents, although it can probably be explained by the limited sensitivity of computed tomography to detect slow diffusion of the contrast agents through mild blood-brain barrier defects. It was concluded that PET is more sensitive than contrast-enhanced computed tomography in the determination of barrier disruption in stroke patients, and that the combined use of PET and computed tomography offers the best chance of detecting these abnormalities in patients with completed stroke.

Temporal Extremes of Cerebral Ischemia

Transient Ischemic Attacks

Only a limited number of PET studies address the issue of transient ischemic attacks (TIAs).[24, 39, 50, 51] Undoubtedly there will be great variability in the PET results from patients with transient ischemic events due to the varying mechanisms of their occurrence. Possible mechanisms for brief ischemic symptoms include diminished perfusion reserve, with ischemia and clinical symptoms produced by further reductions in perfusion pressure (decreased $CMRO_2$ with increased oxygen extraction fraction and decreased cerebral blood flow); small completed infarcts, with rapid resolution of clinical symptoms (eg, lacunes); and ischemia produced by emboli that either recanalize or move to smaller vessels, with resolution of clinical symptoms. Initial studies demonstrated normal cerebral blood flow and oxygen extraction fraction following TIA.[24, 39] Other preliminary studies, however, demonstrated various patterns, including coupled reductions of flow and metabolism or flow-metabolism uncoupling, with either high or low oxygen extraction.[50] Larger numbers of subjects with identified causes of TIA will have to be examined with PET to determine the spectrum of pathophysiologic problems associated with these ischemic events.

Chronic Persistent Reductions in Cerebral Perfusion

States of chronic persistent elevations in oxygen extraction fraction must be less common, since they have only occasionally been reported.[31, 52] Wise and coworkers[31] reported patients having increased oxygen extraction fractions, including one case in which blood pressure manipulations resulted in changes in blood flow and oxygen extraction fraction but no response in oxygen utilization. Baron and colleagues[52] demonstrated that surgical revascularization procedures can reverse chronic persistent underperfusion of the brain with downward correction of the preoperatively increased oxygen extraction fraction and increases in the preoperatively reduced cerebral blood flow (Fig. 15–7). Similar results demonstrated by other groups are discussed in the section on extracranial-intracranial bypass procedures.[53, 54] It is likely that in these states, typically found with internal carotid or proximal middle cerebral artery occlusions, the occurrence of vasodilation and increases in oxygen extraction fraction reflect the maximal use of the ischemia-prevention reserve of the brain in dealing with diminished cerebral perfusion.[17]

Effects of Stroke at Distant Sites

A universal finding in PET studies of stroke has been the observation that abnormalities of flow and metabolism can occur at sites distant from the ultimate structural lesion produced by brain ischemia. These sites include (1) subcortical zones ipsilateral to cortical lesions, (2) cortical zones ipsilateral to subcortical lesions, (3) diffuse and focal abnormalities of the contralateral cerebral hemisphere, and (4) abnormalities in the contralateral cerebellum. These distant effects appear to be truly functional and are generally without macroscopic correlates (Fig. 15–8).[55, 56]

Contralateral Hemisphere

Coupled decreases in CBF and $CMRO_2$ have been found in the hemisphere contralateral to a supratentorial infarct.[26, 30, 39, 57] Discrete mirror foci are typically seen early (less than 2 weeks), and the matched reductions in flow and metabolism can be profound. These mirror foci may reflect disconnection of transhemispheric (callosal) fiber systems.[26, 30] More diffuse reductions in contralateral hemispheric flow and metabolism correlate with decrements in the patient's level of consciousness and tend to reflect generalized reductions in metabolism throughout the brain.[17, 26, 30]

Cortical-Subcortical Zones

Ischemic lesions of cortical zones have been reported to cause reductions in metabolic activity in subcortical (caudate, thalamus) regions.[38, 39, 57] The reverse situation—that is, deep thalamic or basal ganglia infarcts producing ipsilateral cortical metabolic or flow suppressions—has also been reported (see Figs. 15–6 and 15–8).[39, 57, 58] Various causes for these cortical-subcortical interactions have been proposed, including compression-induced ischemia, wallerian degeneration, functional disconnections, occlusion of deep selective end arteries (eg, anterior choroidal), and combinations of all

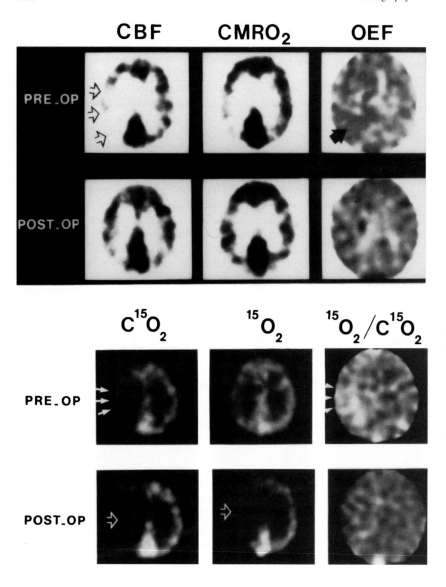

FIGURE 15–7. Cerebral blood flow *(left column)* and cerebral metabolic rate for oxygen *(middle column)* and oxygen extraction *(right column)* in two patients studied before and after extracranial–intracranial bypass. *(A)*, Preoperative positron emission tomography (PET) studies in a patient with a left internal carotid occlusion and focal transient ischemic attacks showed diminished cerebral blood flow in a region corresponding to that indicated by the patient's clinical symptoms. There was a mild decrease in oxygen metabolism and an increase the oxygen extraction fraction consistent with viable though jeopardized tissue. After bypass surgery *(post-op)*, all variables measured by PET returned to normal, and the transient ischemic attacks stopped. *(B)*, Patient with identical clinical and angiographic findings as the patient in *part A*, showing decreased blood flow, a mild decrease in oxygen utilization, and an increased oxygen-extraction fraction preoperatively. Following extracranial–intracranial bypass, the patient had a persistent neurologic deficit. Both blood flow and oxygen utilization are reduced further than in the preoperative study. These findings are indicative of infarction. Postoperative angiogram exhibited nonpatency of the bypass. (From Baron JC, Bousser MH, Rey A, et al.: Reversal of focal "misery-perfusion syndrome" by extra–intracranial arterial bypass in hemodynamic cerebral ischemia. *Stroke.* 1981;12:454. Reproduced with permission. Copyright 1981 American Heart Association, Inc.)

these factors. As yet, few data are available as to the temporal sequence of these cortical-subcortical interactions, nor are there specific data about stoichiometric relationships at these distant sites.

Cerebellum

Baron and coworkers[59] were the first to point out that supratentorial infarctions in the carotid territory can produce matched flow and oxygen metabolism reductions in the contralateral cerebellar hemisphere (Fig. 15–9). These workers coined the term *crossed-cerebellar diaschisis*.[59, 60] These studies, which measured cerebral blood flow and $CMRO_2$, indicated that the phenomenon occurred transiently and early (less than 2 months) and could be seen with either large or small cerebral infarctions. Lenzi and associates[25] reported that the phenomenon may become more exaggerated more than 50 days following the stroke ictus,[26, 30] that it did not occur with small infarcts, and that it was more likely to occur with lesions of the parietal cortex. The magnitude of the flow reductions ranged from 19 to 27 percent; for oxygen utilization, the range was 16 to 25 percent. Glucose metabolism was reduced by approximately 22 percent.[57] Since these

initial studies, a large number of reports have described this phenomenon following both ischemic infarction and hemorrhagic lesions of the putamen.[39, 57, 61–64]

The temporal course of crossed-cerebellar diaschisis is unsettled, as is the importance of the site of the infarction in producing the phenomenon. Martin and Raichle[63] studied 16 patients and noted decreases in cerebellar blood flow and oxygen utilization with both frontal and parieto-occipital infarctions. They found that parieto-occipital infarcts produced flow and metabolism reductions of lesser magnitude than frontal infarctions; frontal infarctions produced asymmetric suppressions in cerebellar hemispheric flow and metabolism, with the contralateral hemisphere having the greatest reduction in these values. These investigators could find no relationship between the effects on the cerebellum and the size of the infarct, motor abnormalities, or the timing of the study following the stroke ictus. By contrast, Kushner and colleagues,[65] who studied patients having both stroke and brain tumors, found a significant association between contralateral cerebellar reductions in LCMRglc and lesions in the parietal lobe.

This interesting phenomenon of crossed-cerebellar flow and metabolism suppression represents an example of PET's

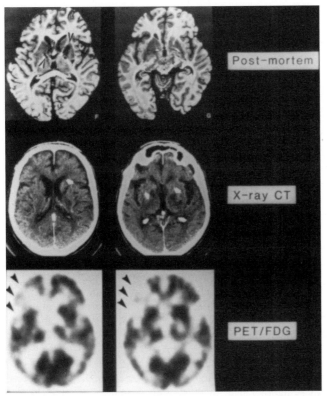

FIGURE 15–8. Structural versus functional anatomy. Images obtained with three different methods from a patient with multi-infarct dementia. The patient underwent computed tomography *(center row)* and positron emission tomography (PET) studies of glucose utilization with (^{18}F) fluoro-2-deoxy-D-glucose *(bottom row)* on the same day. The patient died seven days later of nonneurologic causes, and gross and microscopic evaluation of the brain *(top row)* was performed. Both forms of structural imaging (computed tomography and postmortem) and the metabolic study with PET demonstrated multiple small infarctions of deep structures of the brain (striate body, putamen, thalamus, and internal capsule). Neither structural imaging technique demonstrated abnormalities of the cortex. PET, however, demonstrated widespread abnormalities of frontal cortex, particularly on the left. These distant effects probably represent disruption of afferent and efferent fiber systems between the frontal cortical areas and the subcortical zones, most likely resulting from small subcortical infarcts seen structurally and metabolically. (From Metter EJ, Mazziotta JC, Itabashi HH, et al.: Comparison of glucose metabolism, X-ray CT, and postmortem data in a patient with multiple cerebral infarcts. *Neurology.* 1985;35:1695; with permission.)

ability to demonstrate functionally anatomic connections between the cerebral hemispheres and the posterior fossa. Similar results have been described in patients with supratentorial tumors.[66, 67]

PET versus CT

Ackerman and coworkers[19] reported that PET could identify the site of ultimate infarction earlier than CT if the lesion exceeded 2.5 to 3 cm^2.[19–22] This finding was subsequently supported by other observations and extended to include the fact that PET-identified lesions are typically larger in size than the ultimate macroscopic abnormality seen with computed tomography.[39]

Baron and associates[45] compared computed tomography with PET in 17 patients with cerebrovascular disease. They found decreased attenuation values on computed tomography in regions with reductions in flow or oxygen utilization. In addition, there was a positive correlation between contrast enhancement with iodinated compounds and relative reductions in cerebral blood flow (these were not hyperemic regions, since absolute blood flow was reduced). They concluded that relative increases in flow had a minor direct effect on contrast enhancement, but that these increases in flow might exaggerate leakage of iodinated compounds from the vascular space through the already damaged blood-brain barrier.

Clinical-PET Correlations

Ackerman and colleagues[21, 22] coined the term *clinicophysiologic correlations.* This term accurately describes the contribution of PET studies to the clinical management of patients with stroke.[21] The concept fulfills the goal of unraveling the temporal sequence of pathophysiologic events that result in brain infarction. The studies thus far described demonstrate that (1) oxygen utilization predicts tissue viability; (2) if this parameter drops below specific thresholds, it is unlikely that there will be a rapid return of neurologic function; and (3) a structural lesion will ultimately be seen in the area with computed tomography.[20, 22] The CBF value seems to be of less clinical significance during the postinfarction period. Therefore, the most reliable predictors of clinical outcome are oxygen extraction fraction and oxygen utilization.[20–22]

The correlation of clinical phenomena with PET values has been examined by a number of investigators. Lenzi and coworkers[26] showed that reductions in the patient's level of consciousness correlated with metabolic rates in the hemisphere contralateral to the stroke. In addition, low oxygen utilization and flow values for the posterior fossa and contralateral hemisphere were more likely to be found in patients with impaired consciousness at the time of the scan.[26] In

FIGURE 15–9. Crossed-cerebellar diaschisis. Tomographic images of cerebral blood flow *(CBF)* and cerebral metabolic rate of oxygen *(CMRO$_2$)* at the level of the basal ganglia *(bottom row)* and the cerebellum *(top row)* in a patient with a 4-day-old infarction in the territory of the left middle cerebral artery. The ischemic region is clearly seen at the upper brain levels *(bottom two images at left)* as an area of greatly reduced CBF and CMRO$_2$. Note also cerebellar asymmetry of CBF and CMRO$_2$, the *right side* showing reduced values relative to the *left side*. This functional asymmetry had no counterpart on the computed tomography scan. Values are mL/min/100 g for CBF and CMRO$_2$.

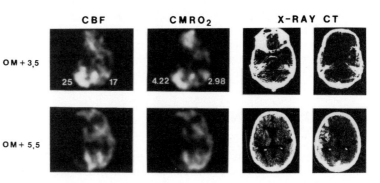

patients having a good clinical outcome, the core of the infarct never had an oxygen utilization value of less than 56 μmol O_2/min/100 g or less than 40 percent of the contralateral hemisphere. In patients with poor clinical outcomes, cerebral blood flow was consistently less than 20 ml/min/100 g, and all patients with flow values exceeding this threshold had some clinical improvement. Baron and co-workers[68] arrived at similar values in a series of studies in which oxygen utilization and blood flow were determined in terms of tissue viability. These investigators found that no pattern of cerebral blood flow–$CMRO_2$ coupling was specific for tissue outcome, but surviving areas had better preservation of these two parameters and less prominent uncoupling than did areas that ultimately became necrotic.[68]

Ackerman and associates[22] suggested that these clinico-physiologic correlations can be used to classify patients into treatment categories. Patients with low LCBF and very mild reductions in $LCMRO_2$ have viable but ischemic tissue and would benefit from increased perfusion. Such candidates would be selected for endarterectomy or extracranial–intracranial bypass procedures. Patients with intermediate depressions in $LCMRO_2$ have viable but metabolically damaged brain tissue and might benefit from maneuvers designed to minimize cerebral metabolic demands. By contrast, patients with profound decreases in $LCMRO_2$ and decreased oxygen extraction fractions, below threshold values for viability, would be candidates for more conservative therapy. Following classification, follow-up PET studies could monitor the effects of these interventions. Such suggested treatments have to take into account the apparent rapid temporal course of irreversible cerebral events that result from decreased brain perfusion, dictating that any intervention must be performed rapidly.[31]

Extracranial–Intracranial Bypass Procedures

The selective staging of patients with pathophysiologic PET criteria has proved successful in a select subgroup of patients undergoing extracranial–intracranial anastomoses. Initial nontomographic studies demonstrated that flow and oxygen metabolism values can be reversed in certain patients who are carefully selected for such revascularization procedures.[53, 69] In such carefully selected patients studied with PET (see Fig. 15–7), abnormal increases in cerebral blood volume and oxygen extraction fraction and decreases in cerebral blood flow and $CMRO_2$ can be normalized following extracranial–intracranial bypass.[33, 34, 36, 54, 70–73] More recent studies indicate that an increase in cerebral blood volume in the jeopardized vascular territory combined with a normal computed tomography study may be a good predictor of postoperative normalization of some aspects of cerebral hemodynamics.[33, 34, 36, 72–74] Such studies are crucial in the selection of individual patients for revascularization procedures. Criteria for patient selection are presently lacking, and one must rely on clinical and angiographic criteria rather than pathophysiologic measurements of tissue viability.

CONCLUSIONS AND FUTURE PROSPECTS

Positron emission tomography fulfills the requirements stated at the beginning of this chapter. That is, PET has the ability to examine the relationships among blood flow, metabolism, and other physiologic variables as a function of the site of injury, the time course of the injury, and the etiology of the ischemia. These capabilities should not be underestimated, since it is only through the examination of a variety of hemodynamic and biochemical processes that a fundamental understanding of the mechanisms underlying the various pathophysiologic events that occur in cerebrovascular disease can be realized.

Despite the fact that clinical studies with PET have become available only recently, a review of the material thus far reported indicates that substantial progress has already been made. The impact of the contributions that PET may make on the field of cerebrovascular disease research and the clinical diagnosis and management of patients with these disorders remains to be determined. Studies are under way to expand or study in greater detail many of the issues presented above. Most important among these will be a comprehensive evaluation of the temporal sequence of pathophysiologic events that occur during the biochemical and hemodynamic processes leading to reversible and irreversible ischemic damage to the brain. This information can then be applied to select patients for specific therapy, and the outcome of that therapy can be monitored using a truly pathophysiologic perspective obtained with PET. Of interest will be the ability to correlate the complex patterns of abnormalities seen in these patients with clinical signs and symptoms.[55, 56] The finding of distant regions of hypometabolism that appear to represent functional disconnections from a discrete cerebral infarction will be of particular interest, since their presence can be identified and monitored only by functional imaging techniques. The correlation of changing signs and symptoms and perhaps recovery from ischemic injury may be elucidated by comprehensive analyses of the changing patterns of these distant effects.

Although blood flow, volume, and cerebral metabolism of both oxygen and glucose, as well as their respective extraction fractions, are the variables of the most immediate interest in the study of cerebrovascular disease, the ability of PET to determine changes in blood-brain barrier integrity,[75] protein synthesis,[16] neuroreceptor systems,[76–78] and cerebral tissue pH[48, 49] will provide additional biochemical perspectives on the pathophysiology of stroke and its reversible antecedents.

Finally, in areas of brain that appear to be functional yet jeopardized by ischemia, one may use provocative tests to determine the functional reserve of such tissue. Thus, much in the way a cardiologist uses physical exercise to reveal latent abnormalities in coronary perfusion, those interested in cerebrovascular perfusion may use provocative tests for the same goal. Provocative maneuvers may involve either particular drugs or various tasks. Drugs might be employed to augment or reduce brain perfusion or metabolism. Task paradigms can be developed to increase neuronal activity in areas of the brain in which perfusion reserve is low and compensatory mechanisms limited. When stressed, such areas may manifest an inability to augment neuronal activities due to insufficient substrate. These same paradigms could be used to explore the issue of recovery from cerebral infarction. Such information might allow for the development of more pathophysiologically appropriate modes of patient rehabilitation.[79–81]

PET is a complex and expensive tool. Technologic advancements will further improve spatial resolution of these devices in the near future. At the same time, these advances may minimize cost and complexity, making this methodology available to centers and hospitals outside university-based research facilities. Even if these advances do not result in a wider dissemination of PET installations, the fundamental principles and the resultant understanding of the mechanisms underlying various types of cerebrovascular disease that PET will provide should contribute significantly to the diagnosis, management, and therapy of patients suffering from these disorders.

Acknowledgments

Special thanks are extended to all the investigators who so generously contributed their time, data, and comments. Gratitude is expressed to Lee Griswold for photography and artwork and to Anita Powers for preparing the manuscript. This work was partially supported by contract AM 03-76-SF00012, grants R01-6M-248388 and P01-NS-15-654 from the National Institutes of Health, and grant R01-MH-37916-01 from the National Institute of Mental Health. Dr. Mazziotta is the recipient of Teacher-Investigator Award 1K07-0058804-NSPA.

REFERENCES

1. Mazziotta JC: Studies of cerebral function and dysfunction: Positron computed tomography for studies of myocardial and cerebral function. *Ann Intern Med.* 1983;9:333.
2. Phelps ME, Mazziotta JC: Positron emission tomography: Human brain function and biochemistry. *Science.* 1985;228:799.
3. Phelps ME, Mazziotta JC, Huang SC: Study of cerebral function with positron computed tomography. *J Cereb Blood Flow Metab.* 1982;2:113.
4. Phelps ME, Mazziotta JC, Schelbert H: *Positron Emission Tomography and Autoradiography: Principles and Applications for the Brain and Heart.* New York: Raven Press; 1986.
5. Ter-Pogossian MM: Physical aspects of emission CT. In Newton TH, Potts DG, eds. *Radiology of the Skull and Brain: Technical Aspects of Computed Tomography.* St. Louis: CV Mosby; 1981:4372.
6. Hoffman EJ, Phelps ME, Huang SC: Performance evaluation of a positron tomograph designed for brain imaging. *J Nucl Med.* 1983;24:245.
7. Huang SC, Carson RE, Hoffman EJ, et al: Quantitative measurement of local cerebral blood flow in humans by positron computed tomography and ^{15}O-water. *J Cereb Blood Flow Metab.* 1983;3:141.
8. Frackowiak R, Lenzi G, Jones T, et al: Quantitative measurement of regional cerebral blood flow and oxygen metabolism in man using ^{15}O and positron emission tomography: Theory, procedure and normal values. *J Comput Assist Tomogr.* 1980;4:727.
9. Jones T, Chesler DA, Ter-Pogossian MM: The continuous inhalation of oxygen-15 for assessing regional oxygen extraction in the brain of man. *Br J Radiol.* 1976;49:339.
10. Huang SC, Phelps ME, Hoffman EJ, et al: Noninvasive determination of local cerebral metabolic rate of glucose in man. *Am J Physiol.* 1980;238:E69.
11. Phelps ME, Huang SC, Hoffman EJ, et al: Tomographic measurement of local cerebral glucose metabolic rate in humans with (F-18)2-fluoro-2-deoxyglucose: Validation of method. *Ann Neurol.* 1979;6:371.
12. Reivich M, Alavi A, Wolf A, et al: Use of 2-deoxy-D-[1-^{11}C]-glucose for the determination of local cerebral glucose metabolism in humans: Variation within and between subjects. *J Cereb Blood Flow Metab.* 1982;2:307.
13. Sokoloff L, Reivich M, Kennedy C, et al: The [^{14}C]deoxyglucose method for the measurement of local cerebral glucose utilization: Theory, procedure and normal values in the conscious and anesthetized albino rat. *J Neurochem.* 1977;28:897.
14. Phelps ME, Huang SC, Hoffman EJ, et al: Validation of tomographic measurement of cerebral blood volume with C-11 labeled carboxyhemoglobin. *J Nucl Med.* 1979;20:328.
15. Ericson K, Bergstrom M, Eriksson L, et al: Positron emission tomography with ^{68}Ga-EDTA compared with transmission computed tomography in the evaluation of brain infarcts. *Acta Radiol.* 1981;22:385.
16. Phelps ME, Barrio JR, Huang SC, et al: Criteria for the tracer kinetic measurement of protein synthesis in man with positron CT. *Ann Neurol.* 1984;15(1):S192.
17. Frackowiak RS, Wise RJ: Positron tomography in ischemic cerebrovascular disease. *Neurol Clin.* 1983;1:183.
18. Ackerman RH: Positron imaging of stroke disease. In Moossy J, Reinmuth OM, eds. *Cerebrovascular Disease.* New York: Raven Press; 1981:67.
19. Ackerman RH, Alpert NM, Correia JA, et al: Correlations of positron emission scans with TCT scans and clinical course. *Acta Neurol Scand.* 1979;60(72):230.
20. Ackerman RH, Alpert NM, Correia JA, et al: Importance of monitoring metabolic function in assessing the severity of a stroke insult (CBF: An epiphenomenon?). *J Cereb Blood Flow Metab.* 1981;1(1):S502.
21. Ackerman RH, Alpert NM, Correia JA, et al: Positron imaging in ischemic stroke disease using compounds labeled with oxygen-15. *Arch Neurol.* 1981;38:537.
22. Ackerman RH, Alpert NM, Davis SM, et al: Positron emission tomography of stroke patients. In Heiss WD, Phelps ME, eds. *Positron Emission Tomography of the Brain.* New York: Springer-Verlag; 1983:113.
23. Baron JC, Bousser MG, Comar D, et al: Noninvasive tomographic study of cerebral blood flow and oxygen metabolism in vivo. Potentials, limitations and clinical applications in cerebral ischemic disorders. *Eur Neurol.* 1981;20:273.
24. Baron JC, Comar D, Bousser MG, et al: Etude tomographique, chez l'homme, du débit sanguin et de la consommation d'oxygène du cerveau par inhalation continué d'oxygène 15. *Rev Neurol.* 1978;134:545.
25. Lenzi GL, Frackowiak RS, Jones T, et al: CMRO$_2$ and CBF by the oxygen-15 inhalation techniques: Results in normal volunteers and cerebrovascular patients. *Eur Neurol.* 1981;20:285.
26. Lenzi GL, Frackowiak RS, Jones T: Cerebral oxygen metabolism and blood flow in human cerebral ischemic infarction. *J Cereb Blood Flow Metab.* 1982;2:321.
27. Lenzi GL, Jones T, McKenzie CG, et al: Study of regional cerebral metabolism and blood flow relationship in man using the method of continuously inhaling oxygen-15 and oxygen-15 labeled carbon dioxide. *J Neurol Neurosurg Psychiatry.* 1978;41:1.
28. Lenzi GL, Jones T, McKenzie CG, et al: Non-invasive regional study of chronic cerebrovascular disorders using the oxygen-15 inhalation technique. *J Neurol Neurosurg Psychiatry.* 1978;41:11.
29. Baron JC, Comar D, Bousser MG, et al: Patterns of CBF and oxygen extraction fraction (EO$_2$) in hemispheric infarcts: A tomographic study with ^{15}O continuous inhalation technique. *Acta Neurol Scand.* 1979;60(72):324.
30. Lenzi GL, Frackowiak RS, Jones T: Regional cerebral blood flow (CBF), oxygen utilization (CMRO$_2$) and oxygen extraction ratio (OER) in acute hemispheric stroke. *J Cereb Blood Flow Metab.* 1981;1(1):S504.
31. Wise RJ, Bernardi S, Frackowiak RS, et al: Serial observations in the pathophysiology of acute stroke. *Brain.* 1983;106:197.
32. Lassen NA: The luxury-perfusion syndrome and its possible relation to acute metabolic acidosis localized within the brain. *Lancet.* 1966;2:1113.
33. Gibbs JM, Wise RSJ, Leenders KL, Jones T: Evaluation of cerebral perfusion reserve in patients with carotid artery occlusion. *Lancet.* 1984;2:310.
34. Gibbs JM, Wise R, Leenders K, et al: The relationship of regional cerebral blood flow, blood volume, and oxygen metabolism in patients with carotid occlusion: Evaluation of perfusion reserve. *J Cereb Blood Flow Metab.* 1983;3(1):S590.
35. Frackowiak RSF, Wise RSJ, Gibbs JM, Jones T: Positron emission tomographic studies in aging and cerebrovascular disease at Hammersmith Hospital. *Ann Neurol.* 1984;15:S112.
36. Powers W, Martin W, Herscovitch P, et al: The value of regional cerebral blood volume measurements in the diagnosis of cerebral ischemia. *J Cereb Blood Flow Metab.* 1983;3(1):S598.
37. Phelps ME, Huang SC, Hoffman EJ, et al: Cerebral extraction of N-13 ammonia: Its dependence on cerebral blood flow and capillary permeability–surface area product. *Stroke.* 1981;12:607.
38. Kuhl DE, Phelps ME, Kowell AP, et al: Mapping local metabolism and perfusion in normal and ischemic brain by emission computed tomography of ^{18}FDG and ^{13}NH$_3$. *Ann Neurol.* 1980;8:47.
39. Celesia G, Polcyn R, Holden J, et al: 18-F-fluoromethane positron emission tomography determination of regional cerebral blood flow in cerebral infarction. *J Cereb Blood Flow Metab.* 1983;3(1):S23.
40. Ginsberg MD, Reivich M, Giandomenico A, Greenberg JH: Local glucose utilization in acute focal cerebral ischemia: Local dysmetabolism and diaschisis. *Neurology (NY).* 1977;27:1042.
41. Pulsinelli WA, Duffy TE: Local cerebral glucose metabolism during controlled hypoxemia in rats. *Science.* 1979;204:626.
42. Wise R, Rhodes C, Gibbs J, et al: The relationship between oxygen metabolism and glucose utilization in early cerebral infarcts. *J Cereb Blood Flow Metab.* 1983;3(1):S580.
43. Gibbs JM, Rhodes CG, Wise RJ, et al: The relationship of regional cerebral blood flow, oxygen metabolism and glucose metabolism following acute stroke. In Heiss WD, Phelps ME, eds. *Positron Emission Tomography of the Brain.* New York: Springer-Verlag; 1983:234.
44. Baron JC, Lebrun-Grandie P, Collard P, et al: Noninvasive measurement of blood flow, oxygen consumption and glucose utilization in the same brain locus in man by positron emission tomography. *J Nucl Med.* 1982;23:391.
45. Baron JC, Delattre JY, Bories J, et al: Comparison study of CT and positron emission tomographic data in recent cerebral infarction. *AJNR.* 1983;4:536.
46. Siesjo BK: *Brain Energy Metabolism.* New York: Wiley; 1978.
47. Hawkins RA, Phelps ME, Huang SC, et al: Effect of ischemia on quantification of local cerebral glucose metabolic rate in man. *J Cereb Blood Flow Metab.* 1981;1:37.
48. Rottenberg DA, Ginos JZ, Kearfott KJ, et al: Determination of regional cerebral acid-base status using ^{11}C-dimethyloxazolidinedione and dynamic positron emission tomography. *J Cereb Blood Flow Metab.* 1983;3(1):S150.
49. Syrota A, Castaing M, Rougemont D, et al: Tissue acid base balance and oxygen

metabolism in human cerebral infarction studied with PET. *Ann Neurol.* 1983;14:419.

50. Donnan G, D'Alton JG, Chang JY, et al: Alterations in cerebral blood flow (CBF) and metabolism (CMRO$_2$) after transient ischemic attacks. *Neurology (NY).* 1983;33(2):115.

51. Rougemont D, Baron JC, Lebrum-Grandie P, et al: Débit sanguin cerebral et extraction d'oxygène dans les hémiplégies lacunaires. *Pathol Biol.* 1982;30:295.

52. Baron JC, Bousser MH, Rey A, et al: Reversal of focal "misery-perfusion syndrome" by extra-intracranial arterial bypass in hemodynamic cerebral ischemia. *Stroke.* 1981;12:454.

53. Grubb RL, Ratcheson RA, Raichle ME, et al: Regional cerebral blood flow and oxygen utilization in superficial temporal-middle cerebral artery anastomosis patients. *J Neurosurg.* 1979;50:733.

54. Yamamoto YL, Little S, Thompson C, et al: Positron emission tomography following EC–IC bypass surgery. *Acta Neurol Scand.* 1979;60(72):522.

55. Metter EJ, Mazziotta JC, Itobashi H, et al: Comparison of glucose metabolism, x-ray CT, and postmortem data in a patient with multiple cerebral infarcts. *Neurology.* 1985;35:1695.

56. Metter EJ, Riege WH, Hanson W, et al: Correlation of metabolic and language abnormalities in aphasia. *Ann Neurol.* 1981;10:102.

57. Heiss WD, Pawlik G, Wagner R, et al: Functional hypometabolism of noninfarcted brain regions in ischemia stroke. *J Cereb Blood Flow Metab.* 1983;3(1):S582.

58. Metter EJ, Waterlain CG, Kuhl DE, et al: ^{18}FDG positron emission computed tomography: A study of aphasia. *Ann Neurol.* 1981;10:173.

59. Baron JC, Bousser MG, Comar D, et al: "Crossed cerebellar diaschisis" in human supratentorial brain infarction. *Trans Am Neurol Assoc.* 1980;105:459.

60. Baron JC, Bousser MG, Comar D, et al: Crossed cerebellar diaschisis: A remote functional depression secondary to supratentorial infarction in man. *J Cereb Blood Flow Metab.* 1981;1(1):S500.

61. Baron JC, Rougemont D, Soussaline F, et al: Positron tomographic investigation in humans of the local coupling among CBF, oxygen consumption, and glucose utilization. *J Cereb Blood Flow Metab.* 1983;3(1):S242.

62. Martin WR, Raichle ME: Cerebellar metabolism and blood flow in supratentorial cerebral infarction. *J Cereb Blood Flow Metab.* 1983;3(1):S584.

63. Martin WR, Raichle ME: Cerebellar blood flow and metabolism in cerebral hemisphere infarction. *Ann Neurol.* 1983;14:168.

64. Kanaya H, Endo H, Sugiyama T, et al: Crossed cerebellar diaschisis in patients with putaminal hemorrhage. *J Cereb Blood Flow Metab.* 1983;3(1):S27.

65. Kushner M, Alavi A, Reivich M, et al: Contralateral cerebellar hypometabolism following cerebral insult: A positron emission tomographic study. *Ann Neurol.* 1984;15:425.

66. DiChiro G, DeLaPaz RL, Brooks RA, et al: Glucose utilization of cerebral gliomas measured by [^{18}F]fluorodeoxyglucose and positron emission tomography. *Neurology (NY).* 1982;32:1323.

67. Patronas NJ, DiChiro G, Smith BH, et al: Depressed cerebellar glucose metabolism in supratentorial tumors. *Brain Res.* 1984;291:93.

68. Baron JC, Rougemont D, Bousser MG, et al: Local CBF, oxygen extraction fraction (OEF), and CMRO$_2$: Prognostic value in recent supratentorial infarction in humans. *J Cereb Blood Flow Metab.* 1983;3(1):S1.

69. Grubb RL, Ratcheson R, Raichle M, et al: Regional cerebral blood flow and oxygen utilization in superficial temporal-middle cerebral artery anastomosis patients. *Acta Neurol Scand.* 1979;60(72):502.

70. Baron JC, Rey A, Guillard A, et al: Noninvasive tomographic imaging of cerebral blood flow and oxygen extraction in superficial temporal to middle cerebral artery anastomosis. In Meyer JS, Lechner H, Reivich M, eds. *Cerebral Vascular Disease 3.* Amsterdam: North-Holland Elsevier; 1980:58.

71. Baron JC, Rey A, Guillard A, et al: Non-invasive tomographic imaging of cerebral blood flow (CBF) and oxygen extraction fraction (OEF) in superficial temporal artery to middle cerebral artery (STA-MCA) anastomosis. *Excerpta Medica.* 1981;3:58.

72. Martin WR, Baker RP, Herscovitch P, et al: The selection of patients for extracranial-intracranial bypass surgery: Hemodynamic and metabolic criteria. *Neurology (NY).* 1982;32(2):A89.

73. Powers WJ, Martin WR, Herscovitch P, et al: Hemodynamic results of cerebral bypass surgery measured by positron emission tomography. *J Nucl Med.* 1983;24:P108.

74. Powers WJ, Martin WR, Herscovitch P, et al: Extracranial-intracranial bypass surgery: Hemodynamic and metabolic effects. *Neurology (NY).* 1984;34:1168.

75. Jarden JO, Dhawan V, Kearfott KJ, Rottenberg DA: Measurement of brain/tumor capillary permeability using ^{82}Rb and positron emission tomography. *Ann Neurol.* 1984;16:131.

76. Frost JJ, Dannals RF, Ravert HT, et al: Imaging opiate receptors with positron emission tomography. *J Nucl Med.* 1984;25:P73.

77. Garnett ES, Firnau G, Nahmias C: Dopamine visualized in the basal ganglia of living man. *Nature (Lond).* 1983;305:137.

78. Wagner HN, Burns HD, Dannals RF, et al: Imaging dopamine receptors in the human brain by positron tomography. *Science.* 1983;22:1264.

79. Mazziotta JC, Phelps ME: Human sensory stimulation and deprivation: PET results and strategies. *Ann Neurol.* 1984;15(1):S50.

80. Mazziotta JC, Phelps ME, Halgren E: Local cerebral glucose metabolic responses to audio-visual stimulation and deprivation: Studies in human subjects with positron CT. *Hum Neurobiol.* 1983;2:11.

81. Mazziotta JC, Phelps ME, Carson RE, et al: Tomographic mapping of human cerebral metabolism: Auditory stimulation. *Neurology (NY).* 1982;32:921.

CHAPTER 16

SPECT Scanning in Cerebrovascular Disease

ROY L. TAWES, JR., ROBERT J. LULL, and PAUL LIZOTTE

Single photon emission computed tomography (SPECT) scanning produces images of the brain that contain unique and clinically important information about cerebral function and blood flow that can significantly affect diagnosis and prognosis.[1-4] This is particularly true when SPECT scanning is used to measure regional cerebral blood flow (rCBF) and its response to standardized vasodilatory stress. When performed in conjunction with intravenous acetazolamide (Diamox), SPECT scanning provides unique and clinically important information about both regional cerebral flow reserve and collateral flow sufficiency in patients who are being considered for carotid endarterectomy.[5] This type of functional information can be used by the vascular surgeon for patient diagnosis, surgical planning, clinical management, and prognostic risk stratification.

As experience is gained with SPECT imaging of rCBF function and flow reserve, such studies become an increasingly important component of the modern management of patients with cerebrovascular disease. The ability to clearly define the location and size of vascular beds in the brain at risk for ischemia and infarction provides unique information that is useful in a variety of vascular surgical candidates. SPECT images of cerebrovascular function at the tissue level complement the anatomic information provided by ultrasonography, computed tomography (CT), magnetic resonance imaging (MRI), and angiography.[1, 3, 6] Sometimes, the functional information provided by SPECT scanning is of greater significance than the information from these other anatomic imaging modalities in the management of vascular surgical patients.

Brain perfusion SPECT studies appear to be following the same pattern that is clinically well established for myocardial perfusion SPECT in the heart. Under this paradigm, rCBF SPECT will likely assume significantly greater importance than other imaging modalities in case selection for carotid endarterectomy surgery, similar to the important role cardiac SPECT now plays in the surgical management of coronary artery disease.[7] Of the many parallels between coronary and carotid atherosclerotic disease as discovered by SPECT evaluation (Table 16–1), perhaps the most significant is the fact that flow reserve decreases in vascular beds supplied by a critically stenosed artery before the onset of frank ischemia or infarction. The basic process triggered by progressive luminal narrowing is reflex vasodilation of the involved vascular bed in response to decreased flow and local hypoxia. The resultant decreased pressure and resistance of the involved vascular bed encourage collateral flow. The capacity to maintain flow by this regional vasodilatory mechanism is the flow reserve of that region.[8-12] However, when maximum vasodilation has occurred, this mechanism can no longer increase flow in the regional vascular bed in response to further luminal narrowing. Such regions have exhausted their flow reserve and are at risk for ischemia or infarction. Many terms have been used to describe this pathophysiologic state but all are essentially equivalent (Table 16–2).

Regions with decreased vascular flow reserve can be detected with SPECT scanning techniques with the use of pharmacologic vasodilation stress (dipyridamole in the heart; acetazolamide in the brain).[13-15] Those regions with an abnormal vasodilation stress response are at increased risk for

TABLE 16–1. Cardiac and Brain SPECT Parallels

Parallel Feature	Heart	Brain
Images regional tissue blood flow	Yes	Yes
Blood flow and metabolism linked	Usually	Usually
Radiopharmaceutical localization		
Redistributing tracer pattern:	Thallium-201	I-123-IMP
Early uptake = blood flow		
Late uptake = tissue viability		
Fixed microsphere-like pattern:	Tc-99m-MIBI	Tc-99m-HMPAO
Uptake = blood flow		Tc-99m-ECD
No significant redistribution		
Exercise stress imaging	Treadmill stress studies	Activation studies using:
		Sensory stimulation
		Task performance
Pharmacologic stress imaging	Dipyridamole (Persantine)	Acetazolamide (Diamox)
	Adenosine (Adenocard)	CO_2 Inhalation
	Dobutamine	(No Equivalent Drug)
Complimentary PET imaging		
PET perfusion agent	N-13-Ammonia	0-15-H_2O
PET metabolism agent	F-18-FDG	F-18-FDG
Complimentary anatomic imaging		
Angiography	Artery anatomy; % occlusion	Artery anatomy; % occlusion
Ultrasonography	Valve lesion; contractility	Screen for carotid disease
Computed tomography	Small clinical role	Large clinical role
Magnetic resonance imaging	Small clinical role	Large clinical role

PET, positron emission tomography.

TABLE 16–2. Equivalent Terms in Common Use

Decreased cerebral vascular flow reserve
Decreased cerebral vascular capacitance
Decreased cerebral vasodilatory reserve
Decreased cerebral collateral flow
Brain-at-risk (for ischemia or stroke)
Ischemic brain

ischemia and infarction.[16] A SPECT pattern of regional brain ischemia may allow significant additional risk stratification beyond mere estimation of the degree of carotid luminal narrowing, just as an ischemic stress response in the heart predicts risk of adverse cardiac events independent of the degree of coronary stenosis.[37] In the future, complete assessment of an occluding carotid artery lesion will not only require a detailed description of carotid anatomy and flow but will often also require study of rCBF reserve at the tissue level, which is a measure of the hemodynamic consequences of the arterial stenosis and the adequacy of collateral flow to the region at risk.

IMAGING TECHNIQUE

SPECT is a widely available nuclear medicine imaging technique that utilizes standard gamma camera detectors mounted on rotating gantries to image the regional distribution of commonly used gamma emitting radiotracer drugs (radiopharmaceuticals) in the patient.[1, 17] As the gamma camera obtains views at multiple angles around the patient, the information is digitized and reconstructed by computer as a three-dimensional image representing the amount of radiotracer drug at each point within the organs being imaged. The images produced by SPECT systems may be displayed either as standard coronal, transverse, and sagittal plane slices or as volumetric displays of the entire reconstructed data set.[1, 3, 6]

Imaging by SPECT requires excellent gamma camera detector performance; stable gantry design; utilization of proper uniformity, linearity, and energy correction maps; continuous quality control; and attention to technical details.[1] Brain SPECT is often acquired using 64 views in a 360-degree circular orbit around the patient's head. Each image is acquired for 30 seconds and digitized to a 128 × 128 pixel matrix. Total scan time is 32 minutes. If a multidetector SPECT camera is used, the image detail can be improved by increasing the number of views to 128 with no increase in total acquisition time. The use of specialized collimators (eg, high-resolution fan beam) can significantly improve the resolution of the reconstructed image to nearly match the resolution achieved by positron emission tomography (PET) systems.[17] Computer processing uses a filtered back projection reconstruction technique with an appropriate level Butterworth filter and Chang attenuation correction. An external reference system can be employed to facilitate exact correlation between functional SPECT and anatomic CT or MRI images.[3]

Although quantitative measurement of absolute rCBF is possible with several SPECT techniques and radiopharmaceuticals, most clinical studies use semiquantitative analysis by comparing radiotracer activity in symmetrical anatomic regions, or by calculating the ratio of activity in a region to global brain activity, cerebellar activity, or a population dataset of normalized rCBF values.[6] SPECT color-coded digital image display systems provide reliable detection of small relative changes in rCBF in normalized comparison image study sets.[17]

The patient environment at the time of intravenous radiopharmaceutical injection should be controlled to minimize ambient stimulation.[3, 17] Intravenous access should be obtained at least 5 minutes before the injection, and the patient should remain in a dimly lit, quiet room for 5 to 10 minutes after the injection. This injection environment should be duplicated as much as possible for serial comparison studies in the same patient.

Compared with PET scanning, SPECT is available in virtually all hospitals, is less expensive, uses radiopharmaceuticals that are available at all times for emergency studies, and is capable of the gamma energy discrimination needed for simultaneous dual isotope imaging of baseline and stress results, providing exact anatomic comparison.[17, 18] On the negative side, SPECT does have less inherent image resolution, is less easily quantified for absolute measurements, and does not use any radiopharmaceutical that directly measures metabolism as PET does with the tracer F-18-flurodeoxyglucose (FDG). Fortunately, SPECT radiopharmaceuticals for measuring rCBF also provide adequate metabolic information for clinical needs, since flow and metabolism are coupled in the normal brain and in most diseases of the brain.[3, 4]

RADIOPHARMACEUTICALS

The many radiopharmaceuticals developed for brain imaging have recently been reviewed.[4, 19] Those commonly used for evaluation of rCBF are listed in Table 16–3. All of these agents are lipid-soluble and thus pass the blood-brain barrier and lipid cell membrane. Their distribution in the brain is proportionate to regional blood flow, which can be imaged with SPECT and measured either as semiquantitative uptake ratios or as absolute blood flow (mL/min) per 100 g of brain tissue.

Xenon-133 (Xe-133). This lipophilic inert radiotracer can be administered either as a gas by inhalation or as a saline solution by intra-arterial injection.[4, 10] Absolute measurement of rCBF can be made by analysis of the exponential rates of tissue clearance of Xe-133, which is proportional to blood flow and the blood-to-brain partition coefficient for Xe-133.[10] The Xe-133 technique has been validated with the use of a variety of probes and imaging systems in numerous laboratories around the world and has become the clinical gold standard for quantifying rCBF.[1] By these techniques, the average resting basal state cerebral blood flow is approximately 50 mL/min per 100 g of brain.[20, 21]

Iodine-123-Iodoamphetamine (I-123-IMP). Iodoamphetamine can be labeled with I-123 and used to image and quantify rCBF. I-123-IMP has a very high first-pass extraction rate (>92%) and is initially distributed in the brain in proportion to blood flow but gradually redistributes to viable brain cells in proportion to the number of their amphetamine receptors.[1, 4, 19] A significant reservoir of I-123-IMP in the

TABLE 16–3. SPECT Radiopharmaceuticals

Radiopharmaceutical	Energy, keV	Half-Life	Localization	Advantages	Disadvantages
Xe-133 Saline solution (artery injection) Gas (inhalation)	80	5.4 day	Lipid soluble Blood-brain partition coefficient Exponential washout	Gold standard for clinical quantitation of rCBF Repeat studies possible within short time (20–30 min)	Poor image quality Regulatory requirements Not at most hospitals Dedicated instruments
I-123-IMP (Iodoamphetamine) (Iofetamine) (Spectamine)	159	13 hr	Lipid soluble Binds amphetamine receptors 92% first pass extraction	Quantitation of rCBF possible Correlates with Xe-133 rCBF Best image contrast Delayed images show ischemia "fill-in" Allows simultaneous dual isotope studies	Expensive Not marketed in USA Changing brain activity Lung is activity reservoir Doses must be ordered daily from supplier
Tc-99m-HMPAO (Hexamethylpropylene amine oxime) (Exametazine) (Ceretec)	140	6 hr (Generator produced)	Lipid soluble d/l—HMPAO diffuses into brain cells Converted to insoluble form and binds in cells 15% early back diffusion Fixed marker of rCBF acts like microspheres	Readily available as kit 24 hours a day Stable (hours) kit now approved by FDA Allows delayed imaging of rCBF at time of injection May be used in dual isotope studies Excellent imaging	Original kit formulation must be used within 30 minutes of preparation Underestimates rCBF at high flow rates
Tc-99m-ECD (Ethylenediylbis-L-cysteine diethylester) (Bicisate) (Neurolite)	140	6 hr (Generator produced)	Lipid soluble ECD diffuses into brain cells 1,1-ECD is enzymatically converted to polar form and trapped in brain cells Fixed marker of rCBF acts like microspheres	Readily available as kit Allows delayed imaging of rCBF at time of injection May be used in dual isotope studies Excellent imaging Kit preparation is stable for hours after preparation Better image contrast than with Tc-99m-HMPAO	Underestimates rCBF at high flow rates Enzyme defect in hypoxic brain may limit cellular trapping and uncouple as a flow marker (eg, zone of "luxury perfusion" near a cerebral infarct)

lungs aids this redistribution process. This capacity to localize initially according to flow and subsequently redistribute to tissue based on viability rather than flow parallels the characteristic distribution of thallium-201 (Tl-201) in the myocardium (Plate 16–1). Indeed, it has been shown that early and 4-hour redistribution images of I-123-IMP can be used to distinguish ischemic but viable brain from infarcted brain,[4] just as Tl-201 does in the heart.

Iodine-123-hydroxymethyl iodobenzyl propane diamine (I-123-HIPDM) is another amine radiopharmaceutical that is very similar to I-123-IMP in uptake and distribution in the brain but was never made commercially available for routine clinical use. This tracer is essentially an equivalent to I-123-IMP for clinical brain rCBF SPECT imaging.[2, 4]

I-123-IMP has been used for absolute quantification of rCBF, and results correlate well with Xe-133 measurements.[4] However, since arterial blood sampling is required for such absolute quantification, most clinical studies have utilized semiquantitative ratios as a measure of rCBF. With modern imaging systems, the 159 keV photon from I-123 can be electronically distinguished from the 140 keV photon of Tc-99m, thus allowing simultaneous imaging of both radiotracers with exact anatomic slice alignment.[1]

The I-123 used to label IMP requires special cyclotron production to avoid contamination with I-124, which can interfere with image quality and increase radiation dose to the patient.[4] The need for daily preparation and distribution of this agent is expensive. Although I-123-IMP is currently not available in the United States, efforts to again make this agent available should soon be successful. A great deal of work is being done in Japan and Europe, where I-123-IMP continues to be available.[19, 22]

Technetium-99m-Hexamethyl-Propylene Amine Oxime (Tc-99m-HMPAO). This agent can be prepared by adding Tc-99m, which is readily available 24 hours a day from a Mo-Tc Generator, to a lyophilized kit containing HMPAO. The original kit formulation required use within 30 minutes of preparation because of a tendency to convert from the lipid-soluble D/L isomer to the lipid-insoluble meso form of HMPAO.[4] A more stable kit formulation has been developed that allows use hours after preparation and has recently received approval from the Food and Drug Administration (FDA) for commercial sale. The D/L form of Tc-99m-HMPAO rapidly diffuses into the brain cells in proportion to blood flow. Approximately 85 percent is converted to an insoluble form, which binds in the cells. The other 15 percent back-diffuses into the blood during the first few minutes, which accounts for some underestimation of rCBF at high flow rates, compared with Xe-133 or I-123-IMP.[4, 15] The irreversibly bound portion of the Tc-99m-HMPAO is distributed in the brain according to rCBF at the time of tracer injection in a manner analogous to the distribution of intra-arterial microspheres. Scanning can be delayed several hours and still provide an image of rCBF as it was at the time of intravenous radiopharmaceutical injection. Because a higher dose of Tc-99m can be used, image quality with this agent is generally superior to that obtained with either Xe-133 or I-123-IMP SPECT.[3]

Technetium-99m-Ethylenediylbis-L-Cysteine (Tc-99m-ECD).
This is a new radiopharmaceutical that was recently granted
FDA approval for brain rCBF imaging. Like HMPAO, lipid-
soluble Tc-99m-ECD is prepared from a kit and enters the
brain cell where the 1,1 enantiomer is enzymatically converted to a polar form, which is trapped in the cell.[4, 13] Brain
distribution of Tc-99m-ECD is proportionate to that of rCBF
at the time of injection and acts, via intracellular trapping,
as a fixed marker of rCBF that parallels quantitative Xe-133
results.[4, 19] Like Tc-99m-HMPAO, Tc-99m-ECD also tends
to underestimate rCBF at high flow rates. However, Tc-99m-
ECD tends to produce better image contrast than HMPAO
and has better stability, allowing injection up to 6 hours
after kit preparation.[4] Tc-99m-ECD has also shown a characteristic uncoupling of its brain uptake from rCBF in "luxury
perfusion" zones of evolving strokes.[4, 13, 18] This appears to
occur in regions where cellular hypoxia is sufficient to cause
enzyme dysfunction as well as increased flow from loss of
normal vascular tone. In these regions, Tc-99m-ECD activity
may be decreased in spite of increased perfusion. Unlike
HMPAO, which localizes in proportion to increased "luxury
perfusion" flow, Tc-99m-ECD may be a better indicator of
decreased cellular metabolism in regions where injury causes
metabolism and flow to become uncoupled.[18]

Although each of these radiopharmaceuticals has both
advantages and disadvantages, all have been used successfully in a clinical setting. However, for all practical purposes,
Tc-99m–labeled HMPAO and ECD are the agents of choice
for most clinical circumstances when absolute quantification
of rCBF is not required. When simultaneous dual isotope
SPECT is needed, I-123–labeled IMP (when again available
in the United States) can be used in conjunction with one of
the Tc-99m agents. Although Xe-133 distribution and washout can be imaged and successfully quantified using slightly
modified multidetector SPECT equipment, the image resolution is poor because of the low energy photons. Also, restrictive regulatory requirements for using Xe-133 gas discourage
routine clinical use.

RECENT ADVANCES

During the past few years, there have been significant
improvements in both the imaging instruments and techniques used for SPECT studies of the brain. The development of multidetector SPECT cameras with two to four
detector heads, combined with the use of focusing collimators that have been specially designed for high-resolution
brain SPECT imaging, represents a significant advance.[1, 17]
Multidetector cameras reduce the time required for imaging
and have advanced electronics that provide the superior
image resolution and the energy separation capability needed
for simultaneous dual energy isotope imaging with both
Tc-99m and I-123. The inherent stability of the typical
multidetector camera gantry simplifies required quality control procedures and allows rapid detector rotation.[5] Rapid
detector rotation with continuous acquisition allows complete sampling of all imaging angles every 15 seconds,
with each 15 second acquisition segment being added to a
cumulative study if there has been no patient motion (Fig.
16–1). Segments with patient motion can be discarded. This
type of rapid sequential imaging technique greatly enhances
the ability to obtain meaningful SPECT images in patients

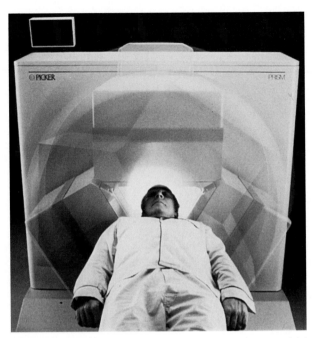

FIGURE 16–1. Multidetector SPECT camera allows rapid sequential imaging to study neurologically impaired patients who are unable to cooperate.
Systems such as this triple head camera (PRISM 3000) provide image
quality that nearly matches that of PET scans and yet have the advantage
of multiple energy windows for simultaneous dual energy tracer studies.
(Courtesy of Picker International.)

with neurologic disorders who are uncooperative but should
not be sedated.[1, 2]

Some SPECT multidetector systems provide capability for
true attenuation correction, which may enhance the calculation of absolute rCBF values using either of the Tc-99m–
labeled agents. The ability to correct for attenuation and
obtain absolute measurement of rCBF together with excellent image resolution was previously available only with
PET imaging. However, the modern multidetector SPECT
camera can now rival PET capability both in image quality
and in obtaining quantitative measurement of rCBF. Compared with PET, SPECT is widely available in most hospitals, less expensive, and allows simultaneous imaging and
exact registration of both stress and baseline studies by using
dual isotope energy discrimination. Although PET has the
ability to directly measure regional cerebral metabolism of
glucose as well as rCBF, SPECT provides similar results,
since metabolism and blood flow remain coupled in the
majority of diseases affecting the brain as well as in normal
brain.[3] Even the new specific neuroreceptor PET radiopharmaceuticals are being duplicated by analogous agents designed for SPECT imaging.[4] Discoveries made in PET research and clinical facilities usually lead to the development
of new SPECT-compatible radiopharmaceuticals that accomplish the same task in a routine clinical setting.[4, 19] Thus,
clinical SPECT imaging of the brain will continue to grow
in its capacity to provide important and unique information
about regional cerebral function.

ACETAZOLAMIDE STRESS STUDIES

Regional changes in blood flow normally occur in the
brain because of increased or decreased neuronal activity.

Both PET and SPECT have been used to demonstrate cortical regions of increased metabolism and perfusion in response to specific mental tasks or other activation stimuli.[11, 17] Perfusion may be increased independent of neuronal metabolism and activity by pharmacologic intervention. In cerebrovascular disease, regions of brain at greatest risk for ischemia or infarction are those that have already lost vascular flow reserves and are thus incapable of responding to pharmacologic vasodilatory challenge. The vascular beds in these regions are maximally dilated and cannot respond to the stimulus of the potent cerebral pharmacologic vasodilator acetazolamide (Diamox).[3, 9, 17] Uncompromized cerebral vascular beds remain capable of a normal vasodilatory response to standard acetazolamide stress. SPECT studies injected during both basal flow state and at the time of maximum vasodilation response to acetazolamide are ideal for demonstrating regions of the brain that fail to show a normal increase in rCBF because of diminished flow reserve.[5, 8, 9, 15, 22] The presence, location, and size of such abnormalities provide important information about collateral flow and the functional impact at the tissue level of complex multivessel atherosclerotic occluding lesions.[3, 6, 16] Acetazolamide stress SPECT provides unique information about tissue perfusion that is not available from MRI, CT, or Doppler ultrasonography. The typical findings of abnormal cerebral flow reserve are demonstrated in Figure 16–2 and Plate 16–2. However, depending on the baseline flow status and underlying pathophysiology, a number of different patterns can be seen. The common clinical patterns seen on acetazolamide stress studies are summarized in Table 16–4.

Although carbon dioxide can be given directly by inhala-

TABLE 16–4. Acetazolamide Stress SPECT Patterns

Baseline rCBF	Acetazolamide rCBF	Interpretation
Normal	Normal	No evidence for vascular flow abnormality, indicates adequate collateral flow.
Normal	Decreased	Decreased flow reserve suggests actual or potential ischemia and increased risk for transient ischemic attack and stroke.
Decreased	Defect size unchanged	Decreased flow and flow reserve indicates fixed cerebral necrosis with no surrounding ischemic brain at risk for extension of infarct zone.
Decreased	Defect size larger	Fixed cerebral infarct surrounded by ischemic brain at risk for extension of the infarct zone.
Decreased	Normal or improves	Decreased flow but normal flow reserve seen in regions of cortical denervation from remote stroke and dementia of the Alzheimer's type.
Increased	No change	Loss of vascular responsiveness with maximal vasodilation in stroke zone of "luxury perfusion."

tion as a vasodilatory stimulus, this is impractical in a busy clinical setting. Acetazolamide is now the standard agent used for producing vasodilation of the cerebral vascular bed without increasing metabolism or neural activity.[5, 8, 9, 11, 14, 17] Acetazolamide acts as a potent cerebrovascular dilator by increasing carbon dioxide levels in the brain via inhibition of carbonic anhydrase in circulating red blood cells. The standard procedure utilizes 1 g of acetazolamide intravenously. The maximum degree of vasodilation is usually achieved within 20 to 30 minutes after injection. SPECT radiopharmaceuticals should be administered at the time of peak vasodilation when assessing rCBF response to acetazolamide stress. The side effects of mild parathesias and lightheadedness are common but spontaneously disappear without treatment and are usually well tolerated by patients.[9, 23] Table 16–5 summarizes the most common clinical uses for acetazolamide stress SPECT scanning.

Ideally, the acetazolamide stress study should be per-

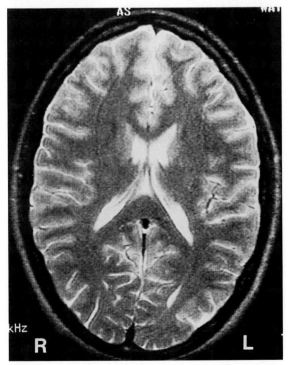

FIGURE 16–2. The normal MRI scan of a 58-year-old man with transient ischemic attacks. See Plate 16–2 for SPECT scans of this patient. (From Montz JM, Deutsch G, Kahn SH: Regional cerebral blood flow changes in stroke imaged by Tc-99m HMPAO SPECT with corresponding anatomic image comparison. *Clin Nucl Med.* 1993;18:1079.)

TABLE 16–5. Clinical Uses of Acetazolamide Stress SPECT

Identify vascular beds with decreased vascular flow reserve, indicating increased risk for ischemia or infarct.

Enhance sensitivity for small infarcts by visualizing surrounding areas of diminished vascular reserve.

Distinguish ischemia (decreased flow with acetazolamide) from denervation (increased flow with acetazolamide) as cause of low rCBF surrounding stroke necrosis zone on baseline SPECT study.

Assess functional reserve flow from collateral routes prior to carotid endarterectomy, permanent balloon occlusion, or surgical ligation.

Distinguish multi-infarct dementia (rCBF defects stay decreased with acetazolamide) from Alzheimer's disease (rCBF defects increase flow with acetazolamide).

formed as soon as possible after the baseline study. Two methods are used to avoid interference from the activity of the baseline study. One technique uses a low dose of Tc-99m-HMPAO (5 mCi) for the baseline SPECT study and a high dose (20 mCi) injected at peak Diamox vasodilation effect for the stress SPECT study.[6, 12] The other technique uses Tc-99m-HMPAO injected at baseline rest conditions and I-123-IMP injected at peak acetazolamide stress.[17] Dual energy image acquisition produces both baseline and stress study images simultaneously and with exact spatial registration. An example of the elegant results from a triple-head detector capable of dual energy SPECT is seen in Plate 16–3, which shows a large peri-infarct region of decreased cerebrovascular flow reserve.

CLINICAL APPLICATIONS

Brain SPECT imaging has many proven clinical applications that are unrelated to cerebrovascular disease.[1–3, 17] For example, epilepsy seizure foci can be demonstrated as zones of increased rCBF when radiopharmaceutical injection is made during or shortly after ictus.[2, 4, 24] Studies of rCBF, when the radiopharmaceutical is injected interictally, show decreased rCBF at the site of the seizure locus. Characteristic patterns of altered rCBF have also been described in SPECT studies of dementia, cocaine abuse, and acquired immunodeficiency syndrome (AIDS) encephalopathy.[2, 4, 17] SPECT utilizing other radiopharmaceuticals has proved useful in distinguishing tumor from infection and in distinguishing recurrent brain tumor from radiation necrosis.[4, 17] SPECT imaging research with radiolabeled neuroreceptor agents shows great promise in the diagnosis and management of common psychiatric disorders such as depression, schizophrenia, and panic attacks.[2, 4, 17] However, in keeping with the focus of this text, we will elaborate only on those clinical applications of potential interest to the cerebrovascular surgeon in which rCBF plays a significant diagnostic or prognostic role.

Early Stroke. Defects in rCBF occur immediately after a nonhemorrhagic stroke and are best visualized by SPECT cerebral perfusion imaging during the first hours after the event. CT and MRI imaging, which visualize anatomic changes occurring hours to days later, are less sensitive than SPECT for demonstrating the location and size of the cortical defect in the immediate post-stroke period.[2, 6] This very early diagnostic information will be of greater clinical importance in the era of more aggressive stroke therapeutic strategies utilizing vascular surgery, percutaneous catheter angioplasty, and thrombolysis in the acute setting in attempts to salvage viable but ischemic brain tissue.[3, 25]

Subacute and Chronic Stroke. Patients with mild nonhemorrhagic stroke may benefit from the prognostic information provided by SPECT analysis of rCBF flow reserve. Patients with significant atherosclerotic carotid artery narrowing and evidence of decreased flow reserve have significantly increased risk for subsequent stroke compared with those with similar carotid narrowing but without demonstrable regions of compromised flow reserve.[3, 6, 16] Comparison of the volume of brain affected by SPECT flow abnormality to the volume showing anatomic change on CT or MRI can provide helpful prognostic information about the probability of significant functional recovery following a stroke.[3] SPECT can

demonstrate zones of diaschisis caused by loss of input stimulus from the stroke, which are marked by neuronal hypoactivity and decreased rCBF.[26] These zones show normal or increased vascular reactivity to acetazolamide stress.[3, 15] Such information might be useful for planning recovery therapy appropriate for an individual's potential as well as for alleviating uncertainty about potential for recovery. Typical examples of acetazolamide SPECT studies can be seen in a patient showing a fixed infarct with no surrounding abnormality (Fig. 16–3 and Plate 16–4) and in a patient with surrounding viable, perfused, and potentially recoverable brain tissue that is just denervated (Fig. 16–4 and Plate 16–5). These patients' response to acetazolamide is in sharp contrast to the findings in patients with decreased vascular flow reserve (see Fig. 16–2 and Plate 16–2) and increased risk for stroke extension during future hemodynamic events.

Diagnostic Evaluation. Recent efforts have focused on preventing strokes by more aggressive diagnostic evaluation and therapy in patients presenting with symptoms that suggest transient episodes of cerebral ischemia.[25] After eliminating nonvascular causes, the initial focus of the diagnostic evaluation is properly on identifying possible sources of emboli or locating critically stenotic atherosclerotic lesions in major cerebral arteries, depending on the clinical findings. However, the anatomy of a carotid artery stenosis, as measured by the degree of stenosis as seen on arteriogram or duplex Doppler ultrasonogram, does not always correlate with the hemodynamic significance of the lesion.[22] Vasodilation, autoregulatory mechanisms, and collateral circulation

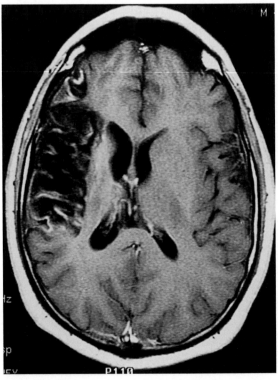

FIGURE 16–3. MRI scan of a patient who suffered a right middle cerebral artery stroke. See Plate 16–4 for SPECT scans of the same patient. (From Montz JM, Deutsch G, Kahn SH: Regional cerebral blood flow changes in stroke imaged by Tc-99m HMPAO SPECT with corresponding anatomic image comparison. *Clin Nucl Med.* 1993;18:1079.)

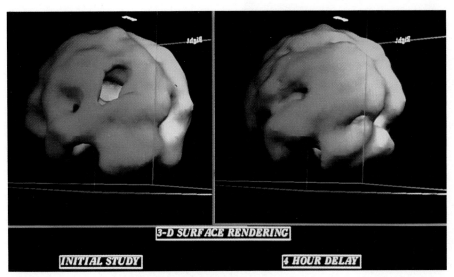

Plate 16–1. Early and 4-hour delayed three-dimensional surface-rendered display of I-123-IMP in a patient with transient ischemic attacks. The rCBF lesion on the early study "fills-in" on the delayed redistribution image—a typical ischemia pattern. (Courtesy of Michael Devous, PhD.)

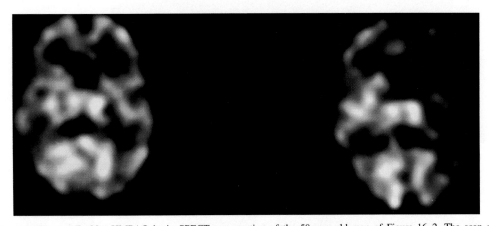

Plate 16–2. Low-dose pre-Diamox Tc-99m-HMPAO brain SPECT scan section of the 58-year-old man of Figure 16–2. The scan shows no significant defects in perfusion *(left)*. With Diamox stress, the repeat high-dose Tc-99m-HMPAO brain SPECT scan *(right)* demonstrates a large region of decreased rCBF to the left frontal, temporal, and parietal lobes. This indicates a loss of vascular flow reserve in the distribution of the left internal carotid artery. (From Mountz JM, Deutsch G, Kahn SH: Regional cerebral blood flow changes in stroke imaged by Tc-99m HMPAO SPECT with corresponding anatomic image comparison. *Clin Nucl Med.* 1993; 18:1079.)

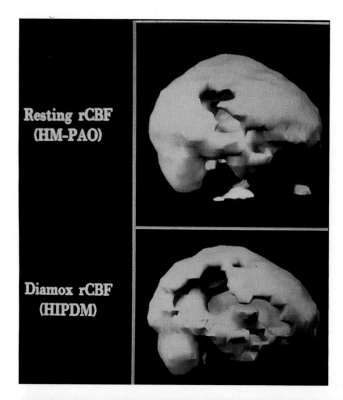

Resting rCBF (HM-PAO)

Diamox rCBF (HIPDM)

Plate 16–3. Three-dimensional surface-rendered images of dual isotope SPECT studies in a stroke patient showing a right frontoparietal rCBF defect that enlarges during Diamox vasodilatation. The enlarged zone represents peri-infarct regions of decreased vasodilatory reserve which is at increased risk for infarction. The resting baseline study used Tc-99m-HMPAO, which remains fixed and does not change in response to subsequent Diamox stress. The stress study used I-123-HIPDM (an amine similar to IMP), which was injected 20 minutes after the Diamox stress test (1 gr IV). Both image studies were acquired simultaneously immediately after administration of I-123-HIPDM, allowing exact anatomic registration for optimal comparison. (From Holman BL, Devous MD Sr: Functional brain SPECT: The emergence of a powerful clinical method. *J Nucl Med.* 1992; 33:1893.)

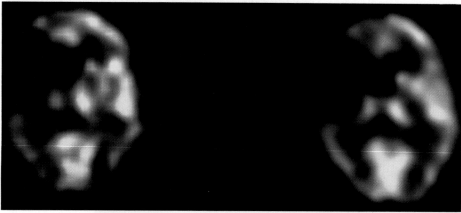

Plate 16–4. Baseline and Diamox stress SPECT scans of the patient shown in Figure 16–3 show similar defects nearly equal in volume to the infarct zone. There are no areas of decreased flow reserve signifying ischemia. (From Mountz JM, Deutsch G, Kahn SH: Regional cerebral blood flow changes in stroke imaged by Tc-99m HMPAO SPECT with corresponding anatomic image comparison. *Clin Nucl Med.* 1993; 18:1075.)

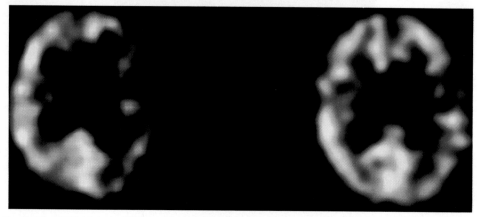

Plate 16–5. The baseline Tc-99m-HMPAO brain SPECT scan *(left)* of the patient shown in Figure 16–4 demonstrates a relatively large area of hypoperfusion involving the territory of the left middle cerebral artery. The Diamox stress Tc-99m-HMPAO brain SPECT scan *(right)* shows a reduction in the size of the perfusion defect, which more nearly equals the defect size observed on MRI (see Fig. 16–4). Normal flow reserve in the large peri-infarct abnormality seen on the baseline SPECT study indicates that the flow decrease was caused by denervation (cortical diaschisis) rather than vascular compromise, which could pose increased risk. This patient showed above-average functional recovery during physical therapy. (From Mountz JM, Deutsch G, Kahn SH: Regional cerebral blood flow changes in stroke imaged by Tc-99m HMPAO SPECT with corresponding anatomic image comparison. *Clin Nucl Med.* 1993; 18:1080.)

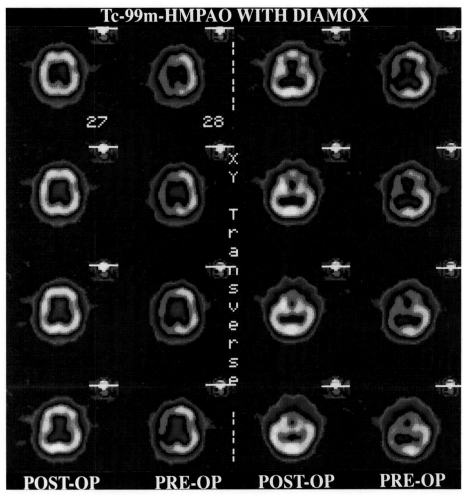

Plate 16–6. Comparison of preoperative and postoperative Tc-99m-HMPAO Diamox stress rCBF images in a patient with TIAs who underwent carotid endarterectomy. Complete normalization of the significant right hemisphere abnormality can be seen, which signified decreased vascular flow reserve on the preoperative study. At surgery, reduced mean stump pressure of 36 mm was measured, and an internal carotid bypass shunt was inserted before the endarterectomy. The normal postoperative study demonstrates that endarterectomy has re-established adequate flow to restore normal vascular capacitance. (Courtesy of Dr. Herb Alexander.)

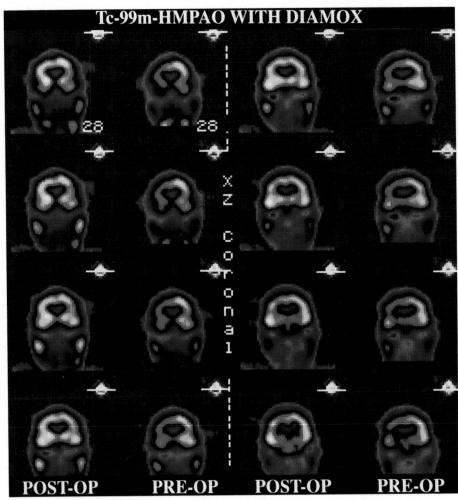

Plate 16–6. *Continued.*

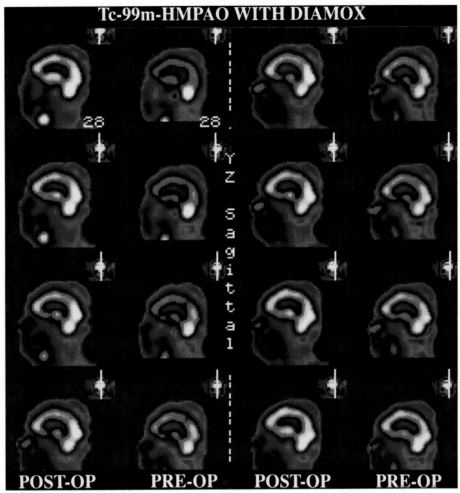

Plate 16–6. *Continued.*

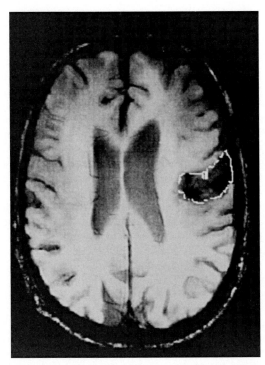

FIGURE 16-4. The MRI scan of a 77-year-old white male taken 1 month after a cerebrovascular accident causing aphasia and marked right-sided sensory and motor defects. The scan demonstrates low signal intensity in the left temporal and parietal lobes, which represents the cerebral infarction. See Plate 16–5 for SPECT scans of the same patient. (From Montz JM, Deutsch G, Kahn SH: Regional cerebral blood flow changes in stroke imaged by Tc-99m HMPAO SPECT with corresponding anatomic image comparison. *Clin Nucl Med.* 1993;18:1080.)

all play important roles. Therefore, physiologic data regarding rCBF can be beneficial in case selection for carotid endarterectomy, as well as for assessing potential stroke risk and results of the surgical procedure.[3, 16, 17, 20]

When significant atherosclerotic lesions are present in the carotid arteries, SPECT images can be used to define the cortical location affected and to assess the impact of anatomic carotid artery stenosis on rCBF and metabolic function at the tissue level.[3, 12] SPECT evaluation is particularly important when the TIA symptoms suggest a hemodynamic cause.[12] Even when there is no detectable flow abnormality in the baseline SPECT study, a repeat study with acetazolamide stress may unmask regions of diminished flow reserve that may be at increased risk for subsequent ischemia or infarction (see Fig. 16–2 and Plate 16–2). Thus, a combination of anatomic imaging of the stenotic carotid arteries and functional imaging of rCBF and flow reserve in the affected vascular beds is ideally needed to fully define the status and risk of a TIA patient's atherosclerotic cerebrovascular disease prior to therapeutic interventions such as carotid endarterectomy.

Carotid Endarterectomy. SPECT images of rCBF can be useful not only for selection of patients most likely to benefit from carotid endarterectomy but also to identify those patients who may need special surgical bypass precautions because of demonstrated lack of collateral flow reserve on acetazolamide stress SPECT study.[5, 23] The presence of decreased flow reserve in the distribution of a significantly

occluded carotid artery has been reported to predict low stump pressures at surgery.[5]

In our own series (submitted for publication) of 74 sequential patients undergoing carotid endarterectomy for significant TIA symptoms, all 48 patients with decreased rCBF on preoperative acetazolamide stress SPECT images demonstrated abnormal low stump pressures below 50 mm mean pressure (mean value was 26 mm with a range of 9 to 37 mm mean pressure). Each of these patients had an intraluminal carotid shunt placed during surgery to assure adequate cerebral flow during endarterectomy. An additional six patients with a history of stroke also had abnormal preoperative acetazolamide stress SPECT results and were electively shunted. All 20 patients with a normal preoperative acetazolamide stress SPECT study had stump pressures above 50 mm mean pressure, and therefore shunts were not used during endarterectomy. These 20 patients had uneventful surgery and recovery.

Our experience with preoperative SPECT studies during acetazolamide stress demonstrated 100 percent overall accuracy for predicting which patients had inadequate collateral flow as measured by abnormally decreased carotid stump pressures.[27] This is a significantly better result than the experience reported by Vorstrup and coworkers[5] using a technique of Xe-133 by inhalation. Postoperative acetazolamide stress SPECT studies on the 48 patients with no history of prior stroke in whom shunts were used demonstrated improved rCBF to the hypoperfused (ischemic) area that was seen preoperatively. A typical example of the scan results in one of these patients is shown in Plate 16–6. The study shows complete restoration of cerebrovascular capacitance. These studies were done in a community hospital setting with a standard single-head detector and no special equipment. Although not elegant, the studies provided very useful information. Thus SPECT imaging was able to confirm that functional reserve and vascular reactivity were restored to normal in these patients following successful carotid endarterectomy.

In our experience, acetazolamide stress SPECT results were far more helpful than CT brain scans in the preoperative and postoperative evaluation of patients with TIA symptoms and significant carotid artery stenosis amenable to carotid endarterectomy. Both SPECT and CT were performed before and after surgery on the first 30 patients in our series. CT was normal in all but two patients with prior strokes. Acetazolamide stress SPECT studies were abnormal in 20 of the 28 patients without prior stroke and became normal on the postoperative study in all 20 of these patients following successful carotid endarterectomy. Since CT brain studies added no additional useful information to the functional SPECT imaging results, CT scans were no longer performed after the first 30 patients, being replaced by SPECT scans in the preoperative evaluation of our TIA patients with significant carotid lesions. Patients with normal preoperative acetazolamide stress SPECT results may be experiencing symptoms as a result of emboli rather than as a result of a hemodynamic ischemia.

Extracranial-Intracranial (EC-IC) Bypass. The same principles discussed above concerning the use of SPECT rCBF studies in evaluating patients for carotid endarterectomy can also be applied to case selection for EC-IC bypass surgery.[23, 27] Again, acetazolamide stress SPECT studies supplement anatomic definition of an arterial lesion by revealing the hemodynamic significance of the lesion on rCBF and functional reserve in the vascular bed it supplies. SPECT brain scans have not been systematically used in this surgical population.[23, 28] Perhaps increased use of such functional information in the future will provide improved risk assessment and better case selection for optimal surgical outcomes from this procedure.

Predicting Carotid Artery Ligation Risk. Patients with a variety of lesions (congenital and acquired; vascular, traumatic, or neoplastic) require permanent occlusion or ligation of the ipsilateral internal carotid artery for adequate therapy. Temporary balloon occlusion of the carotid artery is usually performed as a test of collateral flow adequacy through the circle of Willis and to define the type and extent of neurologic deficit, if any, that may follow the planned permanent occlusion.[29, 30] The temporary occlusion is usually continued for 15 to 45 minutes but is stopped if the patient develops any change in neurologic status. If there has been no change in neurologic status following temporary balloon occlusion, the patient is presumed to have adequate collateral circulation to tolerate permanent occlusion. Unfortunately, between 10 and 20 percent of patients who remain asymptomatic during temporary occlusion develop severe permanent neurologic defects within hours to several days following permanent occlusion.[29] Thus, clinical evaluation alone during temporary balloon occlusion is inadequate for predicting the neurologic outcome following permanent sacrifice of the internal carotid artery.

Several published series point out the value of SPECT rCBF studies in evaluating these patients.[31–35] Either Tc-99m-HMPAO or Tc-99m-ECD can be administered intravenously during the temporary balloon occlusion test and imaged with SPECT 1 to 2 hours later, after all catheters have been removed. It is important to wait at least 20 minutes after the onset of balloon occlusion before radiotracer injection to allow time for collateral flow to become fully established. The occlusion should be maintained for at least 5 to 10 minutes after the injection while radiopharmaceutical localization occurs. The results of the balloon occlusion SPECT study are compared with a baseline SPECT study. When decreased flow is seen in patients with no overt symptoms during trial occlusion, it indicates inadequate collateral flow and increased risk for critical reduction in rCBF after permanent occlusion of the internal carotid artery.[32–34] These patients should be considered at increased risk for delayed cerebral ischemia or infarction and should be re-evaluated for alternate surgical or interventional treatments that spare the internal carotid. Some authors consider a SPECT abnormality developing during balloon occlusion to be an indication for performing an EC-IC bypass to establish better collateral flow before permanent carotid occlusion occurs.[33] Others have emphasized the need for using standardized quantitative indices for optimum evaluation of these patients.[30, 35] Although not yet reported, the simultaneous use of both acetazolamide stress and temporary balloon occlusion at the time of Tc-99m-HMPAO injection might further enhance the sensitivity of SPECT for detecting compromised collateral flow in the ipsilateral hemisphere.

Vasospasm After Subarachnoid Hemorrhage. Cerebral vasospasm is the chief cause of morbidity and mortality in patients surviving an initial subarachnoid hemorrhage.[36] This complication occurs in 25 to 40 percent of such patients.[37, 38] Brain perfusion SPECT is valuable for evaluating delayed cerebral ischemia caused by vasospasm after subarachnoid hemorrhage.[37, 38] Lewis and colleagues[36] describe a series of 40 patients studied with both transcranial Doppler ultrasonography and SPECT perfusion studies. SPECT results in this series proved more reliable in predicting clinically significant spasm and outcome than did transcranial Doppler. SPECT was able to identify critical perfusion reduction from vasospasm before the onset of clinical abnormalities, thus allowing early treatment.[38] SPECT may also be used to monitor for improved perfusion after therapeutic intervention to reverse the vasospasm.[38]

Multi-Infarct Dementia versus Alzheimer's Disease. SPECT cerebral perfusion studies show characteristic patterns that help to distinguish patients with dementia from multiple infarcts caused by cerebrovascular disease from those with dementia from deteriorated neuronal function but without vascular abnormality, such as in Alzheimer's and Pick's diseases.[2, 3, 17] Again, acetazolamide stress SPECT studies may assist in this distinction. Although Alzheimer's patients may have low baseline rCBF compared with age-matched norms, this is presumably a consequence of decreased neuronal activity, which lowers metabolic demands and reduces blood flow. Unless incidental vascular disease is present, patients with Alzheimer's dementia have normal vascular reactivity and flow reserve demonstrated as increased activity on acetazolamide SPECT images.[3] On the other hand, the multi-infarct dementia patient also has decreased rCBF on baseline study but should show regions of abnormal decreased activity in response to acetazolamide because vascular reactivity and flow reserve have been compromised by the underlying severe cerebrovascular disease.[3]

FUTURE ROLE OF SPECT SCANNING

SPECT scanning provides physiologic information about rCBF and better defines the hemodynamic significance of an anatomic lesion of the carotid artery. Acetazolamide stress SPECT studies further define the collateral supply and flow reserve of the affected vascular bed. SPECT scanning is currently markedly underutilized in terms of its potential for adding a significant new clinical dimension to the evaluation of patients for carotid endarterectomy or other cerebrovascular procedures. However, the many parallels between brain and cardiac SPECT predict the likelihood that brain SPECT will follow the same paradigm as cardiac SPECT in providing unique functional information, leading to improved risk stratification and better patient management. Modern multi-detector SPECT instruments, improved imaging techniques, and new radiopharmaceuticals continue to increase the clinical reliability and utility of SPECT.

SPECT scanning is very well tolerated by patients and can be performed on an outpatient basis. The small tracer quantity of radiopharmaceutical administered intravenously has no side effects and gives only a small radiation dose. SPECT images of rCBF are easier to obtain than xenon (nonradioactive) CT studies, are better tolerated by patients, and demonstrate better image detail resolution. Also, the higher doses of xenon required for CT visualization cause significant nonlinear increases in rCBF,[39] whereas the trace quantities of radiopharmaceuticals used for SPECT scanning do not alter the physiologic parameter (rCBF) being measured.

As the clinical utilization of carotid endarterectomy increases in response to favorable outcome studies, SPECT scanning will be used more frequently by cerebrovascular surgeons for case selection and as an important functional adjunct to the detailed anatomic evaluation of the occluding arterial lesion. In many patients with TIA symptoms due to vascular disease, SPECT will displace brain CT, which is usually normal in those without a prior stroke history and provides no information about vascular reserve or collateral flow sufficiency.

REFERENCES

1. Devous MD Sr: Instrumentation, radiopharmaceuticals, and technical factors. In VanHeertum RL, Tikofsky RS, eds. *Cerebral SPECT Imaging,* 2nd Ed. New York: Raven Press; 1995;3.
2. Holman BL, Devous MD Sr: Functional brain SPECT: The emergence of a powerful clinical method. *J Nucl Med.* 1992;33:1888.
3. Mountz JM, Deutsch G, Kuzniecky R, et al: Brain SPECT: 1994 update. In Freeman LM, ed. *Nuclear Medicine Annual 1994.* New York: Raven Press; 1994;1.
4. Saha GB, MacIntyre WJ, Go RT: Radiopharmaceuticals for brain imaging. *Semin Nucl Med.* 1994;24:324.
5. Vorstrup S, Boysen G, Brun B, et al: Evaluation of the regional cerebral vasodilatory capacity before carotid endarterectomy by the acetazolamide test. *Neuro Res.* 1987;9:10.
6. Mountz JM, Deutsch G, Khan SH: Regional cerebral blood flow changes in stroke imaged by Tc-99m HMPAO SPECT with corresponding anatomic image comparison. *Clin Nucl Med.* 1993;18:1067.
7. Machac J, Vallabhajosula S: Cerebral versus myocardial stress perfusion imaging: Role of pharmacological intervention in the diagnostic assessment of flow reserve. *J Nucl Med.* 1994;35:41. Editorial.
8. Oku N, Matsumoto M, Hashikawa K, et al: Carbon dioxide reactivity by consecutive Technetium-99m-HMPAO SPECT in patients with a chronically obstructed major cerebral artery. *J Nucl Med.* 1994;35:32.
9. Sullivan HG, Kingsbury TB IV, Morgan ME, et al: The rCBF response to Diamox in normal and cerebrovascular disease patients. *J Neurosurg.* 1987;67:525.
10. Madsen PL, Holm S, Herning M, et al: Average blood flow and oxygen uptake in the human brain during resting wakefulness: A critical appraisal of the Kety-Schmidt technique. *J Cereb Blood Flow Metab.* 1993;13:646.
11. Tikofsky RS, Hellman RS: Brain single photon emission computed tomography: Newer activation and intervention studies. *Semin Nucl Med.* 1991;21:40.
12. Levine RL, Lagreze HL, Dobkin JA, et al: Cerebral vasocapacitance and TIAs. *Neurology.* 1989;39:25.
13. Nakagawara J, Nakamura J-i, Takeda R, et al: Assessment of postischemic reperfusion and Diamox activation test in stroke using ^{99m}Tc-ECD SPECT. *J Cereb Blood Flow Metab.* 1994;14:S49.
14. Burt RW, Witt RM, Cikrit D, et al: Increased brain retention of Tc-99m HMPAO following acetazolamide administration. *Clin Nucl Med.* 1991;16:568.
15. Matsuda H, Higashi S, Kinuya K, et al: SPECT evaluation of brain perfusion reserve by the acetazolamide test using Tc-99m HMPAO. *Clin Nucl Med.* 1991;16:572.
16. Yonas H, Smith HA, Durham SR, et al: Increased stroke risk predicted by compromised cerebral blood flow reactivity. *J Neurosurg.* 1993;79:483.
17. Devous MD Sr: SPECT functional brain imaging. In Kramer EL, Sanger JJ, eds. *Clinical SPECT Imaging.* New York: Raven Press; 1995;97.
18. Tsuchida T, Nishizawa S, Yonekura Y, et al: SPECT images of Technetium-99m-Ethyl Cysteinate Dimer in cerebrovascular diseases: Comparison with other cerebral perfusion tracers and PET. *J Nucl Med.* 1994;35:27.
19. Walovitch RC, Miletich RS: Radiopharmaceuticals for SPECT brain imaging of perfusion and receptors. In Kramer EL, Sanger JJ, eds. *Clinical SPECT Imaging.* New York: Raven Press; 1995;129.
20. Lassen NA: Normal average value of cerebral blood flow in younger adults is 50 mL/100 g/min. *J Cereb Blood Flow Metab.* 1985;5:347.
21. Lammertsma AA: Noninvasive estimation of cerebral blood flow. *J Nucl Med.* 1994;35:1878.
22. Hoshi H, Ohnishi T, Jinnouchi S, et al: Cerebral blood flow in patients with Moyamoya disease evaluated by IMP SPECT. *J Nucl Med.* 1994;35:44.
23. Vorstrup S, Brun B, Lassen NA: Evaluation of the cerebral vasodilatory capacity by the acetazolamide test before EC-IC bypass surgery in patients with occlusion of the internal carotid artery. *Stroke.* 1986;17:1291.
24. Jeffery PJ, Monsein LH, Szabo Z, et al: Mapping the distribution of amobarbital sodium in the intracarotid Wada test by use of Tc-99m HMPAO with SPECT. *Radiology.* 1991;178:847.
25. Moore WS: Carotid endarterectomy for prevention of stroke. *West J Med.* 1993;159:37.
26. Feeney DM, Baron J-C: Diaschisis. *Stroke.* 1986;17:817.
27. Vostrup S, Lassen NA, Henriksen L, et al: CBF before and after extracranial-intracranial bypass surgery in patients with ischaemic cerebrovascular disease studied with Xenon-133 inhalation tomography. *Stroke.* 1985;16:616.
28. The EC-IC Bypass Study Group: Failure of extracranial-intracranial arterial bypass to reduce the risk of ischemic stroke. *N Engl J Med.* 1985;313:1191.
29. Eskridge JM: The challenge of carotid occlusion. *AJNR Am J Neuroradiol.* 1991;12:1053.
30. Askienazy S, Lebtahi R, Meder J-F: SPECT HMPAO and balloon test occlusion: Interest in predicting tolerance prior to permanent cerebral artery occlusion. *J Nucl Med.* 1993;34:1243.
31. Palestro CJ, Sen C, Muzinic M, et al: Assessing collateral cerebral perfusion with technetium-99m-HMPAO SPECT during temporary internal carotid occlusion. *J Nucl Med.* 1993;34:1235.
32. Mathews D, Walker BS, Purdy PD, et al: Brain blood flow SPECT in temporary balloon occlusion of carotid and intracerebral arteries. *J Nucl Med.* 1993;34:1239.
33. Walker BS, Matthews D, Batjer H, et al: Detection of cerebral hypoperfusion during trial carotid occlusion with reversal following extracranial-intracranial bypass prior to permanent occlusion. *Clin Nucl Med.* 1994;19:499.
34. Moody EB, Dawson RC III, Sandler MP: ^{99m}Tc-HMPAO SPECT imaging in interventional neuroradiology: Validation of balloon test occlusion. *AJNR Am J Neuroradiol.* 1991;12:1043.
35. Monsein LH, Jeffery PJ, van Heerden BB, et al: Assessing adequacy of collateral circulation during balloon test occlusion of the internal carotid artery with ^{99m}Tc-HMPAO SPECT. *AJNR Am J Neuroradiol.* 1991;12:1045.
36. Lewis DH, Hsu S, Eskridge J, et al: Brain SPECT and transcranial Doppler ultrasound in vasospasm-induced delayed cerebral ischemia after subarachnoid hemorrhage. *J Stroke Cerebrovasc Dis.* 1992;2:12.
37. Lewis DH, Eskridge JM, Newell DW, et al: Single-photon emission computed tomography, transcranial Doppler ultrasound, and cerebral angioplasty for post-traumatic vasospasm. *J Neuroimag.* 1993;3:252.
38. Lewis DH, Eskridge JM, Newell DW, et al: Brain SPECT and the effect of cerebral angioplasty in delayed ischemia due to vasospasm. *J Nucl Med.* 1992;33:1789.
39. Matthews D: SPECT evaluation of cervical occlusion. *J Nucl Med.* 1994;35:1556. Letter to Editor.

CHAPTER 17

Computed Electroencephalographic Topographic Brain Mapping

SAMUEL S. AHN, PETER Y. YOUN, SHELDON E. JORDAN, and MARC R. NUWER

Computed electroencephalographic topographic (CET) brain mapping is a sophisticated computer-based method for the analysis and two-dimensional display of electrical brain activity. The electroencephalographic (EEG) data are recorded from 16 to 32 surface electrodes on the patient's scalp. A computer amplifies and analyzes the frequency-amplitude spectra, employing an interpolating algorithm to generate 256 to 4000 additional data points. The frequency-based amplitude distributions derived from such calculations are color coded and represented as a two-dimensional topographic image, which is then displayed on a computer monitor or printer. Several CET brain-mapping systems are now commercially available (Fig. 17–1), and a considerable volume of clinical and basic quantitative EEG studies have been published (Plates 17–1 and 17–2).

The principal advantages of CET brain mapping include the following: (1) it monitors cerebral circulation and function rather than imaging anatomy; (2) it is noninvasive, utilizing neither radioisotopes nor radiation; (3) the equipment is more compact and portable than the standard EEG machine; (4) although the CET brain-mapping equipment is not inexpensive (approximately $100,000), the cost per test is relatively low—similar to a standard EEG test ($400), half the cost of a computed tomography (CT) scan, and one third the cost of a magnetic resonance imaging (MRI) scan; (5) CET brain mapping can monitor changes over time with a temporal resolution of seconds; and (6) for a nonspecialist, the color-coded images are easier and quicker to interpret than the paper tracings of a standard EEG.

HISTORY

For decades, clinical electroencephalographers have been mentally constructing field maps of EEG data and sketching these images on paper in order to understand complicated field structures. In 1935, Adrian and Yamagiwa[1] reported the first topographic description of the human EEG. Then, in 1951, Walter and Shipton[2] developed a 22-channel toposcope that displayed EEG frequency and phase characteristics on a collection of small cathode-ray tubes. These early topographic display mechanisms possessed a host of technical problems and required numerous recording electrodes, specially trained clinical interpreters, and expensive, cumbersome equipment.

With the advent of microcomputer technology, research investigators were able to convert EEG data more readily into clinically applicable topographic images. In 1969, Estrin and Uzgalis[3] presented the first computer-generated, automated topographic display of EEG patterns. In 1971, Lehmann[4] introduced a 48-channel topographic map using a general-purpose computer, displaying the electrical field at one instant of time across the scalp. In 1973 and 1975, Gotman and colleagues[5, 6] used multichannel power spectral analysis to display EEG patterns topographically in a Cannonogram and determined that delta power, derived from one of the four classic EEG frequency bands, was the most valuable EEG parameter in evaluating cerebral ischemia. In 1978, Matsuoka and associates[7] used the square root of average power as an equivalent potential over a given frequency band and displayed a map by interpolating the values between the scalp electrodes. They applied topographic mapping of EEG power data to the functional evaluation of the effects of dexamethasone in patients with brain tumors. In 1979, Duffy and associates[8] displayed the EEG and evoked potential data as color-coded images in dyslexic children. Two years later, Duffy and associates[9] combined Student's t-test with topographic brain mapping to yield a map of brain activity that differentiated normal from abnormal areas of the brain, thus providing lateralizations appropriate to neurologic symptoms and signs. These developments all led to the current brain-mapping machinery, which uses color-coded, topographic displays that emphasize the amplitude spectrum.

The application of CET brain mapping to assess cerebrovascular disease has only recently been investigated. In 1980 and 1984, van Huffelen and colleagues[10, 11] performed quantitative EEG analysis on 20 patients, all of whom had normal

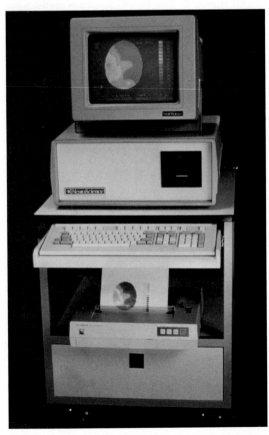

FIGURE 17–1. A commercially available computed encephalographic topographic brain-mapping system. Note the monitor, computer, keyboard, and printer on a portable cart.

EEG tests by standard visual inspection despite a history of transient ischemic attacks (TIAs) or mild cerebrovascular accidents. These patients could be separated from 50 normal controls with an 80 percent specificity and a 70 percent sensitivity, despite normal routine EEGs. In 1984, Yamakami and associates[12] performed serial preoperative and postoperative CET brain maps on 32 patients with cerebral ischemia who underwent superficial temporal artery–to–middle cerebral artery bypass and then correlated these results with clinical outcome and serial cerebral blood flow studies obtained by the ^{133}Xe inhalation method. These investigators found that patients with only TIAs had normal preoperative CET brain maps, whereas patients with stroke had abnormal images; furthermore, bypass surgery did not reverse the abnormal CET brain maps of the stroke patients. Additionally, Nagata and associates[13] compared the results of CET brain mapping, ^{133}Xe regional cerebral blood flow studies, CT scans, and angiograms of 32 patients who had strokes or TIAs. In contrast to the findings of Yamakami and associates,[12] they found that seven of 10 patients with TIAs had abnormal preoperative CET brain maps even after the neurologic deficits had abated. The brain map abnormalities resolved after extracranial–intracranial bypass operations. Furthermore, these brain map abnormalities, particularly increased slow-wave activity, could be reproduced postoperatively by transient compression of the superficial temporal artery. In 1986, Culebras and associates[14] reported that CET brain mapping was useful in identifying oligemic hemispheric regions of the brain. Five of 10 patients with angiographically documented occlusive carotid artery disease developed transient slow-wave activity in cerebral regions angiographically suspected of poor perfusion when their necks were placed in a hyperextended position (presumably due to a compromise of vertebral circulation). Three of four patients who subsequently underwent carotid endarterectomy demonstrated resolution of this transiently provoked electric alteration.

In 1982, Nagata and associates[15] performed CET brain mapping on patients with chronic cerebral infarction and reported that the topographic focus of increased slow-wave activity, particularly delta activity, corresponded significantly to the low-density areas on CT as well as to the ischemic lesions provided by regional cerebral blood flow studies. In 1984, van Huffelen and associates[11] compared a set of five quantitative EEG parameters to CT scans of 20 patients with minor cerebral ischemia. They found a 72 percent abnormality rate using quantitative EEG criteria, whereas CT revealed abnormality in only 10 percent of these patients. In 1987, Nuwer and associates[16] found normal CT scans in 8 of 16 patients (50%) who had mild stroke and whose quantitative EEG studies demonstrated focal electrical abnormalities on topographic maps. The patients with normal CT scans either demonstrated marginal ischemia with fluctuating neurologic symptoms or were tested within 2 to 3 days of symptom onset. Based on the results of these and other topographic EEG studies in cerebrovascular disease, CET brain mapping appears to correlate well with lesions found on CT as well as with the results of regional cerebral blood flow measurements.[17, 18]

In addition, CET brain mapping in cerebrovascular disease has been compared with positron emission tomography (PET), which permits quantitative tomographic measurements of cerebral energy metabolism. In 1984, Buchsbaum and associates[19] performed quantitative EEG mapping studies on six normal volunteers and reported good correlation between EEG power spectra and regional cerebral glucose metabolism. Rosen and colleagues[20] evaluated the predictive value of quantitative EEG studies in determining potential postischemic cortical impairment in rats. They found that quantitative EEG measurements could provide reasonably accurate prognostic information about brain energy metabolism, indicating the extent of brain cell damage and death resulting from ischemia. In 1989, Nagata[21] compared topographic EEG power parameters with those of cortical CBF and cerebral metabolic rate of oxygen, which were provided by PET, in patients with unilateral cerebral infarction. He showed that delta and theta activities correlated negatively with cerebral blood flow and cerebral metabolic rate of oxygen, whereas alpha activity correlated positively. These investigators demonstrated that the relative availability, repeatability, specificity, and low cost of CET brain mapping represent distinct advantages over PET scans.

Recently, we found CET brain mapping to be an accurate, sensitive, and useful monitor of cerebral circulation and function in patients with stroke and those having carotid endarterectomy.[16, 22] Our experience using CET brain mapping is described in the following section.

PATIENT POPULATION AND METHODS

Twenty consecutive patients with well-documented clinical histories of stroke underwent simultaneous standard EEG and CET brain mapping within 60 days of their events. Seventeen of these patients had a CT scan within 2 days of the event, and four patients had an MRI scan. Patients included 9 males and 11 females, with ages ranging from 56 to 82 years and a median age of 67 years.

A separate, although partially overlapping, group of 46 consecutive patients underwent simultaneous EEG and CET brain mapping before, during, and 6 to 8 hours after carotid endarterectomy.[22] Four of these patients were included in the stroke group described above.

Routine 16-lead EEG was obtained using the bipolar and referential montages standard for the laboratory. Computed EEG analysis was recorded by 28-channel acquisition, with scalp electrodes placed according to the international 10–20 system. A band-pass filter of 0.5 to 40 Hz was used to exclude artifacts and account for normal EEG variants. Fast Fourier transform was performed in five bands: 0.5 to 4.0 Hz (delta), 4.1 to 8.0 Hz (theta), 8.1 to 12.0 Hz (alpha), 12.1 to 16.0 Hz (beta 1), and 16.1 to 30.0 Hz (beta 2). Color was coded for the amount of amplitude spectrum in a given frequency band. Spectral edge, the 97.5 percentile of the EEG amplitude spectrum, was also displayed in a color-coded topographic map. Data between each of the 28 EEG electrode sites were filled in by interpolation using an inverse square coefficient for the nearest four electrodes, generating 4096 points of data. Thus, the entire scalp was represented as an oval, two-dimensional, color-coded image on the computer monitor.

In order to monitor for artifacts (eg, eye and muscle movements, lead misplacement), the raw EEG waveforms

TABLE 17–1. Correlation of Noninvasive Tests and Previous Stroke

	N	Abnormal Findings Corresponding to Previous Stroke	
	N	N	%
Previous stroke	20	—	—
CET brain mapping	20	17	85*
Standard electroencephalogram	20	3	15*
Computed tomography	17	7	41†
Magnetic resonance imaging	4	3	75
Physical examination	20	11	55

*$P < 0.01$.
†$P < 0.05$.
CET, computed electroencephalographic topographic; N, number.

and CET brain maps were simultaneously presented on the computer monitor in a real-time fashion. Each frequency band was analyzed separately in epochs of 2.5 seconds, and topographic maps were updated after each epoch. Alternatively, instead of examining individual epochs, the clinician could average across the entire acquisition period, examining approximately 10 minutes of artifact-free EEG in the five frequency bands. Data were stored on magnetic disks for off-line analysis.

All EEG and CET brain-mapping studies were performed by registered EEG technologists and interpreted independently by two clinical neurologists specializing in EEG frequency analysis. One neurologist was aware of the patients' clinical data, and the other neurologist was not. Focal abnormalities of either test were ascertained using a criterion of 50 percent asymmetry during more than 50 percent of the session, seen at more than one adjacent electrode site, and not accounted for by artifacts or normal variant waveforms in the accompanying EEG tracing.

Carotid endarterectomy was performed in the standard fashion. Carotid artery back-pressures were measured according to the method of Moore and Hall.[23] Each patient received a detailed neurologic examination preoperatively, immediately after carotid endarterectomy, 4 to 6 hours postoperatively, the following morning, and as indicated.

RESULTS

Results of the 20 stroke patients are depicted in Table 17–1. CET brain mapping detected focal abnormalities in areas of the brain corresponding to the stroke deficits in 17 of 20 patients (85%). Abnormalities included increased delta or decreased alpha power seen asymmetrically over the involved region.[16] By contrast, routine EEG detected corresponding abnormalities in only 3 of these 20 patients ($P < 0.01$) and was less able to lateralize the area of abnormality. Furthermore, the region of cortical impairment was more clearly defined by CET brain mapping when both it and the routine EEG were abnormal. CT scan demonstrated the strokes in 7 of 17 patients (41%) and MRI scan in three of four patients (75%). Neurologic examination at the time of the EEG revealed clinically detectable residual deficits in 11 of 20 patients (55%). Plates 17–3 through 17–8 depict some illustrative cases.

Table 17–2 outlines the results of preoperative and intraoperative CET brain mapping and standard EEG in the 46 patients undergoing carotid endarterectomy. Seven of 16 asymptomatic stenotic patients (44%), 5 of 11 patients with amaurosis fugax (45%; Plate 17–9), and 8 of 12 patients with TIAs (67%; Plate 17–10) had abnormal preoperative CET brain maps, suggestive of subclinical cerebral dysfunction. Routine EEG detected only 8 of these 20 focal abnormalities (17%). A detailed neurologic examination revealed subtle impairment of higher cortical functions in at least 50 percent of these patients. Four of seven patients with previous stroke (57%) had abnormal preoperative brain mapping, whereas standard EEG detected only two of these abnormalities (28%). (These seven patients experienced mild strokes with minimal residual deficits.) Overall, preoperative CET brain mapping was abnormal in 24 of 46 patients (52%), whereas routine EEG revealed abnormalities in only 10 of 46 patients (22%).

One patient underwent a carotid endarterectomy on the basis of an abnormal preoperative CET brain map. This patient presented with a cortical TIA, but his carotid duplex scan and angiogram were unremarkable (Fig. 17–2A). CT and MRI scans along with routine EEG were also normal. However, CET brain mapping revealed ischemic changes in an area of the brain that corresponded to his symptoms (see Plate 17–10). Surgical exploration revealed an irregular ulcerative plaque at the carotid bifurcation, and the patient's symptoms of TIA resolved postoperatively (see Fig. 17–2B).

Intraoperatively, during the time of carotid cross-clamping, CET brain mapping revealed ischemic changes in 23 of the 46 patients (Plates 17–11 and 17–12; see Table 17–2). Standard EEG detected abnormalities in only 13 of these 46 patients (28%). Interestingly, patients who had previous

TABLE 17–2. Results of Preoperative and Intraoperative CET Brain Mapping and Standard 16-Lead EEG in 46 Patients Undergoing Carotid Endarterectomy

Indication for Surgery	Abnormal Preop CET Brain Mapping			Abnormal Preop EEG		Change in Intraop CET Brain Mapping		Change in Intraop EEG	
	N	N	%	N	%	N	%	N	%
Asymptomatic	16	7	44	2	12	8	50	5	31
Amaurosis fugax	11	5	45	2	18	4	36	1	9
Transient ischemic attack	12	8	67	4	33	5	42	2	17
Stroke	7	4	57	2	28	6	86	5	71
Total	46	24	52	10	22	23	50	13	28

CET, computed electroencephalographic topographic; EEG, electroencephalogram; N, number.
Adapted from Ahn SS, Jordan SE, Nuwer MR, et al: Computed electroencephalographic topographic brain mapping. *J Vasc Surg.* 1988; 8:247; with permission.

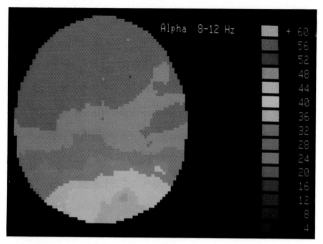

PLATE 17-1. Computed encephalographic topographic brain mapping of a normal patient. Note the symmetry.

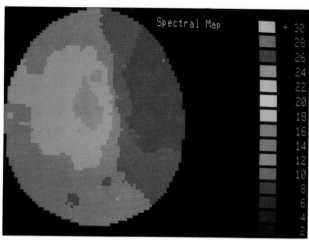

PLATE 17-2. Computed encephalographic topographic brain mapping of a rhesus monkey whose right middle cerebral artery was ligated experimentally. Note the decreased amplitude of brain electrical activity *(dark blue)* in the right frontal and parietal lobes.

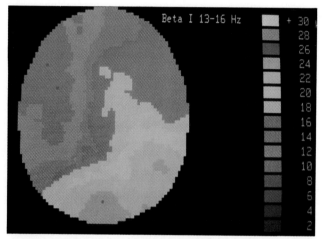

PLATE 17-3. Image of a patient with an occlusion of the left middle cerebral artery and right hemiplegia. Note the decreased amplitude of beta (fast frequency) activity in the left frontal and parietal lobes.

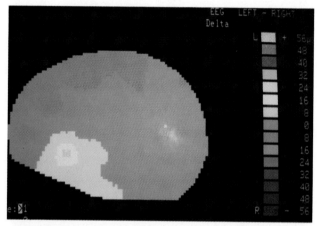

PLATE 17-4. Image of the left hemisphere minus the right hemisphere of a patient with a nonfluent aphasia from an embolic stroke. Note the increased delta (slow frequency) activity *(yellow)* in the left inferior frontal area.

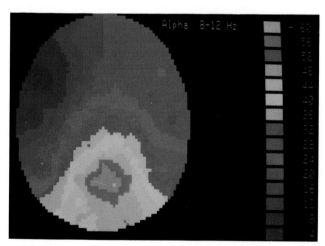

PLATE 17-5. Computed encephalographic topographic brain mapping of a patient with an occlusion of the left internal carotid artery, residual right hemiplegia, and expressive aphasia. Note the decreased amplitude of alpha (fast frequency) activity in the left frontal parietal areas, which are the areas of the distribution of the left middle cerebral artery.

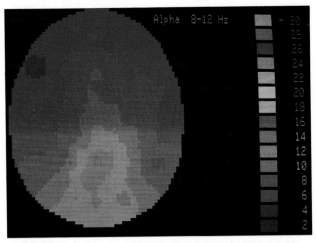

PLATE 17-6. Computed encephalographic topographic brain-mapping image of a patient with bilateral internal carotid artery occlusion and residual quadriplegia. Note the decreased amplitude of alpha activity in the front and parietal lobes bilaterally.

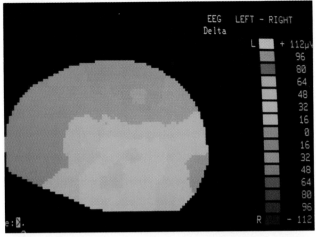

PLATE 17-7. Image of the left hemisphere minus the right hemisphere in a patient with an occlusion of the inferior branc' vessel of the left middle cerebral artery and Wernicke's aphasia. Note the increased delta activity in the left temporal area.

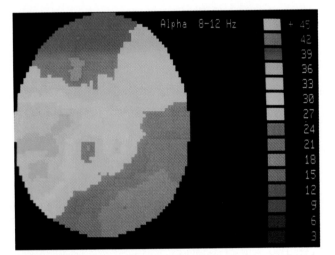

PLATE 17-8. Image of a patient with acute left homonymous hemianopia. Note the decreased alpha activity in the right occipital lobe. A detachable balloon was released inadvertently and embolized into the right posterior cerebral artery during an attempted percutaneous balloon embolization of a basilar artery aneurysm.

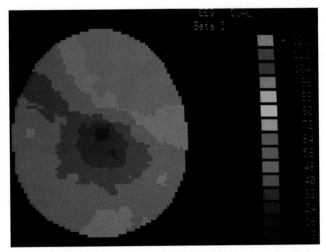

PLATE 17-9. Example of an abnormal preoperative computed encephalographic topographic brain mapping in a patient with a tight left carotid stenosis and amaurosis. Note the decreased beta activity in the left frontal lobe. The large central blue area is an artifact of a vertex reference electrode. A more careful, repeat neurologic examination revealed the presence of a Babinski reflex of the right foot and possible mild short-term memory loss.

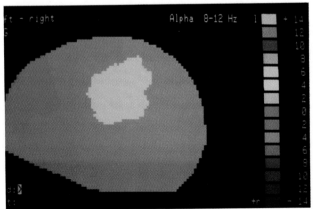

PLATE 17-10. A, Computed encephalographic topographic brain map of a patient presenting with multiple left hemispheric transient ischemic attacks. Standard electroencephalographic and magnetic resonance imaging scans showed no abnormalities. See Figure 17-2 for other views of the same patient.

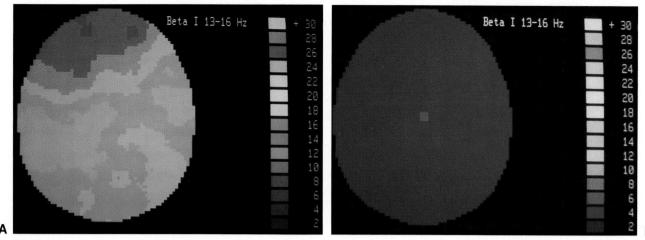

PLATE 17-11. *A,* Preoperative computed encephalographic topographic (CET) brain mapping of a patient who experienced right hemispheric transient ischemic attacks and tight stenosis of the right internal carotid artery, previously occluded left internal carotid artery, and an occluded left vertebral artery. *B,* Intraoperative CET brain mapping of the same patient when the right carotid artery was clamped. This patient's brain was entirely dependent on the right carotid artery, as indicated by the marked decreased amplitude of beta activity in the entire brain. A shunt was inserted expeditiously, and the CET brain-mapping image promptly reverted to the preoperative image.

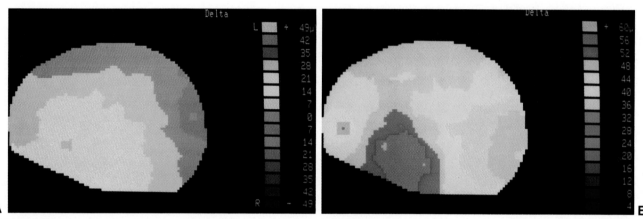

PLATE 17-12. *A,* Intraoperative computed encephalographic topographic (CET) brain mapping of the left hemisphere minus the right hemisphere during carotid cross-clamping. Note the increased delta activity in the left frontal and parietal lobes. *B,* Postoperative CET brain mapping of the same patient. Note the persistent, increased delta activity in the right frontal lobe. This activity corresponded to a new expressive aphasia during the postoperative period. See Figure 17-3 for an angiogram of the same patient.

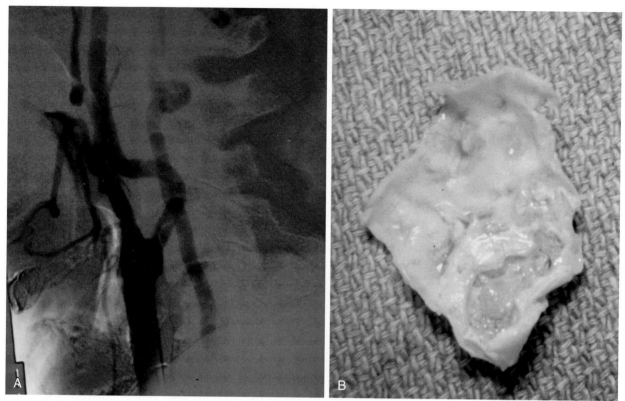

FIGURE 17–2. *A,* Angiography of a patient presenting with multiple left hemispheric transient ischemic attacks revealed essentially normal carotid bifurcation. Echocardiogram and Holter monitor results were also normal. *B,* Intraoperative photograph of the complex ulcerative plaque found at the carotid bifurcation in this patient. See Plate 17–10 for a computed encephalographic topographic brain map of the same patient.

stroke (six of seven) were more likely to develop intraoperative brain-map changes than patients without stroke (17 of 39; $P < 0.05$). Eighteen of the 23 patients who exhibited ischemic changes on CET brain mapping during carotid cross-clamping were shunted. Seventeen of the 18 patients demonstrated complete resolution of their abnormal intraoperative brain-map changes, and all these patients awoke without any new neurologic deficits. One patient demonstrated only partial resolution of his intraoperative brain-map change and awoke with a new, although transient, neurologic deficit. His postoperative CET brain map showed a small ischemic area in the right parietal lobe, corresponding to a new constructional apraxia that resolved within 2 days. This transient neurologic deficit was attributed to a presumed embolic event during shunt placement. Three weeks postoperatively, a repeat neurologic examination and CET brain map were normal.

Five patients were not shunted despite abnormal intraoperative CET brain maps. Four of these five patients, whose carotid artery back-pressures were greater than or equal to 40 mm Hg, demonstrated resolution of their ischemic changes after the carotid artery was reopened. All four patients awoke without any new neurologic deficits.

The remaining patient did not receive an intraoperative shunt because the internal carotid artery was found to be completely occluded at the time of surgery (Fig. 17–3). The preoperative duplex scan and angiogram had inaccurately revealed a "string sign" of the left internal carotid artery. Postoperatively, CET brain mapping revealed a persistent abnormality in the left frontal lobe (see Plate 17–12), and

the patient demonstrated an expressive aphasia that lasted 2 days. Retrospectively, we postulated that the widely patent and enlarged external carotid artery must have contributed significant blood flow to the brain and thus should have been shunted during carotid cross-clamping.

The two neurologists interpreting the standard EEG and CET brain-mapping studies disagreed on two of the 138 EEG results (combining all preoperative, intraoperative, and postoperative tests) and on four of the 138 CET brain-mapping results. The blinded neurologist interpreted these studies as negative or normal, and the unblinded neurologist viewed these test results as abnormal. Later, when the first neurologist became aware of the patients' clinical data, he agreed with the second neurologist. For purposes of this chapter, the interpretation of the unblinded neurologist was used, since most neurologists are aware of the patient's clinical data when interpreting an EEG or brain-map study.

DISCUSSION

Computed electroencephalographic topographic brain mapping appears to be much more accurate than the standard 16-lead EEG. Its specificity was 100 percent and its sensitivity 85 percent in the 20 stroke patients. There were only three false-negative results using CET brain mapping, in contrast to 17 false-negative results based on the standard EEG. Indeed, numerous quantitative EEG studies have reported abnormal test results in 85 to 95 percent of cerebrovascular disease populations, compared with the 45 to 70

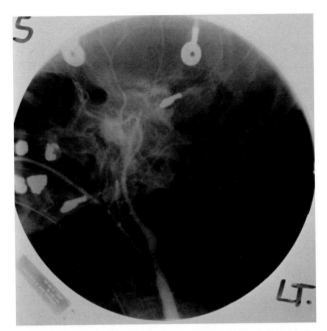

FIGURE 17–3. Intraoperative carotid angiogram of the left hemisphere minus the right hemisphere during carotid cross-clamping. Note the completely occluded internal carotid artery and the widely patent and dilated external carotid artery, which must have contributed significant blood flow to the brain through collateral vessels. Retrospectively, this internal carotid artery should have been shunted during the carotid cross-clamping to prevent the ischemic event. See Plate 17–12 for other views of the same patient.

percent abnormality rate usually detected from visual inspections of routine EEGs.[11, 24–26] CET brain mapping also appears to be more sensitive than the CT scan (85% vs. 41%; $P < 0.05$).

The superior accuracy of CET brain mapping in the assessment of cerebrovascular disease can be attributed to the following. First, CET brain mapping reflects cerebral perfusion and function; the CT scan detects anatomic changes. Jackel and associates[27] reported that quantitative EEG tests became abnormal immediately upon occurrence of cerebral ischemia, whereas CT scans did not become abnormal until 2 to 3 days later. This demonstrates that neuroimaging studies, particularly CT scans, can be normal when the degree of cerebral ischemia is enough to cause cortical impairment but not sufficient to cause frank infarction. Moreover, studies using PET have clearly illustrated that functional derangements can exist in the absence of any structural abnormality, a late consequence of ischemia (see Chapter 15).

Second, the CET brain-mapping system collects electrical activity data from 28 points, whereas standard EEG uses only 16 points. Thus, CET brain mapping utilizes more raw information for evaluation and interpretation than the standard EEG. Furthermore, CET brain mapping amplifies the five EEG bands while muting background activity and artifacts. The ability to average maps over time, to color code amplitude, and then to display the brain electrical data in a simple two-dimensional image greatly simplifies interpretation while highlighting subtle changes that the human eye may not detect in a standard EEG waveform.

The CET brain-mapping system is also more compact and portable than the standard EEG machine. CET brain map-

ping can be performed at the patient's bedside or in the intensive care unit, operating room, or angiography suite. Furthermore, the data are stored on small computer disks, which are far easier to store and retrieve than the bulky paper EEG tracings.

The cost of conducting a CET brain-mapping study is relatively low—similar to the standard EEG, half the cost of a CT scan, and one third the cost of an MRI scan. The only other noninvasive method of evaluating cerebral function, the PET scan, is much more costly, not readily available, not portable, and requires the use of radioisotopes.

The potential applications of CET brain mapping to evaluate patients with cerebrovascular disease are quite varied. One application may involve the detection of cortical impairment in patients in whom routine EEGs are normal. Another may be the monitoring of patients who are at high risk for cerebrovascular disease, such as subarachnoid hemorrhage patients at risk for vasospasm.[26] To date, we have found CET brain mapping to be beneficial in (1) confirming our clinical diagnosis of a recent or past stroke, (2) detecting subclinical strokes in patients presenting with amaurosis fugax or TIAs, (3) selecting appropriate candidates for carotid endarterectomies and monitoring the adequacy of collateral circulation during the procedure, and (4) documenting subtle postendarterectomy neurologic deficits. Our preliminary data further suggest that CET brain mapping can differentiate truly asymptomatic patients from those patients with subclinical ischemia or infarction (see Table 17–2); the ability to make this stratification may enhance our knowledge of the natural history of cerebrovascular disease. For example, one could postulate that patients with silent TIAs demonstrating an abnormal CET brain map have a worse natural history (ie, progression to frank stroke) than truly asymptomatic patients.

Thus, we demonstrated the superiority of CET brain mapping over standard 16-lead EEG for identifying subtle, focal neurologic changes in patients with stroke and concluded that CET brain mapping is a sensitive preoperative monitor that may detect subclinical electrical dysfunction in asymptomatic patients or in those with amaurosis fugax or TIAs. Furthermore, we suggested that CET brain mapping may accurately monitor the adequacy of collateral circulation in patients during carotid cross-clamping and, when used in combination with carotid back-pressure measurements and standard EEG, may enhance the accuracy of the decision whether to shunt a patient during carotid endarterectomy.[22]

In 1990, Elmore and associates[28] performed 65 carotid endarterectomies, using brain maps as the sole neurologic criterion for determining placement of an intraluminal shunt. Forty-three patients (66%) demonstrated abnormal preoperative brain maps. However, only 23 of the 65 patients (36%) had experienced a previous cerebrovascular accident, indicating a high incidence of silent perfusion defects. Ten patients (15%) developed ischemic changes intraoperatively during carotid cross-clamping (all resolved after shunt placement). In contrast to our study,[22] Elmore and associates[28] reported that stroke patients did not demonstrate a higher incidence of intraoperative ischemic changes during cross-clamping than nonstroke patients. However, patients with an abnormal preoperative brain map developed ischemic changes significantly more frequently during cross-clamping than did those with normal preoperative brain maps. (This is not predictive of which patients will need a shunt, for only 23 percent of the patients with an abnormal preoperative brain map developed ischemic changes on their intraoperative brain maps.) Given these findings, it is reasonable to shunt not on the basis of an abnormal preoperative brain map but rather on the basis of ischemic changes that occur at the time of cross-clamping. Hence, CET brain mapping proved to be a sensitive and readily reliable means of monitoring cerebral perfusion during carotid endarterectomy.

DISADVANTAGES OF COMPUTED ELECTROENCEPHALOGRAPHIC TOPOGRAPHIC BRAIN MAPPING

There are a variety of problems in performing CET brain mapping. First, the application of 28 scalp leads is laborious, requiring 1 to 2 hours of the technician's time. Furthermore, maintaining their placement during endotracheal anesthesia is particularly challenging, causing more inconvenience to the patient as well. Loose electrodes could cause reproducible changes in a topographic map that may be misinterpreted as abnormalities. Since the value of CET brain mapping is only as good as its raw data input, all types of artifact (eg, from eye and eyelid movement, electrocardiogram, muscle movement, loose electrodes, leakage, aliasing) should be minimized. The development of a quick-fitting and secure scalp electrode will greatly facilitate the clinical application of CET brain mapping.

Second, the initial cost of the CET brain mapping equipment is significant—approximately $100,000, with an average charge of $400 per patient for the preoperative, intraoperative, and postoperative monitoring and the neurologist's review of the brain maps. However, if one can prevent even one intraoperative stroke, the equipment will quickly pay for itself.

Third, the results of the tests can vary, depending on the neurologist's interpretation of the images and prior knowledge of the patient's clinical data, as seen in our experience. Additionally, clinicians who perform and interpret these tests need to have a solid understanding of traditional polygraph EEGs, as well as additional knowledge and skills required to run and interpret the statistical and EEG computer-processing techniques. The record must be manually reviewed for artifacts, normal variance, abnormal transients, and confounding clinical factors.[26] Further developments of the computer to make the data available in a more objective form are currently under investigation and should be available in the near future.

Fourth, CET brain mapping may be too sensitive. We reported that four of five patients with intraoperative brain-map changes did not receive shunts but had complete resolution of their changes after the carotid artery was reopened.[22] Further, these patients awoke without any new neurologic deficits postoperatively. However, this study clearly shows that subtle and transient neurologic deficits can be detected by CET brain mapping but missed entirely by standard 16-lead EEG, which appears to detect only gross neurologic abnormalities.

In addition, we showed that 50 percent of patients had evidence of ischemia by CET brain mapping at the time of cross-clamping. In contrast, Elmore and associates[28] showed that only 15 percent of their patients developed ischemia with cross-clamping. This difference may be explained by the fact that in Elmore's series, brain-map changes classified as new ischemia required pre-existing abnormalities to have significant amplitude asymmetry that extended into an additional frequency band or that expanded in spatial distribution into another region of the brain. We defined new ischemia based only on an amplitude asymmetry criterion. Further investigations combining CET brain mapping, neuroimaging studies, and sophisticated clinical information obtained through cognitive or psychometric testing are needed, particularly in following up a series of patients through carotid endarterectomy, to shed more light on the subject of silent cerebral ischemia that may be unidentified by the standard EEG.

Fifth, CET brain mapping is generally nonspecific with respect to the type of pathology. Although it seems to be good at assessing the presence and lateralization of an abnormality, CET brain mapping is unable to differentiate ischemic cerebrovascular disease from intracranial hemorrhage, tumor, or head trauma.[29, 30] Furthermore, CET brain mapping may not detect transient changes such as epileptic spikes, which standard EEG is better equipped to monitor.

CONCLUSION

Although there are still controversies concerning various aspects of data acquisition, statistical interpretation, and spatial resolution, CET brain mapping appears to be a sensitive, reliable, readily interpretable, and noninvasive monitor of cerebral perfusion and function.[31–33] Moreover, a growing body of scientific literature suggests that CET brain mapping can contribute significantly to the understanding of the pathophysiology underlying cerebrovascular disease, ischemia, and infarction.[34] CET brain mapping can document the presence of a clinically apparent or perhaps even a subclinical stroke, help select patients who are likely to benefit from bypass surgery or endarterectomy, enhance our ability to monitor the adequacy of collateral circulation during carotid artery cross-clamping, help determine whether a patient should be shunted during carotid endarterectomy, and monitor the results of surgical procedures with increased accuracy. Because of these capabilities, CET brain mapping may differentiate specific subcategories of patients, and the ability to classify patients correctly in subgroups may enhance future randomized studies into the basic processes involved in cerebrovascular disease. Further research will clarify and confirm the clinical applicability of this rapidly growing technology that combines computer and electrophysiology.

REFERENCES

1. Adrian ED, Yamagiwa K: The origin of the Berger rhythm. *Brain.* 1935;58:323–351.
2. Walter WG, Shipton HW: A new toposcopic display system. *Electroencephalogr Clin Neurophysiol.* 1951;3:281–292.
3. Estrin T, Uzgalis R: Computerized display of spatio-temporal EEG patterns. *IEEE Trans Biomed Eng.* 1969;16:192–196.
4. Lehmann D: Multichannel topography of human alpha EEG fields. *Electroencephalogr Clin Neurophysiol.* 1971;31:439–449.
5. Gotman J, Skuce DR, Thompson CJ, et al: Clinical application of spectral analysis and extraction of features from electroencephalograms with slow wave in adult patients. *Electroencephalogr Clin Neurophysiol.* 1973;35:225–235.

6. Gotman J, Gloor P, Ray WF: A quantitative comparison of traditional reading of the EEG and interpretation of computer-extracted features in patients with supratentorial brain lesions. *Electroencephalogr Clin Neurophysiol.* 1975;38:623–639.

7. Matsuoka S, Aragaki Y, Numaguchi K, Ueno S: Effect of dexamethasone on electroencephalograms in patients with brain tumors. *J Neurosurg.* 1978;48:601–608.

8. Duffy FH, Burchfiel JL, Lombroso CT: Brain electrical activity mapping (BEAM): A method for extending the clinical utility of EEG and evoked potential data. *Ann Neurol.* 1979;5:309–321.

9. Duffy FH, Bartels PH, Burchfiel JL: Significance probability mapping: An aid in the topographic analysis of brain electrical activity. *Electroencephalogr Clin Neurophysiol.* 1981;51:455–462.

10. van Huffelen AC, Poortvliet DCJ, van der Wulp CJM: Quantitative electroencephalography in cerebral ischemia: Detection of abnormalities in "normal" EEGs in patients with acute unilateral cerebral ischemia. In Lechner H, Aranibar A, eds. *EEG and Clinical Neurophysiology.* Amsterdam: Excerpta Medica;1980:125–142.

11. van Huffelen AC, Poortvliet DCJ, van der Wulp CJM: Quantitative electroencephalography in cerebral ischemia: Detection of abnormalities in "normal" EEGs. In Pfurtscheller G, Jonkman EJ, Lopes da Silva FH, eds. Brain ischemia: Quantitative EEG and imaging techniques. *Prog Brain Res.* 1984;62:29–50.

12. Yamakami I, Yamaura A, Nakamura T, Isobe K: Non-invasive follow-up studies of stroke patients with STA-MCA anastomosis: Computerized topography of EEG and 133-Xenon inhalation rCBF measurement. In Pfurtscheller G, Jonkman EJ, Lopes da Silva FH, eds. Brain ischemia: Quantitative EEG and imaging techniques. *Prog Brain Res.* 1984;62:107–112.

13. Nagata K, Yunoki K, Araki G, et al: Topographic electroencephalographic study of ischemic cerebrovascular disease. In Pfurtscheller G, Jonkman EJ, Lopes da Silva FH, eds. Brain ischemia: Quantitative EEG and imaging techniques. *Prog Brain Res.* 1984;62:271–286.

14. Culebras A, Kline MD, Ross GS, et al: Quantitative EEG mapping of cerebral ischemia. *Neurology.* 1986;36(1):321.

15. Nagata K, Mizukami M, Araki G, et al: Topographic electroencephalographic study of cerebral infarction using computed mapping of the EEG (CME). *J Cereb Blood Flow Metab.* 1982;2:79–88.

16. Nuwer MR, Jordan SE, Ahn SS: Evaluation of stroke using EEG frequency analysis and topographic mapping. *Neurology.* 1987;37:1153–1159.

17. Tolonen U, Sulg IA: Comparison of quantitative EEG parameters from four different analysis techniques in evaluation of relationships between EEG and CBF in brain infarction. *Electroencephalogr Clin Neurophysiol.* 1981;51:177–185.

18. Nagata K, Tagawa K, Shishido F, et al: Topographic EEG correlates of cerebral blood flow and oxygen consumption in patients with neuropsychological disorders. In Duffy FH, ed. *Topographic Mapping of Brain Electrical Activity.* Boston: Butterworths; 1986:357–370.

19. Buchsbaum MS, Kessler R, King A, et al: Simultaneous cerebral glucography with positron emission tomography and topographic electroencephalography. In Pfurtscheller G, Jonkman EJ, Lopes da Silva FH, eds. Brain ischemia: Quantitative EEG and imaging techniques. *Prog Brain Res.* 1984;62:263–270.

20. Rosen I, Smith ML, Rehncrona S: Quantitative EEG and evoked potentials after experimental brain ischemia in the rat: Correlation with cerebral metabolism and blood flow. In Pfurtscheller G, Jonkman EJ, Lopes da Silva FH, eds. Brain ischemia: Quantitative EEG and imaging techniques. *Prog Brain Res.* 1984;62:175–203.

21. Nagata K: Topographic EEG mapping in cerebrovascular disease. *Brain Topogr.* 1989;2:119–126.

22. Ahn SS, Jordan SE, Nuwer MR, et al: Computed electroencephalographic topographic brain mapping. *J Vasc Surg.* 1988;8:247–254.

23. Moore WS, Hall AD: Carotid artery back-pressure. A test of cerebral tolerance to temporary carotid occlusion. *Arch Surg.* 1969;99:702–710.

24. Niedermeyer E: Cerebrovascular disorders and EEG. In Niedermeyer E, Lopes da Silva FH, eds. *Electroencephalography.* Baltimore: Urban & Schwarzenberg; 1982:233–254.

25. Kopruner V, Pfurtscheller G, Auer LM: Quantitative EEG in normals and in patients with cerebral ischemia. In Pfurtscheller G, Jonkman EJ, Lopes da Silva FH, eds. Brain ischemia: Quantitative EEG and imaging techniques. *Prog Brain Res.* 1984;62:51–84.

26. Nuwer MR: The development of EEG brain mapping. *J Clin Neurophysiol.* 1990;7:459–471.

27. Nagata K, Dhaduk V, Hooker M, et al: Computed EEG topography in acute stroke. *Neurology.* 1987;37(1):364.

28. Elmore JR, Eldrup-Jorgensen J, Leschey WH, et al: Computerized topographic brain mapping during carotid endarterectomy. *Arch Surg.* 1990;125:734–737.

29. Mies G, Hoppe G, Hossmann KA: Limitations of EEG frequency analysis in the diagnosis of intracerebral diseases. In Pfurtscheller G, Jonkman EJ, Lopes da Silva FH, eds. Brain ischemia: Quantitative EEG and imaging techniques. *Prog Brain Res.* 1984;62:85–103.

30. Jerrett SA, Corsak J: Clinical utility of topographic EEG brain mapping. *Clin Electroencephalogr.* 1988;19:134–143.

31. Rodin EA: Some problems in the clinical use of topographic EEG analysis. *Clin Electroencephalogr.* 1991;22:23–29.

32. Welch JB: Topographic brain mapping: Uses and abuses. *Hosp Pract [Off].* 1992;27:163–168, 171, 175.

33. Klotz JM: Topographic EEG mapping methods. *Cephalalgia.* 1993;13:45–52.

34. Nuwer MR: Quantitative EEG. II. Frequency analysis and topographic mapping in clinical settings. *J Clin Neurophysiol.* 1988;5:45–85.

CHAPTER 18

Role of the Vascular Laboratory in the Diagnosis and Management of Patients With Cerebrovascular Disease

WESLEY S. MOORE

The noninvasive vascular laboratory has experienced rapid growth in technology, availability, and utilization during the past 15 years for the diagnostic evaluation of patients with cerebrovascular disease. Subsequent chapters will deal, in depth, with individual methods of testing. The objective of this chapter is to provide an overview with respect to the use of a vascular laboratory in the diagnosis and management of patients with both suspect and proven lesions of the cerebrovascular system.

A wide variety of tests are available in the vascular laboratory that are designed to assess the capacity of the carotid artery system to deliver blood flow to the brain. These tests can be divided into two major categories: indirect tests and direct tests.

INDIRECT TESTS OF CAROTID CIRCULATION COMPETENCE

The tests in this category explore patterns of pressure and flow in branches of the carotid system in order to infer the presence or absence of a hemodynamically significant lesion affecting blood flow to the internal carotid artery. These tests include documenting the collateral relationships between the external and internal carotid arteries by assessing the direction of blood flow about the orbit. This test is based on the fact that when the internal carotid artery becomes hemodynamically compromised, branches of the external carotid artery become collateral contributors to the intracranial circulation via their anastomotic connections with branches of the ophthalmic artery about the orbit. Other categories of indirect testing depend on the fact that the ophthalmic artery is a branch of the internal carotid artery, and the hemodynamics of the ophthalmic artery will parallel changes that occur in the internal carotid artery. For example, a hemodynamic compromise in one carotid artery will slow waveform propagation to the ophthalmic artery and reduce pressure in the ophthalmic artery when compared with the opposite side, assuming the opposite side is distal to an otherwise normal carotid circulation.

DIRECT TESTS OF CAROTID CIRCULATION COMPETENCE

Direct tests include methods of visualizing the carotid bifurcation and studying, by waveform analysis, the patterns of blood flow in the common carotid, external carotid, and internal carotid arteries. These tests include B-mode imaging, Doppler imaging, and spectral analysis. Duplex Scanning, particularly color flow, has become the standard for carotid artery noninvasive testing. Magnetic resonance angiography, either alone or in combination with duplex scan-

ning, has also made an important contribution to noninvasive testing. Magnetic resonance angiography is particularly helpful in providing imaging of the intracranial circulation. It is less helpful in assessing stenosis of the carotid bulb, since it tends to overestimate stenosis by one or two deciles. This is due to signal dropout secondary to turbulence.

It is important to point out that all tests in the vascular laboratory are designed to determine the presence of a flow- or pressure-reducing lesion in the carotid circulation. No test has yet proved accurate in assessing the presence of a nonstenotic ulcerative lesion, with the possible exception of high-resolution B-mode imaging. Thus, when a report comes back from the laboratory indicating a normal study, it is important to keep in mind that the report simply refers to the fact that there is not a pressure- or flow-reducing lesion in the carotid artery. It does not rule out the presence of an ulcerative lesion that may be an embolic source.

The spectrum of vascular laboratory utilization is broad, ranging from nonutilization to abusive practices such as mass population screening programs set up in busy shopping centers. I attempt to give a balanced viewpoint as to the effective use of the noninvasive laboratory for the evaluation of patients with suspected cerebrovascular disease. The use of a vascular laboratory for clinical evaluation can be divided into five general categories: evaluation of asymptomatic patients suspected of having a critical arterial stenosis, use in patients with symptoms typical of carotid artery disease, use in patients with atypical symptoms, follow-up evaluation of patients after operation, and use of the laboratory in clinical investigation.

Asymptomatic Patients

The noninvasive laboratory has had its most obvious impact on the evaluation of patients suspected of harboring critical carotid artery stenosis in the absence of symptoms. Concern about carotid artery stenosis usually arises when a bruit is heard over the carotid bifurcation or in a patient presenting for evaluation and found to have one or more risk factors for carotid artery disease. In the past, cerebral angiography was the only method of evaluating these patients. Yet only 20 to 30 percent of patients with carotid bruit were ultimately found to have a stenosis of hemodynamic importance. Furthermore, 60 percent of patients with angiographically proven stenoses did not have a bruit on physical examination.[1-3] Therefore, had bruit been the only method of identifying patients with carotid stenosis, a large number of patients would have been subjected to angiography in the absence of a significant lesion. Of perhaps greater concern is the fact that many patients with carotid artery stenosis would not have been identified because of the absence of the physical finding of a bruit.

Noninvasive testing offers a satisfactory solution to this clinical problem. Patients with carotid bruit or at risk of having a hemodynamically significant carotid stenosis because of known associated risk factors can be adequately screened by a variety or combination of noninvasive tests. These tests offer an overall accuracy in excess of 90 percent for identifying or ruling out hemodynamically compromising lesions of the carotid artery. In this setting, only those patients with abnormal tests in the vascular laboratory need be referred for angiographic study. This practice has greatly reduced the number of negative angiographic studies when evaluating asymptomatic patients.

The major limitation of the vascular laboratory, in this setting, has been the failure to identify carotid artery ulceration in the absence of a hemodynamically significant stenosis. Since most tests are a measure of pressure- or flow-reducing lesions, a nonstenotic ulcer can escape detection. However, recent reports of high-resolution B-mode ultrasound scanning suggest that some ulcers may be identified. In addition, B-mode evaluation of carotid artery plaque may offer some insight into plaque composition, hence the potential risk of plaque breakdown with thromboembolic complication. It is anticipated that as the technology continues to improve, the limitation of ulcer identification will be overcome.

Patients With Symptoms Typical of Carotid Artery Disease

It can be argued that patients with hemispheric or monocular symptoms are clearly candidates for arteriography and could easily bypass the noninvasive laboratory. There is additional information, however, as well as some advantages to be gained from a noninvasive evaluation of a patient with typical carotid artery symptoms. First, the type of arteriogram may be determined on the basis of information gained in the vascular laboratory. For example, if a high-grade stenosis in the carotid bifurcation is identified by noninvasive means, the technique for arteriography requested for that patient may be limited to an arch aortogram. If the indirect tests are negative or the direct tests suggest a low-profile plaque, perhaps with an ulcer, a selective carotid angiogram with the possibility of multiple oblique views is indicated. The objective of this type of an angiogram is to look for an irregular or ulcerative lesion in the absence of a significant stenosis. In addition, careful intracranial visualization is required to look for pathology of the carotid siphon as well as the branches of the carotid artery.

The final advantage in having noninvasive data available on patients with typical symptoms is that this information provides an excellent comparison when postoperative studies are obtained. It enables the clinician to confirm the technical result of an operation as compared with the preoperative baseline, as well as provides a basis for long-term follow-up in the early detection of recurrent carotid stenosis.

Patients With Atypical Symptoms

In patients presenting with global cerebral ischemic symptoms without localized findings, multiple extracranial arterial stenoses may be the cause. In addition, a large number of differential diagnoses are related to diffuse organ dysfunction, such as cardiac pathology or pathology of the vestibular system. Although tests to rule out alternative diagnoses are

indicated, routine angiography in this group of patients provides a low yield of significant arterial pathology. The noninvasive laboratory provides a safe, rapid, and cost-effective method of screening for significant arterial pathology, and its use leads to better patient selection for angiographic evaluation.

Postoperative Follow-up Examination

Although carotid endarterectomy is a durable operation, an incidence of recurrence may require therapeutic intervention. The diagnosis of recurrent carotid stenoses may be made by waiting for symptoms, or the condition may be anticipated by periodic noninvasive testing during follow-up visits. My own practice is to test the patient during the first postoperative visit, then twice yearly for the next year, and finally during an annual visit thereafter.

The incidence of recurrent carotid stenosis ranges from 5 to 10 percent. The literature is not clear on the indication for reoperation in the absence of symptoms. Nonetheless, the identification of recurrence appears to be worthwhile, and the decision about prophylactic reoperation must be made on an individual basis.

Clinical Investigation

The vascular laboratory is currently used to screen patients for angiography; the information derived from these studies is used as an approximation of the contrast image. In recent years, it has been recognized that angiography is not the gold standard we thought it was. There are many instances in which the angiogram underestimates the extent of a lesion. Angiography can miss significant plaque surface abnormalities and provides no information concerning plaque characteristics and composition. Nor does it tell us anything about the hemodynamics of blood flow or the potential dynamic pathology of thromboembolism. Physiologic testing in the vascular laboratory has the potential of expanding diagnostic information concerning arterial pathology and can explore a dimension beyond the capability of contrast angiography. During the next few years, we can anticipate research to yield techniques for evaluating plaque composition, surface morphology, thromboembolic potential, and specific hemodynamic data not currently available with anything short of surgical exploration and direct examination of pathologic specimens.

The noninvasive laboratory, through research efforts, is poised to leap beyond its current role of anticipating angiographic information; it will provide important data for clinical decision making that the angiogram can only approximate.

CAROTID ENDARTERECTOMY WITHOUT ANGIOGRAPHY

An increasing number of publications suggest that the decision to perform carotid endarterectomy can be made without invasive contrast angiography.[4–8] Some state that a carotid duplex scan with or without color flow, if performed in a validated laboratory, can provide sufficient information to proceed with surgery in patients who are appropriately selected and found to have stenoses of hemodynamic significance. There are several risks involved with this approach, however. First, important lesions at the level of the aortic arch, as well as intracranial stenoses, will be missed. Second, there is a small but finite incidence of very high-grade stenoses being interpreted as total occlusion by duplex scanning.[9–11] Some centers have sought to overcome these limitations by adding magnetic resonance angiography to the database obtained with a carefully performed duplex scan.[12] This can document the intracranial circulation and determine whether there are important lesions involving the carotid siphon or stem of the middle cerebral artery. Finally, the magnetic resonance angiogram also provides an assessment of the carotid bifurcation. If the duplex scan and the magnetic resonance angiogram are in substantial agreement with respect to the carotid bifurcation, and if the magnetic resonance angiogram shows no intracranial lesion that would contraindicate the use of carotid endarterectomy, the decision to proceed with carotid endarterectomy in the absence of a contrast angiogram appears to be reasonably sound. By-passing invasive contrast angiography avoids the complications associated with that procedure, avoids the discomfort associated with an invasive diagnostic study, and substantially reduces the cost of patient evaluation.

It is important to point out that if a decision is made to use duplex scanning as the only test before carotid endarterectomy, the laboratory in which the duplex scan is performed plays a pivotal role. The accuracy of its determinations must be validated by a careful comparison of its noninvasive test results with a series of patients in which contrast angiography has been performed. Subsequent validation can be obtained by comparing the duplex scan data with the lesions found at the time of operation. It should also be pointed out that the study obtained with duplex scanning must be of excellent quality and must be consistent with the patient's history and physical findings. If the duplex scan is not of good diagnostic quality, this is an indication for a contrast angiogram. Furthermore, if there is evidence that the patient has aortic arch occlusive disease, as documented by a difference in arm blood pressures or questionable quality of common carotid artery pulsation, this is an indication for a contrast evaluation of the aortic arch. Finally, if the patient's symptoms are inconsistent with the duplex scan evaluation, a contrast angiogram must be performed. If the patient has active symptoms, and the duplex scan is interpreted as showing a total occlusion of the internal carotid artery, this may represent a very high-grade stenosis that will benefit from carotid endarterectomy. A cross-check of the duplex scan data must be obtained with either a contrast angiogram or perhaps a magnetic resonance angiogram.

As more and more centers begin to use duplex scanning, with or without magnetic resonance angiography, as an alternative to preoperative contrast angiography, it will be important to carefully audit the surgical findings and outcome, since potential errors and abuses of this practice may have important impacts on patient management.

REFERENCES

1. Moore WS, Bean B, Burton R, Goldstone J: The use of ophthalmosonometry in the diagnosis of carotid artery stenosis. *Surgery.* 1977;82:107.
2. Malone JM, Bean B, Laguna J, et al: Diagnosis of carotid artery stenosis: Comparison of oculoplethysmography and Doppler superorbital examination. *Ann Surg.* 1980;191:347.
3. Ziegler DK, Zileli T, Dick A, et al: Correlation of bruits over the artery with angiographically demonstrated lesions. *Neurology (NY).* 1971;21:860.
4. Moore WS, Ziomek S, Quiñones-Baldrich WJ, et al: Can clinical evaluation and noninvasive testing substitute for arteriography in the evaluation of carotid artery disease? *Ann Surg.* 1988;208:91.
5. Farmilo RW, Scott DJ, Cole SE, et al: The role of duplex scanning in the selection of patients for carotid endarterectomy. *Br J Surg.* 1990;77:388.
6. Gelabert HA, Moore WS: Carotid endarterectomy without angiography. *Surg Clin North Am.* 1990;70:213.
7. Dawson DL, Zierler RE, Strandness DE Jr, et al: The role of duplex scanning and arteriography before carotid endarterectomy: A prospective study. *J Vasc Surg.* 1993;18:673.
8. Chervu A, Moore WS: Carotid endarterectomy without angiography. *Ann Vasc Surg.* 1994;8:296.
9. Bornstein NM, Beloev ZG, Norris JW: The limitations of diagnosis of carotid occlusion by Doppler ultrasound. *Ann Surg.* 1988;207:315.
10. Mattos MA, Hodgson KJ, Ramsey DE, et al: Identifying total carotid occlusion with color-flow duplex scanning. *Eur J Vasc Surg.* 1992;6:204.
11. Bridgers SL: Clinical correlates of Doppler/ultrasound errors in the detection of internal carotid artery occlusion. *Stroke.* 1989;20:612.
12. Turnipseed WD, Kennell TW, Turski DA, et al: Magnetic resonance angiography and duplex imaging: Noninvasive tests for selecting symptomatic carotid endarterectomy candidates. *Surgery.* 1993;114:643.

CHAPTER 19

Ocular Pneumoplethysmography

WILLIAM GEE, JAMES F. REED III, ALICE E. MADDEN, and ROBERT L. SMITH

The two basic elements of hemodynamics are pressure and flow. Winsor[1, 2] pioneered the clinical application of pneumatic plethysmography to the study of these two elements in the extremities. His most important contribution was the description of systolic pressure gradients between the lower and upper extremities when lesions of hemodynamic consequence were present in the main arterial channels of the lower extremities. Borrás and associates[3] explored the relationship of the ophthalmic systolic pressure to the brachial systolic pressure in the human. They cannulated the supraorbital artery and passed a catheter in the direction of its junction with the ophthalmic artery. This was accompanied by retrograde catheterization of the brachial artery at the antecubital fossa. Simultaneous recording of the ophthalmic systolic pressure (OSP) and brachial systolic pressure (BSP) documented a gradient in normal individuals characterized by the formula

$$OSP = 73 + 0.28 \ BSP.$$

As will be seen, this formula closely approximates that determined by noninvasive techniques.

The noninvasive measurement of ophthalmic artery pressures received broad clinical acceptance following the report of Bailliart[4] on compression ophthalmodynamometry. The essence of this technique is the elevation of intraocular pressure by increasing tension in the corneoscleral shell by externally compressing it, while simultaneously visualizing the retinal arterial system for pulsatile flash-filling of the vessels. The onset of flash-filling characterizes the diastolic pressure, and sustained emptiness of the vessels typifies the systolic pressure. The relationship between the variable degrees of extrinsic ocular compression and intraocular pressure results in a nomogram that defines this association. A major limitation of this method was the requisite that the longitudinal axis of the instrument had to pass through the center of the eye. Any angulation of the instrument footplate from a 90-degree perpendicular to the curvature of the sclera would result in error.

Kukán[5] was cognizant of the inherent error associated with other than axisymmetric application of the Bailliart ophthalmodynamometer. He reasoned that a circular eyecup applied to the ocular sphere with a vacuum would always apply an axisymmetrical load and that an outward distortion of the corneoscleral shell would have the same effect as an inward distortion of it—increased tension in the corneoscleral envelope and elevation of the intraocular pressure. He experimented with a variety of eyecup sizes and found that small (6–8 mm) eyecups required very high vacuums to achieve the desired elevation of intraocular pressure.

Galin and colleagues[6] elaborated on the Kukán investigation. They standardized the eyecup used; it was hemispheric in shape, with a 12 mm inside and 14 mm outside diameter. They constructed a graph relating the scleral vacuum applied to the intraocular pressure obtained, as determined by applanation tonometry. The suction ophthalmodynamometer control was attached directly to the ophthalmoscope, which allowed simultaneous regulation of the device and retinal observation by a single individual. During this same period,

Best and coworkers[7] were assessing the use of standard pressure transducers that were coupled to fluid pathways and connected by suction to the sclera via the standard suction ophthalmodynamometer eyecups. The experimental apparatus was binocular, and the scleral vacuum used was that which resulted in the greatest amplitude of the ocular pulse wave observed. The most important observation they made was that the ocular pulse wave, like a peripheral (extremity) pulse wave, had a shorter anacrotic ascent and a longer catacrotic descent. In normal patients, the catacrotic segment was devoid of the notch typically observed in the peripheral pulse wave in association with aortic valve closure.

A variety of experimental devices were developed over a 5-year period. The first clinical ocular pneumoplethysmograph (OPG-Gee) underwent a 1-year investigational evaluation (1972–1973), under human experimentation protocol, at the University of California–San Francisco. As a result of this assessment, the device was accepted for standard clinical use at that institution, and the first clinical report documented the observations of the evaluation.[8] Two early reports describe the instrument design.[9, 10] Subsequent animal experiments have resulted in a mathematical analysis of the scleral vacuum–intraocular pressure relationship and its effect on the fluid dynamics of the eye.[11, 12]

BIOMECHANICS

An eyecup with an inside diameter equal to one half the outside diameter of the eye is placed on the eye, followed by the application of a variable vacuum to the eyecup-eye interface. This is associated with three stress resultants as secondary to two displacements and one rotation. Figures 19–1 and 19–2 are graphic representations of these six factors. In Figure 19–1, the rotation β of the normal to the shell element, the radial displacement W in the θ direction, and the displacement V in the ϕ direction are matched (see Fig. 19–2) by the transverse shear stress resultant Q, the membrane stress resultant N_θ, and the membrane stress resultant N_ϕ, respectively. The most important of these elements is the radial displacement W in the θ direction. The pulsatile variation in this displacement is volume-calibrated by the instrument, and it is an essential to the calculation of ocular blood flow.

An unexpected observation in the report from Chen and associates[12] is clarified by Figure 19–3. The two half-globes, separated by the vertical axis, differ in that the left global half-shell has twice the thickness of the right global half-shell. Both half-shells have eyecups with inside diameters equal to one half the outside diameter of the respective half-shells. Although it will be intuitively recognized that the thinner (right) half-shell will deform with greater ease than will the thicker (left) half-shell, the thinner half-shell encompasses a greater noncompressible mass than does the thicker one. Overall, the same scleral vacuum applied to both results in the same intraocular pressure in both half-globes.

The horizontal axis in Figure 19–3, which passes through the center of both eyecups, is defined as the 0–180-degree diameter. The rim of the eyecup impacts the globe at a

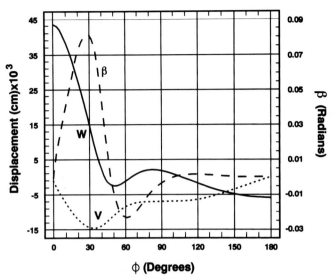

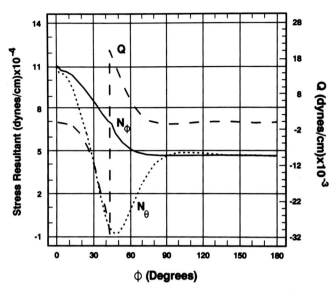

FIGURE 19–1. Graphic representation of the factors involved in calculating ocular blood flow. *Dashed line* represents rotation β; *solid line*, displacement W; *dotted line*, displacement V. (From Chen C, Reed JF III, Rice DC, et al: Biomechanics of ocular pneumoplethysmography. *J Biomech Eng.* 1993;115:231–238; with permission of the American Society of Mechanical Engineers.)

FIGURE 19–2. Graphic representation of the factors involved in calculating ocular blood flow. *Dashed line* represents stress resultant Q; *solid line*, stress resultant N_ϕ; *dotted line*, stress resultant N_θ. (From Chen C, Reed JF III, Rice DC, et al: Biomechanics of ocular pneumoplethysmography. *J Biomech Eng.* 1993;115:231–238; with permission of the American Society of Mechanical Engineers.)

radius 30 degrees removed from the axis of symmetry. As demonstrated by Chen and coworkers,[12] the maximum bending moments and strains are encountered just beyond this 30-degree radius, at approximately 40 degrees from the zero axis.

The practical application of the foregoing is seen in Figure 19–4. When an eyecup has an inside diameter that is one half the outside diameter of the eye on which it is placed, the eyecup always covers 6.7 percent of the surface area of the eye. Conversely, the total surface area of the eye is 14.9 times that covered by the eyecup. The latter factor is essential to the formula for the calculation of ocular blood flow.[13]

OCULAR ANATOMY AND PHYSIOLOGY

Anatomy

The globe has a weight range of 7 to 8 g (mean 7.5 g) and a specific gravity range of 1.0 to 1.1 (mean 1.05).[14]

Division of the two extremes of weight by the mean specific gravity results in a volume range of 6.7 to 7.6 mL (mean 7.15 mL). The outside diameter of the globe, by in vitro measurements, has a range of 23.5 to 24.5 mm (mean 24 mm).[14] If the volume of the globe is calculated from the formula

$$V = 4/3 \ \pi r^3,$$

the volume range is 6.8 to 7.7 mL (mean 7.25 mL). The two means of the volume of the globe, as calculated from two sets of physical measurements, agree within 0.1 mL. In vitro measurement of the inside diameter of the globe has a mean of 22 mm, reflecting a combined thickness of the sclera, choroid, and retina of 1 mm.[14] In vivo ultrasound measurements of the anterior-posterior diameters of 7500 eyes demonstrated an average diameter of 23.65 mm.[15] Other methods of in vivo measurement of eye size involve radiographic

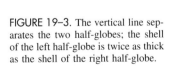

FIGURE 19–3. The vertical line separates the two half-globes; the shell of the left half-globe is twice as thick as the shell of the right half-globe.

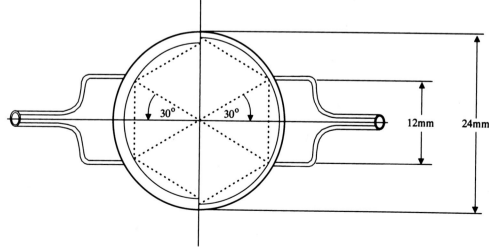

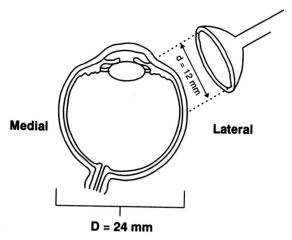

Medial   **Lateral**

D = 24 mm

FIGURE 19–4. The geometry of the surface area of the eye and of the surface area of the eye covered by the eyecup. A is the surface area of the eye; a, the surface area of the eye under the eyecup.

$A = 4\pi r^2 = 1809.56 \text{ mm}^2$
$a = 0.5\pi D [D - (D^2 - d^2)^{0.5}] = 121.22 \text{ mm}^2$
$a/A = 0.067$
$A/a = 14.9$

(From Gee W, Reed JF III: Ocular pneumoplethysmographic evaluation of carotid lesions: Gee method. In Ernst CB, Stanley JC, eds. *Current Therapy in Vascular Surgery*, 2nd ed. Philadelphia: BC Decker; 1991;20–24; with permission of Mosby-Year Book, Inc.)

projection.[16, 17] The average of the anterior-posterior and transverse diameters in 110 eyes as determined by computed tomography was 28.5 mm.[18] By appropriate calculations, this diameter would define a weight of 12.7 g, 69 percent greater than the mean of 7.5 g by in vitro measurement. It appears that radiographic projection methods of in vivo measurement of eye dimensions are of questionable validity.

The globe can be divided conveniently into two compartments: vascularized and nonvascularized. The cornea, lens, vitreous body, and aqueous content are nonvascularized. The remaining tissue, the shell of the globe, is vascularized. The surface area of this hollow sphere of 1 mm thickness is calculated from the formula

$$A = 4 \pi r2 = 1810 \text{ mm.}^2$$

The surface area multiplied by the thickness results in a tissue volume of 1.8 mL. The tissue volume multiplied by a specific gravity of 1.05 results in a tissue weight of 1.9 g, which is approximately 25 percent of the total weight of the eye.

Although the foregoing analysis may seem quite laborious, these calculations are essential to the application of ocular pneumoplethysmography (OPG). When the wide variation in body weight among adult humans is considered, the adult human eye is of remarkably uniform size. This factor is a major element in the precision with which OPG can be performed.

Physiology

The normal intraocular pressure of 10 to 20 mm Hg (mean 15 mm Hg) is maintained by the oculovascular fluid dynamics coupled with a minimal degree of elasticity of the sclera. Forced closure of the eyelids elevates the intraocular pressure to 50 mm Hg.[19] Simply rubbing the eye elevates

this pressure to 150 to 250 mm Hg.[19] Blowout fractures of the orbit must be associated with extreme elevations of the intraocular pressure, yet the globe itself is rarely ruptured, and intrinsic ocular damage is frequently minimal.

PREPARATION FOR THE TEST

Although technical proficiency in test performance is readily achieved, evaluation of the eye history requires considerable clinical judgment.

History of Systemic Conditions

The technologist interviews the patient and reviews the chart, recording pertinent information regarding symptoms of the present neurologic illness, particularly those that suggest hemispheric, monocular, or vertebrobasilar arterial insufficiency. If the referring physician has noted brachiocephalic arterial bruits, these are also recorded.

Allergies, especially to plastics or local anesthetic agents, are noted. The rare patient who is allergic to plastics should be carefully questioned prior to the OPG test, since the plastic eyecups may irritate the conjunctiva. A history of allergy to local anesthetics should also prompt further inquiry. Most such patients describe reactions suggestive of epinephrine effect, which is present in many local anesthetics. We perform a simple check, first asking the patient to swallow to clear the mouth of all saliva. With the head tilted slightly forward and the tip of the tongue touching the hard palate, the patient breathes through the mouth, maintaining dryness under the tongue. Two or three drops of the ophthalmic anesthetic 0.5 percent proparacaine are placed on the floor of the mouth; within 30 to 45 seconds, anesthesia is noted. If no erythema is observed in the anesthetized area, a conjunctival reaction is unlikely.

On several occasions, patients who professed a history of allergic reactions to local anesthetics subsequently received intravenous lidocaine in large amounts for cardiac problems, without reaction. Intravenous lidocaine for cardiac use has no preservatives, and the sterile solution is prepared with hydrochloric acid in water for injection, with the pH adjusted to a range of 6 to 7 by the addition of sodium hydroxide. Standard preparations of this drug are in concentrations of 1, 2, and 4 percent. A 1 percent solution of cardiac lidocaine applied to the eye has achieved adequate anesthesia in 3 to 5 minutes, whereas 0.5 percent proparacaine can achieve adequate anesthesia in less than 1 minute.

Eye History

If the patient has been treated for any eye problem other than simple refractive errors, the ophthalmologist is immediately notified. Frequently, the eye disease as described by the ophthalmologist is quite different from the history related by the patient, and here the judgment of the technologist is most important. Although the OPG test is rarely contraindicated, certain circumstances require caution.

Eye Trauma

Eye trauma, other than minor injuries such as corneal abrasion, may temporarily contraindicate the test, especially if the trauma included globe puncture, retinal disruption (tearing, hole, separation), or ciliary injury. Vitreous hemorrhage or hyphema are also considered temporary contraindications. However, if 6 months have elapsed since injury and if the ophthalmologist concurs, the test can be performed safely.

Eye Surgery

Eye surgery, particularly if it included partial- or full-thickness incision of the globe, is a temporary contraindication to the test, although, with the concurrence of the ophthalmologist, the test can be performed 6 months postoperatively. This also applies to cataract extraction and prosthetic lens implantation. We reported our experience of 115 OPG tests in such patients.[20] Since this report, our total experience has increased to 1036. None of these OPG tests had any adverse effects on the operated eyes. Despite the safety of the OPG test in this circumstance, it remains the policy of our vascular laboratory to obtain telephone concurrence of the ophthalmologist.

Eye Disease

Glaucoma, diabetic retinopathy, and vitreous separation do not ordinarily contraindicate the OPG test. Many of these patients have been studied uneventfully, but only with the concurrence of the ophthalmologist. Diabetic retinopathy associated with neovascular proliferation, however, raises concern regarding the OPG test, especially if the disease process has been associated with microhemorrhages requiring laser coagulation. Interestingly, hemorrhage control by coagulation elsewhere in the body, including the brain, incorporates local tissue pressure elevation for temporary tamponade of the hemorrhage, in order to improve the function of the coagulating mechanism. Thus, elevation of the intraocular pressure during the OPG test may actually be beneficial in patients with diabetic retinal microhemorrhage. As with standard ophthalmodynamometry, a history of spontaneous retinal detachment in either eye ordinarily contraindicates OPG, even in the nonaffected eye. Radial keratotomy is also an absolute contraindication to the test.

Patient Instructions

Most patients have some anxiety at the initial testing, and a careful choice of words is important in giving instructions. The patient should be informed that dimming of vision, including complete loss of vision for several seconds, may be noted. The patient is also informed of the possibility of a scleral ecchymosis. Needless anxiety may result from the use of the words "blind" and "hemorrhage" in describing these two phenomena to the patient. In fact, a spontaneous scleral ecchymosis can occur with no more than a sneeze. These spontaneous ecchymoses, like those induced by the OPG, resolve without therapy in several days. They occur infrequently (3% incidence) and are the result of a ruptured conjunctival vessel. We have noticed no higher incidence or increased severity of scleral ecchymosis in patients who were anticoagulated at the time of the test.

Test Procedure

The manufacturer of the OPG provides a complete set of instructions regarding alignment of the instrument prior to use. This technique should be practiced until it can be performed proficiently before applying the instrument to a patient.

The patient is initially placed in the sitting position. Upper garments are removed, as necessary, for precise measurement of both brachial blood pressures. Brachial blood pressure values should be measured in the standard fashion, with arm cuff and stethoscope. If Doppler arterial pressures or pressures derived from direct arterial lines are recorded, the criteria for OPG interpretation to be described will be seriously distorted. A difference of 10 mm Hg or more between the two standard BSP values should be carefully noted. The blood pressure cuff is replaced on the arm with the higher BSP, and the patient is placed in the supine position. The electrocardiogram electrodes are placed on the right arm and on both legs. Several drops of 0.5 percent proparacaine ophthalmic solution are instilled in each eye. The patient is informed that coldness or a slight stinging sensation of the eyes may be noted. Before placement of the eyecups, the eyes should be carefully wiped with a facial tissue, from medial to lateral, with the eyes closed. This forces excess drops and tear accumulations out of the eyes, avoiding aspiration of this fluid into the pneumatic tubing of the instrument.

The eyecups are maintained in accordance with the recommendations of the *Morbidity and Mortality Weekly Report* of August 30, 1985.[21] The transducer head is positioned over the face of the patient, with the pneumatic tubing and attached eyecups hanging at a level on a transverse plane midway between the bridge and the tip of the nose. The eyecups on either side should reach a point midway between the lateral canthus of the eye and the front of the ear (Fig. 19–5). The examiner grasps both eyecups simultaneously

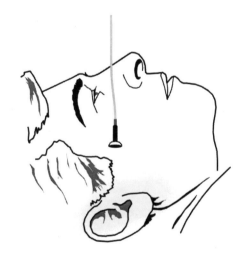

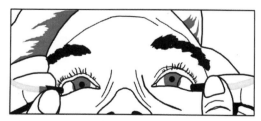

FIGURE 19–5. Composite drawing of location of eyecups prior to placement on the eyes *(top)* and after placement *(bottom)*. The eyecups are located inferolaterally and abut or slightly overlap the respective limbi (outer margin of the iris) bilaterally.

between the thumbs and forefingers, resting the fourth digit of each hand on the malar areas of the patient in order to steady both systems and retract the lower lids downward. The patient is instructed to look up, which automatically raises the upper lids. The eyecups are placed on the inferolateral sclerae, and the patient is instructed to look at the white disk on the bottom of the transducer head. At this point, some precision is required to locate the eyecups over the inferolateral quadrants of the sclerae, with the medial border of each cup abutting or slightly overlapping the respective limbus (see Fig. 19–5).

Once both eyecups have been properly positioned, the foot switch is activated. The operator must maintain a slight pressure on the eyecups to ensure a seal, until sufficient vacuum has been induced to secure them. We perform the initial test at a 300 mm Hg vacuum. When the maximum vacuum (either 300 mm Hg in approximately 3 seconds or 500 mm Hg in approximately 5 seconds) has been achieved, the vacuum pump automatically shuts off. Initiation of the recording starts the degradation of the scleral vacuum over 25 to 30 seconds, depending on the initial maximum vacuum achieved. Thus, the entire test is completed in 28 to 40 seconds, as determined by the maximum vacuum.

The remainder of the test is automatically sequenced by the instrument. As the vacuum decreases, pulses may or may not be noted in either or both eyes. If a pulse wave is noted immediately in either eye, the instrument can be recycled by depressing the 500 mm Hg switch and repeating the test cycle. In less than 5 percent of patients, an ocular pulse is noted immediately in either eye, even at the 500 mm Hg level.

Most patients can control their eye blinking during the test, which is best done with the eyes open and the gaze fixed. In the occasional patient who is unable to control blinking, the test may be repeated with the eyes closed. This eliminates the blink artifact but usually causes an eye motion artifact due to the loss of gaze fixation. The latter artifact is more acceptable than a blink artifact.

Immediately upon completion of the OPG test, and with the patient remaining in the supine position, the brachial blood pressure is again measured in the arm on which the cuff was previously replaced. Ordinarily, only this single measurement is made. However, if the BSP measured in the sitting position differed by 10 mm Hg or more, both brachial blood pressures in the supine position are also determined. The single supine BSP, or the higher of these two pressures if both are measured, is the measurement used for correlation with both OSP, as determined by the OPG.

CALCULATION OF OCULAR HEMODYNAMICS

Ophthalmobrachial Systolic Pressure Index

The relationship of the OSP and BSP was described in a previous report.[22] Briefly, a regression of the OSP on BSP results in a mean represented by the formula

$$OSP = 55 + 0.43 \ BSP.$$

The standard error of estimates ($S_{y.x}$) was 8 mm Hg. The mean minus two $S_{y.x}$ results in the formula

$$OSP = 39 + 0.43 \ BSP.$$

The line characterized by the latter formula has been our demarcation separating normal (above) from abnormal (on or below) BSP-OSP coordinates over the past 12 years. In order to simplify the expression of the BSP-OSP coordinate and simultaneously eliminate the need for a graph to characterize it, the BSP-OSP coordinate can be expressed as the ophthalmobrachial systolic pressure (OBSP) index, with the formula

$$OBSP = OSP - 39 - 0.43 \ BSP.$$

Any positive OBSP index falls above the line of demarcation. All OBSP indexes that are zero (on the line of demarcation) or negative (below the line of demarcation) are considered abnormal. This component of ocular hemodynamics has been applied in a large series of patients described elsewhere.[23] Equally important is the appendix of that report, which contains the statistical explanation of our preference of the OBSP index to the simple expression of an OSP-BSP ratio. Briefly, if the OSP were equal to the BSP in normal circumstances, then a simple OSP-BSP ratio would be an acceptable method of relating the two measurements. However, the OSP does not equal the BSP under normal circumstances, as was demonstrated by Borrás and associates[3] by direct intra-arterial measurements in 15 human subjects. A comparison of their direct data and our indirect data is contained in Table 19–1. Despite the small sample size of the direct data, there is agreement in the two sets of observations over a BSP range from 100 to 200 mm Hg.

Calculation of Ocular Blood Flow

The formula for the calculation of ocular blood flow (OBF), which includes a calibration factor of mm^3/10 mm pen deflection, a volume conversion factor mL/1000 mm^3, the heart rate (HR/min), the maximum ocular pulse amplitude (OPA) in millimeters, and the globe-eyecup surface area factor of 14.9, as previously defined, is as follows:

$$OBF = \underbrace{\frac{HR}{min} \times OPA \ mm}_{\text{Variable Factors}} \times \underbrace{\frac{mm^3}{10 \ mm} \times \frac{mL}{1000 \ mm^3} \times 14.9}_{\text{Constant Factors}}$$

Where elements common to the numerator and denominator are canceled, and the remainder of the three constant factors is expressed as a decimal, the formula can be expressed in this fashion:

$$OBF = HR \times OPA \times 0.00149 = mL/min.[13]$$

The instrument measures a segment of the change in the total ocular volume with each cardiac cycle. Some portion of the total ocular volume, at the end of each ocular wave, is the residual ocular blood volume. We have elected to characterize the pulsatile change of the total ocular volume during a 1-minute interval as the net ocular blood flow. The distinction of blood flow versus blood volume has received considerable attention in the area of cerebral hemodynamics.[24–28]

TABLE 19–1. Measurement of OSP-BSP Relationship by Direct and Indirect Methods

	Regression Formula	BSP = 100 mm Hg	BSP = 200 mm Hg
Gee[22]	OSP = 55 + 0.43 BSP	OSP = 98 mm Hg	OSP = 141 mm Hg
Borrás et al[3]	OSP = 73 + 0.28 BSP	OSP = 101 mm Hg	OSP = 129 mm Hg

BSP, brachial systolic pressure; OSP, ophthalmic systolic pressure.

CLINICAL APPLICATION

Ocular and Cardiac Hemodynamics

The relationship between ocular and cardiac hemodynamics has been explored under a variety of circumstances. One major difference is between OBF during ventricular pacing and OBF during atrioventricular sequential pacing.[29] We recently enlarged on a previous report in which the OBF, with and without intra-aortic balloon counterpulsation, was described.[30, 31] OBF demonstrated a 25 percent reduction during the counterpulsation. This does not imply a reduction of the cardiac index but more likely a redistribution phenomenon, which has been suggested by animal investigations in which a 10 percent reduction of cerebral blood flow during intra-aortic balloon counterpulsation was associated with increased visceral blood flow and no change in cardiac index.[32] A recent report describes the effect of cardiac rhythm irregularity on the ocular pulse amplitude.[33] In a related study, the cardiac index in relation to the OBF was examined.[34] An understanding of these phenomena is essential to proper interpretation of OPG tests.

Ocular Hypoperfusion

One study reported 18 patients who underwent temporal artery biopsies for the assessment of giant-cell arteritis.[35] Half had negative biopsies. The other nine had giant-cell arteritis confirmed by biopsy. The mean of the OBF plus or minus the standard deviation in the nine patients with positive biopsies was 0.40 (± 0.17) mL/minute, whereas those patients with negative biopsies had a mean OBF of 1.27 (± 0.35) mL/minute.

A recent example illustrates the profound changes in ocular hemodynamics associated with the therapy of giant-cell arteritis. A 76-year-old woman presented with the single symptom of transient intermittent left eye blindness for 1 week and a single episode of transient bilateral blindness the

TABLE 19–2. Serial Ocular Hemodynamics in Giant-Cell Arteritis

	OBSP		OBF	
Day*	Right	Left	Right	Left
1†	−22.3	−28.3	0.12	0.12
5	−9.2	−6.2	0.38	0.48
39	−4.1	−28.1	1.37	1.07
494‡	10.2	7.2	1.02	1.07
840	25.0	3.0	1.02	0.91

*Note the progressive improvement from day 1 through day 494, with some deterioration on the left at day 840.
†See Fig. 19–6.
‡See Fig. 19–7.
OBF, ocular blood flow rate; OBSP, ophthalmobrachial systolic pressure.

day prior to her initial visit. The patient was devoid of other symptoms suggestive of giant-cell arteritis. Steroid therapy was immediately initiated. The admission sedimentation rate was markedly elevated, and temporal artery biopsy on the day following admission confirmed giant-cell arteritis. Carotid duplex ultrasound demonstrated moderate right and mild left carotid bifurcation atherosclerosis. Table 19–2 summarizes the serial ocular hemodynamics observed in this patient. Figure 19–6 (day 1) demonstrates the extremely low ocular pulse amplitudes initially noted. The test results shown in Figure 19–7 were obtained approximately 16.5 months after the initial test. Both the OBSP index and OBF were within normal limits. The patient recently returned without eye symptoms but with a pruritic sensation in both temporal areas, 840 days after her initial presentation. Some deterioration of the left ocular hemodynamics was demonstrated. Repeat carotid duplex ultrasound showed no change.

Our observations related to giant-cell arteritis with ophthalmic artery involvement have been confirmed by other investigators using an instrument quite similar to the OPG, the oculo-oscillo-dynamograph (OODG-Ulrich).[36] They found the OODG to be a very sensitive indicator of the success or failure of steroid therapy as well as an early detector of relapse, which helped avoid their sequelae. They emphasized the noninvasive nature, simplicity, and repeatability of the test.

Ocular Hyperperfusion

Whereas ocular hypoperfusion characterizes giant-cell arteritis with ophthalmic artery involvement, ocular hyperperfusion has been described in some patients following carotid reconstructions, especially when the repaired vessels are associated with contralateral carotid occlusions.[37] In order to provide a control series for the 2331 carotid reconstructions reviewed for the assessment of postoperative ocular hyperperfusion, we examined the data from 701 procedures previously reported.[38] In the latter report, each carotid artery was arteriographically categorized in one of three ways: O, total occlusion; S, severe stenosis, where the residual lumen was 50 percent or less in two planes or 33 percent or less in a single plane, as compared with the normal lumen diameter in a more distal segment of the vessel with parallel walls; or N, neither total occlusion nor severe stenosis. In these 701 carotid repairs, four groups of patients were formed, according to the status of the carotid artery ipsilateral (i) and contralateral (c) to the side of reconstruction. The first group was identified as N_i-N_c (110 operations); the second group as S_i-N_c (415 operations); the third group as S_i-S_c (114 operations); and the last group as S_i-O_c (62 operations). Of the four groups, the S_i-O_c group had the lowest average OBF bilaterally before operation and the highest average OBF bilaterally after operation. On the side of operation, the mean

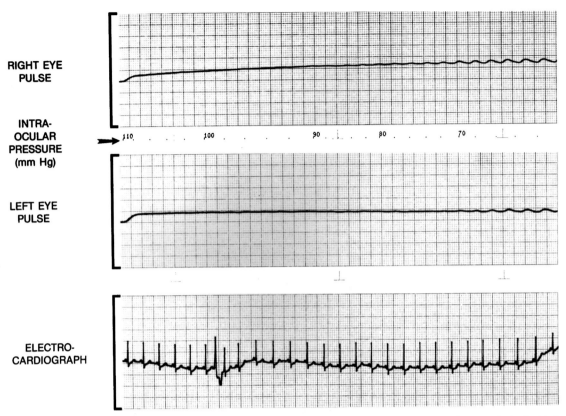

RIGHT EYE PULSE

INTRA-OCULAR PRESSURE (mm Hg)

LEFT EYE PULSE

ELECTRO-CARDIOGRAPH

FIGURE 19–6. Ocular pneumoplethysmographic test results from a patient with giant cell arteritis on day 1. These results were obtained with the instrument available from 1985 to 1992.

postoperative OBF plus three standard deviations equaled 4.13 mL/minute. This figure was selected as the demarcation point: a higher postoperative OBF on the side of operation would be considered ocular hyperperfusion.

Of the 2331 carotid reconstructions reviewed, there were 11 patients (12 procedures) in which the postoperative OBF on the side of operation exceeded 4.13 mL/minute. These patients were divided into three groups: five patients in the S_i-N_c group, three patients in the S_i-S_c group, and four patients in the S_i-O_c group. One patient underwent repair of severe bilateral carotid lesions at different times and was included in the S_i-S_c group at the first operation and the S_i-N_c group at the second operation. Figures 19–8 and 19–9 are the respective preoperative and postoperative OPG test results from one of the patients in the S_i-O_c group. The preoperative OBF of 0.93 mL/minute on the side of operation was the lowest observed in the 12 procedures. The postoperative OBF of 5.38 mL/minute on the side of operation was the highest noted in the 12 procedures, and it is 428 percent greater than the preoperative flow. Tables 19–3, 19–4, and 19–5 contain the preoperative and postoperative OBF data from the side of operation in the S_i-N_c, S_i-S_c, and S_i-O_c groups, respectively,

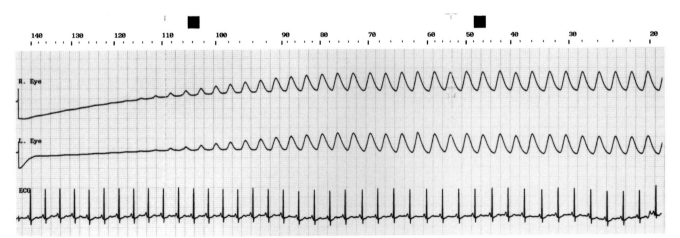

FIGURE 19–7. Ocular pneumoplethysmographic test results on day 494 from same patient represented in Figure 19–6. The numerical scale at the top of the record is the declining intraocular pressure in millimeters of mercury. These results were obtained with the instrument available in 1993.

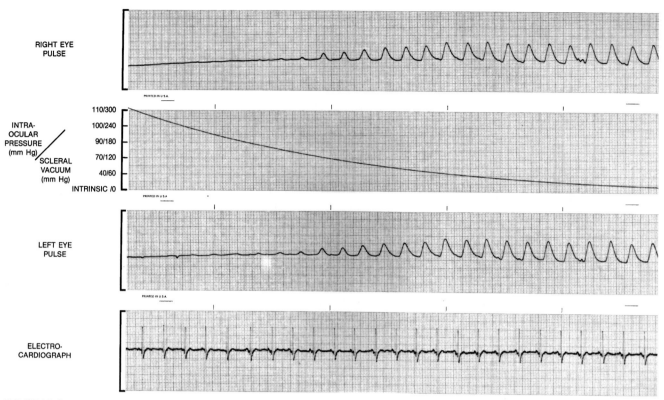

FIGURE 19–8. Preoperative ocular pneumoplethysmographic test results from one of the four S_i-O_c patients with severe stenosis of the proximal left internal carotid artery and total occlusion of the right (see text for description of patient groups). The right and left ocular blood flows are 0.86 and 0.93 mL per minute, respectively. The right and left ophthalmic systolic pressures are 91 and 94 mm Hg, respectively. The ophthalmobrachial systolic pressure (OBSP) indices were −22.0 and −19.0 mm Hg, respectively. The OBSP indices are calculated from the respective ophthalmic systolic pressures (OSP) and the brachial systolic pressure (BSP) with the formula OBSP = OSP − 39.0 − 0.43 BSP, as described by Gee and associates.[23] That article also contains the explanations for our preference of the OBSP index over the OSP/BSP ratio. These results were obtained with the instrument available from 1978 to 1984. (From Nicholas GG, Hashemi H, Gee W, Reed JF III: The cerebral hyperperfusion syndrome: Diagnostic value of ocular pneumoplethysmography. *J Vasc Surg.* 1993;17:690–695; with permission from Mosby-Year Book, Inc.)

for both patients and controls. All the data comparisons were done with one-way analysis of variance, Student *t* tests, or paired *t* tests. Because of the large numbers of statistical tests performed, statistical significance was set at $P < 0.01$. Data are reported as means ± SEM. If the data from the S_i-N_c and S_i-S_c groups are combined, the OBF improvement as a result of carotid reconstruction was 148 percent for the eight patients and 35 percent for the 529 controls. Thus, the improvement for the patients was 4.2 times as great as that for the controls. In the S_i-O_c group, the OBF improvement for the four patients was 267 percent, or 4.3 times the 64 percent improvement in the 62 controls.

The most important element of these distinctions is the outcome of the 12 operations. All four patients in the S_i-O_c group developed profound symptoms of cerebral hyperperfusion. Two of the four had associated intracerebral hemorrhages that were fatal. Another patient died after ipsilateral hemispheric infarct and persistent coma. The last of the four patients had fully recovered, at the time of discharge 9 days after surgery, from a profound ipsilateral hemispheric insult. In contrast, only one of the eight patients in the other two groups had any findings suggestive of cerebral hyperperfusion syndrome, and these were mild and transient.

Carotid Reconstruction

The control series of 701 carotid reconstructions cited in the preceding section was expanded by an additional 1294

carotid reconstructions, for a total of 1995 operations. Seven categories of patients were established, based on the previously described preoperative arteriographic findings (N, S, or O) and the character of the lesion on the side of operation. The data are presented in Table 19–6. Within each group of patients, the differences between the mean OBSP and OBF (side operated versus side opposite) and the differences between the mean OBSP and OBF (preoperative versus postoperative) were evaluated using a paired *t* test. The data are reported as means plus or minus standard deviations. Due to the large number of statistical tests, a Bonferroni adjusted significance level of 0.01 was used to control for experiment-wise error and to reduce the possibility of detecting spurious differences.

N-N Patients. Arteriography in these 316 patients demonstrated no lesions of hemodynamic consequence in either carotid hemisystem. All patients had hemispheric or monocular symptoms or both, appropriate to the side of carotid endarterectomy. There were 146 right and 170 left carotid repairs. The preoperative and postoperative data for the right and left subgroups were analyzed separately, with the expectation that no significant difference existed between the two subgroups, which was confirmed. The collective data for the two subgroups appear first in Table 19–6.

N-O Patients. Arteriography in these 64 patients demonstrated no lesions of hemodynamic consequence on the side of operation, but all had contralateral carotid occlusions. All

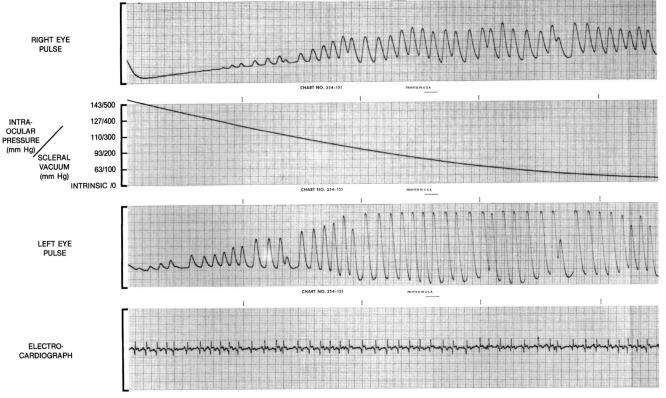

FIGURE 19-9. Postoperative ocular pneumoplethysmographic test results from the same patient represented in Figure 19-8 after left carotid endarterectomy. The right and left ocular blood flow rates are 2.63 and 5.38 mL per minute, respectively. The ophthalmic systolic pressures are 127 and 140 mm Hg, respectively. The ophthalmobrachial systolic pressure indices are −6.6 and 6.4 mm Hg, respectively. The latter figures reflect the occluded right internal carotid artery and the now-patent left internal carotid artery. These results were obtained with the instrument available from 1978 to 1984. (From Nicholas GG, Hashemi H, Gee W, Reed JF III: The cerebral hyperperfusion syndrome: Diagnostic value of ocular pneumoplethysmography. *J Vasc Surg.* 1993;17:690–695; with permission of Mosby-Year Book, Inc.)

patients had hemispheric or monocular symptoms or both, appropriate to the side of carotid endarterectomy. The data from this group appear second in Table 19-6.

S-N Patients. Arteriography in these 992 patients demonstrated ipsilateral carotid stenoses of hemodynamic consequence and contralateral patent vessels. There were 504 right and 488 left carotid endarterectomies. The preoperative and postoperative data from the right and left subgroups were analyzed separately, with the expectation that no significant difference existed between the two subgroups, which was confirmed. The collective data for the two subgroups appear third in Table 19-6.

S-S Patients. Arteriography in these 272 patients demonstrated bilateral carotid stenoses of hemodynamic consequence. Of these 272 patients, 112 (41%) underwent repair of the contralateral severe stenoses at later dates. The preoperative and postoperative data from the second operations were comparable to the data in the S-N group and are not reported. The data from the first operations appear fourth in Table 19-6.

S-O Patients. Arteriography in these 171 patients demonstrated ipsilateral carotid stenoses of hemodynamic consequence and contralateral carotid occlusions. The data from this group appear fifth in Table 19-6.

TABLE 19-3. Ocular Blood Flow Rate* in S_i-N_c Group†
Carotid Lesions

	Patients (n = 5)	Control‡ (n = 415)	P Value
Preoperative	1.81 ± 0.22	1.16 ± 0.02	0.0004
Postoperative	4.46 ± 0.12	1.54 ± 0.03	< 0.0001
P value	< 0.0001	< 0.0001	

*Measured in mL/minute.
†See text for description of study groups.
‡The control data have been modified from those originally reported.[38] The constant used in the previous study was 0.0016 but was recently modified slightly, to 0.00149.[13] All data in this table were calculated using the corrected constant of 0.00149.
From Nicholas GG, Hashemi H, Gee W, Reed JF III: The cerebral hyperperfusion syndrome: Diagnostic value of ocular pneumoplethysmography. *J Vasc Surg.* 1993; 17:690–695; with permission of Mosby-Year Book, Inc.

TABLE 19-4. Ocular Blood Flow Rate* in S_i-S_c Group†
Carotid Lesions

	Patients (n = 3)	Control‡ (n = 114)	P Value
Preoperative	1.90 ± 0.12	1.15 ± 0.05	0.0155
Postoperative	4.75 ± 0.19	1.66 ± 0.07	< 0.0001
P value	0.011	< 0.0001	

*Measured in mL/minute.
†See text for description of study groups.
‡The control data have been modified from those originally reported.[38] The constant used in the previous study was 0.0016 but was recently modified slightly, to 0.00149.[13] All data in this table were calculated using the corrected constant of 0.00149.
From Nicholas GG, Hashemi H, Gee W, Reed JF III: The cerebral hyperperfusion syndrome: Diagnostic value of ocular pneumoplethysmography. *J Vasc Surg.* 1993; 17:690–695; with permission of Mosby-Year Book, Inc.

TABLE 19–5. Ocular Blood Flow Rate* in S_i-O_c Group† Carotid Lesions

	Patients (n = 4)	Control‡ (n = 62)	P Value
Preoperative	1.29 ± 0.21	1.09 ± 0.06	NS
Postoperative	4.73 ± 0.32	1.79 ± 0.09	< 0.0001
P value	0.006	< 0.0001	

*Measured in mL/minute.

†See text for description of study groups.

‡The control data have been modified from those originally reported.[38] The constant used in the calculation of ocular blood flow in the previous report was 0.0016 but was recently modified slightly, to 0.00149.[13] All data in this table were calculated using the corrected constant of 0.00149.

NS, not significant.

From Nicholas GG, Hashemi H, Gee W, Reed JF III: The cerebral hyperperfusion syndrome: Diagnostic value of ocular pneumoplethysmography. *J Vasc Surg.* 1993;17:690–695; with permission of Mosby-Year Book, Inc.

O-N Patients. This group must be distinguished from the previously described N-O group. The N-O group underwent repairs on the side of the patent carotid arteries. Arteriography in the 50 patients in the O-N group demonstrated ipsilateral carotid occlusions and contralateral carotid patency. Of the 50 patients, 24 underwent bypass of occluded common carotid arteries; 19 with internal carotid occlusions had endarterectomies of ipsilateral severe external carotid stenoses; and seven with internal carotid occlusions underwent ipsilateral external carotid–to–internal carotid (EC–IC) bypasses. The data from this group appear sixth in Table 19–6.

O-O Patients. Arteriography in these 18 patients demonstrated bilateral carotid occlusions. Of the 18 patients, seven had bypass of common carotid occlusions; eight with internal carotid occlusions underwent endarterectomies of ipsilateral severe external carotid stenoses; and three with internal carotid occlusions had ipsilateral EC–IC bypasses performed. The data from this group appear last in Table 19–6.

Table 19–7 summarizes the percentage improvements in the OBSP and OBF means, side operated and side opposite, in the seven patient groups. As expected, the percentage OBSP mean improvements closely paralleled the percentage OBF mean improvements, with one exception. In the O-O group, on the side operated, the OBF mean improvement was considerably greater than the OBSP mean improvement, 80 percent versus 53 percent. This phenomenon illustrates the value of repressurization of collateral routes in the presence of bilateral main channel arterial occlusions, in which hypoperfusion rather than embolic events predominates as the cause of symptoms.

The preoperative and postoperative OBSP means, side operated and side opposite, for the seven groups are depicted graphically in Figure 19–10. Similarly, the OBF data are demonstrated graphically in Figure 19–11. It is readily apparent that the preoperative OBSP and OBF means on the side of operation progressively decline as the severity and multiplicity of the carotid lesions increase.

Regressions of the means of the OBF data from Table 19–6 on the respective OBSP data means, side operated and side opposite, preoperative and postoperative, are contained in Figures 19–12 and 19–13. The slopes of the regressions, preoperative and postoperative on the side opposite, and preoperative on the side operated, are identical, 0.013, and the correlation coefficients for these three slopes vary between 0.936 and 0.992. However, the slope of the regression of the postoperative data on the side operated is quite different, 0.006, and the correlation coefficient of 0.484 is weak. It is unlikely that identical slopes for three of the four regressions are a coincidence. All the postoperative OPG tests were performed within several days of operation, prior

TABLE 19–6. Preoperative and Postoperative Ocular Hemodynamics

Operations (n)	Status	Arteriogram Side of Operation	Side Opposite	OBSP (mm Hg)* Side of Operation	Side Opposite		OBF (ml/min)* Side of Operation	Side Opposite	
316	Preoperative	N	N	12.4 ± 9.5	13.1 ± 9.4	P < 0.001	1.31 ± 0.51	1.35 ± 0.51	P < 0.001
	Postoperative			11.7 ± 10.0	12.5 ± 8.7	P < 0.001	1.45 ± 0.52	1.47 ± 0.51	P = 0.080
				P = 0.368	P = 0.406		P < 0.001	P < 0.001	
64	Preoperative	N	O	11.4 ± 8.3	−8.7 ± 12.4	P < 0.001	1.34 ± 0.46	1.04 ± 0.35	P < 0.001
	Postoperative			10.5 ± 12.6	−8.4 ± 12.6	P < 0.001	1.56 ± 0.71	1.14 ± 0.48	P < 0.001
				P = 0.953	P = 0.987		P = 0.801	P = 0.869	
992	Preoperative	S	N	0.2 ± 12.3	11.3 ± 9.1	P < 0.001	1.16 ± 0.47	1.35 ± 0.52	P < 0.001
	Postoperative			10.3 ± 10.5	11.7 ± 8.8	P < 0.001	1.56 ± 0.60	1.51 ± 0.54	P < 0.001
				P < 0.001	P = 0.967		P < 0.001	P < 0.001	
272	Preoperative	S	S	−8.1 ± 14.3	−3.2 ± 13.7	P < 0.001	1.06 ± 0.48	1.15 ± 0.47	P < 0.001
	Postoperative			6.6 ± 11.1	0.1 ± 12.8	P < 0.001	1.60 ± 0.69	1.34 ± 0.52	P < 0.001
				P < 0.001	P < 0.001		P < 0.001	P < 0.001	
171	Preoperative	S	O	−11.1 ± 13.4	−18.4 ± 14.8	P < 0.001	1.04 ± 0.46	0.95 ± 0.43	P < 0.001
	Postoperative			5.3 ± 12.4	−12.4 ± 14.3	P < 0.001	1.65 ± 0.71	1.20 ± 0.57	P < 0.001
				P < 0.001	P < 0.001		P < 0.001	P < 0.001	
50	Preoperative	O	N	−17.8 ± 17.8	5.2 ± 9.0	P < 0.001	0.96 ± 0.38	1.36 ± 0.46	P < 0.001
	Postoperative			−4.2 ± 14.8	8.6 ± 8.5	P < 0.001	1.40 ± 0.60	1.54 ± 0.58	P = 0.027
				P < 0.001	P = 0.020		P < 0.001	P = 0.079	
18	Preoperative	O	O	−24.6 ± 9.8	−23.2 ± 10.7	P = 0.603	0.81 ± 0.38	0.95 ± 0.38	P = 0.020
	Postoperative			−7.6 ± 14.3	−16.1 ± 16.0	P = 0.013	1.46 ± 0.60	1.19 ± 0.36	P = 0.010
				P < 0.001	P = 0.112		P < 0.001	P = 0.015	

*All data are presented as mean ± one standard deviation.

N, patent carotid artery; O, occluded carotid artery; OBF, ocular blood flow rate; OBSP, ophthalmobrachial systolic pressure index; S, severely stenosed carotid artery.

TABLE 19–7. Ocular Hemodynamic Improvement

Operations (n)	Arteriogram		OBSP Increase, mm Hg (%)		OBF Increase, mL/min (%)	
	Side of Operation	Side Opposite	Side of Operation	Side Opposite	Side of Operation	Side Opposite
316	N	N	NS	NS	0.14 (11)	0.12 (9)
64	N	O	NS	NS	NS	NS
992	S	N	9.1 (28)	NS	0.40 (34)	0.16 (12)
272	S	S	14.7 (46)	3.3 (9)	0.54 (51)	0.19 (17)
171	S	O	16.4 (51)	6.0 (10)	0.61 (59)	0.25 (26)
50	O	N	13.6 (43)	NS	0.44 (46)	NS
18	O	O	17.0 (53)	NS	0.65 (80)	NS

N, patent carotid artery; NS, not significant; O, occluded carotid artery; OBF, ocular blood flow; OBSP, ophthalmobrachial systolic pressure index; S, severely stenosed carotid artery.

to discharge from the hospital. It is probable that the relative postoperative oculovascular hyperdynamics on the side of operation do not persist. This hypothesis could not be investigated, as few patients return to the hospital for serial postoperative assessment. However, the data in Table 19–6 do suggest that any element of autoregulation of choroidal blood flow is limited in the circumstances described.

In the N-N group of patients, arteriography demonstrated no carotid lesions of hemodynamic consequence. Under these circumstances, carotid repair would not be expected to result in any improvement of ocular hemodynamics. The observations related to the N-N group in Tables 19–6 and Table 19–7 confirm that there was no improvement of the OBSP index as a result of operation. However, modest bilateral OBF improvement was observed, and this improvement was significant. The probable explanation is that cardiac hemodynamics were improved in these patients immediately before, during, and after the operations as a result of the intensive management of these patients while hospitalized. It is reasonable to assume that some small portion of the postoperative improvement of OBF observed in the other six groups is similarly attributable.

As reported by Bill,[39] the combined blood flow of the choroid, iris, ciliary body, and retina in the anesthetized rabbit was 1056 mg/minute, or approximately 1.06 mL minute. Chen and colleagues[12] reported the average diameter

of the rabbit eye to be 18.36 mm. Our preoperative observations in the N-N group of patients indicated an average bilateral OBF of 1.33 mL/minute. The ratio of the diameters of the rabbit and human eyes (0.77) closely approximates the ratio of the OBFs of the rabbit and human eyes (0.80). Also, the preoperative OBF average of 1.33 mL/minute in our N-N group of patients is comparable to the average of 1.27 mL/minute in nine patients without giant-cell arteritis, as reported by Bosley and associates.[35]

ASYMPTOMATIC SEVERE CAROTID STENOSIS

The problem of asymptomatic severe carotid stenosis is presently the subject of a federally funded study.[40] The original intent of the OPG, when used with proximal common carotid compression, was to noninvasively predict the fate of a cerebral hemisphere if a severe carotid stenosis was allowed to progress to total occlusion.[8, 41] Two reports document the close agreement of the noninvasively obtained collateral OSP with the internal carotid back pressure (stump pressure) measured operatively.[8, 41] In patients undergoing carotid ligation without graft replacement, it has been shown that stump pressures of less than 60 mm Hg are usually associated with stroke, that those between 60 and 68 mm Hg may be associated with stroke, but that those of 70 mm Hg or greater had no associated strokes.[42]

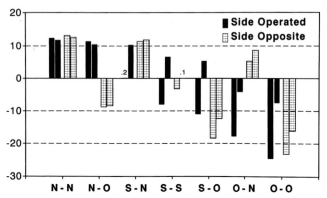

FIGURE 19–10. Graphic representation of the preoperative and postoperative ophthalmobrachial systolic pressure (OBSP) means (mm Hg) from the seven groups listed in Table 19–6. The preoperative OBSP index mean on the side that was operated on in the S-N group and the postoperative OBSP index mean on the opposite side in the S-S group are too small to be seen graphically. They are represented numerically (0.2 and 0.1, respectively).

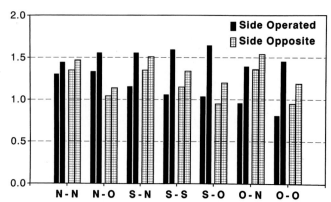

FIGURE 19–11. Graphic representation of the preoperative and postoperative ocular blood flow rate means (mL/min) from the seven groups listed in Table 19–6.

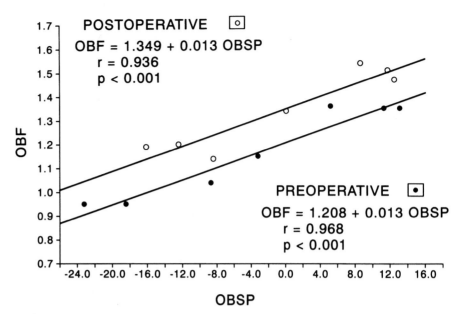

FIGURE 19–12. Regression of ocular blood flow (OBF) (mL/min) on ophthalmobrachial systolic pressure index (OBSP), preoperatively and postoperatively, on the side opposite the side of operation.

Lehigh Valley Hospital has been a participant in the Asymptomatic Carotid Atherosclerosis Study since its inception in 1987.[40] The study protocol did not include a provision for assessing patients with the OPG and proximal common carotid compression. However, some patients with asymptomatic severe carotid stenoses have been clinically managed outside of the study. The principal reason for noninclusion has been lack of patient-institution proximity. The following is a case report of the management of one of these patients.

A 67-year-old member of the cardiology staff of this institution had been serially followed for an asymptomatic right carotid bruit. This individual had recently retired from clinical practice and moved to another state. His most recent return for reevaluation documented considerable deterioration of the right ocular hemodynamics by OPG, and the carotid duplex insonation suggested progression from a very severe to a preocclusively stenosed proximal right internal carotid artery. He had undergone coronary artery balloon

arterioplasties on several occasions but presently had no cardiac symptoms. Prophylactic operation was considered, but the physician-patient asked if there was some method of assessing his risk if the lesion was allowed to progress to total occlusion. The carotid duplex insonation had confirmed that the lower cervical segment of the right common carotid artery was devoid of detectable atherosclerosis. The patient accepted a repeat OPG test in conjunction with carotid compression, the results of which are shown in Figure 19–14. The right collateral OSP is less than 70 mm Hg. Figure 19–15 is the arteriogram, which confirmed the preocclusive proximal right internal carotid stenosis. As predicted by the preoperative OPG test with carotid compression, the operative systolic stump pressure was less than 70 mm Hg. It was 55 mm Hg. The operation was uneventful, and the patient has remained asymptomatic in the 2-year interval.

For many patients, the anxiety associated with the nonoperative management of asymptomatic severe cartoid stenosis

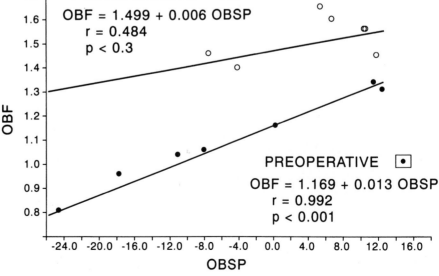

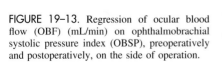

FIGURE 19–13. Regression of ocular blood flow (OBF) (mL/min) on ophthalmobrachial systolic pressure index (OBSP), preoperatively and postoperatively, on the side of operation.

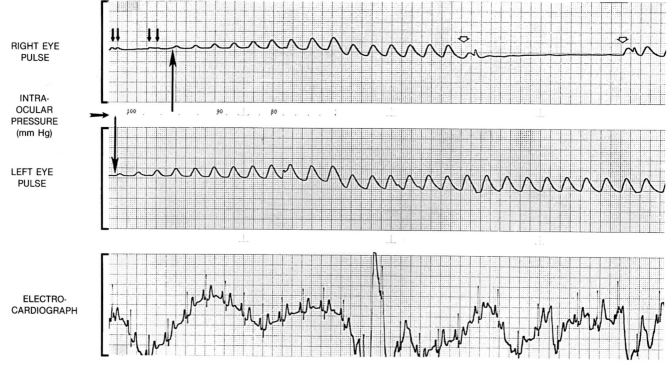

FIGURE 19–14. Results from an ocular pneumoplethysmographic test with right common carotid compression to determine the collateral ophthalmic systolic pressure (COSP). In the right eye pulse channel, four *small arrows* point to recording artifacts. The two *long arrows* in the right and left eye pulse channels point to the respective initial eye pulses. The intraocular pressure (IOP) at which the first right eye pulse was observed was 94 mm Hg, whereas that at which the left eye pulse was observed was 101 mm Hg. In the IOP channel, each 10 mm Hg is separated by four *dots*, which denote intervals of 2 mm Hg. Note that the numbers and dots cease at the 70 mm Hg mark. In the right eye pulse channel, the two *arrowheads* are located at the beginning and end of the right common carotid compression, during which no right eye pulse is detected, which indicates that the COSP is less than 70 mm Hg. The duration of the carotid compression was 8 seconds, at a paper speed of 10 mm per second.

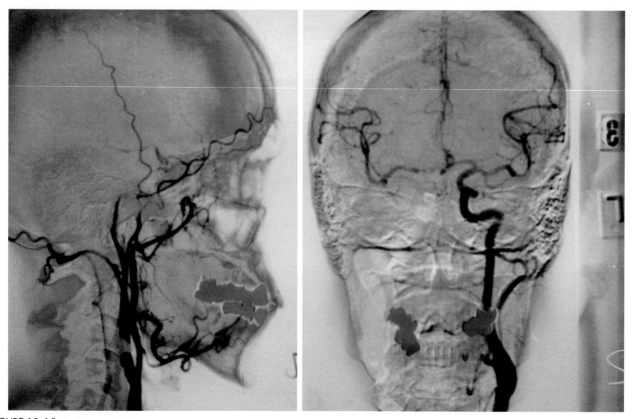

FIGURE 19–15. Composite of the arteriogram in the patient whose tests results are shown in Figure 19–14. On the *left* is the right lateral projection, which demonstrates the preocclusive proximal right internal carotid stenosis. Note that the ophthalmic artery and the distal interval carotid artery are being filled from the external carotid artery, prior to the arrival of dye in the internal carotid artery. On the *right* is the anterior-posterior projection of the selective left carotid arteriogram. The left internal carotid artery fills both anterior cerebral arteries and both middle cerebral arteries.

is considerable. The effect of this continued anxiety should not be minimized.

OBSERVATIONS

Two recent editorials summarize a broad survey of instruments designed to assess the extracranial and intracranial arterial system.[43, 44] One stated:

It is . . . clear that both arteriography and ultrasonography have a variability that make them less than perfect for determining the degree of stenosis.

Is there a possible solution to this dilemma? It is our opinion that lesions that reach a threshold of 50 percent or greater stenosis (75% area-reducing stenosis), regardless of the method of measurement, should prompt consideration for intervention.[43]

It is precisely this degree of stenosis that 2 decades of OPG work has focused on. Others have suggested that the economics of screening patients for carotid lesions of hemodynamic consequence dictate the use of OPG for this purpose.[45]

REFERENCES

1. Winsor T: Influence of arterial disease on systolic blood pressure gradients of the extremity. *Am J Med Sci.* 1950;220:117–126.
2. Winsor T: *Peripheral Vascular Disease.* Springfield, IL: Charles C. Thomas; 1959.
3. Borrás A, Méndez MS, Martínez A: Ophthalmic/brachial artery pressure ratio in man. *Am J Ophthalmol.* 1969;67:684–688.
4. Bailliart P: La pression arterielle dans les branchesde l'artere centrale de la retine, nouvelle technique pour la determiner. *Ann Ocul.* 1917;154:648–666.
5. Kukán F: Ergebnisse der blutdruckmessungen miteinem neuen ophthalmodynamometer. *Z Augenheilkd.* 1936;90:160–191.
6. Galin MA, Baras I, Cavero R: Ophthalmodynamometry using suction. *Arch Ophthalmol.* 1969;81:494–500.
7. Best M, Kelly TA, Galin MA: The ocular pulse—technical features. *Acta Ophthalmol (Copenh).* 1970;48:357–368.
8. Gee W, Mehigan JT, Wylie EJ: Measurement of collateral cerebral hemispheric blood pressure by ocular pneumoplethysmography. *Am J Surg.* 1975;130:121–127.
9. Gee W, Smith CA, Hinsen CE, Wylie EJ: Ocular pneumoplethysmography in carotid artery disease. *Med Instrum.* 1974;8:244–248.
10. Gee W, Smith CA, Hinsen CE: Ocular pneumoplethysmography and method of operation. Patent no. 3, 911, 903. Washington, DC: US Government Printing Office; 1975.
11. Gee W, Oller DW, Homer LD, Bailey RC: Simultaneous bilateral determination of the systolic pressure of the ophthalmic arteries by ocular pneumoplethysmography. *Invest Ophthalmol Vis Sci.* 1977;16:86–89.
12. Chen C, Reed JF III, Rice DC, et al: Biomechanics of ocular pneumoplethysmography. *J Biomech Eng.* 1993;115:231–238.
13. Gee W, Reed JF III: Ocular pneumoplethysmographic evaluation of carotid lesions: Gee method. In Ernst CB, Stanley JC, eds.: *Current Therapy in Vascular Surgery,* 2nd ed. Philadelphia: BC Decker; 1991:20–24.
14. Duke-Elder S, Wybar KC: The anatomy of the visual system. In Duke-Elder S, ed. *System of Ophthalmology,* Vol. 2. St. Louis: CV Mosby; 1961:80–81.
15. Hoffner KJ: Biometry of 7500 cataractous eyes. *Am J Ophthalmol.* 1980;90:360–368.
16. DiChiro C: Angiographic topography of the choroid. *Am J Ophthalmol.* 1962;54:232–237.
17. Hahn FJ, Chu WK: Ocular volume measured by CT scans. *Neuroradiology.* 1984;26:419–420.
18. Crow W, Guinto FC Jr, Amearo E, Stewart K: Normal in-vivo eye dimensions by computed tomography. *J Comput Assist Tomogr.* 1982;6:708–710.
19. Miller D: Pressure of the lid on the eye. *Arch Ophthalmol.* 1967;78:328–330.
20. Gee W: Ocular pneumoplethysmography after lens implantation. *J Cataract Refract Surg.* 1988;14:417–420.
21. Recommendations for preventing possible transmission of human T-lymphotropic virus type III/lymphadenopathy-associated virus from tears. *MMWR.* 1985;34:533–534.
22. Gee W: Carotid physiology with ocular pneumoplethysmography. *Stroke.* 1982;13:666–673.
23. Gee W, Lucke JF, Madden AE: Collateral compensation of severe carotid stenosis. *Eur J Vasc Surg.* 1989;3:297–301.
24. Gibbs JM, Wise RJS, Leenders KL, Jones T: Evaluation of cerebral perfusion reserve in patients with carotid-artery occlusion. *Lancet.* 1984;1:310–314.
25. Powers WJ, Raichle ME, Grubb RL: Positron emission tomography to assess cerebral perfusion (letter). *Lancet.* 1985;1:102–103.
26. Gibbs JM, Wise RJ, Leenders KL, et al: Cerebral hemodynamics in occlusive carotid-artery disease (letter). *Lancet.* 1985;1:933–934.
27. Leblanc R, Tyler JL, Mohr G, et al: Hemodynamic and metabolic effects of cerebral revascularization. *J Neurosurg.* 1987;66:529–535.
28. Schroeder T: Hemodynamic significance of internal carotid artery disease. *Acta Neurol Scand.* 1988;77:353–372.
29. Gee W: Ocular pneumoplethysmography in cardiac pacing. *PACE.* 1983;6:1268–1272.
30. Gee W, Smith RL, Perline RK, Gallagher HS: Assessment of intra-aortic balloon pumping by ocular pneumoplethysmography. *Am Surg.* 1986;52:489–491.
31. Reed JF III, Gee W, Witham MG: Ocular pneumoplethysmography in IABC. In Quaal SJ, ed. *Comprehensive Intraaortic Balloon Counterpulsation,* 2nd ed. St. Louis: CV Mosby; 1993:165–170.
32. Oster H, Stanley TH, Olsen DB, et al: Regional blood flow after intra-aortic balloon pumping before and after cardiogenic shock. *Trans Am Soc Artif Intern Organs.* 1974;20:721–723.
33. Bosley TM, Cohen MS, Gee W, et al: Amplitude of the ocular pneumoplethysmography waveform is correlated with cardiac output. *Stroke.* 1993;24:6–9.
34. Saha M, Muppala MR, Castaldo JE, et al: The impact of cardiac index on cerebral hemodynamics. *Stroke.* 1993;24:1686–1690.
35. Bosley TM, Savino PJ, Sergott RC, et al: Ocular pneumoplethysmography can help in the diagnosis of giant-cell arteritis. *Arch Ophthalmol.* 1989;107:379–381.
36. Ulrich C, Ulrich W-D, Ulrich D: Funktionsdiagnostische behandlungskontrolle der arteriitis temporalis. *Fortschr Ophthalmol.* 1990;87:667–670.
37. Nicholas GG, Hashemi H, Gee W, Reed JF III: The cerebral hyperperfusion syndrome: Diagnostic value of ocular pneumoplethysmography. *J Vasc Surg.* 1993;17:690–695.
38. Gee W, Perline RK, Madden AE: Physiology of carotid endarterectomy with ocular pneumoplethysmography. *J Vasc Surg.* 1986;4:129–135.
39. Bill A: Circulation in the eye. In Renken EM, Michel CC, eds. *The Cardiovascular System, Vol. IV, Pt. 2.* Bethesda: American Physiological Society; 1984:1001–1034.
40. The Asymptomatic Carotid Atherosclerosis Study Group: Study design for randomized prospective trial of carotid endarterectomy for asymptomatic atherosclerosis. *Stroke.* 1989;20:844–850.
41. Cooke PA, Gee W, Wylie EJ: The competence of the circle of Willis in extracranial cerebrovascular atherosclerosis. *S Afr J Surg.* 1975;13:7–14.
42. Ehrenfeld WK, Stoney RJ, Wylie EJ: Relation of carotid stump pressure to safety of carotid ligation. *Surgery.* 1983;93:299–305.
43. Hobson RW II, Strandness DE Jr: Carotid artery stenosis: What's in the measurement? *J Vasc Surg.* 1993;18:1069–1070.
44. Ackerman RH, Candia MR: Identifying clinically relevant carotid disease. *Stroke.* 1994;25:1–3.
45. Fisher FS, Riles TS, Oldford F: Is ocular pneumoplethysmography (Gee) a cost-effective screening test for asymptomatic carotid occlusive disease? *J Vasc Technol.* 1993;17:135–139.

CHAPTER 20

Duplex Scanning and Spectral Analysis

TED R. KOHLER, R. EUGENE ZIERLER, and D. E. STRANDNESS, JR.

Although many noninvasive tests for carotid artery disease are sensitive enough for screening purposes, all have limitations. Indirect tests such as periorbital Doppler and ocularplethysmography detect distant effects of pressure-reducing lesions. Although they reliably diagnose these high-grade lesions, they cannot detect less severe disease and fail to differentiate near from total occlusions.[1] Direct tests image arteries, measure flow velocities within them, or both. For example, ultrasound B-mode imaging visualizes calcified plaque but cannot reliably distinguish among noncalcified plaque, thrombus, and flowing blood. Therefore, its accuracy for measuring high-grade stenoses or detecting total occlusions is poor. At the other extreme, continuous-wave Doppler used alone is accurate for detecting high-grade stenoses but is inaccurate for diagnosing mild degrees of narrowing.[2–4] Ultrasonic duplex scanning, first described at the University of Washington in 1974,[5–7] overcomes these problems. The duplex scanner combines a real-time B-mode ultrasound imager with a pulsed Doppler flow detector and spectrum analyzer. It can accurately classify carotid disease ranging from mild wall irregularity to total occlusion. This chapter outlines the theoretical and practical aspects of this technique and reviews its advantages, limitations, and research applications.

DUPLEX THEORY AND INSTRUMENTATION

The duplex scanner uses ultrasound for both imaging and flow-velocity measurement. The ultrasound beam is backscattered by interfaces between tissues of different acoustic impedances. The amplitude of the backscattered signal is displayed as shades of gray along an image line, corresponding to the path of the ultrasound beam. Multiple ultrasonographic beams from a rotating scan head or linear array transducer are displayed side-by-side to produce a two-dimensional image of the tissues in the neck. Arteries are recognized by the pulsation of the echoes from the arterial wall. The pulsed Doppler detects frequency shifts from the moving blood cells in the lumen. Blood cells moving toward the Doppler probe shift the frequency upward, and those moving away shift it downward. Blood velocity and frequency shift are related by the Doppler equation

$$F_d = F_o\ 2v\ \cos\ \theta/c$$

where F_d is the Doppler-shifted frequency, F_o is the ultrasound transmitting frequency, v is the blood cell velocity, θ is the angle between the ultrasound beam and the direction of blood flow, and c is the constant speed of sound in tissue. The Doppler beam is represented on the B-mode image as a white line (Fig. 20–1), permitting measurement of the angle θ. Thus, blood velocity can be estimated for a given transmitting frequency by measuring F_d and θ.

The pulsed Doppler permits selection of velocity information from a discrete three-dimensional region in the scan plane known as the sample volume. The pulsed Doppler

crystal acts alternatively as transmitter and receiver; it transmits a short pulse of ultrasound and then waits a specific period of time before acting as receiver. Because ultrasound travels through tissues with a constant velocity, the length of time between transmission and reception determines the distance traveled by the received signal. Since the ultrasound pulse must make the probe-to-probe round-trip during the waiting interval, the depth from which the beam was reflected and the velocity data obtained represent half this distance. The waiting interval can be adjusted to change the sample volume depth. Varying the length of time the receiver is open alters the size of the sample volume. The sample volume is indicated by a dot on the white line representing the Doppler path on the B-mode image (Fig. 20–2). Thus, the duplex scanner provides accurate velocity information from known locations along visualized arteries.

The superficial location of the extracranial carotid system permits the use of relatively high ultrasound-transmitting frequencies, which produce high-resolution images. The initial version of the duplex scanner contained three 5-mHz ultrasound transducers mounted on a rotary wheel, which provided the sector B-mode image. A movable, single-gated 5-mHz pulsed-Doppler transducer was located on the side of the scan head, with the Doppler beam aligned in the same plane as the B-mode image. Because separate B-mode and Doppler transducers were used, time-sharing circuitry was needed to avoid interference between the two systems during simultaneous acquisition of B-mode and Doppler data. As it was difficult to keep the Doppler beam properly aligned in the B-mode image plane, the system was redesigned to use the same ultrasound transducers for both imaging and Doppler functions. Newer, linear array transducers do not use a rotating scan head. Their ultrasonographic beams are steered electronically. They have the disadvantage of a larger footprint and poorer lateral resolution. The duplex scanner holds the B-mode image in memory and displays it while one of

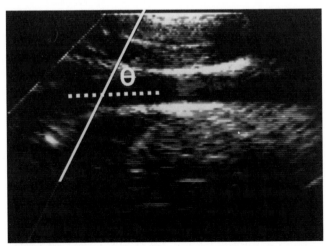

FIGURE 20–1. B-mode image of the common carotid artery with the Doppler beam represented by a *solid white line*, permitting measurement of the angle θ between the Doppler beam and the axis of the artery *(broken line)*.

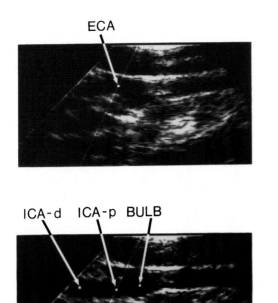

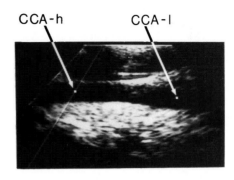

FIGURE 20–2. Standard recording sites. External carotid artery *(ECA)*, internal carotid artery proximal *(ICA-p)* and distal *(ICA-d)*, the carotid bulb *(BULB)*, and the low *(CCA-l)* and high *(CCA-h)* common carotid artery. The Doppler beam is represented by a *white line* and the sample volume by a *dot* on that line.

the transducers functions as the pulsed Doppler. The operator can then alternate between imaging and Doppler functions. This system permits accurate placement of the pulsed Doppler sample volume within the imaged vessels to evaluate local flow patterns. A Doppler pulse-repetition frequency of 19.2 kHz is used, facilitating detection of Doppler shifts of up to 9.6 kHz. The sample volume is approximately 3 mm³ at a focal point of 2 cm.

SPECTRAL ANALYSIS

Because blood cells within the sample volume travel at many different velocities, the Doppler-shifted signal is a composite of frequency components, each corresponding to a particular velocity. The amplitude of each component is proportional to the number of blood cells traveling at its corresponding velocity. Interpretation of the Doppler-shifted signal requires measurement of both the amplitude and frequency of each component, a technique referred to as spectral analysis. The examiner performs a rudimentary form of spectral analysis when listening to the Doppler signal. Pitch is proportional to velocity (frequency), loudness (amplitude) to the number of blood cells traveling at a particular velocity, and the pureness of the tone to the uniformity of the flow pattern (laminar versus turbulent flow).

For carotid studies, more sophisticated signal processing is performed with a spectrum analyzer. Using a fast Fourier transform, this instrument displays the frequency and amplitude content of the Doppler-shifted signal. Typically, the signal is analyzed for frequencies ranging from reverse flow of 3 kHz to forward flow of 7 kHz. With a standard 5-mHz probe and Doppler angle of 60 degrees, this corresponds to reverse flow of 92 cm/second and forward flow of 216 cm/second. The fast Fourier transform determines the frequency

composition in 100-Hz intervals (or bins) and analyzes the signal 400 times per second. The data are displayed graphically, with frequency on the ordinate and time on the abscissa. The amplitude of the signal in each frequency bin is displayed as a shade of gray (Fig. 20–3). Real-time spectral analysis is possible with dedicated microprocessors. Digitized data are stored for ensemble averaging and further computer analysis.

When the vessel narrows, velocity must increase to main-

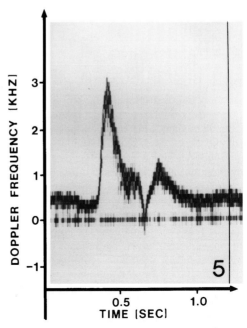

FIGURE 20–3. Typical spectral waveform showing time on the abscissa and frequency on the ordinate, with amplitude indicated by shades of gray.

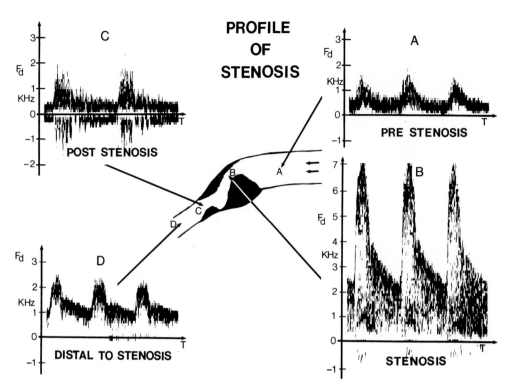

FIGURE 20–4. Spectral waveforms associated with a significant stenosis. The proximal waveform is blunted because of decreased flow. Increased frequency is noted in the stenosis; spectral broadening is evident in all waveforms.

tain constant flow. Thus, the frequency shift of the backscattered signal from a region of stenosis increases as the diameter decreases. Turbulence develops immediately downstream from the stenosis and causes a widening of the frequency band, called spectral broadening (Fig. 20–4). These two features—spectral broadening and increased frequency—provide the basic criteria for classification of carotid artery stenosis. Because flow velocity is inversely proportional to lumen area and therefore to diameter squared, appreciable increases in frequency do not occur until the diameter becomes narrowed by 50 percent. Spectral broadening is a more sensitive indicator of less severe stenosis.

COLOR-FLOW IMAGING

Real-time color-flow imaging is an alternative to spectral waveform analysis for displaying the pulsed Doppler information obtained by duplex scanning.[8] In contrast to spectral analysis, which evaluates the entire frequency and amplitude content of the signal at a selected sample site, color-flow imaging provides a single estimate of the Doppler-shifted frequency or flow velocity for each site within the B-mode image. Thus, spectral waveforms actually contain more information on flow patterns at each individual site than do color-flow images. The main advantage of the color-flow display is that it presents simultaneous flow information on the entire image, even though the amount of data for each sample site is reduced. Spectral waveforms contain a range of frequencies and amplitudes, allowing determination of flow direction and spectral parameters such as mean, mode, peak, and bandwidth. The color assignments for the color-flow image are based on flow direction and a single mean or average frequency estimate for each site in the B-mode image plane. Consequently, the peak Doppler frequency

shifts or velocities shown by spectral waveforms are generally higher than the frequencies or velocities indicated by color-flow imaging.

Because color-flow imaging is based on pulsed Doppler ultrasound, it is subject to the same physical limitations as spectral waveform analysis of pulsed Doppler signals. For example, since the Doppler frequency shift depends on the angle θ in the Doppler equation, color assignments in the color-flow image will be accurate only if this angle is properly adjusted and remains constant along the length of a vessel. Unfortunately, blood vessels are seldom straight, so different colors may represent either true velocity changes or variations in the frequency shift resulting from changes in the Doppler angle. This potential source of error should always be considered when interpreting color-flow images. Aliasing is a pulsed Doppler artifact that occurs in both spectral waveform analysis and color-flow imaging. An aliased spectral waveform shows an abrupt loss of the waveform peak, with the missing portion appearing below the baseline as flow in the reverse direction. When aliasing is present in a color-flow image, high-velocity jets are assigned colors that indicate flow in the direction opposite to arterial flow. Theoretically, aliasing should be more common with color-flow imaging than with spectral waveform analysis, since relatively low pulse repetition frequencies are required to generate color-flow images.

In a color-flow image, shades of two or more distinct colors, usually red and blue, indicate the direction of flow relative to the ultrasound scan lines. A color bar near the image illustrates the particular color scale being used. The display is generally set up by the examiner to show flow in the arterial direction as red and flow in the venous direction as blue. Variations in the Doppler-shifted frequency or flow velocity are then indicated by changes in color, with lighter shades typically representing higher flow velocities. The specific features of color-flow images vary considerably among the commercially available duplex scanning instruments; however, a single sample volume pulsed Doppler and spectrum analyzer are always available for a detailed evaluation of flow patterns at selected arterial sites.

A complete color-flow image includes the color-coded Doppler information superimposed on the real-time B-mode image. Because of the extremely large amount of Doppler and B-mode information needed to produce color-flow images, they are acquired at relatively slow frame rates. Consequently, some of the rapid variations in flow velocity that occur during the cardiac cycle may not be accurately displayed. For example, if it takes approximately 33 milliseconds to generate each frame of a color image (30 frames per second), flow transients with time constants near 20 milliseconds, such as those occurring at the onset of systole, will not be reliably detected. This can result in temporal and spacial distortion in the color-flow image.

METHOD

The basic examination technique is the same for both color-flow imaging and standard duplex scanning. The examination takes approximately 30 minutes and is performed with the patient supine, head turned away from the side being studied. Longitudinal scans of the carotid artery are most useful. Spectral data can almost always be obtained from an artery, even if calcified, by approaching the vessel from many different angles. Wall calcification is generally confined to the proximal portion of the internal carotid artery, so a Doppler signal will be detectable distal to the calcified area. The examination is particularly difficult in patients with short necks, in patients who cannot cooperate by lying still, and in those with very tortuous vessels. The common carotid artery is first identified low in the neck. Moving distally, the carotid bulb is recognized as a slight dilatation in the artery near the upper border of the thyroid cartilage. The external carotid artery is generally anteromedial to the internal carotid, and the bifurcation can usually be visualized if time is taken to scan in various planes. The internal jugular vein, easily identified because it collapses with slight compression, serves as a point of reference, lying lateral to the common and internal carotid arteries. These structures can be identified by their characteristic flow patterns and appearance on the B-mode image.

One of the principal limitations of the standard approach to carotid duplex scanning is the small region of the arterial lumen that can be evaluated at any one time. To obtain complete information on flow patterns throughout the B-mode image, the single pulsed Doppler sample volume must be moved serially to various sites. Even with extreme diligence on the part of the examiner, flow disturbances that are confined to a small section of the vessel may be overlooked. Furthermore, it is more difficult to appreciate the complex three-dimensional features of flow in the carotid bifurcation with the single sample volume technique than it is with color-flow imaging. The color-flow image can be useful for locating the vessels, particularly when kinks, coils, or other anatomic variants are present. Although the color-flow image may also be helpful for identifying flow disturbances, some high-velocity jets may not be apparent on the color-flow

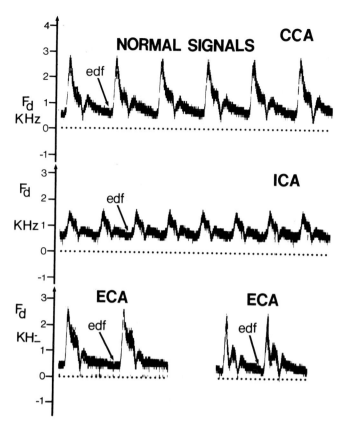

FIGURE 20–5. Normal spectral waveforms from the common *(CCA)*, internal *(ICA)*, and external *(ECA)* carotid arteries. The Doppler-shifted frequency *(F_d)* is displayed on the ordinate. The end-diastolic frequency *(edf)* is demonstrated.

image because the colors are based on a mean Doppler frequency estimate rather than the true peak systolic frequency.

Spectral waveforms are routinely obtained from the low common, the proximal and distal internal, and the external carotid arteries (see Fig. 20–2). In addition, the maximum flow disturbance, which occurs at the site of the tightest stenosis, is always recorded. The vertebral and subclavian arteries are also studied, with particular attention to the direction of flow, patency, tortuosity, and presence of flow disturbances. There are no formal criteria for classifying the severity of vertebral artery disease by duplex scanning.

The common carotid waveform resembles that of the internal carotid, which normally receives 70 percent of the common carotid blood flow (Fig. 20–5). Diastolic flow in the common carotid is usually above zero. When the internal carotid artery is occluded, the ipsilateral common carotid artery waveform resembles that of the external carotid artery[9] (Fig. 20–6).

The normal internal carotid artery waveform has a narrow systolic upstroke and a sharp peak (Figs. 20–5 and 20–7). The maximum velocity is less than 4 kHz (120 cm/s), and the area under the peak is clear. Flow is above zero at all times. This quasi-steady pattern of forward flow throughout the entire cardiac cycle is typical of arteries supplying low-resistance beds such as the brain, kidney, and muscle groups following exercise or ischemia. Normally, flow from center-stream sites produces a narrow band of frequencies during

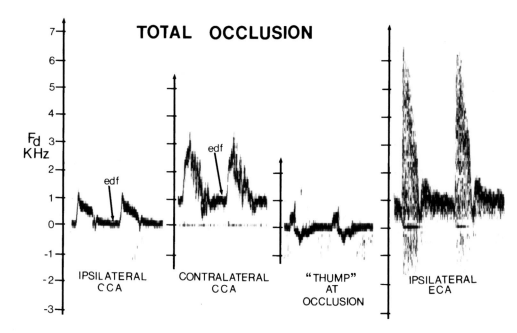

FIGURE 20–6. Spectral waveforms associated with internal carotid artery occlusion. There is no flow in the distal internal carotid artery. CCA, common carotid artery; ECA, external carotid artery; edf, end-diastolic frequency; F_d, Doppler-shifted frequency.

flow acceleration that widens during flow deceleration. Atherosclerotic plaques cause flow disturbances and a broader band of frequencies referred to as spectral broadening—the main feature used to detect minimal disease. Because the normal external carotid artery supplies a relatively high resistance bed, its waveform resembles the triphasic signal typical of peripheral arteries with reversed or near-zero flow in diastole (see Fig. 20–5).

Criteria for classifying internal carotid artery disease according to the degree of luminal narrowing were established by comparing duplex studies with angiograms (Table 20–1). With minimal decreases in luminal diameter (1 to 15% stenosis), spectral broadening is noted in the downslope of the systolic peak and in early diastole (Fig. 20–8). When the artery is narrowed by 16 to 49 percent, spectral broadening is present throughout systole (Fig. 20–9), and the clear area beneath the systolic peak is completely obliterated. The

systolic peak frequency remains below 4 kHz (140 cm/s). The peak systolic frequency in the stenosis exceeds 4 kHz when the diameter is reduced by 50 percent or more (Fig. 20–10). Stenoses greater than 80 percent have an end-diastolic frequency (edf) exceeding 4.5 kHz (140 cm/s).[10] Marked spectral broadening is always associated with lesions of this severity (Fig. 20–11).

The recently completed North American Symptomatic Carotid Endarterectomy Trial and the European Carotid Surgery Trial demonstrated the efficacy of carotid endarterectomy for stroke prevention in patients with transient ischemic attacks or previous stroke and a 70 percent or greater stenosis by conventional angiography.[11–13] Moneta

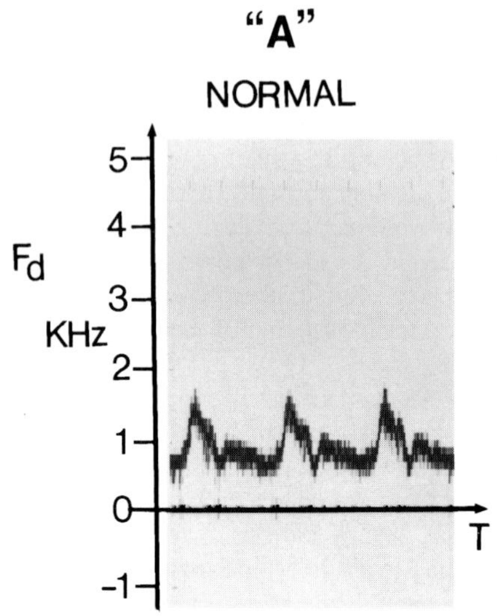

"A"

NORMAL

FIGURE 20–7. The normal internal carotid artery spectral waveform. F_d, Doppler-shifted frequency.

TABLE 20–1. Criteria for Classification of Internal Carotid Artery Disease

Angiographic Reduction in Luminal Diameter (%)	Doppler Spectra Criteria
0	Peak frequency < 4 kHz
	No spectral broadening*
1–15	Peak frequency < 4 kHz
	Spectral broadening in downslope of systole
	Clear area under the systolic peak
16–49	Peak frequency < 4 kHz
	Spectral broadening throughout systole
	Loss of the clear area beneath the systolic peak
50–79	Peak frequency > 4 kHz
	End-diastolic frequency < 4.5 kHz
80–99	End-diastolic frequency > 4.5 kHz
100	No flow in the internal carotid artery
	Lower than usual diastolic flow in the ipsilateral common carotid artery (flow to zero)
	Increased flow in the ipsilateral external carotid artery
	Increased flow in contralateral common carotid artery

*Presence of flow separation in the bulb appears to be particularly characteristic of "young normals."

" B "
1-15 %

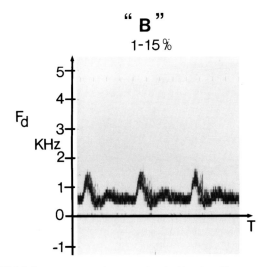

FIGURE 20–8. Spectral waveform associated with a 1 to 15 percent diameter-reducing lesion of the internal carotid artery. F_d, Doppler-shifted frequency.

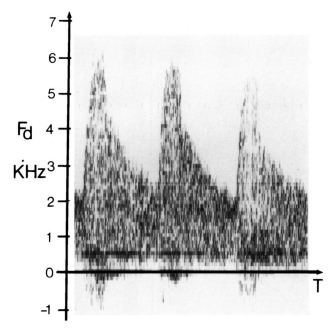

FIGURE 20–10. Spectral waveform associated with a 50 to 79 percent diameter-reducing lesion of the internal carotid artery. F_d, Doppler-shifted frequency.

and colleagues recently modified the classification scheme to determine the presence or absence of a 70 percent or greater diameter reduction. Using receiver-operator characterisics analysis of several velocity criteria, they found that a peak systolic velocity in the internal carotid artery of more than four times that of the common carotid artery had an overall accuracy of 88 percent for this determination. In a prospective, blinded validation of this method, duplex scanning identified a greater than 70 percent stenosis with an overall accuracy of 90 percent (sensitivity 91%, specificity 90%, positive predictive value 86%, and negative predictive value 94%) in the 168 patent carotid arteries that were studied.[14]

When the internal carotid artery is occluded, no flow is detectable in the imaged vessel. Flow may be increased in the ipsilateral external and contralateral common carotid

arteries. On the side of the occlusion, diastolic velocity in the common carotid artery often goes to zero[9, 15] (see Fig. 20–6). When the common carotid artery is occluded, the internal carotid artery may remain patent by retrograde filling

" C "
16-49%

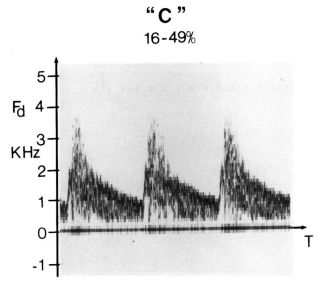

FIGURE 20–9. Spectral waveform associated with a 16 to 49 percent diameter-reducing lesion of the internal carotid artery. F_d, Doppler-shifted frequency.

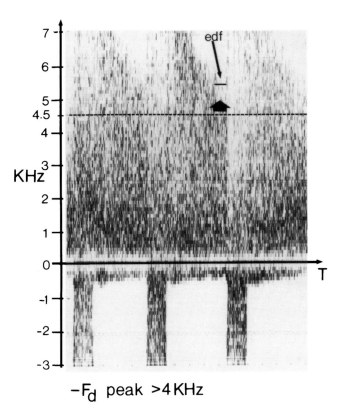

$-F_d$ peak >4 KHz

FIGURE 20–11. Spectral waveform associated with an 80 to 99 percent diameter-reducing lesion of the internal carotid artery. F_d, Doppler-shifted frequency.

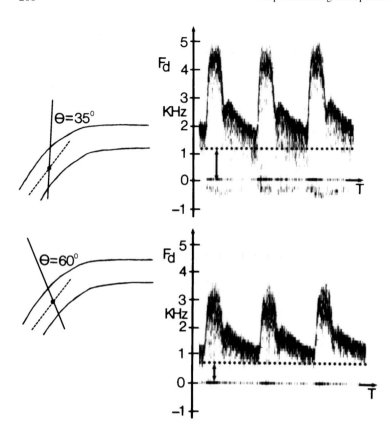

FIGURE 20–12. Changes in Doppler angle *(θ)*, in this case because of difficulty establishing the true axis of flow in a tortuous artery, which causes dramatic changes in the spectral waveform. F_d, Doppler-shifted frequency.

from the external carotid system as the "face feeds the brain." Duplex studies are uniquely suited for diagnosis of this uncommon but clinically important situation.

Many laboratories attempt to assess the degree of cartoid narrowing and the characteristics of the carotid plaque based on the B-mode image, with varying degrees of success.[16–18] Although the sonographic appearance of a plaque may correlate qualitatively with its histologic composition, the clinical relevance of this information is controversial.[19] Lipid is generally the least echogenic component of an atherosclerotic plaque, but as the collagen content of a plaque increases relative to its lipid content, echogenicity also increases. Whereas predominantly fibrous plaques produce a homogeneous B-mode image, focal deposits of thrombus or lipid can produce a more heterogeneous appearance. Calcified atherosclerotic plaque is extremely echogenic and causes bright echoes with acoustic shadows. The appearance of heterogeneity correlates most closely with clinical outcome and most likely represents intraplaque hemorrhage.[20] It is observed more frequently in symptomatic than in asymptomatic patients.[21]

Since ulcerated plaque at the carotid bifurcation is commonly regarded as a source of cerebral emboli, there has been considerable interest in the sonographic evaluation of plaque surface characteristics. Although some favorable results have been reported, the overall reliability of B-mode imaging for the detection of ulcerated atherosclerotic plaque has generally been poor.[18, 21, 22] Interpretation of the B-mode image is most accurate for lesions of minimal to moderate severity and least accurate for high-grade stenoses or occlusions.[17] It is often difficult to estimate the size of the arterial lumen from a B-mode image because the acoustic properties of noncalcified plaque, thrombus, and flowing blood are

similar. In addition, acoustic shadows from calcified plaques may prevent complete visualization of the arterial wall and lumen. These limitations are largely overcome by the addition of pulsed Doppler information and classification of disease severity based on the degree of flow disturbance produced by a particular lesion.

SPECIAL TECHNICAL CONSIDERATIONS

Because changes in the angle between the Doppler beam and the direction of blood flow directly influence the spectral waveforms, a standard angle of 60 degrees is used (Fig.

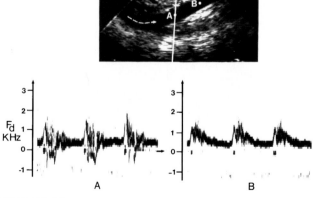

FIGURE 20–13. Flow abnormalities associated with tortuosity. F_d, Doppler-shifted frequency.

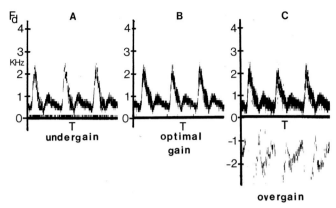

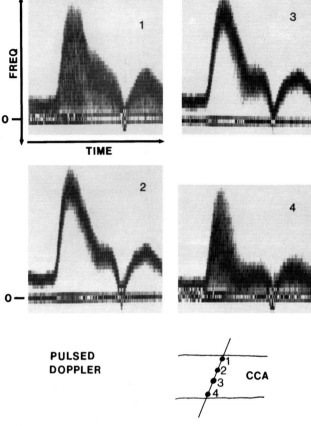

FIGURE 20–14. Proper gain adjustment is shown by clear systolic peaks without shadowing (B).

20–12). Variations of only 2 degrees from this angle change the frequency shift by 6 percent. Precise measurement of this angle is particularly difficult in tortuous vessels. Tortuosity also causes flow disturbances and spectral broadening, further confounding classification of disease in these arteries (Fig. 20–13).

Artificial increases in spectral broadening may result when the Doppler gain is too high. If the gain is too low, the systolic peak may be obscured (Fig. 20–14). Improper placement of the sample volume near the vessel wall, where the velocity gradient is steep, will also produce spectral broadening that may be misinterpreted as an indication of disease (Fig. 20–15). This problem has been lessened by using a smaller sample volume (3 mm^3). Movement associated with respiration may cause a relative shift of the sample volume toward the vessel wall while the B-mode image is frozen on the screen (Fig. 20–16). The examiner must make every effort to obtain the most normal spectral waveform possible from each location, eliminating artifacts due to respiratory variation, tortuosity, or improper placement of the sample volume.

In the carotid bulb, momentum carries flow forward, leaving a nearly stagnant area between center-stream flow and the wall of the expanded vessel. This area is referred to as a flow-separation zone. Because hydrostatic pressure is lower

PULSED DOPPLER

FIGURE 20–15. Spectral waveforms obtained by moving the sample volume in steps from the near to the far wall. Those from center stream (2, 3) have very uniform flow, while those near the wall (1, 4) show marked spectral broadening due to steep velocity gradients at the wall. CCA, common carotid artery; FREQ, frequency.

where blood velocity is higher (Bernoulli principle), pressure differentials develop between the rapidly flowing blood and the relatively stagnant zone. This situation results in helical flow patterns and reverse-flow components in the posterolateral bulb (Fig. 20–17). These secondary flow patterns have been observed in model carotid systems using pulsatile flow[23, 24] and in duplex scans across the carotid bulb of

FIGURE 20–16. Increased spectral broadening due to respiratory artifact in the common carotid artery as the sample volume (sv) moves toward the wall. F_d, Doppler-shifted frequency.

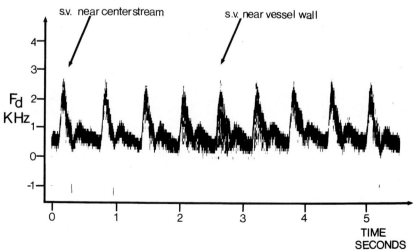

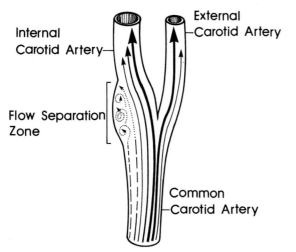

FIGURE 20–17. Flow separation and secondary flow patterns occur in the posterolateral bulb.

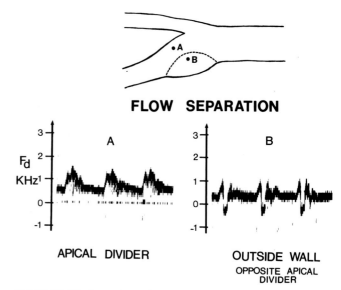

FIGURE 20–18. Spectral waveforms from the apical divider *(A)* and from the zone of flow separation *(B)*. F_d, Doppler-shifted frequency.

young normal volunteers[25] (Fig. 20–18). Flow separation and recirculation are less pronounced and less common in older subjects, perhaps due to decreased distensibility of the carotid artery.[26] Understanding these complex yet totally normal patterns is essential for distinguishing normal from minimally diseased carotid bulbs. When the sample volume is placed in the area of flow separation, a distinct and reproducible pattern of flow reversal and spectral broadening is detected (see Fig. 20–18). Before flow separation was recognized as a normal pattern, these findings were attributed to minor degrees of disease; they are now recognized, however, as characteristic of a normally configured carotid bulb. The arterial wall segment adjacent to the flow-separation zone is subjected to very low, oscillating shear forces, yet is the site of greatest atherosclerosis.[27, 28] Because atherosclerotic plaque usually develops first in the posterolateral bulb, filling in of this region leads to loss of flow separation. Absence of

a flow-separation zone is therefore a sensitive indicator of minimal disease and is noted before spectral broadening develops in the center-stream signal.

When both the external and internal carotid arteries are diseased, it may be difficult to distinguish between them on the basis of either their B-mode images or their spectral waveforms. The external carotid artery waveform can be identified using intermittent compression of the superficial temporal artery in front of the ear. By altering flow in the external carotid artery, this maneuver produces sharp spikes in its spectral waveform (Fig. 20–19).

RESULTS

Standard selective arteriograms were used as the reference standard for validation studies. Duplex results were cross-

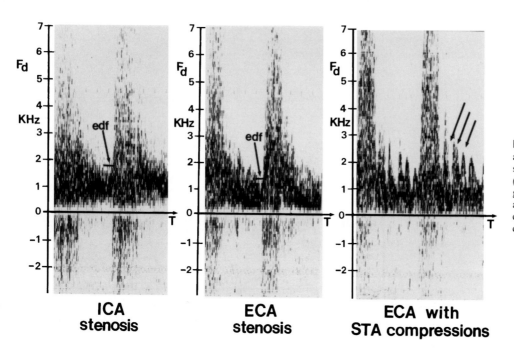

FIGURE 20–19. Superficial temporal artery *(STA)* compressions produce spikes on the external carotid artery *(ECA)* spectral waveform, distinguishing it from the internal carotid artery *(ICA)*. edf, end-diastolic frequency; F_d, Doppler-shifted frequency.

tabulated with angiogram readings and the kappa statistic used to determine the extent of agreement between the two methods.[29, 30] This statistic takes into account agreement that might occur by chance alone and ranges from + 1 for perfect agreement to zero for random association and − 1 for systematic disagreement. It is particularly useful when comparing the extent of agreement in two different cross-tabulations. Evaluations of other noninvasive tests often report only the sensitivity and specificity for determining whether a lesion is hemodynamically significant (50 percent or greater stenosis). Because duplex examinations can detect even minimal narrowing, the sensitivity and specificity for distinguishing totally normal arteries from those with any degree of narrowing were also calculated.

Initial evaluation of the prototype duplex scanner (January 1978 to December 1979) yielded a kappa statistic of 0.534 (Table 20–2).[31, 32] This value improved to 0.813 with the development of shorter focal length transducers with a smaller sample volume[33] and additional experience in obtaining and interpreting the spectral waveforms (Table 20–3).[34] It is unlikely that any noninvasive test will achieve better agreement with arteriography, as even this gold standard has considerable variability.[35–37] The kappa value for agreement between a single angiographer's two readings of the same arteriograms is 0.711 and between two different angiographers' readings of the same arteriograms is only 0.568.[32]

The duplex examination had a sensitivity of 99 percent (4 of 280 angiographically abnormal internal carotid arteries interpreted as normal) and a specificity of 84 percent (9 of 56 angiographically normal arteries read as diseased). For detecting greater than 50 percent lesions, the sensitivity was 94 percent (8 of 139 lesions greater than 50% on angiography read as less than 50% by duplex), and the specificity was 98 percent (four lesions less than 50% on angiography read as greater than 50% by duplex). Of 39 angiographically occluded sides, only one was not interpreted as occluded by duplex scanning, and of 39 sides interpreted as occluded by duplex scanning, only one was open by angiography. Because the Doppler is very sensitive, it may occasionally detect flow in an artery that is not visualized on arteriography. However, Doppler may fail to detect very low flow in nearly occluded lesions. We currently recommend angiography to determine patency of arteries found to be occluded

TABLE 20–2. Cross-Tabulation of Initial Results With the Prototype Duplex Scanner and Angiography

Angiographic Diameter Reduction (%)	Duplex Scanning					
	Normal	1–15%	16–49%	50–99%	100%	Total
0	4	3	4	—	—	11
10	3	9	8	—	—	20
10–49	4	12	52	20	2	90
50–99	—	3	10	84	6	103
100	—	—	2	12	32	46
Total	11	27	76	116	40	270

kappa = 0.534 ± 0.039

Modified from Langlois Y, Roederer GO, Chan A, et al: Evaluating carotid artery disease: The concordance between pulsed Doppler/spectrum analysis and angiography. *Ultrasound Med Biol.* 1983;9:51. Copyright 1983, with kind permission from Elsevier Science Ltd, The Boulevard, Langford Lane, Kidlington OX5 1GB, UK.

TABLE 20–3. Cross-Tabulation of Recent Results of Duplex Scanning and Angiography

Angiographic Diameter Reduction (%)	Duplex Scanning					
	Normal	1–15%	16–49%	50–99%	100%	Total
0	47	9	—	—	—	56
1–15	4	49	8	—	—	61
16–49	—	14	62	4	—	80
50–99	—	1	7	91	1	100
100	—	—	—	1	38	39
Total	51	73	77	96	39	336

kappa = 0.813 ± 0.024

Modified from Roederer GO, Langlois YE, Chan AW, et al: Ultrasonic duplex scanning of extracranial carotid arteries: Improved accuracy using new features from the common carotid artery. *J Cardiovasc Ultrason.* 1982;1:373; with permission.

by duplex scanning if the patient has recent, ipsilateral hemispheric symptoms.

Determining the extent of spectral broadening, particularly when it is less than complete, is somewhat subjective and therefore involves considerable interobserver variability. For this reason, most of the variability of duplex scanning lies in the classification of disease within the less than 50 percent stenosis categories. The most important clinical decision, however, is whether a lesion is "critical," or causing a greater than 50 percent diameter reduction. This decision depends on the measurement of peak frequency, which is much more objective than spectral broadening. This critical decision can be made accurately and with minimal variability from one examination to the next in the same patient, even when different technologists perform the studies.

Although duplex examinations are highly accurate for determining the extent of arterial narrowing, they give no information about plaque morphology or collateral circulation. Although some investigators use B-mode imaging to assess the extent of ulceration and detect intraplaque hemorrhage,[38, 39] the relative importance of hemodynamic versus morphologic factors in the pathogenesis of stroke is currently an issue of considerable debate. There is little doubt, however, that high-grade stenosis is a marker for significantly increased risk of stroke. Long-term duplex studies of asymptomatic patients suggest that progression from the 50 to 79 percent to the 80 to 99 percent stenosis category is associated with a particularly high risk for stroke or occlusion.[40] This finding provides a rational basis for selection of asymptomatic patients for carotid endarterectomy.

Accurate duplex scanning depends on a high degree of technical skill both in performing the study and in interpreting the results. A minimum training period of 2 months is generally required for the technologist to become proficient. Up to a year may be required for the trainee to become comfortable studying tortuous vessels and identifying flow separation or unusual conditions involving reversal of external carotid or vertebral artery flow. Prior experience with ultrasound imaging reduces this training period.

Color-flow imaging offers several potential advantages over the standard approach to duplex scanning. By visualizing areas of flow within a B-mode image, the branches of the carotid bifurcation are more easily identified. The color-flow image also expedites recognition of localized flow disturbances and should shorten the time required to perform an examination. However, since there are currently no definitive color criteria for classification of stenosis severity, spectral waveforms must still be used to determine the extent of carotid disease. Color-flow imaging can facilitate spectral waveform analysis by allowing optimal positioning of the pulsed Doppler sample volume at sites of disease.

The value of color-flow imaging for the assessment of carotid artery disease was evaluated by a study conducted in two vascular laboratories, one with a color-flow imaging instrument and the other with a standard duplex scanner.[41] A total of 307 internal carotid arteries were evaluated by color-flow imaging and arteriography, and 206 internal carotid arteries were evaluated by a standard duplex scan and arteriography. Perfect agreement between the duplex scan result and the arteriogram was achieved in 87 percent of the color-flow examinations and 80 percent of the standard duplex scans. In addition, significantly fewer arteries were overclassified by one disease category when color-flow imaging was used. Although this study supported the overall accuracy of both duplex techniques, there was a strong trend toward improved diagnostic results with color-flow imaging. This difference was attributed to more precise placement of the pulsed Doppler sample volume when the color-flow image was used as a guide. It should be emphasized, however, that the accuracy of standard carotid duplex scanning is already quite good, and the additional value of color-flow imaging in routine carotid testing may be relatively small. Color-flow imaging is most likely to be helpful in selected patients who have atypical arterial anatomy or suspected internal carotid artery occlusion.

CLINICAL APPLICATIONS

Unlike angiography, which is painful and expensive and has occasional complications, duplex scanning is safe and relatively inexpensive. It is ideal for screening patients and following disease progression because it locates lesions anatomically and categorizes them into six levels of stenosis ranging from normal to occlusion. Duplex scanning has provided important information on the natural history of carotid disease,[42] the development of restenosis following endarterectomy[43–46] (Fig. 20–20), the extent of carotid disease in patients undergoing coronary artery bypass,[47] and the progression of disease on the side contralateral to an occlusion or endarterectomy.[48] Similar techniques of pulsed Doppler and spectral analysis can also be used for intraoperative assessment of carotid endarterectomy.[49]

Since duplex scanning has become a reliable method for determining the degree of carotid stenosis, many clinicians have questioned the need for preoperative angiography. Several studies have suggested that angiography is not necessary when a high-quality duplex scan can demonstrate an appropriate lesion in a symptomatic patient.[50–58] Dawson and coworkers[59, 60] reported that duplex scanning is diagnostic in approximately 95 percent of cases. Diagnostic errors occurred in the following situations: (1) disease was not limited to the distal common carotid artery or bifurcation in four patients; (2) it was not possible to obtain satisfactory Doppler signals to estimate the degree of stenosis in one patient; and (3) an internal carotid occlusion could not be distinguished from a high-grade stenosis in two patients. Each of

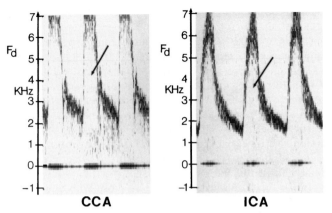

FIGURE 20–20. Spectral waveform from an artery that has developed stenosis following endarterectomy. Spectral broadening is absent under the systolic peak *(arrow)* in this form of smooth stenosis, unlike in stenosis due to atherosclerosis. CCA, common carotid artery; ICA, internal carotid artery; F_d, Doppler-shifted frequency.

these conditions was evident when the duplex scan was performed, so the need for further testing was apparent as soon as the study was completed. Conventional angiography supplies the necessary anatomical information in these cases, but it may be supplanted by other, noninvasive methods such as magnetic resonance angiography.

CONCLUSION

Ultrasound duplex scanning for carotid artery disease combines an ultrasound B-mode image with pulsed Doppler flow detection. This provides both anatomic and hemodynamic information and permits accurate classification of internal carotid artery narrowing. The technique is safe and rapid and carries no significant risk. Unlike other noninvasive tests, it locates the anatomic point of stenosis and detects the entire range of disease from minimal narrowing to total occlusion. Duplex scanning is a powerful tool for studying the natural history of treated and untreated carotid occlusive disease.

Acknowledgment

The authors gratefully acknowledge Jean Primozich and David Phillips for providing the illustrations and Louise Murphy for preparing the manuscript.

REFERENCES

1. Lye CR, Sumner DS, Strandness DE Jr: The accuracy of the supraorbital Doppler examination in the diagnosis of hemodynamically significant carotid occlusive disease. *Surgery.* 1976;73:42.
2. Barnes RW, Rittgers SE, Putney WW: Real-time Doppler spectrum analysis. *Arch Surg.* 1982;117:52.
3. Brown PM, Johnston KW, Kassam M, Cobbold RSC: A critical study of ultrasound Doppler spectral analysis for detecting carotid disease. *Ultrasound Med Biol.* 1982;8:515.
4. Brown PM, Johnston KW, Douville Y: Detection of occlusive disease of the carotid artery with continuous wave Doppler spectral analysis. *Surg Gynecol Obstet.* 1982;155:183.
5. Blackshear WM Jr, Phillips DJ, Thiele BL, et al: Detection of carotid occlusive disease by ultrasonic imaging and pulsed Doppler spectrum analysis. *Surgery.* 1979;86:698.

6. Blackshear WM Jr, Phillips DJ, Chikos PM, et al: Carotid artery velocity patterns in normal and stenotic vessels. *Stroke*. 1980;11:67.

7. Phillips DJ, Powers JE, Eyer MK, et al: Detection of peripheral vascular disease using the duplex scanner III. *Ultrasound Med Biol*. 1980;6:205.

8. Kremkau FW: Principles and pitfalls of real-time color flow imaging. In Bernstein EF, ed. *Vascular Diagnosis*. St. Louis: Mosby-Year Book;1993;90.

9. Bodily KC, Phillips DJ, Thiele BL, Strandness DE Jr: Noninvasive detection of internal carotid artery occlusion. *Angiology*. 1981;32:517.

10. Roederer GO, Langlois YE, Jager KA, et al: A simple spectral parameter for accurate classification of severe carotid disease. *Bruit*. 1984;8:174.

11. North American symptomatic carotid endarterectomy trial collaborators: Beneficial effect of carotid endarterectomy in symptomatic patients with high-grade carotid stenosis. *N Engl J Med*. 1991;325:445.

12. European carotid surgery trialists' collaborative group: European carotid surgery trial: Interim results for symptomatic patients with severe (70–99%) or with mild (0–29%) carotid stenosis. *Lancet*. 1991;337:1235.

13. Mayberg MR, Wilson SE, Yatsu F, et al: Carotid endarterectomy and prevention of cerebral ischemia in symptomatic carotid stenosis. Veterans Affairs Cooperative Studies Program 309 Trialist Group. *JAMA*. 1991;266:3289.

14. Moneta GL, Edwards JM, Chitwood RW, et al: Correlation of North American symptomatic carotid endarterectomy trial (NASCET) angiographic definition of 70% to 99% internal carotid artery stenosis with duplex scanning. *J Vasc Surg*. 1993;17:152.

15. Breslau PJ, Fell G, Phillips DJ, et al: Evaluation of carotid bifurcation disease. The role of common carotid artery velocity patterns. *Arch Surg*.1982;117:58.

16. Comerota AJ, Cranley JJ, Katz ML, et al: Real-time B-mode carotid imaging. A three-year multicenter experience. *J Vasc Surg*. 1984;1:84.

17. Hennerici M, Reifschneider G, Trockel U, Aulich A: Detection of early atherosclerotic lesions by duplex scanning of the carotid artery. *J Clin Ultrasound*. 1984;12:455.

18. O'Donnell TF, Erdoes L, Mackey WC, et al: Correlation of B-mode ultrasound imaging and arteriography with pathologic findings at carotid endarterectomy. *Arch Surg*. 1985;120:443.

19. Reilly LM: Importance of carotid plaque morphology. In Bernstein EF, ed. *Vascular Diagnosis*. St. Louis: Mosby-Year Book; 1993;333.

20. Reilly LM, Lusby RJ, Hughes L, et al: Carotid plaque histology using real-time ultrasonography: Clinical and therapeutic implications. *Am J Surg*. 1983;146:188.

21. Lusby RJ, Ferell LD, Ehrenfeld WK, et al: Carotid plaque hemorrhage: Its role in production of cerebral ischemia. *Arch Surg*. 1982;117:1479.

22. O'Leary DH, Holen J, Ricotta JJ, et al: Carotid bifurcation disease: Prediction of ulceration with B-mode US. *Radiology*. 1987;162:523.

23. Ku DN, Giddens DP: Pulsatile flow in a model carotid bifurcation. *Arteriosclerosis*. 1983;3:331.

24. Motomiya M, Karino T: Flow patterns in the human carotid artery bifurcation. *Stroke*. 1984;15:50.

25. Phillips DJ, Greene FM Jr, Langlois Y, et al: Flow velocity patterns in the carotid bifurcations of young, presumed normal subjects. *Ultrasound Med Biol*. 1983;9:39.

26. Reneman RS, van Merode T, Hick P, Hoeks APG: Flow velocity patterns in and distensibility of the carotid artery bulb in subjects of various ages. *Circulation*. 1985;17:500.

27. Fox JA, Hugh AE: Localization of atheroma: A theory based on boundary layer separation. *Br Heart J*. 1966;28:388.

28. Zarins CK, Giddens DP, Bharadvaj BK, et al: Carotid bifurcation atherosclerosis: Quantitative correlation of plaque localization with flow velocity profiles and wall shear stress. *Circ Res*. 1983;53:502.

29. Cohen J: A coefficient of agreement for nominal scales. *Educ Psychol Meas*. 1960;20:37.

30. Fleiss JL: Measuring nominal scale agreement among many raters. *Psychol Bull*. 1971;76:378.

31. Fell G, Phillips DJ, Chikos PM, et al: Ultrasonic duplex scanning for disease of the carotid artery. *Circulation*. 1981;64:1191.

32. Langlois Y, Roederer GO, Chan A, et al: Evaluating carotid artery disease: The concordance between pulsed Doppler/spectrum analysis and angiography. *Ultrasound Med Biol*. 1983;9:51.

33. Knox RA, Phillips DJ, Breslau PJ, et al: Empirical findings relating sample volume size to diagnostic accuracy in pulsed Doppler cerebrovascular studies. *J Clin Ultrasound*. 1982;10:227.

34. Roederer GO, Langlois YE, Chan AW, et al: Ultrasonic duplex scanning of extracranial carotid arteries: Improved accuracy using new features from the common carotid artery. *J Cardiovasc Ultrason*. 1982;1:373.

35. Chikos PM, Fisher LD, Hirsch JH, et al: Observer variability in evaluating extracranial carotid artery stenosis. *Stroke*. 1983;14:885.

36. Brown PM, Johnston KW: The difficulty of quantifying the severity of carotid stenosis. *Surgery*. 1982;92:468.

37. Croft RJ, Ellam LD, Harrison MJG: Accuracy of carotid angiography in the assessment of atheroma of the internal carotid artery. *Lancet*. 1980;1:997.

38. Katz ML, Comerota AJ, Cranley JJ: Characterization of atherosclerotic plaque by real-time carotid imaging. *Bruit*. 1982;6:17.

39. O'Donnell TF, Erdoes L, Mackey WC, et al: Correlation of B-mode ultrasound imaging and arteriography with pathologic findings at carotid endarterectomy. *Arch Surg*. 1985;120:443.

40. Roederer GO, Langlois YE, Jager KA, et al: The natural history of carotid arterial disease in asymptomatic patients with cervical bruits. *Stroke*. 1984;15:605.

41. Londrey GL, Spadone DP, Hodgson KJ, et al: Does color-flow imaging improve the accuracy of duplex carotid evaluation? *J Vasc Surg*. 1991;13:659.

42. Chan A, Beach KW, Martin DC, Strandness DE Jr: Carotid artery disease in NIDDM diabetes. *Diabetes Care*. 1983;6:562.

43. Bodily KC, Zierler RE, Marinelli MR, et al: Flow disturbances following carotid endarterectomy. *Surg Gynecol Obstet*. 1980;151:77.

44. Zierler RE, Bandyk DF, Thiele BL, Strandness DE Jr: Carotid artery stenosis following endarterectomy. *Arch Surg*. 1982;117:1408.

45. Thomas M, Otis SM, Rush M, et al: Recurrent carotid artery stenosis following endarterectomy. *Ann Surg*. 1984;200:74.

46. Roederer GO, Langlois Y, Chan ATW, et al: Postendarterectomy carotid ultrasonic duplex scanning concordance with contrast angiography. *Ultrasound Med Biol*. 1983;9:73.

47. Breslau PJ, Fell G, Ivey TD, et al: Carotid arterial disease in patients undergoing coronary artery bypass operations. *J Thorac Cardiovasc Surg*. 1981;82:765.

48. Roederer GO, Langlois YE, Lusiani L, et al: Natural history of carotid artery disease on the side contralateral to endarterectomy. *J Vasc Surg*. 1984;1:62.

49. Zierler RE, Bandyk DF, Thiele BL: Intraoperative assessment of carotid endarterectomy. *J Vasc Surg*. 1984;1:73.

50. Blackshear WM Jr, Connar RG: Carotid endarterectomy without angiography. *J Cardiovasc Surg*. 1982;23:477.

51. Ricotta JJ, Holen J, Schenk E, et al: Is routine angiography necessary prior to carotid endarterectomy? *J Vasc Surg*. 1984;1:96.

52. Crew JR, Dean M, Johnson JM: Carotid surgery without angiography. *Am J Surg*. 1984;148:217.

53. Flanigan DP, Schuler JJ, Vogel M, et al: The role of carotid duplex scanning in surgical decision making. *J Vasc Surg*. 1985;2:15.

54. Walsh J, Markowitz I, Kerstein MD: Carotid endarterectomy for amaurosis fugax without angiography. *Am J Surg*. 1986;152:172.

55. Thomas GI, Jones TW, Stavney LS, et al: Carotid endarterectomy after Doppler ultrasonographic examination without angiography. *Am J Surg*. 1986;151:616.

56. Moore WS, Ziomek S, Quiñones-Baldrich WJ, Machleder HI: Can clinical evaluation and noninvasive testing substitute for arteriography in the evaluation of carotid artery disease? *Ann Surg*. 1988;208:91.

57. Goodson SF, Flanigan DP, Bishara RA, et al: Can carotid duplex scanning supplant arteriography in patients with focal carotid territory symptoms? *J Vasc Surg*. 1987;5:551.

58. Geuder JW, Lamparello PJ, Riles TS, et al: Is duplex scanning sufficient evaluation before carotid endarterectomy? *J Vasc Surg*. 1989;9:193.

59. Dawson DL, Zierler RE, Kohler TR: Role of arteriography in the preoperative evaluation of carotid artery disease. *Am J Surg*. 1991;161:619.

60. Dawson DL, Zierler RE, Strandness DE Jr, et al: The role of duplex scanning and arteriography before carotid endarterectomy: A prospective study. *J Vasc Surg*. 1993;18:673.

CHAPTER 21

Transcranial Doppler Ultrasonography

J. DENNIS BAKER and ANNE M. JONES

A major emphasis in noninvasive vascular testing has been placed on the evaluation of the cerebrovascular circulation. Ideally, techniques should provide for assessment from the aortic arch to the main cerebral branches. Although some early Doppler recordings of these vessels were made intraoperatively or in children with open fontanelles, the standard noninvasive investigations were limited to the level of the ophthalmic artery. Ultrasound techniques were developed in the 1950s for echoencephalography, but the strong attenuation of ultrasound by the bony skull precluded the intracranial detection of blood flow by conventional Doppler detector systems with transmission frequencies of 4 to 10 mHz.

The development of 2 mHz directional, pulsed Doppler detectors provided the appropriate tool for transcranial examinations. In 1982, Aaslid and coworkers[1] published the first report on clinical use of transcranial Doppler ultrasonography. They demonstrated the feasibility of detecting velocity signals from the anterior, middle, and posterior cerebral arteries. All recordings were made through the temporal area, where the skull is thinnest. Vessel identification was based on sample volume depth. flow direction, and probe orientation. Recordings of the posterior cerebral arteries (PCAs) from the temporal window proved to be difficult, however. This limitation led to use of the transorbital approach to record from the distal internal carotid artery (ICA) and foramen magnum for easier access to the posterior circulation.[2, 3]

EXAMINATION TECHNIQUE

Transtemporal Approach

The temporal window is above the zygomatic arch, anterior to the ear, providing access to the middle cerebral, anterior cerebral, internal carotid, and proximal posterior cerebral arteries. The thickness of the temporal bone is affected by age, sex, and race, with an inadequate or impenetrable temporal window often found in patients who are elderly, female, or black.[4] In most cases, the problem results from hyperostosis of the temporal bone. Although a number of investigators report failure rates in the 2 to 5 percent range, some centers with a high proportion of black patients report problems in at least 10 percent of studies.[5] Failure to insonate the temporal bone is not always bilateral, so it may be possible to evaluate branches contralateral to a usable window.

After the best temporal window is located, the examination is initiated with the sample volume depth at 55 to 65 mm (measured from the transducer surface on the skull); this depth offers the greatest likelihood of insonating the cerebral vessels. The bifurcation of the terminal ICA into the middle cerebral artery (MCA) and anterior cerebral artery (ACA) occurs at a depth of approximately 60 to 65 mm and is the most reproducible and reliable intracranial landmark. The bifurcation signal is a unique bidirectional waveform, with the MCA signal displayed above the baseline (indicat-

ing flow toward the transducer) and the ACA signal displayed below the baseline (flow toward the midline, away from the transducer). Once the bifurcation signal has been identified, it is used as a reference for identification of the other segments of the circle of Willis, insonated through the temporal window.

The MCA is the largest intracranial vessel, and the one most reliably insonated with transcranial Doppler (Fig. 21–1). The course of the main trunk can be routinely traced for at least 20 to 30 mm before branching occurs. Failure to locate and trace the course of the MCA removes the most reliable and repeatable intracranial landmark. After the course of the MCA is documented, the sample volume is again positioned at the level of the terminal ICA bifurcation. The A-1 (precommunicating) segment of the ACA, from the origin to the junction with the anterior communicating artery (ACoA), follows a lateral course and is the only segment of the ACA that can be routinely identified with transcranial Doppler. Beginning at a depth of 65 mm, the ACA signal is followed to the midline, at a depth of 75 to 80 mm. Under normal conditions, the ACA flow direction is away from the transducer, toward the midline. At the level of the midline, the A-2 through A-5 segments of the ACA take an abrupt superior course around the genu of the corpus callosum, becoming inaccessible to transcranial Doppler insonation. The ACoA is located at the level of the midline and connects the paired ACAs. When the ACoA is functional, carrying collateral flow from one hemisphere to the other, it can be identified by transcranial Doppler. If it is not functional, the signal cannot be distinguished from the two ACA signals converging at a depth of 75 to 80 mm, because of the size of the sample volume and integration into the stronger ACA signals.[6] At this depth, the paired ACAs are both insonated, creating another bidirectional signal, with the ipsilateral ACA flow away from the transducer and the contralateral ACA signal toward the transducer. Recognition of normal ACA flow patterns is critical, as collateralization from one hemisphere to the other causes both ACA segments to demonstrate flow in the same direction, toward the collateralized hemisphere. Flow velocities in the ACA should be less than those in the MCA.

The temporal approach affords access to at least two, and occasionally three, additional segments: the terminal ICA, the proximal PCA, and the terminal segment of the basilar artery (basilar tip). Identification of these segments again relies on the ICA bifurcation landmark. The transducer is angled inferiorly to locate the ICA signal just proximal to the bifurcation. Because of the unfavorable angle of insonation, the waveform is usually damped or blunted, but the information is useful to document the presence and direction of flow in the ICA and screen for poststenotic turbulence, which is often noted distal to an intracranial ICA stenosis.

After completing the assessment of the anterior circulation, the proximal PCA is evaluated. After the ICA bifurcation landmark is localized, the transducer is angled posteriorly and slightly inferiorly, in the same horizontal plane. The PCA signal is identified at a depth of 65 to 75 mm, as it rises from the terminal basilar artery at the level of the

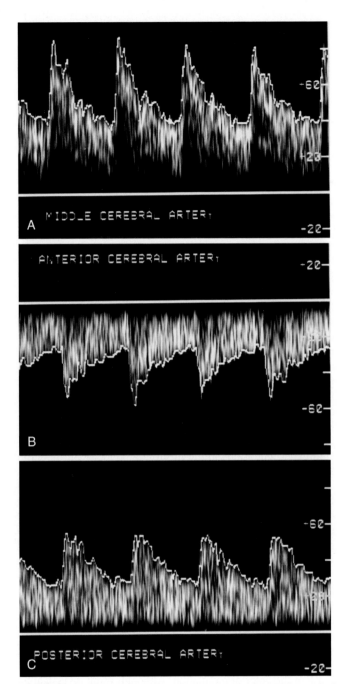

FIGURE 21-1. Normal transcranial Doppler signals. *A*, Middle cerebral artery: 53 cm/second mean velocity. *B*, Anterior cerebral artery: 34 cm/second mean velocity. Tracing below baseline indicates flow away from transducer. *C*, Posterior cerebral artery: 38 cm/second mean velocity.

midline. The P-1 (precommunicating segment) of the PCA is traced from its origin to the junction of the posterior communicating artery (PCoA) at a depth of about 55 mm. The P-2 segment of the PCA extends from the PCoA to the posterior aspect of the midbrain, a course that is usually unfavorable to Doppler insonation. Due to the close proximity of the MCA and PCA, the loss of a PCA signal at a depth of 55 mm helps differentiate it from the MCA, which can routinely be traced to 35 to 45 mm. The PCoA is rarely insonated in isolation and is not routinely insonated unless it is functional. The basilar tip may be insonated at a depth of 75 to 80 mm.[3, 6, 7]

Suboccipital (Transforamenal) Approach

Transcranial Doppler evaluation of the intracranial vertebral arteries and the basilar artery is accomplished by insonating through the natural opening at the base of the skull, the foramen magnum. The paired vertebral arteries enter the skull through the foramen and course superiorly to the level of the pontomedullary junction, where they join to form the basilar artery. This is a unique anatomic configuration, in that two small arteries join to form a larger one.

With the transducer placed at the midline, just below the inion, the sample volume is set at a depth of 55 to 65 mm. The thickness of the soft-tissue layer over the craniocervical junction is highly variable, affecting the depth at which insonation is achieved.[6, 7] The course of the vertebral and basilar arteries can be highly variable, and each vertebral artery should be individually traced from the point of entry though the foramen magnum to the level of the basilar artery. The flow direction of the vertebral arteries is away from the transducer. At the level of the upper medulla, the waveform characteristics may change, indicating the confluence of the two vertebral arteries to form the basilar artery. The mean flow velocity increases only slightly. The course, length, and size of the basilar artery are variable. It can usually be insonated from 80 to 85 mm to a depth of 120 mm. Flow direction, like that of the vertebrals, is cephalad. Because the basilar is often tortuous or deviates from the midline, the examiner must be diligent if the course is to be documented. As the depth increases, the attenuation of the Doppler signal also increases and may limit the ability to reliably assess the terminal basilar artery.

Transorbital Approach

The transorbital approach is used to evaluate the ophthalmic artery and the intracranial ICA (carotid siphon).[2, 5] The patient is instructed to stare to the opposite side to minimize eye movement during the examination. The transducer is placed over the closed eyelid, and only slight pressure is required if sufficient gel is applied. The ophthalmic artery is insonated at a depth of 35 to 50 mm and is traced to the ICA at a depth of 55 to 80 mm. Flow direction in the ophthalmic artery is toward the transducer. The transition from the ophthalmic artery to the ICA can be distinguished by the vessels' waveform patterns: the ophthalmic artery has a high-resistance signal, with minimal flow in diastole, and the ICA has a low-resistance pattern, with continuous diastolic flow. The flow direction of the ICA varies according to the segment insonated. The genu signal is bidirectional, due to the S-shaped curvature at that level. Proximal to the genu, in the parasellar region, flow direction is toward the transducer. Flow direction in the distal, supraclinoid segment is away from the transducer. Careful, gentle angulation of the transducer is required to assess all segments accurately. In order to prevent unnecessary ultrasound exposure to the eye, power levels should be decreased to 10 percent of the maximum.

INTERPRETATION OF RESULTS

The interpretation of transcranial Doppler examinations relies on many of the parameters discussed for vessel identi-

TABLE 21–1. Intracranial Artery Identification Criteria and Range of Normal Velocities

Artery	Window	Depth	Flow Direction Relative to Transducer	Mean Velocity, cm/sec (Mean ± 1 SD)
MCA	Temporal	35–65 mm	Toward	62 ± 12
ACA	Temporal	60–80 mm	Away	51 ± 12
ICA	Temporal	60–65 mm	Toward	Varies
PCA	Temporal	55–80 mm	Toward	41 ± 9
VA	Occipital	55–85 mm*	Away	36 ± 9
BA	Occipital	>85 mm*	Away	39 ± 9
OA	Orbital	40–55 mm	Toward	21 ± 5
ICA siphon	Orbital	55–80 mm	Toward/away†	47 ± 14

*Varies with thickness of soft-tissue layer.

†Varies with position of sample volume in siphon region.

ACA, anterior cerebral artery; BA, basilar artery; ICA, internal carotid artery; MCA, middle cerebral artery; OA, ophthalmic artery; PCA, posterior cerebral artery; VA, vertebral artery.

fication: flow direction, flow velocity, insonation depth, intra-arterial "hierarchy," and waveform characteristics. Correct vessel identification is critical to the accurate interpretation of Doppler results. For that reason, some practitioners rely heavily on the results of common carotid compression maneuvers to identify vessels and assess their response to proximal compression. Indeed, von Reutern and von Budingen[6] suggest that only the MCA can be reliably identified without compression of an extracranial cerebral artery (common carotid or vertebral). Compression maneuvers have not been widely used in the United States for vessel identification.

A range of expected mean flow velocities has been established (Table 21–1).[1, 8, 9] These values should be used as guidelines for interpretation, keeping in mind that variations of up to 25 percent can be considered normal. Before interpretation of the data, the patient's age, hematocrit, blood pressure, and cardiac and extracranial status should be known. It is well known that velocity decreases with age and increases with a low hematocrit.[3, 10, 11] In addition, metabolic factors such as hyperventilation (which decreases velocity) and hypoventilation (which increases velocity) may affect results, if only temporarily. Finally, the presence of a proximal or distal obstruction may alter intracranial hemodynamics, waveform characteristics, and the response to common carotid compression maneuvers. With these factors in mind, it is helpful to review mean flow velocities and compare them with those in the contralateral vessels, noting any significant side-to-side or intra-arterial asymmetry. As noted by Adams and colleagues,[12] when making side-to-side comparisons, the standard deviation between the two sides is generally 10 to 13 percent; therefore, a difference of more than 25 percent may indicate an abnormality. As a precaution, it is always advisable to repeat an examination to determine whether the asymmetry is real or due to technique.

Under normal conditions, the MCA demonstrates the highest mean flow velocity. It is the most reliably insonated of the cerebral arteries due to its favorable insonation angle and high flow volume. The normal value is 62 ± 12 cm/second, (although many institutions double the standard deviation to 24, which considerably broadens the definition of "normal"). The A-1 segment of the ACA is the most reliably insonated segment of that branch, with a normal value of 51 ± 12 cm/second. The P-1 segment of the PCA can be insonated from its origin, at the tip of the basilar

artery, to a depth of approximately 55 mm. Mean flow velocities in the PCA are slightly less than those in the ACA, at 40 ± 10 cm/second. Because the ICA normal values are unreliable, usually only the presence, quality, and direction of flow are evaluated. Flow velocities in the posterior circulation are normally less than those in the anterior circulation. Although some side-to-side asymmetry is expected in the vertebral system (with left usually dominant), the normal vertebral artery mean flow velocity is 36 ± 9 cm/second; and that in the basilar artery is only slightly higher, at 39 ± 10 cm/second. In the presence of severe extracranial or intracranial disease of the anterior circulation, significant alterations in the mean flow velocity are noted in the posterior circulation due to collateral effects.

The pulsatility index and resistivity index have been used for the quantitative description of Doppler waveforms in different parts of the circulation. Although commercial TCD units may compute one or both of these indexes, they have not been widely accepted in the interpretation of intracranial velocity signals.

Other interpretation parameters are the side-to-side asymmetry and velocity "hierarchy" previously mentioned. The MCA velocities should be the highest, followed by those of the ACA. An ACA velocity more than 25 percent higher than that of the MCA may indicate ACA hypoplasia, stenosis, or collateral effects. The same conditions may be present if the velocities in the posterior circulation are greater than those in the anterior circulation. Although some investigators have reported the use of intra-arterial ratios, the ACA-MCA ratio is the only one that has proved to be reliable in the assessment of intracranial pathology. If the ACA-MCA ratio is greater than 1.2, it is considered abnormal.[5]

Detection of the functional intracranial collaterals that can develop with severe stenosis adds to the overall assessment. The most common collateral system is through the ACoA, which links the two cerebral hemispheres via ACAs. High-velocity flow will be noted at the level of the midline, with increased flow velocity and flow reversal in the involved ACA. The collateralized MCA usually demonstrates mean flow velocities within the normal range, although the posterior vessels may also display increased velocities due to collateral effects. Although the posterior circulation can supply the anterior circulation, the ACA-ACoA collateral pathway is the most common.

LIMITATIONS

The two greatest technical limitations of transcranial Doppler are inexperience of the examiner and inadequate insonation windows. Vessel misidentification is a serious limitation of the "blind" or nonimaging techniques. Such errors can occur for a number of reasons, including unknown intracranial or extracranial pathology, anatomic variants, collateral flow patterns, or poor technique. When the examiner assesses the basal cerebral arteries, the flow velocity hierarchy should be noted, since disruption of this hierarchy may indicate collateral effects, a pathologic condition, or incorrect vessel identification. Fortunately, accuracy and confidence increase with experience. It is hoped that improved instrumentation will streamline the learning curve and improve insonation success rates. However, some patients will have a skull anatomy that results in incomplete or suboptimal evaluation. The percentage of patients who undergo inadequate insonation depends on the patient mix studied; laboratories whose patient groups include large numbers of elderly women and black persons will have a higher proportion of problem cases.[4]

APPLICATIONS

Since its introduction, transcranial Doppler has been used to study many clinical problems. Currently, the technique is most accepted for the detection of severe intracranial stenosis and the evaluation of collateral circulation in patients with transient ischemic attacks and strokes and for the assessment of cerebral artery vasospasm after subarachnoid hemorrhage.[13, 14] Many other applications have been described, but these have not yet achieved wide acceptance and should be considered in the developmental stage.

Detection of Occlusive Lesions

Early in the clinical experience, investigators evaluated transcranial Doppler as a screening technique for advanced stenosis of the cervical portion of the ICA. Many patients with severe stenosis or occlusion of this branch have a decrease in the ipsilateral MCA velocity compared with that of the opposite side; in the case of stenosis, this asymmetry is abolished if the patient undergoes endarterectomy. The major limitation when using transcranial Doppler to screen for cervical lesions is the wide variability of this asymmetry, resulting from different degrees of collateral development distal to the ICA lesion. Babikian[13] found that severe ICA stenosis produced significant intracranial changes detected by transcranial Doppler in only 45 percent of cases. In a study of the clinical value of transcranial Doppler for evaluating extracranial carotid disease, Cantelmo and associates[15] found that this method alone was a poor screening test and that its addition to other noninvasive tests did not enhance the overall results. Investigators have studied the pulsatility index, among others, but none has acceptable sensitivity in the detection of extracranial disease. In view of the excellent information that can be obtained with duplex scanning of the carotid bifurcation, it seems inappropriate to use transcranial Doppler to screen for extracranial disease.

Although intracranial lesions are infrequent causes of cerebral ischemia, these can be caused not only by atherosclerosis but also by different types of vasculitis. A major focus of transcranial Doppler studies has been the detection of severe lesions in these arteries. Intracranial stenosis is recognized by a 25 percent or greater focal increase in velocity, poststenotic turbulence and damping of the spectral waveform, and low-frequency baseline energy, often referred to as a bruit. These findings may be accompanied by collateral effects (increased velocity or change in flow direction in other intracranial vessels). At the point of maximum stenosis, mean flow velocities of 80 to 100 cm/second indicate a greater than 60 percent stenosis (Fig. 21–2).[7] Lesions creating a less than 60 percent stenosis are rarely detected by transcranial Doppler. Spencer and Whisler[2] reported a sensitivity of 73 percent and a specificity of 95 percent in the detection of stenosis of the intracranial portion of the ICA. The velocity increase produced by stenosis may be similar to that resulting from vasospasm, so it is important to consider the clinical context of the examination. Although there is an increase in peak velocity with decreasing residual lumen, the variability among patients does not permit a definition of the severity of the lesion. An occlusion of the main trunk can sometimes be diagnosed by the absence of Doppler signals at the depth at which the contralateral vessel

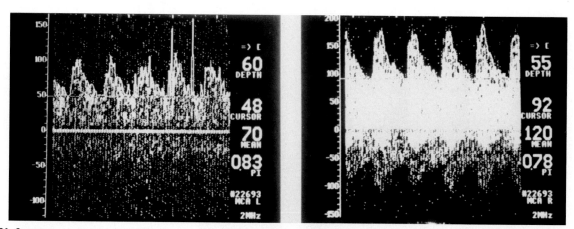

FIGURE 21–2. Middle cerebral artery (MCA) stenosis. *A,* Left MCA tracing with mean velocity of 70 cm/second. *B,* Right MCA with increased velocity at the site of stenosis and a mean velocity of 120 cm/second. Note that different scales are used for the two recordings. (Courtesy of Dr. N. A. Martin.)

is detected. There has been only limited experience in the detection of stenosis in the ACA.

Focal lesions in the basilar or vertebral arteries are likewise identified by increased peak velocity. Early reports suggest that anterior circulation studies are more accurate than those of the posterior circulation. Problems may be caused by both the presence of diffuse disease and the higher frequency of congenital variations in the vertebrobasilar system. Transcranial Doppler can be used to document a subclavian steal, in which retrograde flow occurs in a vertebral artery on the side of a tight stenosis or occlusion proximal to the vertebral origin. In some patients, the reverse flow occurs only with arm exercise. For an optimal evaluation, a recording of the vertebral artery flow is made after exercise or during the period of reactive hyperemia induced by 3 minutes of arterial occlusion with a blood pressure cuff.

Detection of Vasospasm

Detection of severe arterial vasospasm, such as can occur following subarachnoid hemorrhage, is important for patient management, since an intracranial operation performed in the presence of vasospasm carries a substantially higher risk of complication. A major problem in planning treatment is that the onset and the duration of severe spasm are both quite variable. The noninvasive character of transcranial Doppler permits repeated examination of these patients to monitor vascular changes.

Most of the published studies have focused on the assessment of MCA velocities, correlating these with findings on contrast angiograms. The characteristics of vasospasm found with transcranial Doppler are similar to those of stenosis: decreased diastolic flow proximally; focal areas of narrowing, with increased velocity; and poststenotic turbulence. Vasospasm is generally present if mean flow velocities exceed 120 cm/second (Fig. 21–3). MCA velocities in this range are usually associated with at least a 25 percent decrease in lumen diameter, as seen on arteriography. In angiographic correlations, sensitivities have ranged between 78 and 85 percent, specificities between 85 and 98 percent.[16–18] Velocities in excess of 200 cm/second are considered indicative of severe vasospasm.[19, 20] One cannot reliably use a ratio between the two sides as a criterion, since there can be spasm in the hemisphere contralateral to the subarachnoid hemorrhage (although usually of a lesser magnitude). Higher velocities are associated with more advanced spasm, but the variability precludes a precise definition of spasm severity. False-negative results can occur with severe disease, when Doppler velocities may be in the normal or subnormal range. Also, absence of increased velocity in the main MCA does not exclude focal spasm in peripheral branches. Newell and coworkers,[21] however, concluded that this is not a significant limitation; only 7.5 percent of the patients in their series had involvement limited to distal segments with no abnormality in the MCA.

Developing Applications

Monitoring Cerebral Perfusion During Carotid Endarterectomy

Many surgeons do not routinely use intraoperative shunting when performing carotid endarterectomy; they prefer to use this adjunct selectively. Patients with inadequate collaterals have been identified by a variety of techniques, including intracranial angiograms, measurement of ICA back pressure, and electroencephalography or brain mapping. Transcranial Doppler is an appealing technique because it can provide continuous assessment of MCA flow. A major problem in using this technology during carotid operations, however, is obtaining a consistently optimal recording. The narrow width of the ultrasound beam at distances of 5 to 8 cm, combined with the small size of the target vessel, makes probe position critical. Some initial studies were performed with the examiner holding and adjusting the transducer throughout the procedure. This requires reaching up under sterile drapes—a challenge when the monitoring extends for 30 to 60 minutes. Different headbands have been designed to hold the probe in

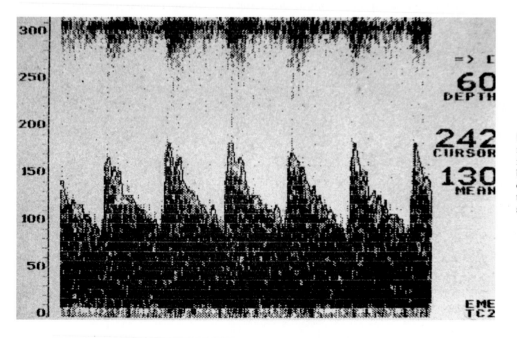

FIGURE 21–3. Vasospasm of the middle cerebral artery; mean velocity is 130 cm/second. Note the similarity between the waveforms produced by chronic stenosis (in Fig. 21–2) and those produced by transient vasospasm.

a fixed position, but these can be knocked out of alignment by the operating team or the anesthesiologist. Some groups have resorted to box or cage devices to protect the headband and transducer from accidental displacement. In spite of these efforts, monitoring problems occur in a substantial proportion of patients. Bass and colleagues[22] reported an inability to obtain a suitable signal in 13 percent of operations and an inability to maintain probe position in another 27 percent. In contrast, in a study of 130 operations, Jansen and coworkers[23] found that monitoring throughout the procedure was achieved in 95 percent of cases. The role of routine TCD monitoring for cerebral ischemia during carotid endarterectomy remains to be defined.

Embolus Detection

The detection of bubbles in the circuit of a cardiopulmonary bypass machine was the first application of Doppler ultrasonography for the detection of emboli. The transit of a bubble or a small solid element through the ultrasound beam produces a distinctive transient signal that is superimposed on the signal from the moving blood. In an analysis of 91 patients undergoing transcranial Doppler monitoring during carotid endarterectomy, Spencer and associates[24] found transient signals compatible with air bubbles in 63 percent of cases. In addition, similar transient signals were detected in 26 percent of patients at times when bubbles were unlikely. These were interpreted as being particle emboli, either atheromatous debris or platelet aggregates. Two patients developed these signals during common carotid artery compression. Particle and bubble emboli had similar frequency characteristics, but the bubbles usually produced a signal with much higher amplitude. Although some patients developed symptoms thought to be associated with emboli, many remained asymptomatic. Several authors advocate the use of continuous transcranial Doppler monitoring during endarterectomy to detect emboli, but there is no substantial evidence to justify this recommendation. Recent experimental investigations have focused on more detailed analysis of the transient signals in order to provide better definition of the size and composition of emboli. Another research area is the development of automated signal identification systems. In addition to intraoperative applications, monitoring for emboli is being evaluated as a tool in stroke prevention, but clinical application will require further development of the equipment.

Cerebrovascular Reactivity

The intracranial circulation normally has a wide range of autoregulation. Increases in carbon dioxide partial pressure (pCO_2) result in increased flow, and decreases in pCO_2 result in decreased flow. Initially, assessment of vascular reactivity was performed using radiotracer techniques, but transcranial Doppler provides a simpler approach.[25, 26] Changes in vasoactive status are caused by changes in pCO_2. Vasoconstriction is produced by hyperventilation, and vasodilation is produced by prolonged breath holding or by breathing gas with an increased CO_2 content. Vasodilation can also be produced by the intravenous injection of 1 g of acetazolamide. Studies of autoregulation using both transcranial Doppler and radiotracer blood flow measurement techniques have shown a positive correlation between the methods.[27] Patients

with low-flow brain infarction or conditions limiting arterial inflow, such as tight stenosis or occlusion of the ICA, have a reduced degree of autoregulation. The main interest in measuring vasoreactivity is to define subsets of patients who may be at increased risk of stroke either with carotid clamping during endarterectomy or with progression of advanced carotid stenosis. Prospective studies are required to define the clinical value of these measurements.

Other Applications

Transcranial Doppler is being investigated for use in a wide range of clinical problems, including detection of increased intracranial pressure, definition of brain death, detection of arteriovenous malformations and monitoring of their endovascular treatment, assessment of intracranial balloon dilation for vasospasm, and thrombolytic therapy. The scope of transcranial Doppler will be expanded if it proves useful in any of these applications in multiple prospective studies.

CONCLUSION

The value of nonimaging transcranial Doppler has been established in the serial assessment of patients in vasospasm, the assessment of collateral flow patterns, and the localization of intracranial stenosis. It is essential that an extracranial evaluation be performed in conjunction with the intracranial assessment so that extracranial pathology can be recognized and evaluated. The portability of equipment is a significant advantage in many settings, making transcranial Doppler the modality of choice in the intensive care unit or operating room. However, the limitations of the nonimaging system are well documented: anatomic variations may result in misinterpretation of data, placement of the Doppler sample volume is not precise, the learning curve is steep, and the acceptance level among practitioners is low. In the past several years, there has been increasing use of color-coded duplex scanners to perform transcranial studies. This technique provides the advantage of more accurate identification of vessels. In addition, more accurate velocity measurements are possible because of the ability to estimate the angle on insonation. Further experience with scanning studies will be needed to define the roles of imaging and nonimaging techniques.

REFERENCES

1. Aaslid R, Markwalder T-M, Nornes H: Noninvasive transcranial Doppler ultrasound recording of flow velocity in the basal cerebral arteries. *J Neurosurg.* 1982;57:769.
2. Spencer MP, Whisler D: Transorbital Doppler diagnosis of intracranial arterial stenosis. *Ultrasound Med Biol.* 1986;17:916.
3. Arnolds BJ, von Reutern G-M: Transcranial Doppler ultrasonography: Examination technique and normal reference values. *Ultrasound Med Biol.* 1986;12:115.
4. Eden A: Letter to the editor: Transcranial Doppler ultrasonography and hyperostosis of the skull. *Stroke.* 1988;19:1445.
5. Katz ML, Comerota AJ: Transcranial Doppler: A review of technique, interpretation and clinical applications. *Ultrasound Quarterly.* 1991;8:241.
6. von Reutern G-M, von Budingen HJ: Ultrasound Diagnosis of Cerebrovascular Disease: Doppler Sonography of the Extra- and Intracranial Arteries, Duplex Scanning. New York: George Thieme; 1993.
7. Ringelstein EB: A practical guide to transcranial Doppler sonography. In Weinberg J, ed. *Noninvasive Imaging of Cerebrovascular Disease.* New York: A. Liss; 1989:75.
8. Harders A: *Neurosurgical Applications of Transcranial Doppler Sonography.* Vienna: Springer-Verlag; 1986.

9. Otis SM, Ringelstein EB: Principles and applications of transcranial Doppler sonography. In Bernstein EF, ed. *Recent Advances in Noninvasive Diagnostic Techniques in Vascular Disease*. St. Louis: CV Mosby; 1990.

10. Grolimund P, Seiler RW: Age dependence of the flow velocity in the basal cerebral arteries—a transcranial Doppler ultrasound study. *Ultrasound Med Biol*. 1988;14:191.

11. Brass LM, Pavlakis SG, DeVivo D, et al: Transcranial Doppler measurements of the middle cerebral artery—Effect of hematocrit. *Stroke*. 1988;19:1466.

12. Adams RJ, Nichols FT, Hess DC: Normal values and physiological variables. In Newell D, Aaslid A, eds. *Transcranial Doppler*. New York: Raven Press; 1992.

13. Babikian VL: Transcranial Doppler evaluation of patients with ischemic cerebrovascular disease. In Babikian VL, Wechsler LR, eds. *Transcranial Doppler Ultrasonography*. St. Louis: CV Mosby; 1993:87.

14. Wechsler LR: Role of transcranial Doppler ultrasonography in clinical practice. In Babikian VL, Wechsler LR, eds. *Transcranial Doppler Ultrasonography*. St. Louis: CV Mosby; 1993:305.

15. Cantelmo NL, Babikian VL, Johnson WC, et al: Correlation of transcranial Doppler and noninvasive tests with angiography in the evaluation of extracranial carotid disease. *J Vasc Surg*. 1990;11:786.

16. Grolimund P, Seiler RW, Aaslid R, et al: Evaluation of cerebrovascular disease by combined extracranial and transcranial Doppler sonography. *Stroke*. 1987;18:1018.

17. Lindegaard K-F, Nornes H, Bakke SJ, et al: Cerebral vasospasm after subarachnoid hemorrhage investigated by means of transcranial Doppler ultrasound. *Acta Neurochir*. 1988;42:81.

18. Sloan MA, Haley EC Jr, Kassell NF, et al: Sensitivity and specificity of transcranial Doppler ultrasonography in the diagnosis of vasospasm following subarachnoid hemorrhage. *Neurology*. 1989;39:1514.

19. Hutchison K, Weir B: Transcranial Doppler studies. *Can J Neurol Sci*. 1989;16:411.

20. Seiler RW, Newell DW: Subarachnoid hemorrhage and vasospasm. In Newel DW, Aaslid R, eds. *Transcranial Doppler*. New York: Raven Press; 1992.

21. Newell DW, Grady MS, Eskridge JM, Winn HR: Distribution of angiographic vasospasm after subarachnoid hemorrhage: Implications for diagnosis by transcranial Doppler ultrasonography. *Neurosurgery*. 1990;27:574.

22. Bass A, Krupski WC, Schneider PA, et al: Intraoperative transcranial Doppler: Limitations of the method. *J Vasc Surg*. 1989;10:549.

23. Jansen C, Vriens EM, Eikelboom BC, et al: Carotid endarterectomy with transcranial Doppler and electroencephalographic monitoring. *Stroke*. 1993;24:665.

24. Spencer MP, Thomas GI, Nicholls SC, Sauvage LR: Detection of middle cerebral artery emboli during carotid endarterectomy using transcranial Doppler ultrasonography. *Stroke*. 1990;21:415.

25. Ringelstein EB, Sievers C, Ecker S, et al: Noninvasive assessment of CO_2-induced cerebral vasomotor response in normal individuals and patients with carotid artery occlusions. *Stroke*. 1988;19:963.

26. Markus HS, Harrison MJG: Estimation of cerebrovascular reactivity using transcranial Doppler, including the use of breath-holding as the vasodilatory stimulus. *Stroke*. 1992;23:668.

27. Dahl A, Lindegaard K-L, Russell D, et al: A comparison of transcranial Doppler and cerebral blood flow studies to assess cerebral vasoreactivity. *Stroke*. 1992;23:15.

CHAPTER 22

Indications for Angiography and Basis for Selecting the Type of Angiographic Study

WESLEY S. MOORE

INDICATIONS FOR ANGIOGRAPHY

Since angiography is an invasive study that carries some risk, moderate cost, and discomfort, the decision to recommend the study must be carefully considered. It is no longer justifiable to do an angiogram solely for purposes of information if that information will not influence the therapeutic decision. History, physical examination, and noninvasive studies have reached such a level of sophistication that angiography should provide few diagnostic surprises. An angiogram is therefore usually performed after a decision is made for some therapeutic intervention, usually surgery. Confirmation of the specific lesion and its relationship to the overall arterial anatomy is a primary requirement for preoperative assessment; angiography should essentially be considered a preoperative study. Under these circumstances, the indications for arteriography are generally for surgery (see Parts VI, VII, and VIII for a detailed discussion). For purposes of this introductory review, the indications can be divided into three major categories: territorial symptoms, global ischemic symptoms, and asymptomatic but critical arterial lesions.

Territorial Symptoms

Transient or fixed monocular and hemispheric events represent the least controversial indication for angiography. The likelihood of finding a lesion in the carotid artery distribution is extremely high, once a cardiac source has been reasonably ruled out. Supporting evidence for carotid artery disease by noninvasive investigation is only confirmatory and not mandatory. On occasion, a negative noninvasive study in a patient with anterior circulation symptoms is confusing to the unsophisticated clinician who fails to recognize that embolization of arterial origin can occur from an ulcerated plaque in the absence of a hemodynamically significant stenosis.

Symptoms in the territory of the vertebrobasilar system can be evaluated only by angiography. The indications for surgery, and therefore angiography, are based on the severity of symptoms and resultant patient discomfort or disability.

Global Ischemic Symptoms

As global ischemic symptoms are relatively nonspecific for cerebrovascular disease, there should be confirmatory noninvasive evidence of a hemodynamically significant lesion, usually in the carotid distribution. If symptoms are disabling and noninvasive studies suggest significant disease, the decision to proceed with preoperative angiography is reasonable.

Asymptomatic Critical Arterial Lesions

Although the indications for carotid endarterectomy remain controversial, there is mounting evidence that patients with stenoses greater than 75 percent are at high risk for neurologic events. When a surgeon can offer prophylactic operation with a risk of less than 3 percent, clearly operation as well as preoperative angiography are indicated.

At the present time, the noninvasive identification of nonstenotic ulceration is inexact. If the resolution of B-mode ultrasonography improves or alternative techniques are developed to define plaque surface morphology, including ulceration, clearly this would represent another indication for angiography.

SELECTION OF ANGIOGRAPHIC STUDY

If the magnitude of angiographic assessment had no effect on risk, it would be easy to recommend routine total visualization of the extracranial and intracranial cerebral circulation. This would require an arch study in two projections, anteroposterior and lateral projections of the extracranial and intracranial carotid circulation using selective injections, and selective subclavian-vertebral artery injections to define the vertebrobasilar system. Unfortunately, the risks of cerebral angiography increase with contrast volume, number of individual injections, and proximity of the catheter tip to a critical atheromatous plaque, such as a carotid bifurcation lesion.

A selective angiographic study, tailored to answer the major clinical question, is a reasonable alternative to panangiography. Limiting the angiographic study should reduce the incidence of angiographic complications. A careful assessment of the patient's history, physical findings, and noninvasive data will enable the clinician to select the angiographic study that will define the important areas of pathology, provide the critical information, and expose the patient to the least risk. This section explores the advantages, disadvantages, and various indications for each angiographic technique. Finally, a clinical algorithm is provided to match individual patient problems with the most appropriate angiographic study.

Digital Intra-Arterial Arch Angiography

Advantages
    Good resolution of those structures adequately seen on an arch study
    Low contrast volume
    Can be done with a small-caliber catheter
    Is suitable for outpatient study
Disadvantages
    Similar limitations as those of conventional arch study
    Overlap of multiple vascular structures
Primary Indications
    Confirmation of high-grade stenoses with or without ulceration

Good visualization of arch vessels and, to a lesser degree, of vertebral arteries

Conventional Arch Study

Advantages
  Good visualization of all extracranial anatomy when two oblique projections are used
  Relatively safe
Disadvantages
  Inadequate visualization of intracranial anatomy
  May miss significant ulcerative lesions in the absence of high-grade stenosis
  Requires relatively large volume of contrast material
  Requires relatively large-bore arterial catheter, hence inpatient hospitalization
Primary Indications
  Visualization of the primary branches of the aortic arch
  Confirmation of high-grade stenoses in the carotid circulation

Selective Carotid or Subclavian–Vertebral Injections

Advantages
  Optimum visualization of the intracranial anatomy
  Detailed visualization of the carotid bifurcation with multiple views as necessary
  Optimum visualization of vertebrobasilar system and orifices of vertebral arteries
  Relatively low volume of contrast material
Disadvantages
  Most dangerous angiographic procedure in atherosclerotic patients
  Time-comsuming
  Does not visualize the aortic arch and its primary branches
Primary Indications
  Suspected intracranial pathology
  Identification of carotid ulcerative lesions
  Optimum visualization of vertebral artery orifices and vertebrobasilar system in patients with suspected posterior circulation ischemic events

ALGORITHMS FOR SELECTION OF ANGIOGRAPHIC STUDY BASED ON CLINICAL PRESENTATION

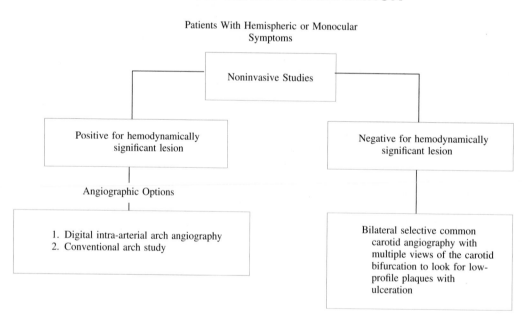

Patients With Nonspecific or Global Ischemic
Symptoms

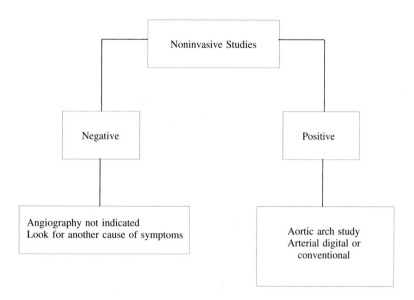

Patients With Symptoms of Vertebrobasilar
Insufficiency

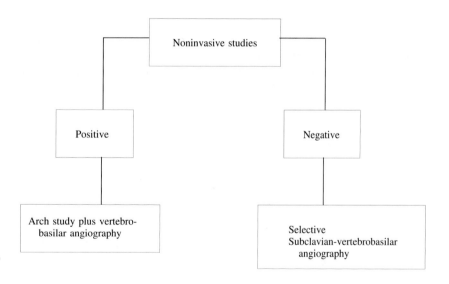

Asymptomatic Patients

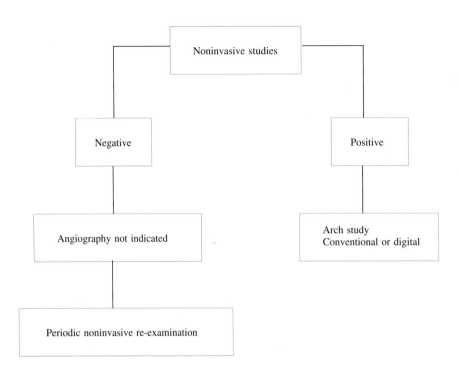

CONCLUSIONS

Angiography is indicated only when it will influence a therapeutic decision. Angiography is usually considered a preoperative examination. The various angiographic tech- niques carry different degrees of patient risk, with the more detailed and complete studies carrying the highest rates of complication. Angiographic risk can be reduced by tailoring the angiographic procedure to the specific patient on the basis of clinical presentation and noninvasive assessment.

CHAPTER 23

Aortic Arch Studies and Selective Arteriography

ANTOINETTE S. GOMES

Visualization of the aortic arch and carotid vessels can be accomplished by selective carotid arteriography, arch aortography with film-screen subtraction, or digital arterial or intravenous subtraction angiography. The angiogram should define the vascular abnormalities in the vessels supplying the symptomatic region. In carotid disease, the asymptomatic side should be evaluated as well. When vertebrobasilar symptoms are present, these vessels should be evaluated. Angiography should define critically stenotic or occluded brachiocephalic vessel origins or vessels, the carotid bifurcation in two projections, and, when indicated, the intracranial circulation.

The selection of a given imaging modality is determined by physician preference, patient status, and available radiographic equipment. In general, conventional film-screen arteriography provides images with the highest resolution. Digital subtraction techniques have lower resolution but increased contrast sensitivity. Digital intravenous studies, although relatively noninvasive, require large volumes of contrast material. Digital arterial studies allow the use of low volumes of dilute contrast material.

PATIENT PREPARATION

Arteriography may be performed on an inpatient or outpatient basis. When performed as an outpatient procedure, adequate facilities should be available for patient observation for 4 to 6 hours after the study. High-risk or elderly patients may be managed as outpatients if appropriate follow-up can be provided.

Informed consent should be obtained prior to all arteriographic studies. Pertinent medical history regarding allergies, renal function, and cardiac status should be elicited. The procedure should be explained to the patient by experienced personnel so that patient fears are allayed.

The currently used contrast agents have systemic physiologic effects on the kidneys, heart, and central nervous system. Because these agents are potentially nephrotoxic, baseline laboratory studies of serum creatinine should be obtained. To avoid potential problems with bleeding, a serum prothrombin time and partial thromboplastin time may be necessary in selected patients. All patients should receive hydration prior to arteriography. This may be accomplished by oral or intravenous (IV) fluid administration. An IV line of dextrose and half-normal or dextrose and quarter-normal saline should be in place during the study. Sedation of the patient is advised prior to the arteriogram. A variety of drugs may be used. Midazolam (Versed) 1 to 2 mg IV and fentanyl citrate (Sublimaze) 50 to 75 μg IV, or midazolam and morphine sulfate 2 to 4 mg IV, provide adequate sedation and analgesia. Intravenous Demerol should be avoided as it may cause hypotension. Oversedation should be avoided. Electrocardiographic monitoring should be used and the patient's blood pressure should be monitored during the examination. Elderly patients in sinus rhythm may tolerate arch injections better if they are given 0.4 mg of atropine IV to counteract any contrast-induced bradycardia and hypotension. In lengthy procedures, 3000 units of low-dose heparin may be given IV to retard thrombosis.[1]

Patients with a prior history of allergy to contrast agents should have pretreatment. In patients with a history of prior mild urticaria, 50 mg of intramuscular diphenhydramine (Benadryl) prior to the study is adequate. Patients with a prior history of severe allergic reactions should be treated with 50 mg of prednisone orally for three doses beginning 18 hours prior to the study and 50 mg of diphenhydramine 1 hour before the study.[2] Cimetidine, a histamine H_2-receptor antagonist, can also be administered. For patients with a documented prior anaphylactoid-type reaction, anesthesia standby is advisable. Low-osmolar contrast agents (discussed later) should be used in patients with a history of allergy to contrast agents, multiple allergies, or asthma.

PATIENT MANAGEMENT FOLLOWING ARTERIOGRAPHY

After angiography, a sterile dressing should be applied to the puncture site. The patient should be kept flat for 3 to 6 hours after the arteriogram is completed. The longer interval is preferred if multiple catheter changes have been made during the study or if the patient is hypertensive. Sandbags may be applied to the groin to remind the patient to remain still. They may be useful in hypertensive patients or in patients with a coagulopathy.[3] In cooperative normotensive patients, they are not required.[4]

Patients should have their IV fluids continued at least during the period of observation. At many institutions, it is customary to start systemic intravenous heparin therapy during the immediate postarteriography period in patients found to have a high-grade carotid stenosis.[4, 5]

RADIOGRAPHIC CONTRAST AGENTS

The radiographic contrast agents used today are derivatives of triiodobenzoic acid. They can be separated into two classes: conventional high-osmolar (ionic) contrast agents and the newer low-osmolar (nonionic and ionic dimers) contrast agents. The ionic compounds are either sodium or meglumine salts. Contrast agents are available in a variety of concentrations. Medium contrast agents (350 to 370 mg iodine/mL) are used for arch studies. Low-concentration contrast agents (282 to 300 mg iodine/mL) are used for selective injections or digital subtraction angiography studies. Of the conventional high-osmolar agents, low-concentration iothalamates (eg, Conray 60) and pure methylglucamine salts are better tolerated by the brain.[6, 7] Currently, however, the newer low-osmolar agents are preferred for arch and intracranial studies because they are better tolerated by the central nervous system.

The currently used agents have systemic effects, but these effects are less severe with low-osmolar agents. In high concentrations, the agents have toxic reversible effects on blood vessels and their contents. Endothelial damage, red blood cell hemolysis, crenation, and intravascular sludging of red cells with impaired circulation can occur.[8, 9] Contrast agents can also exert a direct chemotoxic effect on parenchymal cells, related to the amount of contrast material that crosses endothelial capillary lining cells. The hypertonicity of the contrast agents activates the endothelial pinocytotic vesicles, permitting transport of the contrast macromolecules into perivascular spaces.[10]

Contrast agents exert a direct chemotoxic effect on the brain. Repeated injections of a contrast agent cause "tight junctions" (closely apposed cellular surfaces in the capillary endothelium of the brain) to open, permitting direct contact of the contrast macromolecule with the glial cell.[11] Experimental studies indicate that the more lipophilic the contrast agent, the greater the degree of transport across the endothelial cells of the blood-brain barrier.[12] The contrast agent causes a shifting of the oxygen dissociation curve to the left, increased hemoglobin-oxygen affinity, and tissue hypoxia. Convulsions and other neurologic sequelae may follow intracerebral injection of contrast agents, particularly in patients with underlying cerebral ischemia.[7, 12]

Contrast agents can produce bradycardia and systemic hypotension. These effects are mediated through vagus nerve and vasomotor centers. The effect can be blocked by atropine, but a central effect persists.[13] Following injection of a contrast agent into the root of the aorta, there is typically an initial elevation of blood pressure followed by blood pressure depression for the next 30 seconds.[14]

The contrast agents are excreted by glomerular filtration.[15] In normal kidneys, they produce transient decreased renal blood flow, increased renal vascular resistance, and decreased tubular function.[15–17] In patients with preexisting renal disease, transient worsening of renal function may occur or contrast-induced acute tubular necrosis with anuria may result.

Patients with preexisting renal disease or advanced age (greater than 70 years), those receiving large volumes of contrast material, and patients with diabetes mellitus and cardiac disease are at increased risk for developing acute renal dysfunction following arteriography.[18–21] Dehydration is also an aggravating factor.[22, 23] The likelihood of a patient's developing postangiographic acute renal dysfunction has been shown to be related to the total volume of contrast material received. Postarteriographic renal dysfunction may not manifest for 48 to 72 hours following the arteriogram.[24] Renal failure usually resolves spontaneously within 7 days, but in a small percentage of cases, it may be permanent, requiring dialysis.[18]

In high-risk patients, the risk of postarteriographic renal dysfunction should be weighed against the need to perform high-volume multisystem arteriography at one sitting. Major operations in high-risk patients should be scheduled with consideration of the possibility of a delayed onset of renal dysfunction.

The newer contrast agents with a dimeric on nonionic structure have lower osmolality than conventional agents and produce less patient discomfort and hemodynamic alteration.

They are believed to be less toxic overall than conventional ionic agents.

REACTIONS TO CONTRAST MEDIA

Reactions to contrast agents vary in type and severity, ranging from mild nausea or hot flush to progressively severe cutaneous, respiratory, and cardiovascular reactions, which can be life-threatening.[25] Mild reactions require no treatment. Severe reactions are anaphylactoid in nature and mimic immunoglobin E (IgE)–mediated hypersensitivity, presenting as urticaria, rhinitis, angioedema, bronchospasm, and hypotension. With the high-osmolar ionic contrast agents, anaphylactoid reactions occur in approximately 2 percent of patients.[26, 27] A large recent study demonstrated that severe and potentially life-threatening adverse reactions occur much less often in patients receiving low-osmolar agents than in those receiving high-osmolar (ionic) agents (0.04% versus 0.22%).[28] It is generally accepted that patients who have had prior adverse reactions to contrast media have an increased risk of reaction on subsequent exposure, and with ionic agents, this risk may exceed 30 percent.[2] Patients with a history of hypersensitivity, such as hay fever, asthma, food allergies, or iodine hypersensitivity, are twice as likely to have a reaction to contrast agents than are those with no history of allergy. Sensitivity testing is not sufficiently predictive to be of use and is no longer recommended.[25, 29] Patients with mild urticarial reactions respond to diphenhydramine. Severe anaphylactoid reactions with angioedema, larynogospasm, or hypotension require prompt treatment with epinephrine and steroids and vigorous supportive or resuscitative treatment.

In patients with a prior history of severe reactions to contrast agents in whom repeat studies are required, pretreatment with steroids, as described previously, and the use of low-osmolar agents are recommended.

TECHNIQUE OF ARTERIOGRAPHY

Aortic Arch Studies

Arch aortography can be performed using large-film serialography or digital subtraction angiography when adequate equipment is available. Centers with large field-of-view image intensifiers rely almost solely on digital subtraction angiography. Arch aortography is usually performed via a percutaneous femoral artery approach. A pigtail catheter (5 to 8 French) with multiple side holes capable of rapid delivery of high volumes of contrast material is used. Alternatively, an end-hole catheter with multiple side holes may be used. A vascular sheath may be used when multiple catheter exchanges are anticipated. In patients in whom the femoral arteries are not accessible, an axillary percutaneous approach can be used. Typically, the catheter is positioned just proximal to the origin of the innominate artery.

Using large-film serialography, 50 to 60 mL of 350 or 370 mg iodine/mL contrast medium is delivered with power injection at 28 to 35 mL/second over 1 to 1.5 seconds. Cut films using a rapid film changer are obtained at a rate of three or four per second initially for 3 seconds with late

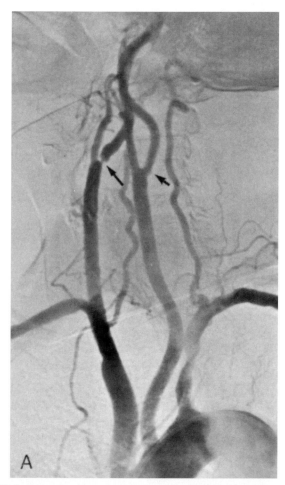 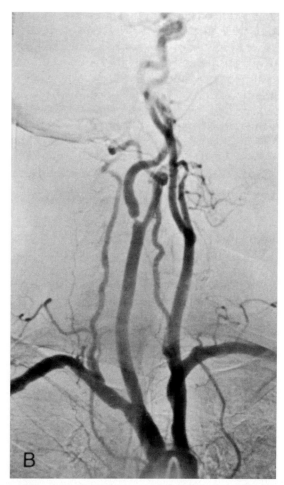

FIGURE 23–1. Subtraction films of a typical aortic arch study. *A,* Right posterior oblique projection shows origin of brachiocephalic vessels. Atherosclerotic plaques are seen in both proximal subclavian arteries. A high-grade stenosis is present at the origin of the right internal carotid artery *(long arrow)* and a shallow plaque with ulceration is identified at the origin of the left internal carotid artery *(short arrow). B,* Left posterior oblique projection shows similar findings. The cervical and petrous portions of the carotid artery are seen.

films, for a total duration of 6 seconds. Two projections are obtained: the left posterior oblique and the right posterior oblique. Selected films are then chosen for film-screen subtraction. This technique provides good visualization of the origin of the brachiocephalic vessels, the carotid bifurcation, and the precavernous portion of the carotid arteries. (Fig. 23–1).

When digital subtraction angiography techniques are used, the field of view of the image intensifier should be of sufficient size to cover the area of interest. Twenty to 40 mL of 300 mg iodine/mL contrast medium is injected at 20 to 25 mL/second over 1 to 1.5 seconds through a 5 French pigtail or high-flow end- and side-hole catheter. When vessel overlap prevents optimal visualization of the carotid bifurcation or a lesion is not seen contrary to noninvasive findings, a selective carotid artery injection should be performed.

Selective Carotid Artery Studies

Selective carotid artery injections are also usually performed via the femoral artery approach. Typically, small 5 French catheters with a preselected preformed shape are used for selective catheterization of carotid and vertebral arteries. In the evaluation of disease of the carotid bifurca-

tion, the catheter is positioned in the common carotid artery. When visualization of the smaller intracranial vessels is required, selective internal carotid injections are used. Depending on clinical symptoms, a vertebral artery injection may or may not be performed.

When large-film serialography is used, common carotid artery injections are performed using power injections of approximately 10 mL of 300 or 320 mg iodine/mL contrast medium delivered at 7 mL/second over 1 to 1.5 seconds, with filming extended to 12 seconds. Longer filming sequences may be necessary when subclavian steal syndromes are present. Filming of the neck is performed in the frontal and lateral projections, and magnification techniques are used (Fig. 23–2). Subtractions may also be performed. Selective internal carotid injections are performed using 7 to 9 mL of contrast power injected at 6 mL/second, with filming extended to 12 seconds. Filming is done in the anteroposterior and lateral projections. In some cases, additional special views may be required for visualization of intracranial vessels.

Currently, most selective carotid artery injections are performed using digital subtraction angiography, as this allows the use of smaller volumes of contrast material. For visualization of the extracranial portion of the carotid, hand

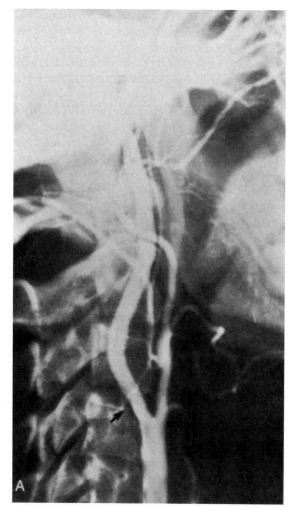
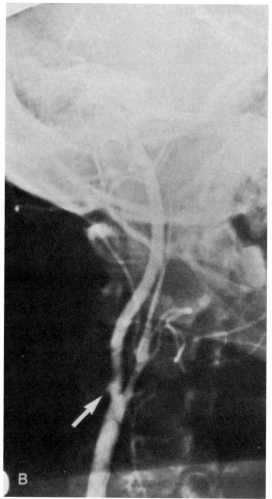

FIGURE 23–2. Typical selective right carotid artery injection. *A,* Lateral view shows mild smooth narrowing of right internal carotid artery origin *(arrow).* *B,* Frontal view with the head turned to the left shows a shallow ulcer laterally *(arrow).*

injections may be adequate. Filming in two orthogonal projections is indicated. The use of a C-arm or parallelogram allows the selection of orthogonal views that are optimal for the anatomy. With digital subtraction techniques, vascular calcifications may be subtracted and not seen, thus both subtracted and nonsubtracted images should be analyzed.

When the femoral artery approach cannot be used, an axillary approach using preformed catheters is employed. Direct carotid artery puncture using a thin-walled needle was once a primary method of performing carotid arteriography. This method was associated with an estimated 10 percent risk of subintimal injection,[30] which could produce narrowing of the arterial lumen sufficient to cause temporary or permanent neurologic sequelae. The technique is now rarely used, as noninvasive techniques such as magnetic resonance angiography can frequently be used to obtain sufficient information to confirm the diagnosis.

ANATOMY

The brachiocephalic vessels and the aorta arise from eight primitive vascular arches that connect the anteriorly located arterial trunk with the posteriorly positioned paired aortas. Persistence of some portions of these arches and involution

of others result in the normal arch. Failure of involution of these primitive vessels produces anomalies. Normally the aorta arches to the left, a persistence of the left fourth primitive arch. If the right fourth arch persists instead, it will arch to the right. Cervical arches (the result of persistence of the third cervical arch rather than the fourth) arise unusually high. They may be located in the thoracic outlet or extend up into the neck. They are often associated with anomalous brachiocephalic branch origins.

The first branch off the normal aortic arch is the innominate artery, the second branch is the left common carotid artery, and the third is the left subclavian artery. A variety of brachiocephalic artery origin anomalies are seen. There may be as many as six separately arising vessels from the arch (both subclavians, the carotids, and the vertebrals) or a single trunk or other combinations. Commonly seen anomalies are a common origin of the left carotid artery and the innominate artery, a high origin of the innominate artery (to the left of the trachea), and an anomalous origin of the left vertebral artery from the aorta. The right subclavian artery may arise distal to the left subclavian artery and pass behind the esophagus to reach the arm. Rarer anomalies are the right subclavian artery arising directly from the aorta proximal or just distal to the right carotid artery, the right vertebral artery

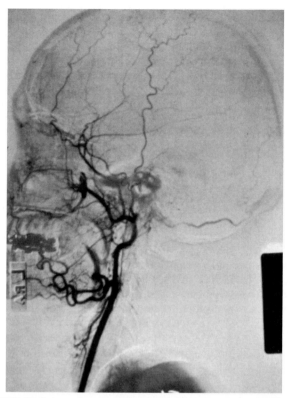

FIGURE 23–3. Selective external carotid artery injection. This patient has an arch anomaly involving congenital absence of the left internal carotid artery. Injection of the left "common" carotid artery shows only filling of the external carotid artery. The absence of the left internal carotid artery branches permits good visualization of the external carotid artery branches.

arising from the aorta, the external carotid artery arising from the aorta, variations in the level of the common carotid artery bifurcation, a bicarotid trunk, absence of the common carotid artery, duplication of vessels, and origin of the vertebral arteries from the carotid arteries. Uncommon anastomoses between the carotid artery and the basilar artery can occur as a result of the presence of remnants of primitive vessels, such as persistent trigeminal, acoustic, or hypoglossal arteries.[31]

CAROTID ARTERIES: NORMAL ANATOMY

The common carotid is encased within the carotid sheath with the jugular vein and vagus nerve. The carotid artery usually bifurcates at the level of the fourth cervical vertebra. The external carotid artery usually arises medial and anterior to the internal carotid artery. In approximately 15 percent of individuals, the external carotid artery originates lateral to the internal carotid artery.[32] This variation is more common (3:1) on the right. The branches of the external carotid artery can be divided into those that arise anteriorly and posteriorly (Fig. 23–3).[33] Anteriorly directed branches are the superior thyroid, lingual, facial, and internal maxillary arteries. The posteriorly directed branches are the ascending pharyngeal, posterior auricular, and occipital arteries. The superficial temporal artery terminal branch continues superiorly along the main axis of the external carotid artery. The superior thyroid supplies the thyroid and parathyroid. The occipital

artery (the second branch in order of origin) feeds arteriovenous malformations and anastomoses with muscular branches from the subclavian, vertebral, and external carotid artery, providing important collaterals in brachiocephalic occlusive disease.

The ascending pharyngeal artery supplies the pharynx and prevertebral muscles. The lingual and facial arteries supply facial structures and the tongue. The internal maxillary artery terminal branches take part in important anastomoses with the ophthalmic artery in occlusive intracranial disease. The middle meningeal branch of the internal maxillary artery often feeds meningiomas or dural arteriovenous malformations. The temporal branches of the external carotid arteries are often biopsied in temporal arteritis. The superficial temporal artery can anastomose with the superior branch of the ophthalmic artery, and the facial artery can anastomose with the inferior branch of the ophthalmic artery. These anastomoses become important collateral channels when either the external or internal carotid arteries are occluded.

The internal carotid artery can be divided into five segments: cervical, petrous, precavernous, intracavernous, and supraclinoid (Fig. 23–4).[33] The cervical segment begins at the bifurcation of the common carotid artery and extends to the carotid canal at the base of the skull. It usually lies

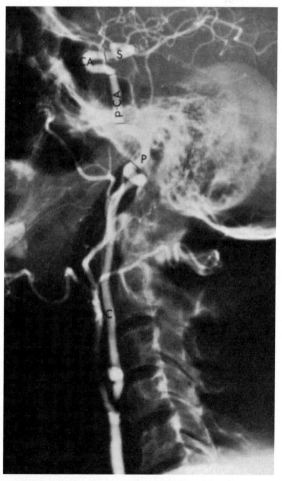

FIGURE 23–4. Selective carotid artery injection showing segments of carotid artery. C, cervical; P, petrous; p-CA, precavernous; CA, cavernous; S, supraclinoid. A high-grade stenosis is seen at the origin of the left internal carotid artery.

lateral and posterior to the external carotid artery. The petrous segment extends from the base of the skull to the apex of the petrous bone. It consists of a vertical portion of about 1 cm and a horizontal portion of 3 to 4 cm. The precavernous segment begins at the apex of the petrous bone and ends just lateral to the lower border of the dorsum sellae. The intracavernous segment begins at the lower border of the dorsum sellae, passes forward in the carotid sulcus, and ends medial to the anterior clinoid process. The cavernous segment (siphon) is S-shaped. The internal carotid artery leaves the cavernous sinus as it passes under the anterior clinoids to become an intradural structure. The supraclinoid segment of the internal carotid artery begins after passing through the dura and continues until it bifurcates into the anterior and middle cerebral arteries. The supraclinoid segment gives rise to the ophthalmic, posterior communicating, and anterior choroidal arteries. The ophthalmic artery supplies the orbit and the meninges on the floor of the anterior cranial fossa. Important anastomoses occur between terminal branches of this vessel and those of the internal maxillary artery. The middle meningeal artery may occasionally originate from the ophthalmic artery.

Each vertebral artery arises from the ipsilateral subclavian artery and ascends in the upper six vertebral transverse foramina to penetrate the dura at the level of the foramen magnum. In obstructive disease, muscular branches from the cervical portion form collaterals with terminal branches of the external carotid artery, costocervical and thyrocervical branches of the subclavian artery, and muscular branches of the contralateral vertebral artery. Radicular branches arising from the cervical portion join the spinal artery. Additional spinal branches arise from the vertebral arteries just before they fuse to form the basilar artery. In addition, meningeal branches supplying the dura arise from the distal extracranial vertebral arteries. The posterior inferior cerebellar artery arises from the vertebral artery, usually above the foramen magnum. The basilar artery gives rise to the anterior inferior cerebellar arteries and the superior cerebellar artery. The basilar artery then bifurcates terminally into two posterior cerebral arteries.

ANGIOGRAPHIC FINDINGS

Atherosclerotic Disease

Angiographic findings in atherosclerosis include stenosis or occlusion, ulceration, and emboli. Atherosclerosis may manifest as tortuosity, elongation, and dilation of vessels. Atheromatous lesions characteristically occur at vessel branches or bifurcations. Common sites include the common carotid bifurcation, origin of the internal carotid arteries, origin of the vertebral arteries from the subclavian artery, origins of the anterior and middle cerebral arteries, and origin of the brachiocephalic arteries from the aortic arch. The external carotid arteries may also be involved, but this involvement is less significant unless the artery is serving as a collateral to the intracranial circulation because of accompanying occlusion of the internal carotid artery. In a review of 300 aortocranial angiograms, Blaisdell and associates[34] noted that 33 percent of angiographically demonstrated lesions were intracranial. The remaining 67 percent were

extracranial, with 38 percent of those lesions located at the carotid bifurcation, 20 percent at vertebral artery origins, and 9 percent at the origin of branches of the aortic arch. A similar distribution was reported by Hass and colleagues[35] following a review of 4748 arteriograms. Atherosclerotic changes and symptomatic carotid artery disease can also develop as a result of injury from external radiation following treatment of cervical tumors.[36]

Observed stenoses correlate imprecisely with cerebral blood flow. Stenoses are usually described as a percentage of the normal vessel diameter. Stenoses of greater than 65 to 75 percent are regarded as hemodynamically significant lesions.[37, 38] Ulceration is seen as irregularity of the vessel wall or a penetrating niche (Figs. 23–5 and 23–6).[39] Thrombosis or embolization can superimpose on stenotic plaques. False-negative results occur when the ulcer is too small to be seen well or when the ulcerated plaque is filled with clot. False-positive angiograms occur when the intima is pitted or when a plaque has an irregular contour but is lined with intima. The misdiagnosis rate in carotid artery ulceration disease is estimated at 10 to 50 percent.[40] The ability to

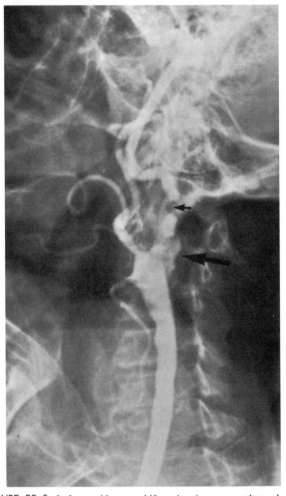

FIGURE 23–5. Left carotid artery bifurcation in severe atherosclerotic disease. Selective left common carotid artery injection shows plaque formation in the distal common carotid artery, with ectasia and a large irregular ulcer of the carotid bulb and the proximal left internal carotid artery *(long arrow)*. A 60 to 70 percent stenosis is also seen in the proximal left internal carotid artery *(short arrow)*. A 50 to 60 percent stenosis is present at the origin of the left external carotid artery.

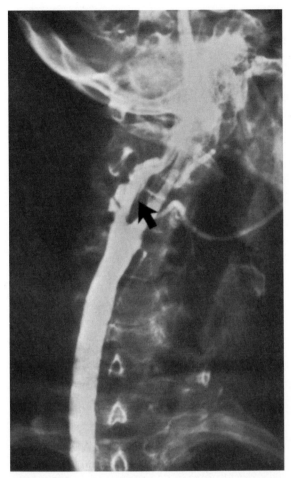

FIGURE 23–6. Left common carotid artery injection shows a large ulcerated plaque and associated linear lucency *(arrow)* consistent with dissection of left internal carotid artery. The dissection occurred spontaneously.

image in optimized oblique or angled projections using a C-arm or parallelogram and digital subtraction techniques should reduce interpretation error.

Emboli may be distinguished if they partly occlude a vessel, or if they are seen early and their convex contour can be seen. When seen later, only an abrupt change in caliber or a zone void of an artery may signify occlusion, and the embolus cannot be identified conclusively.[41, 42] Retrograde filling of a vessel and arteriovenous shunting are also signs of cerebrovascular obstruction. Over time, the embolus may fragment and move distally or shrink and undergo alteration in contour. If occlusive disease is seen in one area, the circulation proximal and distal to that area and the circulation in the remaining brachiocephalic vessels should be evaluated.

Collateral flow induced by intracranial vascular occlusion may result in a steal phenomenon, such as subclavian steal syndrome induced by a subclavian artery stenosis proximal to a patent vertebral artery (Fig. 23–7). Collateral flow to the affected upper extremity is frequently retrograde down the vertebral artery, with consequent siphoning off of blood flow from the basilar artery and posterior fossa circulation.

Vasculitis

A variety of entities can produce inflammatory or secondary changes of the cerebral blood vessels. These include bacterial and viral infectious processes (such as tuberculosis), irradiation, and chemicals (intravenous drugs). Changes can also be caused by a specific vasculitis, such as polyarteritis nodosa, giant-cell arteritis, systemic lupus erythematosus, rheumatoid arthritis, Wegener granulomatosis, or Takayasu arteritis, and by dysproteinemia and chronic recurrent trauma. These entities can sometimes be distinguished pathologically by the anatomic site involved, the histologic findings, or the infecting organism. More often, however, the nonspecific findings of luminal narrowing or occlusion and vessel irregularity may be observed. Often focal areas of dilatation or spasm or aneurysm formation are seen. Tuberculous or fungal meningitis often manifests as smooth tapered narrowing of the supraclinoid carotid artery or other large vessels at the base of the brain.[43]

Temporal (granulomatous) arteritis characteristically involves the carotid and vertebral arteries as they pierce the dura, with sparing of intracranial vessels. The temporal arteries are frequently involved.[44] Pathologically, the findings are inflammatory cells with disruption of elastica and intimal proliferation. The angiographic appearance is one of smooth segmental stenosis. The disease typically presents in older patients manifesting with malaise, fever, and headache. Although the arteritis usually burns itself out within 6 months to 2 years, residual arterial narrowing, blindness, and cerebral ischemia may persist. Aneurysms may occur with bacteremia and systemic lupus erythematosus and have rarely been reported intracranially with polyarteritis nodosa.[45] Arterial beading and small vessel occlusions on cerebral arteriograms have been seen in drug-abuse patients taking methamphetamine.[46]

Takayasu arteritis is a panarteritis that primarily involves the brachiocephalic vessels but can affect the aorta or any of its primary branches. Cranial vessels are spared. Fusiform narrowing of blood vessels over a variable length occurs (Fig. 23–8). Symptoms of fever, malaise, and elevated sedimentation rate are present in the early systemic phase. These symptoms may be absent, and presenting clinical symptoms are often related to cerebral ischemia.[47]

Fibromuscular Dysplasia

Fibromuscular dysplasia or hyperplasia is an angiopathy of unknown etiology that occurs more commonly in women. Several histologic types have been described, including intimal fibroplasia, medial fibroplasia, and perimedial dysplasia.[48] Although the renal arteries are involved most frequently, lesions occur in other vessels and have been identified in 0.7 percent of cerebral angiograms.[49] Fibromuscular dysplasia is the most common nonatheromatous disease of the internal carotid artery. In medial fibroplasia, a string-of-beads pattern with areas of heaped-up intima and media (arterial narrowing) alternating with areas of medial destruction (localized aneurysms) is most often seen (Fig. 23–9). The areas of the internal carotid artery most often involved are the middle and upper portions of the internal carotid arteries, areas more distal than those affected by atherosclerosis. Other cephalic vessels, including the middle cerebral artery, may be involved.[50] Approximately 30 percent of patients with cervical involvement have associated intracranial aneurysms.[51] Intracranial emboli have been reported occasionally.

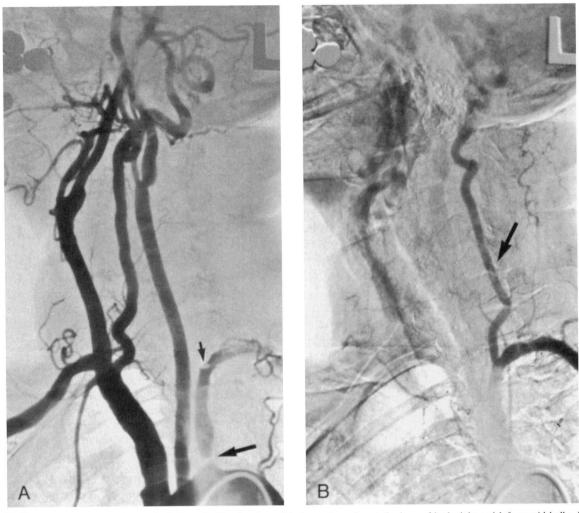

FIGURE 23–7. Subclavian steal syndrome. *A,* Arch study film showing mild plaque formation at the base of both right and left carotid bulbs. There is a high-grade stenosis at the origin of the left subclavian artery *(long arrow).* A lucency from nonopaque blood is seen at the origin of the left vertebral artery, which does not become opaque on initial films *(short arrow).* The left subclavian artery shows faint antegrade filling. *B,* Delayed film of arch injection shows retrograde filling of left vertebral artery *(arrow)* with drainage into the left subclavian artery.

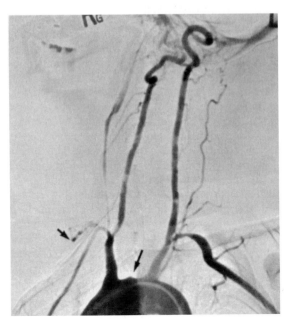

FIGURE 23–8. Takayasu disease in a young woman who presented following a left-sided cerebrovascular accident. Arch injection shows diffuse narrowing of a long segment of the right internal carotid artery. There is occlusion of the left common carotid artery at its origin *(long arrow).* The right subclavian artery is occluded proximally *(short arrow)* and the left subclavian artery is narrowed just distal to the vertebral artery.

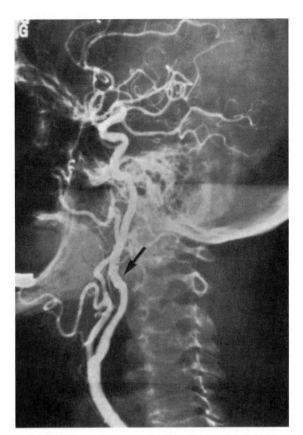

FIGURE 23–9. Selective right common carotid artery injection shows the typical string-of-beads appearance of fibromuscular dysplasia of the right internal carotid artery *(arrow)*. Similar changes were seen in the left internal carotid artery.

Trauma

Arteriography plays a primary role in the evaluation of penetrating or blunt cervical trauma. Carotid artery injury may occur as a result of direct compression or traumatic stretching about bony protuberances at the fracture site. In addition, extreme extension-rotation of the head may cause stretching of the internal carotid artery against the first cervical vertebral body, injuring the vessel just below the base of the skull.[52] Spontaneous intimal dissection in the absence of trauma can also occur (see Fig. 23–6).

In severe dislocations of the cervical spine, the vertebral arteries may be trapped and stretched or sustain local injury (Fig. 23–10). Basal skull fractures may result in injury to

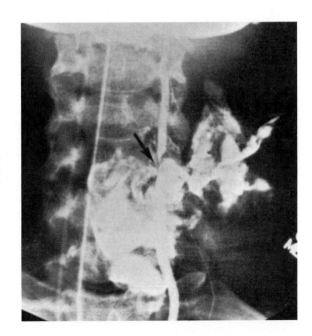

FIGURE 23–10. Trauma in a 22-year-old man who presented with a wound to the left neck. Selective left vertebral artery injection in frontal projection shows massive extravasation of the contrast medium. Narrowing is seen in the left vertebral artery at the site of laceration *(arrow)*.

the cavernous portion of the internal carotid artery. These injuries can cause mural dissection with subintimal or intramural hemorrhage at the site of injury, resulting in a narrowed lumen or occlusion.[53]

Other injuries that occur are spasm, subintimal tears with or without clot formation, and false aneurysm. Intravascular thrombus may propagate proximally and distally at the site of spasm or injury. Emboli may originate at the site of vessel injury or stenosis, and an embolic stroke may announce the presence of a significant vascular injury. Stenotic or occluded injured brachiocephalic vessels may result in stroke. If adequate collaterals are available, occlusion of carotid or vertebral arteries may be asymptomatic. A vertebral artery tear or disruption of the cavernous carotid may result in an arteriovenous fistula.

Miscellaneous Lesions

Elongation, tortuosity, or kinking of the internal carotid artery is seen in approximately 16 to 20 percent of adult carotid arteriograms. These changes can be congenital in origin or secondary to atherosclerosis. Excessive kinking can compromise blood flow.[54] Extrinsic compression of the cervical arteries can compromise cerebral blood flow. Compression of the vertebral artery by bony spurs or hyperostosis can occur as the artery passes through the vertebral canal. Tumors can encase the carotid artery and invade the wall, also producing compression.

Extracranial carotid artery aneurysms are uncommon lesions. The majority are due to atherosclerosis. Other causes include trauma and prior carotid surgery. The majority occur at the bifurcation of the common carotid artery. Angiographically, those involving the bifurcation are fusiform, and those occurring at other sites are saccular.[55]

COMPLICATIONS OF ANGIOGRAPHY

Various types of complications are associated with cerebral studies. These include systemic reactions secondary to medications or contrast agents used in the study, local complications related to the vessel puncture or catheter placement, and neurologic complications.

Contrast reactions have already been discussed. Hematoma formation is the most frequent complication at the puncture site. Although unsightly and painful, hematomas are usually self-limiting. If neurologic deficit occurs as a result of compression of adjacent nerves by hematoma, surgical evacuation and repair of the vessel are necessary. Rarely, chronic pain at the site of puncture indicates formation of a post-traumatic fistula that also requires treatment. Loss of pulse at the site of puncture may be due to spasm or to thrombus. If the absent pulse is due to spasm, application of heat to the contralateral extremity or administration of oral vasodilators may result in return of the pulse. Thrombus formation at the site of catheter puncture may progress to complete occlusion with embarrassment of circulation, requiring operative embolectomy.

Complications may occur at the site of injection with subintimal injections of contrast material. Small subintimal injections may heal spontaneously, but they may lead to complete occlusion of the vessel. Emboli may occur when fragments of clot within the catheter are discharged during injection. They may also result from dislodgment of thrombus or atherosclerotic material adherent to diseased vessel wall. A survey of angiographic complications showed a significant difference in the overall complication rate among transfemoral, transaxillary, and translumbar approaches, with femoral arteriography having the lowest incidence and axillary the highest.[56]

Multiple studies have addressed the incidence of complications of cerebral angiography.[5, 57–63] A survey of complications of cerebral arteriography in 5000 consecutive cerebral arteriograms by Mani and coworkers[61–63] revealed the following findings: The overall incidence of complications was 1.4 percent (68/5000). Complications were transient in 1.2 percent and permanent in 0.1 percent. Of the total complications, 0.8 percent were central nervous system complications, and 0.4 percent were local or systemic. Mortality was 0.02 percent.[61]

Total complication rates were significantly higher in training hospitals (3.4%) than in nontraining hospitals. In nontraining hospitals, the highest complication rates were in patients diagnosed as having vascular occlusive disease (1.2%), arteriovenous malformation or aneurysm (1.9%), and post-traumatic or postoperative conditions (1.3%). The total complication rate in patients with cerebrovascular occlusive disease was significantly higher than the rate in patients with suspected tumor, headache, or seizure.[62]

In their study, Mani and Eisenberg[63] showed that the complication rate of aortic arch injections (alone or in combination with the carotid) was the same as that of carotid injections alone.

Another prospective study of 1517 cerebral studies by Earnest and associates[5] consisted of 1453 transfemoral selective studies, 36 direct carotid angiograms, 2 axillary studies, and 26 aortic arch plus selective studies. They observed an overall incidence of complications of 8.5 percent; the overall incidence of neurologic complications was 2.6 percent. The incidence of neurologic complications in patients referred for evaluation of cerebrovascular disease (exclusive of tumor, subarachnoid hemorrhage, arteriovenous malformation, or seizures) was 4.2 percent, with 0.6 percent of these being permanent deficits. Mortality was 0.06 percent. Recent stroke and frequent transient ischemic attacks were associated with a statistically significant increase in the incidence of neurologic complications.

It appears that patients with disorders associated with reduced cerebral perfusion are more likely to have neurologic complications of angiography than those with normal cerebral blood flow. Hypotension by reducing cerebral perfusion is particularly dangerous. The exact method by which complications occur when there is reduced perfusion is uncertain. Hypoxia might potentiate the toxic effect of the contrast agent, transient displacement of blood by the contrast agent could reduce oxygenation below a critical level, vascular spasm might be induced or aggravated by the contrast medium, or the contrast osmolarity could induce aggregation of formed elements in the blood. Emboli may result from dislodgment of thrombus or atherosclerotic plaque adherent to a diseased vessel wall. Emboli may also occur when fragments of clot within the catheter are discharged during injection of contrast material or saline.

SELECTION OF ARCH AORTOGRAPHY VERSUS SELECTIVE CAROTID ARTERIOGRAPHY

The decision to perform an arch study or a selective carotid study in patients being examined for cerebrovascular disease is often a matter of controversy. There are some who believe that selected carotid studies should be performed in all patients studied for cerebrovascular disease,[64] but others recommend arch studies with selective carotid studies as needed.[65]

When intracranial disease is suspected, a three-vessel carotid study is required. When the examination is for vasculitis, such as Takayasu disease, which involves the brachiocephalic vessels, arch studies are required. An arch study is indicated in patients with suspected vertebrobasilar disease, as it demonstrates vertebral origins (Fig. 23–11). It is also indicated in postoperative patients undergoing evaluation for carotid-to-carotid or similar grafts (Fig. 23–12) and in patients in whom collateral patterns of flow, such as in subclavian steal syndrome, must be defined.

With regard to patients with suspected carotid bifurcation disease, arguments against the use of an arch study alone are that it may not provide optimal visualization of high cervical lesions, it is inadequate for visualization of small intracranial vessels, and it requires larger volumes of contrast material. In the past, the unavailability of small French-size pigtail catheters meant that if a large catheter was used for the arch, a large catheter would have to be used for the selective carotid injections, which is undesirable.[66, 67] The use of a femoral artery vascular sheath allows the safe exchange of catheters of varying size and configuration, rendering this argument obsolete. Another argument is that most plaques lie posteriorly in the carotid artery and a true lateral view, not usually obtained in an arch study, is needed.

The advantages of arch studies are as follows: Atherosclerotic plaques and lesions at the origins of the brachiocephalic vessels are readily identified before prolonged catheter manipulation is performed (Fig. 23–13). Arch studies can be performed rapidly, and with good radiographic technique and subtraction, the bifurcation and the high cervical portion of the carotid are adequately seen in most cases (Fig. 23–14).[31, 65] In patients with suspected high-grade stenosis on noninvasive studies, an arch study may obviate the need for selective studies. Although patients with nonatherosclerotic disease tolerate selective arteriography well, selective injection into occluded or tightly stenosed carotid arteries is associated with a significantly higher risk of neurologic

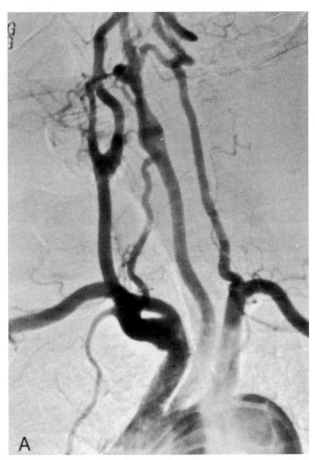

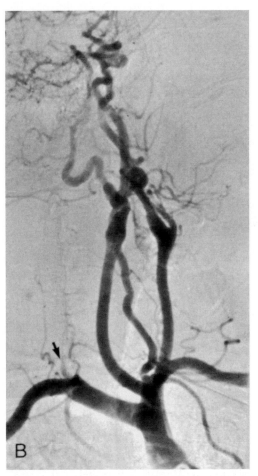

FIGURE 23–11. Positional occlusion of the right vertebral artery. *A,* Arch injection in right posterior oblique projection shows filling of all brachiocephalic vessels, including the right and left vertebral arteries. *B,* The left posterior oblique projection, with the head turned to the left, shows that the right vertebral artery is transiently occluded *(arrow).* This finding was not associated with symptoms. The occlusion is at the entrance of the artery into the transverse canal. Compression of the artery is probably caused by the long muscle of the neck and scalene muscle groups.

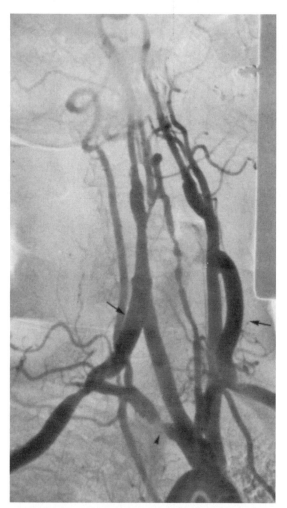

FIGURE 23–12. Left posterior oblique view of aortic arch study in a patient with bilateral carotid to subclavian Dacron bypass grafts *(arrows)* placed for a left subclavian occlusion, which was seen on right posterior oblique projection, and a right subclavian stenosis *(arrowhead)*. Bilateral carotid endarterectomies were also performed.

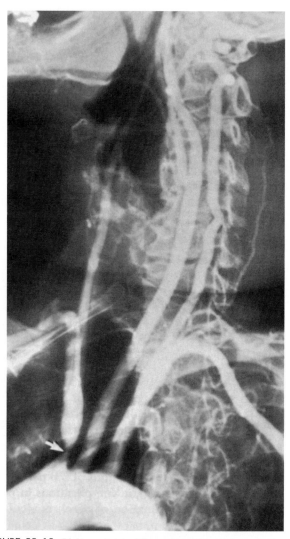

FIGURE 23–13. Right posterior oblique view of an arch study shows a high-grade stenosis at the origin of the innominate artery *(arrow)*.

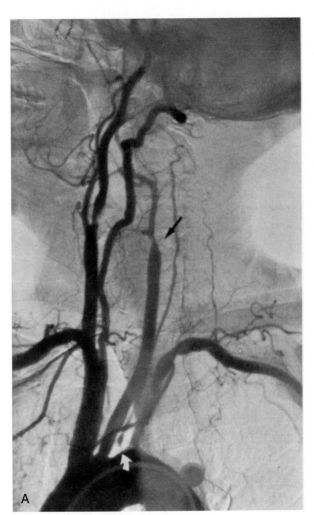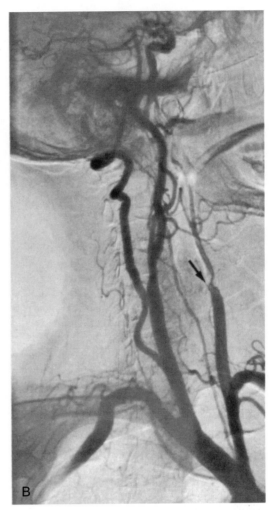

FIGURE 23–14. Arch study. *A,* Right posterior oblique view shows a lesion at the origin of the right internal carotid artery. The left internal carotid artery is completely occluded at its origin *(black arrow).* The left vertebral artery shows a high-grade stenosis at its origin *(white arrow). B,* Left posterior oblique projection shows similar findings.

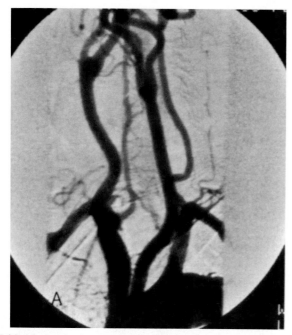 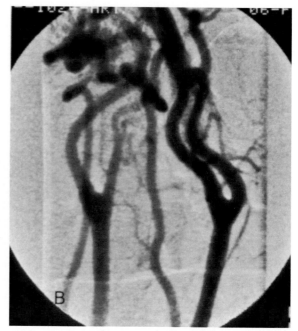

FIGURE 23–15. Arterial digital subtraction angiography study. *A,* Arch injection in the right posterior oblique projection with imaging on 10 inch field size provides good visualization of brachiocephalic vessel origins and carotid bifurcation. *B,* Left posterior oblique projection of arch injection with 6 inch field size confirms a normal carotid bifurcation.

complications than in patients with other diseases such as tumor, subarachnoid hemorrhage, aneurysm, arteriovenous malformation, or seizures.[5] This may be due to the prolonged exposure of the vessel wall to the contrast agent. With selective injections, brachiocephalic origins are not seen, and the likelihood of disrupting atherosclerotic material is present. In a study from Duke University,[31] 8 percent of a series of 350 patients studied for extracranial disease had significant intracranial pathology outlined by angiography. This study concluded that 85 percent of the patients studied for extracranial occlusive disease could be effectively evaluated by adequate multiple-projection arch studies alone.[31] Similar experience has been shared by other investigators.[65]

The vast majority of patients undergoing evaluation for carotid disease undergo noninvasive testing before arteriography. With modern techniques, small French catheters can be used in arch aortography. If the arch study fails to corroborate the results of noninvasive testing, a selective carotid injection can easily be obtained. In addition, the availability of digital subtraction angiography permits a digital arterial study of the arch to be performed with low volumes of contrast material followed by a selective carotid injection, as needed (Fig. 23–15). In patients in whom the noninvasive study shows a shallow nonobstructing lesion, such as a shallow ulcer, one may choose to proceed directly with a selective study. With modern angiographic techniques, the angiographic study can be designed to fit the patient, taking into consideration the patient's age, renal function, vessel tortuosity, overall clinical stability, and whether the study is performed in the setting of a teaching or nonteaching hospital.

REFERENCES

1. Wallace S, Medellin H, DeJongh D, Gianturco C: System heparinization for angiography. *AJR Am J Roentgenol.* 1972;116:204.

2. Kelly JF, Patterson R, Lieberman P, et al: Radiographic contrast media studies in high risk patients. *J Allergy Clin Immunol.* 1978;62:181.
3. Christenson R, Staab EV, Burko H, Foster J: Pressure dressings and post arteriographic care of the femoral puncture site. *Radiology.* 1976;119:97.
4. Eisenberg RL, Mani RL: Pressure dressings and post angiographic care of the femoral puncture site. *Radiology.* 1977;122:677.
5. Earnest F, Forbes G, Sandak B, et al: Complications of cerebral angiography: Prospective assessment of risk. *AJR Am J Roentgenol.* 1984;142:247.
6. Harrington G, Michie C, Lynch PR, et al: Blood brain barrier changes associated with unilateral cerebral angiography. *Invest Radiol.* 1966;1:431.
7. Hilal S: Hemodynamic responses in the cerebral vessels to angiographic contrast media. *Acta Radiol [Diagn].* 1966;5:211.
8. Bjork L: Effect of angiocardiography on erythrocyte aggregation in the conjunctival vessels. *Acta Radiol [Diagn].* 1967;6:459.
9. Haugen O, Brindle M: Effects of contrast media on blood coagulation. *J Can Assoc Radiol.* 1970;21:146.
10. Karnovsky M, Leventhal M: Some aspects of the structural basis for permeability of small blood vessels. In Hilal S, ed. *Small Vessel Angiography: Imaging, Morphology, Physiology and Clinical Applications.* St Louis: CV Mosby; 1973:117.
11. Rapaport S: Reversible opening of blood brain barrier by osmotic shrinkage of the cerebro-vascular endothelium: Opening up the tight junctions as related to carotid arteriography. In Hilal S, ed. *Small Vessel Angiography: Imaging, Morphology, Physiology and Clinical Applications.* St Louis: CV Mosby; 1973:137.
12. Levitan H, Rapoport SI: Contrast media: Quantitative criteria for designing compounds with low toxicity. *Acta Radiol [Diagn] (Stockh).* 1976;17:81.
13. Fischer HW, Echstein JW, Perret G: Comparison of the cardiovascular effects of contrast media by their circulatory effects. *AJR Am J Roentgenol.* 1961;86:166.
14. Gonzalez L, Stieritz D: Experimental evaluation of sodium methylglucamine iothalamate (MP3064): Cardiovascular responses following proximal aortic injection. *Invest Radiol.* 1967;2:266.
15. Hall J, Childs D Jr: The effect of diagnostic and therapeutic roentgenologic procedures on renal function. *Med Clin North Am.* 1966;50:969.
16. Sherwood T, Lavender J: Does renal flow rise or fall in response to diatrizoate? *Invest Radiol.* 1969;4:327.
17. Talner L, Davidson A: Effect of contrast media on renal excretion of PAH. *Invest Radiol.* 1968;3:301.
18. Port FK, Wagoner RD, Fulton RE: Acute renal failure after angiography. *AJR Am J Roentgenol.* 1974;121:544.
19. Older RA, Miller JP, Jackson DC, et al: Angiographically induced renal failure and its radiographic detection. *AJR Am J Roentgenol.* 1976;126:1039.
20. Pillay V, Robbins P, Schwartz F, et al: Acute renal failure following intravenous urography in patients with long standing diabetes mellitus and azotemia. *Radiology.* 1970;95:633.
21. Gomes AS, Baker JD, Martin-Paredero V, et al: Acute renal dysfunction following major arteriography. *AJR Am J Roentgenol.* 1985;145:1249.
22. Eisenberg RL, Bank WO, Hedgcock MW: Neurologic complications of angiography in patients with critical stenosis of the carotid artery. *Neurology (NY).* 1980;30:892.

23. Talner LB: Does hydration prevent contrast material renal injury? *AJR Am J Roentgenol.* 1981;136:1021.

24. Shafi T, Chou SY, Porush JG, Shapiro WB: Infusion intravenous pyelography and renal failure. *Arch Intern Med.* 1978;138:1218.

25. Witten DM: Reactions to urographic contrast media. *JAMA.* 1975;231:974.

26. Witten DM, Hirsch FD, Hartman GW: Acute reactions to urographic contrast media: Incidence, clinical characteristics and relationship to history of hypersensitivity states. *AJR Am J Roentgenol.* 1973;119:832.

27. Shehadi WH: Adverse reactions to intravascularly administered contrast media. A comprehensive study based on a prospective survey. *AJR Am J Roentgenol.* 1975;124:145.

28. Katayama H, Yamaguchi K, Kozuka T, et al: Adverse reactions to ionic and nonionic contrast media: A report from the Japanese Committee on the Safety of Contrast Media. *Radiology.* 1990;175:621.

29. Fischer HW, Doust VL: An evaluation of pretesting in the problem of serious and fatal reactions to excretory urography. *Radiology.* 1972;103:497.

30. Saltzman GF: Circulation through the anterior communicating artery studied by carotid angiography. *Acta Radiol.* 1959;52:194.

31. Johnsrude IS: Aortic arch and brachiocephalic angiography. In Johnsrude IS, Jackson DC, eds. *A Practical Approach to Angiography.* Boston: Little, Brown; 1987:385.

32. Teal JS, Rumbaugh CL, Bergeron RT, Segall HD: Lateral position of the external carotid artery: A rare anomaly? *Radiology.* 1973;108:77.

33. Kido DK, Baker RA, Rumbaugh CL: Normal cerebral vascular anatomy. In Abrams HL, ed. *Abrams Angiography Vascular and Interventional Radiology.* Boston: Little, Brown; 1983:231.

34. Blaisdell FW, Hall AD, Thomas AN, et al: Cerebrovascular occlusive disease: Experience with panarteriography in 300 consecutive cases. *Calif Med.* 1965;103:321.

35. Hass WK, Field WS, North RR, et al: Joint study of extracranial arterial occlusion. II. Arteriography, techniques, sites and complications. *JAMA.* 1968;203:961.

36. Elerding SC, Fernandez RN, Grotta JC, et al: Carotid artery disease following external cervical irradiation. *Ann Surg.* 1981;194:609.

37. May AG, Van de Berg L, DeWeese JA, Rob CG: Critical arterial stenosis. *Surgery.* 1963;54:250.

38. Berguer R, Hwang NHC: Critical arterial stenosis—a theoretical and experimental solution. *Ann Surg.* 1974;180:39.

39. Chase NE: Radiographic diagnosis of the ulcerated plaque. In McDowell MD, Fletcher H, Brennan RW, eds. *Cerebral Vascular Disease.* New York: Grune & Stratton; 1972:253.

40. Edwards JH, Kricheff IL, Riles T, Imparato A: Angiographically undetected ulceration of the carotid bifurcation as a cause of embolic stroke. *Radiology.* 1979;132:369.

41. Ring BA: Diagnosis of embolic occlusions of smaller branches of the inferior cerebral arteries. *AJR Am J Roentgenol.* 1966;97:575.

42. Rumbaugh CL, David DO, Gilson JM: Fate of experimental autologous emboli. *Am J Surg.* 1969;35:823.

43. Greitz T: Angiography in tuberculous meningitis. *Acta Radiol [Diagn].* 1964;2:369.

44. Harrison C: Giant cell or temporal arteritis: A review. *J Clin Path.* 1948;1:197.

45. Leonhardt ET, Jacobson H, Ringqvist OT: Angiographic and clinicophysiologic investigation of a case of polarteritis nodosa. *Am J Med.* 1972;53:242.

46. Citron BP, Halpern M, McCarrow N, et al: Necrotizing angiitis associated with drug abuse. *N Engl J Med.* 1970;283:1003.

47. Lande A, Berkmen Y: Aortitis: Pathologic, clinical and arteriographic review. *Radiol Clin North Am.* 1976;14:219.

48. Stanley JC, Gewertz BL, Bove EL: Arterial fibrodysplasia: Histopathologic character and current etiologic concepts. *Arch Surg.* 1975;110:56.

49. Houser WO, Baker HL Jr, Sandok BA, Holley KE: Cephalic arterial fibromuscular dysplasia. *Radiology.* 1971;101:605.

50. Ellias WS: Intracranial fibromuscular hyperplasia. *JAMA.* 1971;218:254.

51. Osborn AG, Anderson RE: Angiographic spectrum of cervical and intracranial fibromuscular dysplasia. *Stroke.* 1977;8:617.

52. Momose KJ, New PFJ: Nonatheromatous stenosis and occlusion of the internal carotid artery in its main branches. *AJR Am J Roentgenol.* 1973;118:550.

53. New PFL, Momose KJ: Traumatic dissection of the internal carotid artery at the allantoaxial level secondary to non-penetrating injury. *Radiology.* 1969;93:41.

54. Quattlebaum JK Jr, Wade JS, Whiddon CM: Stroke associated with elongation and kinking of the carotid artery: Long-term followup. *Ann Surg.* 1973;177;572.

55. Mokri B, Piepgras DG, Sundt TM Jr, Pearson BW: Extracranial internal carotid artery aneurysms. *Mayo Clin Proc.* 1982;57:310.

56. Hessel SJ, Adams DF, Abrams HL: Complications of angiography. *Radiology.* 1981;138:273.

57. Codden DR, Krieger HP: Circumstances surrounding complications of cerebral angiography: Analysis of 546 consecutive cerebral arteriograms. *Am J Med.* 1958;25:580.

58. Hass WK, Fields WS, North RR, et al: Joint study of extracranial arterial occlusion. II. Arteriography, techniques sites and complications. *JAMA.* 1968;203:961.

59. Wishart DL: Complications in vertebral angiography as compared to nonvertebral cerebral angiography in 447 studies. *AJR Am J Roentgenol.* 1971;113:527.

60. Olivecrona H: Complications of cerebral angiography. *Neuroradiology.* 1977;14:175.

61. Mani RL, Eisenberg RL, McDonald EF, et al: Complications of catheter cerebral arteriography: Analysis of 5,000 procedures. I. Criteria and incidence. *AJR Am J Roentgenol.* 1978;131:861.

62. Mani RL, Eisenberg RL: Complications of catheter cerebral arteriography: Analysis of 5,000 procedures. II. Relation of complication rates to clinical and arteriographic diagnosis. *AJR Am J Roentgenol.* 1978;131:867.

63. Mani RL, Eisenberg RL: Complications of catheter cerebral arteriography: Analysis of 5,000 procedures. III. Assessment of arteries injected, contrast medium used, duration of procedures, and age of patient. *AJR Am J Roentgenol.* 1978;131:871.

64. Goldstein SJ, Fried AM, Young B, Tibbs PA: Limited usefulness of aortic arch angiography in the evaluation of carotid occlusive disease. *AJR Am J Roentgenol.* 1982;138:103.

65. Eisenman J, Jenkin C, Pribram H, et al: Evaluation of the cerebral circulation by arch aortography supplemented by subtraction technique. *AJR Am J Roentgenol.* 1972;115:14.

66. Mani RL: Computer analysis of factors associated with thrombus formation observed on pullout angiograms. *Invest Radiol.* 1975;10:378.

67. Kerber CW, Cromwell LD, Drayer BP, Bank WO: Cerebral ischemia. I. Current angiographic techniques, complications and safety. *AJR Am J Roentgenol.* 1978;130:1097.

CHAPTER 24

Magnetic Resonance Angiography of Cerebrovascular Disease

CHARLES M. ANDERSON

Magnetic resonance angiography (MRA) is a noninvasive technique that has been applied to a variety of vascular diseases of interest to surgeons, including peripheral occlusive disease and deep venous thrombosis. MRA is particularly well suited to the study of vessels in the brain and neck because of the relatively fast velocity of blood in the carotid and cerebral arteries, the availability of high-sensitivity imaging coils for the head and neck and the fact that the head can be held motionless for many minutes. Typical neurologic applications of MRA include the screening of extracranial carotid and vertebral arteries for stenosis and dissection and imaging of intracranial vessels to reveal stenosis, occlusion, aneurysms, vascular malformations, and dural venous thrombosis.[1, 2] The resolution of MRA is not as fine as that of conventional angiography, so MRA is not used for the imaging of vessels affected with vasculitis or of very small vessels.

The principal advantage of MRA over conventional x-ray angiography is that it is noninvasive. Catheter angiography carries a 1 to 4 percent incidence of stroke and a nonnegligible incidence of renal failure or adverse reaction to the contrast medium.[3, 4] Complications associated with MRA are exceptionally rare. In addition, the cost of MRA is a fraction of that of catheter angiography. As a result of these advantages, the use of conventional angiography has declined significantly wherever MRA is available.

Magnetic resonance angiography competes with other noninvasive imaging techniques, notably Doppler ultrasonography and computed tomographic (CT) angiography.[5] This competition is particularly keen in the imaging of the carotid bifurcation. The relationship between these methods in the diagnostic algorithm is a matter of continuing debate, with each technique showing steady improvement. The debate is further complicated by the fact that it is often not clear what parameters of vascular disease are most predictive of the outcome of the disease. Doppler depends strongly on blood velocity and patterns of blood flow for diagnostic imaging, CT angiography is purely a measure of lumen morphology, and the appearance of vessels on MRA reflects both blood flow and lumen morphology. In the absence of definitive guidelines, each medical center continues to use the tools with which it has the most experience. As surgeons become more sophisticated in their ability to interpret MRA studies, they will be likely to choose MRA instead of x-ray angiography, or to use MRA to confirm an unexpected finding on Doppler ultrasonography.

OVERVIEW OF MAGNETIC RESONANCE ANGIOGRAPHIC TECHNIQUES

Magnetic resonance angiography is a form of magnetic resonance imaging (MRI) and is based on cross sectional images of the body acquired with ordinary MRI equipment and without the use of contrast agents. MRA is not a single method or imaging sequence; rather, it is a term used to describe any method that depicts blood and blood vessels.

Numerous such methods have been proposed, each exploiting some physical property of blood to achieve vessel contrast.[6] Although this may seem confusing, an understanding of neuroangiography is made more manageable by the fact that virtually all studies of the brain and neck rely on a single method: time-of-flight.[7] The second most common approach is the phase contrast method.[8] Between them, these two methods encompass nearly all common clinical applications.

Both time-of-flight and phase contrast rely on blood movement to generate image contrast. Conventional angiography, by comparison, creates an image of the opacified intravascular space. Often these two images are the same, but important differences can arise in cases of disorderly flow, very slow flow, or when the main streamline of flow does not follow the contours of the vessel. Therefore it is important to have a general understanding of the mechanism of MRA when interpreting magnetic resonance angiograms.

Time-of-Flight

The time-of-flight method generates an image in which material that enters the area of interest has more signal than does stationary material.[9] For example, carotid blood is bright in the neck because it enters from the thorax. Stationary tissue is dark because the area of the neck that is being imaged is repeatedly pulsed by a radio wave, which has the effect of suppressing or "saturating" the magnetic signal from the stationary tissue. Blood in the thorax is not subjected to this radio wave and maintains its full magnetization. As this blood rushes into the area of stationary tissue, it appears bright against a dark background.

When blood dwells in the imaged area, it too becomes gradually saturated by the radio wave pulses. Therefore, blood is brightest where it enters and gradually becomes darker as it traverses the area. This places a limit on the length of a vessel that can be imaged at one time. In order to image an extended segment of the artery, one must repeat the image acquisition at several points along the course of the vessel so that saturation of the blood by the radio wave is avoided.

The time-of-flight method requires the application of sufficient radio wave pulses to suppress the stationary background tissue without excessively saturating the arriving blood. This is accomplished by adjusting the repetition time, which defines the time between each pulse, and changing the flip angle, which defines the amplitude of each pulse. Long repetition times and small flip angles avoid saturation of blood at the expense of incomplete suppression of background signal. This choice of parameters would be favored if blood flow were slow or if the area of acquisition were large. Fast blood flow, by comparison, would allow the selection of shorter repetition times and larger flip angles.

The time-of-flight sequence can be run either as a two-dimensional or as a three-dimensional acquisition. These two variants have very different properties, with the result that two-dimensional time-of-flight is normally preferred for some applications and three-dimensional for others.

The two-dimensional time-of-flight acquisition is composed of numerous thin slices, usually placed perpendicular to the vessel being studied (Fig. 24–1).[10] After the first slice has been completed, one moves to an adjacent location and begins the next slice. This continues until a stack of sequentially acquired slices is accumulated that spans the area of interest. Blood vessels appear as bright disks where they enter each slice. When the slices are stacked up and viewed from the side, an angiogram is formed. A special algorithm is employed to calculate this projection, called the "maximum intensity projection,"[11] which helps maintain vascular contrast despite the presence of overlying background tissue.

With the three-dimensional time-of-flight approach, a

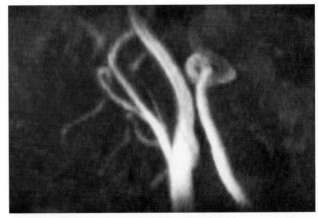

FIGURE 24–2. Three-dimensional time-of-flight magnetic resonance angiographic technique. Sixty-four 1 mm thick transverse partitions through the carotid bifurcation are combined in a maximum intensity projection. The sections are much thinner than those in Figure 24–1, resulting in better resolution.

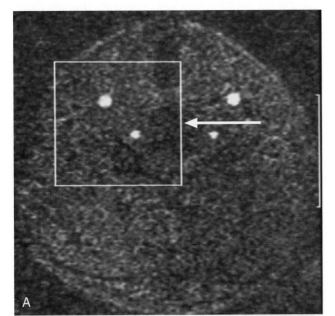

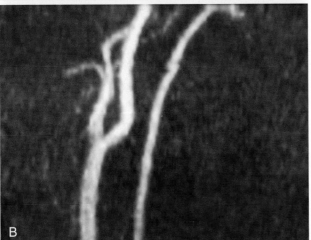

FIGURE 24–1. Two-dimensional time-of-flight magnetic resonance angiographic technique. A, A 3 mm thick, single transverse section through the neck shows the right and left common carotid arteries and vertebral arteries. The jugular venous signal has been removed by a saturation band placed superior to this slice. The *long arrow* indicates the direction of projection. B, A maximum intensity projection of 36 contiguous transverse slices like those in part A calculated from a lateral orientation. Only the structures within the box in part A are included in the projection, thereby eliminating overlap from the left carotid bifurcation.

group of very thin contiguous slices is acquired all at once (Fig. 24–2).[12] The time required to cover an area is approximately the same with either the two-dimensional or three-dimensional approach. Three-dimensional time-of-flight provides much finer resolution, especially in that the slices can be less than a millimeter thick, whereas slices acquired through two-dimensional time-of-flight are rarely less than 2 mm thick. The three-dimensional approach can therefore be viewed from any vantage point with equal resolution, which is beneficial when overlapping vessels are being studied, or the neck of an aneurysm is being searched for. Turbulent flow artifacts are less pronounced in three-dimensional acquisition. The important advantage of two-dimensional time-of-flight is that it provides significantly better contrast in the case of slow flow, such as that encountered beyond a tight stenosis or in the dural venous sinuses. This is because blood must traverse a thick imaging slab to effect inflow contrast in three-dimensional time-of-flight and therefore is likely to become saturated (Fig. 24–3) but need only enter a single thin slice when two-dimensional time-of-flight is used.

The best features of two-dimensional and three-dimensional time-of-flight can be combined in a hybrid approach called multiple overlapping thin slab acquisition (MOTSA).[13] In this approach, a series of three-dimensional time-of-flight areas are acquired, each one consisting of only 10 to 20 slices, and each set overlapping the previous set (Fig. 24–4). As a result of the narrow width of the areas, blood saturation is reduced.

The signal from jugular blood, which flows in the opposite direction to blood in the carotid arteries, can be eliminated from the acquisition by the application of a "saturation band" superior to the acquired slices.[14] Venous blood passing through the band is saturated before it enters the area being imaged and does not give rise to inflow signal. In the same way, blood traveling up the neck can be eliminated by an inferiorly placed saturation band. The bands can be used not only to remove overlapping vessels from the angiogram but also to determine the direction of flow. For example, if a vertebral artery is missing from the image when a superior saturation band is in place, the slice could be reimaged without a saturation band or with an inferior band. If the

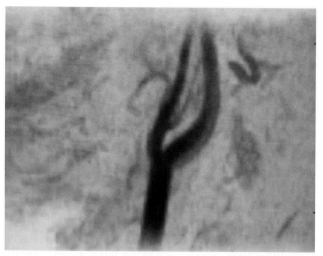

FIGURE 24–3. The effect of saturation on blood signal in the three-dimensional time-of-flight technique. The image is video-reversed (black on white rather than white on black), so that inflow of blood appears dark, as it does on digital subtraction angiography. The angiographic contrast is very strong at the bottom of the image, where blood enters the three-dimensional slab, but fades at the top as a result of progressive saturation of blood magnetization in the radio wave field. The repetition time is 30 milliseconds and the flip angle is 30 degrees. In Figure 24–2, by comparison, which shows less blood saturation, the repetition time is 35 ms and the flip angle is 20 degrees.

vessel appears on the repeated image, subclavian steal phenomenon is present; if not, the vessel is occluded.

Some technical advances that improve vascular contrast in time-of-flight acquisition but are beyond the scope of this chapter are gating to systole, so that inflow contrast is maximized[15]; gating to diastole, so that turbulence is minimized[16]; variation of the flip angle across a three-dimensional time-of-flight slab, so that the influence of blood saturation on vessel contrast is minimized[17]; and magnetization transfer, a technique for further suppression of parenchymal brain background signal.[18]

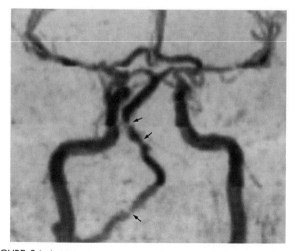

FIGURE 24–4. Multiple overlapping thin slab acquisition magnetic resonance angiographic technique. An anteroposterior projection is calculated from four overlapping three-dimensional time-of-flight slabs, depicting the distal vertebral and carotid arteries, the basilar artery, and the proximal cerebral arteries. The left vertebral artery is occluded. Many severe stenoses of the right vertebral and basilar arteries are noted *(arrows)*.

Phase Contrast

The physical concepts involved in phase contrast are significantly more complex than those involved in time-of-flight. Despite this obstacle, the important points of phase contrast can be understood without resorting to detailed physics.[19]

The phase contrast method produces an image of blood motion rather than of blood inflow. Vascular contrast is achieved by the principle that the direction or "phase" of the magnetic moment is altered in tissue or fluid that moves during the application of a pair of magnetic field gradients. The resulting phase shift is proportional to the velocity of the substance.[20] If the phase at each point is then displayed as an image, a map of velocity is obtained (Fig. 24–5). Note that only motion along the field gradient results in a phase shift. Motion in other directions is ignored. One can choose the velocity encoding direction to be in any direction, independent of the orientation of a slice. The pixel amplitudes on such an image can be read as velocities directly. For these reasons, phase contrast is a popular technique for flow quantitation.

If an angiogram is required, flow must be measured in all three orthogonal directions by running the sequence three times, with the field gradient oriented along each of the three spatial axes. Then the velocities of the three acquisitions are combined to form a single image, which reflects the magnitude of blood flow but not its direction. This angiographic image has been called the "speed" image. The entire pro-

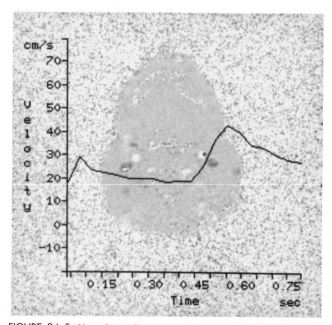

FIGURE 24–5. Use of two-dimensional phase contrast velocity maps to derive blood velocities. A transverse slice through the neck is shown. The flow-encoding gradient direction is across the slice (ie, craniocaudal). The acquisition is triggered to occur during the peak systole phase. Blood flow up the neck in the common carotid arteries is bright, whereas flow down the neck in the jugular veins is dark. Stationary tissues appear medium gray. Note that the motion of the cerebrospinal fluid around the spinal cord is visible. Superimposed on the image is a plot of blood velocity of the left common carotid artery for the entire cardiac cycle, derived from a series of images obtained every 40 milliseconds. The region-of-interest described by the plot is indicated by a small circle in the middle of the left common carotid artery.

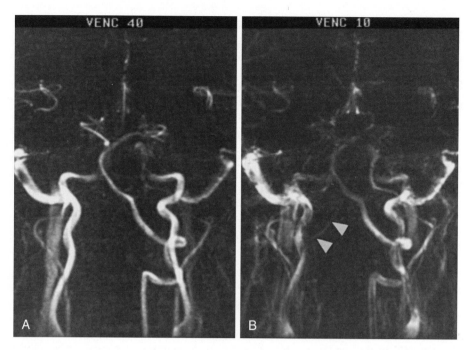

FIGURE 24–6. Effect of Venc on vessel contrast in two-dimensional phase contrast magnetic resonance angiography. *A,* A thick coronal slab is obtained of the distal neck vessels and circle of Willis with a 40 cm/second velocity-encoding gradient. Fast-flowing proximal vessels are well seen, although the image is relatively insensitive to distal, slower vessels. *B,* The same acquisition repeated with a 10 cm/s encoding. Now the slow-flowing vessels, including a right vertebral artery *(arrowheads),* which was suspected to be occluded based on the image in part *A,* are more apparent. The proximal high velocity vessels, however, show alias artifact and have inhomogeneous intensity. (Courtesy of P. Turski.)

cess can be automated so that the angiogram is obtained in a single lengthy acquisition.

The phase contrast angiogram appears different from a time-of-flight angiogram in several respects. Stationary background signal is completely eliminated in phase contrast, but not in time-of-flight.[21] Therefore, nonvascular bright signal, such as hemorrhage, would be invisible on a phase contrast image. Blood saturation effects are a much greater problem with the time-of-flight method than with phase contrast. Disorderly flow leads to artifacts that are often greater in phase contrast than in time-of-flight.

A phase-contrast image, like a time-of-flight image, can be acquired either in a two-dimensional or a three-dimensional form. When velocities are required, a two-dimensional phase contrast approach is used. In that case, a single thin slice perpendicular to the vessel is selected, with velocity encoding across the thickness of the slice. For rapid scout images, a two-dimensional phase contrast image can be acquired as a single, very thick slice with one or three encoding directions. Three-dimensional phase contrast, the acquisition of which requires 8 to 15 minutes, is generally reserved for high-resolution, rotatable angiograms.

A unique feature of phase contrast is that the amplitude of the velocity-encoding gradient pair can be varied to make the sequence sensitive to a range of velocities. This parameter is called the "Venc" and is expressed as the highest velocity correctly encoded by the sequence. Blood traveling at velocities that exceed the Venc appear erroneously slow in velocity or reversed in direction. This is called "aliasing." For example, if a Venc of 100 cm/second is chosen (100 cm/s corresponds to a 180-degree phase shift; −50 cm/s corresponds to −90-degree phase shift), then blood flowing at 200 cm/s will appear motionless (200 cm/s corresponds to 360 degrees, which is the same direction as 0 degrees). Blood vessels whose velocities are much smaller than the Venc will appear very weak on the image. Since it may not be possible to effectively image the entire vascular tree with a single Venc, a common strategy is to run the sequence

twice, first with a large Venc (about 80 cm/s) to visualize large proximal vessels, then with a small Venc (about 20 cm/s) to visualize distal vessels or veins (Fig. 24–6).

Some technical advances that improve vessel contrast in phase contrast are the availability of Vencs that can be independently chosen in each direction, as well as Vencs that change during the cardiac cycle (ie, large during systole, small during diastole).[22]

Strengths and Limitations of the Noninvasive Techniques

The common artifacts of MRA and Doppler ultrasonography are very different. In situations in which MRA is unsuccessful, Doppler ultrasonography may be feasible, and vice versa. For example, a high carotid bifurcation might be inaccessible to the ultrasonographic transducer but present no impediment to MRA. It is useful to summarize the merits of each technique to help elucidate the complementary nature of these modalities.

Doppler equipment is widely available, portable, and can be used with patients who cannot be transported or who need special monitoring. Doppler is inexpensive, although the cost advantage is not great now that the costs of computed tomography and MRI have dropped dramatically.[23] Doppler provides a measure of blood flow and flow patterns, which might be predictive of embolic events or of graft failure, although it is not yet clear how these factors should be incorporated into surgical decisions. Doppler is usually employed in the neck and has limited application in the mediastinum and brain. Complicating factors include the presence of tandem lesions, dense plaque calcification, a short neck, tortuous vessels, or a recent endarterectomy. These factors rarely pose a problem in the use of CT angiography or MRA (although weakly calcified plaques can be mistaken for opacified lumen on a CT angiogram). Most important, Doppler depends on the skill of the technologist rather than the skill of the physician, whereas with MRA, the opposite is true.

Computed tomographic angiography provides a view of the vascular space that is nearly free of blood flow artifacts. This feature will likely permit precise stenosis quantification, although there are as yet no clinical trials to confirm this expectation. As with x-ray angiography, a large iodine contrast bolus is necessary, although it can be administered from a peripheral vein. The field-of-view of CT angiography is chiefly limited by the number of slices that can be acquired during the peak of a contrast bolus. Therefore only one vessel segment can be acquired per imaging session. Postprocessing to form a rendered angiogram from the transverse slices is time-consuming but requires less skill and training than does the performance of Doppler ultrasonography.

Magnetic resonance angiography can assess the heart, aortic arch, carotid bifurcation, and circle of Willis, can measure blood flow rates, and can image brain parenchyma to look for old and recent ischemic events, all in one imaging session (albeit a lengthy one). It is not operator-dependent, which is a criticism of Doppler. The chief problem confronting MRA is disorderly or ''turbulent'' blood flow,[24] usually encountered in the region in which blood flow decelerates beyond a critical lesion, leading to randomization of the phases of magnetic moment and a loss of blood signal. This pattern of blood flow can result in an exaggeration of the apparent degree of stenosis. The problem is more marked with the two-dimensional than the three-dimensional time-of-flight method and with phase contrast than with time-of-flight. It is especially pronounced in two-dimensional phase contrast, since the voxel volumes are quite large. Surgical clips, dental devices, and other pieces of metal can lead to a local change in the magnetic field, which can cause a dark defect in the image. This defect may obscure a portion of a vessel. Patient motion is the most common cause of image degradation and blurring. Motion is generally a greater problem with the three-dimensional than with the two-dimensional time-of-flight method.

THE EXTRACRANIAL CAROTID ARTERIES

Measurements of Carotid Bifurcation Stenosis

Recent multicenter trials, notably the North American Symptomatic Carotid Endarterectomy Trial (NASCET),[25] the European Carotid Surgery Trial (ECST),[26] and the Asymptomatic Carotid Atherosclerosis Study (ACAS),[27] have concluded that the risk of stroke is correlated with the degree of arterial stenosis of the proximal internal carotid artery (ICA) as measured from conventional contrast angiograms.[28] These trials did not assess the ability of noninvasive imaging to predict those patients at risk for stroke. MRA and CT angiography were not included in the study designs. A Doppler ultrasonogram was obtained for many patients in the NASCET study, but there was little standardization in the protocol for those measurements.[29] Standardized Doppler ultrasonography was included in the ACAS trial, but these results have yet to be announced. Therefore, the predictive value of noninvasive testing is assumed but not proved by an outcome trial.

The lack of good outcome data can be addressed in two ways. First, new multicenter studies could be undertaken to determine whether the parameters measured by noninvasive testing are as or more predictive of stroke than is x-ray angiography. These parameters might include the cross sectional lumen area at the lesion, the elevation of blood velocity as a result of the lesion, the presence of turbulent flow, or the size of the plaque. A more specific test for stroke risk would be desirable, since many patients with narrow lumen diameters as measured by x-ray do not subsequently suffer a stroke. For example, in the ACAS study, only 10 percent of patients with stenoses exceeding 60 percent went on to have a stroke. Clearly factors other than vessel diameter contribute to the probability of stroke. Unfortunately, no large-scale outcome studies of MRA are under way.

A second way to address the lack of outcome data is to prove that MRA is highly correlated with measurements made by x-ray angiography. If x-ray angiography is predictive of stroke, then so is MRA. In fact, numerous such comparisons have been made.[30–46] These experiments are difficult to summarize, since each had its own experimental design.[47] The studies evaluated a variety of imaging techniques, especially two-dimensional and three-dimensional time-of-flight. They employed different cut-off values to define severe stenoses. Some studies categorized the severity of stenosis by ''eyeball'' estimation, others by objective measurement of diameters from the film.[48] In each of these studies, all discrepancies were arbitrarily attributed to an error in MRA.

One consistent finding was that MRA was exceptionally sensitive for the detection of stenotic disease. The chief difficulty encountered by the investigators was that the degree of stenosis often appeared exaggerated. This resulted from disorderly blood flow within and beyond a stenosis. Of those publications within the last year that sought to identify a 70 to 99 percent stenosis, Turnipseed and colleagues[49] found a 100 percent sensitivity and 88 percent specificity, Sitzer and colleagues[40] a 73 percent sensitivity and 86 percent specificity, Laster and colleagues[43] a 93 percent sensitivity and 97 percent specificity, Mittl and colleagues[45] a 92 percent sensitivity and 76 percent specificity (worst error was a 64% stenosis thought to be >70%), and Anderson and colleagues[46] a 92 percent sensitivity and 95 percent specificity. The tendency to overestimate disease was especially problematic when signal in the vicinity of a stenosis disappeared altogether so that the vessel appeared interrupted, a phenomenon often called a ''flow gap.'' Patients with evidence of flow gaps were assigned to the surgical category of 70 percent or greater stenosis, although some lesions of less than 70 percent stenosis could result in flow gap.[33, 39, 45] This finding has led some authors to advocate the use of MRA as a screening procedure for the presence of stenosis but not as a definitive replacement for x-ray angiography.[1, 50]

The tendency to overestimate stenosis has been addressed by three recent studies in which the degree of stenosis was measured based on individual slices rather than rendered angiographic projections. These slices were either the original transverse sections or were reformatted sections longitudinal to the vessel (Fig. 24–7). On individual slices, the plaque could often be visualized directly (Fig. 24–8). Anderson and coworkers[46] found that three patients who were

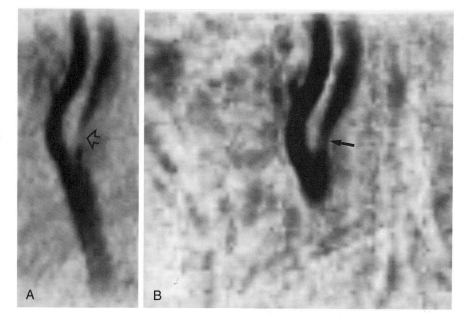

FIGURE 24–7. Use of reformations to improve lumen conspicuousness. *A,* A three-dimensional time-of-flight acquisition of a carotid bifurcation shows an apparent critical stenosis of the proximal internal carotid artery *(open arrow). B,* The same data are used to calculate a single interpolated section in the plane of the bifurcation. Now the stenosis is seen to be much less severe *(arrow).*

judged to have flow gaps based on readings from rendered projections were incorrectly placed in the surgical category but none were incorrectly categorized when their stenoses were measured from source images. Huston and coworkers[39] discovered that specificity for a 50 percent stenosis improved from 67 percent to 86 percent when the stenosis was measured from source images. DeMarco and associates[44] found that interpretation from source images eliminated the overall tendency to overestimate stenosis. A *t*-test showed significant differences between projected MRA and x-ray angiography but no significant difference between source-image MRA and x-ray angiography.

When compared with Doppler, MRA has demonstrated similar accuracy in identifying surgical candidates by the NASCET recommendation, some studies finding MRA slightly better,[36, 37, 39] others finding a small advantage to Doppler.[34, 38, 40] These differences are probably not significant and may be related to details in the experimental protocols. Pan and associates[51] compared the findings of Doppler, MRA, and x-ray angiography with diameters measured from endarterectomy specimens and discovered that Doppler and MRA each correlated better with the endarterectomy specimen than did x-ray angiography. This discrepancy was attributed to the fact that the smallest diameter was often missed by x-ray angiography when the stenosis was elliptical or complex in shape. An increasing number of investigators are advocating the use of Doppler, with MRA confirmation, in lieu of x-ray angiography for the selection of endarterectomy candidates.[49, 52] If Doppler and MRA agree and explain the patient's symptoms, x-ray angiogram is not performed.

Flow volume rates as derived by phase contrast angiography compare well with rates derived by Doppler ultrasonog-

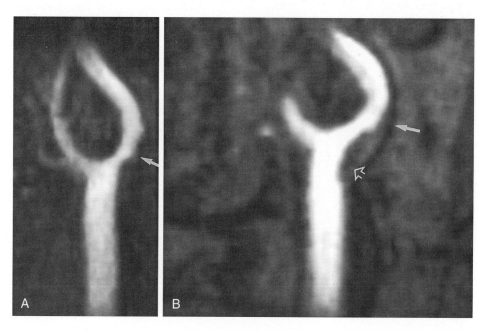

FIGURE 24–8. Visibility of plaque on individual sections. *A,* A three-dimensional time-of-flight acquisition of a carotid bifurcation shows narrowing and irregularity of the proximal internal carotid artery *(arrow).* (The image is not video-reversed.) *B,* A section in the plane of the bifurcation, interpolated from the three-dimensional data, shows the muscular wall of the carotid artery as a thin dark line *(arrow).* A plaque appears gray *(open arrow).*

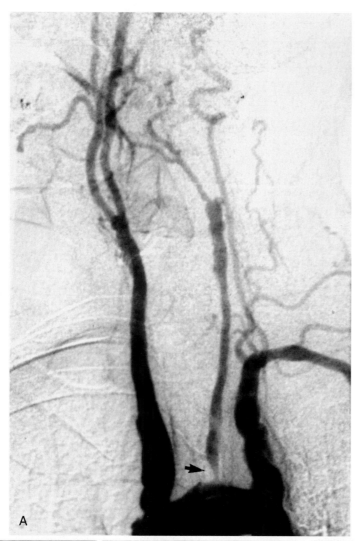

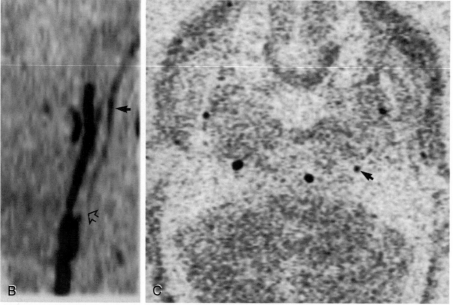

FIGURE 24–9. Patent internal carotid artery detected by magnetic resonance angiography but not by conventional angiography. *A,* A conventional angiogram shows apparent occlusion of the left internal carotid artery. The examination was suboptimal as a result of injection into the ascending aortic arch rather than selectively in the common carotid artery, which was necessitated by a proximal left common carotid artery stenosis *(arrow). B,* A two-dimensional time-of-flight magnetic resonance angiogram of the left carotid bifurcation reveals a patent internal carotid artery *(arrow).* Interruption of the signal in the proximal internal carotid artery *(open arrow)* results from disturbed blood flow beyond the stenosis. *C,* The identity of the patent vessel is confirmed by inspection of a two-dimensional section at the level of the carotid canals, which shows reduced, but present, left internal carotid artery signal *(arrow).* A color Doppler examination also revealed a patent internal carotid artery.

raphy,[53] although it is uncertain how this information should be incorporated into the surgical decision.

Occlusion of the Internal Carotid Artery

The differentiation between near and complete occlusion is important because revascularization procedures of the chronically occluded ICA are ineffective. Recent publications comparing two-dimensional time-of-flight and conventional angiography show complete concordance in the identification of ICA occlusion, but the total number of patients in these studies was only several hundred.[39, 44, 46, 49] This distinction cannot be made by means of three-dimensional time-of-flight angiography. As a result of saturation of blood signal in the distal ICA, blood flow beyond a critical stenosis may not be visible on three-dimensional time-of-flight.

Rarely, in two situations, occluded vessels may appear patent on MRA. A large, dominant vasovasorum collateral vessel may be mistaken for a patent ICA, a very rare phenomenon. Also, clot in a recently thrombosed vessel might appear bright (after several weeks it becomes very dark). This appearance has been described in deep venous thrombosis and could potentially affect carotid studies as well. It can be identified by the application of an inferior saturation band and reacquisition of a two-dimensional time-of-flight slice. The vessel should disappear if it is patent.

The best way to detect a patent ICA is by transverse two-dimensional time-of-flight slices at the level of the carotid canal in the base of the skull. At this location, the vessel can be positively identified and can be differentiated from, for example, an ascending pharyngeal branch of the external carotid artery. Lack of flow at this level implies an occlusion at the bifurcation, since there are no branches of the ICA between these points. Reverse flow in the ICA is very rare. Therefore, absence of the ICA on MRA is almost always

the result of occlusion rather than a steal phenomenon. Reverse flow can be discovered by repeating a two-dimensional time-of-flight slice without the superior saturation band. The ability of two-dimensional time-of-flight to determine occlusion and three-dimensional time-of-flight to avoid turbulence artifact have led some to advocate the use of both two-dimensional and three-dimensional time-of-flight in the standard carotid protocol.[1, 46, 53–55]

Until the advent of color-coded Doppler, sonography was often incapable of detecting a compromised but patent ICA. New studies are warranted to document the improvement in Doppler ultrasonography for this indication. A recent study showed that MRA was more accurate than ultrasonography.[45] X-ray angiography is generally accurate but can fail if a nonselective arch injection is made (Fig. 24–9) or if an insufficient volume of contrast agent is used.[56] Although none of the modalities is infallible, they are each fairly accurate, and one may assume a correct diagnosis if two of the techniques agree.

Other Carotid Diseases

Carotid artery dissection is characterized by a hemorrhage in the carotid wall, often with narrowing of the lumen as a result of mass effect or an initial flap. The hemorrhage may involve just the media or may extend to the adventitia. The site of dissection is often distal to the accessible range of an ultrasonographic transducer. MRA can be very helpful in locating a dissection by detecting a focal change in the caliber of the lumen.[57] The absence of stenosis, however, does not rule out this disease. The diagnosis of dissection is more often made by identifying the hemorrhage on transverse spin-echo magnetic resonance images (Fig. 24–10). The use of fat-saturation sequences prevents bright hemorrhage from being mistaken for bright fat.

Carotid ulcers have been implicated as a potential nidus

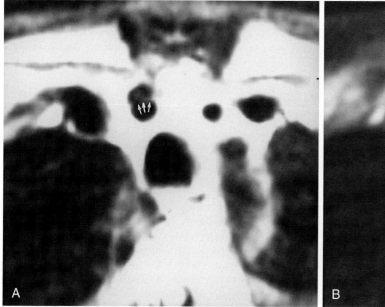
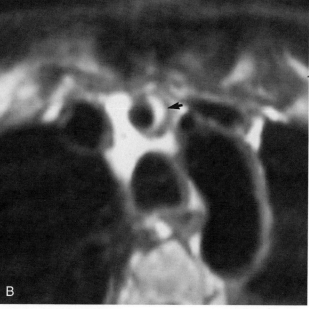

FIGURE 24–10. Dissection detected by magnetic resonance imaging. *A,* A T1-weighted spin-echo image through the proximal bracheocephalic artery shows an intimal flap *(arrows). B,* A section slightly higher in the neck shows a bright signal in the false lumen, which represents clot *(arrow).* Because there was no stenosis, findings on the magnetic resonance angiogram (or x-ray angiogram) did not accurately delineate the extent of the disease.

for emboli formation. Several studies have sought to correlate the presence of ulcers with the incidence of stroke, with varying success. The identification of ulcers on conventional angiograms is not a simple matter.[58] The space between two adjacent plaques can mimic an ulcer, and vice versa. Furthermore, even if an ulcer is correctly recognized, the status of the endothelial layer is unknown. MRA is no better than x-ray angiography and is often less able to visualize an ulcer if blood flow in the crater is slower than flow in the main lumen. For the time being, and until outcome trials have demonstrated a benefit to the identification of ulcers, there is little interest in this entity among magnetic resonance angiographers.

The composition of plaque has also been proposed as an etiologic factor of stroke. Again, this theory has not been consistently supported by clinical studies. High-resolution MRA of endarterectomy specimens, correlated with histology sections, have shown unique appearances for different constituents of plaque, including calcium, fat, hemorrhage (Fig. 24–11), and fibrosis.[59] Display of this level of anatomic detail is best performed with voxels that are less than 0.3 mm across, a resolution that is not practically attainable in situ. Perhaps with a new generation of neck imaging coils, this type of plaque characterization can be achieved.

For fibromuscular hyperplasia, MRA is not the study of choice unless the findings are pronounced. The undulations of the carotid wall may be smaller than the slice thickness or may be mistaken for slice misregistration in two-dimensional time-of-flight angiography. Three-dimensional time-of-flight provides a more accurate portrayal, but the greater rate of inflow in the center of the vessel in comparison to blood

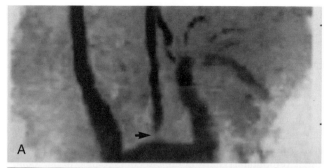
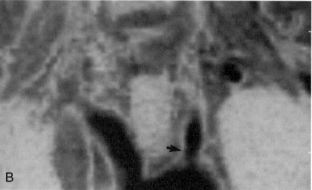

FIGURE 24–12. Multiple overlapping thin slab acquisition magnetic resonance angiographic technique of the aortic arch. *A,* A four-slab overlapping transverse three-dimensional time-of-flight acquisition of the aortic arch of the patient shown in Figure 24–9 again shows stenosis at the origin of the left common carotid artery *(arrow). B,* A coronal section interpolated from the three-dimensional data better depicts the degree of stenosis *(arrow).*

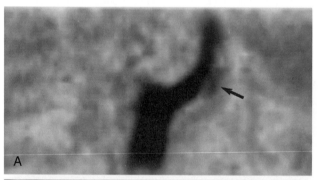
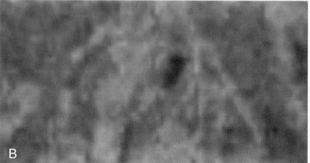

FIGURE 24–11. Plaque characterization by magnetic resonance angiography. *A,* An interpolated section through a carotid bifurcation shows signal adjacent to the lumen and within a plaque *(arrow). B,* The acquisition is repeated, but with a saturation band below the slab so that the flowing blood signal is removed. The structure adjacent to the lumen is not altered, indicating that it represents a plaque hemorrhage rather than an ulcer.

flow near the wall can cause the undulations to be underappreciated.

The Aortic Arch and Carotid Origins

Proximal lesions of the carotid artery are suspected when the waveform during a Doppler study is delayed and dampened. Proximal lesions of the subclavian arteries are suspected when vertebral arterial flow is reversed on the ipsilateral side of the neck. These are indirect signs, however, because the clavicles prevent an ultrasonographic transducer from inspecting the aortic arch directly.

Magnetic resonance angiography of the aortic arch is performed by a series of transverse MOTSA three-dimensional time-of-flight slabs (Fig. 24–12).[44] As is the case with carotid bifurcation lesions, the residual lumen and mural plaque are best seen on the original unprojected slices, or slices reformatted longitudinal to each vessel. A superior saturation band is applied to remove venous signal. This has the undesired effect of removing from the image downgoing arteries, such as the axillary artery, and, if a subclavian steal is present, evidence of reversed vertebral flow.

Magnetic resonance angiography can be used to confirm graft patency in the proximal carotid and subclavian arteries. This determination can be made more conveniently by Doppler, unless the graft passes behind the trachea or originates in the mediastinum.

Magnetic resonance angiographic protocols do not call for imaging of the aortic arch on every patient because of the excessive time that would be required to change coils, reposition the patient, and acquire images from the arch, bifurcation, and brain. Instead, arch views are selectively performed on those patients with signs of proximal disease as shown by Doppler, or who have unilateral reduced common carotid artery inflow as shown on a three-dimensional time-of-flight angiogram of the bifurcation.

CEREBRAL VASCULAR DISEASE

Arterial Occlusive Disease

Images of the petrous carotid, siphon, circle of Willis, proximal cerebral, and distal vertebral and basilar arteries can be acquired simultaneously by a MOTSA three-dimensional time-of-flight using the head coil. This study is often requested in symptomatic patients who have normal carotid bifurcations as shown by Doppler or who are thought to have basilar insufficiency or other posterior circulation symptoms. Stenotic and occlusive lesions of the major vessels are visible by this technique. Sites that are commonly affected are the confluence of the vertebral arteries, the middle basilar artery, the siphons, and the points of bifurcation of the cerebral arteries.[60-62] The resolution of the technique is too low for small, terminal, arterial branches; therefore, occlusions of these vessels are not commonly visible. Likewise vasculitis is not well depicted. A recent study comparing MRA and x-ray angiography of 131 patients showed an 85 percent and 88 percent sensitivity and a 96 percent and 97 percent specificity for detection of stenoses in the intracranial internal carotid and middle cerebral arteries, respectively.[63]

The availability of MRA has dramatically reduced the number of catheter angiograms performed for suspected occlusive disease of the distal vertebral and basilar arteries (see Fig. 24–4) and for basilar dolocoectasia, and those performed to delineate branches of the basilar artery that may come in contact with the fifth or seventh cranial nerves in patients with hemifacial spasm and trigeminal neuralgia.[64] Use of MRA is desirable, since selective studies of vertebral arteries are particularly prone to causing complications from, for example, dissection or release of emboli. The ascendancy of MRA has been so swift that few studies have been performed to define the concordance of MRA and x-ray angiography. Such studies are not forthcoming because x-ray angiography is now rarely performed in addition to MRA.[65] MRA opens up a new and more relevant area of research, however. Now that posterior circulation screening can be done without the fear of complications, the relationship between the myriad symptoms thought to be evidence of vertebrobasilar disease can be correlated with anatomic studies, thereby rendering the clinical diagnosis more specific.

When interpreting vertebral studies, one should keep in mind anatomic variations, such as dominance of one vessel or the termination of a vessel at the posterior inferior cerebellar artery, with the contralateral vertebral artery supplying the basilar artery.

Caution is also warranted when the carotid siphons are studied. Here, flow changes direction several times in rapid succession, leading to unusual velocity profiles and to the so-called flow displacement artifact. Different software implementations of time-of-flight angiography suffer from this

artifact to varying degrees. Before interpreting siphon pathology on a routine basis, the angiographer should test the sequence on normal volunteers.

The circle of Willis provides a ready path for collateral perfusion of the brain in the event of reduced flow in a carotid or vertebral artery. The surgeon may wish to know the direction of flow in the circle in order to learn the hemodynamic significance of a lesion, to judge whether an infarct could have resulted from a lesion in a certain vessel, or to assess what portion of the brain is at risk during a surgical procedure. The direction of flow in, for example, the posterior communicating artery or the A1 segment of the anterior cerebral artery can be determined by acquiring transverse two-dimensional phase contrast slices with flow encoding in the right-left, then in the anteroposterior, directions.[66] Alternatively, one can place a saturation band over one of the vessels of the neck while acquiring a three-dimensional time-of-flight angiogram of the circle. Any cerebral vessel that disappears from the image can be judged to be fed by that saturated vessel.[67]

Magnetic resonance angiography has greatly aided the diagnosis of pediatric cerebrovascular diseases such as sickle cell anemia, Williams and other vascular syndromes, and stroke. The brisk cerebral flow encountered in children permits excellent magnetic resonance angiograms, with the result that the prevalence of the use of x-ray angiography in infants and young children has been considerably reduced.[68] Transcranial Doppler ultrasonography is also of value in children as a means of quantifying basilar and cerebral artery flow. It does not provide the anatomic information available by MRA, nor is it as accurate in flow quantification.[69] It is portable and inexpensive, however, and can be conveniently used for patients who cannot be transported to the magnetic resonance suite.

Cerebral Aneurysms

Magnetic resonance angiography has become a common screening technique for the presence of cerebral aneurysms in patients with subarachnoid hemorrhage. Small aneurysms are routinely visualized by this technique, so long as each individual section is carefully scrutinized.[70] Aneurysms of the distal cerebral arteries are often overlooked as a result of saturation effects. Fortunately, distal aneurysms are rare in the absence of infection or trauma. Despite the widespread use of this test, the sensitivity of MRA for detection of aneurysms has not been confirmed by a large trial. An early study found a sensitivity of just 86 percent, but the quality of cerebral MRA has progressed since then as a result of magnetization transfer, ramped excitation, and high resolution imaging.[71] A second study failed to inspect individual sections.[72] A more definitive study is indicated before the use of x-ray angiography for the detection of aneurysm is abandoned. MRA must prove itself to be a very sensitive test, since the chance of rupture of an untreated aneurysm is great.[73]

The search for intracranial aneurysms should extend as proximal as the origins of the posterior inferior cerebellar artery and as distal as the trifurcation of the middle cerebral arteries. This can be done best with the MOTSA technique. Reformatted sections and rotated projections can be calculated from the MOTSA acquisition to reveal the aneurysm

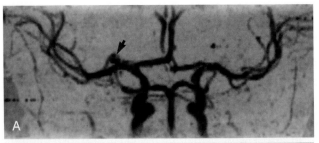

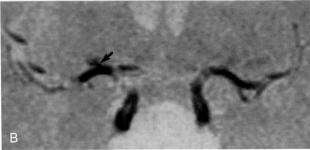

FIGURE 24–13. Demonstration of the neck of an intracranial aneurysm. *A,* A four-slab overlapping transverse three-dimensional time-of-flight acquisition reveals an aneurysm at the trifurcation of the right middle cerebral artery *(arrow). B,* An interpolated section shows the neck of this aneurysm *(arrow).* Note that, unlike with conventional angiography, the orientation of the view can be selected retrospectively.

neck and to plan embolization or clipping procedures (Fig. 24–13). The three-dimensional capabilities of MRA can complement a catheter angiogram by discriminating a tortuous vessel from a true aneurysm and by disclosing the orientation of the neck of the aneurysm. Overlying vessels can be cropped from the calculated projection.

Magnetic resonance imaging acquisitions can augment the examination. For example, a late-echo–gradient-echo sequence helps to locate hemorrhage,[74, 75] whereas a conventional spin-echo examination can delimit edema or mass effect or disclose a thrombosed giant aneurysm that was not

visible by angiographic techniques. MRI by itself is not a reliable method of finding aneurysms because there are gaps between the slices and because an aneurysm can be mistaken for a tortuous vascular loop.

The pulsatile behavior of an aneurysm can be displayed by a cine gradient-echo[76] or cine phase contrast acquisition.[21] This consists of a series of images obtained with cardiac triggering so that flow throughout the cardiac cycle is displayed in a movie loop. Such a study reveals the compliance or expansion of the aneurysm during systole—a behavior that is related to the presence of headache and brain edema. The jet of flow entering the lesion can also be studied, which also helps to define the location and size of the aneurysm neck. Measurements of aneurysm pulsatility may one day prove to be predictive of aneurysm growth or rupture.

Vascular Malformations

Vascular malformations, such as arteriovenous malformations (AVMs) and cavernous angiomas, introduce a shunt between arteries and veins. They are recognized on CT and MRI studies by their dilated and often tortuous system of draining veins. The site of arteriovenous communication, which may be multiple, is termed the nidus. The goal of an imaging examination is to locate the nidus and define its size for radiation therapy or resection, identify feeding vessels, and roughly quantitate the amount of shunting in order to gauge the success of embolization. Some medical centers make extensive use of MRA in the assessment of AVMs, whereas others exclusively use x-ray angiography.

The volume and location of the nidus are best measured from three-dimensional time-of-flight sections performed with external fiduciary markers, while hemorrhage, which might help locate a subtle malformation, is best seen by gradient-echo MRI. If the degree of shunt is small, the use of two-dimensional time-of-flight angiography (Fig. 24–14) or enhancement with gadolinium will better reveal the veins. The source of perfusion is often identified on phase contrast

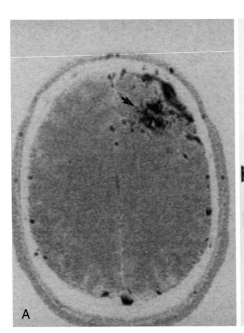

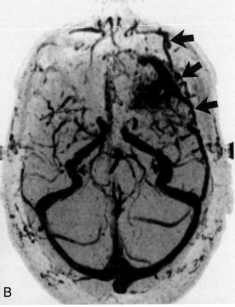

FIGURE 24–14. Two-dimensional time-of-flight magnetic resonance angiogram of an intracranial arteriovenous malformation. *A,* A transverse two-dimensional time-of-flight section through the nidus of an arteriovenous malformation *(arrow). B,* Projection of a series of two-dimensional time-of-flight sections reveals draining veins *(arrows).*

MRA, but conventional angiography remains the best way to define these feeding vessels. Phase contrast can categorize the flow rate as slow or fast,[77] and flow volumes to a large malformation can be measured.[78] Spinal AVMs are often difficult to recognize in MRI without gadolinium enhancement. Likewise, MRA of spinal AVMs should be performed with gadolinium enhancement because saturation effects can hide the draining veins.

Another route for arteriovenous communication is through a carotid cavernous fistula. On three-dimensional time-of-flight angiograms, this is characterized by bright signal within the cavernous sinus resulting from the inflow of unsaturated blood.

Venous Thrombosis

Cerebral venous thrombosis results from dehydration, hypercoagulable states, tumor, and infection. Venous filling defects may not be visible on x-ray angiography as a result of incomplete opacification. Partial and complete thromboses, as well as tumor invasion of the dural sinuses, are better evaluated by MRA.[79] Flow within the deep cerebral veins and dural sinuses is conspicuous on a series of two-dimensional time-of-flight slices (Fig. 24–15). Because inflow contrast is greatest if the slices are perpendicular to the direction of flow, the full sagittal sinus can be studied by a set of coronal slices to visualize the vertex and a set of transverse slices to study the occiput. To make the diagnosis of dural venous thrombosis, each slice is examined for the presence of a filling defect. Spin-echo images are useful to detect infarcts, which may be hemorrhagic, and to define the relationship of veins to tumor, if present. Phase contrast MRA can be employed to confirm the lack of motion if a recently thrombosed clot is suspected to be bright[80]; however, this possibility is usually obvious on the spin-echo sequence by the lack of flow-void phenomenon.

NECESSITY OF CLINICAL TRIALS

Publications in MRA have often centered on technical issues rather than clinical trials. This is understandable since the method has evolved rapidly as a result of improvements in hardware and software. Still, much more effort must be directed toward intermodality comparisons and outcome studies of larger numbers of patients. For example, there are no statistically significant studies to assess the accuracy of aneurysm detection, yet this is a common indication for performing MRA. Investigators must go beyond simple comparisons of MRA and x-ray angiography to learn what capabilities MRA might have that exceed the abilities of catheter angiography. For example, one can assess flow patterns and lumenal cross section area by MRA, but the clinical significance of these measures has not been explored.

Despite the need for additional data, it is already clear that MRA has a role to play in the assessment of cerebrovascular disease. It has already greatly reduced the number of conventional angiograms performed and will likely displace even more such studies in the future. As surgeons learn to interpret these examinations, they should keep foremost in mind the precept that "MRA is not x-ray angiography." That is to say, a magnetic resonance angiogram is not intended to

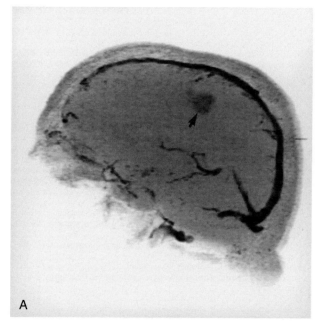

A

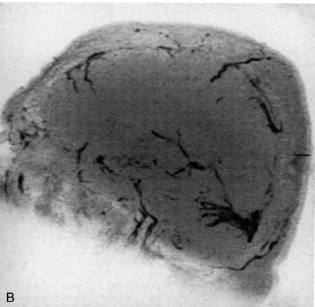

B

FIGURE 24–15. Sagittal sinus thrombosis. *A,* Lateral projection of a two-dimensional time-of-flight magnetic resonance angiogram shows a normal sagittal sinus in patient with an intracranial tumor. The tumor becomes enhanced when gadolinium is injected *(arrow). B,* In another patient who is stable after drainage of subdural hematomas, the sagittal sinus is nearly occluded.

look precisely like an x-ray angiogram, but rather displays a wealth of information regarding blood velocities and flow patterns. Some day this information may prove essential for predicting the course of vascular disease.

REFERENCES

1. Atlas SW: MR angiography in neurologic disease. *Radiology.* 1994;193:1.
2. Turski PA: Intracranial magnetic resonance angiography and stroke. *In* Anderson CM, Edelman RR, Turski PA, eds. *Clinical Magnetic Resonance Angiography.* New York: Raven Press; 1993;181.
3. Hankey GJ, Warlow CP, Sellar RJ: Cerebral angiographic risk in mild cerebrovascular disease. *Stroke.* 1990;21:209.

4. Grzyska U, Freitag J, Zeumer H: Selective arterial intracerebral DSA: Complication rate and control of risk factors. *Neuroradiology.* 1990;32:296.

5. Rubin GD, Dake M, Napel SA, et al: Three-dimensional spiral CT of the abdomen: Initial clinical experience. *Radiology.* 1993;186:147.

6. Anderson CM: What is MRA? *In* Anderson CM, Edelman RR, Turski PA, eds. *Clinical Magnetic Resonance Angiography.* New York: Raven Press; 1993;1.

7. Gullberg GT, Wehrli FW, Shimakawa A, et al: MR vascular imaging with a fast gradient refocussing pulse sequence and reformatted images from transaxial sections. *Radiology.* 1987;165:241.

8. Dumoulin CL, Hart HJ: Magnetic resonance angiography. *Radiology.* 1986;161:717.

9. Bradley WG, Waluch V: Blood flow: Magnetic resonance imaging. *Radiology.* 1985;154:443.

10. Keller PJ, Drayer BP, Fram EK, et al: MR angiography with two-dimensional acquisition and three-dimensional display. *Radiology.* 1989;173:527.

11. Rossnick S, Laub G, Braeckle R: Three-dimensional display of blood vessels in MRI. In Proceedings of the Institute of Electrical and Electronic Engineers: Computers in Cardiology. New York: Institute of Electrical and Electronic Engineers; 1986;193.

12. Masaryk TJ, Modic MT, Ross JS, et al: Intracranial circulation: Preliminary clinical experience with three-dimensional (volume) MR angiography. *Radiology.* 1989;171:793.

13. Parker DL, Yuan C, Blatter DD: MR angiography by multiple thin slab 3D acquisition. *Magn Reson Med.* 1991;17:434.

14. Felmlee JP, Ehman RL: Spatial presaturation: A method for suppressing flow artifacts and improving depiction of vascular anatomy in MR imaging. *Radiology.* 1987;164:559.

15. Selby K, Saloner D, Anderson CM, et al: Cardiac cycle-specific data acquisition in MR angiography. *J Magn Reson Imaging.* 1992;2:637.

16. Saloner D, Selby K, Anderson CM: MRA studies of arterial stenosis: improvements by diastolic acquisition. *Magn Reson Med.* 1994;31:196.

17. Purdy DE, Cadena G, Laub G: The design of variable tip angle slab selection (TONE) pulses for improved 3D MR angiography. In Book of Abstracts: Society of Magnetic Resonance in Medicine 11th Annual Meeting. Berkeley, Calif: Society of Magnetic Resonance in Medicine. 1992;882. Abstract.

18. Edelman RR, Ahn SS, Chien D: Improved time-of-flight MR angiography of the brain with magnetization transfer contrast. *Radiology.* 1992;184:395.

19. Dumoulin CL: Phase contrast magnetic resonance angiography. *Neuroimaging Clin North Am.* 1992;2:1.

20. Moran PR: A flow velocity zeugmatographic interlace for NMR imaging in humans. *Magn Reson Imaging.* 1982;1:97.

21. Huston J, Rufenacht DA, Ehman RL, et al: Intracranial aneurysms and vascular malformations: Comparison of time-of-flight and phase contrast MR angiography. *Radiology.* 1991;181:721.

22. Korosec FR, Mistretta CA, Turski PA: ECG-optimized phase contrast line-scanned MR angiography. *Magn Reson Med.* 1992;24:221.

23. Atlas SW, Edelman RR: Magnetic resonance angiography. *Radiology.* 1993; 189(P):54. Abstract.

24. Urchuk S, Plewes D: Mechanism of flow induced signal loss in MR angiography. *J Magn Reson Imaging.* 1992;2:453.

25. Barnett HJM: North American symptomatic carotid trial collaborators. Beneficial effect of carotid endarterectomy in symptomatic patients with high-grade carotid stenosis. *N Engl J Med.* 1991;325:445.

26. European Carotid Surgery Trialist's Collaborative Group: MRC European carotid surgery trial: Interim results for symptomatic patients with severe (70–99%) or with mild (0–29%) carotid stenosis. *Lancet.* 1991;337:1235.

27. Executive Committee for ACAS: Endarterectomy for Asymptomatic Carotid Artery Stenosis. *JAMA.* 1994;273:1459.

28. Barnett HJM, Warlow CP: Carotid endarterectomy and the measurement of stenosis. *Stroke.* 1993;24:1281. Editorial.

29. Hobson RW, Strandness DE: Carotid artery stenosis: What's in the measurement? *J Vasc Surg.* 1993;18:1069. Editorial.

30. Litt AW, Eidelman EM, Pinto RS, et al: Diagnosis of carotid artery stenosis: Comparison of 2DFT time-of-flight MR angiography with contrast angiography in 50 patients. *AJR Am J Radiol.* 1991;156:611.

31. Masaryk AM, Ross JS, DiCello MC, et al: 3DFT MR angiography of the carotid bifurcation: Potential and limitations as a screening examination. *Radiology.* 1991;179(3):797.

32. Wilkerson DK, Keller I, Mezrich R, et al: The comparative evaluation of three-dimensional magnetic resonance for carotid artery disease. *J Vasc Surg.* 1991;14:803.

33. Heiserman J, Drayer B, Fram E, et al: Carotid artery stenosis: Clinical efficacy of two-dimensional time-of-flight angiography. *Radiology.* 1992;182:761.

34. Polak JF, Bajakian RL, Oleary DH, et al: Detection of internal carotid artery stenosis: Comparison of MR angiography, color Doppler sonography, and arteriography. *Radiology.* 1992;182(1):35.

35. Kido DK, Panzer RJ, Szumowski J, et al: Clinical evaluation of stenosis of the carotid bifurcation with magnetic resonance angiographic techniques. *Arch Neurol.* 1991;48(5):484.

36. Anderson C, Saloner D, Lee R, et al: Assessment of carotid artery stenosis by MR angiography: Comparison with x-ray angiography and color-coded Doppler ultrasound. *AJNR Am J Neuroradiol.* 1992;13:989.

37. Mattle HP, Kent KC, Edelman RR, et al: Evaluation of the extracranial carotid arteries: Correlation of magnetic resonance angiography, duplex ultrasonography, and conventional angiography. *J Vasc Surg.* 1991;13(6):838.

38. Riles T, Eidelman E, Litt A, et al: Comparison of magnetic resonance angiography, conventional angiography and duplex scanning. *Stroke.* 1992;23:341.

39. Huston J, Lewis B, Wiebers D, et al: Carotid artery: Prospective blinded comparison of two-dimensional time-of-flight MR angiography with conventional angiography and duplex US. *Radiology.* 1993;186:339.

40. Sitzer M, Furst G, Fischer H, et al: Between-method correlation in quantifying internal carotid stenosis. *Stroke.* 1993;24:1513.

41. Buijs PK, Klop RB, Eikelboom BC, et al: Carotid bifurcation imaging: Magnetic resonance angiography compared to conventional angiography and Doppler ultrasound. *Eur J Vasc Surg.* 1993;7:245.

42. Blatter DD, Bahr AL, Parker DL, et al: Cervical carotid MR angiography with multiple overlapping thin slab acquisition: comparison with conventional angiography. *AJR Am J Radiol.* 1993;161:1269.

43. Laster RE, Ackern JD, Halford HH, et al: Assessment of MR angiography versus arteriography for evaluation of cervical carotid bifurcation disease. *AJNR Am J Neuroradiol.* 1993;14:681.

44. DeMarco JK, Nesbit GM, Wesbey GE, et al: Prospective evaluation of extracranial carotid stenosis: MR angiography with maximum intensity projections and multiplanar reformation compared with conventional angiography. *AJR Am J Radiol.* 1994;163:1205.

45. Mittl RL, Broderick M, Carpenter JP, et al: Blinded reader comparison of magnetic resonance angiography and duplex ultrasonography for carotid artery bifurcation stenosis. *Stroke.* 1994;25:4.

46. Anderson CM, Lee RL, Levin DL, et al: Measurement of internal carotid artery stenosis from source MR angiograms. *Radiology.* 1994;193:219.

47. Bowen BC, Quencer RM, Margosian P, et al: MR angiography of occlusive disease of the arteries in the head and neck: current concepts. *AJR Am J Radiol.* 1994;162:9.

48. Fox J: How to measure carotid Stenosis. *Radiology.* 1993;186:316.

49. Turnipseed WD, Kennell TW, Turski PA, et al: Magnetic resonance angiography and duplex imaging: Noninvasive tests for selecting symptomatic carotid endarterectomy candidates. *Surgery.* 1993;114:634.

50. Masaryk T, Obuchowski N: Noninvasive carotid imaging: Caveat emptor. *Radiology.* 1993;186:325.

51. Pan XM, Saloner D, Reilly LM, et al: Assessment of carotid artery stenosis by ultrasonography, conventional angiography, and magnetic resonance angiography: Correlation with ex vivo measurement of plaque stenosis. *J Vasc Surg.* 1995; 21:82.

52. Polak J, Kalina P, Donaldson M, et al: Carotid endarterectomy: Preoperative evaluation of candidates with combined Doppler sonography and MR angiography. *Radiology.* 1993;186:333.

53. Levine RL, Turski PA, Holmes KA, et al: Comparison of magnetic resonance volume flow rates, angiography, and carotid Dopplers. *Stroke.* 1994;25:413.

54. Pan XM, Anderson CM, Reilly LM, et al: Magnetic resonance angiography of the carotid artery combining two- and three-dimensional acquisitions. *J Vasc Surg.* 1992;16:609.

55. Goldberg HI, Atlas SW, Mishkin MM, et al: Comparison of high resolution 3D and 2D time-of-flight MR angiography of carotid artery bifurcation stenosis. *Radiology.* 1993;189(P):242. Abstract.

56. Batt M, Avril G, Bozzetto C, et al: Atheromatous pseudo-occlusive stenosis of the internal carotid. *J Mal Vasc (Paris).* 1993;18:233.

57. Levy C, Laissy JP, Raveau V, et al: Carotid and vertebral artery dissections: Three-dimensional time-of-flight MR angiography and MR imaging versus conventional angiography. *Radiology.* 1994;190:97.

58. Eikelboom BC, Riles TR, Mintzer R, et al: Inaccuracy of angiography in the diagnosis of carotid ulceration. *Stroke.* 1983;14:882.

59. Yuan C, Tsuruda JS, Beach KN, et al: Techniques for high-resolution MR imaging of atherosclerotic plaque. *J Magn Reson Imaging.* 1994;4:43.

60. Fujita N, Hirabuki N, Fujii K, et al: MR imaging of middle cerebral artery stenosis and occlusion: Value of MR angiography. *AJNR Am J Neuroradiol.* 1994;15:335.

61. Warach S, Li W, Ronthal M, et al: Acute cerebral ischemia: Evaluation with dynamic contrast-enhanced MR imaging and MR angiography. *Radiology.* 1992;182:41.

62. Wiznitzer M, Ruggiere PM, Masaryk TJ, et al: Diagnosis of cerebrovascular disease in sickle cell anemia by magnetic resonance angiography. *J Pediatr.* 1991;118:657.

63. Korogi Y, Takahashi M, Mabuchi N, et al: Intracranial vascular stenosis and occlusion: Diagnostic accuracy of three-dimensional, Fourier transform, time-of-flight MR angiography. *Radiology.* 1994;193:187.

64. Tien RD, Wilkins RH: MRA delineation of the vertebro-basilar system in patients with hemifacial spasm and trigeminal neuralgia. *AJNR Am J Neuroradiol.* 1993;14:34.

65. Wentz KU, Rother J, Schwartz A, et al: Intracranial vertebrobasilar system: MR angiography. *Radiology.* 1994;190:105.

66. Davis WL, Turski PA, Gorbatenko KG, et al: Correlation of cine MR velocity measurements in the internal carotid artery with collateral flow in the circle of Willis: Preliminary study. *Radiology.* 1993;3:603.

67. Edelman RR, Heinrich PM, O'Reilly GV, et al: Magnetic resonance imaging of flow dynamics in the circle of Willis. *Stroke.* 1990;21:56.

68. Vogl TJ, Balzer JP, Stemmler J, et al: MR angiography in children with cerebral neurovascular diseases. *AJR Am J Radiol.* 1992;159:817.

69. Siebert JJ, Miller SF, Kirby RS, et al: Cerebrovascular disease in symptomatic and asymptomatic patients with sickle cell anemia: Screening with duplex transcranial Doppler US—correlation with MR imaging and MR angiography. *Radiology.* 1993;189:457.

70. Ross JS, Masaryk TJ, Modic MT, et al: Intracranial aneurysms: Evaluation by MR angiography. *AJNR Am J Neuroradiol.* 1990;11:449.

71. Ross JS, Ruggiere PM, Tkach JA: High resolution, magnetization transfer saturation, variable flip angle, time-of-flight angiography of the intracranial vasculature. *Radiology.* 1992;185(P):225. Abstract.

72. Korogi Y, Takahashi M, Mabuchi N, et al: Intracranial aneurysms: Diagnostic accuracy of three-dimensional, Fourier transform, time-of-flight MR angiography. *Radiology.* 1994;193:181.

73. Wiebers DO, Torner JC, Meissner I: Impact of unruptured intracranial aneurysms on public health in the United States. *Stroke.* 1992;23:1416.

74. Bradley WG: MR appearance of hemorrhage in the brain. *Radiology.* 1993;189:15.

75. Yamada N, Imakita S, Nishimura T, et al: Evaluation of the susceptibility effect on gradient echo phase images in vivo: A sequential study of intracranial hematoma. *Magn Reson Imaging.* 1992;10:559.

76. Tsuruda J, Halbach VV, Higashida RT, et al: MR evaluation of large intracranial aneurysms using cine low flip angle gradient refocussed imaging. *AJNR Am J Neuroradiol.* 1988;9:415.

77. Petereit DG, Mehta MP, Turski PA, et al: Treatment of arteriovenous malformations with stereotactic radiosurgery employing both magnetic resonance angiography and standard angiography as a database. *Int J Radiat Oncol Biol Phys.* 1993;25:309.

78. Marks MP, Pelc NJ, Ross MR, et al: Determination of cerebral blood flow with a phase contrast cine MR imaging technique: Evaluation of normal subjects and patients with arteriovenous malformations. *Radiology.* 1992;182:467.

79. Johnson BA, Fram EK: Cerebral venous occlusive disease: Pathology, clinical manifestations and imaging. *Neuroimaging Clin North Am.* 1992;2:769.

80. Nadel L, Braun IF, Kraft FA: Intracranial vascular abnormalities: Value of phase imaging to distinguish thrombus from flowing blood. *AJR Am J Radiol.* 156;373.

V

Medical Management

CHAPTER
25

Medical Management of Carotid Territory Transient Ischemic Attacks

WILLIAM M. FEINBERG

For a patient with a transient ischemic attack (TIA) in the carotid territory, the choice of therapy is often considered a simplistic one—medicine versus surgery. In reality, however, all these patients must receive medical management; the choice is whether to use medical therapy alone or in conjunction with carotid endarterectomy. Medical therapy, in a broad sense, includes treatment of risk factors, antithrombotic therapy for patients who do not undergo endarterectomy, and antithrombotic therapy following endarterectomy. The choice of therapy depends on the patient's underlying risk factors and the specific cause of the TIA.

The fact that medicine and surgery are not an either/or choice was illustrated by the Mayo Asymptomatic Carotid Endarterectomy Study.[1] Patients with asymptomatic carotid stenosis were randomly allocated to receive either carotid endarterectomy or 80 mg of aspirin per day. Aspirin use was discouraged in the surgical group. After 30 months of recruitment, only 71 patients had been entered into the study, but the study was terminated because there had been eight myocardial infarctions in the surgical group and none in the medical group ($P = 0.0037$). Management must consider the patient's overall health status as well as specific therapy aimed at the cerebral circulation.

Patients with carotid territory ischemic symptoms have traditionally been evaluated and managed differently than patients with vertebrobasilar ischemia. Indeed, this book has a separate chapter for the management of vertebrobasilar insufficiency (see Chapter 27). Part of the reason for the difference in management has been that, until recently, the noninvasive evaluation of the extracranial carotid territory was much easier and more reliable than that of the posterior circulation. Also, because of the availability of carotid endar-

terectomy, there is a certain urgency inherent in the treatment decision that is not present for patients with vertebrobasilar symptoms. However, the pathologic processes in the two circulations are identical, and it may not make sense to consider management separately.[2] Although this chapter focuses on carotid territory symptoms, many of the comments on medical therapy are applicable to posterior circulation ischemia.

DIFFERENTIAL DIAGNOSIS OF CAROTID TERRITORY TRANSIENT ISCHEMIC ATTACKS

A TIA is a syndrome with diverse causes. Proper diagnosis is crucial to choosing the appropriate therapy. The various pathologic causes, the clinical spectrum of carotid TIAs, and the clinical and diagnostic evaluation of patients are reviewed in other chapters in this book and will not be discussed in detail here. It is important to remember, however, that TIAs may precede strokes of all types (Table 25–1).[3–7] TIAs are most common in patients with extracranial carotid disease but may also be seen in patients with cardioembolic stroke or lacunar infarction.[3–7] Less common causes of TIA include hypercoagulable states, arterial dissection, arteritis, and drug use. The medical management of a carotid TIA begins with a careful history, physical exam, and diagnostic evaluation to determine the source of the TIA and guide therapy.

TABLE 25–1. Transient Ischemic Attacks Preceding Various Cerebrovascular Syndromes*

Series, Year†	Atherothrombosis	Embolism	Lacuna	Hematoma	SAH
Harvard Stroke Registry[3]	50	23	11	8	7
Michael Reese Stroke Registry[6]	41.5	11	NA	NA	NA
Stroke Data Bank[4]	20	13	13	3	1
Lausanne Stroke Registry[5]	29	30	14	6	NA
UCSD Stroke Registry[7]	23	12	12	NA	NA

*Numbers represent the percentage of each stroke type preceded by transient ischemic attack.
†For full bibliographic information, see reference list at end of chapter.
NA, not available; SAH, subarachnoid hemorrhage.

246

MEDICAL THERAPY FOR RISK REDUCTION

All patients with TIAs should be evaluated for the presence of stroke risk factors. These risk factors are discussed in detail in Chapter 6 and are reviewed briefly here in relation to the management of patients with TIAs. Patient management should include treatment of risk factors in addition to specific stroke prevention therapy such as surgery or antithrombotic medication.

Hypertension

Hypertension is the most powerful, prevalent, and treatable risk factor for stroke.[8–10] Both systolic and diastolic blood pressure are independently related to stroke incidence. In the Framingham Study, the age-adjusted relative risk of stroke in hypertensive individuals was 3.1 for men and 2.9 for women.[8] Even patients with borderline hypertension have an approximately 50 percent increased stroke risk.[8] Isolated systolic hypertension, which is common in the elderly, also considerably increases stroke risk.[11]

A large number of prospective, randomized, primary prevention trials have documented substantial reductions in stroke risk with control of hypertension. An analysis of 14 treatment trials representing over 37,000 hypertensive patients indicated that an average diastolic blood pressure reduction of 6 mm Hg produced a 42 percent reduction in stroke incidence.[12] Recently, the Systolic Hypertension in the Elderly Program trial found that individuals over the age of 60 with isolated systolic hypertension (greater than 160 mm Hg), randomly assigned to receive antihypertension medication, had a 36 percent reduction in stroke compared with those assigned to the placebo group.[13]

The benefit of treating hypertension after a stroke has occurred is less clearly documented. No prospective randomized trials have been performed, and nonrandomized studies have produced conflicting results.[14–16] However, given the magnitude of hypertension as a stroke risk factor, it seems sensible to treat hypertension, including isolated systolic hypertension, in all TIA patients.

Cigarette Smoking

Several large studies have clearly indicated that cigarette smoking substantially increases the risk of stroke.[8, 17–19] In general, most studies have documented relative risk values of 1.5 to 2, and the risk of stroke increases with the number of cigarettes smoked. It is also clear that cessation of smoking dramatically reduces stroke risk. Data from the Framingham Study, the Nurses Health Study, and the Honolulu Heart Program have shown that smoking cessation can promptly reduce stroke risk.[17, 18, 20] Although no prospective studies have specifically assessed the effects of smoking cessation after a TIA, a strong recommendation to stop smoking should be part of the management of every TIA patient.

Blood Lipids

Increased levels of serum cholesterol and triglycerides are independently related to the development of coronary artery disease[21] but the relationship to stroke is less clear. High stroke rates have been noted in families with hyperlipidemias. In addition, serum lipid levels have been related to carotid artery atherosclerosis in a variety of ultrasonographic and angiographic studies.[22] However, no prospective trials have indicated that medical therapy to reduce excessive blood lipid levels can reduce the risk of stroke. A recent meta-analysis of randomized, controlled trials found that cholesterol lowering was not associated with a significant reduction in stroke mortality or morbidity in middle-aged men.[23] Thus the need to aggressively lower blood cholesterol in TIA patients specifically for stroke prevention is not clear. Medications for hyperlipidemia reduce the risk of coronary artery disease, and cholesterol lowering may be recommended in these patients for reasons other than stroke reduction.[24]

Alcohol Consumption

The relationship between alcohol use and stroke is complex. Heavy alcohol use, either on a daily basis or with binge drinking, has been related to excess stroke risk.[25, 26] Light or moderate alcohol consumption may have no effect or a mild protective effect.[27, 28] Moderate consumption also appears to raise high-density lipoprotein cholesterol and lower the risk of atherosclerotic heart disease.[29, 30] Although prospective trials have not been conducted, it is reasonable to counsel patients with TIAs to reduce heavy alcohol intake.

Diabetes

Several trials have indicated that diabetes is an independent risk factor for ischemic stroke.[31, 32] Whether tight control of blood glucose in diabetic patients will reduce the increased stroke risk in diabetics is unknown.

Oral Contraceptives

Several studies have indicated an increased risk of stroke in women who take oral contraceptives.[33–36] The increased stroke risk associated with oral contraceptive use occurs primarily in women over the age of 35, particularly those who smoke or have other cardiovascular risk factors. The risk of stroke is highest with high-estrogen oral contraceptives. Although there have been no prospective randomized trials, it is likely that discontinuation of oral contraceptives will diminish stroke risk. One large study showed that individuals who discontinued oral contraceptives had no higher risk of stroke than those who had never used these agents.[37] In a young woman with a TIA, discontinuation of oral contraceptives should be considered.

Postmenopausal Estrogen Use

The cardiovascular risk associated with postmenopausal estrogen replacement has been controversial. In the Framingham Study, women reporting postmenopausal estrogen use had more than a twofold increased risk for cerebrovascular disease.[38] However, in the 10-year follow-up of 50,000 women in the Nurses Health Study, current use of postmenopausal estrogen was associated with a reduction in the incidence of coronary heart disease and cardiovascular mortality and was not associated with any change in the risk of stroke.[39] Recently, a follow-up of the National Health and Nutrition Examination Survey cohort found that postmenopausal hormone use in white women was associated with a 31 percent *decrease* in stroke incidence and a 63 percent reduction in stroke mortality.[40] The weight of evidence suggests that postmenopausal estrogen use does not increase stroke risk and may lower the risk, so there is no need to discontinue postmenopausal hormone therapy in TIA patients.

Physical Activity

Exercise may exert a beneficial effect on risk factors for atherosclerotic disease by reducing blood pressure, increasing high-density lipoprotein cholesterol levels, lowering low-density lipoprotein cholesterol levels, and improving glucose tolerance. No prospective trials have addressed the relationship between physical activity and stroke risk, but because of these benefits, it is reasonable to encourage increased physical activity in sedentary individuals with TIAs.

ANTITHROMBOTIC THERAPY FOR TRANSIENT ISCHEMIC ATTACKS

Antiplatelet Agents

Over the past decades, evidence has accumulated from rigorous clinical trials proving that antiplatelet agents are effective in the prevention of stroke in high-risk patients. Numerous randomized, double-blind, placebo-controlled trials have evaluated the use of various antiplatelet agents for the secondary prevention of stroke after TIA or minor stroke. These trials have shown a consistent, moderate decrease in stroke risk with the use of antiplatelet agents.

Aspirin

Aspirin (acetylsalicylic acid) is the standard medical therapy used for prevention in patients threatened with stroke. Aspirin inhibits platelet function and likely exerts its clinical effect by blocking cyclooxygenase and decreasing the production of thromboxane and its metabolites. Aspirin was approved by the U.S. Federal Drug Administration for use in cerebrovascular disease on the basis of two seminal studies, one reported by the Canadian Cooperative Study Group[41] and one by Fields and collaborators.[42]

The Canadian Cooperative Study Group evaluated 585 patients (69% men) who had threatened stroke. Patients were randomly assigned to receive 1300 mg of aspirin per day, 800 mg of sulfinpyrazone per day, a combination of both, or a placebo. Aspirin use reduced the risk of stroke or death by 31 percent. There was a significant 48 percent reduction in the risk of stroke or death in men, but no significant risk reduction was detected in women. In retrospect, the gender difference in the response to aspirin was probably due to the small number of women studied and the fact that women who have experienced TIAs have less risk of stroke than men.[43] No beneficial effect was noted with the use of sulfinpyrazone alone, and no additional benefit was seen when it was used in combination with aspirin.

The U.S. trial enrolled 178 patients (66% men) with carotid distribution TIAs in a double-blind, placebo-controlled trial of aspirin for stroke prevention.[42] Patients were randomly assigned to receive either 1300 mg of aspirin daily or a placebo. There was no statistically significant difference in the absolute endpoints of mortality rate or the rate of cerebral and retinal infarction between the group receiving aspirin and the group receiving placebo. Eleven of 88 aspirin-treated patients (13%) had strokes compared with 14 of 90 in the placebo group (16 percent). In post hoc analysis, aspirin use was statistically superior to placebo in the combined endpoints of rates of mortality, cerebral infarction, and retinal infarction in patients with multiple TIAs and in those with carotid artery stenosis greater than 50 percent or ulceration in the artery appropriate to symptoms.

A number of subsequent studies have supported a beneficial effect of aspirin.[44–47] Some negative studies were probably too small to show any benefit of aspirin.[43] Although most of these studies found a trend toward reduced stroke risk in patients treated with aspirin, in some studies it was only with a combination of endpoints—including TIA, stroke, myocardial infarction, and death—that a statistically significant benefit for aspirin was demonstrated. Taken together, these studies provide solid evidence for a moderate beneficial effect of aspirin in reducing stroke risk in patients with previous stroke or TIA.

The optimal dosage of aspirin for stroke prevention is controversial. Most of the early trials used 975 to 1300 mg/day. Since 1987, three large trials have suggested a benefit at doses lower than those used in the original studies. The United Kingdom Transient Ischemic Attack Trial was the first placebo-controlled multicenter trial to compare two doses of aspirin, 1200 mg/day and 300 mg/day.[48] The study enrolled 2435 patients (73% men) who were observed for a mean of 4 years. Aspirin use (both doses combined) decreased the risk of the combined endpoints of myocardial infarction, major stroke, or death by 15 percent, compared with placebo. There was a 7 percent (nonsignificant) reduction in the risk of disabling stroke or vascular death. There was no significant outcome difference between the two doses of aspirin, but the event rate was low, and this could have been a type II (β) error. Upper gastrointestinal symptoms were more common with the higher dose of aspirin than with the lower dose. The incidence of gastrointestinal bleeding was 3 percent for 300 mg aspirin and 5 percent for 1200 mg aspirin, but this difference was not statistically significant.

The Dutch TIA trial enrolled 3131 patients with TIA (one third) or minor stroke and compared a carbaspirin calcium dose of 30 mg/day to a dose of 283 mg/day.[49] There was no placebo group. There was no difference in the endpoint events of TIA or stroke between the two aspirin doses. The 30 mg dose of carbaspirin calcium caused fewer gastrointestinal side effects. The Swedish Aspirin Low-Dose Trial (SALT) enrolled 1360 patients with TIA or minor stroke to receive either aspirin 75 mg/day or placebo.[50] It found an 18 percent reduction in stroke or death for the low-dose aspirin group compared with the placebo group. Neither the Dutch TIA trial nor the SALT trial compared low-dose aspirin to larger doses of aspirin such as those used in earlier TIA trials.

Although controversy remains regarding the optimal dosage of aspirin to prevent stroke,[51] presently there is no compelling evidence that higher or lower doses are more efficacious. In view of the slightly lower incidence of side effects with lower doses and the possibility of increased compliance, many investigators recommend 325 mg/day as an initial dose.

Dipyridamole and Other Antiplatelet Agents

The combination of aspirin, which is a cyclooxygenase inhibitor, and dipyridamole, which is a cyclic nucleotide phosphodiesterase inhibitor, theoretically offers a pharmacologic advantage. But of the three trials that have compared this combination with the use of aspirin alone, none has shown any benefit from the addition of dipyridamole. The Tolouse Study in 1982 evaluated 440 patients (85% men) with TIAs.[52] No statistically significant difference was found in outcome measures among groups receiving 900 mg/day of aspirin, aspirin plus dihydroergotamine, aspirin plus dipyridamole and dihydroergotamine, or dihydroergotamine alone. The French "AICLA" trial studied 604 patients (67% men) with TIAs (16%) or small strokes (84%).[53] Patients were randomized to receive aspirin 1000 mg/day, aspirin combined with dipyridamole 225 mg/day, or placebo. There was a 42 percent reduction in the risk of stroke with aspirin compared with placebo. The effect of aspirin was similar in men and women. No added benefit was noted with dipyridamole. The American-Canadian Cooperative Study evaluated 890 patients (67% men) with carotid distribution TIAs.[54] There was no significant difference in the rate of stroke or retinal infarction in patients on aspirin compared with patients on aspirin plus dipyridamole. There was no difference in the incidence of fatal or nonfatal myocardial infarction between the two groups.

The European Stroke Prevention Study compared 975 mg/day of aspirin plus 225 mg/day of dipyridamole against placebo among 2500 patients with TIAs (33%), reversible ischemic neurologic deficits (7%), or stroke (60%).[55] Overall, there was a 33 percent reduction in the risk of stroke and death, and a 38 percent reduction in the risk of stroke only, for those assigned to active treatment.

In the only trial comparing dipyridamole (400 to 800 mg/day) alone to placebo, there was no evidence of any benefit of dipyridamole.[56] Another antiplatelet agent, suloctidil, was examined in a Canadian study in patients with a recent thromboembolic stroke.[57] The study showed no benefit for suloctidil but was stopped early because of suloctidil's hepatotoxicity.

Ticlopidine

Ticlopidine hydrochloride is a new antiplatelet agent that has recently been approved in the United States for prevention of stroke in patients with TIA or minor stroke. Its antiplatelet action is distinct from that of aspirin or dipyridamole, and it does not affect cyclooxygenase. Two large multicenter randomized trials have evaluated the efficacy of ticlopidine in patients with cerebrovascular disease.

The Canadian American Ticlopidine Study evaluated ticlopidine's efficacy for reducing the incidence of recurrent nonfatal stroke, nonfatal myocardial infarction, and vascular death in patients who had experienced a recent moderate to severe atherothrombotic (74%) or lacunar (26%) stroke (no TIAs were included).[58] A total of 1053 patients were admitted to the study between 1 week and 4 months after the qualifying stroke and randomly assigned to 250 mg of ticlopidine twice a day or to placebo. According to an intention-to-treat analysis, the relative risk reduction for the cluster of vascular events was 23.3 percent. Benefits were observed in both men and women.

The Ticlopidine-Aspirin Stroke Study compared the efficacy of ticlopidine and aspirin in reducing the incidence of stroke and death in patients with recent TIA or minor stroke.[59] Fifty-six centers in the United States and Canada evaluated 3069 patients randomly assigned to receive either 250 mg of ticlopidine twice a day or 650 mg of aspirin twice a day. According to an intention-to-treat analysis, the overall risk reduction at 3 years for fatal and nonfatal stroke was 21 percent in favor of ticlopidine; the risk of stroke and all causes of death was reduced by 12 percent for ticlopidine versus aspirin. A post hoc intent-to-treat analysis found that the relative risk reduction was greatest in the first year after study entry.

Diarrhea was the most frequent side effect in those receiving ticlopidine, occurring in 12.5 percent of patients. Neutropenia was more common in the ticlopidine groups of both of the previously mentioned studies and occurred in 2.4 percent of patients. The neutropenia was severe in 0.8 percent but was reversible in all patients. The severe neutropenia occurred within 90 days of starting therapy. When ticlopidine was released in the United States, it was accompanied by the recommendation to obtain a complete blood count with differential every 2 weeks for the first 3 months of therapy. The decision whether to use aspirin or ticlopidine needs to be individualized in each patient. Weighing the slight benefit of ticlopidine against the incidence of side effects, the need for hematologic monitoring, and the increased cost, many neurologists believe that aspirin is appropriate as initial antiplatelet therapy in most cases (Table 25–2).[60–62] Ticlopidine is a useful alternative, particularly in those patients who cannot take aspirin or who continue to have symptoms despite aspirin therapy.

Antiplatelet Trialists' Collaboration

The Antiplatelet Trialists' Collaboration compiled the results of completed, randomized trials of antiplatelet agents and performed a meta-analysis looking at efficacy in reducing ischemic vascular events. The original 1988 report was based on 25 trials involving 29,000 patients with TIA, stroke, unstable angina, or myocardial infarction. The primary antiplatelet drug was aspirin, but the analysis included trials of sulfinpyrazone, dipyridamole, and various combinations of antiplatelet agents. The initial analysis reported a 15 percent reduction of vascular death and a 30 percent reduction of stroke and myocardial infarction with antiplatelet medication.[63]

This group of investigators has now compiled results of 101 completed, randomized trials involving 101,302 patients with coronary, cerebral, and peripheral vascular atherosclerotic disease or other high-risk vascular conditions.[64] All patients received antiplatelet therapy for at least 1 month. Seven antiplatelet drug regimens were studied, including aspirin, ticlopidine, dipyridamole, sulfinpyrazone, suloctidil,

TABLE 25–2. Patient Selection and Recommended Use of Antithrombotic Agents in Patients With TIAs

Event	Recommended Therapy	Therapeutic Options
TIA*	Aspirin, 325 mg/day† or 1300 mg/day‡	Aspirin, 30–1300 mg/day§ or ticlopidine, 250 mg bid‡
TIA* if patient is aspirin-intolerant or if TIA occurs on aspirin therapy	Ticlopidine, 250 mg bid‡	Warfarin (INR 2–3)¶
Crescendo TIA*	—	Intravenous heparin (aPTT 1.5–2.0), aspirin, 325–1300 mg/day or ticlopidine, 250 mg bid after aspirin loading at 325 mg¶

*Carotid endarterectomy is indicated for angiographically documented symptomatic ipsilateral carotid stenosis ≥ 70 percent, unless surgery is contraindicated. Anticoagulation is indicated if a definite cardiac source of embolism is identified.
†Experts disagree about whether 325 mg aspirin per day offers as much benefit as higher doses.
‡Supported by large randomized controlled trials.
§Supported by randomized, controlled trials with high rates of false-positive or false-negative errors.
¶Supported by nonrandomized cohort studies or case series.
aPTT, activated partial thromboplastin time; bid, twice daily; INR, International normalized ratio; TIA, transient ischemic attack.
From the American Heart Association Medical/Scientific Statement: Guidelines for the management of a transient ischemic attack. *Circulation.* 1994;89:2950. Reproduced with permission. ©1994 American Heart Association.

and the combinations of aspirin plus dipyridamole and aspirin plus sulfinpyrazone. The most widely used antiplatelet agent was 160 to 325 mg of aspirin daily.

In patients with a history of TIA or stroke, the overview analysis found that antiplatelet therapy resulted in a 23 percent risk reduction for the occurrence of nonfatal stroke compared with placebo. There was a 22 percent risk reduction for the cluster of vascular events encompassing nonfatal stroke, nonfatal myocardial infarction, and vascular death. The overview analysis also found significant risk reductions for death from any cause, nonfatal myocardial infarction, and the outcome cluster of vascular death or death from unknown cause (Table 25–3).[64] The relative benefit of antiplatelet therapy was similar in men and women, and in patients younger and older than 65 years. The relative benefit of antiplatelet therapy was also remarkably constant in hypertensive and nonhypertensive patients, and in diabetic and nondiabetic patients.[64]

This comprehensive meta-analysis provides further support for a beneficial effect of antiplatelet agents in patients who have had TIAs or minor strokes.

Anticoagulants

Although oral anticoagulants have been used for decades to prevent stroke in patients with TIAs, there are no conclusive data supporting their use. The number of TIA patients included in clinical trials of anticoagulants is only a fraction of the number studied with antiplatelet agents. Four randomized[65–68] and six nonrandomized[69–74] studies have evaluated oral anticoagulant therapy for TIAs. The randomized trials were performed about 30 years ago and included only 178 patients altogether.[65–68] No significant benefit was demonstrated for warfarin compared with placebo. Three more recent studies compared warfarin with aspirin alone or in combination with dipyridamole. Aggregate data in 501 patients who had TIAs showed no significant difference in the rate of cerebral infarction or death among the patient groups.[75–77] Eriksson[78] also randomly assigned 188 TIA patients to a combination of aspirin and dipyridamole or heparin followed by warfarin. He found no significant difference in the rate of stroke or death between the two groups. Recurrent TIAs or amaurosis fugax was more frequent in the antiplatelet-treated group, particularly in the first 2 months after the onset of TIAs.

Based on these inconclusive data, there is no evidence to recommend the routine administration of anticoagulants to patients with TIAs. The small number of patients studied leaves open the possibility of a type II (β) error. A prospective randomized trial has recently been initiated to compare aspirin and warfarin in these patients, and it is hoped that this study will provide definitive data.

Anticoagulants are indicated in one specific group of patients—those with cardioembolic TIAs. A prospective trial recently demonstrated anticoagulants to be very effective in preventing recurrent stroke in patients with atrial fibrillation who have had a TIA or minor stroke (see later discussion). This emphasizes the need for a complete evaluation of each TIA patient, with therapy based on the cause of the TIA and the patient's underlying risk factors.

Therapy for Subtypes of Transient Ischemic Attacks

The prospective randomized trials of antiplatelet agents were not designed to evaluate their effectiveness for specific TIA subtypes or TIAs with specific causes. Except for cardioembolic TIAs, there is no compelling evidence that different therapies are appropriate for TIAs with specific causes or occurring in specific vascular territories. Post hoc

TABLE 25–3. Risk Reduction in Patients With Previous Transient Ischemic Attack or Stroke: Antiplatelet Therapy vs. Control

Event	Odds Reduction ± SD, %
Nonfatal stroke, nonfatal myocardial infarction, or vascular death	22 ± 4
Vascular death or death from unknown cause	14 ± 7
Death from any cause	16 ± 6
Nonfatal stroke	23 ± 6
Nonfatal myocardial infarction	36 ± 11

SD, standard deviation.
From the Antiplatelet Trialists' Collaboration: Collaborative overview of randomized trials of antiplatelet therapy. I. Prevention of death, myocardial infarction, and stroke by prolonged antiplatelet therapy in various categories of patients. *Br Med J.* 1994;308:81; with permission.

subgroup analyses found that antiplatelet agents are effective in vertebrobasilar TIAs as well as those in the carotid circulation.[79–81] Based on nonrandomized case-control studies and anecdotal evidence, some authors have recommended anticoagulation for TIAs caused by stenotic disease of the intracranial vessels.[82] No prospective trials have studied antithrombotic therapy in small vessel occlusive (lacunar) disease. A subgroup analysis in the French AICLA trial suggested a benefit of aspirin in these patients.[53]

There is general agreement that most patients with stroke or TIA due to cardiac embolism should be treated with anticoagulants. Until recently, this has been based on case-control studies of secondary prevention and extrapolation from randomized, controlled, primary prevention studies in atrial fibrillation[83, 84] and coronary artery disease.[85] The recently reported European Atrial Fibrillation Trial provides compelling evidence for the use of anticoagulants in this group. The study compared warfarin (International Normalized Ratio, 2.5–4.0), aspirin (300 mg/day), and placebo in 1007 patients with nonrheumatic atrial fibrillation and TIAs (23% of patients) or small strokes (77%).[86] There was a 66 percent reduction in subsequent stroke with anticoagulation compared with placebo. Aspirin was less effective than warfarin, with a 14 percent reduction in stroke compared with placebo. Since atrial fibrillation accounts for about half of cardiac embolisms,[87] this study provides further support for anticoagulation in patients with cardioembolic TIAs.

Management of Recent or Frequent Transient Ischemic Attacks

Considerable controversy remains about the proper management of patients with recent or frequent TIAs. Some physicians advocate immediate intravenous administration of heparin for high-risk patients with recent TIAs; in patients with TIAs of increasing severity, frequency, or duration ("crescendo TIAs"); and as an interim medical measure while patients are evaluated before surgery or as maintenance medical therapy (see Table 25–2).[88, 89] However, no randomized trial of adequate size has evaluated heparin use in any of these clinical situations. A small prospective study enrolled 55 patients within 1 week of carotid or vertebrobasilar TIA. Patients received either 1300 mg/day of aspirin or intravenous heparin. Recurrent TIAs occurred in 30 percent of 27 patients assigned to heparin and in 25 percent of patients given aspirin for a mean of 6 days. One patient (4%) in the heparin group had a stroke, compared with four (14%) aspirin-treated patients.[90] The small number of patients studied precludes any definitive recommendations regarding intravenous heparin use in patients with recent TIAs.

Summary

Effective antithrombotic therapy is available to reduce stroke risk in patients with TIAs or mild strokes. The choice of agent depends on the cause of the TIA as well as the patient's associated medical conditions. Antiplatelet agents have been proved effective in a number of randomized, controlled trials and are the first-line treatment for TIAs in most patients (see Table 25–2). Anticoagulants may be indicated in patients with a definite cardiac source for their

TIAs. The value of anticoagulation in patients with recent or frequent TIAs remains uncertain.

ANTIPLATELET THERAPY FOLLOWING CAROTID ENDARTERECTOMY

The role of antiplatelet agents following carotid endarterectomy has not been comprehensively studied. Aspirin might be of value either to prevent perioperative strokes or to decrease the late stroke rate after successful surgery. Aspirin also may reduce the rate of coronary events in these patients.

In the first randomized aspirin trial in the United States, patients in the surgical arm were randomized to receive either 1300 mg of aspirin per day or placebo, started within 5 days of endarterectomy and followed for at least 6 months. There were fewer strokes or deaths in the aspirin-treated group, but the number of events was very small.[91] In another small randomized trial, Kretschmer and associates[92] reported a decreased mortality rate in endarterectomy patients treated with aspirin 1000 mg/day, compared with placebo. The stroke rate was not reported. A Danish trial of "very-low-dose aspirin" randomly allocated patients after carotid endarterectomy to receive either aspirin, 50 to 100 mg/day, or placebo after endarterectomy. No significant difference in stroke or survival was shown between the two groups. However, treatment was not begun until 1 to 12 weeks after surgery.[93] Recently, Lingblad and colleagues[94] compared 75 mg/day of aspirin, begun before surgery, with placebo in patients undergoing endarterectomy. They found a decrease in intraoperative or perioperative stroke in patients treated with aspirin ($P = 0.01$) and a trend toward decreased mortality in the aspirin group ($P = 0.12$). In another randomized trial, the combination of 325 mg of aspirin per day and 75 mg of dipyridamole three times a day did not reduce the incidence of restenosis following endarterectomy.[95]

The North American Symptomatic Carotid Endarterectomy Trial reported some interesting nonrandomized observations. In patients with 70 to 99 percent stenosis undergoing endarterectomy, the ipsilateral stroke rate at 30 days was 2.1 percent, 1.1 percent, 6.5 percent, and 7.8 percent in patients receiving 1300 mg, 650 mg, 325 mg, and no aspirin, respectively.[51] These data raise the possibility that higher-dose aspirin is more effective in preventing perioperative stroke than low-dose aspirin.

Although the status of aspirin's usefulness in decreasing perioperative or postoperative stroke is unresolved, the data regarding coronary events are clearer. The data of the Mayo Asymptomatic Carotid Endarterectomy Trial[1] discussed at the beginning of this chapter are relevant here. In this trial, which compared surgery with medical management for asymptomatic carotid stenosis, aspirin use was discouraged in the surgery group. The trial was stopped early because of the very high myocardial infarction rate in the surgical group. The Antiplatelet Trialists' Collaboration found a 36 percent reduction in myocardial infarction and a 16 percent reduction in vascular death in patients with stroke or TIA treated with antiplatelet agents (see Table 25–3).[64]

In summary, the benefit of antiplatelet therapy to prevent perioperative complications, including stroke, in carotid endarterectomy remains unresolved. However, antiplatelet therapy decreases the incidence of cardiovascular events and improves survival in these patients and can be recommended for this reason. The optimal dose of aspirin is uncertain.

CONCLUSION

Medical management of patients with TIAs in the carotid territory includes reduction of risk factors as well as antithrombotic therapy. In some patients, management may include carotid endarterectomy. Effective therapy is available to reduce the risk of stroke. A patient with a TIA should be carefully evaluated in an attempt to identify the source of the TIA and associated stroke risk factors. With this information, the physician can make a rational decision regarding therapy. The choice of antithrombotic agent depends on the specific etiology of the TIA as well as the patient's associated medical conditions and general health status.

Acknowledgment

The author thanks José Biller, MD, and Gregory W. Albers, MD, for their helpful advice about this manuscript.

REFERENCES

1. Mayo Asymptomatic Carotid Endarterectomy Study Group: Results of a randomized controlled trial of carotid endarterectomy for asymptomatic carotid stenosis. *Mayo Clin Proc.* 1992;67:513.
2. Caplan LR: Vertebrobasilar disease: Should we continue the double standard of managing patients with brain ischemia? *Heart Disease and Stroke.* 1993;2:377.
3. Mohr JP, Caplan LR, Melski JW, et al: The Harvard Cooperative Stroke Registry: A prospective registry. *Neurology (Minneap).* 1978;28:754.
4. Foulkes MA, Wolf PA, Price TP, et al: The Stroke Data Bank: Design, methods, and baseline characteristics. *Stroke.* 1988;19:547.
5. Bogousslavsky J, Van Melle G, Regli F, for Lausanne Stroke Registry Group: The Lausanne stroke registry: Analysis of 1,000 consecutive patients with first stroke. *Stroke.* 1988;19:1083.
6. Caplan LR, Hier DB, D'Cruz I: Cerebral embolism in the Michael Reese stroke registry. *Stroke.* 1983;14:530.
7. Rothrock JR, Lyden PD, Brody ML, et al: An analysis of ischemic stroke in an urban southern California population. *Arch Intern Med.* 1993;153:619.
8. Wolf P, Cobb J, D'Agostino R: Epidemiology of stroke. In Barnett HJM, Mohr JP, Stein BM, Yatsu FM, eds. *Stroke—Pathophysiology, Diagnosis, and Management.* New York: Churchill Livingstone; 1992:3.
9. Welin L, Svardsudd K, Wilhelmsen L, et al: Analysis of risk factors for stroke in a cohort of men born in 1913. *N Engl J Med.* 1987;317:521.
10. Boysen G, Nyboe J, Appleyard M, et al: Stroke incidence and risk factors for stroke in Copenhagen, Denmark. *Stroke.* 1988;19:1345.
11. Colandrea M, Friedman G, Nichaman M: Systolic hypertension in the elderly: An epidemiologic assessment. *Circulation.* 1970;41:239.
12. Collins R, Peto R, MacMahon S, et al: Blood pressure, stroke, and coronary heart disease. Part 2. Short-term reductions in blood pressure: Overview of randomized drug trials in their epidemiological context. *Lancet.* 1990;335:827.
13. SHEP Cooperative Research Group. Prevention of stroke by antihypertensive drug treatment in older persons with isolated systolic hypertension. *JAMA.* 1991;265:3255.
14. Meissner I, Whisnant JP, Garraway WM: Hypertension management and stroke recurrence in a community (Rochester, Minnesota, 1950–1979). *Stroke.* 1988;19:459.
15. Hypertension Stroke Cooperative Study Group: Effect of antihypertensive treatment on stroke recurrence. *JAMA.* 1974;229:409.
16. Beevers DG, Fairman MJ, Hamilton M, Harpur JE: Antihypertensive treatment and the course of established cerebral vascular disease. *Lancet.* 1973;1:1407.
17. Abbott R, Yin Y, Reed R, Yano K: Risk of stroke in male cigarette smokers. *N Engl J Med.* 1987;315:317.
18. Colditz G, Bonita R, Stampfer M, et al: Cigarette smoking and risk of stroke in middle-aged women. *N Engl J Med.* 1988;318:937.
19. Shinton R, Beevers G: Meta-analysis of relation between cigarette smoking and stroke. *Br Med J.* 1989;298:789.
20. Wolf P, D'Agostino R, Kannel W, et al: Cigarette smoking as a risk factor for stroke. *JAMA.* 1988;259:1025.
21. Iso H, Jacobs D, Wentworth D, et al: Serum cholesterol levels and six-year mortality from stroke in 350,977 men screened for the multiple risk factor intervention trial. *N Engl J Med.* 1989;320:904.
22. Tell GT, Crouse JR, Furberg CD: Relation between blood lipids, lipoproteins, and cerebrovascular atherosclerosis: A review. *Stroke.* 1988;19:423.
23. Atkins D, Psaty BM, Koepsell TD, et al: Cholesterol reduction and the risk of stroke in men: A meta-analysis of randomized, controlled trials. *Ann Intern Med.* 1993;119:136.
24. Expert panel on detection, evaluation, and treatment of high blood cholesterol in adults: Summary of the second report of the National Cholesterol Education Program (NCEP) expert panel on detection, evaluation, and treatment of high blood cholesterol in adults (Adult Treatment Panel II). *JAMA.* 1993;269:3015.
25. Gorelick P: The status of alcohol as a risk factor for stroke. *Stroke.* 1989;20:1607.
26. Kozararevic D, Vojvodic N, Dawber T, et al: Frequency of alcohol consumption and morbidity and mortality. The Yugoslavian cardiovascular disease study. *Lancet.* 1980;1:613.
27. Camargo CA Jr: Moderate alcohol consumption and stroke: The epidemiologic evidence. *Stroke.* 1989;20:1611.
28. Palomäki H, Kaste M: Regular light-to-moderate intake of alcohol and the risk of ischemic stroke: Is there a beneficial effect? *Stroke.* 1993;24:1828.
29. Moore RD, Pearson TA: Moderate alcohol consumption and coronary artery disease: A review. *Medicine (Baltimore).* 1986;65:242.
30. Gaziano JM, Buring JE, Breslow JL, et al: Moderate alcohol intake, increased levels of high-density lipoprotein and its subfractions, and decreased risk of myocardial infarction. *N Engl J Med.* 1993;329:1829.
31. Abbott R, Donahue R, MacMahon S, et al: Diabetes and the risk of stroke. The Honolulu Heart Program. *JAMA.* 1987;257:949.
32. Barrett-Connor E, Khaw K: Diabetes mellitus: An independent risk factor for stroke? *Am J Epidemiol.* 1988;128:116.
33. Longstreth W, Swanson P: Oral contraceptives and stroke. *Stroke.* 1984;15:747.
34. Stadel B: Oral contraceptives and cardiovascular disease. *N Engl J Med.* 1981;305:672.
35. Vessey M, Lawless M, Yeates D: Oral contraceptives and stroke: Findings in a large prospective study. *Br Med J.* 1984;289:530.
36. Collaborative group for the study of stroke in young women: Oral contraceptives and stroke in young women. *JAMA.* 1975;231:718.
37. Stampfer M, Willett W, Colditz G, et al: A prospective study of past use of oral contraceptive agents and risk of cardiovascular diseases. *N Engl J Med.* 1988;319:1313.
38. Wilson P, Garrison R, Castelli W: Postmenopausal estrogen use, cigarette smoking, and cardiovascular morbidity in women over 50. *N Engl J Med.* 1985;313:1038.
39. Stampfer M, Colditz G, Willett W, et al: Postmenopausal estrogen therapy and cardiovascular disease. *N Engl J Med.* 1991;325:756.
40. Finucane FF, Madans JH, Bush TL, et al: Decreased risk of stroke among postmenopausal hormone users: Results from a national cohort. *Arch Intern Med.* 1993;153:73.
41. Canadian cooperative study group: A randomized trial of aspirin and sulfinpyrazone in threatened stroke. *N Engl J Med.* 1978;229:53.
42. Fields WS, Lemak NA, Frankowski RF, et al: Controlled trial of aspirin in cerebral ischemia. *Stroke.* 1977;8:301.
43. Dyken ML: Transient ischemic attacks and aspirin, stroke, and death: Negative studies and type II error (editorial). *Stroke.* 1983;14:2.
44. Reuther R, Dornhof W: Aspirin in patients with cerebral ischemia and normal angiograms or nonsurgical lesions. In Breddin K, Dornhof W, Loew D, eds. *Acetylsalicylic Acid in Cerebral Ischemia and Coronary Heart Disease.* Stuttgart: FK Shattauer Verlag; 1978:97.
45. Candelise L, Landi G, Perrone P, et al: A randomized trial of aspirin and sulfinpyrazone in patients with TIA. *Stroke.* 1982;13:175.
46. Sorenson PS, Pederson H, Marquardsen J, et al: Acetylsalicylic acid in the prevention of stroke in patients with reversible cerebral ischemic attacks—a Danish cooperative study. *Stroke.* 1983;14:15.
47. Briton M, Helmers C, Samuelsson K: High dose acetylsalicylic acid after cerebral infarction: A Swedish co-operative study. *Stroke.* 1987;18:325.
48. UK-TIA study group: United Kingdom Transient Ischaemic Attack (UK-TIA) aspirin trial: Final results. *J Neurol Neurosurg Psychiatry.* 1991;54:1044.
49. Dutch TIA trial study group: A comparison of two doses of aspirin (30 mg vs. 283 mg a day) in patients after a transient ischemic attack or minor ischemic stroke. *N Engl J Med.* 1991;325:1261.
50. SALT collaborative group: Swedish Aspirin Low-dose Trial (SALT) of 75 mg aspirin as secondary prophylaxis after cerebrovascular ischemic events. *Lancet.* 1991;338:1345.
51. Dyken ML, Barnett HJM, Easton JD, et al: Low-dose aspirin and stroke: "It ain't necessarily so." *Stroke.* 1992;23:1395.
52. Giraud-Chaumeil B, Rascol A, David J, et al: Prévention des récidives des accidents vasculaires cérébraux ischémiques par les anti-aggrégants plaquettaires. Résultats d'un essai thérapeutique contrôlé de 3 ans. *Rev Neurol (Paris).* 1982;138:367.
53. Bousser MG, Eschwege M, Haguenau JM, et al: AICLA controlled trial of aspirin and dipyridamole in the secondary prevention of athero-thrombotic cerebral ischemia. *Stroke.* 1983;14:5.
54. American-Canadian cooperative study group: Persantine aspirin trial in cerebral ischemia. Part II. Endpoint results. *Stroke.* 1985;16:406.
55. ESPS group: The European Stroke Prevention Study (ESPS). Principal end-points. *Lancet.* 1987;2:1351.
56. Acheson J, Danta G, Hutchinson EG: Controlled trial of dipyridamole in cerebral vascular disease. *Br Med J.* 1969;1:614.
57. Gent M, Blakely JA, Hachinski V, et al: A secondary prevention randomized trial

of suloctidil in patients with a recent history of thromboembolic stroke. *Stroke.* 1985;16:416.

58. Gent M. Blakely JA, Easton JD, et al: The Canadian American Ticlopidine Study (CATS) in thromboembolic stroke. *Lancet.* 1988;2:1211.

59. Hass WK, Easton JD, Adams HP Jr, et al: A randomized trial comparing ticlopidine hydrochloride with aspirin for the prevention of stroke in high-risk patients. *N Engl J Med.* 1989;321:501.

60. Sherman DG, Dyken ML Jr, Fisher M, et al: Antithrombotic therapy for cerebrovascular disorders. *Chest.* 1992;102(suppl):529S.

61. Rothrock JR, Hart RG: Ticlopidine hydrochloride use and threatened stroke. *West J Med.* 1994;160:43.

62. American Heart Association: Guidelines for the management of a transient ischemic attack. *Stroke.* 1994;25:1320.

63. Antiplatelet Trialists' Collaboration: Secondary prevention of vascular disease by prolonged antiplatelet treatment. *Br Med J.* 1988;296:320.

64. Antiplatelet Trialists' Collaboration: Collaborative overview of randomized trials of antiplatelet therapy. I. Prevention of death, myocardial infarction, and stroke by prolonged antiplatelet therapy in various categories of patients. *Br Med J.* 1994;308:81.

65. Veterans Administration cooperative study of atherosclerosis neurology section: An evaluation of anticoagulant therapy in the treatment of cerebrovascular disease. *Neurology.* 1961;11(pt 2):132.

66. Baker RN, Broward JA, Fang HC, et al: Anticoagulant therapy in cerebral infarction: Report on cooperative study. *Neurology.* 1962;12:823.

67. Pearce JMS, Gubbay SS, Walton J: Long-term anticoagulant therapy in transient cerebral ischaemic attacks. *Lancet.* 1965;1:6.

68. Baker RN, Schwartz WS, Rose AS: Transient ischemic attacks: A report of a study on anticoagulant therapy. *Neurology.* 1966;16:841.

69. Fisher CM: The use of anticoagulant in cerebral thrombosis. *Neurology.* 1958;8:311.

70. Siekert RG, Whisnant JP, Millikan CH: Surgical and anticoagulant therapy of occlusive cerebrovascular disease. *Ann Intern Med.* 1963;58:637.

71. Fazekas JF, Alman RW, Sullivan JF: Vertebral-basilar insufficiency. *Arch Neurol.* 1963;8:215.

72. Friedman GD, Wilson S, Mosier JM, et al: Transient ischemic attacks in a community. *JAMA.* 1969;210:1428.

73. Toole JF, Janeway R, Choi K, et al: Transient ischemic attacks due to atherosclerosis. A prospective study of 160 patients. *Arch Neurol.* 1975;32:5.

74. Olsson J, Müller R, Bernell S: Long-term anticoagulant therapy for TIAs and minor stroke with minimum residuum. *Stroke.* 1976;7:444.

75. Olson J, Brechter C, Bäcklund H, et al: Anticoagulant vs. anti-platelet therapy as prophylactic against cerebral infarction in transient ischemic attacks. *Stroke.* 1980;11:4.

76. Burén A, Ygge J: Treatment program and comparison between anticoagulants and platelet aggregation inhibitors after transient ischemic attack. *Stroke.* 1981;12:578.

77. Garde A, Samuelsson K, Fahlgran H, et al: Treatment after transient ischemic attacks: A comparison between anticoagulant drug and inhibition of platelet aggregation. *Stroke.* 1983;14:677.

78. Eriksson SE: Enteric-coated acetylsalicylic acid plus dipyridamole compared with anticoagulants in the prevention of ischemic events in patients with transient ischemic attacks. *Acta Neurol Scand.* 1985;71:485.

79. Sivenius J, Rieffinen PJ, Smets P, et al: The European Stroke Prevention Study (ESPS): Results by arterial distribution. *Ann Neurol.* 1991;29:596.

80. Barnett HJM: The Canadian cooperative study of platelet suppressive drugs in transient cerebral ischemia. In Price T, Nelson E, eds. *Cerebrovascular Disease. Proceedings of the Eleventh Princeton Conference.* New York: Raven Press; 1979:221.

81. Grotta JC, Norris JW, Kamm B, TASS baseline and angiographic data subgroup: Prevention of stroke with ticlopidine: Who benefits most? *Neurology.* 1992;42:111.

82. WASID study group: Warfarin-Aspirin Symptomatic Intracranial Disease (WASID) study (abstract). *Stroke.* 1994;25:273.

83. Laupacis A, Albers GW, Dunn M, Feinberg WM: Antithrombotic therapy in atrial fibrillation. *Chest.* 1992;102(suppl):426S.

84. Albers GW, Sherman DG, Gress DR, et al: Stroke prevention in nonvalvular atrial fibrillation. A review of prospective randomized trials. *Ann Neurol.* 1991;30:511.

85. Cairns JA, Hirsh J, Lewis HD, et al: Antithrombotic agents in coronary artery disease. *Chest.* 1992;102(suppl):456S.

86. European atrial fibrillation study group: Secondary prevention in non-rheumatic atrial fibrillation after transient ischaemic attack or minor stroke. *Lancet.* 1993;342:1255.

87. Cerebral embolism task force: Cardiogenic brain embolism—the second report of the cerebral embolism task force. *Arch Neurol.* 1989;46:727.

88. Sandok BA, Furlan AJ, Whisnant JP, Sundt TM Jr: Guidelines for the management of transient ischemic attacks. *Mayo Clin Proc.* 1978;53:665.

89. Miller VT, Hart RG: Heparin anticoagulation in acute brain ischemia. *Stroke.* 1988;19:403.

90. Biller J, Bruno A, Adams HP Jr, et al: A randomized trial of aspirin or heparin in hospitalized patients with recent transient ischemic attacks: A pilot study. *Stroke.* 1989;10:441.

91. Fields WS, Lemak NA, Frankowski RF, Hardy RJ: Controlled trial of aspirin in cerebral ischemia. Part II. Surgical group. *Stroke.* 1978;9:309.

92. Kretschmer G, Pratschner T, Prager M, et al: Antiplatelet treatment prolongs survival after carotid bifurcation endarterectomy: Analysis of the clinical series followed by a clinical trial. *Ann Surg.* 1990;211:317.

93. Boysen G, Soelberg Sørensen P, Juhler M, et al: Danish very-low-dose aspirin after carotid endarterectomy trial. *Stroke.* 1988;19:1211.

94. Lingblad B, Persson N, Takolander R, Bergqvist D: Does low-dose acetylsalicylic acid prevent stroke after carotid surgery? A double-blind, placebo-controlled randomized trial. *Stroke.* 1993;24:1125.

95. Harker LA, Bernstein EF, Dilley RB, et al: Failure of aspirin plus dipyridamole to prevent restenosis after carotid endarterectomy. *Ann Intern Med.* 1992;116:731.

Medical Management of Acute Cerebral Ischemic Stroke

THOMAS BROTT

No proven effective treatment has been developed for acute ischemic stroke.[1] Nonetheless, by the end of this decade we can reasonably expect advances in three general therapeutic strategies. The first strategy is that of arterial recanalization, resulting in restoration of cerebral blood flow to the ischemic brain.[2] The second strategy is that of cellular protection, with the clinical development of drugs that metabolically alter and help protect neurons, glia, and vascular endothelial cells from irreversible ischemic injury. The third strategy is that of urgent patient evaluation and treatment. For the present, an intensive-care approach to the general medical management of the stroke patient, as described in this chapter, provides an opportunity for meaningful intervention. Consensus-based guidelines for medical management are also presented.[1, 3]

INITIAL MANAGEMENT IN THE EMERGENCY DEPARTMENT

The suggested management of the patient with acute ischemic stroke during the first 6 hours after symptom onset is summarized in Table 26–1.[1, 3] Following the arrival of the patient at the emergency department, the examining physician should first assess the patient with ischemic stroke as if he or she were any patient with a potentially life-threatening illness. Airway, breathing, and circulation—the ABCs of resuscitation—come first. In contrast to many patients with hemorrhagic stroke, the ischemic stroke patient usually has a stable airway.[4] The problem of a threatened airway is encountered primarily in patients with extensive infarction in the vertebrobasilar distribution or sustained seizure activity following hemispheric stroke. In those circumstances, intubation should be performed. In other patients, ventilatory function is usually stable and remains stable during the time of the emergency department evaluation. Those patients with pre-existing chronic obstructive airway disease may experi-

ence a mild increase in symptoms. Patients with asthma may have symptoms or signs of minor bronchospasm. Acute treatment is seldom required.

The mean age of ischemic stroke patients is approximately 70, and roughly two thirds are older than 65 years of age. Aging of the lungs leads to losses in elasticity and increased physiologic shunting.[5] The mismatch between ventilation and perfusion results in lower oxygen tensions. Mean arterial oxygen partial pressure (pO_2) declines with each decade of advancing age, and the pO_2 is usually in the 70 to 80 mm Hg range for those over age 65.[5] The ability of cerebral blood vessels to respond to compromises in ventilatory function (eg, a carbon dioxide partial pressure [pCO_2] of 50 mm Hg) is also blunted.[6] Superimposed on the effects of advancing age are the ventilatory effects of focal cerebral injury. Stroke patients have decreased inspiratory power compared with normal subjects.[6] They also have an impaired response to increases in airway resistance.[6] For example, an ischemic cerebral injury that affects the muscle tone and function of upper airway structures could increase resistance to inspiratory or expiratory flow. The stroke patient would be particularly vulnerable. Finally, ventilation may be compromised during sleep in stroke patients.[7]

If arterial blood gas partial pressures are measured, the finding of normal oxygen saturations ($\geq 90\%$) may be misleading. The patient is likely to be aroused during arterial blood sampling. More important, a peripheral oxygen saturation measurement of 90 percent may not accurately reflect conditions within the brain, particularly within the deep white matter. Experimentally, the peripheral arterial pO_2 is much higher than intracerebral pO_2 and does not provide an accurate index of intracerebral pO_2.[8] The intracerebral partial pressures of O_2 and CO_2 have not been measured in patients with acute ischemic stroke.

Because of these expected compromises in ventilatory function reserve, we recommend that stroke patients be treated with supplemental oxygen. We usually administer 2 to 4 L/minute via nasal prongs. Over the last 11 years, none of our patients receiving supplemental oxygen as part of acute treatment protocols have experienced any significant complications, even those with pre-existing chronic obstructive pulmonary disease. We recognize that some investigators recommend supplemental oxygen for patients with suspected hypoxia, but not for all stroke patients.[1]

Cardiac disease is a feature frequently associated with acute ischemic stroke.[9] Atrial fibrillation is present in approximately 20 percent of patients, heart failure occurs in approximately 5 percent, and myocardial infarction occurs in up to 5 percent. Each of these disorders may predispose to stroke. Each may be associated with clinically significant impairment of cardiac function. In addition, a significant percentage of elderly stroke patients who do not have active cardiac disease may have abnormally low cardiac output at the time of symptom onset.[10] Therefore, the cardiac examination of the stroke patient should include attention to the presence of tachypnea, tachycardia, jugular venous disten-

---

TABLE 26–1. Management of Acute Ischemic
Stroke During the First 6 Hours

Correct any compromise of airway, breathing, or circulation.
Monitor vital signs.
Conduct general assessment.
Conduct neurologic examination.
Do not treat elevation in blood pressure in the absence of specific
    indications (eg, myocardial infarction arterial dissection), or
    unless systolic blood pressure is $\geq$ 220 mm Hg or diastolic is
    $\geq$ 120 mm Hg on repeated measurements over 30 to 60
    minutes.
If seizures occur, administer anticonvulsant therapy, including a full
    loading dose of phenytoin.
If a cerebellar infarction is diagnosed, obtain neurosurgical
    consultation. Evidence of brain-stem compression should prompt
    consideration of urgent surgical decompression.

Adapted from McDowell FH, Brott T, Goldstein M, et al: Stroke: The first six
hours. *Stroke Clinical Updates* 1993;4:1, with permission.

tion, peripheral edema, rales, or a third heart sound. If any symptoms or signs suggest the possibility of heart failure, a chest radiograph should be taken. If heart failure is demonstrated, treatment should be administered promptly, but intravascular volume contraction should be avoided if possible. Drops in systemic blood pressure should be minimized.[11] Among the inotropic agents, dobutamine has the advantage of increasing cardiac output without substantially affecting either heart rate or blood pressure. Dopamine may be particularly useful in patients with relative hypotension. Augmentation of cardiac output has already been shown experimentally to result in modest increases in regional cerebral blood flow.[12] In the case of stroke in humans, autoregulation is impaired, and so systemic increases in cardiac output may increase cerebral perfusion in tissues that have been rendered pressure-passive by acute ischemia.[13]

If myocardial infarction is suggested by the patient's history, examination, or electrocardiogram, cardiac consultation should be obtained, and appropriate supportive therapies should be immediately provided (eg, opiate analgesics, antiarrhythmic drugs). More aggressive therapy should be initiated by the cardiologist if indicated. The presence of atrial fibrillation in the absence of myocardial infarction or heart failure usually poses no acute problem. If tachycardia is identified and is preventing optimal cardiac output, appropriate pharmacotherapy should be administered.

INITIAL DIAGNOSIS AND TREATMENT

After the stroke patient has been medically stabilized, a more detailed history and neurologic examination may proceed. An eyewitness description of the stroke onset should be sought, since the history provided by the patient is frequently incomplete or inaccurate. The presence of risk factors should be detected, and unusual causes of stroke such as arterial dissection, venous thrombosis, illicit drug use, or severe medical illness such as hyperosmolar coma should be identified. The physical examination should include several measurements of blood pressure and heart rate, cardiac, neurovascular examination, and neurologic examination, and examination for signs of trauma. The neurologic examination should be detailed enough to address the differential diagnosis presented by the acute ischemic deficit.

The diagnostic evaluations to be carried out on an emergency basis are listed in Table 26–2. A CT scan of the brain should be performed immediately to distinguish ischemic infarction from intracerebral hemorrhage.[1, 3] Computed tomography is preferable to magnetic resonance imaging (MRI) because of the greater ease it provides in examining acutely ill patients and better reliability in the emergency diagnosis of hemorrhagic stroke. The CT scan performed in the first hours after onset of ischemic stroke may allow localization of acute thrombi.[14, 15] Linear foci of increased attenuation, corresponding in size and location to the symptomatic intracranial artery (eg, M1 segment of the middle cerebral artery) frequently signify the presence of intraluminal thrombus.[14–17]

Management of blood pressure elevations in stroke patients should be approached conservatively.[1, 3, 11] Experimentally and in humans, the initial response to cerebral arterial occlusion is focal vasodilation, which results in focally in-

TABLE 26–2. Emergency Diagnostic Evaluation
Computed tomographic (CT) scan of the brain without contrast agent
Electrocardiogram
Chest x-ray
Hematologic studies
Complete blood count
Platelet count
Prothrombin time
Partial thromboplastin time
Serum electrolytes
Blood glucose
Arterial blood gas levels (if hypoxia is suspected)
Renal and hepatic chemical analyses
Lumbar puncture (if subarachnoid hemorrhage is suspected and CT scan shows no abnormality)
Electroencephalogram (if seizures are suspected)

Adapted from Adams HP, Brott T, Crowell T, et al: Guidelines for the management of patients with acute ischemic stroke. A statement for healthcare professionals from a special writing group of the Stroke Council, American Heart Association. *Stroke.* 1994;25:1901. Copyright © 1994 The American Heart Association. Reproduced with permission.

creased cerebral blood volume.[13] The capacity for further autoregulation is lost. Reductions in cerebral perfusion pressure following drops in arterial blood pressure may directly reduce local cerebral flow within the area of irreversible ischemic injury and within areas of potentially reversible injury, the penumbra. This conundrum is frequently amplified in the stroke patient because autoregulation is already blunted in the elderly, and the autoregulatory curve shifts to the right in the setting of chronic hypertension.

Consequently, specific indications for antihypertensive therapy in the first hour after symptom onset are few. Pharmacologic therapy without a specific indication must be avoided. Treatment may be appropriate in the setting of acute myocardial ischemia, heart failure, acute arterial dissection, and selected instances of acute renal failure. Hypertensive encephalopathy would be an indication for treatment but should be diagnosed in patients with acute, focal neurologic deficits suggestive of stroke only if the history is strongly supportive and specific signs such as papilledema are identified.

Spontaneous declines in blood pressure are common in the first hour after stroke onset. In the NIH pilot study of tissue plasminogen activator for stroke,[18] 29 of 74 patients (39%) had an initial systolic blood pressure of more than 160 mm Hg. From the time of the initial blood pressure measurement to the time of treatment (<90 minutes), 27 of those 29 (93%) experienced a decline in blood pressure. The mean decline was 28 mm Hg. Of the 41 patients who had an initial diastolic pressure higher than 90 mm Hg, 34 (83%) had a decline in pressure by the time of treatment. The mean decline was 14 mm Hg. These rapid spontaneous declines in systemic pressure have two important implications. First, antihypertensive therapy is usually unnecessary if treating physicians are willing to defer therapy. Second, and more important, antihypertensive therapy administered in the first hour may be dangerous. Pharmacologic effects superimposed on a spontaneous blood pressure decline could result in an accelerated fall in blood pressure and in focal cerebral perfusion. For the stroke patient, slower and less substantial reductions are preferred. Recent evidence has been reported that suggests that higher blood pressures are associated with a lower risk for stroke-in-progression.[11]

TABLE 26–3. Antihypertensive Treatment in
Acute Ischemic Stroke

1. Systolic blood pressure 180–230 mm Hg and/or diastolic < 120 mm Hg	Do not treat*
2. Diastolic blood pressure > 140 mm Hg, systolic blood pressure slightly increased on repeated measurements 5 minutes apart	(a) Sodium nitroprusside 2 g/kg per minute, may be repeated with double dose after 3–5 minutes
3. Systolic blood pressure > 230 mm Hg or diastolic blood pressure 120–140 mm Hg or both, on repeated measurements 20 minutes apart	(a) Labetalol 10 mg intravenously, may be repeated with double dose after 10 minutes as needed to a maximum of 160 mg† (b) Nifedipine 10 mg sublingually if labetalol is contraindicated

*Adams et al[1] and McDowell[3] (see reference list for full bibliographic information).
†Avoid labetalol in patients with asthma, cardiac failure, severe conduction abnormalities, and bradycardia.

The algorithm in Table 26–3 describes a conservative approach to blood pressure management.[1, 3, 4, 19, 20] Labetalol provides several advantages in use for patients with stroke.[20, 21] The onset of action is within minutes of intravenous administration, which allows antihypertensive effects to begin quickly. Labetalol blocks alpha- and beta-adrenergic receptors and so matches well pathophysiologically with the increases in adrenergic tone that are common in patients with ischemic stroke. Because labetalol also reduces peripheral vascular resistance, cardiac output is not adversely affected.[20, 21] Labetalol does not cause reflex tachycardia or redistribution of coronary blood flow, effects which may complicate the use of sodium nitroprusside.[20, 21] We recommend 10 mg as the initial intravenous dose for stroke patients over the usual initial 20 mg dose,[20] to minimize the probability of abrupt drops in systemic pressure.

We would not recommend nifedipine as acute hypertensive therapy for ischemic stroke patients, despite its popularity. Because oral administration is required, antihypertensive effects are delayed and so are more difficult to assess. The antihypertensive effects are also variable, and, for some stroke patients, the nifedipine can be excessively potent. In a study of 48 patients treated with 20 mg of sublingual nifedipine for urgent hypertension, the mean decline in systolic pressure at 15 minutes was 24 mm Hg, and the mean decline at 30 minutes was 44 mm Hg.[22] Blood pressure declines of this magnitude may severely compromise local cerebral perfusion in areas of acute, focal ischemia.

Low blood pressure is unusual in the setting of acute ischemic stroke[18, 23] and is usually secondary to volume depletion.[10] Other causes, such as myocardial infarction, heart failure, and sepsis, are possible, and so the specific etiology should be sought and appropriate therapy delivered. For volume depletion, glucose-free colloid solutions delivered intravenously are preferred, as discussed later.

If the patient is hyperglycemic, the etiology of the hyperglycemia should also be sought and appropriate therapy initiated, including insulin administration. Hyperglycemia may lower the neuronal threshold for irreversible ischemic injury[11, 24, 25] and perhaps even lower the threshold for hemorrhagic infarction.[26]

The presence of fever in the stroke patient should not be attributed to a central nervous system response. Rather, the etiology should be sought immediately by history, physical examination, and appropriate laboratory studies. In all stroke patients, the presence of fever at the time of admission should prompt consideration of herpes simplex encephalitis as a potential explanation for the patient's focal neurologic symptoms. Emergency lumbar puncture, MRI (if available), and electroencephalography may be necessary. Regardless of etiology, attempts should be made to lower elevated temperatures with the administration of antipyretics and fluids if appropriate and the use of a cooling blanket if necessary.[1]

MANAGEMENT AFTER THE FIRST HOURS

More definitive diagnostic evaluation may proceed after the stroke patient has been medically stabilized, evaluated neurologically, and studied with computed tomography. For cerebrovascular diagnosis, conventional cerebral arteriography has the advantage of high diagnostic yield if performed early but the disadvantage of patient risk, high cost, and limited 24-hour availability. With regard to diagnostic yield, Fieschi and colleagues[27] described the arteriographic findings of 80 patients studied within 6 hours of symptom onset. Arterial occlusions were identified in 61 patients (76%), which correlated with the acute symptoms; 42 patients had intracranial occlusions; 8 patients had extracranial occlusions; and 11 patients had ipsilateral occlusions of both the extracranial internal carotid artery and the middle cerebral artery (trunk). Wolpert and colleagues[28] reported arteriographic findings from a study of tissue plasminogen activator in which a baseline arteriogram was completed within 8 hours of symptom onset. Of 139 patients, 112 (80.6%) had a complete occlusion in a vessel appropriate for the presenting symptoms. Among the 93 patients who received the tissue plasminogen activator, 62 patients (67%) had occlusion of the middle cerebral artery stem or of one of the middle cerebral artery branches. Unfortunately, one of the 139 patients studied arteriographically sustained procedure-related cerebral infarction.

Because of the potential risk of cerebral arteriography[29] and because the results do not usually alter acute treatment, we suggest that arteriography should be reserved in most instances for patients enrolled in well-designed clinical trials. The high frequency of identifiable occlusive clot in patients with ischemic stroke[28] does hold promise for magnetic resonance angiography (MRA).[30] This methodology can identify acute occlusions in vessels the size of the anterior, middle, and posterior cerebral artery trunks.[31] Resolution in imaging branch disease is improving and MRA is safe. Although expensive, MRA is considerably less expensive than conventional arteriography. Magnetic resonance machines are now available that allow better access to and are better tolerated by sick patients. The future holds out the potential for emergency MRA to localize cerebral arterial occlusions and for emergency MRI to identify early ischemic changes within brain tissue.[32] These latter MRI techniques, diffusion- and perfusion-weighted imaging, may become widely available within the next 5 years and could allow emergency assessment of brain tissue viability.

Currently, noninvasive alternatives to cerebral angiography are available for emergency cases. Doppler ultrasonography of the internal carotid artery can be performed within 24 hours of symptom onset at most hospitals. The degree of internal carotid artery stenosis can be measured with acceptable reliability,[33] even in acutely ill patients with severe neurologic deficits. Knowledge that one or both internal carotid arteries are occluded or severely stenosed may help guide treatment decisions or suggest a need for cerebral angiography. The same knowledge may later assist in judgments regarding patient positioning, the pace of patient mobilization, or the vigor of physical therapy.

Transcranial Doppler sonography may be obtained during the first 24 hours at selected hospitals, and satisfactory insonation may be possible for 80 to 90 percent of patients examined.[34, 35] If an occlusion or stenosis is identified, the vessel may be studied serially so as to detect spontaneous recanalization. Fieschi and colleagues[27] examined 15 patients with middle cerebral artery occlusion with serial transcranial Doppler, and recanalization was demonstrated in 10 (67%). The sensitivity of transcranial Doppler in experienced hands may be 75 percent or higher for hemodynamically significant middle cerebral artery stenosis or occlusion.[34]

Relatively noninvasive intracranial assessment is also possible with single photon emission computed tomography (SPECT).[36] The availability of improved radiopharmaceutical agents[37] allows assessment of regional cerebral blood flow on an emergency basis. The SPECT image obtained with the new agents reflects regional cerebral blood flow during the minutes immediately following the injection of agent. Stroke patients can be injected for SPECT in the emergency department. After the emergency department evaluation and CT scan have been completed, the patient can then be taken to the nuclear medicine department. The SPECT images obtained at that time will reflect regional cerebral blood flow as it was in the emergency department. For small numbers of patients, serial SPECT studies have already been reported that allow assessment of acute intervention (thrombolytic therapy) by providing measures of regional cerebral blood flow before and after treatment.[38, 39]

GENERAL MANAGEMENT

Following evaluation in the emergency department, admission of the stroke patient to an intensive care unit setting is warranted if the patient is potentially unstable or at risk for progression of symptoms.[40] Special care units designated for stroke have been advocated,[1, 41] but benefits of stroke units have been documented only recently. Indredavik and colleagues[42] randomly assigned 220 patients with acute stroke either to treatment in a specialized stroke unit or to treatment in a general medical ward. At 6 weeks, 56 percent of the stroke unit patients had returned home, compared with 33 percent of the general medical patients ($P = .0004$); and at 6 weeks, mortality was 7 percent for the patients treated in the stroke unit and 17 percent for the general medical patients ($P = .027$). These results are encouraging and, if replicated, would justify expanded development of dedicated stroke units.

In hospitals without a stroke unit, admission of the stroke patient to an intensive care unit provides substantial potential benefits. Most important, more nurses are available than in a regular medical department. One nurse is usually responsible for only two patients instead of five to ten. Comprehensive nursing care of airway, oxygenation, and cardiovascular status become realistic. Neurologic assessments are possible on a frequent basis, and so progression of symptoms and signs can be detected promptly. Cardiac monitoring is always available. Pulse oximetry is usually available and allows accurate measurements of oxygenation while the patient is awake or asleep.

When the patient is moved from the emergency department to a special care unit or to the general medical unit, supportive care measures should continue. Supplemental oxygen via nasal prongs at 2 to 4 liters per minute is justifiable, as detailed earlier, despite the cost. After the patient is no longer bedridden, supplemental oxygen may be discontinued. Until the patient is alert and demonstrates adequate swallowing skills, oral feedings should be postponed.[1] For certain patients, detailed evaluation of chewing and swallowing, including fluoroscopic evaluation, may be necessary.[1]

Because most stroke patients do not take fluids orally during the first hours after stroke, administration of a relatively iso-osmolar solution is preferred. Solutions containing glucose are rarely indicated, as they may accelerate the development of cerebral edema and may be associated with elevations in serum glucose concentrations, which may be harmful to potentially viable neurons in the penumbra of the infarction.[11, 24, 25] Therapeutic volume expansion remains controversial. Randomized clinical trials have shown therapeutic volume expansion to be ineffective,[43–45] but initiation of therapy was delayed beyond several hours in the great majority of studies.[46] Volume expansion, therefore, was not accomplished for many hours after stroke onset. An alternative to formal volume expansion therapy would be liberal administration of intravenous fluids during the first hours after stroke onset, which would perhaps supplement cardiac output and cerebral blood flow, particularly in patients with volume contraction. After 12 to 24 hours, fluid administration could be cut back to avoid overhydration and the potential to accelerate cerebral edema.

Neurologic function should be assessed frequently, at least hourly if possible. The nursing assessment forms in use at many hospitals are frequently insensitive and cumbersome. Careful serial assessment of one neurologic sign may be more useful. The sign followed should be the finding that is thought most likely to show change if the patient's condition deteriorates or improves. For example, in the patient with a modest left hemiparesis, the drift of the extended left arm will likely increase with any degree of neurologic decline or decrease with neurologic improvement. Serial assessments of the sign will be sensitive to motor change and also to change in the level of consciousness in the patient. If the patient had a more severe hemiparesis, such that the left arm were paralyzed, testing of the arm would no longer be useful. If the patient were still able to move the left leg, ability to move the leg would likely be the function most sensitive to neurologic change. Serial testing of the leg would then be more appropriate. Assessment of a single neurologic sign requires less than 1 minute, so the patient is less likely to become fatigued and the testing is more reliable. Brevity also increases the probability that the nurse will be able to accomplish frequent testing.

Frequent monitoring of neurologic function is not an exercise in futility. Prompt detection of deterioration from any cause is important if the aggressive general therapeutic measures described later can be delivered soon enough to provide benefit. In addition, identification of neurologic deterioration may indicate stroke in progress soon enough to warrant consideration of anticoagulant treatment. Evidence is available to support the use of intravenous heparin in this setting, but opinion among investigators is not uniform.[1] The performance of a rigorous, randomized trial to adequately prove (or disprove) benefit is not likely to be performed in the foreseeable future.

Frequent monitoring also provides the best opportunity to detect seizure activity. Seizures may complicate the course of acute stroke in 15 percent or more of cases.[47–50] The seizures are often partial and are frequently recurrent. The partial seizures are likely to distort the neurologic examination. Partial seizures may also become generalized in the stroke patient and therefore compromise cardiovascular function and adversely affect acid-base metabolism. Prompt treatment with anticonvulsant agents is warranted. Following single seizures during the first hours after symptom onset, therapy with intravenous phenytoin provides the opportunity for rapid onset of action and the opportunity for sustained anticonvulsant effect. The potential for hypotension can be lessened with infusion at less than 50 mg/minute. For status epilepticus, a more aggressive approach is necessary.[1] In the absence of seizures, prophylactic administration of anticonvulsant medication is not recommended.

AGGRESSIVE MANAGEMENT OF CEREBRAL EDEMA AND INCREASED INTRACRANIAL PRESSURE

Cerebral edema develops within hours after onset of cerebral infarction but rarely becomes life-threatening in the first 24 hours after symptom onset. Cerebellar infarction is an exception.[51] If a cerebellar infarction is identified clinically and by CT scan, and the patient is drowsy, neurosurgical consultation should be obtained immediately. If the patient with cerebellar infarction is alert and brain-stem function is preserved, consideration for surgery could be deferred. The level of consciousness and brain-stem function should be monitored at least every 30 minutes. If deterioration is suspected, the CT scan should be repeated urgently, as the development of severe edema may precede clearcut changes in the neurologic examination. If severe edema is identified, emergency surgical removal of the infarcted cerebellar hemisphere should be considered.[52, 53] Suboccipital craniectomy can be performed with little intrinsic morbidity.[53] Surgical decompression of the posterior fossa in the setting of cerebellar infarction and major mass effect is likely to be more effective if it is accomplished prior to fully developed signs of brain-stem compression. This procedure may be combined with ventriculostomy. In some instances, ventriculostomy alone is warranted.[54]

If the edema and posterior fossa mass effect are less dramatic or if the patient is being prepared for surgery, osmotic diuresis with intravenous mannitol, 25 to 50 g every 3 to 5 hours, can be initiated with a maximum dose of 2 g/kg body weight per day.[55] Intravenous furosemide, 20 to 80 mg every 4 to 12 hours, may supplement the effects of mannitol and may be given intravenously. Corticosteroids have not been shown to be effective and may be harmful.[56–58] Replacement fluids should be administered so as to maintain the calculated serum osmolality in the 300 to 320 mOsm/L range.[55] Replacing fluids based on the measured urine output should be done cautiously, with attention to serum osmolality, because input and output measurements are frequently inaccurate. Hypotonic[55] and glucose-containing solutions[24, 25] should be avoided. Hyperventilation can be effective in temporarily decreasing intracranial pressure. Intubation is required, followed by mechanical ventilation. The target pCO_2 is 25 to 30 mm Hg.[55] More aggressive treatment may overly decrease regional cerebral blood flow and exacerbate tissue ischemia.

Cerebral edema does not usually present a major problem in patients with infarctions of the cerebral hemispheres until after the first 24 hours. Larger infarctions may be associated with severe edema and increased intracranial pressure by the second day.[59] Indicators of developing edema include a decline in level of consciousness, loss of spontaneous venous pulsations on funduscopic examination, enlargement of the pupil ipsilateral to the infarcted hemisphere, progression of the focal deficit, or the appearance of corticospinal signs on the side initially unaffected by the stroke. As is the case for cerebellar infarction, the CT or MRI signs of increasing edema associated with cerebral hemispheric infarction may precede clearcut changes in the neurologic examination. Repeat brain imaging 24 to 48 hours after symptom onset may therefore be helpful in patients with major initial neurologic deficits by providing early identification of potentially life-threatening edema. Medical treatment is similar to that described earlier for edema associated with cerebellar infarction.[55]

For a given initial size of cerebral infarction, cerebral edema may be more likely to be life-threatening in younger adults because of the minimal degree of pre-existing atrophy and ventricular enlargement. An infarction involving less than half of the affected hemisphere may result in sufficient edema to lead to early herniation and death because of lack of space within the cranial cavity. Accordingly, for younger patients with large infarctions, measures to minimize cerebral edema should begin within the first 24 to 48 hours. If osmotic diuresis and hyperventilation fail to prevent deterioration, as demonstrated by radiographic or clinical examination, surgical therapy with hemicraniectomy and decompression may be lifesaving and should be considered.[60, 61] Favorable long-term outcomes have been reported following hemicraniectomy and decompression.[61] The quality of life expected in the event of patient survival should be discussed prior to surgery with the family. Even if a life-long focal motor deficit or a life-long aphasia is anticipated, heroic treatment measures may still be warranted.

MANAGEMENT OF MEDICAL COMPLICATIONS

The stroke patient is particularly susceptible to the medical complications of acute illness. Level of consciousness is frequently blunted. Cranial nerve involvement, motor or sensory, affects respiratory status and airway integrity. A stroke patient with hemiparesis has an even greater degree of immobility than that complicating other acute illnesses requiring hospitalization and bed rest. General medical management should begin with measures to maximize patient alertness and mobility. Sedating drugs must be avoided. Measures to encourage adequate (and regular) sleep should be taken. Mobilization should begin as soon as possible, both of the whole patient and of affected muscles and joints.[1]

The respiratory system presents the earliest specific challenge in the medical management of patients with stroke because of airway compromise. Aspiration of oral contents may be detectable by video-fluoroscopy in as many as 50 percent of patients during the initial days after stroke onset.[62] Because the majority of the pneumonias are caused by aspiration, oral feeding should be withheld until the patient has demonstrated both intact swallowing with small amounts of water and intact coughing on command. The gag reflex by itself is not a reliable measure of pharyngeal coordination; in patients with questionable function, formal evaluation of swallowing may be necessary, including study with video-fluoroscopy. Even with the most conservative initiation of feeding, pneumonia may be difficult to prevent and so a high index of suspicion is essential. Traditional symptoms and signs of pneumonias are often lacking, particularly in elderly patients.[63] Any changes suggestive of infection should prompt a sputum evaluation, chest x-ray, blood cultures, and possible serologic testing for viral agents, *Mycoplasma,* or *Legionella.* Empiric antibacterial therapy should be administered until a specific diagnosis is established and antibiotic sensitivities are determined. The importance of these measures is fully justified because pneumonia causes 15 to 25 percent of deaths among stroke patients.[64–66]

The cardiovascular system is also quite vulnerable early in the course of stroke, and cardiovascular complications following stroke account for 10 to 20 percent of acute mortality.[64, 66] Monitoring of cardiac rhythm during the first 24 hours after stroke is recommended. Vital signs should be carefully measured and followed. Increases in heart rate or respiratory rate are sensible to the development of heart failure. The patient should be questioned on a daily basis with regard to chest pain and dyspnea. Examination of the heart and lungs becomes particularly important in stroke patients. Self-report of symptoms is often limited by confusion or disruption of normal language. Any suspicion of cardiovascular deterioration should prompt systematic evaluation and appropriate consultation.

Over the first several days following stroke onset, the development of occult deep vein thrombosis may occur, particularly in hemiplegic patients. Acute pulmonary embolism becomes a major risk and may be the cause of death in up to 25 percent of patients dying from ischemic stroke.[64, 65] Even patients with minor deficits are at risk, and so death from pulmonary embolism may occur in those who otherwise would have had an excellent recovery. The use of pneumatic compression boots is recommended for patients at bed rest, as they have been demonstrated to decrease the risk of deep vein thrombosis.[67] Subcutaneous heparin, 5000 units every 12 hours, should be administered if not neurologically contraindicated. Patients must be questioned closely and on a daily basis with regard to leg pain, chest pain, and dyspnea. Chest pain and dyspnea are experienced by 70 to 80 percent of patients who have not had a stroke but have

documented pulmonary embolism.[68] Therefore, these symptoms should be carefully sought, especially in patients with abnormal language function in whom the reporting of symptoms is difficult to decipher. Any increase in respiratory rate is a red flag because tachypnea is a sensitive sign of pulmonary embolism. In addition, the patient's lower extremities should be examined daily, specifically to detect signs of deep vein thrombosis. Compressive duplex ultrasonography should be performed in patients with suggestive symptoms or signs and in patients at high risk for deep venous thrombosis, such as those with no movement in one or both legs.[69] If pulmonary embolism is suspected, a ventilation-perfusion lung scan should be performed immediately. Pulmonary arteriography is necessary in selected patients. If pulmonary embolism is demonstrated, systemic anticoagulation is indicated with full-dose intravenous heparin for 5 to 10 days to be followed by warfarin for at least 3 months.[68]

Urinary tract infection becomes a risk for the stroke patient within several days after symptom onset. If detected early and properly treated, major morbidity may be avoided. However, urinary tract infection has the potential to become life-threatening and is present in as many as 40 percent of patients who die from stroke.[65] Hospital-acquired urinary tract infections are usually associated with the use of indwelling catheters, and so their use should be avoided when possible.[63] Intermittent catheterization or condom catheterization are safer alternatives. With regard to treatment, prompt antibacterial therapy is important but should be limited to treatment of symptomatic infection.[70]

Decubitus ulcers are common among stroke patients with impaired mobility. At the end of the first week and the weeks following discharge, the skin of the stroke patient is vulnerable to injury. Careful nutritional support, even with tube feedings if necessary, may be important as a general preventive measure. Frequent turning of immobilized patients is the fundamental specific preventive measure. In addition, the skin of the incontinent patient should be kept dry. For patients at particularly high risk for decubitus ulcers, an air-filled or fluid-filled mattress system should be used.[71] If a decubitus ulcer develops, wet-to-dry saline dressings should be applied four times daily. These dressings may provide some degree of débridement and may reduce bacterial colonization.[71] If the decubitus ulcer does not respond to conservative therapy, antibiotic therapy may be justified for several days, preceding definitive surgical débridement.[70, 71]

CONCLUSION

Despite the absence of specific treatments proven effective for acute ischemic stroke, stroke mortality rates continue to decline. The decline cannot be fully explained by the decline in stroke incidence. Rather, falling case-mortality has been documented[68, 69] and may explain a substantial portion of the fall in overall stroke mortality. Strokes that are occurring today may be less severe than those of previous years and so less likely to result in death. However, we prefer the hypothesis that improved care of the stroke patients is responsible for much of this improvement in case mortality. If an intensive-care approach were to be widely applied for acute care of stroke patients, perhaps stroke mortality would improve even further.

REFERENCES

1. Adams HP, Brott T, Crowell R, et al: Guidelines for the management of patients with acute ischemic stroke: A statement for healthcare professionals from a special writing group of the Stroke Council, American Heart Association. *Stroke.* 1994;25:1901.
2. Brott T, Broderick J, Kothari R: Thrombolytic therapy for stroke. *Curr Opin Neurol.* 1994;7:25.
3. McDowell FH, Brott T, Goldstein M, et al: Stroke: The first six hours. *Stroke Clinical Updates.* 1993;4:1.
4. Brott T, Reed R: Intensive care for acute stroke in the community hospital setting: The first 24 hours. *Stroke.* 1989;20:694.
5. Sparrow D, Weiss ST: Pulmonary system. In Rowe JW, Besdine RW, eds. *Geriatric Medicine.* Boston: Little, Brown & Co; 1988;266.
6. McMahon SM, Heyman A: The mechanics of breathing and stabilization of ventilation in patients with unilateral cerebral infarction. *Stroke.* 1974;5:518.
7. Dyken ME, Somers VK, Adams H, et al: Investigating the relationship between sleep apnea and stroke. *Sleep Research.* 1992;21:30. Abstract.
8. Kennealy JA, McLennan JE, Loudon RG, McLaurin RL:Hyperventilation-induced cerebral hypoxia. *Am Rev Respir Dis.* 1980;122:407.
9. Broderick J, Phillips S, O'Fallon W, et al: Relationship of cardiac disease to stroke occurrence, recurrence, and mortality. *Stroke.* 1992;23:1250.
10. Grotta JC, Pettigrew LC, Allen S, et al: Baseline hemodynamic state and response to hemodilution in patients with acute cerebral ischemia. *Stroke.* 1985;16:790.
11. Jorgensen HS, Nakayama H, Raaschou HO, Olsen TS: Effect of blood pressure and diabetes on stroke in progression. *Lancet.* 1994;344:156.
12. Keller TS, McGillicuddy JE, Labond VA, Kindt GW: Modification of focal cerebral ischemia by cardiac output augmentation. *J Surg Res.* 1985;39:420.
13. Frackowiak RSJ: The pathophysiology of human cerebral ischaemia: a new perspective obtained with positron tomography. *Q J Med.* 1985;57:713.
14. Gacs G, Fox AJ, Barnett HJM, Vinuela F: CT visualization of intracranial arterial thromboembolism. *Stroke.* 1983;14:756.
15. Tomsick T, Brott T, Barsan W, et al: Thrombus localization with emergency cerebral computed tomography. *AJNR Am J Neuroradiol.* 1992;13:257.
16. Leys D, Pruvo JP, Godefroy O, et al: Prevalence and significance of hyperdense middle cerebral artery in acute stroke. *Stroke.* 1992;23:317.
17. Pressman BD, Tourje EJ, Thompson JR: An early CT sign of ischemic infarction: Increased density in a cerebral artery. *AJNR Am J Neuroradiol.* 1987;8:645.
18. Broderick J, Brott T, Barsan W, et al: Blood pressure during the first minutes of focal cerebral ischemia. *Ann Emerg Med.* 1993;22:1438.
19. Brott T, MacCarthy EP: Antihypertensive therapy in stroke. In Fisher M, ed. *Medical Therapy of Acute Stroke.* New York: Marcel Dekker, 1989;117.
20. Wilson DJ, Wallin JD, Vlachakis ND, et al: Intravenous labetalol in the treatment of severe hypertension and hypertensive emergencies. *Am J Med.* 1983;75:95.
21. Stumpf JL: Therapy review: Drug therapy of hypertensive crises. *Clin Pharm.* 1988;7:582.
22. Jaker M, Atkin S, Soto M, et al: Oral nifedipine vs oral clonidine in the treatment of urgent hypertension. *Arch Intern Med.* 1989;149:260.
23. Britton M, Carlsson A, DeFaire U: Blood pressure course with acute stroke and matched controls. *Stroke.* 1986;17:861.
24. Plum F: What causes infarction in ischemic brain? The Robert Wartenberg Lecture. *Neurology.* 1983;33:322.
25. Pulsinelli WA, Levy DE, Sigsbee B, et al: Increased damage after ischemic stroke in patients with hyperglycemia with or without established diabetes mellitus. *Am J Med.* 1983;74:540.
26. Broderick J, Hagan T, Brott T, Tomsick T: Hyperglycemia and hemorrhagic transformation of cerebral infarcts. *Stroke.* 1995;26:484.
27. Fieschi C, Argentino C, Lenzi GL, et al: Clinical and instrumental evaluation of patients with ischemic stroke within the first six hours. *J Neurol Sci.* 1989;91:311.
28. Wolpert SM, Bruckmann H, Greenlee R, et al and the rt-PA Acute Stroke Study Group: Neuroradiologic evaluation of patients with acute stroke treated with recombinant tissue plasminogen activator. *AJNR Am J Neuroradiol.* 1993;14:3.
29. Heiserman J, Dean B, Hodak J, et al: Neurologic complications of cerebral angiography. *AJNR Am J Neuoradiol.* 1994;15:1401.
30. Atlas SW: MR angiography in neurologic disease. *Radiology.* 1994;193:1.
31. Korogi Y, Takahashi M, Mabuchi N, et al: Intracranial vascular stenosis and occlusion: Diagnostic accuracy of three-dimensional, fourier transform, time-of-flight MR angiography. *Radiology.* 1994;193:187.
32. Warach S, Wei L, Ronthal M, Edelman R: Acute cerebral ischemia: Evaluation with dynamic contrast-enhanced MR imaging and MR angiography. *Radiology.* 1992;182:41.
33. Castaldo JE, Nicholas GG, Gee W, Reed JF: Duplex ultrasound and ocular pneumoplethysmography concordance in detecting severe carotid stenosis. *Arch Neurol.* 1989;46:518.
34. Petty GW, Wiebers DO, Meissner I: Transcranial Doppler ultrasonography: Clinical applications in cerebrovascular disease. *Mayo Clinic Proc.* 1990;65:1350.
35. Spencer MP, Thomas GI, Nicholls SC, Sauvage LR: Detection of middle cerebral artery emboli during carotid endarterectomy using transcranial Doppler ultrasonography. *Stroke.* 1990;21:415.
36. Giubilei F, Luigi G, Di Piero V, et al: Predictive value of brain perfusion single-photon emission computed tomography in acute ischemic stroke. *Stroke.* 1990;21:895.
37. Andersen AR, Friberg HH, Schmidt JF, Hasselbalch SG: Quantitative measurements of cerebral blood flow using SPECT and 99mTc-d, 1-HM-PAO compared to Xenon-133. *J Cereb Blood Flow Metab.* 1988;8:S69.
38. Overgaard K, Sperling B, Boysen G, et al: Thrombolytic therapy in acute ischemic stroke: A Danish pilot study. *Stroke.* 1993;24:1439.
39. Hanson S, Grotta J, Rhoades H, et al: Value of single-photon emission-computed tomography in acute stroke therapeutic trials. *Stroke.* 1993;24:1322.
40. Duke RJ, Bloch RF, Turpie AGG, et al: Intravenous heparin for the prevention of stroke progression in acute partial stable stroke: A randomized controlled trial. *Ann Intern Med.* 1986;105:825.
41. Langhorne P, Williams BO, Gilchrist W, Howle K: Do stroke units save lives? *Lancet.* 1993;342:395.
42. Indredavik B, Bakke F, Solberg R, et al: Benefit of a stroke unit: A randomized controlled trial. *Stroke.* 1991;22:1026.
43. Italian Acute Stroke Study Group: Haemodilution in acute stroke: Results of the Italian Haemodilution Trial. *Lancet.* 1988;1:318.
44. Scandinavian Stroke Study Group: Multicenter trial of hemodilution in acute ischemic stroke. I. Results in the total patient population. *Stroke.* 1987;18:691.
45. The Hemodilution in Stroke Study Group: Hypervolemic hemodilution treatment of acute stroke: Results of a randomized multicenter trial using pentastarch. *Stroke.* 1989;20:317.
46. Grotta JC: Current status of hemodilution in acute cerebral ischemia. *Stroke.* 1987;18(4):689. Editorial.
47. de Reuck J, Krakel N, Sieben G, et al: Epilepsy in patients with cerebral infarcts. *J Neurol.* 1980;224:101.
48. Cocita L, Favale E, Reni L: Epileptic seizures in cerebral arterial occlusive disease. *Stroke.* 1982;13:189.
49. Olsen TS, Hogenhaven H, Thage O: Epilepsy after stroke. *Neurology.* 1987;37:1209.
50. Gupta SR, Naheedy MH, Elias D, Rubino FA: Postinfarction seizures. A clinical study. *Stroke.* 1988;19:1477.
51. Macdonell RAL, Kalnins RM, Donnan GA: Cerebellar infarction: Natural history, prognosis, and pathology. *Stroke.* 1987;18:849.
52. Chen HJ, Lee TC, Wei CP: Treatment of cerebellar infarction by decompressive suboccipital craniectomy. *Stroke.* 1992;23:957.
53. Heros RC: Surgical treatment of cerebellar infarction. *Stroke.* 1992;23:937.
54. Krieger D, Busse O, Schramm J, et al: German-Austrian Space Occupying Cerebellar Infarction Study (GASCIS): Study design, methods, patient characteristics. *J Neurol.* 1992;239(4):183.
55. Ropper AH, Rockoff MA: Treatment of intracranial hypertension. In Ropper AH, Kennedy SF, eds. *Neurological and Neurosurgical Intensive Care.* Gaithersburg, MD: Aspen Publishers; 1988;23.
56. Bauer RB, Tellez H: Dexamethasone as treatment in cerebrovascular disease. II. A controlled study of acute cerebral infarction. *Stroke.* 1973;4:547.
57. Norris JW, Hachinski VL: High dose steroid treatment in cerebral infarction. *Arch Neurol.* 1976;33:69.
58. Mulley G, Wilcox RG, Mitchell JRA: Dexamethasone in acute stroke. *Br Med J.* 1978;2:994.
59. Ropper AH, Shafran B: Brain edema after stroke. *Arch Neurol.* 1984;41:26.
60. Greenwood J Jr: Acute brain infarction with high intracranial pressure: Surgical indications. *Johns Hopkins Med J.* 1968;122:254.
61. Delashaw JB, Broaddus WC, Kassell NF, et al: Treatment of hemispheric cerebral infarction by hemicraniectomy. *Stroke.* 1990;21:874.
62. Horner J, Massey EW, Riski JE, et al: Aspiration following stroke: Clinical correlates and outcome. *Neurology.* 1988;38:1359.
63. Garibaldi RA, Neuhaus EG, Nurse BA: Infections in the elderly. In Rowe JW, Besdine RW, eds. *Geriatric Medicine.* Boston: Little, Brown & Co; 1988;302.
64. Bounds JV, Wiebers DO, Whisnant JP, Okazaki H. Mechanisms and timing of deaths from cerebral infarction. *Stroke.* 1981;12:474.
65. Brown M, Glassenberg M: Mortality factors in patients with acute stroke. *JAMA.* 1973;224:1493.
66. Silver FL, Norris JW, Lewis AJ, Hachinski VC: Early mortality following stroke: A prospective review. *Stroke.* 1984;15:492.
67. Skillman JJ, Collins RE, Coe NP, et al: Prevention of deep vein thrombosis in neurosurgical patients: A controlled randomized trial or external pneumatic compression boots. *Surgery.* 1978;83:354.
68. Dantzker DR, Tobin MJ: Pulmonary vascular disease. In Andreoli TE, Carpenter CCJ, Plum F, Smith LH, eds. *Cecil Essentials of Medicine.* Philadelphia: WB Saunders, 1990;153.
69. Hyers TM: Venous thromboembolic disease: Diagnosis and use of antithrombotic therapy. *Clin Cardiol.* 1990;13:23.
70. Yoshikawa TT: Pneumonia, UTI, and decubiti in the nursing home: Optimal management. *Geriatrics.* 1989;44:32.
71. Phillips TJ, Gilchrest BA: Skin. In Rowe JW, Besdine RW, eds. *Geriatric Medicine.* Boston: Little, Brown & Co., 1988;144.

CHAPTER 27

Medical Management of Vertebrobasilar Disease

ROBERT J. WITYK and LOUIS R. CAPLAN

In many respects, the treatment of transient ischemic attacks (TIA) or stroke involving the vertebrobasilar circulation parallels that involving the anterior circulation. Optimal management is aided by knowledge of the location and severity of vascular lesions and the presumed mechanism of ischemia. Treatment of cardioembolic or lacunar stroke, for example, is similar in the posterior and anterior circulations. The differences in vascular anatomy between the vertebrobasilar and carotid circulations, however, lead to specific approaches to treatment of patients with large-vessel occlusive disease.

ANTIPLATELET AGENTS

Aspirin and antiplatelet agents have been shown to be effective in a number of studies for the secondary prevention of stroke in patients with TIAs and minor stroke.[1-4] The Antiplatelet Trialists' Collaboration found in a meta-analysis of eight trials (involving patients with a variety of stroke types and locations) that stroke recurrence was reduced 26 percent and significant vascular events were reduced 23 percent with the use of aspirin as compared with placebo.[1] The European Stroke Prevention Study compared the combination of 75 mg dipyridamole and 330 mg aspirin three times a day with placebo in 2500 patients for secondary prevention of stroke or death after an ischemic event.[2] Use of the aspirin and dipyridamole combination reduced the combined risk for stroke and death by 33 percent compared with placebo. A subgroup analysis of 711 patients with symptoms involving the vertebrobasilar circulation revealed a 65.7 percent reduction in subsequent stroke in the treatment group (from a stroke rate of 10.8 percent on placebo to 5.7 percent on medication).[5] Although not statistically significant, the reduction in the rate of stroke and total endpoints was greater for patients with vertebrobasilar disease than for patients with carotid territory disease.[5] Unfortunately, most studies grouped patients with suggestive signs and symptoms under the general term ''vertebrobasilar insufficiency,'' without further characterization. No study of aspirin or any other medication has used angiography to define the type and location of vascular lesion involved.

The optimal dose of aspirin continues to be debated. Doses as small as 40 mg/day will inhibit production of thromboxane A_2 without affecting prostacyclin synthesis and may therefore be of greater benefit than higher doses.[6] A Swedish group showed that a dose of 75 mg of aspirin a day was effective in reducing the risk of subsequent stroke or death compared with placebo.[4] Approximately 14 percent of the 1360 patients entered into the Swedish study had symptoms in the vertebrobasilar circulation. A Dutch trial found no difference in effectiveness between 30 and 283 mg/day of aspirin.[3] An overview of all the aspirin trials, however, suggests that higher doses of aspirin are associated with a greater risk reduction.[7] Higher doses are also associated with increased side effects, particularly gastrointestinal

bleeding. Whether the risk-benefit ratio favors a higher or lower dose is still a matter of debate. Patients have different responses to particular doses of aspirin as assayed by in vitro platelet aggregation studies.[8] It remains to be seen whether routine use of in vitro tests of platelet function will be clinically helpful in determining the appropriate aspirin dose.

Ticlopidine is an antiplatelet agent that acts by inhibiting adenosine diphosphate–mediated platelet aggregation.[9] Unlike aspirin, ticlopidine has no effect on platelet cyclooxygenase. The Canadian American ticlopidine study of 1072 patients with recent atherothrombotic or lacunar stroke found that ticlopidine use reduced the risk for recurrent stroke, myocardial infarction, and vascular death by 30 percent.[10] Approximately one quarter of the patients in the trial had symptoms in the vertebrobasilar circulation. The Ticlopidine-Aspirin Stroke Study Group compared the effects of 500 mg/day of ticlopidine and 1300 mg/day of aspirin in patients with TIA or minor stroke.[11] At 3 years, there was a 12 percent risk reduction in the rate of nonfatal stroke or death and a 21 percent risk reduction in the rate of stroke in patients receiving ticlopidine compared with aspirin. Twenty-five percent of the study population had qualifying events in the vertebrobasilar circulation. A subgroup analysis found a beneficial effect of ticlopidine over aspirin in the 771 patients with symptoms in the vertebrobasilar circulation.[12] In both studies, ticlopidine was associated with a significantly greater incidence of adverse side effects, the most common being diarrhea, nausea, and skin rash.[10, 11] Twelve percent of patients had to discontinue the medication because of side effects. Neutropenia occurred in 2 to 3 percent of patients and was severe in 0.8 percent. The neutropenia resolved in all patients once ticlopidine was discontinued, and current clinical practice requires biweekly cell count determinations for the first 3 months of therapy. Because of the high incidence of side effects, some of which are potentially serious, ticlopidine remains a second-line agent, to be used after aspirin therapy fails or in patients who are aspirin intolerant.[13]

ANTICOAGULANTS

Anticoagulants were first used for the treatment of vertebrobasilar disease in the 1950s. Early reports suggested significantly decreased mortality when anticoagulants were used in patients with clinical signs of basilar thrombosis.[14-16] Whisnant,[15] for example, reported results in 140 patients with progressive symptoms due to vertebrobasilar disease and found that 8.5 percent of patients treated with anticoagulants died, compared with 58.9 percent of patients not receiving anticoagulants.[15] Unfortunately, most of these and other reports of anticoagulant use for vertebrobasilar disease consist of retrospective or nonrandomized studies, and in most cases the vascular lesions were not well defined.[17, 18]

Many clinicians have noted a dramatic reduction in the

261

frequency of vertebrobasilar TIAs with the use of warfarin or heparin.[19] In our experience, patients with hemodynamically significant stenosis of the intracranial vertebral or basilar arteries who have TIAs often respond to anticoagulation, and their spells typically recur once warfarin is discontinued. Given the risks of prolonged warfarin use, the benefit of long-term anticoagulation is uncertain. Anticoagulation with heparin is also used for patients with acute vertebrobasilar stroke, particularly if basilar thrombosis is suspected.[20, 21] This recommendation must be considered conjectural and unproven. The hope is to prevent further thrombosis or propagation of clot, since a large percentage of patients with vertebrobasilar stroke have progression of ischemia for several days.[22, 23] The few randomized, controlled studies of heparin for patients with progressive stroke failed to show a benefit, but the numbers of patients studied were small and the results inconclusive.[24, 25]

Patients with vertebral or basilar artery occlusion who have stabilized are often treated with anticoagulants in the hope of preventing further strokes from artery-to-artery embolism. An occluded extracranial vertebral artery, for example, may be hemodynamically asymptomatic if the other vertebral artery is patent and adequately supplies the basilar artery. A stroke can occur when a clot in the occluded segment embolizes distally, typically to the posterior inferior cerebellar artery, superior cerebellar artery, or top of the basilar artery.[26] Heparin is used initially, and the patient is maintained on warfarin for 4 to 6 weeks, at which point the intraluminal thrombus has presumably organized and become adherent to the vascular wall. The thrombus then poses less of a risk for embolization. Patients with basilar branch occlusion or lacunar stroke in the brain stem who do not have large-vessel occlusive lesions are treated with antiplatelet agents alone.

Anticoagulation is recommended in dissection of the cervical vertebral artery because of the high risk of emboli arising from the disrupted vascular endothelium.[27, 28] Anticoagulants are generally continued for several months, and repeat studies are performed to assess the patency of the affected vessel. Management of intracranial arterial dissection is problematic, because of the risk of subarachnoid hemorrhage.[27, 28] Nevertheless, some patients with disabling TIAs and chronic intracranial vertebral artery dissection can be managed with antiplatelets or anticoagulants or both.

BLOOD PRESSURE MANAGEMENT

Patients with severe stenosis or occlusion of the basilar artery and continued symptoms present a difficult therapeutic challenge. Despite adequate anticoagulation, patients may continue to have disabling TIAs or progressive brain-stem ischemia. An underemphasized aspect of medical management is the need to maintain adequate cerebral perfusion by manipulation of systemic blood pressure and cardiac output. In the setting of acute stroke, patients should be kept supine and well hydrated. Hypotension from dehydration or inappropriate treatment of elevated blood pressure may lead to ischemia in marginally perfused regions of the brain where collateral circulation is inadequate.[29] Patients who are on antihypertensive medications should have their dosages decreased or be temporarily withdrawn. Blood pressure is

frequently elevated with acute stroke but falls spontaneously over the first 48 hours of hospitalization with bed rest.[30] Use of rapidly acting antihypertensive medications such as nifedipine should be avoided because of the risk of precipitous drops in blood pressure. Patients with cardiac failure may need particularly close hemodynamic monitoring when attempts are made to increase blood pressure with hydration. Some desperate clinicians have gone so far as to hold the patient upside down by the ankles during heparinization, and have reported resulting remarkable clinical improvement.[31, 32]

During the patient's recovery and rehabilitation phase, mobilization and ambulation should be done cautiously, with monitoring of orthostatic blood pressure changes. Patients with chronic symptoms from basilar stenosis or occlusion frequently complain of TIAs associated with arising from a chair or walking. Elastic stockings can be used to decrease venous pooling and blunt the hypotensive response to standing. Further improvements in cerebral perfusion can be achieved by adequate hydration and increased salt intake. Refractory patients may require the judicious use of medications such as fludrocortisone to increase intravascular volume and ephedrine as a venoconstricting agent. Both medications can be hazardous in patients with coronary artery disease or congestive heart failure.

THROMBOLYSIS AND INTERVENTIONAL RADIOLOGY

The most exciting new area in the medical treatment of vertebrobasilar occlusive disease is the use of thrombolytic agents and interventional radiologic techniques. Hacke and coworkers[33] reported the outcome of 65 patients with severe brain-stem strokes due to vertebrobasilar thrombosis as demonstrated by angiography. Forty-three patients were prospectively treated with intra-arterial thrombolytic therapy (either urokinase or streptokinase), and 22 patients who received conventional medical therapy, including anticoagulants or antiplatelet agents, were studied retrospectively. Of the 43 patients who received thrombolytic therapy, 19 had arterial recanalization on repeat angiography, and 13 patients survived (10 with favorable clinical outcomes). None of the patients whose vertebrobasilar systems failed to recanalize survived. In comparison, only 3 of the 22 patients receiving conventional therapy survived. Hemorrhagic transformation of the infarction occurred in 9.3 percent of patients receiving thrombolytic therapy. Zeumer and colleagues[34] reported seven patients with acute vertebrobasilar stroke who were treated with intra-arterial urokinase followed by heparin. Four patients recovered, and the remainder either died or were left with severe neurologic deficits. There were no bleeding complications. A number of issues need further study, such as the optimal thrombolytic agent and technique of delivery, the minimum time period between onset of symptoms and administration of therapy, and patient selection.

There are only a few reports of the use of transluminal angioplasty in the vertebrobasilar circulation. In 1980, Sundt and colleagues[35] from the Mayo Clinic reported good angiographic and short-term clinical results in two patients who underwent transluminal angioplasty of high-grade proximal basilar artery stenosis. Both patients had persistent TIAs prior to the procedure despite maximal medical therapy with antiplatelet agents, anticoagulants, or blood pressure manipulation. A subsequent report from the same group was less optimistic.[36] Four additional patients with vertebrobasilar stenosis were treated with angioplasty, and all had major complications, including a new stroke in one patient and death in three patients. Improvements in microballoon and catheter technology have led others to attempt vertebrobasilar angioplasty, with more attention to lesions of the extracranial vertebral artery.[37–39] Higashida and associates[39] reported their results in 41 patients with a variety of atherosclerotic lesions. Most patients underwent angioplasty from a transfemoral approach. Thirty-three patients had stenotic lesions involving the proximal vertebral artery. The majority of patients had improvement in clinical symptoms with angioplasty, and no permanent complications were reported. Three patients had restenosis of the lesion within 6 months of the procedure, and two underwent successful repeat angioplasty. Serious complications occurred, however, in two of five patients treated for distal vertebral artery stenosis and in one of three patients undergoing angioplasty of basilar artery stenosis. The remaining patients, three with distal vertebral artery disease and two with basilar artery stenosis, reportedly had good clinical outcomes. Complications reported in the literature include occlusion of the vessel at the site of angioplasty, distal embolization, arterial dissection, and subarachnoid hemorrhage.[36, 39] Further refinements of technique and concurrent use of thrombolytic agents may improve results, but at this time, the indication for angioplasty of intracranial lesions remains uncertain. Promising results with proximal vertebral artery lesions suggest a possible role for angioplasty in the treatment of patients with intractable symptoms.

REFERENCES

1. Antiplatelet trialists' collaboration: Secondary prevention of vascular disease by prolonged antiplatelet treatment. *Br Med J.* 1988;296:320.
2. ESPS group: The European stroke prevention study (ESPS). *Lancet.* 1987;2:1351.
3. Dutch TIA trial study group: A comparison of two doses of aspirin (30 mg vs. 283 mg a day) in patients after a transient ischemic attack or minor ischemic stroke. *N Engl J Med.* 1991;325:1261.
4. SALT collaborative group: Swedish aspirin low-dose trial (SALT) of 75 mg aspirin as secondary prophylaxis after cerebrovascular ischaemic events. *Lancet.* 1991;338:1345.
5. Sivenius J, Riekkinen PJ, Smets P, et al: The European stroke prevention study (ESPS): Results by arterial distribution. *Ann Neurol.* 1991;29:596.
6. Tohgi H, Konno S, Tamura K, et al: Effects of low-to-high doses of aspirin on platelet aggregability and metabolites of thromboxane A_2 and prostacyclin. *Stroke.* 1992;23:1400.
7. Dyken ML, Barnett HJM, Easton JD, et al: Low-dose aspirin and stroke: "It ain't necessarily so." *Stroke.* 1992;23:1395.
8. Helgason CM, Tortorice KL, Winkler SR, et al: Aspirin response and failure in cerebral infarction. *Stroke.* 1993;24:345.
9. Uchiyama S, Sone R, Nagayama T, et al: Combination therapy with low-dose aspirin and ticlopidine in cerebral ischemia. *Stroke.* 1989;20:1643.
10. Gent M, Easton JD, Hachinski V, et al: The Canadian American ticlopidine study (CATS) in thromboembolic stroke. *Lancet.* 1989;1:1215.
11. Hass WK, Easton JD, Adams HP Jr, et al: A randomized trial comparing ticlopidine hydrochloride with aspirin for the prevention of stroke in high-risk patients. *N Engl J Med.* 1989;321:501.
12. Grotta JC, Norris JW, Kamm B, et al: Prevention of stroke with ticlopidine: Who benefits most? *Neurology.* 1992;42:111.
13. Albers GW: Role of ticlopidine for prevention of stroke. *Stroke.* 1992;23:912.
14. Millikan CH, Siekert RG, Shick RM: Studies in cerebrovascular disease. III. The use of anticoagulant drugs in the treatment of insufficiency or thrombosis within the basilar arterial system. *Staff Meetings of the Mayo Clinic.* 1955;30:116.
15. Whisnant J: *Transactions of the Third Princeton Conference on Cerebrovascular Disease.* Orlando: Grune & Stratton; 1961:156.
16. Siekert RG, Whisnant JP, Millikan CH: Surgical and anticoagulation therapy of occlusive cerebrovascular disease. *Ann Intern Med.* 1963;58:637.
17. Fazekas J, Alman RW, Sullivan JF: Vertebral-basilar insufficiency. *Arch Neurol.* 1963;8:215.
18. Bradshaw P, McQuaid P: The syndrome of vertebrobasilar insufficiency. *Q J Med.* 1963;32:279.
19. Fisher CM: The use of anticoagulants in cerebral thrombosis. *Neurology.* 1958;8:311.
20. Miller VT, Hart RG: Heparin anticoagulation in acute brain ischemia. *Stroke.* 1987;22:7.
21. Estol CJ, Pessin MS: Anticoagulation: Is there still a role in atherothrombotic stroke? *Stroke.* 1990;25:1.
22. Jones HR, Millikan CH, Sandok BA: Temporal profile (clinical course) of acute vertebrobasilar system cerebral infarction. *Stroke.* 1980;11:173.
23. Gautier JC: Stroke-in-progression. *Stroke.* 1985;16:729.
24. Haley EC, Kassell NF, Torner JC: Failure of heparin to prevent progression in progressing ischemic infarction. *Stroke.* 1988;19:10.
25. Duke RJ, Bloch RF, Turpie AGG, et al: Intravenous heparin for the prevention of stroke progression in acute partial stable stroke: A randomized trial. *Ann Intern Med.* 1986;105:825.
26. Caplan LR, Amarenco P, Rosengart A, et al: Embolism from vertebral artery origin occlusive disease. *Neurology.* 1992;42:1505.
27. Hart RG: Vertebral artery dissection. *Neurology.* 1988;38:987.
28. Mokri B, House OW, Sandok BA, et al: Spontaneous dissections of the vertebral arteries. *Neurology.* 1988;38:880.
29. Powers WJ: Acute hypertension after stroke: The scientific basis for treatment decisions (editorial). *Neurology.* 1993;43:461.
30. Wallace JD, Levy LL: Blood pressure after stroke. *JAMA.* 1981;246:177.
31. Fisher CM: The "herald hemiparesis" of basilar artery occlusion. *Arch Neurol.* 1988;45:1301.
32. Mitsias P, Levine S, Lozon J: Acute basilar artery occlusive disease. *Stroke.* 1990;21:503.
33. Hacke W, Zeumer H, Ferbert A, et al: Intra-arterial thrombolytic therapy improves outcome in patients with acute vertebrobasilar occlusive disease. *Stroke.* 1988;19:1216.
34. Zeumer H, Freitag HJ, Grzyska U, et al: Local intraarterial fibrinolysis in acute vertebrobasilar occlusion. *Neuroradiology.* 1989;31:336.
35. Sundt TM Jr, Smith HC, Campbell JK, et al: Transluminal angioplasty for basilar artery stenosis. *Mayo Clin Proc.* 1980;55:673.
36. Piepgras DG, Sundt TM Jr, Forbes GS, et al: Balloon catheter transluminal angioplasty for vertebrobasilar ischemia. In Berguer R, Bauer RB, eds. *Vertebrobasilar Arterial Occlusive Disease.* New York: Raven Press; 1984;215.
37. Courtheoux P, Tournade A, Theron J: Transcutaneous angioplasty of vertebral artery atheromatous ostial stricture. *Radiology.* 1985;27:259.
38. Theron JG: Angioplasty of supra-aortic arteries. *Semin Intervent Radiol.* 1987;4:331.
39. Higashida RT, Tsai FY, Halbach VV, et al: Transluminal angioplasty for atherosclerotic disease of the vertebral and basilar arteries. *J Neurosurg.* 1993;78:192.

VI

Indications for Carotid Endarterectomy in Asymptomatic Patients

CHAPTER
28

The Natural History of Patients With Asymptomatic Carotid Stenosis

N. M. BORNSTEIN and J. W. NORRIS

In spite of the gradual decline in stroke mortality in industrialized countries since the beginning of the century, stroke is still the third leading cause of death and an important cause of disability in the western world.[1] Success in medical and surgical prophylactic treatment for symptomatic carotid disease has been reported,[2–6] but the management of asymptomatic carotid disease is still a matter of debate.[7–10] In light of these controversies, accurate information about the natural history and outcome of asymptomatic carotid disease is critical.

ROLE OF NECK BRUITS

Patients with asymptomatic carotid disease are usually discovered by auscultation of the neck for bruits, but the clinical significance of these remains uncertain. Angiographic studies indicate that for stenoses over 50 percent, the type and location of the neck bruit have some positive predictive value with very high specificity (0.76–0.94) and low sensitivity (0.29–0.76).[11–13] Studies using carotid Doppler question the predictive value of neck bruits, since they are poor localizers of underlying carotid disease and are not reliable enough to predict the presence or absence of carotid stenosis.[14–17] Other studies disagree and report that neck bruits are reliable indicators of underlying carotid artery stenosis.[18–19] When the incidence and severity of carotid stenosis were compared in patients with carotid strokes, carotid transient ischemic attacks, and asymptomatic neck bruits, the presence of neck bruits in the symptomatic groups was striking.[17] In general, neck bruits indicate underlying carotid disease and signify an increased likelihood of stroke but are not sufficient to predict the severity of carotid artery stenosis at the actual site of the bruit.

SPONTANEOUS VASCULAR OUTCOME VERSUS SURGICAL RISKS

The vascular outcome of patients with asymptomatic carotid stenosis (mainly cerebrovascular and cardiovascular events) is a major concern for physicians considering possible medical and surgical measures to prevent stroke. Several prospective outcome studies have been reported, and their results are summarized in Table 28–1. The two population-based studies did not include any imaging evaluation of the carotid bifurcation, so the relationship of the stroke to ipsilateral carotid stenosis was not determined.[20, 21] The later development of noninvasive duplex scanning of the carotid arteries provided both anatomic imaging of the carotid bifurcation and flow velocity information.

Several prospective studies (see Table 28–1) followed hundreds of patients with asymptomatic carotid bruits and stenosis for years using Doppler ultrasonography. They show that stroke risk in asymptomatic patients is related to the severity and progression of carotid stenosis, and that there is a hierarchy of stroke risk with increasing carotid stenosis. The question remains whether medical or surgical therapy, or a combination of both, can prevent stroke in these patients. Their outcome probably depends on an array of prognostic factors, some of which justify surgical intervention and others of which indicate medical therapy.

Surgery is justified only if the risk associated with endarterectomy is less than the risk of spontaneous stroke. Although the reported complication rate from uncontrolled, nonrandomized, selected surgical series is low,[22] aggregate data from several recent multicenter randomized studies showed that the perioperative complication rate is higher than expected, ranging from 4.7 to 10 percent.[23, 24] In the most recently published study, Hobson and coworkers[23] reported that the permanent stroke and death rate within 30 days after randomization was 4.7 percent, including 1.9 percent death, 2.4 percent completed nonfatal stroke, and 0.4 percent stroke due to angiography. In addition, 0.9 percent of the patients had transient ischemic attacks, and 1.9 percent had myocardial infarction. Clearly, carotid endarterectomy is not a harmless procedure.

Uncertainty about the appropriate application of endarterectomy was raised several years ago.[7, 25, 26] Since then, three multicenter trials have established an unequivocal benefit of carotid endarterectomy for *symptomatic* patients with severe

TABLE 28-1. Vascular Outcome in Asymptomatic Patients

| Study* | Patients, n | | | Method | Mean Follow-Up, mo | Outcome | | | | Annual Mortality, % |
| | Male | Female | Total | | | Overall Annual ICE Rate, % | | Ipsilateral, % | | |
						TIA	Stroke	TIA	Stroke	
Heyman and Wilkinson[20]	18	54	72	Bruit	72	NA	2.3	NA	NA	NA
Wolf et al[21]	66	105	171	Bruit	96	0.6	1.5	50	52	5
Hennerici et al[44]	NA	NA	339	Duplex	29	4.6	1	69 combined		7
Roederer et al[62]	110	52	162	Duplex	30	1.4	0.9	83	100	NA
Autret et al[63]	149	93	242	Duplex	29.4	3.2	1.7	35	60	9.6
Norris et al[45]	327	369	696	Duplex	41	3.9	1.2	75 combined		4
Bogousslavsky et al[64]	21	17	38	Duplex	48	9.8	3.3	88	60	7.2
Ford et al[65]	27	43	70	Duplex	48	1.4	1.1	100	33	7.1
Chambers and Norris[18]	212	288	500	Duplex	23	4.3	1.7	75 combined		4
Wiebers et al[47]	245	321	566	Bruit no Doppler	60	0.9	1.5	77 combined		3.6

*For full bibliographic information, see reference list at end of chapter.
ICE, ischemic cerebral event; NA, not available; TIA, transient ischemic attack.

($< 70\%$) carotid artery disease.[4-6] However, the uncertainties surrounding the appropriate application of carotid endarterectomy in *asymptomatic* patients remain unresolved.[9, 10, 27, 28]

The results of the Asymptomatic Carotid Atherosclerosis Study are still pending and may give more comprehensive answers.[29] Until these results are available, many investigators believe that the most prudent course is to avoid carotid endarterectomy in all cases and allow the carotid stenosis to occlude. There may be a subgroup of patients with asymptomatic carotid artery stenosis in which the stroke risk is high enough to warrant surgery, but their identification is controversial. This subgroup of patients can be identified by using transcranial Doppler to assess the cerebral perfusion reserve and the collateral circulation capacity.[30-33] Another method used to identify this subgroup is to determine the vascular dependency of each cerebral hemisphere by compressing the common carotid artery and simultaneously measuring intracranial arterial velocities in each hemisphere by transcranial Doppler or by measuring the vascular reactivity to carbon dioxide inhalation.[34] Using this test to evaluate the cerebral collateral reserve in patients with severe carotid stenosis and to determine the interdependency of each cerebral hemisphere on the remaining patent artery may discriminate between high-risk and non-high-risk patients. Unfortunately, no trial has yet been performed to test these hypotheses, so active intervention on these grounds remains unproven.

NONSURGICAL STRATEGIES

It is obvious that if we could modify the natural history of the disease by nonsurgical means, especially for severe carotid stenosis, the performance of carotid endarterectomy would not be justified. But can the natural history of asymptomatic carotid stenosis be altered? Risk factor changes might directly influence the evaluation of carotid stenosis or indirectly affect patient mortality by simply modifying the natural history of the disease.

Epidemiologic observations indicate that only 25 percent of the overall decline in stroke mortality can be attributed to the treatment of hypertension, so at least three quarters of the decline in stroke mortality in the United States from 1970 to 1980 is due to other factors.[35] Recently, various studies have assessed the relation of asymptomatic carotid atherosclerotic lesions to vascular risk factors. Prati and coworkers[36] found that age, systolic blood pressure, cigarette smoking, and blood levels of high-density lipoprotein cholesterol were strongly associated with the severity of carotid atherosclerosis. In a population-based sample of 100 Finnish men followed over 2 years using B-mode ultrasonography, low-density lipoprotein cholesterol concentrations and pack-years of smoking were the strongest predictors of atherosclerosis progression.[37] Ford and associates[38] noted a significant positive correlation between the plasma total cholesterol and high-density lipoprotein cholesterol ratio and the extent of carotid bifurcation atherosclerosis.

In the Japanese population, Yasaka and colleagues[39] found that smoking, hypertension, low high-density lipoprotein concentration, diabetes mellitus, and hypercholesterolemia were associated with atherosclerosis of the extracranial carotid arteries and the basilar artery. In some studies, the total years of cigarette smoking was the most significant independent predictor of the presence of severe carotid atherosclerosis,[40] and the progression of carotid atherosclerosis may be slower in patients who quit smoking than in those who continue to smoke.[41] From the Lausanne Stroke Registry data, it has been suggested that light to moderate consumption of alcohol is the first factor to be inversely associated with extracranial carotid atherosclerosis.[42] The question of gender, race, and occlusive cerebrovascular disease is intriguing. Angiographic and pathologic investigations indicate that extracranial atherosclerosis is more common in white males, whereas intracranial atherosclerosis is more frequent in blacks and Asians of both sexes.[43]

So far, no significant attempt has been made to assess the direct benefit of lifestyle changes and drugs on the natural history of atherosclerotic lesions in the carotid artery.

MANAGEMENT APPROACHES

Available data suggest that patients with carotid artery stenosis are at an increased risk for subsequent stroke and especially for myocardial infarction.[21, 22, 44, 45] Cardiac and cerebral ischemic risk factors are closely interrelated, and cardiac risks and vascular deaths increase proportionally to the severity of carotid stenosis. In persons with asymptomatic carotid stenosis greater than 75 percent, the risk of vascular death from all causes is 6.5 percent annually.[45] This raises the important question whether screening the population for asymptomatic carotid disease is justified. Is it cost-effective? If yes, who should be screened? How should screening be done? A recent consensus statement attempts to tackle this problem.[46]

The goal of screening is to identify patients who are at risk for stroke and myocardial infarction in order to modify the natural history of the disease by either education (control of risk factors) or medical care (eg, antiplatelet drugs) and to select patients for carotid surgery. Currently, two methods are used to detect potential carotid artery stenosis: clinical auscultation for neck bruits and noninvasive studies of the artery. Cervical auscultation is often included in the physical examination of every patient, especially those with known vascular risk factors. However, although auscultation of neck bruits is recommended,[17, 47] and noninvasive duplex scanning can confirm the presence of significant obstructive lesions, it is of little clinical value if it cannot be followed by an intervention, either medical or surgical, that prevents subsequent vascular events. Until there is more substantial evidence regarding carotid endarterectomy, the effectiveness of screening for carotid artery disease to prevent subsequent stroke will remain in question.

Some, such as the Canadian Task Force,[48-50] argue against routine screening, whereas others recommend a baseline noninvasive study of carotid arteries in patients considered at high risk for extracranial carotid disease.[47, 51] Cost is a major factor. Although about 4 percent of adults have asymptomatic neck bruits, only a small number (<10%) have severe carotid stenosis, and many of these are not even surgical candidates.[46] The estimated cost of performing duplex scanning on all Americans with neck bruits is $200 million, in addition to the cost of subsequent carotid endarterectomy. A careful cost-effectiveness study is needed to resolve this issue, but one should bear in mind that detecting carotid artery disease can prevent the immense costs resulting from vascular diseases, including myocardial infarction and stroke. Also, about one fifth of those "asymptomatic" patients have silent brain infarction that can lead to vascular dementia or disabling stroke.

Another unresolved problem is screening for asymptomatic carotid disease in patients undergoing general surgical procedures. Patients selected for coronary artery and peripheral vascular surgery commonly have arterial disease elsewhere, so the incidence of asymptomatic carotid stenosis is naturally high. Hennerici and coworkers[14] documented the frequency of carotid artery disease in 375 patients with severe peripheral vascular disease, 264 with coronary artery disease, and 1370 from a population without either disease. Carotid artery stenosis greater than 50 percent occurred in 33 percent of those with peripheral vascular disease, 7 percent of those with coronary artery disease, and 6 percent without either disease. Similarly, in the study by Hertzer and associates,[52] half the patients under consideration for peripheral vascular reconstruction had clinical or angiographic evidence of underlying coronary artery involvement.

PROPHYLACTIC PREOPERATIVE CAROTID SURGERY

It is assumed, but unproven, that the presence of asymptomatic carotid artery stenosis increases the risk of perioperative stroke in patients undergoing unrelated operations. Intraoperative hypotension, postoperative dehydration, and hypercoagulability all encourage vascular occlusion or cerebral hypoperfusion.

Does severe carotid stenosis increase the risk for stroke at the time of coronary artery bypass graft and, if so, does preliminary or simultaneous carotid endarterectomy reduce that risk? Despite the apparent importance of this issue, the effect of associated carotid surgery has never been evaluated by a prospective randomized trial. The several nonrandomized studies addressing this issue concluded that asymptomatic patients with or without hemodynamically significant stenosis can safely undergo coronary artery bypass graft without prophylactic carotid surgery.[53-57]

Newman and Hicks,[58] reviewing the data concerning coexistent carotid and coronary artery disease in almost 1500 patients, concluded that patients with coincidental asymptomatic carotid stenosis should not routinely undergo prophylactic carotid endarterectomy. In a similar study, Grabor and Hetzer[59] maintain that asymptomatic patients with unilateral carotid stenosis who present for coronary bypass are best managed first by myocardial revascularization, followed by medical or surgical treatment of the carotid disease. In a more recent case-control study, 54 patients with postoperative stroke or transient ischemic attacks were compared with 54 randomly selected patients.[60] The presence of carotid bruits appeared to increase the risk of stroke after coronary bypass, but the magnitude of this risk (2.9%) was small and comparable to the reported risk of stroke from carotid endarterectomy. Jain and colleagues[61] (without supporting data) recommended routine preoperative screening to identify hemodynamically significant stenosis in patients undergoing peripheral vascular operations and in patients with cervical bruits, because they are at high risk of having tight stenosis of the carotid artery.

CONCLUSION

In spite of the accumulating information on the natural history of asymptomatic carotid stenosis, including the results of several surgical randomized studies, many questions remain about the management of patients with asymptomatic carotid stenosis. It is hoped that American and European prospective, randomized surgical studies that are now under way answer many of these questions. We must continue the effort to identify the subgroups of patients who are at very high risk for stroke, in whom surgical risks might be justified.

REFERENCES

1. Bonita R: Epidemiology of stroke. *Lancet.* 1992;339:342.
2. Easton JD: Antiplatelet therapy in the prevention of stroke. *Drugs.* 1991;42:39.
3. Haynes RB, Sandler RS, Larson EB, et al: A critical appraisal of ticlopidine, a new antiplatelet agent. *Arch Intern Med.* 1992;152:1376.
4. NASCET collaborators. Beneficial effect of carotid endarterectomy in symptomatic patients with high-grade carotid stenosis. *N Engl J Med.* 1991;325:445.

5. European carotid surgery trialists' collaborative group: MRC European carotid surgery trial: Interim results for symptomatic patients with severe (70–99%) or with mild (0–29%) carotid stenosis. *Lancet.* 1991;337:1235.
6. Mayberg MR, Wilson SE, Yatsu F, et al: Carotid endarterectomy and prevention of cerebral ischemia in symptomatic carotid stenosis. *JAMA.* 1991;266:3289.
7. Barnett HJM, Plum F, Walton JN: Carotid endarterectomy—an expression of concern. *Stroke.* 1984;15:941.
8. Field WS: Asymptomatic carotid bruit: Operate or not? *Stroke.* 1978;9:269.
9. Walker MD: Carotid endarterectomy: A little more light at the end of the tunnel (editorial). *Mayo Clin Proc.* 1992;67:597.
10. Barnett HJM, Haines SJ: Carotid endarterectomy for asymptomatic carotid stenosis. *N Engl J Med.* 1993;328:276.
11. Ingall TJ, Homer D, Whisnant JP, et al: Predictive value of carotid bruit for carotid atherosclerosis. *Arch Neurol.* 1989;46:418.
12. Ziegler DK, Zileli T, Dick A, et al: Correlation of bruits over the carotid artery with angiographically demonstrated lesions. *Neurology.* 1971;21:860.
13. Hankey GJ, Warlow CF: Symptomatic carotid ischaemeic events: Safest and most cost-effective way of selecting patients for angiography before carotid endarterectomy. *Br Med J.* 1990;300:1485.
14. Hennerici M, Aulich A, Sandmann W, et al: Incidence of asymptomatic extracranial arterial disease. *Stroke.* 1981;12:750.
15. Howard VJ, Howard G, Harpold GJ, et al: Correlation of carotid bruits and carotid atherosclerosis detected by B-mode real-time ultrasonography. *Stroke.* 1989;20:1331.
16. Lusiani L, Visona A, Castellani V, et al: Prevalence of atherosclerotic lesions of the carotid bifurcation in patients with asymptomatic bruits: An echo-Doppler (duplex) study. *Angiology.* 1985;235:239.
17. Norris JW: Head and neck bruits in stroke prevention. In Norris JW, Hachinski VC, eds. *Prevention of Stroke.* New York: Springer-Verlag; 1991:103.
18. Chambers BR, Norris JW: Clinical significance of asymptomatic neck bruits. *Neurology.* 1985;35:742.
19. Floriani M, Guilini SM, Bonardelli S, et al: Value and limits of "critical auscultation" of neck bruits. *Angiology.* 1988;3911:967.
20. Heyman A, Wilkinson WE: Risk of stroke in asymptomatic persons with cervical arterial bruits: A population study in Evans County, Georgia. *N Engl J Med.* 1980;302:833.
21. Wolf PA, Kannel WB, Sorlie P, McNamara P: Asymptomatic carotid bruit and risk of stroke: The Framingham study. *JAMA.* 1981;245:1442.
22. Freischlag JA, Hanna D, Moore WS: Improved prognosis for asymptomatic carotid stenosis with prophylactic carotid endarterectomy. *Stroke.* 1992;23:479.
23. Hobson RW 2d, Weiss DG, Fields WS, et al: Efficacy of carotid endarterectomy for asymptomatic carotid stenosis. *N Engl J Med.* 1993;328:221.
24. CASANOVA study group: Carotid surgery versus medical therapy in asymptomatic carotid stenosis. *Stroke.* 1991;22:1229.
25. Winslow M, Solomon DH, Chassin MR, et al: The appropriateness of carotid endarterectomy. *N Engl J Med.* 1988;318:721.
26. Brook RH, Park RE, Chassin MR, et al: Predicting the appropriate use of carotid endarterectomy, upper gastrointestinal endoscopy, and coronary angiography. *N Engl J Med.* 1990;323:1173.
27. Barnett HJM, Barnes RW, Robertson JT: The uncertainties surrounding carotid endarterectomy (editorial). *JAMA.* 1992;268:3120.
28. Levy LL: Carotid endarterectomy: When and why (editorial). *JAMA.* 1991;266:3332.
29. Asymptomatic carotid atherosclerosis study group: Study design for randomized prospective trial of carotid endarterectomy for asymptomatic atherosclerosis. *Stroke.* 1989;20:844.
30. Chimowitz MI, Furlan AJ, Jones SC, et al: Transcranial Doppler assessment of cerebral perfusion reserve in patients with carotid occlusive disease and no evidence of cerebral infarction. *Neurology.* 1993;43:353.
31. Ringelstein EB, Sievers C, Ecker S, et al: Noninvasive assessment of CO_2-induced cerebral vasomotor response in normal individuals and patients with internal carotid artery occlusions. *Stroke.* 1988;19:963.
32. Bishop CCR, Powell S, Rutt D, Browse NL: Transcranial Doppler measurements of middle cerebral artery blood flow velocity: A validation study. *Stroke.* 1986;17:913.
33. Powers WJ, Press GA, Grubb RL, et al: The effect of hemodynamic status of the cerebral circulation. *Ann Intern Med.* 1987;106:27.
34. Norris JW, Krajewski A, Bornstein NM: The clinical role of the cerebral collateral circulation in carotid occlusion. *J Vasc Surg.* 1990;12:113.
35. Bonita R, Beaglehole R: Increased treatment of hypertension does not explain the decline in stroke mortality in the United States, 1970–1980. *Hypertension.* 1989;13(suppl I): I-69.
36. Prati P, Vanuzzo D, Casaroli M, et al: Prevalence and determinants of carotid atherosclerosis in a general population. *Stroke.* 1992;23:1705.
37. Salonen R, Salonen JT: Progression of carotid atherosclerosis and its determinants: A population-based ultrasonography study. *Atherosclerosis.* 1990;81:33.
38. Ford CS, Crouse JR, Howard G, et al: The role of plasma lipids in carotid bifurcation atherosclerosis. *Ann Neurol.* 1985;17:301.
39. Yasaka M, Yamaguchi T, Shichiri M: Distribution of atherosclerosis and risk factors in atherothrombotic occlusion. *Stroke.* 1993;24:206.
40. Whisnant JP, Homer D, Ingall TI, et al: Duration of cigarette smoking is the strongest predictor of severe extracranial carotid artery atherosclerosis. *Stroke.* 1990;21:707.
41. Tell GS, Howard G, McKinney WM, Toole JF: Cigarette smoking cessation and extracranial carotid stenosis. *JAMA.* 1989;261:1178.
42. Bogousslavsky J, Van Melle G, Despland PA, et al: Alcohol consumption and carotid atherosclerosis in the Lausanne stroke registry. *Stroke.* 1990;21:715.
43. Caplan LR, Gorelick PB, Hier DB: Race, sex and occlusive cerebrovascular disease: A review. *Stroke.* 1986;17;648.
44. Hennerici M, Hulsbomer H-B, Hefter H, et al: Natural history of asymptomatic extracranial arterial disease: Results of a long-term prospective study. *Brain.* 1987;110:777.
45. Norris JW, Zhu CZ, Bornstein NM, et al: Vascular risks of asymptomatic carotid stenosis. *Stroke.* 1991;22:1485.
46. Consensus statement on the management of patients with asymptomatic lesions. Prepared by the Consensus Group (Prof. A. Nicolaides, chairman) at the International Workshop on Carotid Bifurcation, Cyprus, 1993. *Lancet.* 1993.
47. Wiebers DO, Whisnant JP, Sandok BA, O'Fallan WM: Prospective comparison of a cohort with asymptomatic carotid bruit and a population-based cohort without carotid bruit. *Stroke.* 1990;21:984.
48. Kuller LH, Sutton KC: Carotid artery bruit: Is it safe and effective to auscultate the neck? *Stroke.* 1984;15:944.
49. Canadian Task Force on the Periodic Health Examination: 1984 update. *Can Med Assoc J.* 1984;130:1.
50. Frame PS: A critical review of adult health maintenance. Part 1. Prevention of atherosclerotic diseases. *J Fam Pract.* 1986;22:341.
51. Toole JF, Adams H Jr, Dyken M, et al: Evaluation for asymptomatic carotid artery atherosclerosis: A multidisciplinary consensus statement. *South Med J.* 1988;81:1549.
52. Hertzer NR, Beven EG, Young JR, et al: Coronary artery disease in peripheral vascular patients: A classification of 1000 coronary angiograms and results of surgical management. *Ann Surg.* 1984;199:223.
53. Barnes R: Noninvasive evaluation of the carotid bruit. *Annu Rev Med.* 1980;31:201.
54. Brener BJ, Brief DK, Alpert J, et al: The risk of stroke in patients with asymptomatic carotid stenosis undergoing cardiac surgery: A follow-up study. *J Vasc Surg.* 1987;5:269.
55. Breslau PJ, Feel G, Ivey TD, et al: Carotid arterial disease in patients undergoing coronary artery bypass operations. *J Thorac Cardiovasc Surg.* 1981;82:765.
56. Furlan AJ, Craciun AR: Risk of stroke during coronary artery bypass graft surgery in patients with internal carotid artery disease documented by angiography. *Stroke.* 1985;16:797.
57. Ivey TD, Strandness E, Williams DB, et al: Management of patients with carotid bruit undergoing cardiopulmonary bypass. *J Thorac Cardiovasc Surg.* 1984;87:183.
58. Newman DC, Hicks RG: Combined carotid and coronary artery surgery: A review of the literature. *Ann Thorac Surg.* 1988;45:574.
59. Grabor RA, Hetzer NR: Management of coexistent carotid artery disease. *Stroke.* 1988;19:1441.
60. Reed GL, Singer DE, Picard EH, et al: Stroke following coronary artery bypass surgery. *N Engl J Med.* 1988;319:1246.
61. Jain KM, Hobson RW, Jamil Z, et al: Clinical screening of preoperative patients for carotid occlusive disease by oculoplethysmography. *Am Surg.* 1980;46:679.
62. Roederer GO, Langlois YE, Jager KA, et al: The natural history of carotid arterial disease in asymptomatic patients with cervical bruits. *Stroke.* 1984;15:605.
63. Autret A, Saudeau D, Bertrand PH, et al: Stroke risk in patients with carotid stenosis. *Lancet.* 1987;1:888.
64. Bogousslavsky J, Despland PA, Regli F: Asymptomatic tight stenosis of the internal carotid artery: Long-term prognosis. *Neurology.* 1986;36:861.
65. Ford CS, Frye JL, Toole JF, et al: Asymptomatic carotid bruit and stenosis: A prospective follow-up study. *Arch Neurol.* 1986;43:219.

CHAPTER 29

The Natural History of Asymptomatic Carotid Ulceration

WESLEY S. MOORE

Atheromatous plaques of the carotid bifurcation can be the cause of transient or permanent neurologic dysfunction. This dysfunction can occur by one of two mechanisms. The first mechanism involves progressive narrowing of the arterial lumen. Stenosis will produce flow reduction and lead to thrombosis of the internal carotid artery, with the possibility of thromboembolic propagation. The second mechanism relates to the friable consistency of the atheromatous plaque that produces plaque degeneration, embolization, and ulceration. The finding of an ulcerative plaque in an asymptomatic patient may represent a warning of future symptomatic embolic events. This chapter reviews the natural history of asymptomatic patients who are found to have ulcerative atheromatous lesions at the carotid bifurcation.

DYNAMICS OF PLAQUE DEGENERATION

Atheromatous plaques of the carotid bifurcation can generally be divided into two major categories relating to the consistency of the atheromatous material: hard plaques and soft plaques. A hard atheromatous plaque appears to have a greater proportion of fibrocalcific material, whereas a soft plaque consists of an increased amount of cholesterol salts combined with an admixture of the products of intraplaque hemorrhage. Soft plaques have lesser amounts of fibrocalcific matrix. The differentiation between hard and soft plaque is particularly important with respect to clinical behavior and outcome. The hard plaque enlarges at a slower rate, is less likely to degenerate, and produces symptoms principally through flow reduction or distal thrombosis.

Soft plaques may turn out to have the greater clinical impact because of their propensity to degenerate and release emboli into the cerebral circulation. The degeneration of the soft plaque may be spontaneous or may be accelerated by the sudden occurrence of a hemorrhage within the substance of the plaque.[1–4]

In either event, the thin intimal lining of the plaque ruptures, and the central contents of the plaque discharge into the lumen, leading to the first, or primary, wave of embolization. The embolic fragments consist of a combination of atheromatous and thrombotic debris. Evidence for a primary embolic discharge is the angiographic documentation of a cavity within the plaque, a so-called ulceration.

Once ulceration has occurred, further embolization of atherothrombotic debris from the atheromatous plaque may take place through the open ulcer. In addition, the ulceration itself forms a nidus for stasis and the buildup of platelet aggregate or thrombotic material that can be swept into the arterial stream as a secondary wave of embolization.

NATURAL CLINICAL HISTORY OF THE ULCERATED PLAQUE

Clinical Question

Until the advent of B-mode ultrasonography, the composition of the atheromatous plaque (hard versus soft) could not be determined until surgical removal or autopsy study. Angiography can only demonstrate encroachment on arterial lumen and plaque contour as seen on profile. Therefore, the only angiographic evidence for a plaque that has degenerative capability is the visible presence of ulceration. The presence of ulceration indicates that there has already been an episode of plaque discharge. This may or may not have been associated with symptoms. Once a soft plaque has been identified, as suggested by the angiographic presence of an ulcerative lesion, the following clinical questions arise: What does the future hold for that ulcerative plaque with respect to subsequent embolic and possibly neurologic events? Will the plaque remain relatively quiescent and produce no subsequent symptoms of neurologic dysfunction, or will this soft plaque produce secondary episodes of embolization with increased risk of either transient or permanent neurologic dysfunction?

Retrospective Review

The angiographic examination for patients presenting with symptoms in the distribution of one carotid artery usually involves the visualization of both carotid arteries for sake of completeness. During the course of such a survey, it is not uncommon to detect an ulcerative lesion in the absence of a hemodynamically significant stenosis in the asymptomatic carotid artery. In our early experience, our practice was to observe these lesions and to treat patients expectantly. Thus we were provided with an opportunity to review retrospectively the clinical course of asymptomatic patients with ulcerative lesions of the carotid artery in order to determine their clinical outcome.

To describe the extent of ulceration, and because there might be a relationship between ulcer size and subsequent outcome, we classified the ulcerative lesions into three categories, A, B, and C ulcers. An A ulcer was a minimal lesion; a B ulcer, a larger lesion; and a C ulcer, a large lesion with a compound or cavernous appearance.[5, 6] Although this initial classification was qualitative, we have subsequently developed a technique to quantify this classification of ulcerative lesions using full-size, cut-film angiograms. Once the ulcer is identified in profile, its length and depth are measured in millimeters. The length is then multiplied by the depth in order to express the two-dimensional area of the visible ulcer. If the area measures 10 mm^2 or less, it is an A ulcer. If the ulcer measures between 10 and 40 mm^2, it is categorized as a B ulcer. If the ulcer exceeds 40 mm^2 or has a compound or cavernous appearance, it is categorized as a C ulcer.[7]

Our initial retrospective series consisted of 67 patients found to have asymptomatic ulcerative lesions in 72 carotid arteries with plaques that were not hemodynamically significant. Forty ulcers in 39 patients were categorized as A ulcers. Thirty-two ulcers in 29 patients were categorized as either B or C lesions. Because of the small number of examples, these two lesions were initially combined for analysis. Patients were followed at varying intervals extending to 84 months between the time of arteriography and subsequent analysis. Stroke incidence as a function of time interval was expressed in a life-table format.

Patients with A ulcers appeared to have a benign outcome. One patient experienced a stroke within 1 year of arteriography, and no patients experienced a subsequent stroke when followed up to 84 months. By contrast, of the 29 patients with category B or C ulcers, 10 suffered strokes appropriate to the side of the lesion. Furthermore, none of these strokes was anticipated by warning transient ischemic attacks. The life-table curve documenting stroke incidence appeared to have a bimodal pattern. The first critical interval occurred within 1 year of arteriography, at which time 15 percent of the patients at risk had experienced a stroke. The second critical interval occurred after 54 months, at which time there was a rapid increase in stroke incidence from 25 to 87 percent of patients at risk. If the stroke risk is averaged over the 7-year follow-up period, we can express an annual stroke risk as a function of ulcer size. The annual stroke risk for A ulcers was 0.4 percent per year, and that for combined B and C ulcers was 12.5 percent per year of follow-up.[6]

Study Challenged

In 1980, Kroener and colleagues,[8] from the University of California, San Diego, reviewed their own experience with ulcerated plaques and challenged our observations and recommendations. They reported their experience with 87 nonstenotic ulcerative lesions in 76 patients. Sixty-three ulcers were in the A category and 24 ulcers in the B category. These investigators stated that there were no C ulcers in their series because they elected to operate prophylactically on patients in whom plaque morphology had the characteristic of a C ulcer. They concurred with our report that the A ulcer carries an insignificant risk. However, in their series, B ulcers likewise carried no risk on follow-up.[8]

It is important to note several differences between the report of Kroener and colleagues and our original report. First, their series had no C ulcers, since they elected to operate on all patients with C ulcers prophylactically. Clearly, this removes an important cohort of patients from contention. It is also important to note that the majority of ulcers in their series (63) were in the A group. They only reported on 24 B ulcers, probably representing a sample size that is too small. Finally, at the time that Kroener and colleagues categorized ulcers, they were using our original qualitative description. Therefore, we cannot be certain whether the ulcers they were categorizing as B may in fact have been in the A category.

Study Enlarged and Confirmed

Although the report of Kroener and colleagues could be debated as I have documented, we considered it essential to enlarge our own series in order to determine whether the natural history data remained consistent. Our initial study of 67 patients was taken from the Veterans Administration population in San Francisco between 1966 and 1977. We decided to enlarge the series by carrying out a retrospective study of patients at the University of California, Los Angeles, who had undergone arteriography in whom ulcerative lesions that were asymptomatic and nonstenotic were identified. Between 1972 and 1982, an additional 74 cases of asymptomatic ulcerative lesions of the carotid bifurcation were identified. Thirty-four lesions were in women and 40 in men. These patients were combined with our 67 patients from the San Francisco Veterans Administration Hospital, only four of whom were women. The combined group yielded 141 patients who had appropriate ulcerative lesions in 153 carotid arteries. There were 72 arteries with type A ulceration, 54 arteries with type B ulceration, and 27 arteries with type C ulceration. Follow-up was carried out to 10 years and expressed in life-table format comparing the percentage of patients at risk who were stroke free at progressive intervals up to 10 years. The results of this study demonstrated once again that the A ulceration carried a rather benign prognosis in that only two patients subsequently developed a stroke. However, 10 of 54 patients with type B ulcers and 5 of 27 patients with type C ulcers developed a stroke appropriate to the side of ulceration. None of these strokes was anticipated by the occurrence of TIAs. If the stroke incidence is averaged over the interval of follow-up, a type B ulcer in our series carried a 4.5 percent per year stroke rate, and a type C ulcer carried a 7.5 percent per year stroke rate.[7]

Thus, it would appear that with the addition of a second group of patients, the conclusions remain the same. That is, types B and C ulcerative lesions carry a significant stroke risk when followed expectantly after arteriographic identification. The reasons that these lesions have significant stroke potential are certainly not clear. For example, we do not know the status of the lesions at the time the strokes occurred. These patients were not subsequently examined by either noninvasive techniques or arteriography. It is conceivable that the nonstenotic ulcerative lesion simply progressed over time to high-grade stenosis or occlusion and that this change was followed by the event of cerebral infarction. It is also possible that the ulcerative lesion underwent a period in which there was a repeat discharge of degenerative atheromatous material. In any event, it is clear that the documentation of ulceration by arteriography provides an important marker that identifies a given plaque, and therefore a given patient, as having an increased stroke risk.

RECENT SUPPORTING DATA

There have been no new retrospective or prospective studies of the natural history asymptomatic carotid ulceration. However, a number of studies have provided additional insight with respect to the relationship between plaque ulceration and the symptomatic status of the patient. Ricotta and colleagues[9] examined 84 intact atheroma specimens removed at the time of carotid endarterectomy and correlated these with findings on preoperative angiograms. They demonstrated macroscopic evidence of ulceration in 43 cases (51%). An additional 34 specimens also contained intramural hemorrhage, and 27 showed mural thrombus. The presence of mural thrombus showed a positive correlation with ulceration ($P < .01$). Intramural hemorrhage was also associated with ulceration (25 of 34 specimens). Angiography identified 78 percent of the ulcers that were demonstrated on macroscopic examination (34 of 43; $P = .05$). However, seven ulcerations seen on macroscopic examination were missed by angiography, and there were 18 angiographic false-positive findings. The presence of microscopic ulceration was most common in patients with symptoms of hemispheric ischemia. The authors concluded that microscopic ulceration was an important cause of hemispheric ischemia and that angiography was not a reliable predictor of the presence or absence of microscopic ulceration.[9] The weakness of identifying ulceration by angiography was further documented in a report by Senkowsky and colleagues.[10] They identified 21 patients with symptoms of hemispheric ischemia in whom the angiographic findings were negative, but the B-mode ultrasonogram demonstrated the presence of atheromatous disease in the carotid bulb. The presence of a nonstenotic ulcerative plaque was confirmed at the time of operation. The size of the stenoses ranged from 20 to 50 percent, but ulceration was confirmed in all. The authors concluded that B-mode ultrasonography better defines nonstenotic ulcerative lesions, and the decision to withhold carotid endarterectomy should not be based on the absence of an angiographically proven lesion. Sterpetti and colleagues[11] examined 90 consecutive intact carotid plaques obtained at the time of carotid endarterectomy and compared them with 43 carotid plaques from cadavers in whom a review of the medical history demonstrated no evidence of cerebral ischemia. They showed that ulceration and the presence of mural thrombus were the only morphologic findings statistically correlated with the presence of hemispheric symptoms ($P < .02$). The authors concluded that ulceration of the plaque played a major role in the onset of hemispheric symptoms. They went on to conclude further that the results of their study supported the hypothesis that in the majority of cases, hemispheric symptoms were embolic in nature. Finally, in a derivative analysis of the North American Symptomatic Carotid Endarterectomy Trial control data, Eliasziw and colleagues[12] looked at the importance of carotid plaque ulceration in the development of subsequent stroke among the patients randomly assigned to medical management. They demonstrated that the presence of angiographically proven ulceration and increasing degree of stenosis had a major impact on subsequent neurologic events. Patients with ulceration and a stenosis reducing vessel diameter by 75 percent experienced a 26.3 percent incidence of stroke during a 24-month follow-up. In contrast, if ulceration was present in patients with 95 percent stenosis, the incidence of stroke rose to 73.2 percent during the same follow-up interval. Patients who had varying degrees of stenosis but did not have angiographically proven ulceration had a constant stroke event rate of 21.3 percent irrespective of the degree of stenosis increase. The authors have not yet had the opportunity to examine the implication of plaque ulceration in patients with lesser degrees of stenosis. It will be most interesting to see whether a high stroke event rate persists in lesser degrees of stenosis but in the presence of ulceration.

Although the importance of plaque ulceration in both asymptomatic and previously symptomatic patients appears to be gathering growing support, the preoperative identification of ulceration is undergoing a metamorphosis with respect to the diagnostic studies obtained. There is an increasing tendency not to perform contrast angiography prior to operation. More and more patients are being operated on based on findings seen on duplex scanning. Since the duplex scan includes a B-mode evaluation of the carotid plaque and provides the opportunity to document not only plaques of mixed consistency but also irregular plaques, it is likely that these will be the new criteria for identification of higher-risk lesions.

SUMMARY

Atheromatous plaques can either be hard and relatively stable or soft and subject to degeneration. Soft plaques that degenerate leave a crypt in their center; they can be identified by the presence of ulceration on arteriography. The presence of an ulcerated plaque provides information with respect to subsequent outcome, depending on ulcer size.

Ulcers are classified as type A, B, or C. A ulcers have a benign prognosis, B ulcers mark a patient for stroke risk of 4.5 percent per year of follow-up, and C ulcers carry a stroke risk of 7.5 percent per year of follow-up. Prophylactic operation on category B and C ulcers is justified, provided that the combined morbidity and mortality rate for carotid endarterectomy associated with a given surgeon is less than 3 percent.

REFERENCES

1. Lusby RJ, Ferrell LD, Ehrenfeld WK, et al: Carotid plaque hemorrhage. Its role in the production of cerebral ischemia. *Arch Surg.* 1982;117:1479.
2. Imparato AM, Riles TS, Gorstein F: The carotid bifurcation plaque: Pathologic findings associated with cerebral ischemia. *Stroke.* 1979;10:238.
3. Johnson JM, Kennelly MM, Decesare D, et al: Natural history of asymptomatic carotid plaques. *Arch Surg* 1985;120(9):1010.
4. Geroulakos G, Ramaswami G, Nicolaides A, et al: Characterization of symptomatic and asymptomatic carotid plaques using high resolution real time ultrasonography. *Br J Surg.* 1993;80(10):1274.
5. Eisenberg RL, Nemzek WR, Moore WS, et al: Relationship of transient ischemic attacks and angiographically demonstrable lesions of the carotid artery. *Stroke.* 1977;8:483.
6. Moore WS, Boren C, Malone JM, et al: Natural history of nonstenotic asymptomatic ulcerative lesions of the carotid artery. *Arch Surg.* 1978;113:1352.
7. Dixon S, Pais SO, Raviola C, et al: Natural history of nonstenotic asymptomatic ulcerative lesions of the carotid artery. *Arch Surg.* 1982;117:1493.
8. Kroener JM, Dorn PL, Shoor PM, et al: Prognosis of asymptomatic ulcerating carotid lesions. *Arch Surg.* 1980;115:1387.
9. Ricotta JJ, Schenk EA, Ekholm SE, DeWeese JA: Angiographic and pathologic correlates in carotid artery disease. *Surgery.* 1986;99:284.
10. Senkowsky J, Bell WH III, Kerstein MD: Normal angiograms and carotid pathology. *Ann Surg.* 1990;56:726.
11. Sterpetti AV, Hunter WJ, Schultz RD. The importance of ulceration of carotid plaque in determining symptoms of cerebral ischemia. *J Cardiovasc Surg.* 1991;32:154.
12. Eliasziw M, Streiffler JY, Fox AJ, et al: Significance of plaque ulceration in symptomatic patients with high-grade carotid stenosis: North American Symptomatic Carotid Endarterectomy Trial. *Stroke.* 1994;25:304.

CHAPTER 30

The American Heart Association Consensus Committee Statement Concerning Indications for Carotid Endarterectomy in Asymptomatic Patients

WESLEY S. MOORE

The Stroke Council and the Council on Cardiothoracic and Vascular Surgery of the American Heart Association recognized that there was a database of sufficient proportion and quality that the time was right for the development of a consensus statement concerning the indications for carotid endarterectomy. It was decided to hold a conference to develop such a statement in Park City, Utah, from July 16 to 18, 1993. The Heart Association appointed Wesley S. Moore, MD, as chairman of the committee and charged him with the responsibility of organizing the conference and spearheading the development of a consensus statement for publication.

THE CONSENSUS PROCESS

The committee chairman took the responsibility of identifying experts from several disciplines and developing a framework for the conference that would result in the consensus statement. The committee chairman decided that it was essential to have a common database for review before entering into a discussion concerning individual potential indications for carotid endarterectomy. The database should include information concerning the natural history of patients with various manifestations of carotid bifurcation disease; provide guidelines concerning patient evaluation; discuss available options for medical management together with outcome data; review the literature with respect to results of surgical management; evaluate data from position statements; and, finally, analyze the results to date of prospective randomized trials for both symptomatic and asymptomatic patients. An agenda of topics was developed, and an expert in the field for each topic was identified. Invitations were then sent to each expert requesting his or her participation in the consensus conference. The cadre of experts at the conference included seven neurologists, three neurosurgeons, eleven vascular surgeons, and one representative from the discipline of health care policy. Prior to the conference, each participant provided the chairman with a brief summary of his or her presentation, together with an appropriate bibliography, and the chairman collated all of these statements into a cohesive first-draft manuscript.

The conference was divided into two parts. The first part consisted of the individual presentations from the developed agenda. Following each presentation, there was the opportunity for discussion, questions, and challenges. After all of the presentations had been made, the first draft of the manuscript was read to the entire group. A critique was then carried out on a line-by-line basis, and on-site revisions were carried out until the first part of the statement received uniform approval of the committee (consensus).

Following completion of the first part of the manuscript, a package of 96 potential indications for carotid endarterectomy was distributed to each participant. Each member was then asked to rank each potential indication into one of four categories. The ranking was to reflect the member's understanding from the common database that was presented, but also would reflect the expert's overall understanding of the literature and would clearly reflect his or her opinion concerning the individual indication for operation. Each indication would be scored into one of four categories, which would contain an appropriate allocated point score. Category I was labeled "Proven." This represented the strongest indication for carotid endarterectomy, and in general meant that the data were supported by the results of prospective, randomized trials. Category II was defined as "Acceptable but not Proven." Interpretation of this category meant that entries were generally agreed to be strong indications for carotid endarterectomy, and that the judgment was supported by promising data, but not the type of scientifically certain data that would come from a prospective randomized trial. Category III was defined as "Uncertain." That meant that there were insufficient data to define the risk-to-benefit ratio. Potential indications falling into the "Uncertain" category might well serve as appropriate topics for future prospective, randomized trials. Category IV was defined as "Proven Inappropriate." That meant that there were sufficient data to state that the risk of operation clearly outweighed its benefit.

All committee members scored each of the 96 potential indications for operation, and each indication then underwent a collation of scores, with an analysis that allowed the indication to be ranked into one of the four categories. The indications were then subdivided into categories for symptomatic patients and asymptomatic patients. These indications were then tabulated and constitute the second part of the manuscript.

ASYMPTOMATIC PATIENTS: MANUSCRIPT PART I

Natural History

Review of contemporary literature suggests that there are at least three factors that affect the outcome of patients with asymptomatic lesions of the carotid bifurcation. These include (1) degree of stenosis; (2) progression of stenosis between examination intervals; and (3) presence or absence of ulceration.

Patients with stenosis of the internal carotid artery exceeding 75 percent, as measured by Doppler examination, are reported to be at risk for stroke at the rate of 2 to 5 percent within the first year of observation. Of the patients who develop stroke within the period of observation, 83 percent have no warning symptoms or transient ischemic attacks prior to the stroke.

The coexistence of ulceration within the plaque appeared to be an additional marker for patients who are at increased risk of stroke.

Results of Carotid Endarterectomy: Retrospective Reviews

The statement makes three important points with respect to the rationale for operating on asymptomatic lesions: (1) The lesion must be associated with a demonstrable stroke risk; (2) removal of the lesion must eliminate or reduce the long-term stroke risk; (3) the surgeon who operates on the asymptomatic carotid lesion must have a low rate of perioperative neurologic morbidity and mortality.

Keeping in mind that the retrospective data analysis suggested that the annual stroke event rate in patients with high-grade asymptomatic carotid stenosis varied from 2 to 5 percent per year, a review of six series looking at the follow-up of patients following successful carotid endarterectomy has documented that the stroke event rate after operation has been reduced to 0.7 to 2.0 percent per year. The risk of performing carotid endarterectomy is also quite variable. Recent publications were cited to show that the risk of combined neurologic morbidity and mortality from the operation has ranged from a low of 0.0 percent to a high of 3.8 percent. A paper citing the selection process for participating in the Asymptomatic Carotid Atherosclerosis Study (ACAS), with respect to carrying out a prestudy audit of participating surgeons, yielded an aggregate of 1511 operations performed by prospective participants for asymptomatic carotid stenosis, which yielded a combined operative morbidity and neurologic mortality of 1.7 percent. This is well within the guidelines recommended by the American Heart Association Stroke Council, which stated that the risk for operating on asymptomatic carotid stenosis with respect to stroke morbidity and mortality should be less than 3.0 percent.

Finally, the opportunity to evaluate the efficacy of carotid endarterectomy compared with medical management alone has been provided by the prospective, randomized studies designed to test this hypothesis. The Veterans Administration trial demonstrated that the combined incidence of ipsilateral neurologic events in the surgical group was 8.0 percent, in contrast to 20.6 percent in the medical group. However, events included transient ischemic attack as well as stroke. Although this was the design of the study, many critics expressed concern that transient ischemic attack was not really the important issue compared with stroke. The Veterans Administration trial was not designed, with respect to numbers of patients, to test this hypothesis, but it did demonstrate that, after a 4-year interval, the ipsilateral stroke rate in the surgical group was 4.7 percent, in contrast to 9.4 percent in the medical group. This failed to achieve statistical significance (P value = 0.056) because of the small sample size; and, in addition, when a relatively high mortality rate of 1.9 percent was added, the difference disappeared. At the time of the consensus conference, the results of the ACAS Study were not available. However, while the report of the

study was in galleys and prior to publication, the National Institute of Neurologic Disease and Stroke group (NINDS) issued a clinical advisory (September 28, 1994), which was incorporated into the consensus statement. The advisory indicated that the aggregate risk over 5 years for the primary outcome of stroke was 4.8 percent for patients assigned to receive surgery and 10.6 percent for patients who were treated medically. The relative risk reduction conferred by surgery was 55 percent. Furthermore, the 30-day operative mortality and neurologic morbidity rate related to operation or angiography in the surgical group was 2.3 percent, of which 1.2 percent was accounted for by complications from preoperative angiography.

At this point, all three criteria have been fulfilled, including the important factor of low perioperative neurologic morbidity among patients operated on by surgeons who have participated in the ACAS trial, coming in at essentially 1.2 percent. It was this low perioperative morbidity and mortality rate that permitted the ACAS Study to demonstrate a 55 percent stroke risk reduction, at the 5-year interval, when compared with medical management alone in patients harboring carotid artery stenosis of 60 percent or greater.

ASYMPTOMATIC PATIENTS: MANUSCRIPT PART II

The second part of the manuscript, dealing with the specific indications for carotid endarterectomy, included a major section for asymptomatic patients with carotid artery disease. The statement took into account the issue of surgical risk, which includes both the overall risk factors attributable to the patient and the track record of the operating surgeon. Thus, three categories of surgical risk were identified: perioperative morbidity and mortality of less than 3.0 percent, 3.0 percent to 5.0 percent, and 5.0 to 10.0 percent. Within each of those risk categories, the indications for operation in asymptomatic patients were divided into four categories of indication: "Proven," "Acceptable but not Proven," "Uncertain," and Proven Inappropriate."

Indications for Carotid Endarterectomy

For Patients With a Surgical Risk of Less Than 3 Percent

Proven Indications. None.

On September 28, 1994, the NINDS stated that it was halting the ACAS because of a clear benefit in favor of surgery. Aggregate risk for the primary endpoint of stroke was 10.6 percent at 5 years for patients who were treated medically. Patients who underwent carotid endarterectomy had a 4.8 percent risk of stroke within the same time interval, including perioperative and angiographic complications. The relative risk reduction conferred by surgery was 55 percent. This was statistically significant, with a P value of 0.004 and a confidence interval of 95%. In patients who were randomly assigned to surgical management, the 30-day operative mortality and neurologic morbidity related to operation or angiography was 2.3 percent, of which the neurologic complications of preoperative angiography accounted for 1.2

percent. After the results of the study are published, surgery for asymptomatic, hemodynamically significant carotid stenosis will be redesignated as a proven indication.

Acceptable But Not Proven Indications. This category will move into the Proven category following publication of the ACAS study but, in the meantime, is defined as ipsilateral carotid endarterectomy for stenosis of 75 percent or greater, with or without ulceration, irrespective of contralateral artery status, ranging from new disease to total occlusion of the opposite side.

Uncertain Indications.
- Stenosis of less than 50 percent with a ''B'' or ''C'' ulcer, irrespective of contralateral internal carotid artery status.
- Unilateral carotid endarterectomy with coronary artery bypass grafting (CABG); CABG required with bilateral asymptomatic stenosis of more than 70 percent.
- Unilateral carotid stenosis of more than 70 percent, CABG required; unilateral carotid endarterectomy with CABG.

Proven Inappropriate Indications. None defined.

For Patients With a Surgical Risk of 3 to 5 Percent

Proven Indications. None.

Acceptable But Not Proven Indications. Ipsilateral carotid endarterectomy for stenosis of 75 percent or greater, with or without ulceration but in the presence of a contralateral internal carotid artery stenosis ranging from 75 percent to total occlusion.

Uncertain Indications.
- Ipsilateral carotid endarterectomy for stenosis of 75 percent or greater, with or without ulceration, irrespective of contralateral artery status, ranging from no stenosis to occlusion.
- CABG required; with bilateral asymptomatic stenosis of more than 70 percent, unilateral carotid endarterectomy with CABG.
- Unilateral carotid stenosis of more than 70 percent, CABG required; ipsilateral carotid endarterectomy with CABG.

Proven Inappropriate Indications. None defined.

For Patients With a Surgical Risk of 5 to 10 Percent

Proven Indications. None.

Acceptable But Not Proven Indications. None.

Uncertain Indications.
- CABG required with bilateral asymptomatic stenosis of more than 70 percent; unilateral carotid endarterectomy with CABG.
- Unilateral carotid stenosis of more than 70 percent, CABG required; ipsilateral carotid endarterectomy with CABG.

Proven Inappropriate Indications.
- Ipsilateral carotid endarterectomy for stenosis of 75 percent or greater, with or without ulceration, irrespective of contralateral internal carotid artery status.
- Stenosis of 50 percent or less, with or without ulceration, irrespective of contralateral carotid artery status.

STATEMENT SUMMARY

A consensus conference sponsored by the American Heart Association reviewed the current potential indications for carotid endarterectomy in asymptomatic patients. Twenty-two committee members, representing the disciplines of health care policy, neurology, neurosurgery, and vascular surgery, reviewed the current medical literature and ranked the indications for carotid endarterectomy in asymptomatic patients. The votes for each indication were averaged and ranked by four categories: Proven; Acceptable, but not Proven; Uncertain; and Proven Inappropriate.

From this statement emerges a clear definition of the indications for carotid endarterectomy and the circumstances of surgical risk. This represents the best recommendations by an expert committee at the present time. The statement goes on to conclude that many indications are the subject of ongoing prospective, randomized trials, and that as these trials reach completion, it is likely that recommendations in the document will be subject to change. It was the committee's hope that the document could and should undergo periodic revision.

SUGGESTED READINGS

Moore WS, Barnett HJM, Beebe HG, et al: Guidelines for carotid endarterectomy: A multidisciplinary consensus statement from the ad hoc committee, American Heart Association. *Stroke.* 1995;26:188–201.

Moore WS, Barnett HJM, Beebe HG, et al: Guidelines for carotid endarterectomy: A multidisciplinary consensus statement from the ad hoc committee, American Heart Association. *Circulation.* 1995;91:566–579.

VII

Indications for Carotid Endarterectomy in Symptomatic Patients

<table>
<tr><td>CHAPTER
31</td><td># The Rand Study Positions Concerning Carotid Endarterectomy</td></tr>
</table>

LOUIS R. CAPLAN

The Rand Corporation's publication on carotid endarterectomy contained two parts: a literature review, and ratings by a panel of the appropriateness and necessity of carotid endarterectomy for various indications.

The literature review began with a search using MEDLINE, a computerized database of the National Library of Medicine. The key word *carotid endarterectomy* was searched for in human studies published in English between 1966 and 1991. Ultimately, 362 articles were found, reviewed, and abstracted. Topics included the risk of stroke in patients with carotid artery disease, the efficacy of carotid surgery, surgical complications, and the number of endarterectomies and their cost. This review and the bibliography were sent to the panelists before the panel met.

During a two-day meeting in January 1991, a Delphi panel of nine physicians (two neurologists, one neurosurgeon, three vascular surgeons, and three generalists) rated the appropriateness of various surgical procedures in patients with various clinical presentations who had various arterial lesions and who were estimated to be at various surgical risks. The panelists were instructed to use their own best clinical judgment and to consider an average group of patients presenting in 1990 to an average American physician who performed carotid endarterectomies. Physicians used a 9-point system to rate the appropriateness of surgery: 1, extremely inappropriate; 5, uncertain; and 9, extremely appropriate. Clinical presentations in symptomatic patients included: (1) a single episode of transient ischemic attack (TIA) or amaurosis fugax; (2) multiple carotid TIAs or amaurosis fugax episodes in patients (a) never treated medically, (b) with recurrence since medical treatment started or in whom medical treatment was contraindicated or not tolerated, (c) with no recurrence since medical treatment started 3 months previously, (d) with at least one recurrence since medical treatment started; (3) crescendo carotid TIAs; (4) vertebrobasilar TIAs; (5) atherothrombotic stroke, either more or less than 3 weeks after the stroke, and with mild or moderate severity; and (6) stroke in evolution.

There were four chapters that concerned patients with asymptomatic carotid artery stenosis: (1) asymptomatic, normal stroke risk; (2) asymptomatic, prepared for major elective intra-abdominal or intrathoracic surgery (except coronary artery bypass graft); (3) asymptomatic, prepared for coronary artery bypass graft; and (4) combined carotid artery and coronary bypass surgery. In the first two chapters, the stroke risk was assumed to be low (<3%), and in the last two the stroke risk was elevated (<5% for those prepared for coronary artery bypass graft pre-op, and <8% for those with combined surgeries).

Physicians were asked to rate the appropriateness of operating on the *ipsilateral* or *contralateral* carotid artery in patients with these clinical presentations and with various arterial lesions shown at angiography, including 30 to 49 percent stenosis, with or without small or large ulcers; 50 to 69 percent stenosis, with or without ulcers; 70 to 99 percent stenosis; acute occlusion; and chronic occlusion. Different ratings were given for patients with low surgical risk (<3% stroke and mortality), elevated surgical risk (3–5%), and high surgical risk (5–7%). In instances in which the panel considered an operation appropriate (average rating >6), they were also asked to rate the necessity of the procedure in the same circumstances.

Before coming to the meeting, the panelists had already performed and mailed in preliminary ratings after having reviewed the literature. During the panel meeting, for each chapter, the panel members were first given their prior ratings, both individual and group. After a discussion, the ratings were repeated. These final ratings were then tabulated and analyzed for the degree of agreement. The individual chapters each contained a different clinical presentation. When the panel considered an indication appropriate for carotid endarterectomy (median rating >6; no more than two panelists rated in the 1–3 range), they were asked to rate the necessity of performing the procedure.

RESULTS

Symptomatic Patients

I summarize the data by noting those situations in which the panel consensus was that carotid endarterectomy was indicated. In the first chapter, the clinical presentation was a

TABLE 31–1. Example of Rand Panel Ratings of Appropriateness of Surgery: Clinical Presentation of Carotid Transient Ischemic Attack or Single Episode of Amaurosis Fugax

Appropriateness of Operating Ipsilaterally If Angiography Shows		Low Surgical Risk (<3%)	Elevated Surgical Risk (3–5%)
1a Ipsi:	Chronically occluded	9	9
Contra:	None or 1–49%	1 2 3 4 5 6 7 8 9	1 2 3 4 5 6 7 8 9
		(1.0, 0.0, A)	(1.0, 0.0, A)
1b Ipsi:	Acutely occluded	1 1 4 3	1 1 1 3 1 2
Contra:	None or 1–49%	1 2 3 4 5 6 7 8 9	1 2 3 4 5 6 7 8 9
		(7.0, 1.6, A)	(6.0, 1.7, I)
2a Ipsi:	Chronically occluded	9	9
Contra:	50–99%	1 2 3 4 5 6 7 8 9	1 2 3 4 5 6 7 8 9
		(1.0, 0.0, A)	(1.0, 0.0, A)
2b Ipsi:	Acutely occluded	2 2 5	2 3 2 2
Contra:	50–99%	1 2 3 4 5 6 7 8 9	1 2 3 4 5 6 7 8 9
		(8.0, 1.6, A)	(6.0, 1.6, I)
3 Ipsi:	70–99%	3 6	1 7 1
Contra:	0–99%	1 2 3 4 5 6 7 8 9	1 2 3 4 5 6 7 8 9
		(9.0, 0.3, A)	(8.0, 0.2, A)
4 Ipsi:	70–99%	2 7	1 7 1
Contra:	Occluded	1 2 3 4 5 6 7 8 9	1 2 3 4 5 6 7 8 9
		(9.0, 0.2, A)	(8.0, 0.2, A)
5 Ipsi:	50–69%	2 4 1 2	4 2 1 2
Contra:	0–99%	1 2 3 4 5 6 7 8 9	1 2 3 4 5 6 7 8 9
		(7.0, 0.8, A)	(6.0, 1.0, I)
6 Ipsi:	50–69%	4 2 3	2 2 2 2 1
Contra:	Occluded	1 2 3 4 5 6 7 8 9	1 2 3 4 5 6 7 8 9
		(8.0, 0.8, A)	(7.0, 1.1, I)
7 Ipsi:	30–49%		
Contra:	None or 1–49%	2 1 2 2 1 1	2 2 3 1 1
With or without MR evidence of brain infarct		1 2 3 4 5 6 7 8 9	1 2 3 4 5 6 7 8 9
		(3.0, 1.6, I)	(3.0, 1.2, A)
8 Ipsi:	30–49%		
Contra:	50–99%	1 1 3 1 1 1 1	2 2 3 1 1
With or without MR evidence of brain infarct		1 2 3 4 5 6 7 8 9	1 2 3 4 5 6 7 8 9
		(3.0, 1.4, I)	(3.0, 1.2, A)
9 Ipsi:	30–49%	1 1 1 3 1 2	1 1 3 2 2
Contra:	Occluded	1 2 3 4 5 6 7 8 9	1 2 3 4 5 6 7 8 9
With or without MR evidence of brain infarct		(4.0, 1.6, I)	(3.0, 1.2, I)
10 Ipsi:	50–69% with large ulcerative lesion	3 3 3	1 5 2 1
Contra:	0–99%	1 2 3 4 5 6 7 8 9	1 2 3 4 5 6 7 8 9
		(8.0, 0.7, A)	(7.0, 0.7, A)
11 Ipsi:	30–49% with large ulcerative lesion	4 3 2	1 2 2 3 1
Contra:	0–99%	1 2 3 4 5 6 7 8 9	1 2 3 4 5 6 7 8 9
		(7.0, 0.7, I)	(6.0, 1.1, I)
12 Ipsi:	50–69% with small ulcerative lesion	1 4 1 1 2	1 4 1 3
Contra:	0–99%	1 2 3 4 5 6 7 8 9	1 2 3 4 5 6 7 8 9
		(6.0, 1.1, I)	(5.0, 1.2, I)
13 Ipsi:	30–49% with small ulcerative lesion		
Contra:	0–99%	1 2 4 1 1	4 2 1 1 1
With or without MR evidence of brain infarct		1 2 3 4 5 6 7 8 9	1 2 3 4 5 6 7 8 9
		(5.0, 1.0, I)	(4.0, 1.1, I)

Appropriateness scale: 1, extremely inappropriate; 5, uncertain; 9, extremely appropriate.

The rating bar goes from 1 to 9, indicating the possible responses. The numbers above this line indicate how many panelists provided a particular rating for the indication. For example, in the left column of row 2b, two panelists rated this indication 2, two rated it 7, and five rated it 8. The summary statistics are shown below the number bar. In this example, the median score was 8.0 and the mean absolute deviation from the median (a measure of dispersion) was 1.6.

A, agreement; I, indeterminate (neither agreement nor disagreement); D, disagreement, using the definitions described in the test; MR, magnetic resonance.

single episode of a carotid TIA or amaurosis fugax (Table 31–1). Indications for ipsilateral carotid endarterectomy were: 70 to 99 percent ipsilateral stenosis (contralateral artery 0–99% occluded); 50 to 69 percent ipsilateral stenosis (contralateral artery 0–99% occluded) and low surgical risk; 50 to 69 percent ipsilateral stenosis with a large ulcerative lesion (contralateral artery 50–99% occluded) and low surgical risk. Contralateral carotid endarterectomy was considered to be indicated only when the ipsilateral artery was occluded (contralateral artery 70–99% occluded).

In the second chapter, the clinical presentation was multiple episodes of carotid TIAs or amaurosis fugax, never treated medically. The indications for carotid endarterectomy were the same as those described in the first chapter, except for the addition of ipsilateral artery 30 to 49 percent stenotic with large ulcerative lesion (contralateral artery 0–99% occluded) and low surgical risk. There were no definite indications for surgery on the contralateral artery.

In the third chapter, the presentation was multiple episodes of carotid TIAs or amaurosis fugax, with at least one recurrence since initiation of medical therapy or medical therapy contraindicated or not tolerated. The indications for ipsilateral carotid endarterectomy broadened to include acutely occluded ipsilateral artery (contralateral artery 50–99% occluded) and elevated surgical risk (3–5%); ipsilateral artery 50 to 69 percent stenotic (contralateral artery 0–99% occluded) and elevated surgical risk; and ipsilateral artery 50 to 69 percent stenotic with small ulcerative lesion (contralateral artery 0–99% occluded) and low surgical risk. Contralateral endarterectomy was considered indicated, as described in chapter 1, for an occluded ipsilateral artery (contralateral artery 70–99% occluded) and low surgical risk.

In the fourth chapter, the presentation was multiple episodes of carotid TIAs or amaurosis fugax, with no recurrence since initiation of medical therapy at least 3 months previously. In this case, the only indication for ipsilateral surgery was ipsilateral artery 70 to 99 percent stenotic (contralateral artery occluded) and low surgical risk. The indication for contralateral surgery was the same as that described in chapters 1 and 3.

The fifth chapter clinical presentation was crescendo carotid TIAs. The indications for ipsilateral and contralateral carotid endarterectomy were the same as for chapter 3, except that ipsilateral surgery for ipsilateral 70 to 99 percent stenosis was also judged appropriate, even if the patient had a high surgical risk (5–7%). This category of high surgical risk had not been considered in preceding chapters. Ipsilateral surgery for ipsilateral 30 to 49 percent stenosis with a large ulcerative lesion (contralateral artery 0–99% occluded) and low surgical risk just failed to fulfill appropriate indication criteria.

The sixth chapter concerned the clinical presentation of vertebrobasilar TIAs. Only two indications for operating on the ipsilateral carotid artery were considered: (1) severe uncorrectable vertebrobasilar disease and ipsilateral artery more than 70 percent occluded; and (2) vertebrobasilar TIAs thought to be influenced by more than 70 percent occlusion of the ipsilateral artery. Both were considered at low and elevated surgical risk. The only indication judged appropriate was the second when there was low surgical risk.

Chapter 7 concerned patients with atherothrombotic stroke more than 3 weeks after the stroke—first in the case of a mild stroke, and then in the case of a moderate stroke. The panel considered no indication clearly appropriate in the case of a moderate stroke and no indication appropriate for contralateral carotid surgery when the stroke was mild. For mild stroke, the appropriate indications for ipsilateral carotid endarterectomy were ipsilateral artery 70 to 99 percent stenotic (contralateral artery 0–99% occluded) and low or elevated (but not high) surgical risk; ipsilateral artery 50 to 69 percent stenotic (contralateral artery occluded) and low surgical risk; and ipsilateral artery 50 to 69 percent stenotic with large ulcerative lesion (contralateral artery 0–99% occluded) and low surgical risk.

Chapter 8 concerned patients with atherothrombotic stroke less than 3 weeks after the stroke. The panel did not think that there were any definite indications for either ipsilateral or contralateral carotid endarterectomy. (Chapters 9–12 concerned asymptomatic patients and are not considered here.)

Chapter 13 concerned the clinical presentation of multiple episodes of carotid TIAs or amaurosis fugax, with at least one recurrence since initiation of medical therapy. In all cases, the ipsilateral carotid artery was occluded. The panel did not find any definite indications in that circumstance for external carotid artery surgery.

The last chapter concerned stroke in evolution. The panel thought that all indications considered were appropriate. These were ipsilateral artery more than 70 percent occluded with or without clot at any surgical risk, and less than 70 percent occluded with a clot at any surgical risk.

The panel next considered the *necessity* of carotid endarterectomy in those cases in which it had judged the procedure appropriate. There were five situations in which *ipsilateral* surgery was deemed necessary:

1. Single episode of carotid TIA or amaurosis fugax: ipsilateral artery 70 to 99 percent stenosed (contralateral artery 0–99% occluded), low or elevated surgical risk.

2. Multiple episodes of carotid TIAs or amaurosis fugax, never subjected to medical therapy: any patient with 70 to 99 percent stenosis; or ipsilateral artery 50 to 69 percent stenotic and contralateral artery occluded, but only if low surgical risk.

3. Multiple episodes of carotid TIAs or amaurosis fugax, with at least one recurrence since initiation of medical therapy or medical therapy contraindicated or not tolerated: any patient with 70 to 99 percent stenosis; or ipsilateral artery 50 to 69 percent stenotic, but only if low surgical risk.

4. Crescendo carotid TIAs: ipsilateral artery 70 to 99 percent stenotic (contralateral artery 0–99% occluded) at low or elevated surgical risk but not at high risk (5–7%); or ipsilateral artery 70 to 99 percent stenotic (contralateral artery occluded) at all surgical risks; or ipsilateral artery 50 to 69 percent stenotic, only if low surgical risk.

5. More than 3 weeks after atherothrombotic stroke: ipsilateral artery 70 to 99 percent stenotic (contralateral

---

TABLE 31–2. Indications for Carotid Endarterectomy
When Carotid Stenosis Is 70 to 99%
(Contralateral Artery 0–99% Occluded)

Ipsilateral Surgery
  Carotid TIAs or amaurosis fugax
    Single episode
    Multiple episodes, never on medical therapy
    Multiple episodes with recurrence since medical therapy
    Multiple episodes, no recurrence since medical therapy (only if
      contralateral artery occluded and low surgical risk)
    Crescendo TIAs
  Vertebrobasilar TIAs thought influenced by carotid stenosis
  Mild atherothrombotic stroke >3 weeks previously (surgical risk <5%)
  Asymptomatic (contralateral artery occluded, low surgical risk)
  Stroke in evolution
Contralateral Artery (ipsilateral artery occluded)
  Carotid TIAs or amaurosis fugax
    Single episode
    Multiple episodes, recurrence since medical therapy (low surgical
      risk)
    Multiple episodes, no recurrence since medical therapy (low surgical
      risk)
    Crescendo TIAs (low surgical risk)

TIA, transient ischemic attack.

TABLE 31–3. Indications for Carotid Endarterectomy
When Carotid Stenosis Is 50 to 69%
(Contralateral Artery 0–99% Occluded)*

Carotid TIAs or amaurosis fugax
  Single episode (low surgical risk)
  Multiple episodes, never on medical therapy (low surgical risk)
  Multiple episodes, recurrence since medical therapy
  Crescendo TIAs (surgical risk <5%)
Mild atherothrombotic stroke >3 weeks prior (only if contralateral artery
  occluded and low surgical risk)

*The presence of a large ulcer did not change the panel's ratings.
TIA, transient ischemic attack.

TABLE 31–4. Indications for Carotid Endarterectomy
When Carotid Stenosis Is 30 to 49% With a
Large Ulcerative Lesion

Carotid TIAs or amaurosis fugax
  Multiple episodes, never on medical therapy
  Multiple episodes with at least one recurrence since medical
    therapy (also appropriate to operate on small ulcer)

TIA, transient ischemic attack.

artery 0–99% occluded) if surgical risk is less than 5 percent but not if risk is greater; or ipsilateral artery 50 to 69 percent stenotic and contralateral artery occluded, but only at low surgical risk.

Contralateral surgery was deemed necessary in only one circumstance: multiple episodes of carotid TIAs or amaurosis fugax and at least one recurrence since start of medical therapy or medical therapy contraindicated or not tolerated when the ipsilateral artery is occluded and the contralateral artery has 70 to 99 percent stenosis, but only if there is low surgical risk.

In some circumstances, such as ipsilateral surgery for a chronically occluded artery, the panel rated the operation as extremely inappropriate. In other circumstances, median or average ratings in the 1–3 range indicated that the surgery was definitely inappropriate. In many other circumstances, the panel was divided without a clear consensus; these cases were called indeterminate.

Asymptomatic Patients

In asymptomatic patients at normal stroke risk without pending surgery, the only agreed indication was for 70 to 99 percent stenosis (contralateral artery occluded). The degree of conviction was weaker than for nearly all the indications in symptomatic patients. There were no definite indications in any of the preoperative groups. There were no situations that the panel thought were necessary indications for carotid endarterectomy in asymptomatic patients. In many more situations in the chapters on asymptomatic patients, the panel judged the surgery to be very inappropriate.

DISCUSSION

A Delphi panel is one way to try to arrive at a consensus. The panel was relatively small, and its members came from diverse backgrounds and disciplines. All shared the same data. Surprisingly, there was a great degree of consensus on the appropriateness, and even the necessity, of surgery when there was a severe degree of carotid artery stenosis. Table 31–2 shows the appropriate indications for carotid endarterectomy in patients with stenoses of 70 to 99 percent. With moderate stenosis (50–69%, with or without ulceration) (Table 31–3), and in patients with 30 to 49 percent stenosis with large ulcerative lesions (Table 31–4), there was less agreement. There was also general agreement that surgery was not indicated in patients with minor stenosis and in the vast majority of asymptomatic patients, even those about to undergo major surgery.

CHAPTER 32

The Management of Patients Requiring Coronary Bypass and Carotid Endarterectomy

BRUCE J. BRENER, HOWARD HERMANS, DAVID EISENBUD, DEBRA CREIGHTON, CHRIS BROWN MAHONEY, DONALD K. BRIEF, JOSEPH ALPERT, ROBERT GOLDENKRANZ, JAN HUSTON, and VICTOR PARSONNET

Atherosclerosis commonly affects the coronary and carotid arteries simultaneously. When both arterial systems require surgical repair, should the operations be performed simultaneously or sequentially? Simultaneous carotid and coronary surgery is convenient and cost-effective, but is it safe? If the two procedures are to be performed in stages, which should be done first? Carotid endarterectomy (CEA), performed when the patient has significant coronary artery disease, can result in myocardial infarction and death. Coronary artery bypass graft (CABG) carried out in the presence of carotid disease can lead to stroke. Do the location, distribution, and severity of the various lesions affect the morbidity and mortality associated with either the staged or the simultaneous procedure? Does the presence of cerebral symptoms affect the results?

These questions have been posed repeatedly since 1972, when Bernhard and coworkers,[1] after noting increased morbidity and mortality when performing carotid endarterectomy in patients with coronary artery disease, performed 15 simultaneous procedures with no mortality and a 6.6 percent incidence of stroke. Unfortunately, the surgical literature has been confusing and contradictory concerning the roles of simultaneous and staged procedures.

INCIDENCE OF COMBINED DISEASE

Approximately 5 percent of patients undergoing CABG have asymptomatic but hemodynamically significant carotid disease. In 1987, we reported the results of routine, noninvasive carotid screening of 4047 patients undergoing open-heart surgery.[2] A total of 153 of the patients (3.8%) had carotid lesions that narrowed the lumen by more than 50 percent. Other studies found the prevalence of significant carotid disease in patients undergoing CABG to be between 3 and 18 percent (Table 32–1).[3-12] The variation among studies was probably due to differences in patient populations, noninvasive equipment, and indications for the study (for example, screening all patients undergoing CABG versus studying only patients with bruits or symptoms).

In addition to the patients with asymptomatic carotid stenosis, some patients admitted for CABG reveal prior neurologic symptoms, such as transient ischemic attack or stroke. More often, patients presenting primarily for evaluation of carotid disease are found to have significant coronary disease. There are several lines of evidence supporting this observation. First, routine cardiac catheterization of 506 patients with carotid disease treated at Cleveland Clinic indicated that 35 percent had severe coronary stenosis and occlusion.[13] Second, 60 to 70 percent of patients undergoing CEA had an abnormal electrocardiogram, a history of angina, or a myocardial infarct.[13, 14] Third, 18 percent of patients undergoing carotid surgery had significant coronary disease demonstrated by cardiac catheterization, despite the absence of symptoms or electrocardiographic evidence.[13] Fourth, 15 to 20 percent of patients without overt coronary disease but with carotid stenosis had evidence of coronary ischemia on thallium-201 scintigraphy after exercise or dipyridamole administration.[15] And finally, perioperative and long-term morbidity and mortality following carotid surgery are predominately cardiac in nature.[16, 17]

As a result of the discovery of combined carotid and coronary disease, some patients undergo percutaneous transluminal coronary angioplasty prior to carotid surgery. Others have stable coronary disease requiring only medication and can safely undergo carotid surgery alone. In this chapter we are concerned with patients with coronary disease severe

TABLE 32–1. Prevalence of Carotid Disease in Patients Undergoing Coronary Bypass

Study*	Method of Testing	Number/Total	Percentage
Hennerici et al[4]	CWD, SA	18/264	6.8
Mehigan et al[10]	History, OPG-G, OPG-K	49/874	5.6
Turnipseed et al[3]	CWD, SA	20/170	11.8
Barnes et al[5]	CWD, PD	40/324	12.3
Breslau et al[6]	Duplex, PD, SA	18/102	17.6
Balderman et al[7]	OPG-G	17/500	3.4
Brener et al[2]	OPG-G, OPG-K, PD, duplex	153/4047	3.8
Lusiani et al[9]	Duplex	26/144	18.0
Rostad and Grip[12]	CWD, PD	13/126	10.3
Jausseran et al[11]	Duplex	23/210	10.9
Faggioli et al[8]	Duplex, OPG-G	47/539	8.7
Totals		429/7300	9.9

*For full bibliographic information, see reference list at end of chapter.
CWD, continuous-wave Doppler; OPG-G, oculopneumoplethysmography; OPG-K, pulse-delay oculoplethysmography; PD, periorbital Doppler; SA, spectral analysis.

TABLE 32–2. Incidence of Myocardial Infarction, Stroke, and Death in Patients With No Severe Coronary Disease Undergoing Carotid Endarterectomy

Study*	Patients, n	Incidence of Adverse Events, %		
		MI	Stroke	Death
Cambria et al[21]	203	2.0	1.0†	0.5
NASCET[29]	328	0.9	5.5	0.6
			1.8†	
Rizzo et al[22]	482	0.8	1.5†	0.6

*For full bibliographic information, see reference list at end of chapter.
†Major or permanent stroke.
MI, myocardial infarction; NASCET, North American Symptomatic Endarterectomy Trial.

enough to require CABG who also have significant carotid lesions.

COMBINED CORONARY AND CAROTID DISEASE: PATIENT PROFILE

It has been postulated that patients who undergo both CEA and CABG are older and sicker than patients with isolated coronary disease who require CABG. Our review of the incidence of left main coronary artery disease found no difference between patients undergoing isolated CABG (21 percent) and those with significant carotid disease undergoing CABG (20 percent).[2] Jones and colleagues[18] found no correlation between carotid disease and the presence of unstable angina, history of congestive failure, incidence of triple-vessel disease, mean ejection fraction, or number of patients with three or more bypass grafts. Hertzer and coworkers[19] found that patients with combined disease were more likely to have an American Heart Association class III-IV rating (49 vs. 22%), triple-vessel disease (81 vs. 71%), left main coronary stenosis (23 vs. 13%), and ventricular impairment (72 vs. 56%) than patients of similar age with isolated coronary disease. The 5-year survival rate of patients with combined disease was lower than that of patients with isolated coronary disease (92 vs. 81%).[19] Vermeulen and coworkers[20] found that patients with combined disease were about 10 years older than their counterparts who had isolated coronary disease; the incidence of left main coronary artery disease was 29 percent, triple-vessel disease 80 percent, and class III–IV rating 70 percent. Cambria and associates[21] found that 37 percent of their patients with combined disease had left main coronary disease, whereas only 9.8 percent of routine CABG patients had left main stenosis. Many of these differentiating features were reviewed by Rizzo and coworkers,[22] who found that patients with combined disease had a higher incidence of risk factors such as hypertension, diabetes, and a history of smoking than those undergoing isolated CEA or CABG.

There are two possible explanations for these findings. The first is that in one's effort to avoid the combined operation, one chooses only the sicker patients to undergo it, preferring to perform isolated CEA in those with less cardiac disease. An alternative explanation assumes that patients with combined disease are in fact older and sicker. Does this mean that patients with combined disease are more

likely to suffer stroke, myocardial infarction, and death than those undergoing isolated CABG?

LIKELIHOOD OF STROKE, MYOCARDIAL INFARCTION, AND DEATH IN PATIENTS UNDERGOING ISOLATED CORONARY ARTERY BYPASS GRAFTING OR CAROTID ENDARTERECTOMY

To determine whether combined or staged CABG and CEA is preferable, we need to establish the risk of myocardial infarction, stroke, and death in two groups of patients: those with no known coronary disease undergoing carotid surgery, and those with no carotid disease undergoing CABG. Many studies have documented the incidence of perioperative stroke, myocardial infarction, and death in patients undergoing isolated CEA or CABG.[2, 8–10, 19, 21–28] Results from some of the most recent reports are shown in Tables 32–2 and 32–3.

In two studies, the isolated procedures were not preceded by a prospective uniform screening for coronary disease or carotid stenosis.[21, 22] However, in the judgment of the surgeons, there was no need for simultaneous procedures. In one report, each of the patients undergoing CABG had noninvasive carotid screening; only those with normal studies are included in Table 32–3.[8] Likewise, the North American Symptomatic Carotid Endarterectomy Trial (NASCET),[29] a prospective, randomized trial of carotid endarterectomy versus medical treatment, provided contemporary and accurate data to compare with the results of staged and combined procedures.

Comparison of published results assumes that the same definition of stroke was used in each study and that the identification of stroke was accurate. This may not be the case. Two of these studies were prospective[8, 29] and two were retrospective.[21, 22] The NASCET study indicated that the overall risk of stroke following CEA was 5.5 percent and that the risk of major or permanent stroke was less than 2 percent. The 5.5 percent figure includes all strokes, including contralateral events. But we cannot be sure that all contralateral strokes were enumerated in each of the studies cited. The rate of operative mortality from CEA was less than 1 percent. The risk of stroke following routine CABG was less than 2 percent, and the risk of death was 2 to 4 percent.

TABLE 32–3. Incidence of Myocardial Infarction, Stroke, and Death in Patients With No Known Carotid Disease Undergoing Isolated Coronary Bypass

Study*	Patients, n	Incidence of Adverse Events, %		
		MI	Stroke	Death
Cambria et al[21]	3570	na	0.6†	2.2
Faggioli et al[8]	432	na	1.2	1.8
Rizzo et al[22]	3012	4.7	1.4†	4.0

*For full bibliographic information, see reference list at end of chapter.
†Major or permanent stroke.
MI, myocardial infarction; na, information not available.

Patients With Known Coronary Disease Undergoing Carotid Endarterectomy

It is clear that many patients with coronary disease safely undergo CEA. With improved medical management of coronary disease; appropriate intraoperative monitoring; judicious uses of nitrates, beta blockers, calcium channel blockers, and regional anesthesia; and improved care if myocardial infarction occurs, the need for CABG may be minimized. However, the requirement for CABG still persists in a number of patients, as demonstrated by Bernhard and associates,[1] Urschel and associates,[30] and Ennix and associates.[31] In the latter study, the incidences of myocardial infarction and death in 77 patients with angina undergoing CEA were 15 and 18 percent, respectively. These types of studies, demonstrating the increased risk of myocardial damage during CEA, prompted the use of combined CEA and CABG.

Patients With Known Carotid Disease Undergoing Coronary Artery Bypass Grafting

In general, it is agreed that patients with carotid disease have a greater chance of having a stroke during a CABG procedure than do those with no carotid disease. Although three studies contradict this opinion,[5, 9, 26] most reports indicate that the risk is between 6 and 16 percent. The data from several studies in which the carotid lesion was not repaired are reviewed in Table 32–4. This does not include studies in which CEA was performed subsequent to CABG, a staging strategy that is discussed later. In our own study,[2] the incidence of stroke after isolated CABG was 1.9 percent; the incidence after 64 CABGs in which known carotid stenosis was not repaired was 6.3 percent. If patients with known carotid occlusions were included, the incidence was 9.2 percent ($P = 0.001$). This does not mean that performance of CEA lowers the risk of stroke. That subject remains to be discussed.

OPERATIVE STRATEGIES

It is clear that some patients with combined disease benefit from preoperative balloon angioplasty followed by CEA.

This strategy is useful for patients with symptomatic carotid disease who are found to have single high-grade, threatening coronary lesions. It may be useful in patients found to have high-grade asymptomatic carotid lesions and isolated coronary disease, although this concept requires confirmation. Of course, many patients with stable coronary disease can safely undergo CEA without invasive treatment of the coronary lesions.

The focus of this chapter is the management of patients with carotid disease who require coronary surgery. Three operative strategies have been proposed: Both procedures can be conducted simultaneously. This is convenient for the patient, lowers the cost, and reduces the number of anesthetic experiences. Alternatively, the carotid surgery can be performed first, exposing the patient to a risk of myocardial infarction and death (since the coronary disease is unrelieved). Third, the CABG can be performed first. This should result in the same risk of myocardial infarction and death as the combined procedure, but it may expose the patient to a risk of stroke.

META-ANALYSIS

To attempt to determine the rates of morbidity and mortality associated with selected strategies, a computer-based search of published English-language papers was performed. All papers reporting combined or staged carotid and coronary procedures were analyzed. Data, taken directly from the papers, was abstracted by three of the authors (BJB, HH, DC); in some cases, their interpretations of the data were different from those of the original authors. Most papers were reviewed by more than one person to confirm that the data were abstracted accurately. When several reports from the same institution contained duplicate data, only the most recent paper was selected.[2, 18, 20, 22, 34–41] Patients who received operations other than CEA for extracranial disease (such as aortocarotid bypass, innominate endarterectomy) were excluded from the studies. The following information was tabulated when available: number of patients and procedures; extent of carotid disease (unilateral stenosis, bilateral stenosis, stenosis and occlusion); symptomatic versus asymptomatic carotid disease; and incidence of myocardial infarction, death, stroke, and transient ischemic attack. Strokes were identified as permanent or temporary, major or minor, ipsilateral or contralateral.

Unfortunately, the data were incomplete in most studies. The criteria for myocardial infarction were rarely stated. Because of the wide variation in descriptions of stroke, the distinctions of permanent or temporary, major or minor, and ipsilateral or contralateral were abandoned; all strokes were tallied equally.

Meta-analysis was performed according to standard methods.[56, 57] This statistical technique adjusts for differences in the size of the groups and eliminates certain biases (see appendix). Needless to say, if the data are flawed when entered, the results of the meta-analysis will be skewed.

RESULTS IN THE LITERATURE

Only one paper reported the results of a prospective randomized trial. All other papers were nonrandomized; some

TABLE 32–4. Incidence of Adverse Events in Patients Undergoing Isolated Coronary Bypass With Known Carotid Stenosis

Study*	Patients, n	Incidence of Adverse Events, %		
		MI	Stroke	Death
Barnes et al[5]	40	na	2.5	10.0
Ivey[28]	19	na	15.8	na
Furlan and Craciun[32]	29	na	3.4	na
Lusiani et al[9]	6	0	0	0
Brener et al[2]	64	na	6.3	15.7
Marinelli et al[23]	2	na	100.0	100.0
Schultz et al[26]	50	na	2.0	6.0
Faggioli et al[8]	28	na	14.3	7.1
Johnsson et al[33]	7	na	0	na

*For full bibliographic information, see reference list at end of chapter.
MI, myocardial infarction; na, information not available.

were prospective, and others were retrospective. Fifteen papers compared the results of more than one strategy in the same institution. Thirty-five papers reported the results of 2308 combined cardiac and carotid procedures. There were 15 reports of 407 staged procedures in which the carotid operations were performed first. Six papers were reviewed that reported the results of 213 examples of "reversed" staging, that is, CABG first, CEA second.

Ideally, one would like to study the effect of sequence on comparable groups of patients, controlling for the effects of the extent of coronary and carotid disease and the presence or absence of symptoms. For example, the effect of performing simultaneous versus staged coronary and carotid procedures would be studied in patients with unilateral and bilateral, symptomatic and asymptomatic carotid stenosis, with stable and unstable coronary disease and good and poor ventricular function. No prospective randomized study has been carried out that controls for all these variables.

Prospective Randomized Study

In the only prospective randomized study attempted, 71 patients with asymptomatic unilateral carotid stenosis were assigned to a combined coronary-carotid operation.[19] There were three deaths (4.2%) and two strokes (2.8%), one of which was fatal. Fifty-eight patients with asymptomatic unilateral carotid disease were assigned to have CABG then CEA. As a result of the isolated CABG, there were two deaths (3.4%) and four strokes (6.9%). The difference in the incidence of stroke was not statistically significant ($P = 0.25$), indicating that CEA could not be confirmed to have lowered the likelihood of stroke during CABG. Interestingly, after the delayed CEA, there was another death (1.9%, total 5.3%) and four more strokes (7.5%, total 14.4%). The difference in incidence of stroke in the combined group (2.8%) and the group undergoing staged CABG and CEA (14.4%) was significant ($P = 0.042$). The incidence of stroke in the staged group was higher when the subsequent CEA was done during the same hospitalization as the CABG; the incidence of stroke was lower when the CEA was performed 1 to 2 months after discharge. This study of 129 patients indicates that combined procedures prevent strokes in patients with unilateral asymptomatic carotid stenosis undergoing CABG. However, the stroke rate during the subsequent CEA in the staged group was inexplicably higher than noted in previous reports from the Cleveland Clinic.[17] The combined approach was successful, not necessarily because it reduced the stroke rate during the CABG, but because it eliminated the subsequent CEA.

Staged Procedure: Carotid Endarterectomy First, Coronary Artery Bypass Graft Second

Fifteen studies provided information on the results of staged surgery in which the CEA was performed before the CABG. When patients who require CABG are subjected in an unselected fashion to CEA, one would expect a significant risk of cardiac morbidity and mortality. Studies by Bernhard and colleagues[1] and Ennix and colleagues[31] demonstrated the unacceptably high risk of carotid surgery in patients with severe coronary artery disease and focused attention on the need for careful selection. In modern series of staged procedures in which CEA is done before CABG, careful selection criteria are used to reduce cardiac complications. Patients are carefully monitored, and consequences of myocardial infarction can be minimized by modern medical treatments. CABG can be urgently carried out when necessary.

A modern example of staging in which the CEA is done first is provided in two subgroups in the paper by Hertzer and colleagues.[19] Thirty-three patients underwent "unprotected CEAs." Twenty-four patients with unilateral carotid disease, both symptomatic and asymptomatic, and stable coronary disease were subjected to CEA alone, followed by subsequent CABG. One patient had a stroke following CEA and suffered a fatal myocardial infarction while awaiting a staged CABG (4%). In another group of nine patients with stable coronary disease and bilateral carotid stenosis, there was no cardiac or cerebral morbidity during the preliminary CEA, but two patients died during a subsequent combined operation in which the second CEA and a CABG were performed. This strategy of CEA first, CABG second represents a small fraction (33 of 275, 12%) of the number of patients with combined disease at Cleveland Clinic. Other recent studies by Faggioli and coworkers[8] and Carrel and associates[27] show equally good results in a small number of patients.

This study was combined with the data from 14 other studies and subjected to meta-analysis (Table 32–5). The probability of an adverse effect when patients with carotid and coronary disease underwent CEA followed by a separate CABG was as follows: stroke 0.0530 (5.3%), myocardial infarction 0.1147 (11.5%), death 0.0938 (9.4%). The high rate of cardiac morbidity is probably due to the inclusion of earlier papers. This strategy is useful in only a small number of patients whose coronary disease is stable and mild enough to allow "unprotected" carotid surgery but severe enough to eventually require CABG.

Reversed Staged Procedure: Coronary Artery Bypass Graft First, Carotid Endarterectomy Second

There were only six papers that included data in which the CABG was carried out before the CEA (Table 32–6). If the hypothesis is correct that CEA prevents strokes that would occur during CABG in patients with carotid stenosis, then the reversed staged group should have a higher probability of stroke than either the combined group or the CEA first, CABG second group. Studies by Rosenthal and coworkers[42] and Hertzer and colleagues[19] indicate this trend. In the latter study, the incidence of stroke in 58 patients with unilateral asymptomatic carotid disease (discussed earlier) and 23 with unilateral symptomatic carotid disease who had preliminary "unprotected CABG" was 6.9 and 8.8 percent, respectively. In comparison, the incidence of stroke in 71 patients with unilateral asymptomatic carotid disease (discussed earlier) and 60 patients with unilateral symptomatic carotid stenosis who had combined operations was 2.8 and 8.3 percent, respectively. The difference due to strategy was not statistically significant. This indicates that although patients with carotid and coronary disease had a higher incidence of stroke after CABG than patients with no carotid disease, simultaneous CEA did not lower this increased incidence of stroke. To complete the staging, 81 delayed

TABLE 32–5. Probability of an Adverse Event Following Staged Carotid Endarterectomy and Coronary Bypass

Study*	Number of Patients	Death	MI	TIA	Stroke				
					Total	Temporary	Permanent	Major	Minor
Bernhard et al[1]	15	0.2	0	0.13	0.06	0.06	0	0	0.16
Urschel et al[30]	8	0	0.125	0	0	0	0	0	0
Mehigan et al[10]	24	0.042	0.042	0	0	0	0	0	0
Ennix et al[31]	5	0.8	0.8	0	0.2	0	0.2	0.2	0
Rosenthal et al[42]	14	0.071	0.071	0	0	0	0	0	0
Berkoff and Turnipseed[43]	3	0	0	0	0	0	0	0	0
Ivey[28]	4	0	0	0	0	0	0	0	0
Babu et al[44]	5	0	0	0	0	0	0	0	0
Reul et al[45]	164	0.049	na	0	0.024	na	0.024	0.024	na
Marinelli et al[23]	5	na	na	na	na	na	na	na	na
Newman and Hicks[46]	28	0	0	0	0	0	0	0	0
Schultz et al[26]	46	na	na	na	na	na	na	na	na
Hertzer et al[19]	24	0.04	0	0	0.04	0	0	0.04	0.04
Faggioli et al[8]	17	0	na	0	0	0	0	0	0
Carrel et al[27]	45	0.044	0.088	0	0	0	0	0	0
Meta-Analysis	407	0.0938	0.1147		0.053				

*For full bibliographic information, see reference list at end of chapter.

MI, myocardial infarction; na, information not available; TIA, transient ischemic attack.

CEAs were performed. Five additional strokes occurred during the delayed CEAs, four in the asymptomatic group and one in the symptomatic group, increasing the overall incidence of stroke to 14 percent in the asymptomatic group and 13 percent in the symptomatic group. Thus, the differences due to staging were due primarily to the high incidence of stroke during the subsequent CEA. As pointed out, this finding was unexpected, since the overall incidence of stroke during CEA at Cleveland Clinic has been noted to be under 2 percent.[17]

Because of the weight of the two studies mentioned, the meta-analytic probabilities were as follows: stroke 0.1003 (10%), myocardial infarction 0.0274 (2.7%), and death 0.0358 (3.6%). In patients undergoing staged CABG first, CEA second procedures, the CABG protected against cardiac morbidity and mortality, but the delayed CEA resulted in a higher incidence of stroke.

Combined Carotid Endarterectomy and Coronary Artery Bypass Graft

Thirty-five reports were analyzed (Table 32–7). Seventeen had more than 50 patients, and seven had more than 100

patients enrolled (Table 32–8). Using meta-analytic techniques, we calculated the probabilities of having an adverse effect as follows: stroke 0.0617 (6.2%), myocardial infarction 0.0467 (4.7%), and death 0.0560 (5.6%). Thus the combined group seems to have the same incidence of stroke as the CEA first group and the same mortality as the CABG first group.

RISK OF STROKE, MYOCARDIAL INFARCTION, AND DEATH: COMBINED VERSUS STAGED OPERATIONS

Using the meta-analytic method, we calculated the probabilities of an adverse event occurring (Table 32–9). As noted, the combined group and the CABG first group have approximately the same probability of myocardial infarction and death. The combined group and the CEA first group have approximately the same probability of stroke. The "unprotected CABG" group has a higher probability of stroke, and the "unprotected CEA" group has a higher probability of myocardial infarction and death. The statistical

TABLE 32–6. Probability of an Adverse Event Following Staged Coronary Bypass and Carotid Endarterectomy

Study*	Number of Patients	Deaths	MI	TIA	Stroke				
					Total	Temporary	Permanent	Major	Minor
Bernhard et al[1]	1	0	0	0	0	0	0	0	0
Urschel et al[30]	17	0	0	0	0.059	0	0.059	0.059	0
Ennix et al[31]	84	0.012	0.024	0	0.024	0	0.024	0	0.024
Rosenthal et al[42]	18	0	0	0	0.11	0.11	0	0	0.111
Newman and Hicks[46]	12	0	0	0	0	0	0	0	0
Hertzer et al[19]	81	0.037	0	0	0.135	0	0.135	0.049	0.086
Meta-Analysis	213	0.0358	0.0274		0.1003				

*For full bibliographic information, see references list at end of chapter.

MI, myocardial infarction; TIA, transient ischemic attack.

TABLE 32–7. Probability of an Adverse Event Following Combined Carotid Endarterectomy and Coronary Bypass

Study	Patients, n	Death	MI	TIA	Stroke Total	Temporary	Permanent	Major	Minor
Bernard et al[1]	15	0	0	0	0.066	0.066	0	0	0.066
Urshel et al[30]	8	0	0	0	0	0	0	0	0
Mehigan et al[10]	21	0.048	0	0	0.095	0	0.095	0.048	0.048
Okies et al[47]	16	0.0625	0.0625	0	0.125	0.0625	0.0625	0	0.125
Ennix et al[31]	51	0.059	0.059	0.019	0.019	0	0.019	0.019	0
Rice et al[48]	54	0	0	0	0.038	0.019	0.019	0.038	0
Schwartz et al[49]	73	0.10	0	0.014	0.014	0	0.014	na	na
Hertzer et al[25]	331	0.057	0.063	0	0.090	0.045	0.045	0.024	0.066
Rosenthal et al[42]	24	0	0	0	0	0	0	0	0
Berkoff and Turnipseed[43]	13	0.077	na	0	0	0	0	0	0
Ivey[28]	4	0.25	na	na	0.25	0	0.25	0.25	0
Perler et al[50]	37	0.081	0.027	0	0.027	0.027	0	0	0.027
Babu et al[44]	57	0.048	na	0.032	0.016	0	0.016	0.016	0
Dunn[51]	124	0.048	na	na	0.105	0.065	0.040	na	na
Lord et al[41]	78	0.064	0.03	0.03	0.064	0.051	0.013	0.013	0.051
Matar[52]	32	0	0.031	0	0.031	0	0.031	0.031	0
Reul et al[45]	143	0.042	na	na	0.028	na	na	na	na
Lubicz et al[53]	40	0.05	0	0.05	0.10	0.075	0.025	0.025	0.075
Marinelli et al[23]	12	0	0	0	0	0	0	0	0
Luisiani et al[9]	20	0.10	na	0	0	0	0	0	0
Brener et al[2]	57	0.105	na	0.018	0.07	0.052	0.018	0.018	0.052
Newman and Hicks[46]	10	0	0	0	0.10	0.10	0	0	0.10
Schultz et al[26]	16	na	na	na	0.125	0.063	0.063	0.063	0.063
Minami et al[38]	114	0.018	0	0	0.044	0.026	0.018	0.018	0.026
Jausseran et al[11]	17	0.059	0.059	0	0	0	0	0	0
Cambria et al[21]	71	0.028	0.028	0.014	0.042	0	0.042	0.028	0.014
Hertzer et al[19]	170	0.053	na	0	0.053	0	0.053	0.029	0.012
Duchateau et al[54]	82	0.073	0.037	0.012	0.061	0.012	0.048	na	na
Faggioli et al[8]	2	0	na	na	0	na	na	na	na
Pome et al[55]	52	0	0.076	0.038	0.019	0.019	0	0.019	0
Rizzo et al[22]	127	0.055	0.047	0.016	0.063	0.007	0.055	na	na
Weiss et al[24]	23	0.043	0.086	na	0	0	0	0	0
Carrel et al[27]	52	0.038	0.02	0.02	0	0	0	0	0
Jones[18]	132	0.03	na	na	0.015	0	0.015	na	na
Vermeulen et al[20]	230	0.035	0.017	0.026	0.061	0.03	0.03	0.03	0.03
Meta-Analysis	2308	0.0560	0.0467		0.0617				

MI, myocardial infarction; na, information not available; TIA, transient ischemic attack.

significance of these differences is summarized in Table 32–10.

This analysis must be tempered by the comments made above. It is unlikely that the CEA first, CABG second strategy will be used often, since few patients who require CABG have such stable and mild disease that the CABG can be postponed. The incidence of stroke was lower in the combined group than in the CABG first, CEA second group. But as pointed out, most of the strokes in one large study came during the delayed CEA rather than the unprotected CABG.[19] This is an area that can be studied further. Particularly in patients with asymptomatic carotid disease, the carotid surgery can be postponed for several weeks after CABG. Furthermore, this analysis does not take into account the financial and psychological costs of delaying the second procedure. It is possible that the risk of stroke and myocardial infarction is the same in the combined series and in carefully controlled staged series. In this case, it may still

TABLE 32–8. Probability of an Adverse Event Following Combined Carotid Endarterectomy and Coronary Bypass in Series With Over 100 Patients

Study	Patients, n	Death	MI	Stroke
Hertzer et al[25]	331	0.057	0.063	0.090
Dunn[51]	124	0.048	na	0.105
Reul et al[45]	143	0.042	na	0.028
Minami et al[38]	114	0.018	0	0.044
Hertzer et al[19]	170	0.053	na	0.053
Rizzo et al[22]	127	0.055	0.047	0.063
Vermeulen et al[20]	230	0.035	0.017	0.061

MI, myocardial infarction; na, information not available.

TABLE 32–9. Probability of an Adverse Event According to Meta-Analysis

Procedure	Stroke	MI	Death
Combined CEA and CABG	0.0617	0.0467	0.0560
CEA first, CABG second	0.0530	0.1147	0.0938
CABG first, CEA second	0.1003	0.0274	0.0358

CABG, coronary artery bypass graft; CEA, carotid endarterectomy; MI, myocardial infarction.

TABLE 32–10. Numerical Differences in Probability
of an Adverse Event (P Values)

Procedure	Stroke	MI	Death
CEA first vs. CABG first	−0.047 (0.081)	0.087 (0.012)	0.058 (0.019)
CEA first vs. simultaneous CEA and CABG	−0.009 (0.298)	0.068 (0.021)	0.038 (0.023)
CABG first vs. simultaneous CEA and CABG	0.039 (0.105)	−0.019 (0.179)	−0.020 (0.114)

CABG, coronary artery bypass graft; CEA, carotid endarterectomy; MI, myocardial infarction.

be advisable to perform the operations together to save time and money.

RELATION BETWEEN CEREBRAL SYMPTOMS AND RISK OF STROKE DURING COMBINED OPERATIONS

One might expect that patients with previous stroke or transient ischemic attack would have a higher probability of stroke in the perioperative period than those with no cerebral symptoms (Table 32–11). This was noted in the study by Hertzer and coworkers,[19] in which 2 of 71 (2.8%) asymptomatic patients with unilateral carotid disease who were randomly assigned to receive combined surgery had strokes and 5 of 60 (8.3%) patients with symptomatic unilateral disease who were obliged by protocol to have combined operations had strokes. Despite this apparent difference, there was no statistical significance ($P = 0.17$). In two studies from the Cleveland Clinic, the incidence of perioperative stroke in patients with previous stroke was 20 percent.[19, 25]

Vermeulen and associates[20] demonstrated that the perioperative risk of stroke was increased by a factor of only 1.4 in patients with preoperative transient ischemic attack or amaurosis fugax, but was increased 3.9 times by the presence of preoperative reversible ischemic neurologic deficit or stroke ($P = 0.046$). However, a large study by Hertzer and colleagues[25] showed no difference in perioperative stroke in

158 symptomatic and 173 asymptomatic patients subjected to simultaneous CEA and CABG.

The meta-analytic comparison of stroke in asymptomatic and symptomatic patients was carried out only in patients undergoing simultaneous procedures, since data relating to symptoms in the staged series were scarce. Data from the study by Vermeulen and colleagues[20] could not be included in the meta-analysis because the raw figures were not published. There was no significant difference in the probability of stroke in patients with or without carotid symptoms undergoing simultaneous procedures (0.0932 vs. 0.0723; $P = 0.18$). However, this analysis did not separate patients with transient ischemic attack from those with stroke. It is possible that patients who have had preoperative strokes are more likely to have perioperative strokes.

RELATION BETWEEN BILATERAL CAROTID DISEASE AND RISK OF STROKE DURING COMBINED OPERATIONS

In two series reported by Hertzer and coworkers[19, 25] and in a study by Dunn,[51] patients with bilateral carotid disease undergoing combined operations had a greater likelihood of having strokes than patients with unilateral carotid disease. Data in the large study by Vermeulen and coworkers[20] yielded equivocal results. The presence of bilateral high-grade carotid stenosis was marginally significant in increasing the risk of severe postoperative neurologic events and insignificant in increasing the risk of all neurologic events. The increased risk of bilateral disease was not confirmed by Rizzo and coworkers[22] or others (Table 32–12). However, by using meta-analysis and combining all patients, we found that the probability of having a stroke while undergoing combined carotid and coronary procedures was 0.069 for patients with unilateral disease and 0.1277 for those with bilateral disease ($P = 0.016$). The probability of stroke was even greater if one carotid artery was stenotic and the other was occluded; we found the incidence of stroke to be 29 percent in this high-risk group.[2]

TABLE 32–11. Probability of Stroke in Symptomatic and Asymptomatic Patients Undergoing Combined Carotid Endarterectomy and Coronary Bypass

Study	Patients, n		Probability of Stroke	
	Symptomatic	Asymptomatic	Symptomatic	Asymptomatic
Mehigan et al[10]	26	23	0.38	0.013
Emery et al[36]	17	13	0	0
Ivey[28]	9	0	0.11	—
Berkoff and Turnipseed[43]	13	0	0	—
Perler et al[50]	16	21	0.063	0
Lubicz et al[53]	28	12	0.071	0.167
Hertzer et al[25]	158	173	0.10	0.081
Brener et al[2]	0	57	—	0.070
Minami et al[38]	50	64	0.10	0
Hertzer et al[19]	60	71	0.083	0.028
Rizzo et al[22]	87	40	0.092	0
Weiss et al[24]	9	14	0	0
Meta-Analysis			0.0932	0.0723

TABLE 32–12. Probability of Stroke in Patients With Unilateral and Bilateral Carotid Disease
Undergoing Combined Carotid Endarterectomy and Coronary Bypass

Study	Patients, n		Probability of Stroke	
	Unilateral	Bilateral	Unilateral	Bilateral
Mehigan et al[10]	19	2	0	1.0
Emery et al[36]	29	11	0.069	0
Hertzer et al[25]	216	115	0.069	0.131
Berkoff and Turnipseed[43]	7	7	0	0
Babu et al[44]	43	10	0.043	0
Dunn[51]	78	52	0.077	0.135
Brener et al[2]	35	15	0.057	0
Newman and Hicks[46]	38	3	0	0.333
Hertzer et al[19]	140	30	0.05	0.167
Rizzo et al[22]	52	73	0.077	0.053
Weiss et al[24]	17	4	0	0
Meta-Analysis			0.069	0.1277

Although it is not surprising that the presence of bilateral disease increases the risk of stroke, it remains to be proved that CEA lessens that risk. In the series of Hertzer and colleagues,[19] none of the patients with bilateral carotid disease had an unprotected CABG; that is, a CABG with no CEA. This control group was missing. Nine patients had CEA first (no strokes) followed by combined operation (no strokes, two deaths). Thirty had a combined operation first (two strokes, 6.7%; no deaths) followed by delayed CEA (three strokes, 10%; no deaths). Once again, the incidence of stroke during the delayed CEA is unexpected and significantly affects the conclusions. The incidence of stroke during the combined operation in patients with bilateral carotid disease (6.7%) is not much higher than the incidence of stroke during combined procedures in patients with unilateral disease (5.3%), nor is it significantly different from an unprotected CABG alone in patients with unilateral disease (stroke 5.3%). Thus, the increased risk of stroke in patients with bilateral disease remains to be proved, as does the assertion that CEA lessens that risk.

BIAS

The meta-analytic study of the management of combined coronary and carotid disease is biased in several ways. First, studies in which poor results were obtained from any strategy may remain unpublished. Second, patients subjected to staged procedures may have strokes, myocardial infarctions, or die after the first procedure. Unless the intention-to-treat paradigm is used, these patients who are not subjected to the second procedure may be excluded from the study. This means that the results of staged procedures reported in a retrospective manner will be inappropriately favorable to the staging strategy. Third, papers from the 1970s are included with papers from the 1980s and 1990s. Fourth, there are few studies that distinguish between unilateral and bilateral disease and consider the presence or absence of cerebral symptoms. Fifth, there are few patients in which the CABG is performed first and the CEA second. At the Cleveland Clinic, one of the best sources of data, no patients with bilateral carotid disease underwent CABG alone, because of the opinion that such patients require combined procedures.

Because of these biases, it is not possible to be sure that one timing strategy is better than another. It is clear that patients requiring combined or staged carotid and coronary surgery are different from patients with disease in only one system. Patients with combined disease may be older, and the heart disease may be more advanced. Although they may have a higher risk of stroke, myocardial infarction, and death than patients with disease in only one system, this may not necessarily be related to their carotid arteries alone. For example, these patients may have more advanced disease of the aortic arch, making them more susceptible to emboli. To assess the need for carotid surgery, a control group with delayed CEA will have to be compared with the combined group. Although complex and costly, these studies are best done by randomization.

If a randomized prospective study is done, the intention-to-treat paradigm will be necessary. Specific endpoints will have to be defined and quantified. The extent of coronary and carotid disease as well as the presence or absence of symptoms must be specified, and the risk of angiography should be noted. The experience of the surgeons at multiple centers will also have to be reviewed, and criteria for acceptance established.

CONCLUSION

The management of patients with coronary and carotid disease is complex. Fears concerning the risk of myocardial infarction and stroke are justified, since these patients are older and more seriously compromised than the usual patient undergoing CABG. Patients with symptomatic carotid disease must be treated promptly; delaying carotid surgery by staging may be as dangerous as performing carotid surgery without myocardial revascularization. Carefully selected patients can undergo staged procedures, depending on the severity of disease in each arterial system. However, patients with severe symptoms and disease in both arterial areas may require combined procedures. Although it has not been definitely proved that CEA lowers the risk of stroke during CABG, it may be efficient, cost-effective, and psychologically appealing to perform both procedures simultaneously.

Appendix: Methodology

The general model used is formulated as follows. Let $\Theta_k = \Theta_1, \Theta_2, \ldots \Theta_k$ be the basic parameters. There is no restriction that the basic parameters be independent; some or all of them can be multivariate. Let $\pi(\Theta_k)$ be the joint prior distribution for Θ_k. If all the basic parameters are independent, with prior distributions $\pi(\Theta_i)$, then

$$\pi(\Theta_k) = \prod_{i=1}^{k} \pi_i(\Theta_i)$$

Functional parameters can be denoted as $\Theta_{k+1}, \ldots, \Theta_m$, with the order such that any particular functional parameter, Θ_l, can be written as a function of the basic parameters and other functional parameters that precede it in order. In general,

$$\Theta_l = f_l(\Theta_1, \Theta_2, \ldots, \Theta_k, \Theta_{k+1}, \ldots, \Theta_{l-1})$$

A requirement of the general model is that this ordering be possible. This ordering implies that all functional parameters can, by successive substitutions, be written as functions only of basic parameters. Let Θ_m be the entire set of basic and functional parameters such that $\Theta_m = \Theta_1, \Theta_2, \ldots, \Theta_m$.

Data from the experiments can be represented by $\mathbf{y}_j$, $j = 1 \ldots n$ (variables representing the evidence), where j indexes the jth experiment. The general likelihood function for the jth experiment can be written as

$$L_j(\mathbf{y}_j \mid \Theta_1, \Theta_2, \ldots, \Theta_m)$$

The likelihood for this model can be represented by

$$\mathbf{L} = \prod_{j=1}^{n} L_j(\mathbf{y}_j \mid \Theta_1, \ldots, \Theta_m)$$

which is the product of the likelihood functions. Maximum likelihood estimates can be calculated using this model for parameters.

The particular case for this analysis is a dichotomous outcome model. The outcomes of interest are either success or failure. In this analysis, ''success'' is the occurrence of an adverse health outcome. The adverse health outcomes examined here are stroke, myocardial infarction, and death. The outcome we observe is Θ, or the probability of developing the adverse health outcome (''success''). ''Success,'' or presence of the ith adverse health outcome, is denoted with $y_i = 1$; $y_i = 0$ denotes that the ith adverse health outcome is not present; that is, a ''failure.''

We can represent the number of successes with s, where

$$s = \sum_{i=1}^{n} \mathbf{y}_i$$

and the number of failures with f, where

$$f = \sum_{i=1}^{n} (1 - \mathbf{y}_i).$$

Outcomes are assumed to be independent and identically distributed, and the likelihood function can then be derived from the binomial distribution,

$$L(\mathbf{y} \mid \Theta) \propto \Theta^s (1 - \Theta)^f.$$

This assumes that all individuals are subject to the same probability of success.

The measure of effect used here to examine adverse health outcomes resulting from different operative strategies is the actual probability of occurrence. In all cases, the data available are the reported probability of adverse health outcomes that occur following each operative strategy. The actual probability can be represented by:

$$\epsilon_i = \Theta_i$$

The random effects or hierarchical model is used to perform the meta-analyses that combine information across studies. This model adjusts for the existence of unknown biases that may affect experimental results. If the larger distribution from which all the experimental results are drawn is assumed to be normal, the specific form of the hierarchical distribution function is

$$P(\Theta_j \mid \mu, \tau^2) \propto 1/\tau e^{-(\Theta_3 - \mu)2/2\,\tau2}$$

representing the functional form utilized in this analysis by the FASTPRO program.

As pointed out, the least ambiguous and most meaningful way to describe the effect of any intervention is to present the outcomes of both alternative interventions separately, along with the difference in measures examined in the analysis. The measure used here to compare adverse health outcomes resulting from different operative strategies is the actual difference in probabilities. The data available are used to calculate the occurence across studies for each operative strategy. Differences between operative strategies are then calculated for each adverse health outcome. This calculated difference in probabilities can be represented by:

$$\epsilon_d = \Theta_s - \Theta_d$$

where Θ_s and Θ_d represent probability of the adverse health outcome occurring in each of two different surgical strategies.

REFERENCES

1. Bernhard VM, Johnson WD, Peterson JJ: Carotid artery stenosis: Association with surgery for coronary artery disease. *Arch Surg.* 1972;105:837.
2. Brener BJ, Brief DK, Alpert J, et al: The risk of stroke in patients with asymptomatic carotid stenosis undergoing cardiac surgery: A follow-up study. *J Vasc Surg.* 1987;5:269.
3. Turnipseed WE, Berkoff HA, Belzer FO: Postoperative stroke in cardiac and peripheral vascular disease. *Ann Surg.* 1980;192:365.
4. Hennerici M, Aulich A, Sandmann W, et al: Incidence of asymptomatic extracranial arterial disease. *Stroke.* 1981;12:750.
5. Barnes RW, Liebman PR, Marszalek PB, et al: The natural history of asymptomatic carotid disease in patients undergoing cardiovascular surgery. *Surgery.* 1981;90:1075.
6. Breslau PJ, Fell G, Ivey TD, et al: Carotid arterial disease in patients undergoing coronary artery bypass operations. *J Thorac Cardiovasc Surg.* 1981;82:765.
7. Balderman SC, Gutierrez IZ, Makula P, et al: Noninvasive screening for asymptomatic carotid artery disease prior to cardiac operation. Experience with 500 patients. *J Thorac Cardiovasc Surg.* 1983;85:427.
8. Faggioli GI, Curl GR, Ricotta JJ: The role of carotid screening before coronary artery bypass. *J Vasc Surg.* 1990;12:724.
9. Lusiani L, Visona A, Castellani V, et al: Prospective evaluation of combined carotid and coronary surgery. *Eur J Cardiothorac Surg.* 1987;1:16.

10. Mehigan JT, Buch WS, Pipkin ED, Fogarty TJ: A planned approach to coexistent cerebrovascular disease in coronary artery bypass candidates. *Arch Surg.* 1977;112:1403.

11. Jausseran JM, Bergeron P, Reggi M, et al: Single staged carotid and coronary arteries surgery: Indications and results. *J Cardiovasc Surg.* 1989;30:407.

12. Rostad H, Grip A: Screening of the carotid arteries with Doppler ultrasound in patients with coronary artery disease. *J Oslo City Hosp.* 1988;38:93.

13. Hertzer NR, Young JR, Beven EG, et al: Coronary angiography in 506 patients with extracranial cerebrovascular disease. *Arch Intern Med.* 1985;145:849.

14. O'Donnell TF, Callow AD, Willet C, et al: The impact of coronary artery disease on carotid endarterectomy. *Ann Surg.* 1983;198:705.

15. Boucher CA, Brewster DC, Darling RC, et al: Determination of cardiac risk by dipyridamole-thallium imaging before peripheral vascular surgery *N Engl J Med.* 1985;312:389.

16. Thompson JE, Austin DJ, Patman RD: Carotid endarterectomy for cerebrovascular insufficiency: Long-term results in 592 patients followed up to thirteen years. *Ann Surg.* 1970;172:663.

17. Hertzer NR, Beven EG, O'Hara PJ, Krajewski LP: A prospective study of vein patch angioplasty during carotid endarterectomy: Three-year results for 801 patients and 917 operations. *Ann Surg.* 1987;206:628.

18. Jones EL, Craver JM, Michalik RA, et al: Combined carotid and coronary operations: When are they necessary? *J Thorac Cardiovasc Surg.* 1984;87:7.

19. Hertzer NR, Loop FD, Beven EG, et al: Surgical staging for simultaneous coronary and carotid disease: A study including prospective randomization. *J Vasc Surg.* 1989;9:455.

20. Vermeulen FEE, Hamerlijnck RPHM, Defauw JJAM, Ernst SMPG: Synchronous operation for ischemic cardiac and cerebrovascular disease: Early results and long-term follow-up. *Ann Thorac Surg.* 1992;53:381.

21. Cambria RP, Ivarsson BL, Akins CW, et al: Simultaneous carotid and coronary disease: Safety of the combined approach. *J Vasc Surg.* 1989;9:56.

22. Rizzo RJ, Whittemore AD, Couper GS, et al: Combined carotid and coronary revascularization: The preferred approach to the severe vasculopath. *Ann Thorac Surg.* 1992;54:1099.

23. Marinelli G, Turinetto B, Bombardini T, et al: Surgical approach to combined carotids and coronaries lesions. *Int Angiol.* 1987;6:393.

24. Weiss SJ, Sutter FP, Shannon TO, Goldman SM: Combined carotid operation and carotid endarterectomy during aortic cross-clamping. *Ann Thorac Surg.* 1992;53:813.

25. Hertzer NR, Loop FD, Taylor PC, Beven EG: Combined myocardial revascularization and carotid endarterectomy. *J Thorac Cardiovasc Surg.* 1983;85:577.

26. Schultz RD, Sterpetti AV, Feldhaus RJ: Early and late results in patients with carotid disease undergoing myocardial revascularization. *Ann Thorac Surg.* 1988;45:603.

27. Carrel T, Stillhard G, Turina M: Combined carotid and coronary artery surgery: Early and late results. *Cardiology.* 1992;80:118.

28. Ivey TD: Combined carotid and coronary disease—a conservative strategy. *J Vasc Surg.* 1986;3:687.

29. North American symptomatic carotid endarterectomy trial (NASCET): Beneficial effect of carotid endarterectomy in symptomatic patients with high-grade carotid stenosis. *N Engl J Med.* 1991;325:445.

30. Urschel HC, Razzuk MA, Gardner MA: Management of concomitant occlusive disease of the carotid and coronary arteries. *J Thorac Cardiovasc Surg.* 1976;72:829.

31. Ennis CL, Lawrie GM, Morris GC, et al: Improved results of carotid endarterectomy in patients with symptomatic coronary disease: An analysis of 1,546 consecutive carotid operations. *Stroke.* 1979;10:122.

32. Furlan AJ, Craciun AR: Risk of stroke during coronary artery bypass graft surgery in patients with internal carotid artery disease documented by angiography. *Stroke.* 1985;16:797.

33. Johnsson P, Algotsson L, Ryding E, et al: Cardiopulmonary perfusion and cerebral blood flow in bilateral carotid artery disease. *Ann Thorac Surg.* 1991;51:579.

34. Brener BJ, Brief DK, Alpert JA, et al: A four-year experience with preoperative noninvasive carotid evaluation of two thousand twenty-six patients undergoing cardiac surgery. *J Vasc Surg.* 1984;2:326.

35. Vermeulen FEE: Simultaneous extensive extracranial and coronary revascularization: Long-term follow-up up to 13 years. *Eur J Cardiothorac Surg.* 1988;2:113.

36. Emery RW, Cohen LH, Whittemore AD, et al: Coexistent carotid and coronary artery disease. *Arch Surg.* 1983;118:1035.

37. Minami K, Sagoo KS, Breymann T, et al: Operative strategy in combined coronary and carotid artery disease. *J Thorac Cardiovasc Surg.* 1988;95:303.

38. Minami K, Gawaz M, Ohlmeier H, et al: Management of concomitant occlusive disease of coronary and carotid arteries using cardiopulmonary bypass for both procedures. *J Cardiovasc Surg.* 1989;30:723.

39. Craver JM, Murphy DA, Jones EL, et al: Concomitant carotid and coronary artery reconstruction. *Ann Surg.* 1982;195:712.

40. Lord RSA, Graham AR, Shanahan MX, et al: Combined carotid coronary reconstructions—synchronous or sequential? *Aust N Z J Surg.* 1985;55:329.

41. Lord RSA, Graham AR, Shanahan MX, et al: Rationale for simultaneous carotid endarterectomy and aortocoronary bypass. *Ann Vasc Surg.* 1986;1:201.

42. Rosenthal D, Caudill DR, Lamis PA, et al: Carotid and coronary artery disease: A rational approach. *Am Surg.* 1984;50:233.

43. Berkoff HA, Turnipseed WD: Patient selection and results of simultaneous coronary and carotid artery procedures. *Ann Thorac Surg.* 1984;38:172.

44. Babu SC, Shah PM, Singh BM, et al: Coexisting carotid stenosis in patients undergoing cardiac surgery: Indications and guidelines for simultaneous operations. *Am J Surg.* 1985;150:207.

45. Reul GJ Jr, Cooley DA, Duncan JM, et al: The effect of coronary bypass on the outcome of peripheral vascular operations in 1093 patients. *J Vasc Surg.* 1986;3:788.

46. Newman DC, Hicks RG: Combined carotid and coronary artery surgery: A review of the literature. *Ann Thorac Surg.* 1988;45:574.

47. Okies JE, MacManus Q, Starr A: Myocardial revascularization and carotid endarterectomy: A combined approach. *Ann Thorac Surg.* 1977;23:560.

48. Rice PL, Pifarfe R, Sullivan HJ, et al: Experience with simultaneous myocardial revascularization and carotid endarterectomy. *J Thorac Cardiovasc Surg.* 1980;79:922.

49. Schwartz RL, Garrett JR, Karp RB, Kouchoukos NT: Simultaneous myocardial revascularization and carotid endarterectomy. *Circulation.* 1982;66(suppl I):I-97.

50. Perler BA, Burdick JF, Williams M: The safety of carotid endarterectomy at the time of coronary artery bypass surgery: Analysis of results in a high-risk patient population. *J Vasc Surg.* 1985;2:558.

51. Dunn EJ: Concomitant cerebral and myocardial revascularization. *Surg Clin North Am.* 1986;66:385.

52. Matar AF: Concomitant coronary and cerebral revascularization under cardiopulmonary bypass. *Ann Thorac Surg.* 1986;44:431.

53. Lubicz S, Kelly A, Field PL, et al: Combined carotid and coronary surgery. *Aust N Z J Surg.* 1987;57:593.

54. Duchateau J, Nevelsteen A, Sergeant P, et al: Combined myocardial and cerebral revascularization. *J Cardiovasc Surg.* 1989;30:715.

55. Pome G, Fassini L, Colucci V, et al: Combined surgical approach to coexistent carotid and coronary artery disease. *J Cardiovasc Surg.* 1991;32:757.

56. Sacks HS, Berrier J, Reitman D, et al: Meta-analysis of randomized controlled trials. *N Engl J Med.* 1987;316:450.

57. Eddy DM, Hasselblad V, Shachter R: An introduction to a Bayesian method for meta-analysis: The confidence profile method. *Med Decis Making.* 1990;10:15.

ADDITIONAL READING

Dalton ML, Parker TM, Mistrot JJ, Bricker DL: Concomitant coronary artery bypass and major noncardiac surgery. *J Thorac Cardiovasc Surg.* 1978;75:621.

Morris GC, Ennis CL, Lawrie GM, et al: Management of coexistent carotid and coronary artery occlusive atherosclerosis. *Cleve Clin Q.* 1978;45:125.

Rollinson RD, Toole JF: Management of concomitant, symptomatic surgical lesions of the coronary and carotid arteries. *Surg Neurol.* 1979;11:70.

Mannick J: When to combine bypass with carotid endarterectomy (editorial). *J Cardiovasc Med.* 1983;8:629.

Gravlee GP, Cordell AR, Graham JE, et al: Coronary revascularization in patients with bilateral internal carotid occlusions. *J Thorac Cardiovasc Surg.* 1985;90:921.

Gardner TJ, Horneffer PJ, Michalik RA, et al: Stroke following coronary artery grafting: A ten-year study. *Ann Thorac Surg.* 1985;40:574.

Barnes RW: Asymptomatic carotid disease in patients undergoing major cardiovascular operations: Can prophylactic endarterectomy be justified? *Ann Thorac Surg.* 1986;42:536.

Cosgrove DM, Hertzer NR, Loop FD: Surgical management of synchronous carotid and coronary artery disease. *J Vasc Surg.* 1986;3:690.

Byrne E: The treatment of combined carotid and coronary arterial disease (editorial comment). *Aust N Z J Surg.* 1987;57:587.

Skotnicki SH, Schulte BPM, Leyten QH, et al: Asymptomatic carotid bruit in patients who undergo coronary artery surgery *Eur J Cardiothorac Surg.* 1987;1:11.

Graor RA, Hetzer NR: Management of coexistent carotid artery and coronary artery disease. *Stroke.* 1988;19:1441.

Loop LD: Changing management of carotid stenosis in coronary artery surgery patients. *Ann Thorac Surg.* 1988;45:591.

Yeager RA, Moneta GL, McConnell DB, et al: Analysis of risk factors for myocardial infarction following carotid endarterectomy. *Arch Surg.* 1989;124:1142.

Arom KV, Cohen DE, Strobi FT: Effect of intraoperative intervention on neurological outcome based on electroencephalographic monitoring during cardiopulmonary bypass. *Ann Thorac Surg.* 1989;48:476.

CHAPTER 33

The American Heart Association Consensus Committee Statement Concerning Indications for Carotid Endarterectomy in Symptomatic Patients

WESLEY S. MOORE

The Stroke Council and the Council on Cardiothoracic and Vascular Surgery of the American Heart Association recognized that there was a database of sufficient proportion and quality that the time was right for the development of a consensus statement concerning the indications for carotid endarterectomy. It was decided to hold this conference in Park City, Utah, July 16 to 18, 1993. The Heart Association appointed Wesley S. Moore, MD, as chairman of the committee and charged him with the responsibility of organizing the conference and spearheading the development of a consensus statement for publication.

THE CONSENSUS PROCESS

The committee chairman took the responsibility of identifying experts from several disciplines and developing the framework for the conference that resulted in the consensus statement. The committee chairman decided that it was essential to have a common database for review before entering into a discussion concerning individual potential indications for carotid endarterectomy. The database was to include information concerning the natural history of patients with various manifestations of carotid bifurcation disease, provide guidelines concerning patient evaluation, discuss available options for medical management together with outcome data, review the literature with respect to results of surgical management, evaluate data from position statements, and analyze the results to date of prospective randomized trials with both symptomatic and asymptomatic patients. An agenda of topics was developed, and an expert in the field for each topic was identified. Invitations were then sent to the experts requesting their participation in the consensus conference. The cadre of experts at the conference included seven neurologists, three neurosurgeons, 11 vascular surgeons, and one representative from the discipline of health care policy. Prior to the conference, participants provided the chairman with brief summaries of their presentations, together with an appropriate bibliography. Prior to the conference, the chairman collated all of these statements into a cohesive first draft manuscript.

The conference was divided into two parts. The first part consisted of the individual presentations from the developed agenda. Following each presentation, there was the opportunity for discussion, questions, and challenges. After all the presentations had been made, the first draft of the manuscript was read to the entire group. A critique was then carried out on a line-by-line basis; on-site revisions were carried out until the first part of the statement received uniform approval of the committee (consensus).

Following completion of the first part of the manuscript, a package of 96 potential indications for carotid endarterectomy was distributed to each participant. Each member was then asked to rank that potential indication into one of four categories. The ranking was to reflect the member's understanding from the common database that was presented, but also would reflect the expert's overall understanding of the literature, and each member's opinion concerning the individual indications for operation. Each indication would be scored into one of four categories, which would contain an appropriately allocated point score. Category I was labeled ''proven.'' This represented the strongest indication for carotid endarterectomy and in general meant that the data were supported by the results of prospective randomized trials.

Category II was defined as ''acceptable but not proven.'' Interpretation of this category meant that there was general agreement that it represented a strong indication for carotid endarterectomy that was supported by promising data, but not the type of scientifically certain data that would come from a prospective randomized trial. Category III was defined as ''uncertain.'' That meant that there were insufficient data to define the risk-to-benefit ratio. Potential indications falling into the ''uncertain'' category might well serve as appropriate topics for future prospective randomized trials. Category IV was defined as ''proven inappropriate.'' That meant that there were sufficient data to state that the risk of operation clearly outweighed its benefit.

All committee members scored each of the 96 indications for operation, and each indication then underwent a collation of scores, with an analysis that allowed the indication to be ranked into one of the four categories. The indications were then divided into symptomatic patients and asymptomatic patients. These indications were then tabulated and constituted the second part of the manuscript.

SYMPTOMATIC PATIENTS: PART I

Natural History

The consensus group examined the natural history of symptomatic patients based on retrospective reviews of identifiable patient cohorts and by looking at the control group of the North American Symptomatic Carotid Endarterectomy Trial (NASCET). The consensus group identified symptomatic patients as those presenting with transient or persistent monocular visual loss, hemispheric transient ischemic attacks (TIAs), and ischemic stroke. They also pointed out that it is difficult to assign mechanism-specific stroke risk based on currently available data because there appear to be an increasing number of recognizable factors that may affect subsequent stroke risk that were not considered within the original studies. These factors, often not recognized, include the type of event, the frequency of events, the degree of stenosis of the carotid artery in question, and the plaque characteristics of individual lesions. In spite of these limitations, it was stated that patients with TIAs related to carotid artery lesions are at risk of stroke at the rate of 12 to 13 percent within the first year of onset of symptoms and have a cumulative stroke risk of approximately 30 to 35 percent at the end of 5 years. It was also noted that patients with hemispheric TIAs, recent TIA, increasing frequency of TIA, or high-grade stenosis have stroke rates that are probably higher than those with a remote or single event or a lesser degree of stenosis.

The consensus group stated that patients who have had a stroke continue to be at risk for subsequent stroke at the rate of 5 to 9 percent per year, and approximately 25 to 45 percent have another stroke within 5 years of the original event.

There also is a considerable body of evidence to suggest that plaque characteristics may affect subsequent ischemic events. For example, only 20 to 30 percent of asymptomatic patients had echolucent plaques, in contrast to symptomatic patients, in whom echolucent plaques were present in 70 percent of the cohort. In addition, computed tomographic scanning of patients with carotid plaques demonstrated a 36 percent frequency of cerebral infarction in patients with echolucent plaques but only a 6 percent frequency in patients with echogenic plaques, suggesting that patients with echolucent or heterogeneous plaques are at two to four times greater risk of stroke than those with echogenic plaques.

A review of the control group of the NASCET study demonstrated the importance of another plaque characteristic, namely ulceration. In the absence of angiographic evidence of ulceration, the 2-year stroke event rate was 17 percent, in contrast to a 30 percent 2-year stroke event rate in the presence of ulceration. Finally, the importance of percent stenosis was emphasized in the control group of the NASCET trial. For every 10 percent increase in percent stenosis there was a corresponding increase in subsequent stroke risk.

Results of Endarterectomy for Symptomatic Patients With Carotid Artery Disease

Retrospective Reviews

The consensus committee noted that the cumulative results of carotid endarterectomy (immediate and long-term) with respect to subsequent stroke event rates are influenced by the 30-day operative stroke morbidity and mortality rates. These rates can vary depending on the indication for operation as well as the experience of the operating surgeon and institution. Patients undergoing surgery for transient ischemic attack appear to be at lower risk of perioperative events than those undergoing operation for prior stroke as an indication for endarterectomy. The consensus group reviewed four recent series and noted a range of combined 30-day mortality and stroke morbidity from a low of 2 percent to a high of 6.1 percent. Aggregating these results in a meta-analysis provided a surgical experience of 1498 patients with symptoms of transient ischemic attack or prior stroke and

yielded a combined 30-day operative mortality and stroke morbidity rate of 2.74 percent. Additional information concerning the risk of operation was obtained from the data submitted by prospective surgeons wishing to enter the Asymptomatic Carotid Atherosclerosis Study (ACAS) trial. A review of surgeons successfully admitted to the ACAS trial provided an experience with 5641 carotid endarterectomies performed for a variety of indications with combined operative mortality and stroke morbidity of 2.3 percent.

Late Stroke Risk After Carotid Endarterectomy in Symptomatic Patients

A review of the literature suggests that patients undergoing successful carotid endarterectomy for the indication of TIA have a subsequent stroke risk for ipsilateral hemispheric stroke at the rate of 1 to 2 percent per year. Patients who have had successful carotid endarterectomies for the indication of prior stroke, without perioperative neurologic complication, continue to be at risk for subsequent ipsilateral stroke at the rate of 2 to 3 percent per year.

Results of Carotid Endarterectomy Based on Review of the Prospective Randomized Trials for Symptomatic Patients

Examination of results of the NASCET study of patients with carotid stenosis of 70 percent or greater demonstrated that carotid endarterectomy reduced the cumulative mortality and stroke risk (including perioperative morbidity and mortality) from an event rate of 26 percent in 2 years in those managed without operation to 9 percent in 2 years in those patients undergoing carotid endarterectomy. Similar findings were also noted in the European trial and in the Veterans Administration symptomatic trial.

Carotid Endarterectomy in Special Circumstances

The consensus group also recognized that there were symptomatic patients who might be considered candidates for carotid endarterectomy who did not fall neatly within the categories of TIA and prior stroke. A special evaluation concerning rationale for surgical management, or lack thereof, was presented for each of these.

Acute Carotid Occlusion

The consensus group stated that most patients who had a neurologic deficit associated with acute carotid occlusion are not candidates for carotid endarterectomy. This was principally due to either the severity of their deficit or a delay in diagnosis. They also noted that a few patients, under unusual circumstances, might benefit from emergency surgery by virtue of proximity to a medical center with documented expertise in the management of cerebrovascular disease. Those patients with a mild neurologic deficit associated with an acute carotid occlusion who have undergone a rapid work-up (within hours of the event) might well benefit from emergency surgery. The consensus group also noted that there were not sufficient data to support or to refute this concept and that this might be an important topic for future study or trial. The suggestion of the consensus group was that currently each case be managed on an individual basis.

Evolving Stroke

The consensus group noted a number of publications suggesting improved prognosis with emergency operation; however, they noted that all of these publications were now more than 10 years old, predating current imaging technology and thus making conclusions in this area at the present time impossible. They also noted that this would be an important area for new investigation.

Combined Carotid-Coronary Surgery

The consensus group examined this topic in detail and concluded that the optimal strategy for the management of patients with combined coronary and carotid disease can only be established by a well-designed prospective randomized trial.

Acute Carotid Dissection

The consensus group concluded that this condition was best treated conservatively. They noted that in rare instances, in which focal ischemic symptoms recurred in spite of adequate anticoagulation, surgery might represent an alternative approach.

Analysis of Surgical Risk

The consensus group emphasized the fact that carotid endarterectomy is a prophylactic operation designed to reduce the risk of subsequent stroke and stroke-related death. Clearly, then, the effectiveness of the operation is directly related to the perioperative risk of performing carotid endarterectomy. They noted that operative risk is affected by several factors, including patient selection, selection of the surgeon, and the institution at which the operation is performed.

In addition to factors that affect the patient's general state of health, the specific indication for carotid endarterectomy also has an effect on perioperative complication rates. Retrospective reviews of the literature clearly indicate that the lowest complication rates occur in asymptomatic patients. There appears to be a slight increase in complication rates when the operation is performed for transient cerebral ischemia, and the highest complication rates occur in patients who have had a prior stroke. This is particularly true if the operation is done for acute stroke or if the patient has a major residual deficit at the time the operation is performed.

It is difficult to get a true expression of 30-day morbidity and mortality because the recorded results are quite variable. The lowest rates occur in individual reported series, and the highest rates are reported when community-based audits are carried out. For example, results of five community-based audits have demonstrated that the percentage of patients disabled or dead following carotid endarterectomy ranges from 4.8 percent to 9 percent. The ad hoc committee of the American Heart Association Stroke Council, when reviewing all available reports, made specific recommendations with respect to upper acceptable limits for stroke morbidity and mortality following carotid endarterectomy. For asymptomatic patients, the upper acceptable risk was 3 percent. For patients in whom the operation was being performed for transient cerebral ischemia, the upper acceptable risk was 5 percent. For those patients who had suffered a prior stroke but had made a reasonable recovery and were scheduled for elective operation, the upper acceptable risk was 7 percent. Finally, for those patients who had recurrent stenosis and indication for operation, the upper acceptable risk was 10 percent.

The consensus committee recommended that an institutionally based, computerized registry of the results of carotid endarterectomies within an individual institution be maintained on an ongoing basis. This would require a periodic audit, and in addition, performance standards should be established within a given hospital. When complication rates exceed acceptable limits, an institutional peer-review committee should investigate. If extenuating circumstances cannot be identified, appropriate corrective action should be carried out. This would range anywhere from careful monitoring of the surgeon's subsequent operative procedures to actual revocation of hospital privileges to perform the procedure.

SYMPTOMATIC PATIENTS: PART II

The second part of the manuscript, dealing with specific indications for carotid endarterectomy, included a major section for symptomatic patients with carotid artery disease. The statement took into account the issue of surgical risk, which includes both the overall risk factors attributable to the patient and the track record of the operating surgeon within a given institution. Thus, two categories of surgical risk were identified: perioperative stroke morbidity and mortality of less than 6 percent, and an increased risk ranging from 6 to 10 percent. Within each of these two risk categories, the indications for surgery in symptomatic patients were divided into four categories: "proven," "acceptable but not proven," "uncertain," and "proven inappropriate."

Indications for Carotid Endarterectomy for Symptomatic Patients With a Surgical Risk of Less Than 6.0 Percent

Proven Indications

- Single or multiple TIAs within a 6-month period, or crescendo TIAs in the presence of a stenosis of 70 percent or greater, with or without ulceration, with or without antiplatelet therapy
- Mild stroke within a 6-month period in the presence of a stenosis of 70 percent or greater, with or without ulceration, with or without antiplatelet therapy

Acceptable But Not Proven Indications

- TIA (single, multiple, or recurrent) within a 6-month period in the presence of a stenosis of 50 percent or greater, with or without ulceration, with or without antiplatelet therapy

- Crescendo TIAs in the presence of a stenosis of more than 50 percent, with or without ulceration, with or without antiplatelet therapy
- Progressive stroke in the presence of a stenosis of 70 percent or greater, with or without ulceration, with or without antiplatelet therapy
- Mild stroke in the presence of a stenosis of 50 percent or greater, with or without ulceration, with or without antiplatelet therapy
- Moderate stroke in the presence of a stenosis of 50 percent or greater, with or without ulceration, with or without antiplatelet therapy
- Ipsilateral carotid endarterectomy combined with coronary artery bypass grafting (CABG) in a patient experiencing TIAs, in the presence of unilateral or bilateral stenoses of 70 percent or greater, CABG needed

Uncertain Indications

- TIA (single, multiple, or recurrent) with stenosis of less than 50 percent, with or without ulceration, with or without antiplatelet therapy
- Crescendo TIAs, with or without ulceration, and a stenosis of less than 50 percent
- TIAs in a patient who requires CABG and has a stenosis of less than 70 percent
- Mild stroke with carotid stenosis of less than 50 percent, with or without antiplatelet therapy
- Moderate stroke with carotid stenosis of less than 69 percent, with or without ulceration, with or without antiplatelet therapy
- Evolving stroke with carotid stenosis of less than 69 percent, with or without ulceration, with or without antiplatelet therapy
- Global ischemic symptoms with ipsilateral carotid stenosis of more than 75 percent but with contralateral stenosis of less than 75 percent, with or without ulceration, with or without antiplatelet therapy
- Acute dissection of internal carotid artery with persistent symptoms while on heparin
- Acute carotid occlusion, diagnosed within 6 hours, producing transient ischemic events
- Acute carotid occlusion, diagnosed within 6 hours, producing a mild stroke

Proven Inappropriate Indications

- Moderate stroke with stenosis of less than 50 percent, with patient not on aspirin
- Evolving stroke with stenosis of less than 50 percent, with patient not on aspirin
- Acute internal carotid artery dissection, asymptomatic, with patient on heparin

Indications for Carotid Endarterectomy in Symptomatic Patients With Surgical Risk of 6 to 10 Percent

Proven Indications

None.

Acceptable But Not Proven Indications

- Single or multiple TIAs, within a 6-month period in the presence of a carotid stenosis of 70 percent or greater, with or without ulceration, with or without antiplatelet therapy
- Recurrent TIAs while the patient is on antiplatelet drugs for a carotid stenosis of 50 percent or greater in the presence of ulceration or of 70 percent with or without ulceration
- Crescendo TIAs with a stenosis of 50 percent or greater with or without ulceration, with or without antiplatelet therapy
- Mild stroke in the presence of a stenosis of more than 70 percent with or without ulceration, with or without antiplatelet therapy
- Moderate stroke with a stenosis of more than 70 percent with or without ulceration, with or without antiplatelet therapy
- Evolving stroke in the presence of a stenosis of more than 70 percent with large ulceration

Uncertain Indications

- Single TIA with stenosis of less than 70 percent with or without ulceration, with or without antiplatelet therapy
- Multiple TIAs within 6 months with stenosis of less than 70 percent without antiplatelet therapy, with or without ulceration
- Recurrent TIAs while on antiplatelet drugs with stenosis of less than 70 percent with or without ulceration
- Crescendo TIAs for stenosis of less than 70 percent with or without ulceration, with or without antiplatelet therapy
- Acute carotid occlusion with transient cerebral ischemia
- Acute occlusion with mild stroke
- Acute carotid artery dissection with continued symptoms while the patient is on heparin
- Transient cerebral ischemia secondary to a stenosis of 70 percent or greater, in need of CABG, with or without contralateral stenosis, use of combined surgical operations
- Mild stroke with stenosis of less than 70 percent with or without ulceration, with or without antiplatelet therapy
- Moderate stroke with stenosis of less than 70 percent, with or without ulceration, with or without antiplatelet therapy
- Evolving stroke with stenosis of less than 70 percent with or without ulceration, with or without antiplatelet therapy
- Global ischemic symptoms with an ipsilateral stenosis of more than 75 percent with or without symptoms, irrespective of contralateral artery status, with lesions up to and including contralateral occlusion

Proven Inappropriate Indications

- Single TIA, less than 50 percent stenosis, with or without ulceration, with patient not on aspirin
- Multiple TIAs within 6 months, stenosis less than 50 percent, with patient not on aspirin
- Mild stroke, stenosis less than 50 percent, with patient not on aspirin
- Moderate stroke, stenosis less than 50 percent, with or without ulceration, with patient not on aspirin

- Evolving stroke, stenosis less than 50 percent, with or without ulceration, with patient not on aspirin
- Global ischemic symptoms with stenosis less than 50 percent, with or without ulceration
- Acute dissection of internal carotid artery, no symptoms while patient is on heparin
- Asymptomatic unilateral carotid stenosis of 70 percent or greater, undergoing CABG

STATEMENT SUMMARY

A consensus conference sponsored by the American Heart Association reviewed the current potential indications for carotid endarterectomy in symptomatic patients. Twenty-two committee members, representing the disciplines of health care policy, neurology, neurosurgery, and vascular surgery, reviewed the current medical literature and ranked the indications for carotid endarterectomy in symptomatic patients. The votes for each indication were averaged and ranked by four categories: proven, acceptable but not proven, uncertain, and proven inappropriate.

From this statement emerges a clear definition of the indications for carotid endarterectomy and the circumstances of surgical risk. This represents the best recommendations by an expert committee at the present time. The statement goes on to say that many indications are the subject of ongoing prospective randomized trials and that, as these trials reach completion, it is likely that recommendations in the document will be subject to change. It was the committee's hope that the document could and should undergo periodic revision.

SUGGESTED READINGS

Moore WS, Barnett HJM, Beebe HG, et al: Guidelines for carotid endarterectomy: A multidisciplinary consensus statement from the ad hoc committee, American Heart Association. *Stroke.* 1995;26:188.

Moore WS, Barnett HJM, Beebe HG, et al: Guidelines for carotid endarterectomy: A multidisciplinary consensus statement from the ad hoc committee, American Heart Association. *Circulation.* 1995;91:566.

VIII

Emergency Surgery of the Carotid Artery

CHAPTER
34

The Natural History and Current Status of Carotid Endarterectomy for Stroke Secondary to Acute Carotid Occlusion

HUGH G. BEEBE

Surgeons who perform carotid endarterectomy in the 1990s may treat hundreds of patients without ever operating on one who has suffered an acute stroke with acute ipsilateral carotid artery occlusion. A recent report of 1734 patients undergoing carotid endarterectomy at Massachusetts General Hospital over a 14-year period included only 5 who were operated on for acute carotid artery occlusion.[1] Many physicians regard such patients as inappropriate candidates for surgery, because of experience accumulated in the early days of carotid surgery. In the 1960s, retrospective analysis of urgent carotid endarterectomy for acute stroke showed poor results, with mortality rates in excess of 20 percent. This was confirmed prospectively.

In the 1990s, it is difficult to recognize the relevance of this older experience because so much has changed: selective catheter angiography, brain imaging, duplex scanning, intensive hospital care, technical surgery, and improved surgical training programs are just a few of the factors having a major impact on carotid surgery results. Thus, a renewed interest in a surgical approach to the occluded carotid artery in patients with acute stroke has recently been expressed. There are three theoretical, but unproven, reasons to perform emergency surgery on acute carotid occlusion: to reverse a neurologic deficit, to restore patency of a major cerebral artery before it becomes irretrievably damaged by post-thrombotic changes, and to prevent further late stroke after recovery from the initial clinical event.

This chapter discusses the natural history of and current status of carotid endarterectomy for acute stroke secondary to acute carotid occlusion by examining six questions:

1. What does the modern literature tell us about the course of a patient with acute carotid occlusion resulting in ischemic stroke who is managed nonoperatively?

2. What was the experience with emergency surgery for acute stroke at the beginning of carotid surgery?

3. What is the recent experience in the application of carotid endarterectomy with modern techniques for acute occlusion with stroke?

4. How do current issues of ischemic penumbra, advances in vascular imaging, and experience with emergency reoperation affect surgical judgement?

5. What recommendations are available from current guidelines?

6. What conclusions can be derived from these data?

NONOPERATIVE MANAGEMENT

Hospital care and modern therapeutics have been sufficiently improved over the past 20 years to make interpretation of the existing literature somewhat problematic. Acute carotid thrombosis may result in a wide spectrum of consequences, ranging from an asymptomatic clinical status to coma and death. The prognosis is dependent on the severity of the initial neurologic deficit.[2] Grillo and Patterson[3] described a 25 percent mortality in 23 patients with completed stroke and carotid occlusion. Meyer and colleagues[4] summarized the natural history of acute carotid occlusion from the literature largely of the 1970s.[5-10] They concluded that 2 to 12 percent of patients will make a good recovery, 40 to 69 percent will be disabled by severe neurologic handicaps, and 6 to 55 percent will die from infarction. More recently, Biller and coworkers[11] studied 29 strokes within 12 hours of onset and found that 24 percent of patients showed spontaneous improvement within the first hour following clinical evaluation and half had improved by 18 hours after the onset of stroke.

Apart from wide variation in the clinical impact of carotid artery occlusion, inconsistency among the available literature compounds the issue. There are great differences in patient selection, methods of assessing carotid occlusion, and retrospective methodology, as well as a lack of serial data and short-term follow-up. An examination of three representative studies illustrates the problem.

In 1974, Dyken and associates[12] from Indiana University described the neurologic outcome in patients selected by angiographic criteria. They reviewed 43 patients with complete occlusion of at least one internal or common carotid artery from a total of 279 patients selected for referral to a cerebrovascular disease research unit. Seventy percent of them had suffered strokes, and 21 of these 30 patients had moderate to severe deficits. The investigators provided a detailed explanation of associated arteriosclerotic disease in the remaining three major extracranial vessels at the time of the patients' entry into the study. Unfortunately, no subsequent anatomic data during follow-up were obtained. Eleven percent of the patients had further neurologic symptoms in 17 months. Patients with internal carotid and common carotid artery occlusions were not separately analyzed. Moreover, the time from the onset of stroke to entry into the study was not reported. This illustrates a retrospective study based on anatomic data in a highly selected referral population.

In 1983, Cote and coworkers[13] offered a prospective study of internal carotid artery occlusion in 47 patients with only mild neurologic deficits or none at all. These patients were followed for an average of 34 months. All patients were identified by angiography to have an occlusion of the internal carotid artery and were a subset of patients in the Canadian cooperative study on platelet inhibitory drugs. The stroke rate distal to an occluded internal carotid artery was 5 percent per year. However, 24 patients (51%) continued to experience transient ischemic attacks (TIAs) in the territory of the occluded internal carotid artery, despite the fact that at least half of them were treated with aspirin. Although this study has the advantages of being prospective in nature, having adequate follow-up, and obtaining high-quality anatomic information at the time of study entry, it selected only those patients with minimal clinical neurologic problems and did not provide serial anatomic data during the follow-up interval.

In 1986, Nicholls and colleagues[14] reported their observations in 24 patients who were followed with serial duplex scans as their internal carotid artery stenosis progressed to unilateral occlusion. Four (16%) had TIA symptoms, six (25%) had clinical strokes, and 13 (54%) had no observed clinical symptoms resulting from the occlusion. During the 24-month postocclusion interval, nearly one out of four had further neurologic symptoms that did not correlate with the status of the contralateral artery. These observations illustrate the value of a prospective study that acquires serial anatomic data for both the ipsilateral artery and the contralateral major vessels in correlating clinical data and neurologic examination.

In summary, it can be concluded that an attempt to use historical controls for the evaluation of modern intervention in the management of acute stroke is difficult to the point of impossibility—not to mention the doubtful nature of historical controls in the first place.

It can also be concluded that a severe deficit at the outset of stroke from internal carotid artery occlusion carries a poor prognosis, and the clinical result is not predictable from the status of the remaining extracranial vessels.

EARLY SURGICAL EXPERIENCE

After reviewing the experience and lessons learned during the 1960s, three giants in the field emphatically advised against operations on the carotid artery for acute stroke. William S. Fields, a University of Texas neurologist, was the principal organizer of the Joint Study of Extracranial Arterial Occlusion, which was the best source of information about carotid artery disease management based on prospective and partially randomized data. Fields summarized the lessons learned from observing more than 5000 patients and stated:

A surgical mortality of 50% can be anticipated in patients with recent or acute occlusion of the internal carotid artery with any neurologic deficit if operation is performed during the acute phase of the illness. A significantly higher percentage of such patients will recover with medical treatment.[15]

Several years earlier, Charles G. Rob, whose 1954 report of a successful carotid artery reconstruction had popularized carotid surgery, summarized a dismal experience with urgent carotid endarterectomy for acute completed stroke due to thrombosis of the internal carotid artery.[16] He reported that of 74 patients operated on, 29 percent died, 43 percent were unchanged, and only 28 percent derived any benefit from the procedure. He concluded: "Our results with emergency operations for patients with acute occlusions of the carotid artery causing either progressing or completed strokes have been so bad that we no longer recommend such procedures."

Another major figure with worldwide influence, Edwin J. Wylie of the University of California–San Francisco, sounded a warning in 1964 that intracranial hemorrhage may follow surgical revascularization for the treatment of acute stroke.[17] He and his colleagues reported on nine patients who had urgent operations after acute strokes with varying degrees of neurologic residual. Five of these nine patients died from cerebral hemorrhage.

Taken together, these reports exerted a powerful influence that has persisted as a warning against surgery for acute stroke. It was powerful because an easily understood theoretical pathophysiology could account for the usually delayed postoperative bleeding that resulted in neurologic deterioration or death. The availability of computed tomography (CT) and better means of controlling blood pressure now makes this observation less clearly relevant than it was 25 years ago.

A number of other reports contain variations on this same theme. DeWeese and colleagues[18, 19] reported that of 16 patients operated on within 24 hours of the onset of a completed stroke, eight worsened and seven died. The joint study data reported in 1969 by Blaisdell and coworkers[20] described a 42 percent mortality for operations on totally occluded carotid arteries during acute stroke. Others reported similarly bad outcomes.[21]

Not all reports of surgical management of totally occluded internal carotid arteries were so negative. In 1981, Hafner and Tew[22] described 47 operations for total occlusion of the internal carotid artery. Only 21 percent of these patients had fixed neurologic deficits, but all were described as having classical symptoms of cerebral ischemia. Twelve patients (25%) were operated on less than 1 week after the onset of symptoms. Although the method of reporting makes evaluation of the results difficult, two observations seem particularly important: there were no operative deaths and no neurologic worsening. Also, postoperative arterial patency was assessed by angiography or noninvasive laboratory tests and found to vary as a function of duration of carotid occlusion, as judged by symptoms. Those operated on within 1 week had a 100 percent patency rate, but only 50 percent of arteries operated on 1 month after the onset of symptoms remained open postoperatively.

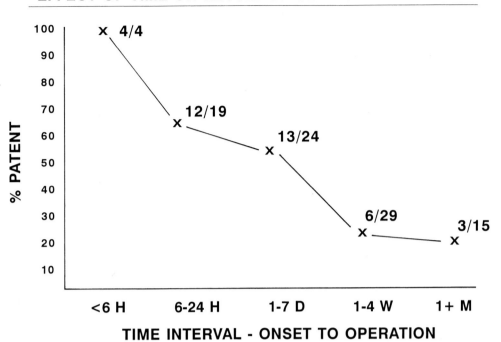

FIGURE 34–1. Graph depicting the decline in immediate postoperative patency with increasing time interval between the onset of symptoms and surgery. D, days; H, hours; M, months; W, weeks. (Modified from Thompson JE, Austin DJ, Patman RD: Endarterectomy of the totally occluded carotid artery for stroke. *Arch Surg.* 1967;95:791; with permission.)

The importance of urgency has been strongly suggested by the observations of two groups that have made major contributions to the understanding of cerebrovascular disease. In 1967, Thompson and associates[23] from Dallas, Texas, reported on the results of 100 operations on totally occluded carotid arteries. Overall, cerebral blood flow was restored by endarterectomy in 39 arteries, but the best anatomic results were clearly obtained in patients operated on within 6 to 12 hours of onset (Fig. 34–1). Occlusions of 2 weeks' duration or more were seldom successfully repaired.

Najafi and colleagues[24] from Chicago described their experience in 53 patients undergoing emergency carotid thromboendarterectomy. Twenty-five of these patients had spontaneous stroke or stroke immediately associated with cerebral angiography. Approximately 50 percent of their patients in this category were improved postoperatively—which is no different from some reports of the natural history of acute carotid thrombosis. No neurologic score was described, and there was no mention of postoperative hemorrhage, but there was a 12 percent associated mortality. The clear implication of this study, as interpreted by the authors, was:

In relation to spontaneous stroke, the most important factor in aiding the selection of patients for or against surgery is the interval between the onset of stroke and the diagnosis of internal carotid occlusion. The general experience indicates that patients with acute stroke of a few hours' duration or longer are not candidates for emergency thromboendarterectomy.

They also concluded that operation was contraindicated in patients with major cerebral deficits such as fixed hemiplegia.

A similar sense of urgency was expressed by Ojemann and associates,[25] whose 1975 study of 21 patients with acute stroke and carotid occlusion reported marked postsurgical improvement in 8 (38%) and death in 3 (14%). They emphasized the importance of expediency but had no control group by which to assess the results of the surgical approach.

The occurrence of postoperative hemorrhage is not unique to operations for acute stroke or on occluded arteries. Massive intracerebral hemorrhage has been described following carotid endarterectomy in patients who were neurologically stable at the time of operation, free of recent symptoms, and being treated for stenosis rather than complete occlusion. Hafner and colleagues[26] documented 10 such patients in 1987 who were studied with modern imaging techniques and suggested that postoperative systemic hypertension was probably a causally related factor.

The net result from these early recorded experiences with urgent surgery was negative. They left the impression that the risk of bleeding into revascularized areas of infarction after emergency surgery for acute stroke with carotid thrombosis was greater than the benefit to the ischemic penumbra.

RECENT SURGICAL EXPERIENCE

Meyer and colleagues at the Mayo Clinic analyzed the experience with 34 patients with acute internal carotid artery occlusion and stroke who underwent emergency revascularization.[4] All patients had profound neurologic deficits preoperatively, including hemiplegia and aphasia. In 94 percent, patency restored. Thirteen patients (38%) made a dramatic recovery, and seven (20%) died.

Several features of this interesting report deserve examination. Despite an emphasis on the concept of reversible ischemia as the basis for urgent endarterectomy, there was no correlation between clinical result and time of ischemia up to 8 to 12 hours. Furthermore, 33 of these 34 patients were already hospitalized with cerebrovascular diagnoses prior to events that prompted consideration of emergency surgery. In nine patients, occlusion occurred within 1 hour of cerebral angiography, and in five patients, acute neurologic change was observed following carotid endarterectomy. Only 15 patients had preoperative angiography in this series. In the majority, the diagnosis of acute carotid occlusion was made clinically. Although many operations were performed after 6 hours, only two of the seven deaths were attributed to hemorrhagic infarction, and in both of those patients the operations were done within 6 hours or less. Balloon catheter thrombectomy was employed in 10 cases; in one patient, distal internal carotid artery damage caused an unsuccessful operation. Furthermore, three cases of documented middle cerebral artery embolus occurred when balloon catheter thrombectomy was employed.

In their analysis, these authors recommended complete angiography prior to surgical intervention, accepting the inherent delay and risk of angiography in association with cerebral ischemia. An exception to this recommendation would be patients with carotid occlusion following endarterectomy. They also stated that their inability to show a correlation between outcome and duration of carotid artery occlusion reflected the complexity of factors involved in cerebral ischemia and infarction.

In 1987, Walters and colleagues[27] from Massachusetts General Hospital included 16 patients with complete internal carotid artery occlusion in a series of 64 emergency carotid endarterectomies. Nine patients (56%) were improved, but it was not possible to correlate preoperative clinical symptoms and the timing of carotid endarterectomy. At least four of 16 (25%) had mild persistent deficits before operation. In the selection of patients for emergency carotid endarterectomy, the level of consciousness and severity of preoperative deficit were weighed. A significantly reduced level of consciousness was a contraindication to surgical treatment.

The most recent description of emergency thromboendarterectomy for symptomatic occluded internal carotid artery is the 1992 report by McCormick and colleagues.[28] In operations on 42 patients—12 of whom had acute new strokes—57 percent of occluded internal carotid arteries were successfully reopened. There were no postoperative deaths in this series. There was no outcome difference between patients with restored patency of the internal carotid artery, and those in whom patency was not restored. Interestingly, no patient in either group had a subsequent stroke during a mean follow-up of 40 months, and the rate of TIA for both groups was comparable to that expected from the natural history of similar patients treated nonoperatively. Little information was given about preoperative neurologic status in this series, but the authors considered profound neurologic deficit a contraindication to operation (Table 34–1).

Welling and colleagues reported on surgical therapy for recent total occlusion of the internal carotid artery in 24 patients.[29] The timing of operation was not clearly stated, but serial duplex scanning was performed postoperatively, establishing the anatomic result. Fifteen of 24 patients (63%) had internal carotid artery patency restored. On serial duplex follow-up at least 45 days postoperatively, four of these 15 (26%) were found to have occluded arteries. This is consistent with other observations relating patency rate to duration of occlusion. For example, Kusunoki and colleagues[30] achieved an 86 percent patency rate for thromboendarterectomy of totally occluded internal carotid arteries when performed within 72 hours of the occlusion, but only a 46 percent patency for those performed after 72 hours.

Sannella[31] described an innovative approach in 1992—treating acute stroke with ipsilateral carotid occlusion by immediate repair of contralateral, hemodynamically significant stenosis when found on arteriography. All 13 patients described had stroke, but not severe deficits, and positive CT scans. They underwent contralateral endarterectomy within 2 to 10 days following the onset of symptoms. Most patients in this series had bilateral stenosis, but four had complete occlusion of the ipsilateral carotid artery. There was no mortality and no postoperative worsening of neurologic status. Detailed neurologic evaluation with appropriate scoring before and after operation was lacking from this report, but gradual neurologic improvement was the general observation during an average follow-up interval of 41 months.

THE CONCEPT OF ISCHEMIC PENUMBRA

Experimental evidence of the existence of reversible ischemia has been provided, suggesting that cerebral tissue should not be regarded as suffering all or no infarction within minutes of vascular occlusion. Tolerance of brain tissue to relative ischemia as determined by collateral flow may provide an opportunity for therapeutic intervention to reverse the ischemic process. Experimental studies in primate models support the notion that 6 hours of ischemia can be reversed without infarction, although there is a risk of subsequent hemorrhage.[32-34] Thus, the term "ischemic penumbra" means neuronal electrical dysfunction, separable from cellular death, resulting from oligemia.

Clinical correlation of this evidence is perhaps most strongly suggested by the experience of emergency middle cerebral or carotid bifurcation embolectomy. Rob[16] called attention to the distinction between spontaneous internal carotid artery thrombosis and an embolus from cardiac origin in 1969. More recently, Meyer and coworkers[35] found that 7 of 20 patients (35%) undergoing emergency middle cerebral artery embolectomy made a dramatic recovery after restora-

Study*	Patients, n	Deficit	Patent Artery, n (%)	Improved, n (%)	Died, n (%)
Meyer et al[4]	34	Severe	32 (94)	13 (38)	7 (20)
Walters et al[27]	16	Mild	16 (100)	9 (56)	1 (6)
McCormick et al[28]	12	Unknown	7 (57)	Unknown	0

TABLE 34–1. Results of Carotid Endarterectomy for Acute Stroke

*For full bibliographic information, see reference list at end of chapter.

tion of flow. This, they believed, supported the concept of reversible ischemic neuronal damage.

An interesting case report illustrates the pathophysiology of the ischemic penumbra concept. McKenzie and colleagues[36] described a patient with a dense hemiplegia, hemisensory loss, gaze disturbance, and hemineglect associated with an impaired level of consciousness. Serial CT scans over 4 days showed no evidence of infarction. Angiography revealed a preocclusive stenosis of the right internal carotid artery with sluggish antegrade flow. After 4 days of persistent dense neurologic deficit, carotid endarterectomy was performed, resulting in improvement within hours of the operation. All neurologic deficit was gone within 3 days.

The recently accumulated experience with thrombolytic therapy is also of interest.[37, 38] An analysis of the safety and efficacy issues surrounding this treatment of acute carotid artery occlusion with stroke is beyond the scope of this chapter. But if such treatment is successful in restoring internal carotid artery patency, and presumably preserving viability and function of some tissue with reversible ischemic injury, the majority of such patients may be found to have an underlying hemodynamically significant stenosis at the origin of the extracranial internal carotid artery. Thus, the extent to which modern thrombolytic therapy is successful will affect the role and timing of carotid endarterectomy in a way not previously experienced. The combination of these two treatments is unfamiliar territory, as evidenced by an examination of the incidence of hemorrhagic infarction associated with successful thrombolysis in acute stroke. Hemorrhagic infarction without clinical deterioration has been detected by follow-up CT in as many as 28 percent of patients.[39] The effect of carotid endarterectomy on such a condition following thrombolysis is unknown.

THE ACCURACY OF MODERN IMAGING

If any emergency surgical treatment of the thrombosed internal carotid artery with acute stroke is truly beneficial, theoretical considerations and the burden of anecdotal clinical evidence strongly suggest that time is of the essence in achieving the best clinical outcome. Therefore, a protocol for assessing a patient's candidacy for emergency surgery should focus on tests that can be done rapidly and yield maximum critical information. Presently, CT scanning of the brain and duplex ultrasound examination of the extracranial carotid artery system appear to be the first line of investigation. It is also theoretically possible that these two tests, taken together, could provide sufficient information for surgical decision making without other more elaborate and riskier procedures, such as angiography. Recently published standards for cerebrovascular noninvasive testing do not mention criteria for establishing the diagnosis of carotid artery occlusion.[40] Transcranial Doppler may be useful as an adjunct to cervical duplex scanning. Giller and associates[41] observed middle cerebral artery velocity changes associated with clinical carotid artery thrombosis occurring at a known time. The accuracy of duplex scanning for establishing the presence of carotid occlusion has varied between 93 and 100 percent. Maiuri and colleagues[42] reported a 95 percent sensitivity in cases confirmed by angiography in a study of

70 patients with complete occlusion of the internal carotid artery.

Apparently, not all internal carotid artery occlusions remain static, however. For example, occasional cases of spontaneous recanalization with restoration of flow have been described.[43] Combe and colleagues[44] in France documented that four of six patients with acute stroke and angiographically observed free-floating clots in the extracranial internal carotid artery demonstrated complete clot lysis after treatment with heparin anticoagulation alone.

Computed tomography of the brain within only a few hours of an acute neurologic deficit cannot be expected to define the full extent of infarction. In the context of emergency surgery for acute stroke, CT scanning has its greatest value in ruling out other conditions such as intracranial hemorrhage or associated mass lesions. Although CT scanning may show early abnormality within 3 hours of the onset of ischemic symptoms, more characteristically, low-density changes are seen between 1 and 3 days following stroke. Still, about half of CT scans done within 3 days after the development of a neurologic deficit do not show areas of cerebral infarction. Inoue and colleagues[45] showed that 25 of 132 patients (19%) with neurologic deficits and normal initial CT scans demonstrated areas of infarction on subsequent scans enhanced by contrast medium injection. It is believed that infarcts that demonstrate early contrast enhancement are apt to be embolic because of early reperfusion, which is not present as often when infarcts are caused by in situ thrombosis.

Dosick and colleagues[46] observed that 171 of 245 patients (70%) with mild to moderate neurologic deficits had negative CT scans on the first day of symptoms. These remained negative when rescanned at 5 days. Of the 30 percent with positive scans, most were detected on the first examination, and only 15 percent at a later time with or without enhancement by contrast injection.

Illustrative Case Report

A 72-year-old man had sudden onset of right hemiparesis and expressive aphasia. He was hospitalized and seen by a neurologist. A CT scan of the brain showed some mild atrophic change but was otherwise normal. On the second hospital day, his neurologic signs were markedly improved; there was only mild weakness of the right hand, and fluent speech returned. A carotid duplex ultrasound examination was performed, which showed that the arterial velocity (systolic/diastolic, measured in centimeters per second) was as follows: right common carotid, 81/11; left common carotid, 53/12; right internal 162/42; and left internal carotid 270/160. B-mode imaging also showed changes consistent with a greater than 90 percent stenosis in the left internal carotid artery.

On the third hospital day, a repeat CT scan of the brain with contrast showed slight low density in the left middle cerebral artery distribution. Vascular surgery consultation was obtained, and an arteriogram was done. This showed complete occlusion of the left internal carotid artery, with filling via ophthalmic branches of the right middle cerebral artery. There was mild stenosis of the right carotid bifurcation (Fig. 34–2A). No operation was performed.

The patient remained hospitalized for the next 20 days

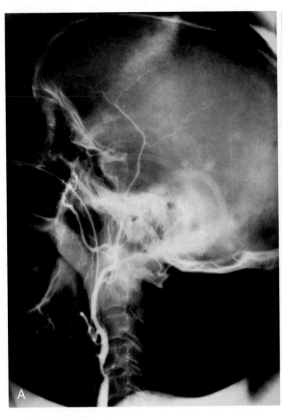
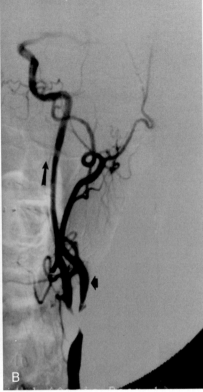

FIGURE 34–2. *A,* Selective left carotid arteriogram performed on the third hospital day, demonstrating thrombosis of the internal carotid artery. Duplex scan evidence obtained 18 hours previously had shown a patent but tightly stenotic artery. *B,* Selective carotid arteriogram repeated on the 23rd hospital day shows a patent left internal carotid artery *(arrows)* with a typical very tight stenosis at its origin.

for abdominal pain, which was thought to be caused by diverticulitis of the sigmoid colon and other problems. His neurologic status was stable and remained improved, though persistent mild right hand weakness was noted.

When his abdominal complaints resolved and he was nearly ready for discharge, he suddenly developed right hemiparesis and aphasia again. A carotid duplex scan was repeated, with an identical interpretation of a patent but severely stenotic left internal carotid artery. On the same day, within several hours, repeat vascular surgery consultation was obtained. Repeat cerebral angiography now showed a patent left internal carotid artery with 99 percent stenosis at its origin and possibly a small amount of adjacent thrombus. The intracranial vessels were visualized, and no occlusion was seen (see Fig. 34–2B). An emergency carotid endarterectomy was performed immediately.

The pathologic specimen showed a severe but typical carotid atheroma, and there was no operative evidence of thrombosis. The patient made a good recovery, and his neurologic deficit resolved within several hours after surgery. A third CT scan of the brain was obtained on the third postoperative day and showed no evidence of infarction or hemorrhage. He was discharged on the fourth postoperative day.

This unusual case illustrates some of the most difficult issues in considering emergency carotid endarterectomy for stroke with carotid occlusion. What is the most reliable method of assessing whether complete occlusion is present? How should the initial neurologic event be classified—as stroke, reversible ischemic neurologic deficit, or possibly TIA if the mild right-hand weakness were missed? Should left carotid thromboendarterectomy have been done on the second day? Did the artery thrombose and then recanalize?

Since the second neurologic event was a right hemiparesis that persisted until the time of emergency surgery within 6 hours of onset, how should the second neurologic event be classified?

ACUTE CAROTID OCCLUSION AND NEUROLOGIC DEFICIT FOLLOWING CAROTID ENDARTERECTOMY

In a sense, the purest model for examining the effect of ischemia duration on neurologic deficit recovery is acute carotid occlusion and neurologic deficit following carotid endarterectomy. This is particularly true if one focuses on those patients who are observed to be neurologically intact following carotid endarterectomy and who subsequently develop an acute neurologic deficit referable to the ipsilateral hemisphere during the early postoperative period. Koslow and colleagues[47] reviewed 22 patients with perioperative stroke and carotid thrombosis. Seventeen were promptly reexplored; of those, 13 (76%) were improved during a 30-day follow-up interval. Only one of five patients with acute stroke and carotid thrombosis treated nonoperatively had a similar result. Similar advice has been offered by Imparato,[48] who stressed the importance of controlling systemic blood pressure, and by others.[49–51] The anecdotal experiences collected in the literature strongly suggest that speed in accomplishing reoperation to restore carotid patency is important.

RECOMMENDATIONS FROM CURRENT GUIDELINES

A recent summary of recommendations for the management of ischemic stroke includes a wide variety of therapeutic options that may be urgently pursued: thrombolytic therapy, calcium channel antagonists, heparin anticoagulation, and at least eight other medical therapies for ischemic stroke.[52] Emergency carotid surgery is conspicuously absent from consideration in that review.

Conversely, Brown and Humphrey[53] discuss carotid endarterectomy and recommendations for the management of various conditions, including ischemic stroke. There is no mention of acute stroke as an indication for emergency carotid endarterectomy in their review.

Perhaps the decade of the 1990s will be known at some future time as the Decade of Guidelines. There is certainly a proliferation of them, and carotid endarterectomy has received a full measure of attention because the operation is extremely common, significantly expensive, and, until recently, not fully accepted as being of proven value. Four sets of guidelines for carotid endarterectomy have recently been promulgated.

In 1990, the Agency for Healthcare Policy and Research (AHCPR) published a health technology assessment report entitled "Carotid Endarterectomy."[54] This federal document, released under the auspices of the U.S. Public Health Service, was formulated on the basis of a literature review that included 130 references analyzed without direct participation by neurologists or vascular surgeons. There is little mention of acute symptoms and carotid artery occlusion, except for a summary of the opinion of the American Association of Neurological Surgeons and the Congress of Neurological Surgeons, whose list of indications for carotid endarterectomy included acute cerebral ischemia due to acute carotid artery occlusion (this was accompanied by the recommendation for individualized therapeutic decisions in such patients). The AHCPR report also quotes the University of California–Los Angeles Section of Vascular Surgery as offering the opinion that outcome comparisons of carotid endarterectomy versus medical management of symptomatic patients with carotid artery occlusion do not clarify whether carotid endarterectomy has any significant beneficial effect. These two opinions were essentially the only mention of acute stroke treated by emergency carotid thromboendarterectomy in the AHCPR guidelines.

In 1988, the Rand Corporation of Santa Monica, California, published an analysis of the appropriateness of carotid endarterectomy by a two-step process.[55] First, a literature review was used to develop a list of 864 possible indications for performing carotid endarterectomy. Then a panel of nationally known experts in the field rated the appropriateness of each indication. On the basis of this expert panel's ratings, the appropriateness of carotid endarterectomy in a random sample of 1302 Medicare patients having carotid endarterectomy 7 years previously in three different geographic areas was examined. This study noted that 7 percent of TIA patients (defined as having neurologic symptoms up to but not beyond 24 hours) underwent carotid surgery of one sort or another for an occluded artery. These were deemed inappropriate.

That report was sufficiently controversial that the Rand Corporation reexamined carotid endarterectomy, this time in association with the Academic Medical Center Consortium and the American Medical Association. The second guideline document, published in 1992, separately reported appropriateness ratings and necessity ratings judged by a panel

of nine experts, including neurologists, neurosurgeons, and vascular surgeons.[56]

In the appropriateness rating scores, several clinical scenarios were relevant, either directly or indirectly, to the role of carotid endarterectomy in acute stroke with carotid artery occlusion. For example, the panel was in agreement that a single episode of carotid TIA and an acutely occluded ipsilateral carotid artery was a moderately strong indication for operation. No comment was made about the timing of the surgical procedure or brain imaging in that evaluation. However, when identical symptoms were associated with only an occluded ipsilateral carotid artery, there was agreement that operation was not indicated with or without magnetic resonance evidence of brain infarction. Presumably, the implication was that this was a chronic occlusion of the ipsilateral carotid artery. Similarly, surgery for multiple episodes of carotid TIA associated with an acutely occluded ipsilateral carotid artery was judged to be strongly indicated, regardless of the application of medical therapy. Although the question of the timing of surgery was not specifically addressed in this evaluation, it was implied that urgent operation was judged appropriate for an acutely occluded ipsilateral artery because of the judgment that operation was strongly indicated for acutely occluded arteries but strongly contraindicated for chronically occluded arteries.

The appropriateness of carotid endarterectomy for atherothrombotic stroke associated with an acutely occluded ipsilateral artery of less than 6 hours' duration was judged indeterminate by the panel, with a weakly positive appropriateness score. If the ipsilateral occluded artery was of 6 hours' duration or greater, however, there was agreement that operation was extremely inappropriate.

The second Rand study then went on to consider the matter of necessity. No operation on an acutely occluded carotid artery for any of the clinical indications was judged to be necessary.

In 1993, the National Stroke Association issued a consensus statement on emergency evaluation and treatment that was sponsored by major neurology and neurosurgical specialty societies and the National Institute of Neurological Disorders and Stroke.[57] In that privately published document, the following consensus guideline was presented:

For the patient who arrives with a continuing neurological deficit due to cerebral ischemia, evidence of the efficacy of immediate surgical removal of obstruction is controversial and unproven. Over the past decade, emergency endarterectomy has been performed in a sizeable number of patients to remove obstruction or open an arterial occlusion but without support of efficacy from carefully controlled randomized studies. Consideration of urgent carotid endarterectomy for recent ischemic stroke generally is limited to conscious patients with: (1) stroke in evolution who have a minimal fixed neurological deficit, or (2) a moderately severe neurological deficit of abrupt onset when surgery can be completed within the first few hours after the onset of deficit. This usually means that patients are only considered for surgery when the deficit has occurred while the patient is in a hospital where expert facilities are available for rapid diagnosis and treatment. However, there is no firm data to mandate this approach.

An ad hoc committee of the Joint Council of the Society for Vascular Surgery and the North American Chapter of the International Society for Cardiovascular Surgery published practice guidelines for carotid endarterectomy in 1992.[58] This multidisciplinary panel, which included representatives from neurology, neurosurgery, and vascular surgery, considered the matter of acute stroke and surgical intervention. Acute stroke was defined as an acute neurologic deficit lasting longer than 24 hours. In advising on appropriate patient evaluation, the panel found that time was the primary determinant:

If the patient reaches the hospital emergency department within an hour of the event or if the patient happens to have been in the hospital for an unrelated problem at the time the event occurs, the patient may be considered a candidate for emergency intervention.

Emergency duplex scanning and either CT or magnetic resonance imaging of the head were recommended. The panel expressed ambivalence about whether the time required to obtain angiography yielded information that made it worthwhile to prolong the preoperative ischemic duration. Medical management of patients with mild to moderate neurologic deficit was recommended as resulting in "quite satisfactory" outcomes. Regarding surgical intervention, these guidelines stated:

Acute stroke has been considered a contraindication to carotid endarterectomy . . . [because] instability of the patient may yield an increased mortality rate as well as the risk of acute reperfusion of an area of infarcted brain that may produce hemorrhage within the substance of the infarct.

Although acknowledging that anecdotal reports of small series of patients have described dramatic recovery after restoration of blood flow in an acutely occluded artery, there was no good control population by which to evaluate these results. The panel concluded, "Until a prospective randomized trial is carried out to compare the results of medical and surgical management, this will remain an unanswered question." Its conclusion was that acute stroke should be considered a contraindication to carotid endarterectomy, with possible exceptions in individual circumstances.

CONCLUSIONS

Consideration of the role of carotid endarterectomy in acute stroke with acute carotid artery thrombosis is a prime example of how difficult it is to make clinical management decisions on the basis of imperfect data. Anecdotal, retrospective, and largely superficial evaluation of dissimilar, selected patient groups has certainly proved that enormous variations between patients and therapeutic approaches exist. Because of the lack of appropriate, contemporaneous controls, it is not possible to conclude that surgical intervention is generally more beneficial than nonsurgical treatment. However, those who have personally observed the dramatic reversal of profound neurologic deficit that occasionally occurs immediately following successful carotid thromboendarterectomy of a completely occluded artery are entitled to conclude that there was a causal relationship. The issue is complex, and available literature is heterogeneous.

Another conclusion seems to be generally supported by the information at hand: if surgery is to be pursued, it should be accomplished as rapidly as possible, because the duration of ischemia is one of the factors that appears to influence outcome. If this is so, it raises two important issues that

need to be resolved before progress can be made in acquiring evidence by which to judge the role of emergency carotid thromboendarterectomy: First, the definition of TIA has traditionally included an arbitrary time interval of 24 hours. Thus, emergency operations done within less than 6 hours will necessarily preclude assigning patients to traditional TIA versus stroke categories. Second, current imaging methods do not permit distinguishing between acute and chronic arterial occlusion on the basis of depiction of anatomic structures. These two factors taken together make it likely that a prospective trial to evaluate emergency carotid thromboendarterectomy for stroke would necessarily include a heterogeneous population that could not be distinguished preoperatively or postoperatively. Chronic occlusions could be identified at operation, but this would mean that the surgical arm of such a trial would include patients who would not be expected to benefit from the treatment. The surgical arm would also include patients whose symptoms might have cleared fully within 24 hours if an operation had not been performed at all. A prospective randomized trial would also need to confront the enormous problem of controlling for the effect on outcome of the status of the collateral circulation provided by other major extracranial vessels.

In general, the present burden of evidence weighs heavily against operation for acute stroke with carotid artery occlusion. Two individual exceptions to this rule seem warranted:

1. A patient who develops a postoperative neurologic deficit after a normal interval following carotid endarterectomy should be considered for immediate return to the operating room.

2. Institutions with a demonstrated high level of expertise in managing cerebrovascular disease provide the setting for occasional emergency operations on patients whose carotid anatomy has been defined previously and who develop sudden neurologic deterioration while under observation in that setting. Even then, it should be noted that the benefit of surgical therapy has not been proved to exceed that offered by nonoperative treatment.

REFERENCES

1. Gertler JP, Blankenstejn J, Brewster DC, et al: Carotid endarterectomy in neurologically unstable patients: Do results justify an aggressive approach? (abstract). J Vasc Surg. 1993;17:1115.
2. Hachinski V, Norris JW: The Acute Stroke. Philadelphia: F. Davis; 1985.
3. Grillo P, Patterson RH: Occlusion of the carotid artery, prognosis (natural history) and the possibilities of surgical revascularization. Stroke. 1975;6:17.
4. Meyer FB, Piepgras DG, Sandok BA, et al: Emergency carotid endarterectomy for patients with acute carotid occlusion and profound neurological deficits. Ann Surg. 1986;203:82.
5. McDowell FH, Potes J, Groch S: The natural history of internal carotid and vertebral-basilar artery occlusion. Neurology (Minn). 1961;11:153.
6. Millikan CH: Clinical management of cerebral ischemia. In McDowell FH, Brennan RW, eds. Cerebral Vascular Disease, Eighth Conference. New York: Grune & Stratton; 1973:209.
7. Jones HR, Millikan CH: Temporal profile (clinical course) of acute carotid system cerebral infarction. Stroke. 1976;7:64.
8. Grillo P, Patterson RH: Occlusion of the carotid artery, prognosis (natural history), and the possibilities of surgical revascularization. Stroke. 1975;6:17.
9. Oxbury JM, Greenhall RC, Grainger KN: Predicting the outcome of stroke: Acute stage after cerebral infarction. Br Med J. 1975;3:125.
10. Norrving B, Nilsson B: Carotid artery occlusion: Acute symptoms and long term prognosis. Neurol Res. 1981;3:229.
11. Biller J, Love BB, Marsh EE, et al: Spontaneous improvement after acute ischemic stroke: A pilot study. Stroke. 1988;19:1216.
12. Dyken ML, Klatte E, Kolar OJ, et al: Complete occlusion of common or internal carotid arteries. Arch Neurol. 1974;30:343.

13. Cote R, Barnett HJM, Taylor DW: Internal carotid occlusion: A prospective study. *Stroke.* 1983;14:898.
14. Nicholls SC, Kohler TR, Bergelin RO, et al: Carotid artery occlusion: Natural history. *J Vasc Surg.* 1986;4:479.
15. Fields WS: Selection of stroke patients for arterial reconstructive surgery. *Am J Surg.* 1973;125:527.
16. Rob CG: Operation for acute completed stroke due to thrombosis of the internal carotid artery. *Surgery.* 1969;65:862.
17. Wylie EJ, Hein MF, Adams JE: Intracranial hemorrhage following surgical revascularization for treatment of acute strokes. *J Neurosurg.* 1964;21:212.
18. DeWeese JA, Rob CG, Satran R, et al: Endarterectomy for atherosclerotic lesions of the carotid artery. *J Cardiovasc Surg.* 1971;12:299.
19. DeWeese JA: Management of acute strokes. *Surg Clin North Am.* 1982;62:467.
20. Blaisdell WF, Clauss RH, Galbraith JG, et al: Joint study of extracranial arterial occlusion. *JAMA.* 1969;209:1889.
21. Bruetman ME, Fields WS, Crawford ES, et al: Cerebral hemorrhage in carotid artery surgery. *Arch Neurol.* 1963;9:458.
22. Hafner CD, Tew JM: Surgical management of the totally occluded internal carotid artery: A ten-year study. *Surgery.* 1981;89:710.
23. Thompson JE, Austin DJ, Patman RD: Endarterectomy of the totally occluded carotid artery for stroke. *Arch Surg.* 1967;95:791.
24. Najafi H, Javid H, Dye WS, et al: Emergency carotid thrombendarterectomy. *Arch Surg.* 1971;103:610.
25. Ojemann RG, Crowell RM, Roberson GH, et al: Surgical treatment of extracranial carotid occlusive disease. *Clin Neurosurg.* 1975;22:214.
26. Hafner DH, Smith RB III, King OW, et al: Massive intracerebral hemorrhage following carotid endarterectomy. *Arch Surg.* 1987;122:305.
27. Walters BB, Ojemann RG, Heros RC: Emergency carotid endarterectomy. *J Neurosurg.* 1987;66:817.
28. McCormick PW, Spetzler RF, Bailes JE, et al: Thromboendarterectomy of the symptomatic occluded internal carotid artery. *J Neurosurg.* 1992;76:752.
29. Welling RE, Cranley JJ, Krause RJ, et al: Surgical therapy for recent total occlusion of the internal carotid artery. *J Vasc Surg.* 1984;1:57.
30. Kusunoki T, Rowed DW, Tator CD, et al: Thromboendarterectomy for total occlusion of the internal carotid artery: A reappraisal of risks, success rate, and potential benefits. *Stroke.* 1978;9:34.
31. Sannella NA: Bilateral severe carotid stenosis or occlusion and computed tomographic scan positive hemispheric stroke with neurologic deficit: Immediate contralateral carotid endarterectomy. *Ann Vasc Surg.* 1992;6:252.
32. Sundt TM Jr, Grant WC, Garcia HJ: Restoration of middle cerebral artery flow in experimental infarction. *J Neurosurg.* 1969;31:311.
33. Watanabe O, Bremer AM, West LR: Experimental regional cerebral ischemia in the middle cerebral artery territory in primates. Part 1. Angioanatomy and description of an experimental model with selective embolization of the ICA bifurcation. *Stroke.* 1977;8:61.
34. Morawetz RB, DeGirolami V, Ojemman RG, et al: Cerebral blood flow determined by hydrogen clearance during middle cerebral artery occlusion in unanesthetized monkeys. *Stroke.* 1978;9:143.
35. Meyer FB, Piepgras DG, Sundt TM Jr, et al: Emergency embolectomy for acute occlusion of the middle cerebral artery. *J Neurosurg.* 1985;62:639.
36. McKenzie RL, Awad IA, Sila CA: Reversal of a dense, persistent, holohemispheric neurological deficit after an endarterectomy of the carotid artery: Case report. *Neurosurgery.* 1991;29:261.
37. Pessin MS, del Zoppo GJ, Estol C: Thrombolytic agents in the treatment of stroke. *Clin Neuropharmacol.* 1990;13:271.
38. Hacke W, del Zoppo GJ, Hirschberg M, eds.: *Thrombolytic Therapy in Acute Ischemic Stroke.* Heidelberg: Springer; 1991.
39. von Kummer R, Hacke W: Safety and efficacy of intravenous tissue plasminogen activator and heparin in acute middle cerebral artery stroke. *Stroke.* 1992;23:646.
40. Thiele BL, Jones AM, Hobson RW, et al: Standards in noninvasive cerebrovascular testing. *J Vasc Surg.* 1992;15:495.
41. Giller CA, Mathews D, Purdy P, et al: The transcranial Doppler appearance of acute carotid artery occlusion. *Ann Neurol.* 1992;31:101.
42. Maiuri F, Gallicchio B, Cinalli G: Diagnosis of carotid artery occlusion by duplex scanning. *Neurol Res.* 1990;12:75.
43. Hoshing H, Takagi M, Takeuchi I, et al: Recanalization of intracranial carotid occlusion detected by duplex carotid sonography. *Stroke.* 1989;20:680.
44. Combe J, Poinsard P, Besancenot J, et al: Free-floating thrombus of the extracranial internal carotid artery. *Ann Vasc Surg.* 1990;4:558.
45. Inoue Y, Takemota K, Yoshikawa N, et al: Sequential computed tomography scans in acute cerebral infarction. *Radiology.* 1980;135:655.
46. Dosick SM, Whalen RC, Gale SS, et al: Carotid endarterectomy in the stroke patient: Computerized axial tomography to determine timing. *J Vasc Surg.* 1985;2:214.
47. Koslow AR, Ricotta JJ, Ouriel K, et al: Reexploration for thrombosis in carotid endarterectomy. *Circulation.* 1989;80:III73.
48. Imparato AM: Recognition and management of acute stroke following carotid endarterectomy. In Ernst CB, Stanley JC, eds. *Current Therapy in Vascular Surgery,* 2nd ed. Philadelphia: BC Decker; 1991:104.
49. Kwaan JH, Connolly JE, Sharefkin JB: Successful management of early stroke after carotid endarterectomy. *Ann Surg.* 1979;190:676.
50. Novick WM, Millili JJ, Nemir P Jr: Management of acute postoperative thrombosis following carotid endarterectomy. *Arch Surg.* 1985;120:922.
51. Beebe HG, Stanley JC: Complications of surgical therapy for cerebral, renal, and splanchnic arterial disease. In Strandness DE, Van Breda A, eds. *Vascular Diseases, Surgical & Interventional Therapy.* New York: Churchill Livingstone; 1994.
52. Marshall RS, Mohr JP: Current management of ischaemic stroke. *J Neurol Neurosurg Psychiatry.* 1993;56:6.
53. Brown MM, Humphrey PRD: Carotid endarterectomy: Recommendations for management of transient ischaemic attack and ischaemic stroke. *BMJ.* 1992;305:1071.
54. Handelsman H: Carotid endarterectomy. AHCPR Health Technology Assessment Reports. 1990.
55. Winslow CM, Solomon DH, Chassin MR, et al: The appropriateness of carotid endarterectomy. *N Engl J Med.* 1988;318:721.
56. Matchar DB, Goldstein LB, McCrory DC, et al: Carotid endarterectomy: A literature review and ratings of appropriateness and necessity. Rand AMCC. 1992.
57. National Stroke Association consensus statement: Stroke: The first six hours; emergency evaluation and treatment. *Stroke: Clinical Updates.* 1993;4:1.
58. Moore WS, Mohr JP, Najafi H: Carotid endarterectomy: Practice guidelines. *J Vasc Surg.* 1992;15:469.

CHAPTER 35

Emergency Surgery for Stroke in Evolution and Crescendo Transient Ischemic Attacks

JERRY GOLDSTONE

Carotid endarterectomy has been widely used for the treatment of cerebral and retinal ischemic attacks for more than 30 years. The results in terms of operative mortality and stroke morbidity rates vary considerably in published reports,[1-3] but the efficacy of this procedure in certain groups of symptomatic patients has recently been documented by randomized prospective clinical trials. Although many factors influence these results, the clinical status of the patient at the time of the operation is perhaps the most important. In general, perioperative morbidity and mortality rates are directly related to the extent of preoperative cerebral dysfunction. For example, when carotid endarterectomy is performed during the acute phase of a severe stroke, the mortality approaches 50 percent. In the Joint Study on Extracranial Arterial Occlusion (EAO study), there was a 42 percent operative mortality when endarterectomy was performed within 2 weeks of an acute, severe stroke.[4] Sundt and colleagues[3] divided their patients into several groups according to medical, neurologic, and angiographic risk factors. The operative morbidity and mortality rates ranged from 1 to 2 percent in those patients with no risk factors to 10 percent in those with neurologic risk factors (ie, unstable deficits, frank stroke). A similar mortality rate (11%) was reported by Najafi and coworkers[5] among 53 patients undergoing emergency carotid endarterectomy.

Correction of acute thrombotic occlusion of the internal carotid artery can usually be accomplished if the operation is performed soon after the occlusion has occurred. Several surgeons have reported dramatic reversal of severe neurologic deficits following such procedures.[5-7] Nevertheless, postoperative strokes have occurred in spite of patent reconstructions.

In 1963, Bruetman and associates[8] called attention to postoperative cerebral hemorrhage, which was documented in six patients out of a total of 900 undergoing surgical treatment for internal carotid artery stenosis or occlusion. These investigators postulated that the cause of these hemorrhagic infarctions was restoration of blood flow into fresh ischemic areas. Shortly thereafter, Wylie and colleagues[9] reported five patients operated on within 3 to 9 days of acute stroke who died of intracranial hemorrhage. Gonzalez and Lewis[10] reported three similar cases of hemorrhagic cerebral infarction after restoration of arterial flow into an area of brain affected by an ischemic infarction.

These reports, including the EAO study, are largely responsible for the long-standing and widely held belief that carotid surgery and even arteriography in the setting of an acute stroke are contraindicated. Most neurologists and vascular surgeons have tended to place into this same high-risk category any patient with a neurologic deficit that is not completely reversible, that is, not a bona fide transient ischemic attack (TIA).

The experimental support for this clinical concept—namely, that reperfusion converts ischemic infarction into hemorrhagic cerebral infarction—was provided by Meyer,[11] who demonstrated ischemic damage to small vessels adjacent to ischemic brain lesions produced by occlusion of middle cerebral arteries in monkeys. The mechanism postulated as being responsible for deterioration in this situation is restoration of flow and pressure into an area of ischemic brain containing permeable capillaries. This converts an ischemic infarct into a hemorrhagic infarct and eventually into a massive hemorrhage into the area of infarction.[8-10, 12] Although it is possible to produce hemorrhagic infarction experimentally by re-establishing flow in an occluded middle cerebral artery, hemorrhagic infarcts can also be produced by arterial occlusion alone.[13, 14] In both situations, hypertension appears to play an important, if not essential, role. In Meyer's study, hemorrhagic brain infarction was associated with anticoagulant administration and wide fluctuations in blood pressure.[11] In many of the clinical case reports cited earlier, wide fluctuations and severe elevations in blood pressure were noted.[5-7]

Although not all the factors involved in the development of hemorrhagic cerebral infarction are clearly understood, it can be produced by cerebral embolization alone, with or without operation. Fisher and Adams[13] analyzed 66 patients with hemorrhagic infarction and found that most of them had embolic occlusion of cerebral arteries. The presence of a soft thrombus at the carotid bifurcation that can easily be dislodged and travel downstream has been encountered by many surgeons during carotid operations. This factor may be as significant as restoration of flow in the production of hemorrhagic infarction.[15, 16]

STROKE IN EVOLUTION

Stroke in evolution, also known as deteriorating stroke, progressing stroke, incomplete stroke, stroke in progression, and ingravescent stroke, describes the temporal profile of strokes with a variety of causes.[17-20] The definition of this type of actively changing neurologic deficit is imprecise, and several symptom patterns can be included in the term. For example, an acute neurologic deficit of mild to moderate degree may, within hours or days of the initial event, progress in a sequential series of acute exacerbations to a major stroke. Alternatively, after the initial episode, the neurologic deficit may improve temporarily only to reappear later, often with more widespread involvement, leading to a pattern of waxing and waning of signs and symptoms that occurs over hours to days, with incomplete recovery.[21] Although some investigators have attempted to set a 24-hour time limit beyond which an evolving stroke becomes, by definition, a completed stroke, progression can occur much later and take much longer to complete.[17, 22]

Crescendo TIAs should be included in the category of deteriorating stroke. These cerebral hemispheric or retinal episodes of transient ischemia, usually lasting a few minutes to hours, leave no residual signs and symptoms between attacks; the attacks abruptly start with several a day or increase in frequency to at least several a day. Alternatively, some authors include in this term TIAs that abruptly increase in severity, although this is a less common pattern. The natural history of crescendo TIAs results in a permanent, moderate to severe deficit in most patients.[18, 23, 24]

Stroke in evolution is probably more frequent than is generally believed.[25, 26] In a series of 179 acute strokes reported by Jones and Millikan,[22] it was the pattern of onset in 29 percent of patients and was even more common in vertebrobasilar than hemispheric strokes. Evolving stroke was also more frequent than sudden onset in the Harvard Stroke Registry.

Since there are several different causes of deteriorating stroke, several different mechanisms are believed to play a role, including extension of thrombus, with obliteration of collaterals or the lumen of a parent vessel (ie, internal carotid); repeated embolization; increase in brain edema; and deterioration in the general condition of the patient (eg, cardiopulmonary, renal). Thus, stroke in evolution cannot be equated with thrombosis in evolution, as was formerly believed. Whatever the mechanism, the diagnosis of deteriorating stroke must be established so that immediate action to stop the progression can be taken. This is mandatory if the clinical outcome is to be altered favorably.

Diagnostic Evaluation

The primary objective of treatment of patients with deteriorating stroke is prevention of cerebral infarction or worsening of infarction, if it has already begun. The concept of an ischemic penumbra—an area of brain that is sufficiently ischemic to be dysfunctional or nonfunctional but not yet irreversibly so—is pertinent in this regard. No known treatment will reverse infarction, once it has occurred. The very nature of deteriorating stroke permits only a limited time to make initial observations and start treatment if this objective is to be achieved.[27] The diagnostic evaluation must therefore proceed on an urgent basis.

Although different types of deterioration can produce the same clinical picture, the diagnosis of deteriorating stroke is best made on clinical grounds, largely from analysis of the patient's history and by repeated physical examination (see Chapter 9). When the neurologic deficit is only mild to moderate and there is no depression in the level of consciousness, the scheme outlined in Figure 35–1 is recommended. A computed tomography (CT) or magnetic resonance imaging (MRI) study should be performed to image the brain. The limitations of CT scans are well known—they may show normal results within the first 24 to 36 hours following cerebral infarction, unless the infarction is hemorrhagic. It is nonetheless an important diagnostic study, because it may identify pathologic causes of symptoms other than extracranial arterial disease, such as intracerebral hematoma, brain tumor, and arteriovenous malformation. Lacunar infarctions are also frequently seen on CT scans.[28] These findings have an important influence on the decision to administer anticoagulants and to proceed with angiography and surgery.

Magnetic resonance imaging is a relatively new and less widely available diagnostic modality. Its main advantage is the ability to discriminate tissue differences in a manner far superior to that afforded by CT. Thus it has superior sensitivity in detecting focal pathologic alterations in tissue. For example, blood-brain barrier breakdown is reported to be manifest almost immediately on MRI; it should therefore be possible to determine whether cerebral infarction has occurred earlier than with other modalities.

If the results of a CT or MRI scan are normal or do not identify a lesion thought to be the cause of the symptoms, the patient should immediately be anticoagulated while the remainder of the workup is in progress. There are few

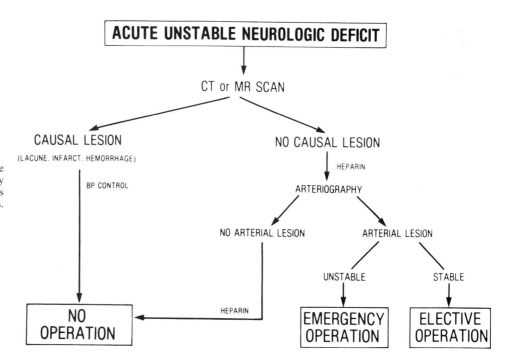

FIGURE 35–1. Algorithm showing the recommended approach for emergency evaluation and treatment of patients with acute unstable neurologic deficits.

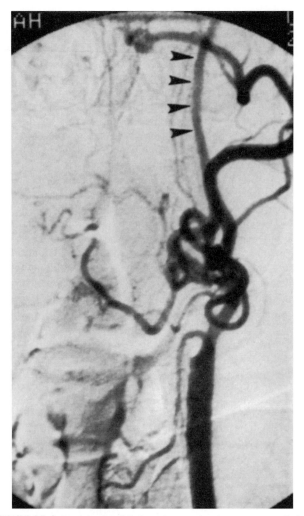

FIGURE 35–2. Intra-arterial digital arteriogram showing apparent occlusion of the proximal internal carotid artery but with opacification of the more distal extracranial internal carotid artery *(arrowheads)*. Patient had a waxing and waning pattern of deteriorating stroke.

and small amounts of contrast medium. Digital subtraction equipment facilitates the study and minimizes contrast volume. Although complete visualization of extracranial and intracranial arteries is desirable, it is prudent to limit the studies in neurologically unstable patients. Therefore, arch and vertebral views are not routinely requested, and occasionally, when a critical lesion is identified that is appropriate to the symptoms, only one carotid system is visualized. It is important to obtain adequate visualization of the carotid bifurcation to ensure that the internal carotid artery is not occluded, since some patients may have apparent occlusion of the origin of the internal carotid on one view but a patent artery confirmed on other projections. This is clearly demonstrated in Figures 35–2 and 35–3. The heparin need not be discontinued for arteriography unless a transaxillary route is required. I have had no significant angiographic complications in my patients.

Patients with deteriorating strokes frequently have critical arterial lesions, which are presumed to be the cause of the clinical problem. Critical arterial lesions have been arbitrarily defined as those producing a 95 percent or greater reduction in the diameter of the internal carotid artery or those associated with thrombus seen on arteriograms to be freely floating within the lumen of the vessel or attached to the vessel wall (Figs. 35–2 through 35–4). These preocclusive and thrombotic lesions are thought to be unstable because of their propensity to become totally occlusive or to embolize. Most patients with the stroke-in-evolution pattern

controlled studies on the efficacy of anticoagulation in acute deteriorating stroke. Baker and coworkers[29] reported a notable reduction in progression of infarction in the anticoagulated group compared with the control group. Although other more recent studies have not substantiated this advantage, they have shown that heparin can be safely administered in this situation without increasing the risk of cerebral hemorrhage.[24, 26, 30, 31] The potential advantages of anticoagulation seem to outweigh the risks in this clinical situation.

Arteriography should be the next diagnostic procedure. Many clinicians are reluctant to subject neurologically unstable patients to angiography, for fear of exacerbating the neurologic deficit. These fears do not appear justified with today's modern angiographic techniques. Even in the EAO study of 20 years ago, the grave complication (stroke) rate was only 0.5 percent overall among 4748 patients subjected to four-vessel cerebral angiography, and in patients with severe neurologic deficits, the stroke rate was only 1 percent.[32] The current angiographic technique at the University of California–San Francisco and at many other institutions involves transfemoral retrograde catheterization and selective carotid injections using small catheters (4 to 5 French)

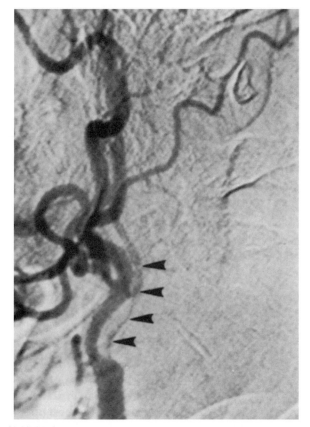

FIGURE 35–3. Intra-arterial digital subtraction arteriogram of same internal carotid artery shown in Figure 35–2. A different projection confirms the patency of the vessel and the preocclusive stenosis of the proximal portion *(arrowheads)*.

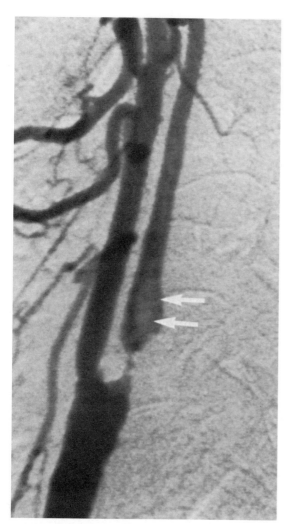

FIGURE 35–4. Intra-arterial digital arteriogram showing a critical carotid artery lesion in a patient with deteriorating stroke. Note the preocclusive stenosis and the intraluminal filling defect, which was due to free-floating thrombus (arrows).

of deteriorating stroke have this type of arterial pathology.[21, 23, 24, 33] Ulcerated nonstenotic atheromatous plaques may release multiple emboli into the bloodstream and cause crescendo TIAs (Fig. 35–5). Although not classified as critical arterial lesions, in this clinical setting, atheromatous plaques have the same surgical significance in patients with crescendo TIAs as in patients with stroke in evolution, and they occur more frequently in patients with crescendo TIAs.

Other diagnostic studies are of dubious benefit. In the typical patient with deteriorating stroke, electroencephalography, cerebrospinal fluid, physical examination, static brain scan, and routine blood tests do not add information useful for decision making. Noninvasive studies employing indirect means, such as periorbital Doppler and oculoplethysmography, may be helpful in identifying a hemodynamically significant stenosis in the appropriate internal carotid artery, but they cannot accurately predict the need for arteriography. Direct noninvasive tests, such as duplex scans of the carotid bifurcation, should be able to identify the types of unstable or critical arterial lesions generally responsible for deteriorating strokes. Some clinicians have adopted duplex ultrasound as the only direct diagnostic means of evaluating the carotid

bifurcation prior to endarterectomy, and its early use in the setting of an unstable neurologic deficit is easily justifiable. A decision not to proceed with angiography might reasonably be made in a patient with a normal duplex scan of the carotid artery, but this would preclude examination of those portions of the carotid system not accessible with current duplex technology.

INDICATIONS FOR EMERGENCY CAROTID SURGERY

Patients with deteriorating stroke (including those with crescendo TIAs) and unstable arterial lesions should undergo carotid endarterectomy as soon as possible, since this provides the best opportunity to prevent progression to a permanent neurologic deficit. If a noncritical arterial lesion is encountered and the neurologic symptoms stabilize with heparin anticoagulation, it is probably better to delay carotid endarterectomy until it is certain that stroke has not occurred and medical risk factors have been thoroughly evaluated and their management optimized.

It must be emphasized that none of the patients my colleagues and I have operated on for deteriorating stroke had severe neurologic deficits—all deficits were either mild or at

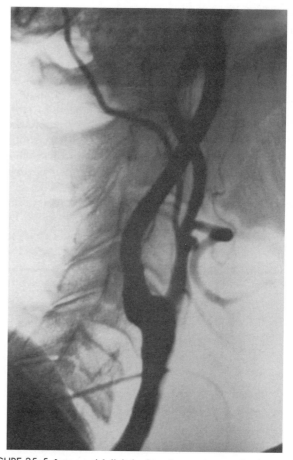

FIGURE 35–5. Intra-arterial digital subtraction arteriogram showing a nonstenotic ulcerated carotid artery in a patient with crescendo transient hemispheric ischemic attacks. This image represents the least severe arteriographic appearance among patients encountered with acute unstable neurologic deficits.

most moderate, and no patient had a depressed level of consciousness.[21, 33, 34] Although it cannot be established with certainty that none of these patients had suffered a preoperative cerebral infarction, it is probable, based on the clinical course and CT scans, that if any infarctions were present, they were small.

This, then, defines a select group of patients who should be considered candidates for emergency carotid endarterectomy. These patients differ considerably from those described in earlier reports.[8–10] Most of the earlier patients had severe neurologic deficits, severe or poorly controlled hypertension, and total occlusion of their carotid arteries. In my opinion, these findings represent contraindications to emergency carotid surgery.

SURGICAL MANAGEMENT OF PATIENTS WITH UNSTABLE NEUROLOGIC DEFICITS

The surgical and anesthetic management recommended for emergency carotid operations is similar to that used in elective operations, including the use of general endotracheal anesthesia. Usually a volatile inhalation anesthetic agent such as isoflurane is used because it increases cerebral blood flow while reducing cerebral oxygen consumption. Arterial carbon dioxide tension is maintained at normal levels. Intraluminal shunts are normally used selectively on the basis of carotid backpressure measurement, except in patients who have had previous ipsilateral stroke. In these patients, shunts are employed regardless of the level of carotid backpressure. In conformity with this policy, a shunt should be used in patients with progressing stroke, because of the uncertainty about the presence of early cerebral infarction. Arterial patches are rarely necessary for closure of primary carotid operations. Assessment of the technical adequacy of the endarterectomy should be accomplished with either intraoperative arteriography or ultrasonic (duplex) scanning. Vigorous control of systemic blood pressure is essential during the entire perioperative period. This requires an intra-arterial catheter for continuous blood pressure monitoring. Anticoagulants are not used postoperatively, but antiplatelet-aggregating agents are routinely administered. Other management protocols (eg, regional anesthesia, electroencephalographic monitoring) with proven records of good results are appropriate, according to individual practitioner and institutional experiences.

RESULTS OF TREATMENT

The surgical results of the EAO study provided no data on the number of patients with fluctuating neurologic deficits. Nevertheless, more than 270 surgically treated cases have been published (Table 35–1).[6, 21, 23, 33–42] In 1964, Young and associates[35] described 100 patients who underwent 118 carotid operations. Included in this group were four patients with progressing stroke. Two (50%) were improved by the operation, one was unchanged, and one died from a myocardial infarction. In the 1965 series by DeBakey and colleagues[36] 38 (61.3%) of 62 patients were improved, another 16 (25.8%) were unchanged, only three (4.8%) worsened, and five (8.1%) died following carotid endarterectomy. The initial experience Moore and I had with 11 emergency operations, published in 1976, was gratifying in that all patients improved dramatically following surgery.[21] This series was enlarged to 28 patients and reported in a subsequent publication, with only one poor result in a patient operated on for crescendo TIAs in whom a brain-stem (pontine) stroke developed on the third postoperative day, resulting in death.[34]

McIntyre and I described an additional 20 patients in another report.[33] Crescendo TIAs were the indication for surgery in 14 of these patients, and six had progressive, or deteriorating, strokes. All had dramatic, prompt, and complete relief of their neurologic deficits following emergency carotid endarterectomy, except for one patient, in whom preoperative arteriography and CT scan were not performed. This patient's crescendo TIAs resulted in a mild fixed deficit subsequently attributed to a lacunar infarction in the internal capsule (documented on postoperative CT scan).

Mentzer and associates[23] retrospectively analyzed the early and late results of 55 patients treated for stroke in evolution and crescendo TIAs. Emergency carotid surgery was performed on 24 of these patients. All seven of those experienc-

TABLE 35–1. Carotid Endarterectomy for Progressing Stroke

Study*	Patients	Improved n (%)	Unchanged n (%)	Worsened n (%)	Death n (%)
Young et al[35]	4	2 (50.0)	1 (25.0)	0 (0.0)	1 (25.0)
DeBakey et al[36]	62	38 (61.3)	16 (25.8)	3 (4.8)	5 (8.1)
Hunter et al[37]	26	20 (76.9)	5 (19.2)	0 (0.0)	1 (3.8)
Rob[6]	74	21 (28.4)	26 (35.1)	15 (20.3)	12 (16.2)
Ojemann et al[38]	10	8 (80.0)	1 (10.0)	0 (0.0)	1 (10.0)
Goldstone and Moore[21]	11	11 (100.0)	0 (0.0)	0 (0.0)	0 (0.0)
Goldstone and Effeney[34]	28	27 (96.4)	0 (0.0)	0 (0.0)	1 (3.6)
Collected Mentzer et al[23]	190	105 (55.2)	48 (25.3)	18 (9.5)	19 (10.0)
Mentzer et al[23]	24	19 (79.2)	4 (16.7)	0 (0.0)	1 (4.2)
McIntyre and Goldstone[33]	20	19 (95.0)	1 (5.0)	0 (0.0)	0 (0.0)
Lenzi et al[39]	22	20 (90.9)	1 (4.5)	0 (0.0)	1 (4.5)
Greenhalgh et al[40]	12	11 (91.7)	0 (0.0)	1 (4.3)	0 (0.0)
Greenhalgh et al[41]	22	19 (86.4)	0 (0.0)	2 (9.1)	1 (4.5)
Gertler et al[42]	52	45 (86.5)	5 (9.6)	2 (3.8)	0 (0.0)

*For full bibliographic information, see reference list at end of chapter.

ing TIAs recovered completely; 12 (70.5%) of the 17 stroke-in-evolution patients were normal or improved, and only one (4.2%) died. These investigators also reviewed all the cases of surgery for fluctuating neurologic deficits published up to 1980. The collated results demonstrated that 55 percent of the patients improved, 25 percent were unchanged from their preoperative status, 10 percent were worse, and 10 percent died.

Lenzi and associates[39] reported their results of emergency carotid operations in 22 patients with crescendo TIAs and progressing stroke. There were no postoperative neurologic complications, but one patient died from a myocardial infarction. Greenhalgh and associates[40] reported a similar experience with 12 patients. All but one patient improved completely or partially, and one patient's deficit progressed to complete hemiplegia. It is of interest that 8 of these 12 patients showed preoperative evidence of cerebral infarction by CT. In a more recent series, Greenhalgh and associates[41] described 22 urgent operations (7%) in a series of 300 carotid endarterectomies. This series included the 12 patients from their previous (1985) publication. Stroke progression was arrested in all 15 patients with progressing stroke; 6 recovered completely, 8 others improved (93.3% improved), and 1 patient suffered an ipsilateral stroke 1 week after initial halting of neurologic progression. Seven patients had crescendo TIAs; five recovered completely, one had a very mild deficit, and one suffered a fatal stroke. Overall, improvement occurred in 86.4% of patients in this series. It is of interest that preoperative CT scans revealed cerebral infarction in 15 of the 18 patients who were so studied.

The most recent report was that of Gertler and coworkers,[42] which described 70 carotid operations in 68 neurologically unstable patients. Seventeen had stroke in evolution, 34 had crescendo TIAs that continued in spite of heparin anticoagulation, and 20 had crescendo TIAs that were controlled by heparin anticoagulation. Using a neurologic event severity scale to evaluate results, the neurologic status of these patients improved in 86.5% and worsened in 3.8%, with no deaths.

The results in all these series are similar, with most patients showing improvement or at least not becoming worse. Nevertheless, the operative morbidity and mortality are higher than for elective carotid operations performed on neurologically stable or asymptomatic patients. However, the risk of nonoperative treatment appears to be even greater. The natural history of stroke in evolution has been studied by Millikan.[43] He reported a series of 204 consecutive patients with the following results: 69 percent became hemiparetic, 5 percent monoparetic, 14 percent died, and only 12 percent returned to normal by 14 days after the onset of symptoms. In the collected series of 263 patients reported by Mentzer and colleagues,[23] 61 (23.2%) were left with no or only mild deficits, 164 (62.4%) had moderate or severe deficits, and 38 (14.5%) died. Although most physicians favor immediate heparinization for patients with progressing stroke, there is limited evidence that anticoagulation is beneficial in this situation.[24, 28–31, 44] Millikan[43] stated that these patients undergo emergency evaluation and operation in an effort to alter the dismal natural history and prognosis of this condition.

The natural history of what have been called crescendo TIAs is less well defined but is believed to be similar to that of stroke in evolution. Mentzer and coworkers[23] described 12 patients with this clinical pattern. Seven were operated on as emergency cases, with complete recovery. Of the five treated non-operatively, only one recovered completely, three became moderately to severely impaired, and one died. In another review, Millikan and McDowell[24] referred to patients "with a cluster of frequent carotid TIAs" and recommended anticoagulation treatment, emergency evaluation, and surgery.

The only data relevant to this topic available from prospective randomized clinical trials are from the North American Symptomatic Carotid Endarterectomy Trial. That study included a subset of 25 patients who had intra-arterial thrombus beyond a severe stenosis. The perioperative or postrandomization stroke rate was 22% in the nine surgically treated patients and 25% in the 16 patients in the medical group. Unfortunately, it is not possible to document the clinical findings that led to randomization in this small subset of patients. Therefore, these data may not be applicable to the neurologically unstable patients discussed in this chapter. In a recently developed multidisciplinary consensus statement on indications for carotid endarterectomy, stroke in evolution in the presence of greater than 70% stenosis with large ulceration, and crescendo TIAs with stenosis of 50% or greater, with or without ulceration, were classified as acceptable but not proven indications for carotid endarterectomy.[45] Nevertheless, until additional data are available, the excellent results associated with emergency carotid surgery reported in several series indicate that the natural history of selected patients with stroke in evolution and crescendo TIAs can be favorably altered by this aggressive therapeutic approach. The timing of surgical intervention is crucial, since the nature of progressing stroke permits only a limited time in which to make the initial observations and initiate treatment. Time will usually be saved if the neurologist and surgeon work together from the beginning.

Neither arteriography nor operation is recommended for patients with severe fixed neurologic deficits, especially when associated with depressed levels of consciousness. Presumably, cerebral infarction has already occurred in these patients. Operations to re-establish flow in a totally occluded internal carotid artery are also not recommended, whether there are symptoms of cerebrovascular insufficiency or not, unless patency and flow can be restored within less than 4 to 6 hours from onset of the occlusion.[5, 37]

Acknowledgments

This work was supported in part by the Pacific Vascular Research Foundation.

REFERENCES

1. West H, Burton R, Roon AJ, et al: Comparative risk of operation and exptectant management for carotid disease. *Stroke.* 1979;10:117.
2. Byer JA, Easton JD: Therapy of ischemic cerebrovascular disease. *Ann Intern Med.* 1980;93:742.
3. Sundt TM, Sandok BA, Whisnant JP: Carotid endarterectomy—complications and preoperative assessment of risk. *Mayo Clin Proc.* 1975;50:301.
4. Blaisdell WF, Clauss RH, Galbraith JG, et al: Joint study of extracranial arterial occlusion. IV. A review of surgical consideration. *JAMA.* 1969;209:1889.
5. Najafi H, Javid H, Dye WS, et al: Emergency carotid thromboendarterectomy: Surgical indications and results. *Arch Surg.* 1971;103:611.
6. Rob CG: Operation for acute completed stroke due to thrombosis of internal carotid artery. *Surgery.* 1969;65:862.

7. Thompson JE, Austin DJ, Patman RD: Endarterectomy of the totally occluded carotid artery for stroke. *Arch Surg.* 1967;95:791.

8. Bruetman ME, Fields WS, Crawford ES, DeBakey ME: Cerebral hemorrhage in carotid artery surgery. *Arch Neurol.* 1963;9:458.

9. Wylie EJ, Hein MF, Adams JE: Intracranial hemorrhage following surgical revascularization for treatment of acute strokes. *Neurosurgery.* 1964;21:212.

10. Gonzalez LL, Lewis CM: Cerebral hemorrhage following successful endarterectomy of the internal carotid artery. *Surg Gynecol Obstet.* 1966;123:773.

11. Meyer JS: Importance of ischemic damage to small vessels in experimental cerebral infarction. *J Neuropathol Exp Neurol.* 1958;17:571.

12. Garcia JH, Lowry SL, Briggs L, et al: Brain capillaries expand and rupture in areas of ischemia and reperfusion. In Reivich M, Hurtig HL, eds. *Cerebrovascular Diseases.* New York: Raven Press; 1983:169.

13. Fisher CM, Adams RD: Special reference to the mechanism of hemorrhagic infarction. *J Neuropathol Exp Neurol.* 1951;10:92.

14. Paulson OB: Cerebral apoplexy (stroke): Pathogenesis, pathophysiology and therapy as illustrated by regional blood flow measurements in the brain. *Stroke.* 1971;2:327.

15. Towne JB, Bernhard VM: The relationship of postoperative hypertension to complications following carotid endarterectomy. *Surgery.* 1980;88:575.

16. Caplan LR, Skillman J, Ojemann R, Fields WS: Intracerebral hemorrhage following carotid endarterectomy: A hypertensive complication? *Stroke.* 1978;9:457.

17. Gautier JC: What is stroke in evolution? In Courbier R, ed. *Basis for a Classification of Cerebral Arterial Diseases,* Vol 1. Amsterdam: Excerpta Medica; 1985:122.

18. Frisch R: Progressing stroke. In Courbier R, ed. *Basis for a Classification of Cerebral Arterial Diseases,* Vol 1. Amsterdam: Excerpta Medica; 1985:127.

19. Gautier JC: Stroke-in-progression. *Stroke.* 1985;16:729.

20. Tadayoshi I, Watanabe M, Nishide M, et al: Pathophysiological aspects of cerebral infarction followed by deteriorating of minor neurological deficits—what is progressing stroke? In Ito Z, Kutsuzawa T, Yasui N, eds. *Cerebral Ischemia—An Update,* Vol 1. Amsterdam: Excerpta Medica; 1983:127.

21. Goldstone J, Moore WS: Emergency carotid artery surgery in neurologically unstable patients. *Arch Surg.* 1976;111:1284.

22. Jones HR, Millikan CH: Temporal profile (clinical course) of acute carotid system cerebral infarction. *Stroke.* 1976;7:64.

23. Mentzer RM, Finkelmeir BA, Crosby IK, Wellons HA Jr: Emergency carotid endarterectomy for fluctuating neurologic deficits. *Surgery.* 1981;89:60.

24. Millikan CH, McDowell FH: Treatment of progressing stroke. *Stroke.* 1981;12:397.

25. Grotta J: The significance of clinical deterioration in acute carotid distribution cerebral infarction. In Reivich M, Hurtig HI, eds. *Cerebrovascular Diseases.* New York: Raven Press; 1983:109.

26. Millikan CH: Treatment of occlusive cerebrovascular disease. In McDowell FH, Caplan LR, eds. *Cerebrovascular Survey Report for the National Institute of Neurological and Communicative Disorders and Stroke.* Bethesda: National Institute of Neurological and Communicative Disorders and Stroke; 1985:149.

27. Carter LP, Yamagata S, Erspamer R: Time limits of reversible cortical ischemia. *Neurosurgery.* 1983;12:620.

28. Lodder J, Gorsselink EL: Progressive stroke caused by CT-verified small deep infarcts; relation with the size of the infarct and clinical outcome. *Acta Neurol Scand.* 1985;71:328.

29. Baker RW, Broward JA, Fang HC, et al: Anticoagulant therapy in cerebral infarction: Report on cooperative study. *Neurology (NY).* 1962;12:823.

30. Haley EC, Kassell NF, Torner JC: Failure of heparin to prevent progressing ischemic infarction. *Stroke.* 1986;17:132.

31. Duke RJ, Turpie AG, Block RF, et al: A randomized controlled trial of heparin in acute partial thrombotic stroke. *Stroke.* 1986;17:133.

32. Hass WK, Fields WS, North RR, et al: Joint study of extracranial arterial occlusion: Arteriography, techniques, sites and complications. *JAMA.* 1968;203:961.

33. McIntyre KE Jr, Goldstone J: Carotid surgery for crescendo TIA and stroke in evolution. In Bergan JJ, Yao JST, eds. *Cerebrovascular Insufficiency.* New York: Grune & Stratton; 1983:213.

34. Goldstone J, Effeney DJ: The role of carotid endarterectomy in the treatment of acute neurologic deficits. *Prog Cardiovasc Dis.* 1980;22:415.

35. Young JR, Humphries AW, deWolfe VG, et al: Extracranial cerebrovascular disease treated surgically. *Arch Surg.* 1964;89:848.

36. DeBakey ME, Crawford ES, Cooley DA, et al: Cerebral arterial insufficiency: One to 11-year results following arterial reconstructive operation. *Ann Surg.* 1965;161:921.

37. Hunter JA, Julian OC, Dye WS, Javid H: Emergency operation for acute cerebral ischemia due to carotid artery obstruction: Review of 26 cases. *Ann Surg.* 1965;162:901.

38. Ojemann RG, Crowell RM, Roberson GH, Fisher CM: Surgical treatment of extracranial carotid occlusive disease. *Clin Neurosurg.* 1975;22:214.

39. Lenzi GL, Rasura M, Ventura M, et al: Surgical treatment of unstable and acute cerebral ischaemia: Indications and results in the light of pathophysiological data. In Courbier R, ed. *Basis for a Classification of Cerebral Arterial Diseases,* Vol 1. Amsterdam: Excerpta Medica; 1985:189.

40. Greenhalgh RM, McCollum CN, Bourke BM, et al: Urgent carotid surgery for progressing stroke: Successful intervention based on a clinical classification. In Courbier R, ed. *Basis for a Classification of Cerebral Arterial Diseases,* Vol 1. Amsterdam: Excerpta Medica; 1985:132.

41. Greenhalgh RM, Cuming R, Perkin GD, McCollum CN: Urgent carotid surgery for high risk patients. *Eur J Vasc Surg.* 1993;7(Suppl A):25.

42. Gertler JP, Blankensteijn JD, Brewster DC, et al: Carotid endarterectomy for unstable and compelling neurologic conditions: Do results justify an aggressive approach? *J Vasc Surg.* 1994;19:32.

43. Millikan CH: Clinical management of cerebral ischemia. In McDowell FH, Brennan RW, eds. *Cerebral Vascular Disease. Eighth Princeton Conference.* New York: Grune & Stratton; 1973:209.

44. Duke RJ, Turpie AG, Bloch RF, Trebilcock RG: Clinical trial of low dose subcutaneous heparin for the prevention of stroke progression: Natural history of acute partial stroke and stroke-in-evolution. In Reivich M, Hurtig HI, eds. *Cerebrovascular Diseases.* New York: Raven Press; 1983:399.

45. Moore WS, ad hoc committee of the American Heart Association: Indications for carotid endarterectomy: A multidisciplinary consensus statement. *Circulation.* In press.

CHAPTER 36

Traumatic Dissection of the Internal Carotid Artery: Conservative Versus Surgical Management

DAVID R. BLATT and ARTHUR L. DAY

Most lesions of the cervical carotid artery are caused by arteriosclerosis, and the majority affect the internal carotid artery at or just above where the common carotid artery bifurcates into internal and external branches. This site usually corresponds to the C-4 vertebral body level, although variations above and below this plane are not uncommon. The natural history of this disease process and its appropriate medical and surgical management have been clarified by several recent studies.

Dissections make up a small group of lesions that affect the cervical carotid artery, most commonly that portion of the internal carotid artery near the skull base, well above the cervical bifurcation. In many instances, the development of this abnormality is clearly related to predisposing factors (eg, trauma, underlying vasculitis), but often the cause remains obscure. This chapter outlines the clinicopathologic features of cervical carotid dissections and clarifies the differences between them and lesions caused by arteriosclerosis.

DEFINITION AND TERMINOLOGY

Extracranial carotid artery dissections, produced when circulating blood penetrates into the wall of the vessel, can be divided broadly into spontaneous and traumatic types, depending on whether there is evidence of obvious penetrating or blunt injury to the vessel. The resultant intramural hematoma extends for a variable distance within the wall of the artery, most often distally toward the skull base, creating a false lumen. The mass effect of the intramural clot may narrow or occlude the true lumen, or the hematoma may rupture back into the original arterial lumen to produce a double channel. The false lumen may also expand toward the adventitia to produce a fusiform aneurysmal dilatation of the vessel (dissecting aneurysm), which may not be apparent on arteriographic studies alone.[1-3]

The terms "pseudoaneurysm" and "false aneurysm" have often been applied inappropriately to these lesions. Dissecting aneurysms are invariably "true" aneurysms because their walls are formed by blood vessel elements. False or pseudoaneurysms are perivascular encapsulated hematomas that communicate with the lumen of the blood vessel. Thus, their walls are not entirely composed of blood vessel elements.[4]

PATHOLOGIC FEATURES

Carotid artery dissections most commonly originate in the high cervical region, 4 to 6 cm distal to the bifurcation (Fig. 36–1). Dissections are classified as traumatic or spontaneous types, based on a clinical history or evidence of obvious head or neck trauma. Although dissections in patients who

have been subjected to obvious blunt or penetrating head or neck injury are easily classified, minor or "trivial" trauma such as coughing, straining, or unusual neck movements cannot always be excluded.

Penetrating injuries are more likely to result in arterial transection, false aneurysm, and arteriovenous fistula. Blunt trauma is responsible for most dissections, although such injuries may cause internal carotid artery thrombosis without dissection.[5] The most common cause of such blunt trauma dissections are motor vehicle accidents that produce abrupt flexion, extension, and rotation of the neck.[1, 5-7] Direct blows to the head and neck, hanging, blunt intraoral trauma, chiropractic manipulation, carotid artery compression, local surgical procedures, arterial needle puncture and catheterization for arteriography or monitoring, basilar skull fractures, and mandibular fractures have also been implicated.

The vessel is presumed to be traumatized by rotation and hyperextension of the neck, which stretches the internal carotid artery against the transverse process of the upper cervical vertebrae or a prominent styloid process.[5, 8-11] Abrupt and severe neck flexion may also impinge the artery between the angle of the mandible and the upper cervical spine.[11] The greater mobility of the cervical spine (and hence a greater degree of stretch or distraction of the carotid artery)

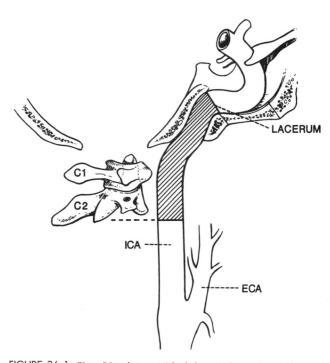

FIGURE 36–1. Site of involvement (*shaded area*). Internal carotid artery (ICA) dissections typically originate several cm above the bifurcation (C1-C2 region), and end at or within the carotid canal. On occasion, the luminal stenosis extends to the region of the foramen lacerum, just before the ICA enters the cavernous sinus. ECA, external carotid artery.

may account for the increased frequency of dissection in younger age groups. The uncoiling of elastic tissue that occurs with age may reduce the chances of stretch injuries to the vessel in older populations.[1]

The common pathologic event leading to carotid artery dissection, whether traumatic or spontaneous, is an intimal tear that allows extension of blood into the vessel wall (Fig. 36–2). In some instances, particularly in the spontaneous type, the initial event may be an intramedial hemorrhage from the vasa vasorum. The intimal tear and communication between the true and false lumina can sometimes be identified in pathologic specimens. The outer or false lumen is often filled with thrombus and covered by variable thicknesses of residual media and adventitia. There is loss of muscle fibers in the media and fragmentation of the internal elastic lamina.[1, 2] Arteriosclerotic changes are rarely seen angiographically, at the time of surgery, or on pathologic examination.[1, 2, 4]

The pathogenesis of spontaneous carotid dissections is unclear in most patients, reinforcing the notion of "trivial" trauma in its development. Ehlers-Danlos and Marfan syndromes and fibromuscular dysplasia are known to be associated with an increased frequency of carotid dissections but are uncommonly identified in traumatic dissections. Cystic medial necrosis in the affected carotid artery was described in early reports, but more recent literature has failed to show any particular microscopic abnormalities in the vessels studied.[4] Approximately 15 percent of patients with spontaneous dissections exhibit fibromuscular dysplasia.[12, 13] This incidence may actually be higher, as the changes produced

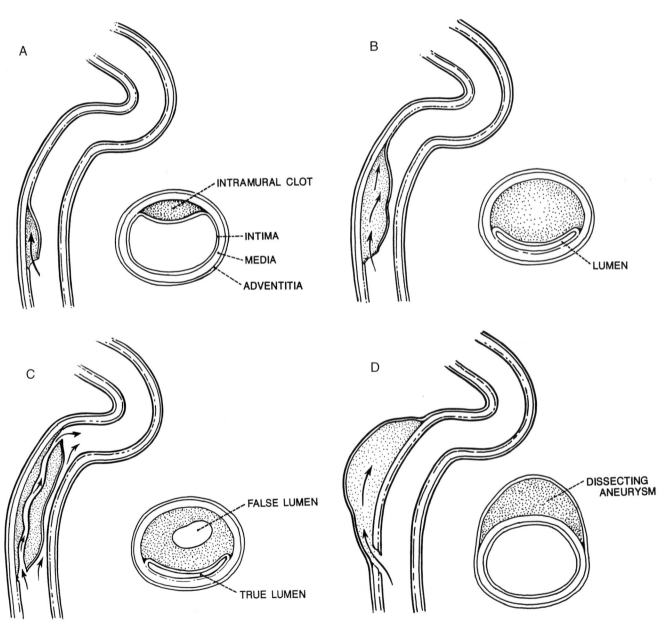

FIGURE 36–2. Pathogenesis (lateral and cross sectional views of the internal carotid artery). *A,* The initial intimal tear and subintimal and intramedial hematoma. *B,* Progression of the hemorrhage, with compromise of the vascular lumen. *C,* Rupture of the intramural hematoma through the intima distally, which establishes a second communication between the false and true lumens. *D,* Extension of hemorrhage toward the adventitia; if the false lumen remains patent, the dissecting aneurysm is visible on arteriography, and the pouch can serve as an embolic source.

by the dissection may distort or obliterate the common angiographic patterns diagnostic of fibromuscular dysplasia. Hypertension and migraine headaches are also found with increased frequency in patients who develop spontaneous dissections; smoking and contraceptive use have an unclear association with this disorder.[4, 13, 14] The pathogenesis of the spontaneous variety is likely to be multifactorial, with a final mechanical event occurring on top of an underlying (and generally previously asymptomatic) vascular abnormality.

The degree of external bulging and the later demonstration of an aneurysmal lumen are presumably related to the severity of the vessel's injury, the depth of extension of the intramural hemorrhage toward or into the adventitia, and the thickness of the remaining outer vessel wall. Significant trauma probably causes greater damage to the artery, and early luminal stenosis progressing to internal carotid artery occlusion is more common with the traumatic type of dissection. The incidence of occlusion is 27 percent in the traumatic type and 17 percent in the spontaneous type.[5, 13] An aneurysmal lumen may not be apparent on initial arteriographic investigation unless the false lumen persists or recanalizes. The demonstration of an aneurysm with a false lumen occurs in 58 percent of traumatic dissections and 37 percent of those classified as spontaneous in origin.[5, 13]

CLINICAL FEATURES

The average age of patients with traumatic dissections is under 35 years; it is around 45 years for those with the spontaneous variety.[1, 4, 5, 7, 12, 13] This age pattern is in clear contrast to arteriosclerotic carotid artery disease, which is typically found in an older age group (over 50 years). Overall, the disease is slightly more common in men, which probably reflects the increased incidence of trauma in younger individuals and in males.[15] The spontaneous type may be slightly more common in females.[13] The disease in uncommon but not rare. The exact incidence is not known, but more than 200 cases have been reported in the literature.

Two common clinical presentations have been recognized: hemicranial headaches associated with a bruit or oculosympathetic paresis, or focal cerebral ischemic symptoms soon after or remote to trauma.[5, 13] Although either type of dissection may produce either class of symptoms, there are clear differences in the frequency and severity of certain symptoms, depending on the presence or absence of obvious preceding trauma.[5, 12, 13]

Patients with spontaneous dissections usually present with unilateral headache confined to the periorbital region, ipsilateral to the arterial abnormality.[4, 13, 15, 16] The pain, which occurs in over 80 percent of spontaneous dissections, is described as steady and nonthrobbing, and it often fluctuates in intensity. Neck pain, scalp tenderness, or diffuse headaches are also occasionally reported. Oculosympathetic paresis is observed in approximately 50 percent of patients with spontaneous dissections.[4, 16] This finding represents an incomplete Horner syndrome caused by disruption of the sympathetic fibers that run in the adventitia of the cervical internal carotid artery. Facial sweating is spared, as these fibers exit at the bifurcation and travel with the external carotid artery.

The presence of multiple, often severe, craniospinal or

systemic injuries may obscure the early signs of traumatic dissection, making early diagnosis difficult. Associated mandibular fractures, neck injuries, and basilar skull fractures may be identified. Ptosis might be masked by periorbital trauma or facial swelling. More than half of patients have a loss of consciousness associated with the initial accident.[5–7] Focal headaches may be attributed to the effects of head injury. A persistently depressed level of consciousness obviously prevents the reporting of headaches and should generally prompt a search for an expanding intracranial clot before the diagnosis of dissection is considered.

Ischemic symptoms appear to be less common and less severe in spontaneous dissections than in traumatic ones.[4] In the majority of cases, the ischemic symptoms are attributable to embolization. In some instances, marked luminal stenosis or occlusion, caused by a large intramural hematoma, may lead to ipsilateral reduction of hemispheric cerebral blood flow, resulting in stroke or transient ischemic attack. With adequate collateral channels to the affected hemisphere, which often occur in younger populations, the obstruction might go unnoticed. If collateral flow is borderline, the development of ischemic symptoms could depend on the patient's hemodynamic status (blood pressure, cardiac output, and intravascular volume).

Nonspecific symptoms such as light-headedness or syncope are uncommon; in contrast to arteriosclerotic disease, amaurosis fugax is infrequent. Focal episodes such as transient ischemic attacks or completed stroke are seen in nearly 60 percent of patients at some time during their clinical course.[4] Spontaneous dissections appear to be responsible for approximately 2.5 percent of all occlusive strokes.[17, 18] The exact incidence of strokes caused by traumatic dissections is unknown.

In spontaneous dissections, ischemic symptoms are usually delayed, following the onset of headache by minutes, days, or even longer. In traumatic cases, the interval between the accident and the onset of ischemic symptoms ranges from less than 1 hour to as long as 10 years. Symptoms that appear weeks to years later are more often related to embolization from clots within a dissecting aneurysm rather than carotid luminal obstruction.[1, 5]

RADIOLOGIC FEATURES

The definitive diagnostic study in the evaluation of carotid dissections is arteriography (Table 36–1). This study should be considered in the presence of an unexplained Horner syndrome, hemicranial headaches centered around the eye, or focal ischemic symptoms, especially in young patients. Arteriography should be contemplated immediately in

TABLE 36–1. Arteriographic Findings: Internal Carotid Artery Dissections

Luminal stenosis typically beginning 4–6 cm above cervical ICA bifurcation	Intimal flap
	Double lumen
Abrupt luminal reconstitution, usually at entrance of ICA into carotid canal; occasionally extending to foramen lacerum	Tapered ICA occlusion
	Slow ICA-MCA flow
	Distal branch occlusions
Extracranial aneurysm	

ICA, internal carotid artery; MCA, middle cerebral artery.

trauma patients when computed tomographic scanning does not explain focal neurologic signs, especially those that develop hours or days after an injury.

Luminal stenosis is the most consistent angiographic finding, typically beginning several centimeters distal to the bifurcation and ending at the skull base where the internal carotid artery enters the petrous bone (Fig. 36–3). The dissection usually appears as a long segment of luminal irregularity and stenosis, with more severe luminal compromise centered at the C-1–C-2 region.[19] Characteristically, abrupt luminal reconstitution occurs at the skull base, where the

bony support offered by the carotid canal entrance likely blocks further extension. Occasionally, the stenosis continues through the petrous segment to the foramen lacerum.[20]

Aneurysms are also frequently identified and are usually localized in the upper cervical and subcranial regions. The lumen of the aneurysm may appear saccular or elongated and fingerlike, paralleling the true internal carotid artery lumen.[20] Intimal flaps are often seen near the proximal end of the aneurysm, and, on occasion, the true and false lumina may also communicate distally (Fig. 36–4).

Slow filling of the middle cerebral artery branches is

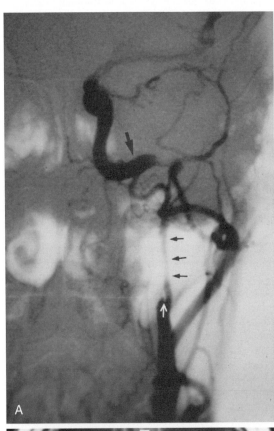

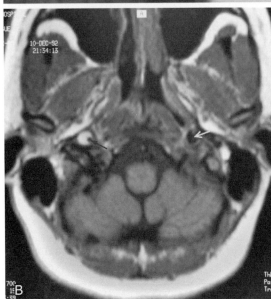

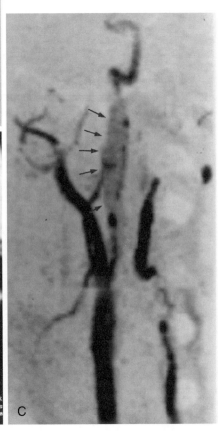

FIGURE 36–3. Case 1. Long-segment internal carotid artery (ICA) stenosis in a patient with bilateral dissections who presented with headache and transient ischemic attacks. *A,* Arteriogram (anteroposterior view) demonstrates severe stenosis (*small arrows*), or "string sign," beginning distal to the ICA bifurcation, with restitution of the vascular lumen in the carotid canal (*large arrow*). An intimal flap is apparent at the proximal end of the dissection (*white arrow*). Note the poor filling of the middle carotid artery branches, probably from washout from flow through other collateral arteries. *B,* Magnetic resonance image (axial view) demonstrates bilateral dissections. On the *left,* an intramural hematoma (high signal abnormality) within the vessel wall is easily seen. The lumen (*dark arrow*) is low-signal (flow void effect) and is markedly narrowed. On the *right,* the intramural clot has resolved (*white arrow*), allowing visualization of the aneurysm lumen. *C,* Magnetic resonance angiogram demonstrates the entire abnormal vessel, with its stenosed lumen and surrounding intramural dissecting aneurysmal bulge (*arrows*) not visible on arteriogram.

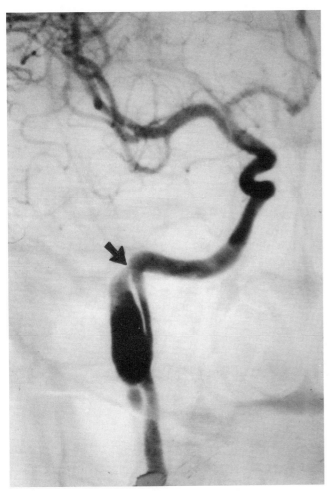

FIGURE 36–4. Case 2. Arteriogram (anteroposterior view) showing a dissection in which the false lumen is re-entering the distal internal carotid artery lumen (*arrow*).

commonly seen in association with tight luminal stenosis. In less severe obstructions, distal branch occlusions related to intracranial embolization can be documented in more than 10 percent of cases (Fig. 36–5).[4, 15] Internal carotid artery occlusion is seen in up to one fourth of cases, usually starting well distal to the carotid bulb and typically tapering to a flame-shaped point (Fig. 36–6). Signs of fibromuscular dysplasia in the ipsilateral internal carotid artery or other cranial or renal vessels, or other subtle luminal irregularities, may also be visualized. Bilateral carotid dissections are identified in up to 25 percent of cases; these are more common among the spontaneous type.[4]

The angiographic appearance of carotid dissections is often dynamic and varies, depending on the severity and extent of the dissection and on the time interval between the onset of the dissection and the performance of the study.[20] An early study may demonstrate a typically located string sign, without an aneurysm lumen, or a complete internal carotid artery occlusion. Later, the true lumen may widen or reopen, with a small bleb at the point of the original intimal tear as the only residual. The likelihood of near complete resolution appears greatest when the trauma is minimal or unsubstantiated (spontaneous type) and when there is no underlying vascular disorder such as fibromuscular dysplasia.

In other cases, the aneurysm lumen may appear where none was apparent on the initial study, presumably as a result of clot lysis within the false channel, combined with persistent flow communication between the two lumina.[9, 20] Complete thrombosis and arteriographic resolution of large aneurysmal sacs are less likely, especially when the trauma has been significant or when the dissection is associated with fibromuscular dysplasia.

Magnetic resonance imaging and magnetic resonance angiography are proving to be excellent tools for imaging carotid dissections, both in establishing the initial diagnosis and in following the progress of treatment.[21–24] These studies have the advantage of demonstrating the dissection noninvasively and can demonstrate the aneurysm even when its lumen is not apparent angiographically. Magnetic resonance imaging can also demonstrate cerebral ischemic changes earlier than computed tomographic scanning, but its use may be limited in acute post-traumatic situations. A normal magnetic resonance imaging investigation does not completely rule out the diagnosis of dissection, and arteriography is still indicated in questionable cases.

Doppler ultrasound may also be useful but is less definitive than magnetic resonance imaging or arteriography.[25] Retinal artery pressures and oculopneumoplethysmography are helpful in determining the presence of an obstructive lesion by demonstrating reduced ocular flows. These studies are most useful for follow-up, as there appears to be a reliable correlation between increasing retinal artery pressures and resolution of luminal stenosis.[26] Intravenous digital subtraction arteriography is not as accurate as arteriography but may also provide useful follow-up data. Computed tomographic scanning is best used following trauma, to differentiate other causes of clinical deterioration such as intracranial hemorrhage.

NATURAL HISTORY

It is now clear that most patients who survive the initial event will do well, especially those with spontaneous dissections. Major infarction is more common in patients with traumatic dissections, and the prognosis for those that present with stroke is not benign.[17, 27] Those patients with a delayed onset of symptoms relative to the development of the dissection, however, have a much more benign presentation and better prognosis.[27, 28] Although two thirds of patients have ischemic symptoms at some point during their clinical course, up to 85 percent progressively improve and have excellent or normal neurologic function.[4, 12] The patient population with dissections is generally young, lacks significant arteriosclerotic disease, and is likely to have good collateral circulation, which protects against further deficits, even in the face of a complete internal carotid artery occlusion.[3] When followed by serial arteriography, stenosis markedly improves or completely resolves in up to 85 percent of cases.[4, 15, 19, 20]

The dissecting aneurysm resolves or decreases in size in two thirds of patients, and rupture rarely (if ever) occurs.[4] Residual aneurysms appear to be more frequent in traumatic dissections or those associated with a vascular disorder such as fibromuscular dysplasia. Delayed or recurrent ischemic symptoms, invariably related to aneurysm persistence, are

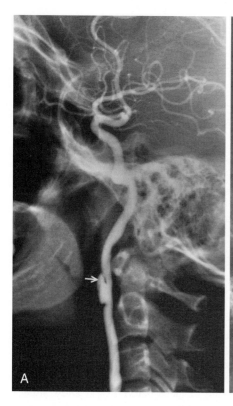
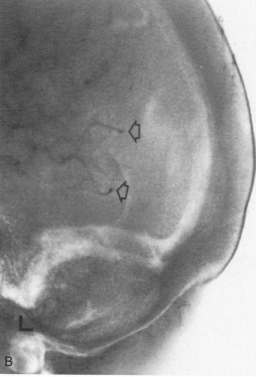

FIGURE 36–5. Case 3. Dissecting aneurysm in a patient with an intracranial embolization. *A*, Arteriogram (lateral view) demonstrates a dissecting aneurysm (*arrow*) at the C1-C2 level. *B*, The emboli have occluded several distal middle carotid artery branches (arrowheads).

uncommon, even though the aneurysm lumen remains patent.

Oculosympathetic paresis resolves less frequently and persists in two thirds of patients. The residual Horner syndrome is usually mild and may go undetected, producing no functional problems. Periorbital headache resolves in up to 95 percent of patients, and its continued presence suggests persistence of the aneurysm. Audible bruits resolve in more than 75 percent of patients, and their long-term presence suggests internal carotid artery occlusion, residual stenosis, or aneurysm.[4]

MANAGEMENT

Considering the benign natural history of most carotid dissections and the propensity for many of the vascular irregularities to improve or resolve with time, the treatment of most lesions is primarily medical (Fig. 36–7). Acutely, major anticoagulation (heparin and coumadin) is the treatment of choice for most patients presenting with hemispheric ischemic symptoms. These drugs are usually maintained for 3 to 6 months and then replaced by antiplatelet medications, to be maintained indefinitely if the affected internal carotid artery remains significantly stenosed or the false lumen persists. Utilization of these medicines may, however, be limited by associated systemic or intracranial injuries.

Surgical therapy may be indicated when ischemic symptoms continue despite best medical treatment or when anticoagulation is inadvisable. The specific type of procedure depends on whether symptoms are caused by reduced hemispheric flow or continued embolization. Intraoperative electroencephalographic monitoring, arteriography, and cerebral blood flow measurements are important adjuvants to the selection of the appropriate procedure and help improve its safety.

Direct thromboendarterectomy should be reserved for those rare cases in which the dissection is confined to proximal portions of the vessel. Adequate distal exposure is difficult and risky, and direct repair is problematic because the vessel wall is often thin and friable. If persistent embolization is suspected, carotid ligation alone may suffice. In patients with compromised hemispheric flow (prior to or as a result of internal carotid artery ligation), resection of the diseased segment followed by interposition graft end-to-end anastomosis, or extracranial–intracranial bypass, may be successful in selected instances.

Experience with interventional neuroradiologic techniques is limited in this disorder. In cases of recurrent embolization from a persistent aneurysm, it may be possible to thrombose the lesion with newly available coils, although such a procedure would not enhance ipsilateral hemispheric flow. Graduated intraluminal dilatation of an obstructed vessel appears to carry unacceptable risks of internal carotid artery restenosis or thrombosis, repeat dissection, or distal embolization.

CONCLUSIONS

The treatment of most cervical carotid dissections is medical therapy. Patients presenting with ischemic symptoms, if seen early after the onset of symptoms, are best treated with major anticoagulation (heparin and coumadin) for 3 to 6 months, followed by conversion to antiplatelet drugs. Patients seen remote from their ischemic symptoms, or those presenting with headache or oculosympathetic paresis, may be observed or treated with antiplatelet drugs. Surgery is reserved for patients with ischemic symptoms refractory to

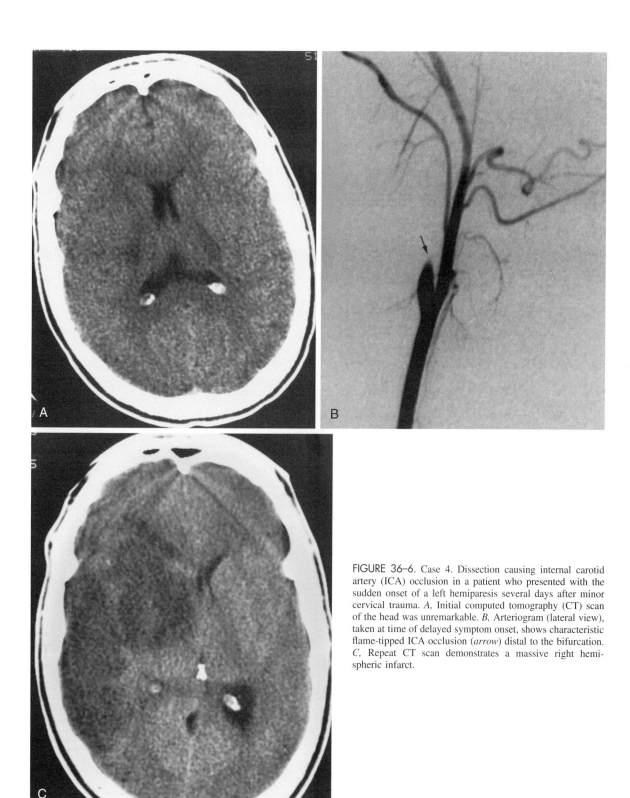

FIGURE 36–6. Case 4. Dissection causing internal carotid artery (ICA) occlusion in a patient who presented with the sudden onset of a left hemiparesis several days after minor cervical trauma. *A,* Initial computed tomography (CT) scan of the head was unremarkable. *B,* Arteriogram (lateral view), taken at time of delayed symptom onset, shows characteristic flame-tipped ICA occlusion (*arrow*) distal to the bifurcation. *C,* Repeat CT scan demonstrates a massive right hemispheric infarct.

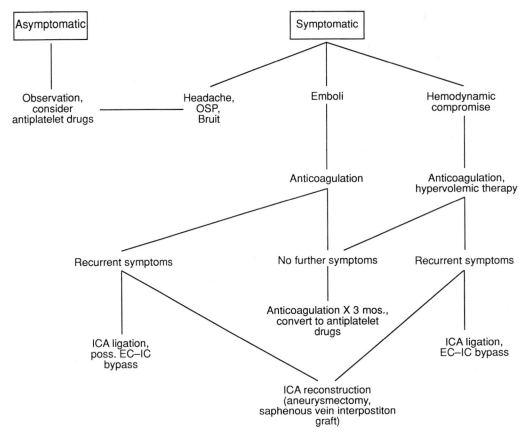

FIGURE 36–7. Treatment algorithm for internal carotid artery dissection. OSP, oculosympathetic paresis; ICA, internal carotid artery; EC–IC, extracranial-intracranial.

medical therapy. Surgical options include carotid ligation alone or combined with an extracranial–intracranial bypass procedure or saphenous vein interposition graft following resection of the diseased segment. Direct approaches with thromboendarterectomy alone are higher-risk procedures and are limited to those uncommon situations in which the dissection arises and is confined to lower regions of the neck.

REFERENCES

1. Batzdorf U, Bentson JR, Machleder HI: Blunt trauma to the high cervical carotid artery. *Neurosurgery.* 1979;5:195.
2. Ehrenfeld WK, Wylie E: Spontaneous dissection of the internal carotid artery. *Arch Surg.* 1976;111:1294.
3. Friedman WA, Day AL, Quisling RG, et al: Cervical carotid dissecting aneurysms. *Neurosurgery.* 1980;7:207.
4. Mokri B: Dissections of cervical and cephalic arteries. In Sundt TM Jr, ed. *Occlusive Cerebrovascular Disease: Diagnosis and Surgical Management.* Philadelphia: WB Saunders; 1987:38.
5. Mokri B, Piepgras DG, Houser OW: Traumatic dissections of the extracranial internal carotid artery. *J Neurosurg.* 1988;68:189.
6. Davis JW, Holbrook TL, Hoyt DB, et al: Blunt carotid artery dissection: Incidence, associated injuries, screening, and treatment. *J Trauma.* 1990;30:1514.
7. Watridge CB, Muhlbauer MS, Lowery RD: Traumatic carotid artery dissection: diagnosis and treatment. *J Neurosurg.* 1989;71:854.
8. Beatty R: Dissecting hematoma of the internal carotid artery following chiropractic cervical manipulation. *J Trauma.* 1977;17:248.
9. Stringer WL, Kelly DL: Traumatic dissection of the extracranial internal carotid artery. *Neurosurgery.* 1980;6:123.
10. Sundt TM, Pearson BW, Piepgras DG, et al: Surgical management of aneurysms of the distal extracranial internal carotid artery. *J Neurosurg.* 1986;64:169.
11. Zelenock GB, Kazmers A, Whitehouse WM, et al: Extracranial internal carotid artery dissections: Noniatrogenic traumatic lesions. *Arch Surg.* 1982;117:425.
12. Hart RG, Easton JD: Dissections of cervical and cerebral arteries. *Neurol Clin.* 1983;1:155.
13. Mokri B, Sundt TM, Houser OW, Piepgras DG: Spontanous dissection of the cervical internal carotid artery. *Ann Neurol.* 1986;19:126.
14. D'Anglejan-Chatillon J, Ribeiro V, Mas JL, et al: Migraine: A risk factor for dissection of cervical arteries. *Headache.* 1989;29:560.
15. Anson J, Crowell RM: Cervicocranial arterial dissection. *Neurosurgery.* 1991;29:89.
16. Fischer CM: The headache and pain of spontaneous carotid disection. *Headache.* 1981;22:60.
17. Bogousslavsky J, Despland PA, Regli F: Spontaneous carotid dissection with acute stroke. *Arch Neurol.* 1987;44:137.
18. Lanzino G, Andreoli A, Di Pasquale G, et al: Etiopathogenesis and prognosis of cerebral ischemia in young adults: A survey of 155 treated patients. *Acta Neurol Scand.* 1991;84:321.
19. Quisling RG, Friedman WA, Rhoton AL: High cervical carotid artery dissection: Spontaneous resolution. *AJNR.* 1980;1:463.
20. Houser OW, Mokri B, Sundt TM, et al: Spontaneous cervical cephalic arterial dissection and its residuum: Angiographic spectrum. *AJNR.* 1984;5:27.
21. Bui LN, Brant-Zawadzki M, Verghese P, Gillan G: Magnetic resonance angiography of cervicocranial dissection. *Stroke.* 1993;24:126.
22. Gelbert F, Assouline E, Hodes JE, et al: MRI in spontaneous dissection of vertebral and carotid arteries: 15 cases studied at 0.5 tesla. *Neuroradiology.* 1991;33:111.
23. Goldberg HI, Grossman RI, Gomori M, et al: Cervical internal carotid artery dissecting hemorrhage: Diagnosis using MR. *Radiology.* 1986;158:157.
24. Sue DE, Brant-Zawadzki MN, Chance J: Dissection of cranial arteries in the neck: Correlation of MRI and arteriography. *Neuroradiology.* 1992;34:273.
25. Sturzenegger M: Ultrasound findings in spontaneous carotid artery dissection: The value of duplex sonography. *Arch Neurol.* 1991;48:1057.
26. Gee W, Kaupp HA, McDonald KM, et al: Spontaneous dissection of internal carotid arteries: Spontaneous resolution measured by serial ocular pneumoplethysmography and angiography. *Arch Surg.* 1980;115:944.
27. Yamada S, Kindt GW, Youmans JR: Carotid artery occlusion due to nonpenetrating injury. *J Trauma.* 1967;7:333.
28. Pozzati E, Giuliani G, Poppi M, Faenza A: Blunt traumatic carotid artery dissection with delayed symptoms. *Stroke.* 1989;20:412.

CHAPTER 37

Blunt and Penetrating Injuries of the Extracranial Cerebral Vessels

MALCOLM O. PERRY

In the United States, trauma is the leading cause of death during the first three decades of life.[1] More than 50 million injuries and 100,000 deaths occur annually; vascular wounds cause many of these deaths and result in severe disability in some of the survivors.[2]

Although major vascular injuries can be encountered in almost any civilian setting, the greatest incidence is in urban areas, where violence is endemic. Penetrating wounds caused by knives and bullets are common, but accidental stab wounds produced by shards of glass or metal projections are also encountered. Several large city hospitals have described their emergency room experience with these wounds; as expected, stab wounds are more frequent, occurring several times more often than shotgun wounds. Many stab wounds are not serious, however, and deeper structures are often spared. This reflects the type of weapon used, usually a small knife, razor, or ice pick.

By contrast, gunshot wounds penetrate deeply, often into the trunk or thorax as well as the neck and extremities, and are likely to result in serious damage. The vessels of the extremities are usually involved, but the more deeply placed, larger arteries are vulnerable to gunshot wounds, and multiple vascular wounds are often encountered in these types of injuries. Any of these wounds can cause lethal bleeding, but obviously death is more common with injuries of major vessels in the chest or abdomen, where early detection and rapid control of hemorrhage are more difficult (Table 37–1).[3, 4]

ETIOLOGY AND MECHANISM OF INJURY

Penetrating injuries producing direct vascular wounds are usually caused by stabbing or bullets traveling at low velocity, and the damage is confined mainly to the wound tract. Lacerations are seen most often with knife wounds, but transections, contusions, or punctures are also encountered (Table 37–2). By contrast, higher-velocity bullets not only damage the neurovascular structures in the wound path but also cause other problems due to their concussive effects. Contusion or even vessel transection may follow the cavitation effects associated with missiles traveling at high veloci-

ties of 1500 to 3000 feet per second (fps). Even if immediate vessel disruption does not occur, mural contusions can result in delayed thrombosis or even necrosis and wall separation, late hemorrhage, and false aneurysm formation.[3]

A high-velocity bullet or metal fragment produces a great deal of tissue damage. A small-caliber bullet traveling at very high speeds (over 3000 fps) can destroy a large volume of flesh and muscle because of its great energy ($E = \frac{1}{2}\,mV^2$). If it strikes bone and all the bullet's energy is dissipated in the target, the destructiveness is appalling. Also, secondary missiles consisting of bullet or shell fragments or bone splinters may be created, and they can produce other wounds. Direct injury and cavitation are accompanied by a powerful suction effect as the blast cavity collapses, drawing surface structures such as clothing and dirt into the wounds. Such destructive effects may not be suspected from inspection of the skin surface, where in some cases rather small entry and exit wounds are seen. But despite these small entry wounds, the interior damage can be extensive, and wide débridement is needed if infection is to be avoided.[3]

Special problems are encountered in the treatment of shotgun wounds. The muzzle velocity of shotgun pellets is similar to that produced by the familiar .22-caliber rifle bullet, approximately 1200 fps. Because of the poor ballistic shape of the spherical pellets, energy losses are rapid and the velocity quickly drops, even over short distances. A large number of pellets may cause widespread damage, however. Close-range wounds are particularly destructive and, although the plastic wadding and fillers used in modern short-shell ammunition cause fewer problems than the older fiber inserts, bits of clothing may be carried into the wound with the missiles. Such foreign bodies further complicate the management of these wounds because they increase the incidence of infection.[4]

Motor vehicle accidents are a major cause of vascular trauma, and accident victims commonly have multiple injuries. Direct vessel trauma occurs, but major arterial or venous wounds are often the result of fractures; this is especially likely to occur near joints, where the vessels are relatively fixed and more vulnerable to shear forces.

The bending and sudden breaking of large, heavy bones release tremendous forces. The damage to soft tissue and neurovascular structures can be extensive—the effects similar to those produced by the cavitation associated with high-velocity bullets. After the bones fall back into near-normal positions, the magnitude of the injuring forces may not be

TABLE 37–1. Distribution of Arterial Injuries in 196 Cases

Artery	Number
Innominate	8
Subclavian	38
Axillary	43
Aorta	11
Common carotid	53
Internal carotid	17
External carotid	19
Vertebral	7

TABLE 37–2. Types of Arterial Wounds

Wound	%
Laceration	51
Transection	38
Puncture	6
Contusion	5

appreciated and the severity of damage may be underestimated.

PATHOPHYSIOLOGY

Although injuries of large arteries can usually be readily identified because of the severe hemorrhage, less extensive wounds may not be evident. Ischemia distal to the area of the injury may not be present, especially when intervening collateral vessels are adequate and hypotension is absent.

The assessment of the adequacy of blood flow based on the detection of distal extremity pulses is limited by normal hemodynamic properties. The pulse wave is a pressure wave, attaining velocities up to 10 m/second as it proceeds distally in the less distensible arteries of the extremities. The pressure wave may be transmitted beyond intimal flaps, via circuitous collaterals or even through limited areas of fresh, soft clot, and reach the distal small arteries. The flow wave, with a velocity of 40 to 50 cm/second, is distinct from the pulse wave, and the physical examination must take this fact into account. With the anatomic provisions for flow through collaterals, and with some injuries limited only to vessel wall damage, it is not surprising that the distal pulses have been found to be relatively normal in up to 20 percent of patients with operatively proven arterial injuries. Such a combination is especially likely with penetrating wounds of the neck and shoulder, where the collateral circulation is abundant.

The detection of Doppler signals and the measurement of distal arterial systolic blood pressure by this or any of a variety of plethysmographic techniques are helpful, but the specificity suffers from related hemodynamic limitations. Subtle abnormalities in these measurements are common, but relatively normal values are also seen, thereby compromising the reliability of these methods for excluding vascular wounds. This is a particular problem in patients with multiple injuries who also have hypotension from other causes.

The tendency for thrombosis to complicate arterial or venous injuries often presents serious problems in diagnosis and management. Clot propagation is not uncommon, especially if hypotension is present and if the time from wounding to definitive care is prolonged. The appearance of ischemia in an extremity initially observed to be normal or only mildly compromised is an ominous finding and may mean that distal thrombosis has occurred. The ultrasonic velocity flow detector may offer substantial assistance in these situations by demonstrating distal arterial patency. In some cases, because of the helical arrangement of vascular smooth muscle, decreases in intraluminal arterial pressure may reach a critical value (30 mm Hg), and the vessel will close. Flow will cease as the lumen collapses, and, with activation of the intrinsic clotting mechanisms, widespread thrombosis supervenes. These problems are obviously more likely to occur when resuscitation is inadequate or when the patient also has cardiopulmonary disease or low-flow states from any cause.

INITIAL EVALUATION

It is now customary for injured patients to be divided into three categories to permit a more precise establishment of priorities.[4] Category I injuries (tension pneumothorax, cardiac tamponade, exsanguinating hemorrhage) are immediate threats to the survival of the patient and are given the highest priority. Category II injuries, which include major fractures, abdominal trauma, and genitourinary trauma in patients with stable vital signs, are serious wounds, but there is usually time for a more extensive evaluation. Category III injuries such as lacerations, simple fractures, and contusions can be managed in a more leisurely fashion.

Injuries of major vessels rarely compete with category I problems but usually take priority over most of the injuries in categories II and III. Obviously, urgent attention is warranted for any vascular injury associated with severe ischemia or continued bleeding.

It is helpful to divide injuries of the neck according to location. Monson and coworkers[5] suggested using three zones for the categorization of these injuries. Zone I includes those penetrating injuries below the sternal notch, zone II the injuries between the sternal notch and the angle of the mandible, and zone III those injuries between the angle of the mandible and the base of the skull. It is evident that penetrating wounds in zone I are likely to damage the great vessels and may even have penetrated the chest and injured the aorta or the heart.[6, 7] Injuries in zone II, although still serious, may be managed in a more direct fashion if the patient does not have a neurologic injury or wounds of the aerodigestive tract.[8] Injuries in zone III require special attention, since exposure of the internal carotid artery in this area is often difficult, and extensive damage to the vessel may not be amenable to repair.[9, 10] Even if the diagnosis is secure, it is often helpful to know the exact location and number of vessel wounds. Arteriography is frequently recommended for penetrating wounds in all three zones, but especially for patients who have wounds in zones I and III and in those with neurologic deficits.[9]

DIAGNOSIS

During an 18-year experience with more than 600 vascular wounds, the value of certain diagnostic features was evaluated.[3] This experience suggests that certain signs and symptoms are helpful in diagnosing arterial wounds, especially when several signs are present. Patients who have a deficit in distal pulses or who have ischemia, a large hematoma, and continuing hemorrhage are likely to have serious vascular wounds, but false-positive normal distal pulses were found in 10 percent of the patients in this series who had operatively proven proximal arterial injuries. Misleading distal pulses were usually seen in patients who had contusions, small arterial lacerations, or injured deep femoral or deep brachial arteries. Minor arterial wounds were not always the only finding in such patients; several almost complete transections of femoral, subclavian, and axillary arteries were found to have normal distal pulses and blood pressures on preoperative examination.

Injuries of the heart and great vessels present special diagnostic problems because of their inaccessibility to direct examination.[11] Hemopneumothorax or mediastinal bleeding is common with penetrating injuries of the chest, even without major vascular wounds.[12] Patients with such injuries may initially be stable, thought to have only parenchymal lung damage or minor venous disruption, but sudden hemodynamic collapse may be the first sign of more severe problems. (Widened mediastinum, cardiac arrest, persistent shock, cardiac tamponade, and recurring hemothorax may indicate serious injuries.)

Brachiocephalic Vessels

Injuries of the intrathoracic aorta and great vessels result in the highest mortality rate of all arterial wounds, often ending in early exsanguination and death.[7, 11, 13] In several studies, many patients were dead on arrival in the emergency room or were in profound hemorrhagic shock when initially seen.[7] As pointed out by Hewitt and colleagues,[6] these injuries present special problems because of the difficulty in making a specific diagnosis and the wide surgical exposure required to obtain control of bleeding. In the report by Flint and associates,[7] 40 percent of 146 patients were in shock when first seen, and Reul and coworkers[11] observed that almost half the patients in their study were hypotensive and that more than 40 percent had other serious wounds. Such combined injuries appear to be a major reason for the lethality of penetrating injuries of the upper chest and root of the neck.

Most major vascular wounds in this area are caused by bullets or stabbing (97 percent of the cases of Flint and associates), but blunt trauma may also be at fault.[7, 12] Multiple injuries are more likely to be caused by gunshot wounds, especially when the wound tract is in an oblique or lateral plane, thus passing through several vessels. Major venous injuries are also common and can seriously compromise efforts to control bleeding. With venous injuries in this area, however, bleeding is not the only risk; with resuscitation and operative manipulation, air embolism can occur.[7]

Certain varieties of blunt trauma are particularly likely to result in vascular injury: steering wheel injuries, deceleration forces, and falls and crushing blows to the chest and root of the neck. Posterior fractures of the first and second rib, for example, are an indication that the chest has been subjected to tremendous forces, and the likelihood of associated serious damage is high.[3]

The diagnosis of vascular injury is obvious in the presence of specific findings such as bleeding, large or expanding hematomas, weak or absent distal pulses, and continued intrathoracic hemorrhage. But in one large series, one third of the patients had no diagnostic signs.[4, 7] Penetrating trauma causes injuries of nearby nerves more frequently here than in other areas, because of the close anatomic relationships of the vessels and the brachial plexus, phrenic nerve, vagus nerves, and even the spinal cord.[12]

Most patients with serious vascular injuries have large hematomas at the base of the neck, widened mediastinum (more than 8 cm in the second interspace on an upright chest radiograph), continued intrathoracic bleeding, or massive hemothorax.[3] Unfortunately, persistent bleeding in the chest may not be apparent until after a period of observation and after more blood loss. Also, a number of patients early after an injury may experience cardiac tamponade or cardiac arrest, especially in the presence of combined injuries.[2] In a few cases, the only early symptom apart from the obvious penetration is refractory hypotension, but when a chest tube is inserted, massive bleeding becomes apparent.

If the injured patient is stable, arteriography may be of great help in precisely defining the extent and location of the injuries. High-quality biplane angiography can be very reliable, but it is also clear that it is not infallible, particularly when vascular wounds in this area are involved.

Several surgeons have observed false-negative studies, perhaps reflecting the difficulties in obtaining the multiple views needed for precision.[3, 4, 7] When preoperative arteriograms can be obtained safely, they may offer information that can materially assist in the conduct of surgery, particularly if special preoperative maneuvers are needed (eg, shunts, cardiac bypass pump, remote catheter control techniques). It has been emphasized by several workers that a delay in required surgery may be dangerous in unstable patients, and if firm indications for immediate operation exist, it is best not to hesitate.[8, 14] If arteriograms are necessary, they can be obtained in the operating room; if sudden collapse ensues, immediate exploration can then be undertaken.

Carotid and Vertebral Arteries

Most wounds of the cervical vessels are caused by penetrating trauma, and the common carotid artery is usually involved.[9] The left carotid artery is injured slightly more often than is the right, perhaps suggesting that more assailants are right-handed. Several reviews have emphasized the special problems encountered in patients with these types of injuries.[9, 15-17] In addition to the vascular injury, major difficulties are caused by neurologic dysfunction. Also, there may be associated wounds of the larynx, esophagus, and trachea, thereby increasing the likelihood of bacterial contamination.

Experience in the management of patients with occlusive extracranial arterial disease has clearly underscored the risks of vascular reconstruction in patients with acute stroke, especially if there are alterations in consciousness or coma. When vascular reconstructions are attempted in these patients, mortality rates of 40 percent and higher are found.[16, 18, 19] This high death rate was thought to be mainly the result of conversion of an anemic cerebral infarct into a hemorrhagic infarct, with subsequent extension of the stroke. It is believed that restoration of normal arterial pressure and flow to the damaged brain can be followed by bleeding into the softened tissue. Recent investigations suggest that microhemorrhage is a part of many cerebral infarctions and that extensive intracerebral bleeding may supervene even without restoration of normal arterial pressure. In fact, it is believed that some lacunar microinfarcts are hemorrhagic. These observations suggest that other factors may be involved in the sudden neurologic deterioration that occurs when vascular reconstruction is performed in patients with acute severe strokes. The precise roles of hypertension, heparinization, anesthesia, and surgery are uncertain, but it seems clear that patients with severe strokes caused by complete occlusion of the carotid artery are poor candidates for vascular reconstruction.[20] Almost all studies report high mortality rates in this group of patients.[17, 21]

Accurate preoperative assessment is essential for the successful management of patients with carotid injuries, since it appears that the eventual outcome depends on the extent of the initial preoperative neurologic deficit. Moreover, a significant number of these patients have other injuries; for example, closed head trauma can distort the diagnostic picture. Such combined problems are particularly confusing when the indications for surgery are being considered. A precise neurologic evaluation is mandatory before extensive vascular repairs are begun in these patients.

The results of several studies strongly support surgical repair of all carotid injuries in patients who have no neurologic deficits or only mild ones.[17, 21, 22] This decision is easier when the arterial injury is bleeding actively, but it may be more difficult when there is complete carotid artery occlusion and no neurologic symptoms have been reported. In this situation, technical problems encountered during surgery could conceivably produce brain damage, although in the reported experience, this has been rare. The risk exists, however, and careful neurologic and arteriographic studies are needed before operation is undertaken in order to assess the danger accurately and formulate the sequence of treatment.

Even an artery depicted on an arteriogram as being completely blocked may prove to be patent at surgery. The slow flow of blood through a small channel may not be visible even on a good arteriogram. Untreated, this lesion is likely to progress to complete occlusion, with occasional extension into the cerebral arteries, thus causing a stroke. Thromboembolic events may also supervene, and middle cerebral artery emboli have been observed in such situations. Although some arterial wounds heal spontaneously, this is not predictable. Delayed development of a false aneurysm is also possible, although such lesions are uncommon. For these reasons,

most surgeons believe that practically all carotid wounds should be repaired if the patient does not have a complete occlusion complicated by an acute severe stroke.[9, 17]

Carotid wounds from blunt trauma may be more difficult to detect and evaluate (Fig. 37–1). Such trauma is not invariably accompanied by telltale bruises and cuts; in fact, about half of patients have no superficial evidence of trauma. Clinical features suggesting the presence of blunt trauma to the carotid artery include Horner syndrome, transient ischemic attack, lucid interval after injury, and limb paresis in an alert patient. Alternatively, there may be no neurologic symptoms even in the presence of severe carotid damage. Hyperextension injuries of the neck are particularly likely to produce extensive stretching, contusion, and intimal damage in the distal internal carotid artery.[20] The artery at this level is fixed by entry into the skull and can be forcibly stretched over the cervical vertebra by hyperextension. This type of stretch injury, or even direct contusion, predisposes to a special sequence of events.[19] Initially there may be no sign of injury and no neurologic symptoms, but as thrombosis of the vessel or intramural hemorrhage occurs, stroke becomes evident. This can be delayed for several hours but is almost always apparent within the first 24 hours. By this time, there is usually complete occlusion of the artery, often with extension of the clot into the head and occasionally even distal embolization. If an initial neurologic problem is suspected, it is often thought to be caused by direct brain damage, that is, a subdural or epidural hematoma, resulting in a delay in making the true diagnosis.

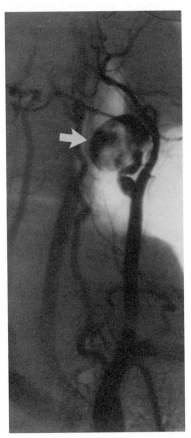 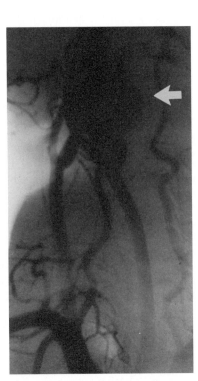 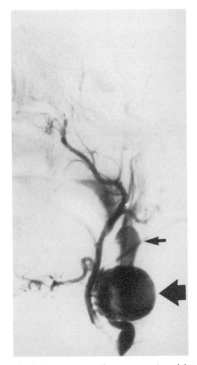

FIGURE 37–1. Blunt trauma to the internal carotid artery as a result of a snowmobile accident caused the false aneurysm (*large arrows*) and intramural dissection (*small arrows*) seen in this panel of radiographs.

Most of these arterial wounds eventually cause specific symptoms, but by then, they may not be reversible. Also, the delay between wounding and the emergence of neurologic symptoms can be protracted. Crissey and Bernstein[23] reported one person in whom 15 years elapsed before the injury was diagnosed, having by then caused a severe carotid stenosis. One patient in the author's series also developed common carotid stenosis and transient attacks of cerebral ischemia more than a year after the carotid contusion (Fig. 37–2).[20]

Although noninvasive vascular tests can be useful in chronic, stable cases, they are not particularly helpful in an acute evaluation. Arteriography is the definitive test, and, when properly employed, it is quite reliable in diagnosing or excluding carotid artery injuries.[10] Moreover, knowing the type and location of the wound preoperatively assists in planning the operation. Since complete exposure of the internal carotid artery requires an extensive surgical dissection, and since some blunt injuries may not be easily detected by examining the exterior of the vessel, the angiogram is helpful. For example, the identification of an acute fistula between the internal carotid artery and the jugular vein permits the surgeon to prepare special techniques for management. If a graft is needed to replace a damaged artery, it is best to know this in advance, have it ready, and thus reduce the carotid occlusion time. If a patient is stable, preoperative cerebral arteriography is recommended, particularly if there are neurologic problems. But if for some reason this cannot be done, an angiogram can be obtained in the operating room. Most penetrating wounds of the midcervical region can be managed adequately without arteriograms, but distal

clots or other injuries near the base of the skull may pose serious problems, and operative arteriography can be helpful.

Adjunctive Methods

Ordinary radiographs may be of some value in the initial evaluation of patients with vascular injuries, since such pictures may disclose the presence of subcutaneous or mediastinal air, features suggesting penetration of the aerodigestive tracts.[8, 14] In other situations, there may be displacement of soft tissues by large hematomas. Unfortunately, on some occasions, even in the presence of serious vascular injuries, ordinary radiographic studies offer little assistance. They cannot be depended on to exclude serious injury.

Recent studies have suggested that computed tomographic (CT) scanning may be of benefit in the assessment of injured patients.[24] Even without the administration of contrast medium, CT can often detect displacement of soft-tissue structures, hematomas, and collections of fluid. In specialized situations in which arterial injury may have resulted in extreme narrowing of an artery (eg, the distal internal carotid), even arteriograms may suggest that the artery is blocked, because blood flow is so sluggish through the narrowed area that it cannot be detected on ordinary studies. Rapid-sequence CT scanning with infusion of contrast medium in such a patient may disclose a patent internal carotid artery. All these studies take some time, however; in hemodynamically stable patients, they may offer valuable information, but it is clear that if the patient is not stable, it is best to proceed immediately to the operating room and complete the diagnostic evaluation during resuscitation. Un-

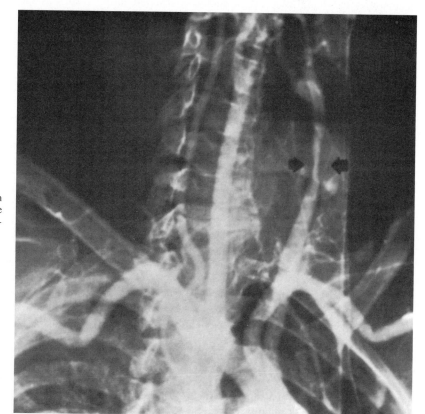

FIGURE 37–2. Stenosis (*arrows*) in the left common carotid artery resulting from an assault and blow to the neck 2 years before the onset of left hemispheric ischemic symptoms.

toward delays in this situation may lead to irreversible deficits, especially if sudden cardiovascular collapse supervenes.

RESUSCITATION

A patient with multiple serious injuries presents dramatically, usually bleeding, pale, apprehensive, short of breath, and often with low blood pressure. Successful resuscitation requires that certain priorities be established and specific plans of treatment be formulated.[4]

In all these circumstances, attention to the airway and control of bleeding must be paramount. When these problems are severe, the need is usually obvious, but a more dangerous situation exists when hypoxia is not recognized, blood loss is slowly increasing, and cardiopulmonary stability has been achieved by compensatory mechanisms. A temporarily stable situation evolves, but when the patient is no longer capable of making the internal adjustments needed, collapse is sudden, and shock may be irreversible.

Once control of the airway has been obtained, the vital signs assessed, and an overall evaluation completed, proper priorities can be set. A rapid physical examination is performed. If external bleeding is present, it is controlled with direct finger pressure, pressure dressings, or pressure on proximal vascular structures. Blind attempts to clamp bleeding vessels located deep in the wound are ineffective and dangerous, often causing further neurovascular damage.[3, 4]

After control of the airway is secured and respiratory assistance initiated, ventilation and lung mechanisms are evaluated. Chest trauma of any type can cause direct lung damage, or a hemopneumothorax may produce severe restrictive respiratory deficiency. If chest tubes are needed to decompress the pleural space, these should be inserted early during the resuscitation, before pressure-assisted ventilation causes more severe mechanical problems by increasing the air leak.

Fluid and blood requirements in trauma patients are often impressive, and adequate intravenous access lines are needed. Large catheters are placed into an uninjured upper and lower extremity, if needed, and carefully secured. During the selection of veins for administering intravenous fluids, the possibility of injury to the innominate vein or superior vena cava should be considered. The lines should be placed to ensure that the fluid and blood can reach the general circulation and not be impeded if that vein must be clamped. One line is committed only for fluid replacement; it is not used for drug administration or anesthetic manipulation. If hemorrhage is severe, the rate of blood replacement will have to be rapid and continuous. Since there may be a need for venous autografts for vascular repair, it is often prudent to preserve the saphenous or cephalic veins, but the treatment of shock must take precedence.

In most cases, a combination of a balanced electrolyte solution and whole blood is chosen for resuscitation. As described by Shires,[1] trauma and shock induce internal shifts of interstitial fluid that respond satisfactorily to appropriate infusion of electrolyte solutions. Blood loss is corrected with blood transfusion, but it is wise not to overtransfuse, especially if chest trauma or cardiac disease is present. In fact, rheologic and oxygen transport studies suggest that a whole blood hematocrit of approximately 30 percent is optimum; further increases in hemoglobin are unneeded and may increase blood viscosity unnecessarily. Few convincing data exist to show that the infusion of colloid solutions (eg, albumin, dextran) is of any additional value; some studies even suggest that giving such colloid solutions may be harmful and increase the likelihood of fluid overload.[3] Also, anaphylaxis has been described in association with the administration of a number of colloid solutions and may be related to the particles rather than the specific substance.

During the general assessment, other wounds of a less serious nature should be protected from further injury and from bacterial contamination. It is easy to forget these patients' vulnerability to infection, and the portal of entry for pathogenic bacteria may well be a relatively minor wound that is heavily contaminated while a dramatic resuscitation is being performed. Contamination can come in many forms, and observation of the routine procedures employed in many emergency rooms discloses a number of opportunities for accidental wound inoculation. Once infection is established, particularly with hospital-based organisms, the spread to other more significant injuries is common, and the results can be disastrous. In fact, the relatively low incidence of fatal infections seen in these patients is surprising and is a tribute to the basic recuperative powers of the individual and to the generally excellent care.

Prophylactic antibiotic administration is considered appropriate in trauma cases. Although this practice is not supported by unequivocal data, it is agreed that antibiotic levels in tissue and blood must be attained preoperatively if the regimen is to be effective.[4] Since wound contamination with trauma is likely, these drugs may be of help in reducing the incidence of infection. This can be of particular importance when separate incisions are to be made for other procedures such as subcutaneous bypass grafting. Broad-spectrum antibiotics are recommended in these situations and are usually given just before surgery and stopped on the second postoperative day.

PREOPERATIVE PREPARATION

As in most cases of cervical trauma, induction of anesthesia must be gentle to prevent the dislodgment of tamponading clots, which might cause recurrence of bleeding. Distal embolization is also possible if induction is rough and causes the patient to lurch and move about. Although it is often appropriate to explore some stab wounds under local anesthesia to determine their depth, once penetration of the platysma muscle is confirmed and a vascular injury suspected, general anesthesia is preferred. A variety of anesthetic agents are effective, and the final choice rests with the anesthesiologist. Drugs likely to cause hypotension are not desirable for obvious reasons and should be avoided. Endotracheal intubation is required in these circumstances, making preoperative knowledge of laryngeal nerve function essential. If a proper evaluation cannot be made before reaching the operating room, the vocal cords can be directly inspected during intubation.

During the initial phases of examination and resuscitation, the need for special monitoring techniques is usually evident. Those patients with minor penetrating wounds of an extremity who are hemodynamically stable often require only routine procedures, especially if they are young and free of intercurrent serious illnesses. By contrast, a patient with multiple injuries and shock or with pre-existing cardiopulmonary problems is certain to need continuous monitoring of vital signs, pulmonary mechanics, and cardiac and cerebral function.[3] Such baseline data are particularly important when resuscitation must include the administration of large amounts of blood and fluids and perhaps vasoactive drugs.

Some estimate of cardiac filling and output is often helpful; clinical signs are of value, but other maneuvers may be needed. A venous catheter for measuring the central venous pressure is helpful, but this measurement can be misinterpreted because of overestimation of its reliability and sensitivity. Measurements of central venous pressure yield one very useful piece of data: an estimate of the ability of the right heart to handle a given load of inflow volume per unit of time. Rapid rises in the central venous pressure afford a clear warning that the right heart is incapable of handling the volume load at that rate, and the infusion should be slowed. No real information about the absolute quantity of intravascular volume is obtained from this monitoring technique if there is any discrepancy between the function of the right and left heart.

When cardiac or pulmonary problems are present and resuscitation is difficult or unsatisfactory, a Swan-Ganz catheter is invaluable. Measurements of pulmonary artery pressure are extremely valuable in guiding fluid administration and in assessing cardiac and pulmonary function. Moreover, if positive end-expiratory pressure is needed to ensure adequate oxygenation, its effect on cardiac function can be followed and any adverse influence of high pressure can be detected early and avoided.

If measurements of cardiac output are needed, these can be performed easily with a Swan-Ganz multilumen catheter in place. Thermistor-computer techniques have simplified these maneuvers, and rapid sequential measurements of cardiac output can be obtained. Mixed venous blood samples can also be drawn, and analysis of these samples for oxygen content and saturation often yields information that may be particularly helpful when cardiac and pulmonary problems arise. Selection of the entry site it important: laceration of a subclavian vein adds another serious injury and, if it is on the same side as an arterial wound, this can be a technical problem. A distal remote vein may be the best place for inserting the catheter.

INCISIONS

The decision regarding surgical exposure is often complex; whether to approach the wound through a thoracotomy or in an extrathoracic route is an important part of management (Fig. 37–3).[5–7] The proximity and number of vital structures in this area are well known, and the danger of combined injuries of the large arteries and veins is apparent. If exsanguination is to be avoided, early operation and vascular control are essential, and several experienced trauma surgeons strongly recommend initial thoracotomy when dealing with suspected vascular wounds in the root of the neck.[6] Some even suggest a median sternal splitting incision for all penetrating wounds below the cricoid cartilage or below C7. Others suggest a more moderate approach, but all agree that if major vascular wounds are strongly suspected, early thoracotomy is needed. Unnecessary thoracotomy may introduce an additional risk; it is therefore recommended by most surgeons that specific plans be formulated and followed, which is easier if the number and location of the vascular injuries are known.

The data reported by Flint and coworkers,[7] Hewitt and associates,[6] and others suggest that when firm signs of major vascular wounds of the root of the neck and upper mediastinum are present, control through a midline sternal splitting incision is best.[11] This approach affords access to the heart, major veins, and great vessels of the arch, except for the origin of the left subclavian artery. This incision can be opened quickly, is usually well tolerated, and is easily closed. It may be extended into the supraclavicular area or into the anterior triangle along the sternomastoid muscle to reach the common carotid artery. For exposure of the intrathoracic portion of the left subclavian artery, many surgeons prefer a separate anterolateral fourth or fifth interspace thoracotomy. At most trauma centers, the sternal splitting incision is usually used because of its simplicity, speed of opening, familiarity to most surgeons, and ready access to the most vulnerable and commonly injured vessels. A limited median sternotomy can be quickly enlarged by extending the original incision or by adding an intercostal incision.

Extrathoracic incisions for managing vascular injuries of the subclavian and common carotid arteries are also useful. In stable patients with isolated, well-defined penetrating injuries, exposure and repair of these vessels can be easily managed with this approach.[5, 12] In selected cases, especially on the left side, injuries of the second and third portion of the subclavian artery may require resection of the medial half of the clavicle for adequate exposure.[7] For example, in patients with penetrating wounds suspected of causing only subclavian injury, the extrathoracic approach is satisfactory and causes little late morbidity. Venous repairs can be performed through these same incisions.

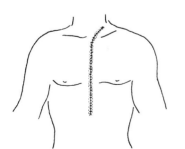
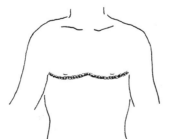
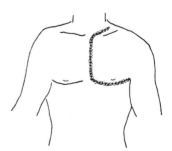

FIGURE 37–3. These incisions are usually satisfactory for exposing arterial wounds in the neck and thoracic outlet. It may be necessary to open the chest to obtain adequate control. These incisions are commonly employed. (See text for further descriptions.)

When exploration is undertaken with a firm clinical diagnosis or after a positive arteriogram, exposure of the injury is usually straightforward, but in other cases, the damage may not be apparent. If bleeding or large hematomas are absent, a thorough exploration is still required. Hematoma in the carotid sheath or in the adventitia of the proximal portion of the vessel is an indication for more extensive exposure. A rather extensive wound can be present in this situation, being effectively tamponaded by the surrounding fascia and the neurovascular sheath, which may have more substance in this region than in others.

CONTROL OF BLEEDING

Most bleeding wounds can be controlled with direct digital pressure. Brisk hemorrhage has usually stopped in patients who have survived to reach the emergency room, but often large hematomas are present, and some bleeding may persist. If the wound is not bleeding, it is best not to disturb it during the early resuscitation, and no attempt should be made to remove foreign bodies or to evacuate clots until a general assessment has been completed. Once the overall examination is completed and initial resuscitation established, specific wound care can be begun. During patient transportation, care should be taken to prevent dislodging clots or causing further damage, especially when there are fractures or embedded foreign bodies. Penetrating objects that are still in the wound must be protected during such transportation or they may cause further damage, perhaps severing adjacent arteries, nerves, or veins not involved in the initial injury. It is best not to extract these instruments until complete control is available, because uncontrollable hemorrhage may occur from the heart or great vessels.

When fatal hemorrhage appears likely to occur in the emergency room, the wound can be extended and clamps applied under direct vision. This has been done successfully in a number of cases in large emergency rooms, where the staff are very experienced. Even thoracotomy can be performed rapidly and safely at these centers.[2] In certain severe cases, patients have been placed on cardiopulmonary bypass in the emergency room before being transported to the operating room for definitive treatment.[2, 6, 11] These are unusual requirements, however, and such maneuvers should be approached with caution, especially by those who are not experienced. A separate indication for emergency thoracotomy may exist when patients are admitted in profound hypovolemic shock. Closed cardiac massage during resuscitation is not likely to be successful in this setting, and open massage is needed. In such circumstances, open cardiac resuscitation can be life saving, warranting an aggressive approach.

Once the injury has been exposed, the clot should be evacuated and the extent of the injury examined. Every effort should be made to avoid fragmenting and dislodging intraluminal clots or extending the damage to the vessel. In patients who have atherosclerotic disease, the arteries may be quite fragile, and it is easy to cause more damage. Repairs are not begun until hemorrhage is arrested. It is wise to pause in the resuscitation to be certain that bleeding has stopped, because even slow bleeding can cause a great deal of unnoticed blood loss over time.

Direct control may be difficult to obtain if the injury has occurred at the confluence of several vessels. In such cases, it may be helpful to insert a balloon-tipped catheter into the vessel, inflate the balloon, and gently retract the catheter. A Foley catheter or a Fogarty catheter to which a three-way stopcock has been attached can be used. These techniques are especially useful in managing penetrating injuries in large vessels of the abdomen or chest, particularly when there are combined injuries of the aorta and major veins. It is possible to repair these lesions carefully in some cases without totally occluding these large vessels, removing the catheter just before tying the final sutures.

Brachiocephalic Vessels

Direct control of bleeding can be accomplished in most situations by the usual techniques—most often by digital pressure. Packing may offer temporary assistance while incisions are widened or additional ones opened, but it cannot be recommended for prolonged use.[11] Lack of complete control and pressure occlusion of other vascular structures are real hazards that can contribute to blood loss and perhaps to ischemic complications.[7]

Once vascular clamps have been applied, standard vascular techniques of repair are satisfactory (Fig. 37–4). With large vessels, lateral repair can often be used, but if the wound cannot be closed without narrowing the artery, patch graft angioplasty is indicated. With more extensive wounds of the great vessels, resection and anastomosis will be required; if the closure cannot be accomplished without tension, an interposition graft is needed. Most surgeons use plastic grafts for repair of these large vessels, although a few surgeons strongly recommend vein grafts, especially if the gastrointestinal or respiratory tract is also injured. Remote bypass techniques may be needed to avoid placing a graft into a field heavily contaminated with bacteria. Subclavian–carotid, axillary–axillary, and carotid–carotid bypasses have been used successfully in a number of cases. Such precautionary procedures may be particularly important when the wound has been caused by erosion from a tracheostomy tube, for example. Infection is extremely likely in this setting.

Temporary shunt procedures to maintain cerebral blood flow while the innominate or common carotid arteries are being repaired are used infrequently. Several reports allude to these maneuvers, but none describes the indications or documents the basis for their use.[7, 17, 22] No statistically valid study has been conducted to clarify this issue, but many trauma surgeons suggest that if there is scant backflow or low back pressure in the distal arteries (<70 mm Hg), insertion of a temporary shunt may be in order. A variety of techniques have been used, including application of inlying tube shunts, combined external and internal shunts, and external shunts.[10]

Major venous wounds in this area are dangerous, as described by several investigators.[6, 7] Multiple injuries are often seen, and control of bleeding is difficult. Although repair of the superior vena cava is an accepted procedure, other veins are sometimes simply ligated. This is particularly common when there are multiple wounds, especially of other major arteries, whose repair often takes precedence. Although a few instances of long-term disability after subclavian vein

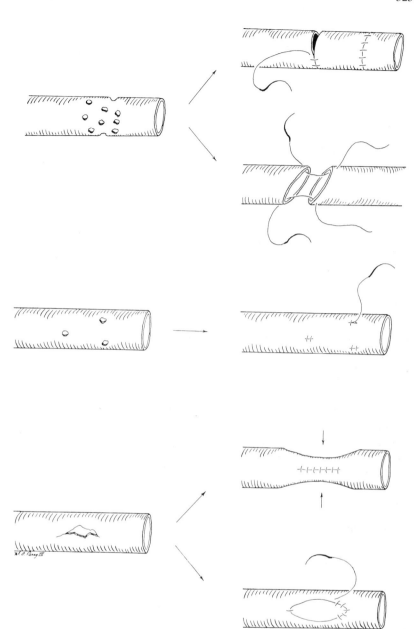

FIGURE 37–4. Standard vascular surgical techniques are used for the repair of brachiocephalic vessels. It is best to complete the débridement before deciding which method of repair is needed. Repairs under tension are contraindicated, and autogenous material is preferred for grafts.

ligation have been described, the true incidence has not been widely appreciated. Several recent reports concerned with vascular injuries in this region note some late venous problems after subclavian vein ligation; others observed little disability. It is not possible from published data to clearly state the indications, risks, outcome, and desirability of venous repair, but several related studies are of interest. Adams and coworkers[25] and Tilney and colleagues[26] described with each passing year of follow-up a progressive increase in the incidence and severity of venous insufficiency after subclavian vein thrombosis. No actual study of this type has been reported, but inferentially, one view suggests that venous repairs are indicated if they will not introduce additional risks. In a study by Rich and associates[27] of popliteal vein trauma, postphlebitic and thromboembolic events were seen less often after vein repairs than after ligation. These same features may be important in the upper extremities in selected cases, but at present, only a general statement supporting venous repairs is appropriate. If obvious venous hypertension is present, destruction of collateral vessels has been identified, and concomitant major arterial injuries exist, venous repair rather than ligation appears to be indicated.

Carotid Artery

Since the investing fascia and the deep cervical fascia are relatively strong structures, bleeding may be contained deep within the neck, and the external evidence of blood accumulation may be modest, although a hematoma is often seen. If the wound has not been accurately identified, wide exposure will be needed for further surgical exploration. The neurovascular structures are approached through the usual carotid incision made along the anterior border of the sternomastoid muscle.[9] Proximal control of the carotid artery is obtained before the area of suspected injury is exposed. Even with a laceration of the artery, gentle digital pressure usually controls bleeding and thus minimizes the time of carotid occlusion. If the injury is in the external carotid, it is controlled with vascular clamps and either repaired or ligated as indicated. Unless there is evidence that the external carotid artery is functioning as a major cerebral collateral, it is usually not grafted or shunted.

More often, the common or internal carotid artery is damaged and should be repaired. Once control of bleeding is obtained, internal carotid artery backflow is assessed. Brisk pulsatile backflow is usually satisfactory evidence of adequate cerebral perfusion, but measurement of carotid stump pressure may be helpful. Pressures greater than 60 or 70 mm Hg are believed to indicate adequate cerebral perfusion. If shunts are needed because of low pressure or scant backflow, a variety of instruments and techniques are used. The simple in-lying 10 French tube shunt advocated by Thompson and Talkington[28] has been used many times, but some of the newer shunts are easier to insert. Most surgeons use systemic heparin when shunts are in place, and anticoagulants are not contraindicated, although it seems more important to heparinize the patient if the distal carotid artery is filled with a stagnant pool of blood. Most studies of shunting and heparinization during operations on carotid injuries have failed to document the need for, and results of, these maneuvers.

Standard vascular techniques are used, but because of the size of the carotid artery and the importance of securing a smooth intimal surface, resection and anastomosis are preferred. This is especially important with blunt trauma, because the mural damage is likely to be extensive. After resection, a repair without tension is required, or graft interposition will be necessary.

Several special maneuvers are helpful in these cases. Sub-stitution of the external carotid for the internal carotid, or use of the external carotid as a patch for the internal carotid, may simplify the repair (see Fig. 37–4). If grafts are needed and a shunt is to be used, the shunt can be placed through the graft prior to insertion and then removed before completing the final anastomosis (Fig. 37–5).

Injuries at the base of the skull are difficult to expose and repair. Division of the digastric muscle and excision of the styloid process may aid the exposure. Subluxation of the mandible can be of assistance in obtaining adequate exposure of the distal internal carotid artery. This maneuver usually requires preoperative placement of dental wires and appliances and must be performed with care to prevent compression of the opposite carotid or other structures.

One method of control and shunting can be very helpful. A No. 4 Fogarty catheter with an attached three-way stopcock is prepared by threading a straight carotid shunt over it (a Pruitt-Inahara shunt is also useful). The catheter is then inserted through a small proximal transverse incision in the common carotid artery and advanced beyond the area of injury. Precise expansion of the balloon controls carotid backflow. If necessary the shunt can be guided beyond the laceration into the distal carotid artery. The balloon is then deflated, and prograde cerebral perfusion is restored. The arterial injury can be repaired accurately and without haste; then the catheters are removed and a completion arteriogram performed before closure of the small access arteriotomy. In this manner, the shunt not only permits a deliberate and disciplined repair but also acts as a stent and reduces the chances of narrowing the artery.

Some of these maneuvers are useful in controlling and repairing acute arterial venous fistulas. If these lesions are known to exist before exploration, the balloon-tipped cathe-

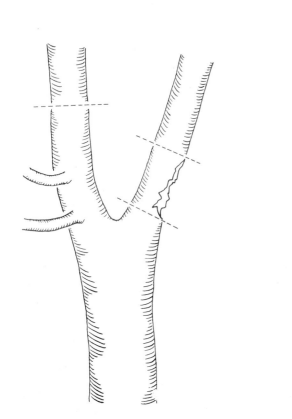

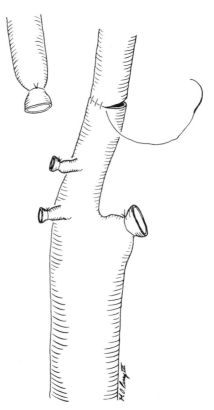

FIGURE 37–5. If the origin of the internal carotid artery is damaged beyond direct repair, the external carotid artery can be used as an arterial autograft.

ter can be inserted from a remote area and advanced to the fistula and then inflated to assist in controlling bleeding.

If resection is required and direct anastomosis is impossible, a saphenous vein graft is preferred to restore continuity (Fig. 37–6). The distal vein from the ankle can be used, or the cephalic vein is satisfactory. Local cervical veins are too fragile for this use. Plastic grafts may be needed in the common carotid artery, especially in large men and hypertensive patients. All injured and devitalized artery must be débrided. If damaged intima is left behind, local thromboembolic events can cause a delayed stroke. This is particularly likely in blunt injuries, where the artery may sustain extensive damage. In this situation, a graft will almost certainly be needed.

When concomitant injuries of the trachea, esophagus, or pharynx are present, and drains are needed, these should be routed away from the repaired artery, and all fascial layers should be closed between the wounds. There is little room for changing the path of the arteries, and local protection will be needed. In a few cases, when heavy contamination is expected to cross the operating field, it may be necessary to redirect the carotid artery through the posterior triangles of the neck and interpose other tissues. This has not been required in the author's experience, however.[9]

With the advent of combined extracranial and intracranial vascular procedures for treating occlusive arterial disease, difficult intracranial injuries of the cerebral arteries may be

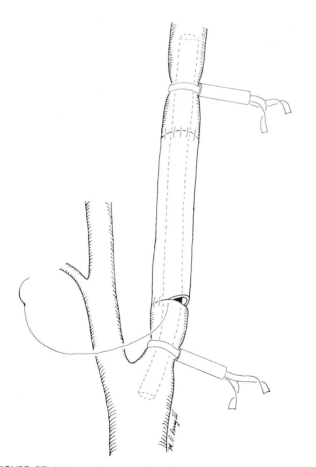

FIGURE 37–6. If a saphenous vein graft is required to restore internal carotid artery blood flow, it can be inserted as shown here, with or without the assistance of an in-lying shunt.

repaired. Injuries of the carotid artery in the petrous bone or the cavernous canal are surgically inaccessible and may require proximal and distal ligation to control bleeding. Alternatively, it may be possible to construct bypasses from the cervical carotid to intracranial vessels and thus preserve adequate cerebral perfusion. Although these are formidable procedures, in special circumstances they may prevent serious neurologic problems caused by carotid ligation.[10, 21]

With the advent of better methods of diagnosis, patient selection, and vascular repair, ligation of the carotid artery is rarely indicated. In a few patients in whom the arterial damage is so extensive that repair cannot be done, ligation may be necessary. If distal backflow and blood pressure are high, carotid occlusion will probably be safe. This is not always true, however, because distal thrombosis of the intracranial carotid artery may lead to stroke. Heparin has been used to control the extent of thrombosis in the distal carotid following proximal ligation.[29] This adjunct may prove useful in selected trauma cases as well. It must be remembered, however, that stroke rates up to 50 percent are to be expected following acute carotid ligation.

If sufficient distal artery is available for pressure measurements, a vascular reconstruction can often be done, perhaps even originating from the subclavian or the opposite carotid artery, if the ipsilateral common carotid artery cannot be used. Also, the extracranial to intracranial techniques can solve the problem of restoring perfusion in selected cases.

It now appears that carotid ligation is needed in only a very small group: patients with complete internal carotid occlusion and severe neurologic deficits, including coma.[9, 17, 21, 22] Revascularization, with repair of all the damaged artery and complete removal of all clots, is seldom possible in a patient who has a totally occluded carotid artery as a result of blunt trauma. It total repair is attempted but not completed, the results are often progressive neurologic deterioration and death. Obviously, restoration of flow through the carotid without clearing the distal artery is dangerous and contraindicated. In these patients, carotid ligation is probably best, especially since it appears that the neurologic damage caused by the occlusion has already occurred, and it is unlikely that delayed disobliteration will reverse fixed deficits.

Vertebral Artery

Bleeding from the vertebral canal can be profuse and difficult to control, especially when the injury is caused by a gunshot wound that has also shattered the cervical vertebrae. Some of the bleeding can be from the multiple vertebral veins that traverse the canal with the artery; these are attached to the periosteum and thus tend to remain open when they are torn. Proximal exposure and control of the artery below C6, where it enters the canal, is often needed in these cases. Backbleeding usually remains fairly brisk because of the extensive collateral circulation, some vessels even reaching the artery in the canal itself. Direct pressure, packing, application of bone wax, proximal ligation, and even distal exposure up to C2 may be needed in rare cases. Balloon catheter control as described in the preceding section can be helpful in recalcitrant cases.

Although the artery can be repaired, even in the bony canal, ligation has been used more often than not.[30] The vertebral arteries are usually paired and join to form the basilar artery, but this is not invariable; occasionally, one vertebral artery may be hypoplastic or may terminate as the posterior inferior cerebellar artery. If the extracranial cerebral architecture in a given patient is known in advance, the repairs can be planned with more accuracy, and unusual problems can be better managed. Arteriography may therefore be of importance in handling patients with vertebral artery injuries.

POSTOPERATIVE CARE

Although any vascular repair is susceptible to bleeding, this is unusual in these patients unless they have multiple injuries or coagulation defects. Drains are not usually employed in isolated vascular wounds, but in selected patients, they may be used for 12 to 24 hours to prevent the accumulation of blood, a technique commonly used in elective carotid surgery. Even with the low incidence of bleeding, this complication should be considered, because the relatively strong cervical fascia can contain blood under pressure and cause acute respiratory difficulties. Elevation of the head and upper body to reduce venous engorgement, adequate hemostasis, selective drainage, and careful observation during the postoperative period usually prevent these problems.

Thromboembolic events are also unusual, but when they occur, serious neurologic problems are likely to ensue. Early identification and treatment are essential if irreversible brain damage is to be avoided. Adequate fluid resuscitation and maintenance of normal systemic blood pressure are important; drugs likely to have a hypotensive effect should therefore be avoided. Frequent evaluation of the hemodynamic and neurologic status of these patients is mandatory. During the early postoperative period, this should be performed every hour, at least for several hours, and then every 4 hours for the first 2 days. Any aberration in the findings is a clear indication for more exact studies. If a buildup of thrombus in the artery is suspected, noninvasive tests may be helpful. Oculoplethysmography, for example, may expose this complication before complete carotid occlusion supervenes, thus allowing time to return the patient to surgery for thrombectomy and repair, but the test may be false-positive. Other noninvasive studies using ultrasound (B-mode scanning, Doppler spectral analysis) can be used to assess patency, although it may be difficult to evaluate vessels in a fresh surgical wound.

High-grade stenosis can be diagnosed in this manner, and patency can also be confirmed. If doubt exists as to the interpretation of the findings, repeat arteriography is indicated. Intracranial views are needed to ascertain whether cerebral arterial embolization has occurred. In some cases, intracranial emboli have been extracted successfully with complete recovery, but these are difficult, requiring close cooperation among vascular surgeons, neurosurgeons, and vascular radiologists. If postoperative carotid thrombosis does occur, immediate carotid disobliteration is indicated and likely to be successful. Correction of the cause of failure may require thorough exploration and operative arteriography, but it is essential to success. Such problems are unusual, but they do happen; they should be treated aggressively in a postoperative patient who appears to be developing a stroke.

TABLE 37–3. Results of Carotid Artery Repair

Group	Degree of Deficit	Patients, n	Complications, n
I	None	49	0
II	Mild	8	1
III	Severe	15	5

In fact, it is probably best not to delay for confirmatory arteriograms but to return the patient to the operating room for exploration and restoration of cerebral perfusion as rapidly as possible.[3]

RESULTS OF TREATMENT

The long-term results of repairing carotid injuries are quite good.[3, 17, 22] In the series reported by Thal and associates,[9] the patients were divided into three groups in order to evaluate treatment. The first and largest group contained those patients with common or internal carotid artery wounds but no neurologic deficits (group I). Group II included those with mild deficits, and group III patients had severe deficits. Among these groups, very few complications arose (Table 72–3). In fact, in the absence of infection problems generated by other injuries, most patients with carotid injuries do very well. False aneurysms and arteriovenous fistulas, often a result of untreated wounds, are rare when the vessels are repaired. False aneurysm as a complication of infection of the repaired artery is seen on rare occasions and presents a formidable problem. Although not supported by unequivocal data, it is widely held that this problem is more likely when plastic prosthetic material has been used in the vascular repair, either as a graft or as patch material. The diagnosis is usually established easily, although reluctantly. Local signs of infection, a draining sinus, bleeding, sepsis, and a mass are often seen. Arteriography confirms the diagnosis, and operative therapy is indicated. Although a few isolated cases of successful cure without removal of the plastic graft have been reported, most false aneurysms require specific antibiotic drainage and removal of all prosthetic material. Reconstruction with autogenous tissue, or rerouting of the vessel through clean tissue planes, is generally satisfactory treatment if the patient has no neurologic deficits.

REFERENCES

1. Shires GT, ed.: Preface. In *Principles of Trauma Care*, 3rd ed. New York: McGraw-Hill; 1985:xi.
2. Feliciano DV, Bitondo CG, Mattox KL, et al: Civilian trauma in the 1980s. *Ann Surg.* 1984;199:717.
3. Perry MO: *The Management of Acute Vascular Injuries.* Baltimore: Williams & Wilkins; 1981.
4. Snyder WH, Thal ER, Perry MO: Peripheral and abdominal vascular injuries. In Rutherford RB, ed. *Vascular Surgery.* Philadelphia: WB Saunders; 1984:460.
5. Monson DO, Saletta JD, Freeark RJ: Carotid vertebral trauma. *Trauma.* 1969;9:987.
6. Hewitt RL, Smith AD, Becker ML, et al: Penetrating vascular injuries of the thoracic outlet. *Surgery.* 1974;76:715.
7. Flint LM, Snyder WH, Perry MO, et al: Management of major vascular injuries in the base of the neck. *Arch Surg.* 1973;106:407.
8. Roon AJ, Christensen N: Evaluation and treatment of penetrating cervical injuries. *J Trauma.* 1979;19:391.
9. Thal ER, Snyder WH, Hays RJ, et al: Management of carotid artery injuries. *Surgery.* 1974;76:955.
10. Fry RE, Fry WJ: Extracranial carotid artery injuries. *Surgery.* 1980;88:581.

11. Reul GJ, Beall AC, Jordon GL, et al: The early operative management of injuries to the great vessels. *Surgery*. 1973;74:862.
12. Lim LT, Saletta JD, Flanigan DP: Subclavian and innominate artery trauma. *Surgery*. 1979;86:890.
13. Smith RF, Elliott JP, Hagaman JH, et al: Acute penetrating arterial injuries of the neck and limbs. *Arch Surg*. 1974;109:198.
14. Narrod JA, Moore EE: Selective management of penetrating neck injuries. *Arch Surg*. 1984;119:574.
15. Bradley EL: Management of penetrating carotid injuries: An alternative approach. *J Trauma*. 1973;13:248.
16. Yamada S, Kindt GW, Youmans JR: Carotid injuries due to non-penetrating injury. *J Trauma*. 1967;7:333.
17. Liekweg WG, Greenfield LJ: Management of penetrating carotid arterial injury. *Ann Surg*. 1978;188:587.
18. Krajewski KP, Hertzer NR: Blunt carotid trauma. *Ann Surg*. 1980;191:341.
19. Jernigan WR, Gardner WC: Carotid artery injuries due to closed cervical trauma. *J Trauma*. 1971;11:429.
20. Perry MO, Snyder WH, Thal ER: Carotid artery injuries caused by blunt trauma. *Ann Surg*. 1980;192:74.
21. Ledgerwood AM, Mullins RJ, Lucas CE: Primary repair vs. ligation for carotid artery injuries. *Arch Surg*. 1980;115:488.
22. Unger SW, Tucker WS, Mrdega MA, et al: Carotid arterial trauma. *Surgery*. 1980;87:477.
23. Crissey MM, Bernstein EF: Delayed presentation of carotid intimal tear following blunt craniocervical trauma. *Surgery*. 1974;75:543.
24. Auh YH, Rubenstein WA, Kazan E: Computed body tomography (with ultrasound correlation) of the trauma patient. In Shires GT, ed. *Principles of Trauma Care*, 3rd ed. New York: McGraw-Hill; 1985:110.
25. Adams JT, McEvoy RK, DeWeese JA: Primary deep venous thrombosis of upper extremity. *Arch Surg*. 1965;9:29.
26. Tilney NL, Griffiths HJG, Edwards EA: Natural history of major venous thrombosis of the upper extremity. *Arch Surg*. 1970;101:792.
27. Rich NM, Hobson RW, Collins GJ, Anderson CA: The effect of acute popliteal venous interruption. *Ann Surg*. 1979;183:365.
28. Thompson JE, Talkington CM: Carotid endarterectomy. *Ann Surg*. 1976;184:1.
29. Ehrenfeld WK, Stoney RJ, Wylie EJ: Relation of carotid stump pressure to safety of carotid artery ligation. *Surgery*. 1983;93:299.
30. Brink BJ, Meier D, Fry WJ: Operative exposure and management of lesions in the vertebral artery. *J Cardiovasc Surg*. 1979;20:435.

IX

Surgical Management of Lesions of the Carotid Artery

Anesthetic Considerations for Carotid Endarterectomy

KATE T. HUNCKE and JORDAN D. MILLER

Anesthetic management of patients undergoing carotid endarterectomy can be a major challenge. Patients with cerebrovascular disease tend to be elderly and have multiorgan system dysfunction. The anesthesiologist is faced with the task of maintaining adequate cerebral perfusion without jeopardizing physiologic function of other diseased organs. These two goals are frequently at odds. For example, elevated arterial blood pressure is utilized to ensure cerebral perfusion, but this leads to increased myocardial wall tension, which may induce myocardial ischemia. It is therefore critical that the nature and severity of other organ system dysfunction be reviewed preoperatively so that rational perioperative management can take place.

PREOPERATIVE EVALUATION

Not surprisingly, the most common medical conditions associated with cerebrovascular disease are hypertension, coronary artery disease, diabetes mellitus, and chronic obstructive pulmonary disease.[1] Evaluation and optimal treatment of these coexisting diseases should be sought during the preoperative visit. A consultation may be necessary to delineate the severity of coexisting disease and to determine whether the patient may benefit from further medical management preoperatively.

Chronic hypertension is present in 60 to 80 percent of patients who undergo carotid endarterectomy and has a major impact on the regulation of cerebral blood flow.[1] Cerebral blood flow is normally kept constant between a mean arterial blood pressure of 50 to 150 mm Hg by a process called autoregulation. Chronic hypertension shifts both the upper and lower limits of autoregulation to higher pressures.[2] Therefore, these patients may need a higher blood pressure to maintain adequate cerebral blood flow.

It is useful to establish the normal blood pressure fluctuation for a given patient, since autoregulation is assumed to occur within this range. Intraoperatively, blood pressure is kept within this range to ensure adequate cerebral blood flow. During the preoperative visit, blood pressure should be measured in both arms, since there may be a discrepancy due to peripheral vascular disease. If available, records from previous office visits and hospitalizations are useful in estab-

lishing normal blood pressure fluctuation. If the patient is admitted on the day of surgery, an attempt is made to keep blood pressure within 20 percent above or below the patient's normal mean blood pressure.

Several studies suggest that perioperative morbidity may be reduced in patients undergoing carotid endarterectomy by adequate treatment of preoperative hypertension. Prys-Roberts and coworkers[3] found that untreated or inadequately treated hypertensive patients were at greater risk of developing intraoperative hypotension and associated myocardial ischemia. In patients with cerebrovascular disease, this may further compromise blood flow to ischemic brain tissue. Asiddao and colleagues[4] discovered that new neurologic deficits and postoperative hypertension were more common in patients with poorly controlled preoperative hypertension, that is, arterial blood pressure greater than 170/95 mm Hg. Although hypertension was not found to affect the rate of permanent neurologic sequelae or myocardial infarction, uncontrolled postoperative hypertension places patients at greater risk of developing myocardial ischemia, cerebral edema, and cerebral infarction. Most clinicians now agree that hypertension must be adequately controlled prior to carotid endarterectomy in order to reduce potentially harmful intraoperative blood pressure fluctuations and transient neurologic deficits.

Antihypertensive medication should be continued throughout the perioperative period to ensure adequate blood pressure control. The pharmacology of all agents must be reviewed to anticipate possible adverse effects under anesthesia, such as decreased sympathetic tone, altered response to vasopressors, sedation, and electrolyte abnormalities. The use of volatile anesthetics in combination with beta blockers or calcium channel blockers leads to additive myocardial depression.[5–7] The dose of inhalation agent should be titrated to the hemodynamic response to avoid a detrimental fall in blood pressure. In contrast, antihypertensive medication withdrawal may stress the cardiovascular system.[8, 9] Abrupt discontinuation of beta blockers, calcium channel blockers, or alpha$_2$ agonist therapy may cause rebound hypertension and myocardial ischemia.[10–14] These drugs in particular should be continued on the day of surgery and in the postoperative period. Diuretics are held the morning of surgery, since the patient has abstained from fluid intake. Hypokalemia is common in these patients due to chronic potassium wasting. There is no adverse outcome associated with serum potassium levels greater than 2.6 meq/dL, as long as maneuvers that would cause further decreases in potassium are avoided intraoperatively.[15] A serum potassium level of 4.0 meq/dL is recommended if arrhythmias are present.

Patients with cerebrovascular disease are prone to concomitant involvement of the coronary arteries. Ischemic heart disease is common in patients with peripheral vascular disease, carotid bruits, or asymptomatic carotid artery occlusion.[16–19] Since the major cause of mortality following carotid endarterectomy is myocardial infarction,[4] a thorough preoperative cardiac evaluation is warranted.

A normal electrocardiogram (ECG) in patients with peripheral vascular disease is not sensitive in ruling out significant coronary artery disease, even if anginal symptoms are absent. In a study by Tomatis and associates,[20] 44 percent of patients who were scheduled for aortoiliac reconstruction were found on angiography to have at least 50 percent stenosis of one or more coronary arteries, and 30 percent had greater than 75 percent stenosis. All these patients had normal ECGs and no cardiac symptoms. When compared with patients with abnormal ECGs, the percentage with significant stenosis was the same for both groups. Another study by Hertzer and colleagues[16] confirmed these findings. This study looked at patients with peripheral vascular disease who had normal ECGs and no history of myocardial disease. They found a 37 percent incidence of at least 70 percent coronary narrowing in one or more coronary arteries.

Since coronary artery disease is common among patients with peripheral vascular disease, further assessment of the coronary anatomy is warranted prior to carotid endarterectomy. Several noninvasive screening tests are available that provide information regarding the severity of coronary atherosclerosis. These studies help identify patients that may benefit from further medical management, invasive cardiac monitoring intraoperatively, or angioplasty of a coronary artery. They also help identify patients who may need staged or simultaneous repair of their coronary arteries.[21]

Exercise testing in patients with risk factors for coronary artery disease has a sensitivity of 70 percent and a specificity of 90 percent.[22] It is highly predictive of postoperative cardiac events when ST changes are characteristic, large, and sustained; occur early in the exercise period; and are associated with below-normal increases in blood pressure.[22–24] Knowledge of the location of the ischemic changes on ECG and the heart rate and blood pressure at which these changes occur is valuable to the anesthesiologist. This provides guidelines for the location of ECG monitoring and acceptable hemodynamic thresholds.

Echocardiography used in conjunction with exercise testing provides information regarding left ventricular function and ejection fraction. Exercise-induced ischemia causes changes in regional wall motion, wall thickening, or both. Identification of these changes is valuable in patients whose ECGs cannot be used as a monitor of ischemia due to the presence of left bundle branch block, left ventricular hypertrophy, mitral valve prolapse, or digoxin therapy.

In patients who are unable to exercise, dipyridamole thallium, Holter monitoring, or dobutamine stress echo may be used to assess the severity of coronary artery disease. In patients undergoing peripheral vascular procedures, dipyridamole thallium imaging was shown to be superior to exercise testing. Studies showed it to be highly sensitive (89–100%) and reasonably specific (53–80%) for detecting significant coronary artery disease.[25, 26] Patients with redistribution on dipyridamole thallium imaging have a high incidence of postoperative ischemic events.[26, 27] Holter monitoring for 24 to 48 hours is effective in evaluating asymptomatic ischemia that may occur with normal daily activity. Raby and colleagues[28] found that the appearance of preoperative ischemia with Holter monitoring showed a high correlation with postoperative cardiac complications such as myocardial infarction, unstable angina, and congestive heart failure. Again, this study has limited value in patients whose ECGs may be uninterpretable due to left bundle branch block, left ventricular hypertrophy, or drug therapy.

Diabetic patients undergoing carotid endarterectomy frequently have evidence of end organ involvement, which has a significant impact on their anesthetic management. These patients are prone to hypertension, coronary artery disease, immune suppression, and autonomic neuropathy. Autonomic neuropathy may manifest as delayed gastric emptying, placing these patients at risk of aspiration during anesthesia. These patients may benefit from preoperative administration of metoclopramide and an H_2 blocker to facilitate gastric emptying and increase gastric pH. Autonomic neuropathy may also manifest as resting tachycardia, loss of beat-to-beat variability with respirations, and orthostatic hypotension. Several studies note that when autonomic neuropathy is present, there is dramatic intraoperative cardiovascular instability, especially during induction of anesthesia.[29–31] A greater increase in blood pressure is reported, followed by significant hypotension after intubation, requiring administration of vasoactive drugs.[29, 30] These patients frequently have small heart-rate changes after the administration of atropine or propranolol.[32, 33] The presence of diabetic stiff joint syndrome can complicate airway management and head positioning. Diabetes can lead to stiffening and contracture of the atlanto-occipital joint. This can limit neck extension and make intubation by direct laryngoscopy difficult.[34] Renal insufficiency is commonly present in long-standing diabetics. Preoperative and postangiographic blood urea nitrogen and creatinine should be obtained to assess the degree of renal dysfunction, since some anesthetics depend on renal clearance.

Occasionally, protamine is used to control excessive postoperative bleeding due to heparin administration. Diabetic patients receiving protamine-containing insulin develop antibodies to protamine. These patients are more likely to suffer an anaphylactic or anaphylactoid reaction if protamine is administered to reverse heparin anticoagulation.[35] A 5 mg test dose of protamine should be given prior to the full reversal dose. Fluids, epinephrine, and bronchodilators should be readily available for treatment of a life-threatening allergic reaction.

The adequacy of blood glucose control should be determined prior to surgery. If blood glucose is poorly controlled, insulin-dependent diabetics are prone to ketoacidosis, whereas maturity-onset diabetics tend to develop nonketotic hyperglycemic coma. It is mandatory that serum glucose and electrolytes be measured preoperatively to rule out these metabolic disturbances. Elective surgery should never be undertaken in the presence of either of these states, since they can lead to serious volume depletion and electrolyte disturbances.

Several studies suggest that elevated blood glucose may have a deleterious effect on neurologic outcome following cerebral ischemia. In a retrospective study of patients surviving cardiac arrest, those who awakened had significantly lower blood glucose levels than those who remained comatose.[36] Among patients who recovered, persistent neurologic deficit was associated with higher blood glucose levels. In another retrospective study of stroke patients, diabetic patients with elevated blood glucose levels greater than 259 mg/dL had significantly worse neurologic outcomes when compared with nondiabetics.[37] Elevated blood glucose in nondiabetics was also associated with worse neurologic outcome.[37] Prospective animal studies confirm these findings. Transient focal ischemia produced significantly larger infarcts in hyperglycemic versus normoglycemic animals.[38]

Tight control of plasma blood glucose is critical perioperatively. Protocols to achieve this goal have ranged from administering half the usual morning insulin dose and starting a dextrose infusion to withholding all insulin therapy.[39, 40] No one regimen is superior to another as long as serum glucose is checked frequently and appropriate adjustments in insulin therapy are made. It is best to leave decisions regarding preoperative insulin administration to the anesthesiologist, since he or she will be responsible for the intraoperative management.

Chronic obstructive pulmonary disease may be present in patients with long tobacco smoking histories. Forty percent of patients presenting for cerebrovascular revascularization had a history of smoking more than 80 packs a year.[41] Consequently, complications of long-term obstructive pulmonary disease such as chronic bronchitis, emphysema, pulmonary hypertension, and cor pulmonale should be suspected, since they can have a significant impact on the anesthetic management. The presence of dyspnea, chronic productive cough, and decreased exercise tolerance suggests the need for preoperative pulmonary function tests and arterial blood gas determination. This will help identify patients who are at increased risk of postoperative pulmonary complications or even respiratory failure. Pulmonary function tests also help identify patients who may benefit from better medical management with the use of bronchodilator therapy, steroids, and/or antibiotics preoperatively.

Intraoperative management of ventilation can be difficult in the presence of chronic obstructive pulmonary disease. These patients have ventilation-perfusion mismatching, which deteriorates further under anesthesia. Due to increased dead-space ventilation, the end tidal carbon dioxide will be lower than arterial carbon dioxide. Because carbon dioxide is important to maintenance of normal cerebral blood flow, intraoperative arterial blood gases are necessary for accurate assessment. These patients can also have intrapulmonary shunting, leading to hypoxia, despite delivery of supplemental oxygen. Patients with chronic obstructive pulmonary disease are more sensitive to respiratory depression from sedatives than are healthy patients. Hypoventilation can have deleterious effects on cerebral blood flow and reduce oxygen delivery to ischemic brain tissue. Hyper-reactive airway response to the endotracheal tube can trigger coughing intraoperatively, which leads to increased venous pressure. This may interfere with adequate cerebral blood flow intraoperatively and may also contribute to hematoma formation during emergence from anesthesia if "bucking" is severe.

PREMEDICATION

Premedication in patients undergoing carotid endarterectomy may help relieve hypertension and tachycardia associated with anxiety. These hemodynamic alterations can precipitate arrhythmias, myocardial ischemia, and even myocardial infarction in patients with coronary artery disease.[42, 43] As previously discussed, hypertension can also increase the risk of a postoperative neurologic deficit.[4] Premedication may also be useful for alleviating pain associated with the placement of invasive monitors, such as an arterial line.

It is equally important to avoid oversedation and hypoventilation. Hypercarbia may shunt blood away from a cerebral tissue supplied by stenotic arteries. In patients scheduled for regional anesthesia, oversedation may interfere with intraoperative neurologic assessment. Long-acting agents are best avoided, since they can produce excessive somnolence postoperatively, which may interfere with neurologic evaluation. This is a problem especially in the elderly, who may have impaired clearance or increased sensitivity to sedatives. The recent availability of flumazenil, a benzodiazepine antagonist, may make benzodiazepines an attractive alternative to propofol for local stand-by sedation.

MONITORING

Routine monitoring for carotid endarterectomy includes pulse oximetry, ECG, blood pressure, respiratory gases, temperature, and, if muscle relaxants are used, a neuromuscular twitch monitor. Preferably, blood pressure is monitored directly with an arterial line. It should be inserted prior to induction, since laryngoscopy can precipitate tachycardia and hypertension. Rapid detection and treatment of this hyperdynamic response may prevent myocardial ischemia. Multiple-lead ECG and ST segment analysis are the preferred monitors for the detection of myocardial ischemia. Most ischemic episodes were found to occur in the lateral precordial leads.[44] A combination of leads V4 and V5 will detect 90 percent of ischemic episodes; if lead II is added, the sensitivity is increased to 95 percent.[44] Since most operating rooms are not equipped to analyze three leads simultaneously, many clinicians choose to monitor lead II and V5. With this technique, the reported sensitivity for ischemia detection is 80 percent,[44] and detection of arrhythmias is maximized with lead II analysis.

Occasionally, the cardiovascular status of a patient may warrant the use of pulmonary artery pressure monitoring or transesophageal echocardiography. In patients who have suffered a recent myocardial infarction, the risk of perioperative reinfarction may be reduced by optimizing the hemodynamic status with a pulmonary artery catheter.[45] When moderate to severe left ventricular dysfunction is present, the pulmonary artery catheter is valuable for guiding medical therapy to maximize cardiac output. Acute increases in pulmonary capillary wedge pressure or the development of V waves may precede ST changes during myocardial ischemia.

However, elevations in pulmonary capillary wedge pressure lack the sensitivity of ST segment analysis.[46] Therefore, the value of pulmonary artery catheter insertion solely for the detection of myocardial ischemia is limited,[47] since significant morbidity may be associated with its insertion.

Transesophageal echocardiography provides useful information regarding left ventricular and valvular function and myocardial ischemia. It appears to be superior to the ECG in detecting myocardial ischemia,[48] and reported complications are rare. In patients undergoing carotid endarterectomy, myocardial ischemia is frequently detected at the time of carotid cross-clamping.[48–51] With transesophageal echocardiography, the incidence of myocardial ischemia was found to be as high as 25 percent. Some clinicians argue that transesophageal echocardiography should be a routine monitor of myocardial ischemia in patients undergoing carotid endarterectomy.[51] Currently, widespread use is limited by the cost ($75,000–$235,000 per unit) and the extensive training required for accurate interpretation. Many clinicians also find that it distracts from other important aspects of patient management. Another limitation is that the probe is rarely inserted prior to induction, since it is uncomfortable and interferes with airway management.

INDUCTION AND MAINTENANCE

There are several reasons that many clinicians prefer general anesthesia over regional anesthesia for carotid endarterectomy. Patient comfort is ensured, allowing surgery to proceed in an unhurried fashion. Lack of head movement may facilitate surgical exposure and prevent dislodgement of an arterial shunt intraoperatively. The airway is secured, decreasing the risk of aspiration secondary to oversedation or loss of consciousness during carotid cross-clamping. Ventilation can be strictly controlled, which is important to maintenance of normal cerebral blood flow. General anesthesia, by decreasing cerebral metabolic oxygen consumption, may offer a mechanism for cerebral protection during ischemia.

It is difficult to state exactly what drugs will be used for the induction and maintenance of anesthesia. The decision is made by balancing the risk of ischemia with the patient's coexisting medical conditions. Avoidance of drugs or techniques that could worsen central nervous system ischemia or exacerbate coexisting disease is obviously a major goal of anesthesia. No outcome data clearly state that any specific technique is superior to another. The advantages and disadvantages of any agent used must be weighed in each clinical circumstance.

Thiopental sodium (Pentothal) is frequently utilized for induction because of its dose-dependent decrease in cerebral metabolic rate of oxygen consumption ($CMRO_2$) and smaller decrease in cerebral blood flow.[52, 53] These advantageous effects may be offset by myocardial depression and decreased peripheral vascular resistance. Use of this agent in patients with certain forms of cardiac disease such as left ventricular dysfunction or aortic stenosis can lead to serious falls in blood pressure that may impair cerebral perfusion. Etomidate is an alternative agent that can be used in this setting. It produces a similar reduction in $CMRO_2$ and cerebral blood flow[54] but a less dose-dependent decrease in

systemic vascular resistance and myocardial contractility.[54] Etomidate is not routinely used for induction because of the high incidence of pain on injection, postoperative nausea and vomiting, and transient adrenal suppression associated with its use. Propofol is another agent that can be used for induction of anesthesia for carotid endarterectomy. Compared with sodium pentothal, propofol produces a similar reduction in $CMRO_2$ and cerebral blood flow.[55] However, it produces a greater degree of myocardial depression and decreased peripheral vascular resistance, which again is a problem for patients with significant cardiac disease and cerebral ischemia.

None of these agents is effective at adequately blunting the hyperdynamic response to laryngoscopy and intubation. Short- or intermediate-acting narcotics such as alfentanil, sufentanil, or fentanyl are frequently used to attenuate this response. Typical doses are fentanyl 3 to 7 µg/kg, sufentanil 0.5 to 1.0 µg/kg, or alfentanil 25 to 50 µg/kg. The narcotic is titrated to respiratory depression prior to induction. Large doses are avoided, since the duration of the procedure is short and respiratory depression or excessive postoperative somnolence is undesirable. In hypertensive patients, a nondepolarizing muscle relaxant is often used instead of succinylcholine to facilitate intubation, since its delayed onset allows a greater depth of anesthesia to be achieved before laryngoscopy. Succinylcholine should also be avoided in patients with a previous denervation injury due to stroke, because of the risk of a hyperkalemic response.[56]

Since stimulation is transient during induction, short-acting vasoactive agents are frequently used to treat the hemodynamic response. Nitroprusside, nitroglycerin, and esmolol have also been used to treat hypertension and tachycardia during induction and surgical stimulation.[43, 57, 58] In patients with evidence of significant coronary artery disease, continuous infusion of nitroglycerin (0.25–1.0 µg/kg minute) has been used as prophylaxis against coronary vasospasm. However, controlled studies have failed to demonstrate a decreased incidence of intraoperative myocardial ischemia during a continuous infusion of nitroglycerin or esmolol,[58–60] even though there was a dose-related decrease in blood pressure or heart rate. Therefore, infusions of nitroglycerin and esmolol should be used mainly for hemodynamic control.

After intubation, anesthesia is usually maintained with 60 percent nitrous oxide, 40 percent oxygen, and a low dose of a volatile agent. This is supplemented with small doses of the previously mentioned narcotics. Rapid control of fluctuations in blood pressure or heart rate, which are common during carotid endarterectomies, can be achieved by adjusting the dose of volatile agents or by administering short-acting vasoactive drugs. Phenylephrine is an $alpha_1$ agonist that is commonly used to correct hypotension intraoperatively. However, a study by Smith and coworkers[61] showed that administration of phenylephrine during carotid endarterectomy to maintain blood pressure was associated with a threefold increase in myocardial ischemia when compared with "light" anesthesia using nitrous oxide, oxygen, and low concentrations of isoflurane of halothane. Low doses of inhalational agents also allow for rapid recovery of consciousness and early assessment of neurologic function in the postoperative period.

Isoflurane is generally selected for the maintenance of

anesthesia, since there is some evidence of cerebral protection associated with its use. Isoflurane is the only volatile agent that can abolish electroencephalographic (EEG) activity at clinically useful concentrations. This corresponds to a 50 to 60 percent reduction in $CMRO_2$.[62, 63] Critical regional cerebral blood flow, defined as the flow below which EEG signs of cerebral ischemia occur, is lower for isoflurane compared with halothane or enflurane.[62] Retrospective data confirmed a decreased incidence of EEG changes in patients undergoing carotid endarterectomy with isoflurane versus enflurane or halothane.[64] This study has been criticized, since it is a historical study that looked at halothane during the early 1970s, enflurane during the mid-1970s, and isoflurane during the early 1980s. It did not control for the severity of cerebrovascular disease, difference in surgical technique, or more advanced intraoperative monitoring of blood pressure, heart rate, temperature, or ventilation. No difference in neurologic outcome was detected, since all patients with EEG changes were shunted. Another study suggested that isoflurane may delay the onset of ischemia, but if the ischemic insult is prolonged beyond 10 minutes, there is no detectable difference in the incidence of ischemia or the cerebral blood flow at which it occurred with either halothane or isoflurane.[65] Animal studies have failed to demonstrate any protective effect of isoflurane on the severity of neurologic deficit or histopathologic change following focal or global ischemia.[66-69] Also of note is that narcotics, when compared with low-dose isoflurane, produced a similar degree of cerebral metabolic suppression when used for carotid endarterectomy.[70, 71]

Regardless of the drugs selected for anesthesia, maintenance of blood pressure within the patient's normal range is critical for ensuring adequate cerebral perfusion. Blood vessels in ischemic brain tissue are considered to be maximally vasodilated and unable to respond to vasomotor stimuli. Perfusion to these areas becomes pressure dependent. Hypotension may lead to cerebral ischemia, and hypertension can cause cerebral edema. Hypotension and hypertension can also cause myocardial ischemia by leading to aberrations in myocardial oxygen supply and demand. Therefore, most clinicians aim to keep the mean arterial blood pressure within 20 percent of the patient's normal blood pressure. The situation is slightly different during carotid cross-clamping, since blood flow to ischemic brain tissue becomes dependent on adequate collateral perfusion. A rise in blood pressure generally occurs at this time, due to increased sympathetic outflow. In order to ensure adequate collateral perfusion, this rise in blood pressure is allowed to occur as long as there are no signs of myocardial ischemia. Indeed, reversal of ischemic EEG changes has been demonstrated by augmenting the mean arterial pressure during carotid cross-clamping.[72-74] Some surgeons require a slight amount of head elevation to facilitate surgical exposure. Venous pooling in the lower extremities can lead to profound falls in blood pressure. Use of support stockings, the ability to elevate the legs with pillows or flexion of the operating room bed, and adequate hydration may help preserve adequate venous return. Vasopressors to treat persistent hypotension due to venous stasis should not be used for prolonged periods, since they may contribute to myocardial ischemia.

Intraoperative surgical stimulation of the carotid sinus can lead to bradycardia and hypotension. This reflex arc involves afferents from the ninth cranial nerve synapsing in the medulla and sending efferent impulses to the vagus. Any hemodynamic changes during manipulation of the carotid sinus should be relayed to the surgeon, who can temporarily halt further dissection. The reflex can then be blocked by injecting the carotid sinus with a small volume of 2 percent lidocaine. Injection may smooth the heart rate and blood pressure fluctuations associated with dissection. Some clinicians argue that blockade of the sinus nerve should not be routinely used, since it may contribute to postoperative hypertension.[74] This seems unlikely, since the half-life of lidocaine is only 90 minutes. The reflex can also be treated by administering atropine or glycopyrrolate. However, these drugs produce tachycardia, which may precipitate myocardial ischemia in patients with coronary artery disease. Furthermore, anticholinergics do not directly treat the withdrawal of sympathetic tone associated with activation of the reflex arc. Patients on beta blockers may require large doses of anticholinergics or beta agonists to prevent bradycardia.[1] Therefore, it is preferable to first inject the sinus nerve.

Control of ventilation intraoperatively has a significant impact on maintenance of cerebral blood flow. Hypercarbia, commonly used in the past for carotid endarterectomy, dilates cerebral blood vessels, potentially increasing blood flow at any given perfusion pressure. It was later discovered that elevated carbon dioxide can lead to a detrimental change in cerebral flow around the ischemic area by a process called intracerebral steal. This is the result of normal cerebral blood vessels vasodilating in response to carbon dioxide and shunting blood away from vessels in ischemic brain tissue that are already maximally vasodilated.[75, 76] Decreased blood flow in the territory of the occluded carotid artery has been documented using hypercarbia.[75] Conversely, hypocarbia as a means of vasoconstricting cerebral vessels and shunting blood into ischemic areas was also proposed. Hypocapnia has been shown to increase regional cerebral blood flow in the ischemic territory.[75, 76] Unfortunately, hypocarbia causes a leftward shift in the oxyhemoglobin disassociation curve, leading to decreased oxygen delivery to ischemic and normal brain tissue. Therefore, most anesthesiologists recommend that normocarbia be maintained intraoperatively.

In the absence of significant blood loss intraoperatively, fluid requirements beyond replacing deficits and maintenance are minimal. Non-dextrose-containing solutions should be used for routine hydration. Fasting patients, due to their neuroendocrine response to surgical stress, usually have a breakdown of glycogen. As a result, normal or mildly elevated blood glucose is common in the perioperative period. If glucose-containing solutions are administered, moderate hyperglycemia often develops, and hyperglycemia is associated with worsening of ischemic brain injury.

CEREBRAL PROTECTION

The question of whether to administer a prophylactic dose of thiopental prior to carotid cross-clamping is the subject of much debate. The ability of barbiturates to reduce cerebral infarction had been documented under a variety of experimental conditions, but some of the results are conflicting. This variability has been attributed to the dose, duration, and timing of administration of the barbiturates.[52] It also depends on the species studies, the duration of vascular occlusion, and the hemodynamic response to barbiturates.[52] Pretreatment with pentobarbital before permanent cerebrovascular occlusion reduced the infarct size in animals but did not improve neurologic outcome in all studies.[77–81] Transient occlusion of a major cerebral vessel in animals introduced the additional problem of reperfusion injury. Extremely high doses of pentobarbital (30–70 mg/kg) or continuous infusion to maintain isoelectric EEG appeared to confer cerebral protection in this setting.[79, 81, 82] However, this dose is associated with detrimental cardiovascular depression that could reduce cerebral blood flow. Based on these data, prophylactic barbiturate therapy has been used for cerebral protection during carotid endarterectomy.[83–85] In one of these studies, relatively small doses of barbiturate were used, with the rationale that the barbiturate was trapped in ischemic tissue during cross-clamping due a low flow state.[85] In an animal study, protection was not conferred with a single small bolus dose of barbiturate.[86] These human studies have also been criticized because they were not randomized and controlled. Only two such studies are available in humans. In one of these studies, improved neurologic outcome was reported in patients undergoing open-heart surgery with normothermia and maintenance of EEG burst suppression.[87] In contrast, a more recent study found no neurologic benefit of barbiturates for open-heart surgery if hypothermia and arterial filters were employed.[88] Patients given barbiturates also had longer times to extubation and greater use of inotropic support due to barbiturate therapy. Based on current evidence, prophylactic barbiturate therapy titrated to EEG burst suppression may have some benefit in patients at high risk for cerebral ischemia during carotid cross-clamping. These patients may require additional invasive monitoring such as pulmonary artery catheterization to guide inotropic support. The risk-benefit ratio of this therapy must be weighed in each clinical circumstance.

Recent literature suggests that even mild hypothermia intraoperatively may confer cerebral protection. In animals, decreases in brain temperature as little as 2 to 4°C are associated with substantial reductions in histologic damage following an ischemic insult.[89–91] This is explained by the fact that the brain's utilization of oxygen can be divided into that used for support of electrophysiologic activity and that used for maintenance of cellular integrity.[92] Hypothermia suppresses energy utilization for both of these functions, but general anesthesia suppresses only electrophysiologic activity. There is evidence that hypothermia also prevents the release of fatty acids and free radicals associated with cellular injury during ischemia.[93, 94]

Mild hypothermia is common under general anesthesia because anesthetics depress metabolic heat production and central thermoregulation. Immediately after induction, vasodilation allows peripheral blood to mix with warm central blood, decreasing body temperature 1 to 2°C. Further falls in temperature occur intraoperatively as body heat is lost to the cool operating room environment. No attempt should be made to warm the patient until after the carotid endarterectomy has taken place, since this degree of hypothermia may offer cerebral protection. Temperatures below 34.5°C should be avoided, however, because they may cause serious side effects, such as peripheral vasoconstriction. Increases in peripheral vascular resistances can lead to metabolic acidosis,

myocardial dysfunction, and inability to reverse muscle relaxants. Postoperatively, hypothermia leads to shivering, which causes a dramatic rise in oxygen consumption, leading to myocardial ischemia. Prior to emergence, active attempts to warm the patient should be undertaken if significant hypothermia is present.

POSTOPERATIVE MANAGEMENT

Blood pressure needs to be as carefully controlled during emergence and postoperatively as it was intraoperatively. Postoperative hypertension causes a threefold increase in the risk of neurologic deficit.[95] Elevated blood pressure can also lead to cerebral edema by increasing perfusion of vessels with impaired autoregulation. The postoperative period places additional stresses on the patient due to pain, bladder distention, temperature changes, and altered respiratory function. This can lead to adverse cardiac outcome secondary to hypertension and tachycardia. Myocardial ischemia is thought to occur more commonly during the postoperative period and persists for 48 hours or longer following noncardiac surgery.[96, 97] If a patient was hypertensive during induction, he or she will tend to be hypertensive during emergence and postoperatively. A continuous infusion of nitroglycerin, nitroprusside, or esmolol is acceptable treatment for postoperative hypertension. If the hypertension is sustained, longer-acting agents such as labetalol, nifedipine, or hydralazine can be instituted. Although much less common, hypotension can occur in the postoperative period. Initial treatment involves crystalloid or colloid infusion to ensure adequate left ventricular filling pressure. If the patient is unresponsive, vasopressor therapy may be necessary.

Patients should be carefully evaluated postoperatively for cranial nerve deficits. High carotid dissection can lead to injury of the facial nerve, resulting in perioral weakness. Damage to the recurrent laryngeal nerve secondary to deep retraction can lead to unilateral vocal cord paralysis. The superior laryngeal nerve, which is responsible for sensation of the hypopharynx above the vocal cords, can be injured during dissection of the medial portion of the carotid artery. Tongue weakness can be the result of damage to the hypoglossal nerve. These types of deficits can impair the patient's ability to handle his or her secretions. This could result in aspiration and may require reintubation for airway protection.

The development of a wound hematoma requires immediate attention. The enlarging neck mass can compress the airway and lead to respiratory failure. As the patient becomes more symptomatic, blood pressure tends to rise, increasing the size of the hematoma. There is evidence that it is best to perform the evacuation under local anesthesia instead of general anesthesia. A small study looked at 15 patients following carotid endarterectomy who developed neck hematomas.[98] Of the eight patients who had evacuation under local anesthesia, none had any perioperative complications. However, there was considerable difficulty with airway management under general anesthesia, which led to myocardial infarctions in two patients and stroke resulting in death in one patient.

Special attention should be paid to patients who have a history of a contralateral carotid endarterectomy, since the carotid body may have been damaged. Chemoreceptors in the carotid body increase ventilation in response to hypoxemia. Patients who have sustained bilateral carotid body injury due to the previous and current carotid endarterectomies are at risk of hypoxemia even after the effects of the anesthetics have waned. Patients need to be carefully observed as they are weaned from routine supplemental oxygen during the postoperative period. Narcotics should be used cautiously in these patients.

CONCLUSION

Careful preoperative assessment and preparation are essential in minimizing the risks associated with carotid endarterectomy. Striving to protect the brain and heart from myocardial ischemia is a major challenge. Early detection and treatment of alterations in blood pressure, heart rate, ventilation, depth of anesthesia, temperature, and blood glucose may help reduce morbidity and mortality associated with this procedure. This requires that adequate monitoring be employed. The success of the anesthetic appears to rely more heavily on the skill of the anesthesiologist at controlling these variables than on the specific agents used. Those who favor general anesthesia argue that it allows for stricter control of these parameters. It also allows one to utilize agents and techniques that may offer cerebral protection during an ischemic insult. Postoperatively, these patients are at continued risk of serious complications and need close observation. As always, the anesthesiologist needs to be prepared to assist in the detection and treatment of perioperative complications.

REFERENCES

1. Jacobs GB, Frost E: The management of cardiovascular disease. In Frost E, ed. *Clinical Anesthesia in Neurosurgery*, 2nd ed. Boston: Butterworth-Heinemann; 1991:184.
2. Strandgaard S, Olesen J, Skinhoj E, et al: Autoregulation of brain circulation in severe arterial hypertension. *Br Med J*. 1973;3:507.
3. Prys-Robert C, Meloche R, Foex P: Studies of anesthesia in relation to hypertension. I: Cardiovascular responses of treated and untreated patients. *Br J Anaesth*. 1971;43:122.
4. Asiddao CB, Donegan TN, Whitesell RL, et al: Factors associated with perioperative complications during carotid endarterectomy. *Anesth Analg*. 1982;61:631.
5. Philbin DM, Lowenstein E: Lack of beta-adrenergic activity of isoflurane in the dogs: A comparison of circulatory effects of halothane and isoflurane after propranolol. *Br J Anaesth*. 1976;48:1165.
6. Schulte-Sasse U, Hess W, Markschies-Hornung A, et al: Combined effects of halothane anesthesia and verapamil on systemic hemodynamics and left ventricular myocardial contractility in patients with ischemic heart disease. *Anesth Analg*. 1984;63:791.
7. Kapur PA, Bloor B, Flacke WE, et al: Comparison of cardiovascular response to verapamil during enflurane, isoflurane or halothane anesthesia in the dog. *Anesthesiology*. 1984;61:156.
8. Houston MC: Abrupt cessation of treatment in hypertension: Consideration of clinical features, mechanisms, prevention, and management of the discontinuation syndrome. *Am Heart J*. 1981;102:415.
9. Hart GR, Anderson RJ: Withdrawal syndromes and the cessation of antihypertensive therapy. *Arch Intern Med*. 1981;141:1125.
10. Brodsky JB, Bravo JT: Acute postoperative clonidine withdrawal syndrome. *Anesthesiology*. 1976;44:519.
11. Bruce DL, Croley TF, Lee JS: Preoperative clonidine withdrawal syndrome. *Anesthesiology*. 1978;51:90.
12. Slogoff S, Keats AS, Ott E: Preoperative propranolol therapy and aorto-coronary bypass operation. *JAMA*. 1978;240:1487.
13. Weber MA: Discontinuation syndrome following cessation of treatment with clonidine and other antihypertensive agents. *J Cardiovasc Pharm*. 1980;2:s73.
14. Houston MA, Hodge R: Beta-adrenergic blocker withdrawal syndromes in hypertension and other cardiovascular diseases. *Am Heart J*. 1988;116:515.
15. Vitez TS, Soper LE, Wong KS, et al: Chronic hypokalemia and intraoperative dysrhythmias. *Anesthesiology*. 1985;63:130.
16. Hertzer NK, Beven EG, Young JR, et al: Coronary artery disease in peripheral vascular patients: A classification of 1000 angiograms and results of surgical management. *Ann Surg*. 1984;199:223.
17. Barnes RW, Liebman PR, Marszalek PB, et al: The natural history of asymptomatic carotid disease in patients undergoing cardiovascular surgery. *Surgery*. 1981;90:1075.
18. Barnes RW, Marszalek PB: Asymptomatic carotid disease in the cardiovascular surgical patients: Is prophylactic endarterectomy necessary? *Stroke*. 1981;12:497.
19. Ropper AH, Wechsler LR, Wilson LS: Carotid bruit and the risk of stroke in elective surgery. *N Engl J Med*. 1982;307:1388.
20. Tomatis LA, Fierens EE, Verbrugge GP: Evaluation of surgical risk in peripheral vascular disease by coronary angiography: A series of 1000 cases. *Surgery*. 1972;71:429.
21. Ivey TD: Combined carotid and coronary disease: A conservative strategy. *J Vasc Surg*. 1986;3:687.
22. Schneider RM, Seaworth JF, Dohrmann ML, et al: Anatomic and prognostic implications of early positive treadmill exercise test. *Am J Cardiol*. 1982;50:682.
23. Dagenais GR, Rouleau JR, Christen A, et al: Survival of patients with strongly positive, exercise electrocardiogram. *Circulation*. 1982;65:452.
24. Cohn PF, Lawson WE: Characteristics of silent myocardial ischemia during out-of-hospital activities in asymptomatic angiographically documented coronary-artery disease. *Am J Cardiol*. 1987;59:746.
25. Leppo J, Plaja J, Gionet M, et al: Noninvasive evaluation of cardiac risk before elective vascular surgery. *J Am Coll Cardiol*. 1987;9:269.
26. Eagle KA, Coley CM, Newell JB, et al: Combining clinical and thallium data optimizes preoperative assessment of cardiac risk before major vascular surgery. *Ann Intern Med*. 1989;110:859.
27. Boucher CA, Brewster DC, Darling C, et al: Determination of cardiac risk by dipyridamole-thallium imaging before peripheral vascular surgery. *N Engl J Med*. 1985;312:389.
28. Raby KE, Goldman L, Creager MA, et al: Correlation between pre-operative ischemia and major cardiac events after peripheral vascular surgery. *N Engl J Med*. 1989;321:1296.
29. Linstedt U, Jaeger H, Petry A: The neuropathy of the autonomic nervous system: An additional risk in diabetes mellitus (in German). *Anaesthetist*. 1993;42:521.
30. Knuttgen D, Weidemann D, Doehn M: Diabetic autonomic neuropathy: Abnormal cardiovascular reactions under general anesthesia. *Klin Wochenschr*. 1990;68:1168.
31. Knuttgen D, Buttner-Belz U, Gernot A, et al: Unstable blood pressure during anesthesia in diabetic patients with autonomic neuropathy (in German). *Anasth Intensivther Notfallmed*. 1990;25:256.
32. Lloyd-Mostyn RH, Watkins PJ: Defective innervation of heart in diabetic autonomic neuropathy. *Br Med J*. 1975;3:15.
33. Ewing DJ, Campbell IW, Clarke BF: Assessment of cardiovascular effects in diabetic autonomic neuropathy and prognostic implications. *Ann Intern Med*. 1980;92:308.
34. Hogan K, Rusy D, Springman SR: Difficult laryngoscopy and diabetes mellitus. *Anesth Analg*. 1988;67:1162.
35. Weiss ME, Nyhan D, Deng ZK, et al: Association of protamine IgE and IgG antibodies with life-threatening reactions to intravenous protamine. *N Engl J Med*. 1989;320:886.
36. Longstreth WT, Inui TS: High blood glucose level on hospital admission and poor neurological recovery after cardiac arrest. *Ann Neurol*. 1984;15:59.
37. Pulsinelli WA, Levy DE, Sigsbee B, et al: Increased damage after ischemic stroke in patients with hyperglycemia with and without established diabetes mellitus. *Am J Med*. 1983;74:540.
38. Nedergaard M: Transient focal ischemia in hyperglycemic rats is associated with increased cerebral infarction. *Brain Res*. 1987;408:79.
39. Walts LF, Miller JD, Davidson MB, et al: Perioperative management of diabetes mellitus. *Anesthesiology*. 1981;55:104.
40. Roizen MF: Anesthetic implications of concurrent disease. In Miller RD, eds. *Anesthesia*, 3rd ed. New York: Churchill Livingstone;1990:793.
41. Frost E: Anesthesia for elective intracranial procedure. *Anesth Rev*. 1980;7:13.
42. Freeman LT, Nixon PG, Sallabank P, et al: Psychological stress and silent myocardial ischemia. *Am Heart J*. 1987;114:477.
43. Coriat P, Baron JF, Natali J, et al: Incidence of myocardial ischemia during carotid endarterectomy. *Int Angiol*. 1986;5:203.
44. London MJ, Hollenberg M, Wong MC, et al: Intraoperative myocardial ischemia: Localization by continuous 12-lead electrocardiography. *Anesthesiology*. 1988; 69:232.
45. Rao TL, Jacobs KM, El-Etr AA: Reinfarction following anesthesia in patients with myocardial infarction. *Anesthesiology*. 1983;59:499.
46. Haggmark S, Hohner P, Ostman M, et al: Comparison of hemodynamic electrocardiographic, mechanical, and metabolic indicators of intra-operative myocardial ischemia in vascular surgical patients with coronary artery disease. *Anesthesiology*. 1989;70:19.
47. Mangano DT: Perioperative cardiac morbidity. *Anesthesiology*. 1990;72:153.
48. Smith JS, Cahalan MK, Benefiel DJ, et al: Intra-operative detection of myocardial ischemia in high risk patients: Electrocardiography versus two-dimensional transesophageal echocardiography. *Circulation*. 1985;72:1015.
49. Ellis JE, Shah MN, Briller JE, et al: A comparison of methods for detection of myocardial ischemia during non-cardiac surgery: Automated ST segment analysis system, electrocardiography, and transesophageal echocardiography. *Anesth Analg*. 1992;75:764.
50. Landesberg G, Erel J, Anner H, et al: Perioperative myocardial ischemia in carotid

endarterectomy under cervical block anesthesia and prophylactic nitroglycerin infusion: A prospective study. *J Cardiothorac Vasc Anesth.* 1993;7:259.

51. Roizen MF: Role of the anesthesiologist in vascular procedures. *J Cardiothorac Vasc Anesth.* 1993;7:257.

52. Shapiro HM: Barbiturates in brain ischaemia. *Br J Anaesth.* 1985;57:82.

53. Hicks RG, Kerr DR, Horton DA: Thiopentone cerebral protection under EEG control during carotid endarterectomy. *Anaesth Intensive Care.* 1986;14:22.

54. Renou AM, Vernhiet T, Macrez P, et al: Cerebral blood flow and metabolism during etomidate anaesthesia in man. *Br J Anaesth.* 1978;50:1047.

55. Ramani R: A dose-related study of the influence of propofol on cerebral blood flow and metabolism. *J Neurosurg Anesthesia.* 1992;4:99.

56. Cooperman LH, Strobel GE Jr, Kennel EM: Massive hyperkalemia after administration of succinylcholine. *Anesthesiology.* 1970;32:161.

57. Menkhaus PG, Reves JG, Kissin I, et al: Cardiovascular effects of esmolol in anesthetized humans. *Anesth Analg.* 1985;64:327.

58. Thompson IR, Mutch WAC, Colligan JD: Failure of intravenous nitroglycerin to prevent intraoperative myocardial ischemia during fentanyl-pancuronium anesthesia. *Anesthesiology.* 1984;61:385.

59. Gallagher JD, Moore RA, Jose AB, et al: Prophylactic nitroglycerin infusion during coronary artery bypass surgery. *Anesthesiology.* 1986;64:785.

60. Cucchiara RF, Benefiel DJ, Matteo RS, et al: Evaluation of esmolol in controlling increased heart rate and blood pressure during endotracheal intubation in patients undergoing carotid endarterectomy. *Anesthesiology.* 1986;65:528.

61. Smith JS, Roizen MF, Cahalan MK, et al: Does anesthetic technique make a difference? Augmentation of systolic blood pressure during carotid endarterectomy: Effects of phenylephrine versus light anesthesia and of isoflurane versus halothane on the incidence of myocardial ischemia. *Anesthesiology.* 1988;69:846.

62. Sundt TM, Sharbrough FW, Piepgras DG, et al: Correlation of cerebral blood flow and electroencephalographic changes during carotid endarterectomy. *Mayo Clin Proc.* 1981;56:533.

63. Messick JM, Casement B, Sharbrough FW, et al: Correlation of regional cerebral blood flow (rCBF) with EEG changes during isoflurane anesthesia for carotid endarterectomy: Critical rCBF. *Anesthesiology.* 1987;66:344.

64. Michenfelder JD, Sundt TM, Fode N, et al: Isoflurane when compared to enflurane and halothane decreases the frequency of cerebral ischemia during carotid endarterectomy. *Anesthesiology.* 1987;67:336.

65. Verhaegen MJ, Todd MM, Warner DS: A comparison of cerebral ischemia flow thresholds during halothane, N_2O and isoflurane, N_2O anesthesia in rats. *Anesthesiology.* 1992;76:743.

66. Sano T, Drummond JC, Patel PM, et al: A comparison of the cerebral protective effects of isoflurane and mild hypothermia in a model of incomplete forebrain ischemia in the rat. *Anesthesiology.* 1992;76:221.

67. Warner DS, Deshpande JK, Wieloch T: The effects of isoflurane on neuronal neurosis following near complete forebrain ischemia in the rat. *Anesthesiology.* 1986;64:19.

68. Nehls DG, Todd MM, Spetzler RF, et al: A comparison of the cerebral protective effects of isoflurane and barbiturates during temporary focal ischemia in primates. *Anesthesiology.* 1987;66:453.

69. Warner D, Zhou J, Ramani R, et al: Reversible focal ischemia in the rat: Effects of halothane, isoflurane, methohexital anesthesia. *J Cereb Blood Flow Metab.* 1991;11:794.

70. Young WL, Prohovnik I, Correl JW, et al: A comparison of the cerebral hemodynamic effects of sufentanil and isoflurane in humans undergoing carotid endarterectomy. *Anesthesiology.* 1989;71:863.

71. Young WL, Prohovnik I, Correl JW, et al: Cerebral blood flow and metabolism in patients undergoing anesthesia for carotid endarterectomy: A comparison of isoflurane, halothane, and fentanyl. *Anesth Analg.* 1989;68:712.

72. Hansebout RR, Blomquist G Jr, Gloor P: Use of hypertension and electroencephalographic monitoring during carotid endarterectomy. *Can J Surg.* 1981;24:304.

73. String ST, Callahan A: The critical manipulable variables of hemispheric low flow during carotid surgery. *Surgery.* 1983;93:46.

74. Elliot BM, Collins GJ Jr, Youkey JR, et al: Intraoperative local anesthetic injection of the carotid sinus nerve: A prospective, randomized study. *Am J Surg.* 1986;152:695.

75. Boysen G, Ladegaard-Pedersen HJ, Henriksen H, et al: The effects of $PaCO_2$ on regional cerebral blood flow and internal carotid arterial pressure during carotid cross clamping. *Anesthesiology.* 1971;35:286.

76. Fourcade HE, Larson CP, Ehrenfeld WK, et al: The effects of CO_2 and systemic hypertension on cerebral perfusion pressure during carotid endarterectomy. *Anesthesiology.* 1970;33:383.

77. Smith AL, Hoff JT, Nielsen SL, et al: Barbiturate protection in acute focal ischemia. *Stroke.* 1974;5:1.

78. Michenfelder JD, Milde JM, Sundt TM: Cerebral protection by barbiturate anesthesia. Use after middle cerebral artery occlusion in Java monkeys. *Arch Neurol.* 1976;33:345.

79. Selman WR, Spetzler RF, Roessmann UR, et al: Barbiturate induced focal ischemia, effects after temporary and permanent MCA occlusion. *J Neurosurg.* 1981;55:220.

80. Hoff JT, Nishimura M, Newfield P: Pentobarbital protection from cerebral infarction without suppression of edema. *Stroke.* 1982;13:623.

81. Levy DE, Brierley JB: Delayed pentobarbital administration limits ischemic brain damage in gerbils. *Ann Neurol.* 1979;5:59.

82. Selman WR, Spetzler RF, Jackson D, et al: Regional cerebral blood flow following middle cerebral artery occlusion and barbiturate therapy in baboons. *J Cereb Blood Flow Metab.* 1981;1:S214.

83. Hicks RG, Kerr DR, Houton DA: Thiopentone cerebral protection under EEG control during carotid endarterectomy. *Anaesth Intensive Care.* 1986;14:22.

84. Spetzler RF, Martin N, Hadley MN, et al: Microsurgical endarterectomy under barbiturate protection: A prospective study. *J Neurosurg.* 1986;65:63.

85. McMeniman WJ, Fletcher JP, Little JM: Experience with barbiturate therapy for cerebral protection during carotid endarterectomy. *Ann R Coll Surg Engl.* 1984;66:361.

86. Gelb AW, Floyd R, Lok P, et al: A prophylactic bolus of thiopental does not protect against prolonged focal cerebral ischemia. *Can Anaesth Soc J.* 1986;33:173.

87. Nussmeier NA, Arlund C, Slogoff S: Neuropsychiatric complications after cardiopulmonary bypass: Cerebral protection by a barbiturate. *Anesthesiology.* 1986;64:165.

88. Zaidan JR, Klochany A, Martin WM, et al: Effect of thiopental on neurologic outcome following coronary artery bypass grafting. *Anesthesiology.* 1991;74:406.

89. Minamisawa II, Nordstrom C-H, Smith M-L, et al: The influence of mild body and brain hypothermia on ischemic brain damage. *J Cereb Blood Flow Metab.* 1990;10:365.

90. Ridenour TR, Warner DS, Todd MM, et al: Mild hypothermia reduces infarct size resulting from temporary but not permanent focal ischemia in rats. *Stroke.* 1992;23:733.

91. Busto R, Dietrich WD, Globus MY-T, et al: Small differences in intraischemic brain temperature critically determine the extent of ischemic neuronal injury. *J Cereb Blood Flow Metab.* 1987;7:729.

92. Michenfelder JD: *Anesthesia and the Brain: Clinical, Functional, Metabolic and Vascular Correlates.* New York: Churchill and Livingston;1988.

93. Busto R, Globus MY-T, Dietrich WD, et al: Effect of mild hypothermia on ischemia induced release of neurotransmitters and free fatty acids in rat brain. *Stroke.* 1989;20:904.

94. Ginsberg MD, Sternau LL, Globus MY-T, et al: Therapeutic modification of brain temperature: Relevance to ischemic brain injury. *Cerebrovasc Brain Metab Rev.* 1992;4:189.

95. Towne TB, Bernhard VM: The relationship of postoperative hypertension to complication following carotid endarterectomy. *Surgery.* 1980;88:575.

96. Fergert G, Hollenberg M, Browner W, et al: Perioperative myocardial ischemia in non-cardiac surgical patients (abstract). *Anesthesiology.* 1988;69:A49.

97. Wong MG, Wellington YC, London MJ, et al: Prolonged postoperative myocardial ischemia in high-risk patients undergoing non-cardiac surgery (abstract). *Anesthesiology.* 1988;69:A56.

98. Kunkel JM, Gomez ER, Spebar MJ, et al: Wound hematoma after carotid endarterectomy. *Am J Surg.* 1984;148:844.

Alternatives to General Anesthesia for Carotid Endarterectomy

THOMAS S. RILES and MARK GOLD

In recent years, there has been a resurgence in the use of local and regional anesthesia for surgical procedures. This renewed interest has been fueled in part by a desire to decrease the recovery and hospitalization time after an operation. In addition, regional anesthesia has been used to minimize the pulmonary and cardiac risks that may be associated with general anesthesia. Most centers now prefer regional anesthesia for vascular reconstructions of the lower extremities.

The use of regional anesthesia for carotid surgery dates back to the earliest carotid endarterectomies. The majority of vascular surgeons today, however, do not perform this operation on awake patients. But since regional anesthesia provides even greater advantages for carotid surgery than for vascular reconstruction of the lower extremities, it is worthwhile for anesthesiologists and vascular surgeons to be familiar with the technique.

For over 30 years, regional anesthesia has been the preferred technique when performing carotid endarterectomy at our institution.[1] In the early years, the main advantage was the ability to monitor the patient's cerebral function during carotid clamping.[2] Knowledge of the patient's neurologic status throughout the surgery permitted the use of selective shunting. Even as more sophisticated monitoring systems became available, we found that an awake patient kept the operation simple and made monitoring reliable. In addition, the technique was easily adapted by newly trained surgeons as they began their own practices away from the medical center. Also, we have found the technique to be useful in elderly patients, because of the shortened recovery period. We believe that regional anesthesia gives us the ability to perform carotid surgery on patients who might otherwise be considered too high risk because of cardiac or pulmonary disease. It is interesting that many patients are relieved to learn that the operation can be performed without general anesthesia, as they are often more concerned about anesthesia than the carotid reconstruction.

Clearly, some patients are not suitable candidates for carotid surgery under regional anesthesia. Relative contraindications include a history of claustrophobia or anxiety. In many cases, these problems can be addressed, but it is a judgment whether the effort is worthwhile if general anesthesia is a suitable alternative. More specific contraindications are those that render the patient unable to cooperate, such as a severe preoperative stroke, involuntary movements, confusion, bronchospasm, and pulmonary congestion.

When we discuss the operation with the patient during the initial consultation, regional anesthesia is presented as a choice. Occasionally, a patient expresses concern that he or she will be unable to cooperate throughout the surgery. It is reassuring to point out that at any time during the operation, if the patient experiences discomfort or anxiety, additional local anesthetic or sedation can be given and, if necessary, general anesthesia can be induced. At the time of admission, the methods of administering the anesthetic and monitoring

the patient are detailed by the anesthesiologist, who will be in constant communication with the operating team.

THE TECHNIQUE OF CERVICAL REGIONAL ANESTHESIA

Although carotid endarterectomy may be performed entirely with local anesthesia, the use of a regional anesthetic reduces the amount of anesthetic agent required and greatly decreases the amount of discomfort experienced by the patient. Essential to the administration of a cervical regional anesthetic is an understanding of the principal pain pathways from the area. The main pathways to the neck pass through nerve roots C2–C4. The distribution of these nerves covers the area from the base of the head down to the clavicle. Overlap of sensation may come from other dermatomes. T2 may innervate the lower neck. This is the next dermatome after C4, as C5–T1 forms the brachial plexus (Fig. 39–1). The third division of the trigeminal nerve provides sensation down to the edge of the mandible and in the region of the upper pole of the incision. Near the midline, there may also be overlap from the contralateral dermatomes. The carotid sheath has additional pain pathways through cranial nerves nine and ten. There are several techniques to block all these pathways. We prefer to directly anesthetize nerve roots C2–C4 and then add additional superficial infiltration along the line of the incision and in the carotid sheath to block the secondary pathways.

The administration of a cervical block begins by carefully identifying and marking the anatomic structures necessary to find the cervical nerve roots and the superficial cervical plexus. The nerve roots emerge superior to the transverse process of each cervical vertebra. In the adult, the larynx overlies cervical vertebrae four through six and is useful to approximate the position of these structures. The notch of the thyroid cartilage marks the upper border of the larynx (C4), and the cricoid cartilage identifies the lower border (C6). Another C6 landmark is the point where the external jugular vein crosses the posterior border of the sternocleidomastoid muscle. With the patient's head turned to the contralateral side, a line can be drawn from the cricoid cartilage to the point where the external jugular vein crosses the muscle, marking the level of C6. A parallel line beginning at the notch of the thyroid cartilage identifies C4 (Fig. 39–2).

To determine the position of the C4 transverse process, the mastoid process is palpated and a mark is made 1 cm posterior. A line is drawn from this point perpendicular to the C4 line. Where the two lines intersect at right angles is the location of the C4 transverse process. The location of C2 and C3 is easily determined once the position of C4 is marked. Using the distance between the C4 and C6 line as a measure, the C2 process is that distance cephalad along the perpendicular line to the mastoid from the C4 point. The C3 process is halfway between C2 and C4 (see Fig. 39–2).

After marking the positions of the transverse process, the

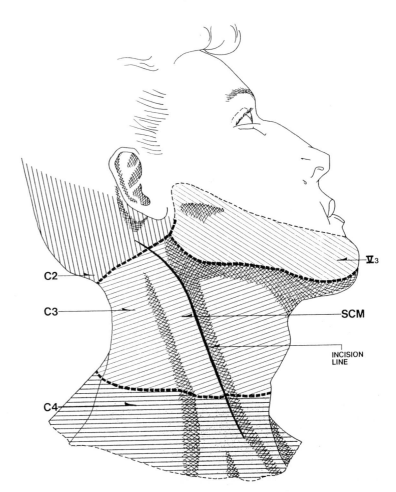

FIGURE 39-1. The zones of innervation of nerve routes C2, C3, C4, and the lower branch of the trigeminal nerve (V_3). The sternocleidomastoid muscle (*SCM*) is shown.

neck is prepped and draped. Using a 22-gauge 1.5-inch needle, the transverse processes are located by entering perpendicular to the skin. The depth varies with the body habitus of the patient. Once bone is located, the needle is pulled back slightly and directed cephalad. This is repeated until the needle is "walked off" the bone. The needle should not be inserted any more than 1 to 2 mm deeper than the bone, as deeper penetration can result in entering the subarachnoid space or the vertebral artery. After a negative aspiration, 5 cc of local anesthetic is injected slowly. This is repeated at the other two transverse processes. It is important to maintain communication with the patient continually, observing for a change in mental status that could occur with an intravascular or intrathecal injection.

The superficial block is performed by injecting local anesthetic along the posterior border of the sternocleidomastoid muscle, particularly along the midpoint of the muscle, where the bulk of the superficial cervical plexus is located (Fig. 39-3). Anesthetic is also injected along the anterior border of the muscle and along the lower border of the mandible to ensure comfort along the line of the incision and to block any overlapping nerve pathways.

A variety of local anesthetics may be used for the cervical block. We have found that mepivacaine in a concentration of 1.5 percent gives an adequate block for approximately 4 hours. Approximately 30 cc of local anesthetic is necessary to block the neck. Since the neck is quite vascular, there may be a good deal of systemic absorption of the anesthetic agent.[3] To decrease the risk of anesthetic toxicity, absorption can be reduced by adding epinephrine in a concentration of 1:200,000. When local anesthetic is used at this volume and concentration, the likelihood of reaching a toxic level is low for an average-size adult. For smaller patients, either the volume or the concentration of the agent must be reduced.

Once the anesthetic is set, the patient's head is rotated to the contralateral side and secured. To keep the drapes off the patient's face and to allow access for the anesthesiologist, an Omni retractor is used to construct a frame over the upper head. A child's squeaker toy is placed in the hand of the patient contralateral to the side of the surgery. So as not to interfere with the movement of the hand, the arterial monitoring line is placed in the radial artery ipsilateral to the operation.

The neck is prepped and draped, and the procedure is performed in the conventional manner. If the patient shows any signs of discomfort, $\frac{1}{2}$ percent lidocaine with epinephrine is infiltrated into the area with a 25-gauge needle. Additional anesthesia is often needed in the carotid sheath and occasionally for the fibers from the baroreceptors of the carotid bifurcation. Before making the arteriotomy, the surgeon test-clamps the internal carotid artery. The patient is asked to count and squeak the toy in the contralateral hand for approximately 2 minutes. If there is no evidence of cerebral ischemia, the operation may proceed without a shunt. If the patient shows signs of monoparesis, aphasia, dysarthria, slowing of mentation, loss of consciousness, or

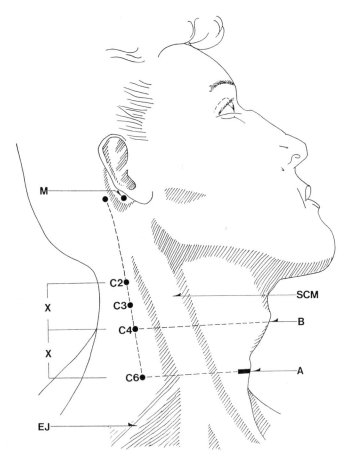

FIGURE 39–2. Landmarks for locating and injecting the nerve routes C2 through C4. Landmarks include the cricoid cartilage (*A*), the thyroid cartilage (*B*), the sternocleidomastoid muscle (*SCM*), the mastoid bone (*M*), and the external jugular vein (*EJ*). C2 is located by measuring the same distance (*x*) cephalad from C4 as determined by the distance caudad to C6. C3 is half the distance between C2 and C4.

confusion, the clamp is removed and preparations are made for shunting.

The vast majority of patients can tolerate the 1½ to 2 hours of surgery with no more than light sedation and periodic reassurance by the surgeon and anesthesiologist. Management of sedation is important during cervical block. The patient must be awake enough to respond to commands, thereby assuring adequate cerebral blood flow. Some sedation may be needed, however, to allow the patient to tolerate the surgery. Small amounts of benzodiazepines, narcotics, or both may be titrated to achieve the desired effect.

Occasionally, especially in elderly patients, benzodiazepines cause disinhibition, resulting in restlessness and confusion. This can be differentiated from inadequate cerebral blood flow by reversing the benzodiazepine with flumazenil. Oversedation with narcotics can be reversed with small doses of naloxone. Caution must be exercised when using naloxone, because rapid administration may result in hypertension and congestive heart failure.

Occasionally, it is necessary to convert to general anesthesia with endotracheal intubation during the operation. Reasons for conversion may include patient discomfort, inability to cooperate, or claustrophobia. Other reasons include unusually difficult anatomy or a prolonged operation. Under these

circumstances, the surgeon may choose to complete the operation with the patient intubated and anesthetized. We have been able to convert to general anesthesia at any point in the operation without difficulty. This is done by first having the surgeon remove unnecessary instruments from the wound and place a sterile towel over the incision. The surgeon keeps his or her hand over the incision to prevent violation of the sterile field while the anesthesiologist folds back the drapes, removes the Omni retractor, and rotates the head to the midline. The patient is then intubated, and anesthesia is induced. Once the endotracheal tube is secured, the head is returned to the rotated position, the drapes are folded back to the head of the table, and the operation proceeds. We occasionally plan the operation in this manner to allow for test clamping of the carotid arteries before the patient is anesthetized in order to determine whether a shunt is necessary.

COMPLICATIONS

It is important that the anesthesiologist and surgeon be aware at all times of the possibility of several potentially serious complications of the cervical block anesthetic. First, as with any local anesthetic, a potential exists for systemic toxic effects, with or without an intravascular injection. The manifestations of a local anesthetic toxicity may be neurologic (sedation, tinnitus, and seizures) or cardiac (con-

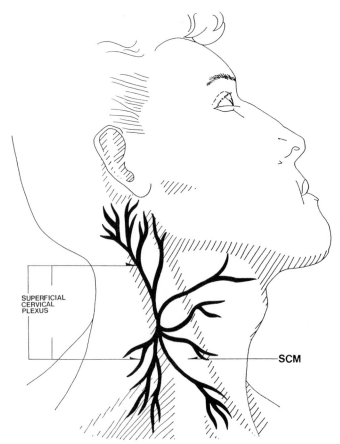

FIGURE 39–3. The superficial cervical plexus radiating from its exit posterior to the sternocleidomastoid muscle (*SCM*).

duction blockade, myocardial depression, arrhythmias, and cardiac arrest).[4–6] The risk of central nervous system toxicity may be reduced by giving the patient intravenous benzodiazepine prior to performing the block. This may raise the seizure threshold.[7, 8] Although the risk is small, it is important that the individuals administering the block be knowledgeable about the management of lidocaine toxicity.

Because of the close proximity of the vertebral arteries, extreme caution must be taken during the injection of the anesthetic agent. With the rich vasculature of the neck, an intravascular injection is a potential risk. It is important to make slow and careful injections with frequent aspirations and to maintain constant verbal communication with the patient, looking for signs of local anesthetic toxicity.

Another potentially serious complication is from an inadvertent intrathecal injection, resulting in a total spinal anesthetic. This may occur from injecting too deeply or from dissection of the anesthetic agent within the sheath of the nerve root back to the subarachnoid space. If this should occur, the patient may develop progressive paralysis of the extremities, become aphasic, and then lose consciousness, with loss of spontaneous responsiveness, within a matter of minutes. It is important to be alert to the possibility of this complication and to observe the patient carefully while blocking the neck. Prompt intubation and adequate ventilation will sustain the patient until the spinal anesthetic wears off. It is possible to continue the operation under general anesthesia if one is certain that the cause of the neurologic symptoms is the intrathecal injection.

An additional complication of cervical block is hematoma formation. This may occur if the needle enters a large blood vessel. Usually local compression alleviates the problem, but occasionally a hematoma will progress. If a hematoma occurs, one must be alert to the possibility of airway compromise.

Advocates of regional anesthesia for carotid surgery have produced large series with low rates of perioperative stroke and death.[1, 9–11] It is difficult to conclude, however, that the good results are directly related to the choice of anesthetic, since the literature contains equally impressive series with general anesthesia.[12–14]

CONCLUSIONS

One obvious advantage of having the patient awake is the ease of monitoring cerebral function during carotid clamping and the early postoperative phase. When the patient is asleep, it is generally agreed that one must routinely use a shunt or rely on some monitoring system (eg, stump pressure, electroencephalogram, evoked potential) to determine when a shunt may be necessary. Although the measurement of carotid stump pressure is a simple technique, the lack of specificity leads to more shunting than is necessary. Electroencephalogram and evoked potential monitoring is far more precise but requires additional equipment and personnel. With the patient awake, the surgeon can be aware of the patient's mental status at all times without relying on machines or technicians.

It is unclear whether regional anesthesia is safer for patients with severe coronary artery disease. Advocates of the technique have argued the point, but good comparative data are not available. In our practice, the incidence of myocardial infarction has been sufficiently low that we prefer regional anesthesia for patients with known cardiac and pulmonary risks. For routine cases, we no longer perform stress testing preoperatively unless general anesthesia is anticipated.

Regional anesthesia for carotid surgery is not for every patient—and not for every surgeon. In our current practice, 82 percent of carotid operations are performed with the patient awake.[1] We do not hesitate to use this technique for patients undergoing reoperation for recurrent carotid disease.[15] We believe that it is a valuable method to have available. As with many types of surgery, the more skills one has for solving patients' problems, the easier the task. Surgeons and anesthesiologists should have the option of performing carotid surgery without general anesthesia, even if only for selected patients.

REFERENCES

1. Riles, TS, Imparato AM, Jacobowitz GR, et al: The cause of perioperative stroke after carotid endarterectomy. *J Vasc Surg.* 1994;19:206.
2. Imparato AM, Ramirez A, Riles TS, Mintzer R: Cerebral protection in carotid surgery. *Arch Surg.* 1982;117:1073.
3. Tucker GT, Moore DC, Bridgenbaugh PO, et al: Systemic absorption of mepivacaine in commonly used regional block procedures in anesthesiology. *Anesthesiology.* 1972;37:277.
4. Wagman IH, deJong RH, Price DA: Effects of lidocaine on the central nervous system. *Anesthesiology.* 1967;28:155.
5. Block A, Covino B: Effect of local agents on cardiac conduction and contractility. *Reg Anaesth.* 1981;6:55.
6. Liu PL, Feldman HS, Giasi R, et al: Comparative CNS toxicity of lidocaine, etidocaine, bupivacaine and tetracaine in awake dogs following IV administration. *Anesth Analg.* 1983;62:375.
7. DeJong RH, Bonin JD: Benzodiazepines protect mice from local anesthetic convulsions and death. *Anesth Analg.* 1981;60:385.
8. Moore DC, Balfour RI, Fitzgibbons D: Convulsive arterial plasma levels of bupivacaine and the response to diazepam therapy. *Anesthesiology.* 1979;50:454.
9. Rich NM, Hobson RW: Carotid endarterectomy under regional anesthesia. *Am J Surg.* 1975;41:253.
10. Connolly JE, Kwaan JHM, Stemmer EA: Improved results with carotid endarterectomy. *Ann Surg.* 1977;186:334.
11. Hafner CD, Evans WE: Carotid endarterectomy with local anesthesia: Results and advantages. *J Vasc Surg.* 1988;7:232.
12. Moore WS, Yee JM, Hall AD: Collateral cerebral blood pressure: An index of tolerance to temporary carotid occlusion. *Arch Surg.* 1973;106:520.
13. Callow AD, Matsumoto G, Baker D, et al: Protection of the high risk carotid endarterectomy patients by continuous electroencephalography. *J Cardiovasc Surg.* 1978;19:55.
14. Towne JB, Bernhard WM: Neurologic deficit following carotid endarterectomy. *Surg Gynecol Obstet.* 1982;154:849.
15. Gagne PJ, Riles TS, Jacobowitz GR, et al: Long-term follow-up of patients undergoing reoperation for recurrent carotid artery disease. *J Vasc Surg.* 1993;18:991.

Standard and Extensile Exposure of the Carotid Artery

LOUIS L. SMITH and J. DAVID KILLEEN

Increased awareness of the association of atherosclerosis at the carotid artery bifurcation and strokes has made carotid thromboendarterectomy one of the most commonly performed surgical procedures in the United States. Modern imaging techniques have demonstrated arterial disease due to a variety of causes occurring proximally in the chest, centrally at the carotid bifurcation, and distally at the base of the skull. Once the anatomy of these vascular lesions is demonstrated, the challenge becomes to find the optimal surgical exposure for correction. The carotid arterial system is unique because of its inaccessibility both proximally and distally and its association with vital cranial nerves in the central portion. It is the purpose of this chapter to review the essential anatomy involved and the commonly employed incisions used in the exposure of the carotid artery in the chest and neck. Optimal exposure is always the hallmark of good surgery.

ANATOMY OF THE CAROTID ARTERY IN THE CHEST AND NECK

The two common carotid arteries differ in their origin and length. The right common carotid artery arises from the brachiocephalic arterial bifurcation, and the left common carotid artery usually arises directly from the aortic arch. The right common carotid artery originates above the sternoclavicular joint in approximately 12 percent of cases.[1] Rarely, the right common carotid artery may arise as a separate branch from the aortic arch or has a common origin with the left common carotid artery. The most common arterial anomaly of the aortic arch branches is a common origin for the brachiocephalic and left common carotid arteries. This anatomic variation occurs in 20 to 25 percent of cases.[2]

Once the left common carotid artery enters the neck, the two carotid vessels have essentially mirror-image courses. The vessels pass obliquely up the neck, covered anteriorly by skin, fat, fascia, and platysma, omohyoid, and sternocleidomastoid muscles. The common carotid artery divides near the upper border of the thyroid cartilage to form the internal and external carotid arteries. This bifurcation is approximately 2.5 cm below the angle of the mandible. Since the aortic arch moves upward with age due to the gradual loss of elasticity with gradual dilatation and lengthening, the carotid bifurcation may be at a higher level in elderly patients. This gradual increase in length results in tortuosity of the carotid vessels.

The exact level of the carotid bifurcation varies from patient to patient, as well as from side to side. A carotid arteriogram is helpful in locating the level of the carotid bifurcation in relation to the angle of the mandible. The carotid arterial wall at the bifurcation demonstrates a thinned media. Arising in the adventitia is the carotid sinus, an extensive network of sensory nerves derived from the glossopharyngeal nerve. This structure functions as a baroreceptor

for the control of systemic blood pressure. The carotid body, which functions as a chemoreceptor, lies posterior to the carotid bifurcation.

The external carotid artery rapidly divides to form the facial and scalp circulations. Several of these facial vessels function as important potential intracerebral arterial collaterals in the event of internal carotid artery occlusion. Distal to the bifurcation, the internal carotid artery assumes a deeper plane, passing posterior to the digastric and stylohyoid muscles and eventually entering the carotid canal in the petrous temporal bone. The artery is at first anterior to the cochlea and the tympanic cavity as it passes through the base of the skull. It is separated from the latter by a thin bony lamella. Anteriorly, it is separated from the trigeminal ganglion by a thin plate of bone. The intracranial internal carotid artery is surrounded by a plexus of small veins and the carotid plexus of nerves derived from the superior cervical ganglion of the sympathetic trunk.

Many vital structures lie in close proximity to the carotid artery. The internal jugular vein lies lateral to the common and internal carotid vessels. The superior and middle thyroid veins cross over the common carotid artery to join the internal jugular vein. The large common facial vein is usually at the level of the carotid bifurcation. The small sternocleidomastoid veins high in the neck overlie the hypoglossal nerve above the carotid bifurcation.

The marginal mandibular branch of the facial nerve sags below the angle of the mandible. It is rarely visualized but is prone to injury by energetic retraction during carotid bifurcation surgery. The greater auricular nerve lies on the sternocleidomastoid muscle posterior to the angle of the mandible (Fig. 40–1). The transverse cervical nerve (C1–C2) arises with the greater auricular nerve from the posterior border of the sternocleidomastoid muscle near its midpor-

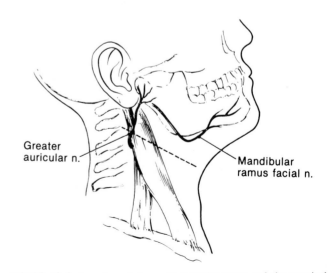

FIGURE 40–1. Location of the great auricular nerve and the marginal mandibular ramus of the facial nerve in relation to the transverse flexion-crease incision for carotid endarterectomy.

tion. It supplies a small triangular area of sensation just below the mandible. Identification and protection of the nerves adjacent to the carotid vessels are of extreme importance. Evans and coworkers[3] reported a 16 percent overall incidence of cranial nerve injury during carotid endarterectomy. They reported the incidence of cranial nerve injury as observed by clinicians as well as speech pathologists. Table 40–1 shows the incidence of cranial nerve injury in two prospective studies.[3, 4] Note that most of these deficits cleared by 6 weeks after surgery.

The vagus nerve lies between the internal jugular vein and the common carotid artery in the lower and mid neck. The sympathetic trunk is located at a deeper level at the base of the neck. The recurrent laryngeal nerve is usually located medial to the common carotid artery, though its course may be aberrant. This latter nerve lies in the tracheoesophageal groove.

The ansa cervicalis crosses the internal jugular vein and common carotid artery just above the omohyoid muscle. The ansa cervicalis nerve joins the descending branch of the hypoglossal nerve; it can be seen lying deep to the cervical fascia in front of the anterior border of the sternocleidomastoid muscle. If the descending branch of the hypoglossal nerve is followed upward, it can be seen joining the hypoglossal nerve above the carotid arterial bifurcation.

The superior laryngeal nerve arises from the vagus nerve posterior to the internal carotid artery and travels lateral to medial to descend by the side of the pharynx. The external branch passes in front of or behind the superior thyroid artery near its origin and supplies the cricothyroid and inferior constrictor pharyngis muscles. The nerve to the carotid sinus ascends from the carotid bifurcation to its origin from the main glossopharyngeal nerve.

SURGICAL EXPOSURE

Proximal Common Carotid Artery

With the widespread use of extra-anatomic revascularization, the need to expose the proximal common carotid artery is infrequent. Trauma or complex reconstructions of multiple aortic arch branches require proximal carotid arterial exposure. A conventional sternal splitting incision offers the best exposure of the superior mediastinum and the origins of the common carotid arteries. Extension of the sternotomy incision along the anterior border of either sternocleidomastoid muscle permits visualization of the right or left common carotid artery, depending on the side of extension. The

entire course of the common carotid artery can be exposed, including the carotid bifurcation. The sternohyoid and sternothyroid muscles should be divided low in the neck to avoid interrupting their innervation. It is important to stay in the midline during the mediastinal dissection to avoid the pleural cavities as well as the right and left lobes of the thymus gland. The left brachiocephalic vein courses from left to right and should be identified, taking care to individually ligate the lowest thyroid vein superiorly and the thymic veins joining the left brachiocephalic vein inferiorly.

During dissection of the origin of the right common carotid artery, the recurrent laryngeal nerve should be identified and protected as it loops around the origin of the right subclavian artery. The left vagus and recurrent laryngeal nerves are avoided by staying close to the adventitia of the left common carotid artery.

Carotid Arterial Bifurcation

The bifurcation of the carotid artery can be exposed by either a transverse flexion crease incision centered over the bifurcation or a more vertical incision placed just anterior to the sternocleidomastoid muscle. The flexion crease incision gives a better cosmetic result, especially if the skin is closed by a running subcuticular suture of fine absorbable suture material. By 6 months, this incision is barely visible. The vertical incision gives greater mobility should proximal or distal extension be necessary, but the more noticeable postoperative scar detracts from this advantage. We have rarely needed a second stepladder incision to expose an atheromatous extension involving the proximal common carotid artery.

Once the skin incision is made, the platysma is incised and the dissection continues deep to this muscle to avoid injury to the marginal mandibular ramus of the facial nerve. Extension and turning the neck away from the side of the operation place the mandibular ramus on tension and increase the possibility of nerve damage by retraction or dissection (see Fig. 40–1). At this point, the common facial vein is located. Following ligation and division, the opening in the deep cervical fascia is developed, and the carotid bifurcation is located by palpation. The carotid sheath is entered by sharp dissection through its several layers until the surgeon is dissecting on the carotid adventitia, as evidenced by the vasa vasorum. This reduces the likelihood of injury to the vagus nerve. The terminal common carotid artery is freed proximal to palpable disease, and a vascular loop is passed around this structure for gentle traction. The superior thyroid artery should be easily visible at this time.

TABLE 40–1. Cranial Nerve Injury During Carotid Endarterectomy

| Study* | Postoperative Nerve Deficits, % | | | | | |
| | Vagus | | Hypoglossal | | Glossopharyngeal | |
	Early	6 Weeks	Early	6 Weeks	Early	6 Weeks
Evans et al[3]						
Clinicians	14.6	4.5	5.6	0	0	0
Speech pathologists	35.0	15.0	11.0	4	1.5	0
Hertzer et al[4]	7.9	1.0	5.4	0	0	0

*For full bibliographic information, see reference list at end of chapter.

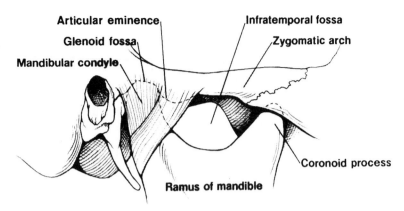

FIGURE 40–2. Anatomy of the temporomandibular joint. The mandibular condyle is subluxated onto the articular eminence but is not dislocated into the infratemporal fossa. (From Fisher DF Jr, Clagett GP, Parker JI, et al: Mandibular subluxation for high carotid exposure. *J Vasc Surg.* 1984;1:727; with permission.)

Verta and colleagues[5] emphasized the importance of staying close to the external carotid artery while encircling this vessel. This precaution reduces the likelihood of injury to the superior laryngeal nerve.

The descending branch of the hypoglossal nerve is usually visualized by this time and can be followed up to its point of origin from the main nerve. An arterial branch from the external carotid artery supplying the sternocleidomastoid muscle is usually encountered at this level. Careful dissection and division of this artery and accompanying veins provide a more generous exposure of the proximal internal carotid artery. Additional exposure of the internal carotid vessel is provided by division of the descending branch of the hypoglossal nerve. The latter nerve can be gently displaced forward, providing a wider view of the internal carotid artery.

The importance of staying on the internal carotid artery adventitia, thereby avoiding injury to the vagus nerve, cannot be overemphasized. This is particularly important in reoperations at the carotid bifurcation, since this nerve may seem to be fused to the internal carotid artery by scar tissue. It is always important to preserve any branches arising from the vagus nerve, as occasionally the recurrent laryngeal nerve is not recurrent but courses directly from the vagus nerve to the larynx.

High Internal Carotid Artery

The high internal carotid artery has been defined as that portion of the vessel cephalad to a line drawn between the tip of the mastoid process and the angle of the mandible. This line is approximately at the upper border of the second cervical vertebra.[6]

One of the advantages of arteriography prior to carotid endarterectomy is the accurate location of the bifurcation in relation to bony landmarks. Furthermore, the extent of the arteriosclerotic involvement can be more accurately assessed. Mock and associates[7] performed dissections on 12 cadavers' 24 carotid bifurcations and documented the level to which surgical dissection could be accomplished by using several standard exposure procedures. They then documented the level to which exposure was accomplished by placing a metal clip and obtaining a lateral radiograph of the neck. In their study, division of the posterior belly of the digastric muscle allowed visualization of the internal carotid artery to the middle one third of the first cervical vertebra.

When exposure is required to the level of the proximal third of the first cervical vertebra, a more extensive surgical procedure must be planned.

In 1984, Fisher and associates[8] reported their experience in managing lesions of the high internal carotid artery in 24 patients using mandibular subluxation. This exposure moves the mandibular condyle forward to the articular eminence (Fig. 40–2) but does not dislocate the mandible. Dental fixation is accomplished by arch bars and wires to maintain this mandibular position during the internal carotid artery reconstruction. General anesthesia via nasal intubation is required and may also improve exposure, since the mouth is closed and the angle of the mandible is therefore further forward.

Exposure of the high internal carotid artery is impaired by the progressive encroachment of the mandibular ramus. The surgeon is literally struggling for exposure in the apex of a triangle. Subluxation of the mandible converts the

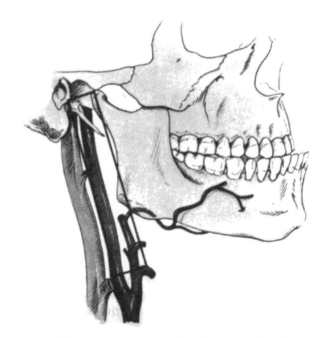

FIGURE 40–3. Mandible in subluxated position, converting the narrow triangular field to a rectangle, thus increasing the width of exposure of the internal carotid artery at the base of the skull. (From Fisher DF Jr, Clagett GP, Parker JI, et al: Mandibular subluxation for high carotid exposure. *J Vasc Surg.* 1984;1:727; with permission.)

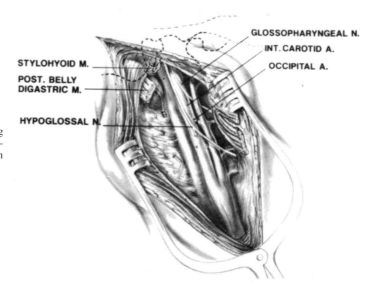

FIGURE 40–4. Exposure of the high internal carotid artery following mandibular subluxation. Note the divided posterior belly of the digastric muscle and the styloid muscles. The occipital artery has also been divided and ligated. See text for details.

narrow triangular field into a rectangle, thus increasing the field of view for dissection of the high internal carotid artery (Fig. 40–3). Small nutrient arteries and veins supplying the sternocleidomastoid muscle are controlled as encountered, and the posterior belly of the digastric muscle is divided. Should additional exposure be necessary, the muscles attached to the styloid process can likewise be sacrificed, along with the styloid process (Fig. 40–4). The underlying facial nerve must be protected from injury. Other nervous structures that require preservation are the cervical sympathetic chain and the glossopharyngeal, superior laryngeal, and spinal accessory nerves.[9] The application of arch bars and wires is time-consuming and a definite drawback in emergency situations, in which time is valuable. Dossa and associates[10] recently reported a simplified technique for maintaining temporary mandibular subluxation. The ipsilateral mandibular bicuspids are cross-wired to the contralateral maxillary bicuspids to maintain the mandibular subluxation. Edentulous patients or individuals with chronic periodontal disease can have temporary mandibular subluxation maintained by the insertion of Steinmann pins into the mandible on the ipsilateral side and into the maxilla on the contralateral side. The protruding portions of the metal pins are then wired to stabilize the subluxated position. This technique for maintaining subluxation of the mandible is simpler and quicker to perform in emergency situations, such as acute traumatic injury to the high internal carotid artery.

Mandibular subluxation with styloidectomy extended the exposure to above the first cervical vertebra in Mock's study.[7] This exposure may be sufficient to suture a simple laceration of the distal internal carotid artery or to remove an extended atheroma, but in our experience, it does not provide sufficient exposure of the high internal carotid artery to resect and reconstruct an aneurysm or to repair an injury requiring an interposition vein graft. In these situations, we employ mandibular fixation and vertical mandibulotomy posterior to the foramen for the inferior alveolar vessels and nerves as described by Wylie and associates.[11]

This exposure also requires general anesthesia via nasal intubation and mandibular fixation by arch bars and wiring. A long oblique incision is made below the angle of the

mandible, extending behind the ear. The mandible is exposed subperiosteally, and vertical division of the ramus of the mandible is carried out posterior to the mandibular foramen, using a power saw. The posterior mandibular segment is rotated out of the way or completely removed by dividing the attached pterygoid muscle. The bone fragment is stored in lactate Ringer's solution. The dissection of the high internal carotid artery proceeds as previously described with mandibular subluxation. Vertical mandibulotomy gives better exposure for very high internal carotid artery lesions.

When the high internal carotid artery reconstruction is completed, the mandibular fragment is replaced into its anatomic location, and the mandible secured by a titanium plate and screws. The arch bars and wires are left in place for 6 weeks. See Chapter 46 for illustrations of this high internal carotid artery exposure.

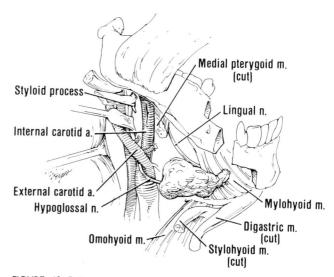

FIGURE 40–5. Lateral mandibulotomy for exposure of the high internal carotid artery by means of step-osteotomy anterior to the mental foramen. See text for details. (From Dichtel W, Miller R, Feciciano D, et al: Lateral mandibulotomy: A technique of exposure for penetrating injuries of the internal carotid artery at the base of the skull. *Laryngoscope.* 1984;94:1140; with permission.)

The emergency exposure of injuries to the high internal carotid artery may require variations of the previously described exposure. Dichtel and associates[12] proposed lateral mandibulotomy as a procedure requiring less preoperative preparation for exposing acute high internal carotid artery injuries at the base of the skull. A stair-step division of the mandible anterior to the mental foramen is employed, allowing outward displacement and upward rotation of the mandible hinged on the temporomandibular joint (Fig. 40–5). The exposure then proceeds as previously described. The mandible is immobilized at the completion of the reconstruction by wiring the stair-step mandibular division and applying arch bars and wiring for 6 weeks.

Angle marginal mandibulectomy has been proposed by Goldsmith and associates[13] to gain additional exposure if required. A rongeur is employed to remove the angle of the mandible posterior to the masseter muscle. Removal of this bony angle provides considerable additional exposure.

A small occluding balloon catheter is helpful in controlling backbleeding from an acutely injured high internal carotid artery while exposure is in progress. The use of a balloon catheter can also eliminate the space required to control backbleeding from the internal carotid artery when distal exposure is limited.

REFERENCES

1. *Gray's Anatomy*, 36th ed. Philadelphia: WB Saunders; 1980.
2. Krayenbuhl HA, Yasargil MG: *Cerebral Angiography*. Philadelphia: JB Lippincott; 1968.
3. Evans WE, Mendelowitz DS, Liapis C, et al: Motor speech deficit following carotid endarterectomy. *Ann Surg*. 1982,196:461.
4. Hertzer NR, Feldman BJ, Beven EG, et al: A prospective study of the incidence of injury to the cranial nerves during carotid endarterectomy. *Surg Gynecol Obstet*. 1980;151:781.
5. Verta MJ Jr, Applebaum EL, McClusky DA, et al: Cranial nerve injury during carotid endarterectomy. *Ann Surg*. 1977;185:192.
6. Blaisdell W, Clauss R, Galbraith J, et al: Joint study of extracranial arterial occlusion. *JAMA*. 1969;1209:1889.
7. Mock CN, Michael PL, McRae RG, Carney EI Jr: Selection of the approach to the distal internal carotid artery from the second cervical vertebra to the base of the skull. *J Vasc Surg*. 1991;13:846.
8. Fisher DF Jr, Clagett GP, Parker JI, et al: Mandibular subluxation for high carotid exposure. *J Vasc Surg*. 1984;1:727.
9. Sweeney P, Wilbourn AJ: Spiral accessory (11th) nerve palsy with carotid endarterectomy. *Neurology*. 1992;42:674.
10. Dossa C, Shepard AD, Wolford GD, et al: Distal internal carotid exposure: A simplified technique for temporary mandibular subluxation. *J Vasc Surg*. 1990;12:319.
11. Wylie E, Stoney R, Ehrenfeld W, Effeney D: Nonatherosclerotic disease of the extracranial carotid arteries. In Egdahl R, ed. *Manual of Vascular Surgery*, Vol 2. New York: Springer-Verlag; 1986:187.
12. Dichtel W, Miller R, Feliciano D, et al: Lateral mandibulotomy: A technique of exposure for penetrating injuries of the internal carotid artery at the base of the skull. *Laryngoscope*. 1984;94:1140.
13. Goldsmith M, Postura D, Jones F: The surgical exposure of penetrating injuries to the carotid artery at the skull base. *Otolaryngol Head Neck Surg*. 1986;95:278.

Carotid Artery Shunt: Argument for Its Routine Use

JAMES M. MALONE and JEFFREY L. BALLARD

The purpose of carotid artery surgery is to eliminate recurrent neurologic symptoms or to prevent stroke. Despite the initial report of Eastcott and associates[1] detailing the surgical repair of a carotid artery lesion in 1954, the proper role of carotid artery surgery is only now finally being clearly defined.[2–4] As the natural history of both symptomatic and asymptomatic carotid lesions becomes less controversial, the risks and benefits of carotid endarterectomy must be carefully analyzed, so that surgeons can adopt the most appropriate criteria for patient selection and the safest surgical techniques and methods of perioperative management.

Owing in part to the fact that a postoperative neurologic deficit is the most feared complication of carotid endarterectomy, no area of carotid artery surgery has been as controversial as the use of the proper techniques for cerebral protection during the critical phase of carotid artery clamping that is necessary to perform carotid endarterectomy. Historical and current methods employed for cerebral protection include the type of anesthesia (eg, regional versus general), induced hypertension, hypercarbia or hypocarbia, and the use of a temporary inlying or outlying intraluminal carotid shunt. Although some surgeons continue to advocate the use of cervical block anesthesia and have reported excellent results with this technique,[5–11] the majority of surgeons prefer general endotracheal anesthesia. Besides providing a motionless operative field, general anesthesia decreases the metabolic demand (oxygen consumption) of brain tissue. The concept that systemic hypertension increases blood flow has been questioned by many investigators.[12–15] Most now believe that the detrimental effects of induced hypertension on myocardial oxygen consumption outweigh the minimal improvement in regional cerebral blood flow in patients with poor collateral circulation. Although the general cerebrovascular effect of hypercapnia made it, at one time, an appealing method of intraoperative management, the current consensus is that although hypercapnia may increase blood flow in the normal brain, it decreases flow to the ischemic brain because of vasomotor paralysis in areas of cerebral ischemia (the so-called reversed Robin Hood phenomenon).[16, 17] In fact, there are data suggesting that because of this cerebral ''steal'' effect, higher cerebral perfusion pressures are required to maintain normal cerebral metabolism with increasing hypercapnia.[18, 19] Hypocapnia, on the other hand, causes cerebrovasoconstriction, which depresses overall cerebral blood flow, reduces potential collateral flow, and probably increases the risk of cerebral ischemia.[15, 18]

Despite a greater understanding of cerebral physiology and a refinement in the techniques of carotid artery surgery, the various maneuvers to protect the brain from ischemia have been used either routinely without reliance on a monitoring technique or selectively with precision monitoring. Generally, normocapnia and normotension (intraoperative blood pressure maintained at average ''normal'' preoperative levels) are maintained to maximize cerebral protection. A consensus has not yet emerged regarding local versus general endotracheal anesthesia, but this issue stirs fewer emotions

among surgeons than the debate over the use of intraluminal carotid artery shunts. At times, the arguments for and against shunting have left the realm of logic and science and bordered on religious philosophy.

The controversy concerning the use of an indwelling shunt during carotid endarterectomy encompasses three main schools of thought, one favoring routine shunting, one no shunting, and one selective shunting. Those surgeons who routinely use shunts,[19–25] most arduously advocated by Javid and colleagues[19] and Thompson and colleagues[20] believe that routine shunting improves surgical results because cerebral protection allows extended operating time and therefore the achievement of the best possible technical result. In addition, routine shunting may decrease the frequency of technical problems associated with the occasional use of a shunt and remove the indecision inherent in the application of the various criteria for selective shunting. Surgeons who do not use shunts, as advocated by Baker and associates[26] and supported by others,[27–31] have emphasized the dangers of shunt-induced thrombosis, embolization, and intimal dissection and have proposed that the physical presence of a shunt impairs satisfactory technical performance of carotid artery surgery. A third group of surgeons, represented by Moore and coworkers,[32] Hays and coworkers,[33] and Sundt and coworkers,[34–36] selectively use an indwelling temporary shunt and base the use of the shunt on criteria according to which an attempt is made to determine either abnormalities in intraoperative cerebral perfusion or in hypoperfusion.[21, 32–41] The selective criteria for shunt use include abnormal intraoperative electroencephalographic findings,[34–36, 38, 39] decreased cerebral blood flow,[34] preoperative neurologic deficit,[32] intraoperative neurologic deficit with test carotid occlusion in awake patients,[5–7, 40, 41] poor backflow bleeding, low internal carotid artery back pressure (stump pressure),[21, 32, 33, 37, 40] and contralateral carotid occlusion.[21, 26, 27]

The hypothesis of this chapter is that routine use of an indwelling intraluminal shunt is the best method for maximizing cerebral protection during carotid endarterectomy and minimizing perioperative neurologic complications.

RATIONALE FOR THE ROUTINE USE OF A SHUNT

Stroke following carotid endarterectomy in as many as one half of cases can be attributed to surgical technique rather than to the type of anesthesia used.[11] Embolization of atheromatous debris or platelet aggregates is probably the most common cause of strokes soon after surgery with or without the use of a carotid shunt. Cortical ischemia (presumably occurring during the period of carotid artery occlusion), thrombosis of the surgical site, intracerebral hemorrhage, and postoperative hyperperfusion syndrome[34] are generally felt to be the other major causes of cortical injury during carotid artery surgical procedures. Although surgical techniques are important, such as the sequence of clamping and unclamping of the carotid artery, the depth and degree of completion of the endarterectomy, direct visualization of the results of endarterectomy, the use of a patch for carotid closure, and postreconstruction technical assessment (ie, angiography, duplex ultrasonography), a well-functioning intraluminal carotid shunt is the most direct way to ensure that cerebral blood flow remains uninterrupted during carotid endarterectomy.

The rationale for the use of an indwelling intraluminal shunt in patients with cerebral hypoperfusion is theoretically appealing and well accepted; however, the difficulty, from a surgical standpoint, is the identification of those patients in whom cerebral hypoperfusion is most likely to occur. According to various authors, one tenth to two thirds of patients undergoing carotid artery surgery require some sort of protective measure during surgery.[5, 12–19, 21, 32–36, 38–41] The ability of neural tissue to recover from an ischemic episode depends on the period of ischemia and the degree of cerebral blood flow. At zero flow, the reversible ischemic period approaches 4 minutes, but cerebral blood flow at 15 mL/100 g per minute in laboratory studies can be tolerated for up to 1 hour when barbiturate anesthesia is applied.[34] Boysen and colleagues[42–44] demonstrated with regional cerebral blood flow studies that flows of less than 18 mL/100 g/min occur in approximately 20 to 25 percent of patients who undergo carotid endarterectomy and are associated with ischemic electroencephalographic changes and neurologic deficits. These data support the concept that a small but significant percentage of patients, ranging from 20 to 35 percent, experience ipsilateral cerebral ischemia during carotid clamping and, therefore, require carotid shunting during surgery. In a publication endorsing no shunting during carotid surgery, Baker and associates[26] identified a group of patients undergoing carotid endarterectomy in whom a carotid shunt would have been appropriate. Eighty-two of 812 patients (10%) had both a contralateral carotid occlusion and a carotid back pressure less than or equal to 50 mm Hg. The rate of permanent deficit was 11 percent when either factor was singly present and 0.9 percent when neither factor was present.[26] In a review of 956 carotid endarterectomies performed under cervical block anesthesia and trial temporary carotid occlusion, Imparato and coworkers[5] documented three factors that increased the perioperative risk of stroke: (1) intolerance to clamping, which increased the risk of stroke fivefold; (2) contralateral carotid occlusion, which increased the risk fourfold; and (3) history of previous stroke, which doubled the risk of perioperative stroke. Data from that study suggest that 416 of 661 patients (63%) meet those criteria and therefore would have been potential candidates for intraluminal shunting. After analysis of the study's data, Imparato and coworkers[5] concluded that total occlusion of the contralateral artery was the major risk factor for intolerance to carotid clamping and therefore perioperative stroke. However, other authors have not found an increased incidence of stroke during carotid endarterectomy contralateral to an occluded carotid artery.[45, 46] Depending on whether one chooses to use intolerance to clamping, the carotid collateral back pressure, the status of the contralateral carotid artery, the neurologic status of the patient, or a combination of those factors as criteria for selecting patients who would

require cerebral protection, the incidence of such patients ranges from 10 percent to more than 60 percent.

It has been suggested by Javid and associates[19] that the insertion time for a routine shunt is generally less than 2 minutes, a period of cerebral ischemia that is unlikely to produce permanent cerebral injury.[34] There is a wide range of time intervals during carotid endarterectomies, however, when the carotid arteries are cross-clamped. The reported average cross-clamp time ranges from 10 to 33 minutes.[26, 28, 29, 47] Although carotid cross-clamp time may not be prolonged or significant for the experienced carotid artery surgeon, cross-clamp time may be important in a training environment in which the general surgery resident or vascular fellow must learn technical perfection in an unhurried fashion. Such considerations further support the routine use of a shunt during carotid endarterectomy.

Objections to the routine use of an intraluminal shunt that are generally raised include difficulty with shunt insertion, the increased potential for cerebral embolization, intimal damage caused by the shunt, and difficulty in exposure of high lesions of the internal carotid artery with the shunt in place. In addition, those surgeons who argue against the routine use of a shunt have suggested that carotid endarterectomy is cumbersome and technically more difficult with a shunt in place. However, in a review of 1800 internal carotid endarterectomies over a 17-year period, Javid and associates[19] reported only 12 instances (0.007%) in which insertion of the shunt was not possible because of proximal or distal extension of the atheroma disease; only four patients (0.002%) in whom the internal carotid artery was too small to permit introduction of the shunt; and rare cases in which distal extension of the atheromatous plaque had to be removed prior to insertion of the distal end of the intraluminal shunt. In addition, Javid and associates reported no instances of intraluminal thrombosis, intimal tear, or dissection. In a report by Browse and Ross-Russell,[22] the Javid shunt could not be used in only 4 of 193 (2%) carotid operations in which its insertion was attempted. Shunt insertion caused arterial damage (common carotid artery dissection) in only one patient. Both reports emphasized that meticulous technique with respect to the surgical procedure itself and in shunt insertion was important in minimizing shunt-induced complications.

In a review of 335 consecutive patients who underwent 390 carotid endarterectomies, Lees and Hertzer[48] reported a dramatic drop in the incidence of neurologic complications when they changed their technique to include normocarbic general anesthesia and routine carotid shunting. In those patients with transient ischemic attacks (TIAs) or asymptomatic carotid stenosis as the indication for surgery, the incidence of stroke decreased from 8 percent to 2.4 percent ($P < 0.01$). In those patients in whom the contralateral carotid artery was either occluded or had a greater than 50 percent stenosis, the incidence of neurologic complications decreased from 11.8 percent to 4.1 percent ($P < 0.02$). Gumerlock and Neuwelt,[49] in a prospective randomized study of the use of intraluminal carotid shunt in 118 consecutive symptomatic carotid endarterectomies, observed a statistically significant ($P = 0.023$) decrease in the perioperative stroke rate in the group of patients in whom a shunt was inserted. Furthermore, there was no increased incidence of complications directly related to the use of a carotid shunt, and, with the exception of cerebral infarction, no significant difference was found in the overall morbidity and mortality between the group receiving shunts and the group without shunts.[49]

In summary, the rationale for the routine use of an intraluminal shunt during carotid artery surgery is based on the following assumptions: (1) a large group of patients is at risk for neurologic complications during carotid artery cross-clamping because of cerebral hypoperfusion; (2) a correlation exists between the time of carotid artery cross-clamping and the neurologic outcome; (3) the use of the shunt does not significantly increase the complication rate or hinder the technical performance of the procedure; and (4) there is so much overlap among the various selective criteria for the use of a shunt that the choice of which selection technique to use is difficult or confusing. Factors that influence the surgical results and the decision to use an intraluminal shunt during carotid endarterectomy also include the patient selection process, the technical proficiency of the surgical team, and the care with which the patient is evaluated neurologi-

cally before and after surgery. The literature supporting the routine use of a shunt suggests that such an approach is appropriate because the benefits clearly outweigh the risks. That conclusion appears to be logical; however, too many variables are probably involved in the cited studies to allow valid comparison between the various published reports. This issue will be addressed in a subsequent section.

TECHNIQUES FOR SHUNT USE

The specific techniques for the performance of carotid endarterectomy are addressed in several chapters in this book, and the interested reader is referred to those chapters. The following paragraphs address only those technical details of the surgical procedure that directly affect the use of a temporary intraluminal shunt.

In general, there are two types of shunts commonly in use: inlying intraluminal shunts and outlying intraluminal shunts (Fig. 41–1). Each type of shunt has its own propo-

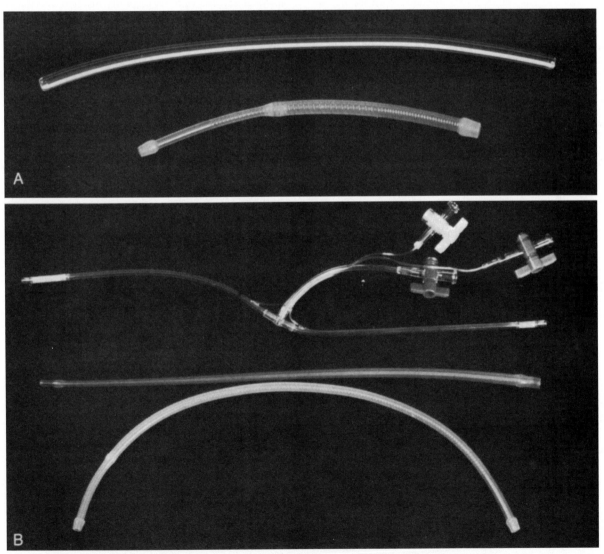

FIGURE 41–1. *A,* The two most common inlying intraluminal shunts: the straight PVC cannula *(top),* and the Heyer-Schulte internal and external carotid shunt (10 cm) *(bottom). B,* The three most common outlying intraluminal shunts: the Pruitt-Inahara carotid shunt *(top),* the USCI Javid carotid bypass shunt *(middle),* and the Heyer-Schulte internal and external carotid (loop) shunt (30 cm) *(bottom).*

nents and detractors. The technique of shunt insertion and removal has usually been considered to be the most important aspect of shunt use, and little emphasis in the literature has been placed on the actual type of shunt. Recent reports in both animal and flow circuit models show differences in flow rate and pressure gradients among various types of shunts.[50, 51] Both flow and pressure gradients across shunts may be particularly important when the collateral flow in the circle of Willis is absent or when a localized area of hypoperfused and vulnerable cerebral cortex exists.[51] Until more data accumulate, the extrapolation of laboratory data regarding flow and pressure differences among shunts to clinical practice is premature, but in the future, such data may assist the surgeon in choosing the appropriate carotid shunt to maximize cerebral blood flow.

For the purposes of further discussion, it is assumed that all operations are performed under general endotracheal normocarbic anesthesia with care taken to maintain the blood pressure at preoperative levels. Prior to carotid artery cross-clamping, intravenous sodium heparin is given in a dose that ranges from 100 to 150 U/kg body weight. Full onset of heparin effect usually takes 3 to 5 minutes. With the use of either an inlying or outlying shunt, certain technical features need to be emphasized, such as gentle manipulation of the carotid bifurcation; adequate arterial exposure; a longitudinal common or internal carotid arteriotomy lateral to the flow divider; meticulous and gentle insertion of the distal end of the shunt into the internal carotid artery; adequate retrograde filling of the shunt to remove air bubbles; careful inspection of the proximal end of the arterial incision to make certain that no debris is present within the lumen; and gentle insertion of the proximal end of the shunt after the intraluminal common carotid pouch is filled with blood, to prevent the

introduction of air bubbles or debris into the shunt. Both types of shunts can be used for external carotid endarterectomy when the internal carotid artery is occluded (Fig. 41–2). The techniques of shunt use in such surgery are generally the same as those for shunt use in the internal carotid artery. We advocate routine post-reconstruction evaluation with either duplex ultrasonography or contrast arteriography. The administration of protamine to neutralize the heparin follows the confirmation of a technically sound carotid endarterectomy.

Inlying Shunt

Before shunt insertion, the patency of the shunt is ensured by its being flushed with heparinized saline solution (1000 U/1000 mL). A heavy suture should be secured around the middle portion of the shunt to later serve as a handle to facilitate shunt removal. The external, internal, and common carotid arteries are sequentially clamped. After a generous arteriotomy is made that completely divides and extends above the most distal point of the plaque in the internal carotid artery, the shunt is carefully inserted into the internal carotid artery. When backflow has been established, the proximal portion of the shunt is placed in the common carotid artery, and both ends are secured in place with Rumel tourniquets. Careful attention should be paid to allow backflow of blood from the internal carotid artery through the shunt. This retrograde flow is used to flush the proximal portion of the common carotid artery so as to remove air and debris prior to unclamping the common carotid artery and allowing antegrade shunt flow.

After the endarterectomy is completed satisfactorily, the arteriotomy is closed over the shunt with the use of the

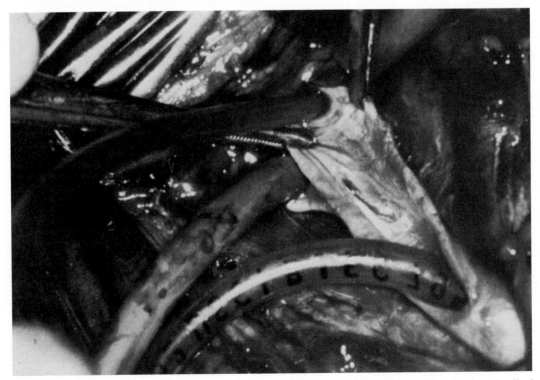

FIGURE 41–2. An intraoperative view of a completed carotid endarterectomy with an outlying shunt in place. Note the clear visualization of the distal endpoint in the internal carotid artery (top left).

surgeon's choice of suture, usually a 6-0 or 7-0 cardiovascular monofilament suture. The endarterectomy can be closed either with two sutures, one starting proximally and one starting distally, or with one suture, whereby a long loop is left in the midportion of the arteriotomy closure. With the two-suture technique, both suture lines progress toward the middle of the arteriotomy and the closure is completed but the sutures are not tied. The suture line is later loosened, the shunt is removed, the arteries are backflushed, and the suture line is secured. Flow is re-established into the external carotid system, and then the internal carotid clamp is removed. Alternatively, the shunt is removed, a partially occluding clamp is placed, and the suture line is completed with partial flow restored to the cerebral circulation. With the single-suture technique, both ends of the suture are secured and the large loop left in the suture line is divided. The shunt is withdrawn (by gentle traction on the shunt ligature), and the suture line is secured after flushing proximally and distally. Regardless of which technique is used, great care must be taken to flush the arterial circulation both proximally and distally after shunt removal to avoid accumulation of embolic debris or air bubbles. If a partially occluding clamp is used (two-suture technique), the internal carotid artery should be temporarily occluded prior to clamp removal so that any residual air or debris will flush into the external carotid circulation.

Using this technique for an inlying shunt during carotid surgery, Schiro and colleagues[25] reported an average operating time of 1 hour and 15 minutes and an average ischemic time for insertion and removal of the shunt of 1.5 minutes.

Another technique we have used to fully visualize a clean distal endpoint in the internal carotid artery and to minimize the extent of the dissection and the length of the arteriotomy is to complete the endarterectomy prior to shunt insertion. Realizing that the ischemic tolerance of neural tissue is at least 4 minutes even at zero flow,[34] we are generally able to complete the endarterectomy (enough to fully visualize both the distal and proximal endpoints) and insert the shunt in well under 4 minutes. With the use of this technique, the shunt can be inserted without the risk of an intimal tear or embolization of atheromatous material by the scooping of debris into the shunt tip. With the shunt in place, meticulous care can then be taken in an unhurried fashion to "fine-tune" the endarterectomy. A two-suture technique is used to close the surgical line. The shunt can be clamped and divided between two small straight hemostats to facilitate its removal through the open arteriotomy. After back-flushing of the internal and common carotid arteries, flow is re-established first into the external carotid system and then into the internal carotid artery.

Outlying Shunt

Proponents of the use of an outlying shunt suggest that technical complaints about the difficulty of carotid surgery around an inlying shunt are obviated by use of an outlying shunt.

Prior to shunt insertion, the patency of the shunt is ensured by its being flushed with heparinized saline solution. The outlying shunt is inserted in the carotid artery in essentially the same manner as the inlying shunt is, with several minor variations. The arteriotomy in the internal carotid artery *must* extend beyond the most distal point of the plaque (see Fig. 41–2). The distal portion of the shunt is placed in the internal carotid artery and secured. Backflow of blood from the internal carotid artery through the shunt is allowed, and the shunt can be left open or occluded. The proximal portion of the shunt is then inserted into the artery, with care taken to evacuate the lumen of the common carotid artery with retrograde shunt flow, or to prograde flow from the common carotid artery in order to avoid embolic complications. The proximal portion of the shunt is then secured and antegrade shunt flow is established. The shunt, if occluded earlier, should be opened slowly and the shunt flow observed for air bubbles or emboli, the presence of which mandate shunt occlusion, back-flushing of the shunt, and forward-flushing of the common carotid artery. Depending on the type of shunt used, the shunt is secured with Rumel tourniquets, Javid clamps, or indwelling balloon catheters (Fig. 41–3). The shunts may be uncoiled and gently retracted out of the surgical field in order to facilitate surgical exposure. Upon completion of the endarterectomy, the arteriotomy is generally closed with two sutures, one placed proximally and one placed distally. The shunt is removed from the carotid artery and the artery is allowed to forward-flush before being clamped. The area of the arteriotomy is gently irrigated with heparinized saline solution, and a small side-biting clamp is placed so that it includes the open portion of the arteriotomy and a small portion of the proximal and distal suture line. Flow is re-established into the external carotid system, and then the internal carotid artery clamp is removed. Closure of the suture line of the endarterectomy is completed, the internal carotid artery is temporarily occluded, and the side-biting clamp is removed. After a few seconds, the internal carotid artery is again reopened to common carotid flow.

ANALYSIS OF PUBLISHED CLINICAL DATA

A total of 2826 carotid endarterectomies performed with no shunt are reviewed in Table 41–1. The temporary stroke rate was 1.8 percent, the permanent stroke rate was 2.1 percent, and the overall neurologic complication rate was 3.9 percent. Table 41–2 lists 3366 carotid procedures performed with routine shunting and demonstrates a temporary stroke rate of 1.4 percent, a permanent stroke rate of 1.1 percent, and an overall neurologic complication rate of 2.5 percent. Similar data for selective shunting during 2131 carotid endarterectomies are shown in Table 41–3. The temporary stroke rate was 1.8 percent, the permanent stroke rate was 1.6 percent, and the total neurologic complication rate was 3.4 percent. Analysis with use of the χ^2 test with continuity correction of the permanent stroke data (Table 41–4) demonstrated a statistically significant difference, in favor of routine shunting, when routine shunting was compared to no shunting ($P = 0.001$). There was a trend toward statistical significance when routine shunting was compared with selective shunting ($P = 0.12$). No statistically significant difference was noted when no shunting was compared with selective shunting with respect to the incidence of permanent stroke. A similar analysis of the incidence of temporary stroke showed no significant difference between

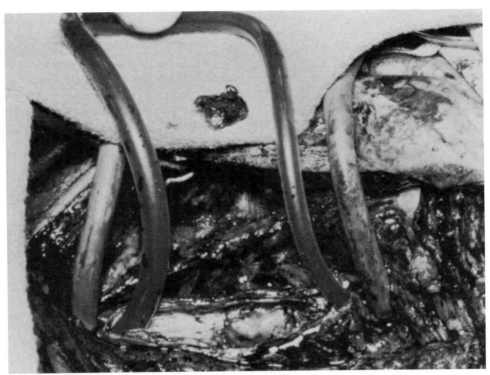

FIGURE 41-3. Intraoperative photograph demonstrating placement of an outlying shunt secured with Rumel tourniquets (top of the head to the right) during an external carotid endarterectomy. Note how easily accessible the carotid artery is with the shunt in place.

no shunting and selective shunting ($P = 0.95$), no shunting and routine shunting ($P = 0.28$), and routine shunting and selective shunting ($P = 0.36$). Analysis of the incidence of total neurologic deficit demonstrated that routine shunting was better than no shunting ($P = 0.003$) or selective shunting ($P = 0.07$). Once again, there was no significant difference between no shunting and selective shunting when total neurologic deficits were compared.

Even though the statistical analysis would suggest that shunts should routinely be used during the performance of carotid endarterectomy, such data analysis has several flaws. A comparison of published surgical series is interesting but probably has limited usefulness because of the following problems: (1) differences in patient populations, the indications for surgery, and methods of patient selection; (2) variations of patient evaluation and management prior to and following surgery; (3) the completeness and accuracy of reporting; (4) the active participation of a neurologist in preoperative and postoperative neurologic evaluation; and (5) no clear and consistent report of the timing of strokes (inoperative or postoperative). In fact, a review similar to the one reported in this chapter, which analyzed many of the same studies, was published as an editorial by Ferguson.[59] The conclusions of that review were that neither intraoperative monitoring nor the use of indwelling shunts is necessary to avoid intraoperative stroke during carotid endarterectomy, and that the best surgical results are achieved with no shunt. Gumerlock and Neuwelt,[49] in a more recent review of similar data, noted the difficulty in comparative data analysis, particularly with respect to the true incidence and definition of temporary and permanent postoperative neurologic deficits.

Such differences in interpretation of published results and in cumulative reviews of published results are difficult if not impossible to reconcile. A careful analysis of the published data suggests, however, that good surgeons in experienced centers are achieving approximately the same results with routine shunting, no shunting, and selective shunting. The message would therefore seem to be that if you are getting good results with your particular choice of cerebral protection, do not change. Excellent results should be the goal of every surgeon performing carotid endarterectomy, and, in fact, such results must be obtained if your patients are to realize the full benefits of carotid artery surgery.

CONCLUSIONS

It is clear that there is a group of patients who require carotid shunting during carotid endarterectomy for cerebral protection. However, the size of that group of patients is not clear. Depending on the criteria used, 10 to 65 percent of patients undergoing carotid artery surgery are candidates for intraoperative cerebral protection. Based on data reviewed in this chapter, there are three groups of patients who require the routine use of a shunt during carotid endarterectomy: patients who have a change in neurologic function while undergoing carotid artery surgery under regional anesthesia; patients with contralateral carotid occlusions and carotid artery backflow pressures less than 50 mm Hg; and patients who have had prior ipsilateral cerebral infarctions, perhaps including the small group of patients with retinal infarctions. The decision to use a routine shunt in patients who do not fall into those three groups would appear to be more a personal preference than a logical scientific conclusion.

TABLE 41-1. Endarterectomies Performed With No Shunt

Study*	Procedures, n	Temporary Stroke, n (%)	Permanent Stroke, n (%)	Total, n (%)
Whitney et al[29]	1197	14 (1.2)	28 (2.3)	42 (3.5)
Baker et al[26]	940	21 (2.2)	23 (2.4)	44 (4.7)
Ott et al[28]	309	6 (1.9)	4 (1.3)	10 (3.2)
Bland and Lazar[52]	280	2 (0.7)†	3 (1)	5 (1.8)
Reddy et al[30]	100	8 (8)	1 (1)	9 (9)
Totals	2826	51 (1.8)	59 (2.1)	110 (3.9)

*For full bibliographic information, see reference list at end of chapter.
†Incomplete data.

TABLE 41-2. Endarterectomies Performed With Routine Use of Shunt

Study*	Procedures, n	Temporary Stroke, n (%)	Permanent Stroke, n (%)	Total, n (%)
Haynes and Dempsey[53]	276	7 (2.5)	4 (1.4)	11 (4)
Nunn[54]	234	7 (3)	4 (1.7)	11 (4.7)
Thompson[55]	516	4 (0.7)	7 (1.3)	11 (2.1)
Javid et al[19]	1951†	18 (0.9)	18 (0.9)	36 (1.8)
Schiro et al[25]	200	3 (1.5)	2 (1)	5 (2.5)
Browse and Ross-Russell[22]	189	9 (4.8)	1 (0.5)	10 (5.3)
Totals	3366	48 (1.4)	36 (1.1)	84 (2.5)

*For full bibliographic information, see reference list at end of chapter.
†Excludes emergency carotid endarterectomies.

TABLE 41-3. Endarterectomies Performed With Selective Use of Shunt

Study*	Procedures, n	Temporary Stroke, n (%)	Permanent Stroke, n (%)	Total, n (%)
Callow et al[56]	186	3 (1.6)	7 (3.8)	10 (5.3)
Baker et al[57]	399	10 (2.5)	4 (1)	14 (3.5)
Hays et al[33]	200	4 (2)	3 (1.5)	7 (3.5)
Moore et al[32]	107	3 (2.8)	1 (1.9)	5 (4.7)
Sundt et al[35]	474	9 (1.9)	12 (2.5)	21 (4.4)
Archie and Feldtman[58]	100	3 (2)	2 (2)	4 (4)
Archie[37]	665	7 (1.1)	4 (0.6)	11 (1.7)
Totals	2131	39 (1.8)	33 (1.6)	72 (3.4)

*For full bibliographic information, see reference list at end of chapter.

TABLE 41-4. Comparison of the Summary Data of Carotid Artery Surgery

Method	Study Reference Number*	Procedures, n	Permanent Stroke, n (%)	Total Neurologic Deficit, n (%)
No Shunt	26, 28, 30, 52	2826	59 (2.1)	110 (3.9)
Routine Shunt	19, 22, 25, 53–55	3366	36 (1.1)	84 (2.5)
Selective Shunt	32, 33, 35, 37, 56–58	2131	34 (1.6)	72 (3.4)

*See numbered reference list at end of chapter.

REFERENCES

1. Eastcott HHG, Pickering GW, Robb C: Reconstruction of internal carotid artery in a patient with intermittent attacks of hemiplegia. *Lancet.* 1954; ii:994.

2. Towne JB, Weiss DG, Hobson RW: First phase report of cooperative Veterans Administration asymptomatic carotid stenosis study—operative morbidity and mortality. *J Vasc Surg.* 1990;11(2):252.

3. NASCET Collaborators: Beneficial effect of carotid endarterectomy in symptomatic patients with high-grade carotid stenosis. *N Engl J Med.* 1991;325(7):445.

4. ECST Collaborative Group: MRC European Carotid Surgery Trial: Interim results for symptomatic patients with severe (70–99%) or with mild (0–29%) carotid stenosis. *Lancet.* 1991;337:1235.

5. Imparato AM, Ramirez A, Riles T, Mintzer R: Cerebral protection in carotid surgery. *Arch Surg.* 1982;117:1073.

6. Hobson RW, Wright CB, Sublett JW, et al: Carotid artery back pressure and endarterectomy under regional anesthesia. *Arch Surg.* 1974;109:682.

7. Connolly JE, Kwann JHM, Stemmer EA: Improved results with carotid endarterectomy. *Ann Surg.* 1977;186:334.

8. Connolly JE: Carotid endarterectomy in the awake patient. *Am J Surg.* 1985;150:159.

9. Whittemore AD: Carotid endarterectomy. An alternative approach. *Arch Surg.* 1980;115:940.

10. Riles TS, Kopelman I, Imparato AM: Myocardial infarction following carotid endarterectomy. A review of 683 operations. *Surgery.* 1979;85:249.

11. Imparato AM: Cerebral protection during anesthesia for carotid and vertebral surgery. In Bernstein EF, Callow AD, Nicolaides AN, Shifrin EG, eds. *Cerebral Revascularisation.* London: Med-Orion; 1993.

12. Waltz AG: Effect of blood pressure on blood flow in ischemic and non-ischemic cerebral cortex: The phenomena of autoregulation and luxury perfusion. *Neurology.* 1968;18:613.

13. Bloodwell RD, Hallman GL, Keats AS, Cooley DA: Carotid endarterectomy without a shunt: Results using hypercarbic general anesthesia to prevent cerebral ischemia. *Arch Surg.* 1968;96:644.

14. Fog M: *Om Piaarteriernes Vasomotoriske Reaktioner.* Copenhagen, Denmark: Munksgaard, 1934; Thesis.

15. Boysen G: Cerebral hemodynamics in carotid surgery. *Acta Neurol Scand.* 1973;52(suppl):1.

16. Youmans JR, Kindt GW: Efficacy of carbon dioxide in the treatment of cerebral ischemia. *Surg Forum.* 1968;19:425.

17. Brawley BQ, Strandness ED, Kelly WA: The physiologic response to therapy in experimental cerebral ischemia. *Arch Neurol.* 1967;17:180.

18. Ferguson GG, Gamache FW: Cerebral protection during carotid endarterectomy: Intraoperative monitoring, anesthetic techniques, and temporary shunts. In Smith RR, ed. *Stroke and the Extracranial Vessels.* New York; Raven Press; 1984;187.

19. Javid H, Ormand CH, Williams SD, et al: Seventeen year experience with routine shunting in carotid artery surgery. *World J Surg.* 1979;3:167.

20. Thompson JE, Talkington CM: Carotid endarterectomy. *Ann Surg.* 1976;184:1.

21. Hertzer NR, Beven EG, Greenstreet RL, Humphries AW: Internal carotid back pressure, intraoperative shunting, ulcerated atheroma, and the incidence of stroke during carotid endarterectomy. *Surgery.* 1978;83:306.

22. Browse NL, Ross-Russell R: Carotid endarterectomy and the Javid shunt: The early results of 215 consecutive operations for transient ischemic attacks. *Br J Surg.* 1984;71:53.

23. Hamann H: Carotid endarterectomy: Prevention of stroke in asymptomatic (stage I) and symptomatic (stage II) patients? *Thorac Cardiovasc Surg.* 1988;36:272.

24. Strawn DJ, Hunter GC, Guernsey JM, Kishore C: The relationship of intraluminal shunting to technical results after carotid endarterectomy. *J Cardiovasc Surg.* 1990;31:424.

25. Schiro J, Mertz GH, Cannon JA, Cintora I: Routine use of a shunt for carotid endarterectomy. *Am J Surg.* 1981;142:735.

26. Baker WH, Littooy FN, Hayes AC, et al: Carotid endarterectomy without a shunt: The control series. *J Vasc Surg.* 1984;1:50.

27. Baker WH, Dorner DB, Barnes RW: Carotid endarterectomy: Is an indwelling shunt necessary? *Surgery.* 1977;82:321.

28. Ott DA, Cooley DA, Chapa L, Coelho A: Carotid endarterectomy without temporary intraluminal shunt. Study of 309 consecutive operations. *Ann Surg.* 1980;191:708.

29. Whitney DG, Kahn EM, Estes JW, Jones CE: Carotid artery surgery without a temporary indwelling shunt: 1917 consecutive procedures. *Arch Surg.* 1980;115:1393.

30. Reddy K, West M, Anderson B: Carotid endarterectomy without indwelling shunts and intraoperative electrophysiologic monitoring. *Can J Neurol Sci.* 1987;14:131.

31. Morowetz RB, Zeiger EH, McDowell HA Jr: Correlation of cerebral blood flow and EEG during carotid occlusion for endarterectomy (without shunting) and neurologic outcome. *Surgery.* 1984;96:184.

32. Moore WS, Yee JM, Hall AD: Collateral cerebral blood pressure: An index of tolerance to temporary carotid occlusion. *Arch Surg.* 1973;106:520.

33. Hays RJ, Levinson SA, Wylie EJ: Intraoperative measurement of carotid back pressure as a guide to operative management for carotid endarterectomy. *Surgery.* 1972;728:953.

34. Sundt TM Jr, Sharbrough FW, Piepgras DG, et al: Correlation of cerebral blood flow and electroencephalographic changes during carotid endarterectomy with results of surgery and hemodynamics of cerebral ischemia. *Mayo Clin Proc.* 1981;56:533.

35. Sundt TM Jr, Houser OW, Sharbrough FW: Carotid endarterectomy: Results, complications and monitoring techniques. *Adv Neurol.* 1977;16:97.

36. Phillips MR, Johnson WC, Scott M, et al: Carotid endarterectomy in the presence of contralateral carotid occlusion. The role of EEG and intraluminal shunting. *Arch Surg.* 1979;114:1232.

37. Archie JP Jr: Technique and clinical results of carotid stump back-pressure to determine selective shunting during carotid endarterectomy. *J Vasc Surg.* 1991;13:319.

38. Baker JD, Gluecklich B, Watson CW, et al: An evaluation of electroencephalographic monitoring during carotid surgery. *Surgery.* 1975;78:787.

39. String ST, Callahan A: The critical manipulable variables of hemispheric low flow during carotid surgery. *Surgery.* 1983;93:46.

40. Kwaan JH, Peterson GJ, Connolly JE: Stump pressure: an unreliable guide for shunting during carotid endarterectomy. *Arch Surg.* 1980;115:1083.

41. Steed DL, Peitzman AB, Grundy BL, Webster MW: Causes of stroke in carotid endarterectomy. *Surgery.* 1982;92:634.

42. Boysen G, Engell HC, Pistolese GR, et al: On the critical lower level of cerebral blood flow in man with particular reference to carotid surgery. *Circulation.* 1974;49:1023.

43. Boysen G, Ladegaard-Pederson HJ, Engell HC: Cerebral blood flow studies during carotid surgery. In Brock M, Fieschi C, Ingvar DH, et al, eds. *Cerebral Blood Flow.* New York; Springer-Verlag; 1969;155.

44. Boysen G, Engell HC, Henriksen H: The effect of induced hypertension on internal carotid artery pressure and regional cerebral blood flow during temporary carotid clamping for endarterectomy. *Neurology.* 1972;22:1133.

45. McKittrick JE, MacLean WB, Lim RA: Carotid endarterectomy in patients with contralateral occlusion: Is the risk increased? *Ann Vasc Surg.* 1989;3:324.

46. Mackey WC, O'Donnell TF Jr, Callow AD: Carotid endarterectomy contralateral to an occluded carotid artery: Perioperative risk and late results. *J Vasc Surg.* 1990;11:778.

47. Baker WH: Indications for operations. Part IV. Emergency carotid surgery, with special emphasis on noninvasive diagnosis and surgical technique. In Baker W, ed. *Diagnosis and Treatment of Carotid Artery Disease.* New York: Futura Publishing; 1979;161.

48. Lees CD, Hertzer NR: Postoperative stroke and late neurologic complications after carotid endarterectomy. *Arch Surg.* 1981;116:1561.

49. Gumerlock MK, Neuwelt EA: Carotid endarterectomy: To shunt or not to shunt. *Stroke.* 1988;19:1485.

50. Aufiero TX, Thiele BL, Rossi JA, et al: Hemodynamic performance of carotid artery shunts. *Am J Surg.* 1989;158:95.

51. Grossi EA, Giangola G, Parish MA, et al: Differences in carotid shunt flow rates and implications for cerebral blood flow. *Ann Vasc Surg.* 1993;7:39.

52. Bland JE, Lazar ML: Carotid endarterectomy without shunt. *Neurosurgery.* 1981;8:153.

53. Haynes CD, Dempsey R: Carotid endarterectomy: Review of 276 cases in a community hospital. *Ann Surg.* 1979;189:758.

54. Nunn DB: Carotid endarterectomy: An analysis of 234 operative cases. *Ann Surg.* 1975;182:733.

55. Thompson JE: Complications of carotid endarterectomy and their prevention. *World J Surg.* 1979;3:155.

56. Callow AD, Matsumoto G, Baker D, et al: Protection of the high risk carotid endarterectomy patient by continuous electroencephalography. *J Cardiovasc Surg.* 1978;19:55.

57. Baker JD, Gluecklich B, Watson CW, et al: An evaluation of electroencephalographic monitoring for carotid study. *Surgery.* 1975;78:787.

58. Archie JP Jr, Feldtman RW: Determinants of cerebral perfusion pressure during carotid endarterectomy. *Arch Surg.* 1982;117:319.

59. Ferguson GG: Intraoperative monitoring and internal shunts: Are they necessary in carotid endarterectomy? *Stroke.* 1982;13:287.

CHAPTER 42

Justification for Routine Nonshunting of the Carotid Artery

WILLIAM H. BAKER

One of the favorite topics of discussion at any meeting of vascular surgeons is the emotional subject of shunting versus nonshunting during a carotid endarterectomy. The surgeons fall into three camps. The first group routinely shunts all patients regardless of any other measurable criteria, stating "why not?—there is no need for selection criteria, placement is easy and promotes facility in using the shunt"; the second group shunts patients selectively based on a variety of anatomic and physiologic measurements, stating "the shunt is sometimes a detriment to an otherwise pleasing technical exercise but occasionally patients require its use"; and the third group never shunts patients, stating that "the shunt is cumbersome and may in fact contribute to technical misadventures, and there is little proof that shunt usage improves the results of a carotid endarterectomy." The purpose of this chapter is to review the rationale for not employing a temporary indwelling shunt during the performance of a carotid endarterectomy.

During the early days of carotid endarterectomy, the operation was usually performed using local anesthesia. Proponents of this method claimed that not only did the anesthesia cause minimal circulatory and respiratory changes, but under local anesthesia the patient could be constantly assessed and changes in neurologic status promptly recognized. Some surgeons grew disenchanted with this method, and in 1963 Wells and associates[1] reported on 66 carotid endarterectomies that were consecutively performed on 56 patients under general anesthesia. One patient in their series died of a hypertensive crisis, one developed a related hemiplegia that cleared within 1 week, and a third patient developed a contralateral neurologic deficit thought to be due to hypotension, anoxia, and failure to maintain anesthesia. Nineteen patients were tested preoperatively with manual carotid compression for 30 to 60 seconds. Interestingly, four patients who became unconscious and developed convulsions during this period of compression tolerated the carotid occlusion with anesthesia for long periods without neurologic sequelae. Such a finding is not unique. Sterling Edwards, writing in a personal correspondence, remembers two patients who were unable to tolerate cross-clamping of the carotid artery during an attempted endarterectomy utilizing local anesthesia. When general anesthesia was administered, the endarterectomy was performed without the use of a temporary indwelling shunt, and the patients experienced no undue neurologic sequelae.

The report by the Houston group popularized the use of general anesthesia for carotid endarterectomy. Wylie and Ehrenfeld[2] reported a stroke rate of 0.9 percent with a 0.5 percent death rate in 219 operations performed in 166 patients under general anesthesia without the use of a temporary indwelling shunt. The patients in this consecutive series fared much better than those in a previous historical control series who received local anesthesia.

These reports underscore the assessment that most patients could undergo endarterectomy quite safely without the use of an indwelling shunt. Nonetheless, an occasional patient

was found to awake from anesthesia and suffer a stroke, which suggested to surgeons and neurologists alike that temporary ischemia was not well tolerated in that patient. This discovery led to numerous attempts on the part of many surgical investigators to select patients who might benefit from temporary shunting during endarterectomy. In this way, the bulk of patients could be operated on without a cumbersome shunt, but a shunt would be used in those patients who were at increased risk.

In 1969, Moore and Hall[3] demonstrated the safety of carotid endarterectomy under local anesthesia but without a shunt if the carotid artery back pressure was greater than 25 mm Hg. In 1973, they reported a series of 107 operations in 78 patients under general anesthesia.[4] In 96 patients with a backflow pressure of more than 25 mm Hg, a shunt was not used and there were no neurologic deficits. The only new stroke was in the shunted patient with backflow pressure of less than 25 mm Hg. Yet in the same city of San Francisco, Hays and coworkers[5] reviewed 297 operations done under general anesthesia and concluded that the safe lower limit of backflow pressure was not 25 mm Hg but 50 mm Hg. In the group of 58 shunted patients who had a low stump pressure, 3 had a temporary and 2 had a permanent neurologic deficit. In those 15 patients with a low stump pressure in whom a shunt was not used, 1 had a temporary and 7 had permanent deficits. Five of these latter seven deficits were of a severe nature. Finally, Hobson and colleagues[6] reported that test occlusion may result in neurologic symptoms even with a back pressure of more than 50 mm Hg. Archie[7] uses a cerebral perfusion pressure (back pressure-jugular venous pressure) of 18 mm Hg to determine the need for a shunt. These reports emphasize that although measurement of the carotid back pressure is of some value in selecting patients for shunt use, there is no universality of agreement concerning the safe level.

Other investigators have suggested that reduced flow is not the only reason for an intraoperative neurologic deficit. Imparato and colleagues[8] reviewed 956 carotid endarterectomies in 661 conscious patients operated on under cervical block anesthesia. Their overall stroke rate was only 2.5 percent. In one half of the 23 patients who suffered perioperative strokes, the stroke was thought to be due to technical problems; one fourth of the strokes were related to intraoperative embolization; one sixth were related to intracranial hemorrhage; and the remainder of the strokes were not directly related to the operative procedure. In this series, 16 of 862 patients who tolerated internal carotid artery clamping experienced a perioperative stroke (1.9%). Temporary shunts were not used in these patients. This rate compares with a stroke rate of 9.9 percent in the 71 patients who did not tolerate internal carotid artery clamping and in whom a shunt was used, which suggests either that the shunt does not totally protect against intraoperative stroke or that the shunt in and of itself contributes to stroke risk.

Rosenthal and associates,[9] from Atlanta, Georgia, compared 818 patients who underwent carotid endarterectomy.

355

In 318 patients who had an intraluminal shunt, 9 (2.8%) had transient deficits and 5 (1.6%) had permanent deficits. Of 274 patients who had no indwelling shunt, 8 (2.9%) had transient deficits and 6 (2.2%) had permanent deficits. In 226 patients, monitoring was done with an electroencephalogram. Shunts were used selectively. Five (2.2%) transient deficits and four (1.8%) permanent deficits occurred in this group. Since there was no significant difference in the incidence of postoperative neurologic deficits between the groups, the investigators could not implicate inadequate collateral cerebral blood flow as the major cause of postoperative stroke. Rather, technical errors that caused carotid thrombosis or cerebral emboli accounted for most of these deficits.

Sundt and coworkers[10] from the Mayo Clinic analyzed 1145 consecutive carotid endarterectomies. Their patients were monitored by electroencephalogram and cerebral blood flow studies. The overall mortality rate was 1.5 percent, major morbidity 1 percent, minor morbidity 1 percent, and transient neurologic dysfunction 2 percent. Intraoperative embolization and postoperative hyperperfusion syndromes were the most common causes of neurologic complications. Their study suggested that hemodynamic events occurred when cerebral autoregulation was paralyzed and that embolism caused most of the deficits. It should be noted that intraoperative ischemia was avoided in their series by the selective use of a temporary indwelling shunt when the electroencephalogram was abnormal or the cerebral blood flow was reduced or both.

In 1982, Steed and coworkers[11] from the University of Pittsburgh presented the results of carotid endarterectomy in 345 patients to the Central Surgical Association. In 96 percent of their patients, carotid occlusion was tolerated under local anesthesia; thus they did not need a temporary indwelling shunt. Of those patients operated on without a shunt, 6 (1.7%) developed prolonged deficits and 15 (4.3%) developed temporary deficits. Twenty of their 21 deficits were thromboembolic, reperfusion phenomena, or related to hypotension. This report underscores that shunting is not required in a vast majority of patients.

The effectiveness of carotid shunting was studied by Gee and colleagues.[12] A Javid shunt was employed in six patients during carotid endarterectomy. An ocular pneumoplethysmograph was applied to the ipsilateral eye of all patients. Measurements were taken after the induction of anesthesia, during the measurement of carotid stump pressures, after the placement of a Javid shunt, and after the procedure was completed. In each patient, the shunt functioned as a vessel with a cross-sectional area stenosis of at least 75 percent. However, use of the shunt elevated the ipsilateral ophthalmic systolic pressure over the level noted during carotid clamping in all cases. Although the shunt improved the margin of safety, it did not provide "normal" carotid flow.

Pearce and associates[13] used the photoplethysmograph to monitor adequate shunt blood flow during carotid endarterectomy. In 13 of 15 endarterectomies, artery cross-clamping of the common carotid resulted in a greater than 30 percent reduction in amplitude of the ipsilateral supraorbital photoplethysmographic waveform. Serious shunt flow reductions requiring correction by shunt repositioning occurred in 3 of the 15 patients. In one instance, the flow occlusion was caused by an upper wound retractor. On at least four occasions, milder flow reductions were corrected by slight changes in retractor position. In addition, the investigators noted interuption of flow from shunt impingement on the arterial wall and kinking of the internal carotid artery above the operative field. They suggest that even with a shunt in place there exists a risk of prolonged unrecognized intraoperative cerebral ischemia.

A temporary indwelling shunt cannot be expected to transform dismal morbidity and mortality statistics into statistics representing a higher plane of accomplishment. Prioleau and coworkers[14] reviewed 240 consecutive patients in whom 317 carotid endarterectomies were performed. The overall incidence of stroke was 10.7 percent and the morality rate 3.2 percent. When a shunt was used, the stroke rate was 12.8 percent, compared with a stroke rate of 8.5 percent when no shunt was used. When the authors standardized the series to eliminate extraneous risk factors, the no-shunt group had a stroke rate of 0.9 percent, but the stroke rate in the shunted group persisted at 9.5 percent. The shunt also did not protect against stroke in those unselected patients who had a high degree of contralateral internal carotid artery stenosis. It was concluded that the intraoperative shunt did not protect against stroke in this setting. Easton and Sherman[15] reviewed the carotid endarterectomies performed in Springfield, Illinois. The overall stroke and death rate was 21.1 percent (48 of 228 patients). Two hundred and four patients received a temporary indwelling shunt. Of these patients, 23 (11%) suffered a stroke and 9 (4%) died. Of those patients who did not have a temporary indwelling shunt, three (7%) had a stroke and four (9%) died. The combined morbidity/mortality rate of these two groups was equal. These two series from the Southeast and the Midwest both underscore that a temporary indwelling shunt is not the primary ingredient of a successful and safe carotid endarterectomy.

Graber and associates[16] from the Tufts University School of Medicine and the Boston Veterans Administration Hospital reported that stroke after carotid endarterectomy was predicted by a preoperative computed tomography scan. Forty-one patients had a preoperative computed tomography scan that showed abnormal results. A shunt was used in 26 of these patients; 5 of those had a postoperative neurologic deficit. A shunt was not used in 15 patients, 4 of whom had a postoperative stroke. In comparison, 66 patients with a normal preoperative scan had only three postoperative neurologic deficits. One of these deficits occurred in the group of 26 patients in whom a shunt was not used. These investigators concluded that a computed tomography scan was sensitive in identifying patients at increased risk for stroke during carotid endarterectomy. Their data suggest that shunting does not protect against stroke in this setting. The small numbers in their series require that further similar studies be performed.

All these data suggest that there are several mechanisms for the production of stroke. One of these mechanisms, namely, intraoperative cerebral hypoperfusion, can at least be partially corrected by the use of a temporary indwelling shunt. The shunt is not foolproof and in fact will not protect against most operation-related strokes, most of which are secondary to technical misadventures. With the attitude that the shunt was of little value, we began in 1970 to perform all carotid endarterectomies without the use of a temporary indwelling shunt. The operations were performed at the University of Iowa Hospitals and Clinics, the Iowa City Veterans Administration Hospital, the Iowa Methodist Medical Center in Des Moines, Iowa (D. Dorner and D. Stubbs), and the Loyola University Medical Center in Maywood, Illinois. In 1984, we published our results of 940 carotid endarterectomies.[17] Six patients (0.6%) died, 17 patients (1.8%) had a permanent neurologic deficit, and 21 patients (2.2%) had temporary neurologic deficits. A correlation of internal carotid artery back pressures and arteriographic data was possible in 783 operations. There were 15 (4.7%) permanent neurologic deficits in 319 patients who had a stump pressure of less than 50 mm Hg. The stroke rate in 464 patients with a stump pressure of more than 50 mm Hg was 1.1 percent ($P < 0.05$). In addition, there was a 9.3 percent stroke rate in the 107 patients who had a contralateral internal carotid artery occlusion. This rate was comparable to a 1.5 percent stroke rate in the 676 patients who had a patent contralateral internal carotid artery ($P < 0.05$). Further analysis of these patients revealed that patients who had both a patent contralateral internal carotid artery and a stump pressure of more than 50 mm Hg had a 0.9 percent risk of permanent neurologic deficit during their carotid endarterectomy. Of the 25 patients with an occluded contralateral internal carotid artery with a stump pressure greater than 50 mm Hg, only 1 (4.0%) had an operation-related permanent neurologic deficit. Although this is not a statistically significant difference, this group should be observed further in this regard. Six (2.5%) of 237 patients with a patent contralateral internal carotid artery but with a low stump pressure had a permanent neurologic deficit. This percentage is not significantly different from that of the first group. But most disturbingly, there were 9 (11%) permanent neurologic deficits in 82 patients who had both an occluded contralateral internal carotid artery and a low stump pressure, making this group at increased risk of stroke during endarterectomy in our series. Assuming that intraoperative cerebral ischemia was responsible for stroke in this group of patients, a temporary indwelling shunt would be expected to decrease the incidence of postoperative stroke. We have operated on 41 such high-risk patients using a shunt since January 1983.[18] Two patients had postoperative internal carotid artery occlusions, two had prolonged ischemia due to technical problems, and two had contralateral strokes. Thus, we continue to have a stroke rate of 14.6 percent despite the use of the shunt. Our statistics and those of other investigators emphasize that a shunt is not a panacea.

The international community likewise finds the benefit of shunting controversial. Halsey,[19] writing for the International Transcranial Doppler Collaborators, reported that severe ischemia occurred in 7.2 percent of their cases. Interestingly, this ischemia cleared spontaneously in about half of the cases. Although shunting protected against stroke in patients with persisting ischemia, the stroke rate was actually higher if a shunt was used and severe ischemia was not present. Sandmann and colleagues,[20] from Düsseldorf, randomly used a shunt in 503 cases. The incidence of postoperative stroke did not differ significantly between the patients shunted (4.2%) and those not shunted (3.3%). Of interest, 10 patients were shunted because of severe alterations in the electroencephalographic and somatosensory evoked potential (SEP) readings. Two of those 10 patients (20%) had a stroke. And

finally, Raithel[21] from Nürnberg reports that he has not used a shunt in carotid surgery since 1975. Of the 7084 carotid reconstructions he has performed between 1984 and 1992, the perioperative morbidity rate was 2.3 percent (1.1% stroke and 1.2% transient neurologic deficit). The operative mortality rate in the total group was 1.3 percent. Thus, operation without a shunt is quite safe in his hands; clearly most strokes during operation are caused by factors other than the shunt.

Regardless of the alleged benefits of the use of a shunt, the question is whether the shunt actually causes harm. There is no doubt that the shunt can ''snowplow'' debris into the carotid flow if it is improperly inserted, and that emboli have been recorded traversing the shunt during an endarterectomy. The major detrimental factor is that the shunt does in fact get in the way of the surgeon during the performance of the operation. Although experienced endarterectomists deny that this occurs, Green and coworkers,[22] from Rochester, New York, reported that technical errors were more common when a shunt was used (5%) than when no shunt was used (0.9%). If this acknowledged center of excellence has problems, the surgeon of lesser experience cannot expect to escape similar difficulties.

The justification for routine nonshunting of the patient undergoing carotid endarterectomy is not difficult. This review of the literature as well as the statistics gleaned from our own series of carotid endarterectomy patients underscores that the most important factor in a safe operation is technical perfection. Avoidance of intraoperative embolization and postoperative carotid occlusion rather than the use or nonuse of the shunt is emphasized at our clinic. Nonetheless, at present, we do indeed use a temporary indwelling shunt in those patients that we consider to be at high risk. Although the use of a shunt has not been shown to reduce neurologic problems in these patients, we have assumed that its use is of benefit. The cynic may suggest that further data are required to prove this point.

REFERENCES

1. Wells BA, Keats AS, Cooley DA: Increased tolerance to cerebral ischemia produced by general anesthesia during temporary carotid occlusion. *Surgery.* 1963;54:216.
2. Wylie EJ, Ehrenfeld WK: Complications and results of surgery. In Wylie EJ, Ehrenfeld WK, eds. *Extracranial Occlusive Cerebrovascular Disease. Diagnosis and Management.* Philadelphia: WB Saunders; 1970;214.
3. Moore WS, Hall AD: Carotid artery back pressure. A test of cerebral tolerance to temporary carotid occlusion. *Arch Surg.* 1969;99:702.
4. Moore WS, Yee JM, Hall AD: Collateral cerebral blood pressure. *Arch Surg.* 1973;106:520.
5. Hays RJ, Levinson SA, Wylie EJ: Intra-operative measurement of carotid back pressure as a guide to operative management for carotid endarterectomy. *Surgery.* 1972;72:593.
6. Hobson RW, Wright CB, Sublett JW, et al: Carotid artery back pressure and endarterectomy under regional anesthesia. *Arch Surg.* 1974;109:682.
7. Archie JP Jr: Technique and clinical results of carotid stump back pressure to determine selective shunting during carotid endarterectomy. *J Vasc Surg.* 1991;13(2):319.
8. Imparato AM, Ramirez A, Riles T, Mintzer R: Cerebral protection in carotid surgery. *Arch Surg.* 1982;117:1073.
9. Rosenthal D, Zeichner WD, Lamis PA, Stanton PE: Neurologic deficit after carotid endarterectomy: Pathogenesis and management. *Surgery.* 1983;94:776.
10. Sundt TM, Sharbrough FW, Piepgras DG, et al: Correlation of cerebral blood flow and electroencephalographic changes during carotid endarterectomy. *Mayo Clin Proc* 1981;56:533.
11. Steed DL, Peitzman AB, Grundy BL, Webster MW: Causes of stroke in carotid endarterectomy. *Surgery* 1982;92:634.
12. Gee W, McDonald KM, Kaupp HA: Carotid endarterectomy shunting. Effectiveness determined by operative ocular pneumoplethysmography. *Arch Surg* 1979;114:720.

13. Pearce HJ, Becchetti JJ, Brown HJ: Supraorbital photoplethysmographic monitoring during carotid endarterectomy with the use of an internal shunt: An added dimension of safety. *Surgery* 1980;87:339.

14. Prioleau WH, Aiken AF, Hairston P: Carotid endarterectomy: Neurologic complications as related to surgical techniques. *Ann Surg* 1977;185:678.

15. Easton JD, Sherman DG: Stroke and mortality rate in carotid endarterectomy: 228 consecutive operations. *Stroke* 1977;8:565.

16. Graber JN, Vollman RW, Johnson WC, et al: Stroke after carotid endarterectomy: Risk as predicted by preoperative computerized tomography. *Am J Surg* 1984;147:492.

17. Baker WH, Littooy FN, Hayes AC, et al: Carotid endarterectomy without a shunt: The control series. *J Vasc Surg* 1984;1:50.

18. Zenni GC, Burke KA, Murchan PM, et al: Carotid shunting in a high risk population. Presented at the 21st World Congress, ISCVS. Sept. 1993; Lisbon, Portugal.

19. Halsey JH Jr: Risks and benefits of shunting in carotid endarterectomy. *Stroke.* 1992;23:1583.

20. Sandmann W, Kolvenbach R, Willere F: Risks and benefits of shunting in carotid endarterectomy. *Stroke.* 1993;24:1098.

21. Raithel D: Current surgical techniques of carotid endarterectomy. In Bernstein EF, Callow AD, Nicholaides AN, Shifrin EG, eds. *Cerebral Revascularization.* Los Angeles: Med-Orion; 1993;301.

22. Green RM, Messick WJ, Ricotta JJ, et al: Benefits, shortcomings, and costs of EEG monitoring. *Ann Surg.* 1985; 201:785.

CHAPTER 43

Selective Shunting of the Carotid Artery: An Overview

WESLEY S. MOORE

In the early experience with carotid endarterectomy, selective shunting was used. Operations were done under local anesthesia, and the patient's tolerance to carotid cross clamping was assessed by speaking to him or her and testing the motor function of the contralateral extremities. Those patients who tolerated trial clamping of the carotid artery went on to have the artery opened and endarterectomy performed without the use of a shunt. Those patients who developed cerebral dysfunction with trial occlusion were identified as needing additional blood flow because of inadequate collateral circulation, and this additional flow was provided by an internal shunt. In reported series in which local anesthesia was used, the need for internal shunts ranges from 10 to 15 percent of patients. Trial clamping under local anesthesia provided the opportunity to perform carotid endarterectomy in 85 to 90 percent of patients without the encumbrance or potential complications associated with the use of an internal shunt.

In spite of the fact that local anesthesia is an excellent method for identifying the patient who requires an internal shunt, the trend has been to perform carotid endarterectomy under general anesthesia. The benefits of general anesthesia include patient comfort, surgeon preference, airway control, increased cerebral blood flow, and decreased cerebral metabolic demand. However, the absence of a conscious response to trial carotid artery clamping was a serious handicap for those surgeons who wished to practice selective shunting, and it led to the practice of routine shunting at many centers.

The advocates of selective shunting point out that the presence of an internal shunt is a handicap in that attention and manipulation are required to keep the shunt out of the surgeon's way during endarterectomy and arteriotomy closure. The visibility of the distal endpoint is compromised by an intraluminal tube. With the shunt in place, proper visualization and testing of the security of the distal endpoint require that the arteriotomy be extended further up the internal carotid artery than would have been required if a shunt had not been employed. If the arteriotomy is not opened further, the surgeon risks failing to recognize an intimal flap at the endpoint. An unrecognized intimal flap can set the stage for thromboembolic complications and increased stroke risk. Other complications inherent with shunt use include the possibility of intimal damage produced by the ''snow plow'' effect that can occur when an intraluminal plastic tube is inserted into the artery. Finally, the possibility of air or atheromatous debris being trapped in the shunt itself, with resultant embolization to the brain following initiation of blood flow, has been documented.

The advocates of routine shunting argue that routine use teaches facility and should reduce the inherent shunt complication rate. By contrast, since only 10 to 15 percent of patients require shunting, why subject 85 to 90 percent of patients to an unnecessary procedure with even small risk, provided that the surgeon can accurately identify the few patients who require shunting? Why not limit the risk of shunting to those patients who actually need the adjunctive measure? These considerations led to the development of methods for identifying those patients who require shunting under general anesthesia. These methods include measurement of internal carotid artery back pressure and continuous electroencephalographic monitoring. Both methods have been shown to be effective and are described in detail in the following two chapters.

The Use of Internal Carotid Artery Back Pressure to Determine Shunt Requirement

WESLEY S. MOORE

DEVELOPMENTAL BACKGROUND

Internal carotid artery back pressure was the first of the currently used methods to determine the need for an internal shunt when performing carotid endarterectomy under general anesthesia. Until 1966, carotid endarterectomy was performed basically in one of two ways: local anesthesia with placement of a shunt in those patients who were intolerant to trial clamping of the carotid artery, or general anesthesia with the routine use of an internal shunt.

When carotid endarterectomy was performed under local anesthesia, it was frequently observed that patients who tolerated trial clamping of the carotid artery were also noted to have more vigorous backbleeding from the internal carotid artery than those who were intolerant of clamping and required an internal shunt. This observation certainly had theoretical merit, since good backbleeding is a sign of good collateral circulation to the ipsilateral hemisphere. Satisfactory collateral circulation to the ipsilateral hemisphere is what makes temporary carotid clamping tolerable.

In 1966, my colleagues and I set about the task of developing a method that would permit the identification of the 10 to 15 percent of patients who require an internal shunt, while taking advantage of the benefits of general anesthesia. We wished to use the apparent correlation between rate of internal carotid artery backbleeding and tolerance to temporary clamping. We posed two questions: (1) How can backbleeding be rapidly quantitated? and (2) Would there be a measurably sharp dividing line below which patients would require a shunt and above which the artery could be clamped with safety? Although it is theoretically possible to cannulate the internal carotid artery, allow the vessel to backbleed into a graduated cylinder, and measure flow rate by comparing volume delivered in a unit of time, this method would be slow and cumbersome.

The next choice involved an assumption that there would be a linear relationship between backflow and back pressure, in which the back pressure would be the hemispheric collateral perfusion pressure reflected in the static column of blood in the proximally clamped internal carotid artery. We then set about to test this hypothesis by comparing internal carotid artery back pressure in a series of patients undergoing carotid endarterectomy under local anesthesia. This allowed us to correlate the patient's conscious response to temporary clamping with the measured value of internal carotid artery back pressure. Of 36 patients undergoing 48 carotid endarterectomies under local anesthesia, 5 patients developed neurologic deficits with temporary clamping that were reversed with the placement of an internal shunt. All five patients had internal carotid artery back pressures of less than 25 mm Hg. Forty-three operations were performed, during which temporary carotid clamping was well tolerated. The internal carotid back pressures in this group of patients ranged from 25 to 88 mm Hg.[1] On the basis of these observations, we were prepared to proceed with the next phase of study, which involved performing carotid endarterectomy under general anesthesia, measuring back pressure, and making a decision concerning shunt requirement based on back pressure measurement. All patients with pressures less than 25 mm Hg were shunted and all patients with pressures greater than 25 mm Hg underwent surgery without a shunt. We analyzed the next group of 78 patients undergoing 107 carotid artery operations and found that this method of selection was quite accurate for those patients who presented with transient ischemic events or asymptomatic lesions as indications for operation. However, the technique was not accurate for patients who had had a previous stroke on the side of the carotid endarterectomy. Four of the 24 patients with back pressures greater than 25 mm Hg and no shunt experienced a temporary worsening of their preoperative neurologic deficit, in contrast to a similar group of patients with prior stroke who were operated on with the use of an internal shunt because of low back pressure. We postulated that patients with prior stroke have a penumbra of viable, marginally perfused brain tissue surrounding an area of infarction. This ischemic penumbra is more sensitive to drops in pressure and flow than in patients without prior infarction who have an intact arterial perfusion system. Thus, we identified one group of patients who represent an exception to the back pressure criteria, those with prior stroke.[2] I continue to use a shunt in these patients routinely.

Since our original and subsequent reports, there have been many reports in the literature that either validate or refute our observations.[3–10] However, studies in which cerebral blood flow is correlated with internal carotid artery back pressure demonstrate that a pressure of 25 mm Hg represents the critical closing pressure for capillary perfusion. Thus a pressure of 25 mm Hg or greater does in fact represent the minimum perfusion pressure that will maintain blood flow sufficient to preserve the viability of brain tissues. I would criticize those reports that refute our data in two ways: the first category of report is those that assume that every postoperative neurologic deficit is related to the ischemia of clamping. Therefore, the authors would claim that if there was an adequate back pressure and a postoperative complication developed, that would be sufficient evidence to refute the back pressure technique. We now know that postoperative deficits represent primarily thromboembolic complications rather than the temporary ischemia associated with carotid clamping.[11] The second area of dispute occurs in those reports of patients who underwent surgery under local anesthesia, which include patients with prior stroke, a known and well-defined exception to the technique. Those reports that state that there is not a good correlation between back pressure and temporary tolerance to clamping have failed to separate out patients who are being operated on for prior stroke, and the exceptions most likely represent that group of patients.

The advent of electroencephalographic (EEG) monitoring has brought forth an additional debate as to the accuracy of back pressure measurement. A study comparing EEG monitoring with back pressure measurement has been reported in which EEG was used as the "gold standard." Investigators report several instances in which patients with low back pressure had normal EEGs and in which patients with high back pressures had abnormal EEGs when the artery was clamped. However, these investigators failed to separate out the patients with prior stroke before carrying out their correlation.[12] It may well be that the EEG will be able to distinguish those patients with prior stroke who require shunting from those who do not. On the other hand, the technique of back pressure measurement remains simple, does not require additional equipment or personnel, and in our hands continues to identify accurately the majority of patients who do not require a shunt. We recently updated our experience in 139 operations using back pressure criteria for shunt selection. This yielded an overall stroke rate of 0.7 percent and a mortality of 0.8 percent in a mixed group of patients, 43 percent of whom were considered to be at high risk for postoperative stroke.[13] It should once again be emphasized that a satisfactory back pressure means that it is safe to clamp the carotid artery and carry out carotid endarterectomy without a shunt in those patients who have not had a prior stroke. There is no guarantee that other complications, unrelated to carotid clamping, will be prevented.

MODIFICATIONS OF BACK PRESSURE MEASUREMENT

Methods for modifying or improving the accuracy of back pressure data have been proposed by Archie.[14] He evaluated the outcome of 665 carotid endarterectomies. He measured mean arterial pressure, back pressure, and internal jugular vein pressure. He defined cerebral perfusion pressure as (back pressure − jugular vein pressure). He also calculated the collateral-to-hemisphere vascular resistance ratio as follows:

$$\text{ratio} = \frac{\text{arterial pressure} - \text{back pressure}}{\text{back pressure} - \text{jugular vein pressure}}$$

He noted that unless these additional confirmation techniques were applied, erroneously high back pressure measurements occurred in 10 to 15 percent of operations. He further concluded that patients with a cerebral perfusion pressure of 18 mm Hg or greater and a back pressure of 25 mm Hg or greater could safely undergo carotid endarterectomy without a shunt.

TECHNIQUE OF BACK PRESSURE MEASUREMENT

After the carotid bifurcation has been suitably mobilized for carotid endarterectomy, I administer 5000 units of heparin intravenously. A 22-gauge needle is bent at a 45-degree angle for placement in the common carotid artery. The needle is connected to rigid pressure tubing (KOBE). The other end of the pressure tubing is passed off to the anesthesiologist for connection to a pressure transducer. The pressure tubing and needle are flushed with heparinized saline solution, and a zero pressure baseline is established at the

level of the carotid artery. The needle is then inserted into the common carotid artery to measure systemic arterial blood pressure and to ensure proper placement by demonstration of a normal, sharp arterial waveform on the monitor. The external carotid artery and common carotid artery are then clamped proximal to needle placement. The pressure in the common carotid artery then equilibrates across the lesion of the internal carotid artery with the pressure in the internal carotid artery distal to the lesion. This pressure, the internal carotid artery back pressure, is essentially equal to the collateral perfusion pressure at the level of the middle cerebral artery (Fig. 44–1).

A question that is frequently asked is whether placement of the needle proximal to the lesion of the internal carotid artery alters the pressure reading. It is important to point out that the pressure being measured is a static pressure, since

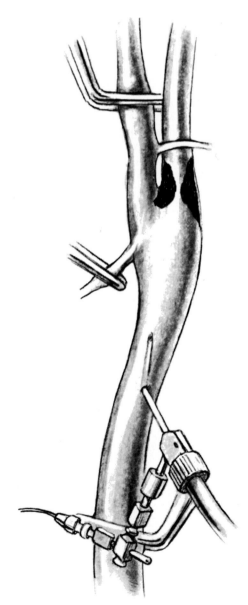

FIGURE 44–1. Artist's concept of the carotid artery bifurcation. A needle is inserted into the common carotid artery. Following the clamping of the common carotid and external carotid artery branches, the internal carotid artery back pressure equalizes across the stenosis and can be measured.

the common and external carotid artery are clamped and no flow is taking place. Under these circumstances, as long as there is an opening through the stenotic lesion, pressure will be equal on both sides.

When the carotid artery is clamped, there is usually a reflex increase in systemic arterial pressure. The anesthesiologist should be asked to note that increase in pressure and to use that as a new baseline for maintaining the patient during carotid clamping. Systemic pressure should not be allowed to fall below that baseline.

SUMMARY

Internal carotid artery back pressure is a good approximation of collateral cerebral perfusion pressure and collateral blood flow. Patients undergoing carotid endarterectomy for the indications of transient ischemic attacks or asymptomatic lesions can demonstrate their need for an internal shunt by an internal carotid artery back pressure of less than 25 mm Hg.

Patients in whom a prior stroke is the indication for carotid endarterectomy, regardless of the degree of recovery or the interval between stroke and operation, represent an exception to the back pressure method for identifying the need for an internal shunt. For this reason, we recommend routine use of an internal shunt in this group of patients.

It has been shown that back pressure measurement is a simple, safe, and accurate method for documenting the need for an internal shunt or the safety of carotid clamping and carotid endarterectomy without a shunt under general anesthesia.

REFERENCES

1. Moore WS, Hall AD: Carotid artery back pressure. A test of cerebral tolerance to temporary carotid occlusion. *Arch Surg.* 1969;99:702.
2. Moore WS, Yee JM, Hall AD: Collateral cerebral blood pressure. An index of tolerance to temporary carotid occlusion. *Arch Surg.* 1973;106:520.
3. Hays RF, Levinson SA, Wylie EJ: Intraoperative measurement of carotid back pressure as a guide to operative management for carotid endarterectomy. *Surgery.* 1972;72:953.
4. Smith LL, Jacobson JG, Hinshaw DB: Correlation of neurologic complications and pressure measurements during carotid endarterectomy. *Surg Gynecol Obstet.* 1976;143:233.
5. Hertzer NR, Beven EG, Greenstreet RL, Humphries AW: Internal carotid back pressure, intraoperative shunting, ulcerated atheroma, and the incidence of stroke during carotid endarterectomy. *Surgery.* 1978;83:306.
6. Hobson RW, Wright CB, Sublett JW, et al: Carotid artery back pressure and endarterectomy under regional anesthesia. *Arch Surg.* 1974;109:682.
7. Lord RS, Graham AR: The validity of internal carotid back pressure measurements during carotid endarterectomy for unilateral carotid stenosis. *Aust N Z J Surg.* 1986;56:493.
8. Gnanadev DA, Wang N, Comunale FL, Reile DA: Carotid artery stump pressure: How reliable is it in predicting the need for a shunt? *Ann Vasc Surg.* 1989;3:313.
9. Forssel C, Takolander R, Bergquist D: Pressure measurements as predictors for perioperative neurologic deficits in carotid surgery. *Eur J Vasc Surg.* 1990;4:153.
10. Beebe HG, Starr C, Slack D: Carotid artery stump pressure: Its variability when measured serially. *J Cardiovasc Surg.* 1989;30:419.
11. Riles JS, Imparato AM, Jacobowitz GR, et al: The cause of perioperative stroke after carotid endarterectomy. *J Vasc Surg.* 1994;19:206.
12. Kelly JJ, Callow AD, O'Donnell TF, et al: Failure of carotid stump pressures. *Arch Surg.* 1979;114:1361.
13. Hunter GC, Sieffert G, Malone JM, Moore WS: The accuracy of carotid back pressure as an index for shunt requirements—A reappraisal. *Stroke.* 1982;13:319.
14. Archie JP Jr: Technique and clinical results of carotid stump back pressure to determine selective shunting during carotid endarterectomy. *J Vasc Surg.* 1991;13:319.

CHAPTER 45

The Use of Electroencephalographic Monitoring to Determine Shunt Requirement

MARC R. NUWER

Electroencephalographic (EEG) monitoring is useful in carotid endarterectomy procedures. Electroencephalography can monitor the brain when the central nervous system is at risk during surgery, reassuring the surgical team that the brain remains adequately perfused and well oxygenated and suffers no focal impairment. Such testing is now commonly used in patients undergoing carotid endarterectomy. Similar EEG monitoring is also used in other procedures on the heart or great vessels, including clipping of intracranial aneurysms. When ischemia is detected by electroencephalogram, strong consideration should be given to the use of a vascular shunt to restore adequate cerebral perfusion during the procedure. Conversely, when an EEG fails to detect significant ischemia upon clamping, the patient might be spared the use of a shunt. Recording techniques for electroencephalography in the surgical suites are derived from the routine procedures used for electroencephalography in the outpatient setting.

TECHNIQUES FOR USE

The patient is set up for operating-room monitoring in the same manner as is used for a routine electroencephalography.[1] It is common to apply the standard 22 electrodes in the so-called 10-20 electrode placement system (the International System), which includes the 16 parasagittal and temporal chain electrodes and three midsagittal electrodes, one at each ear and a ground electrode. At some institutions, a subset of these is used. It is preferable to monitor 16 to 21 channels, since that number gives adequate access to the entire hemisphere ipsilateral to the clamping site, as well as access to a "control hemisphere." Use of eight channels over the ipsilateral hemisphere gives a minimal sampling of the EEG from the various portions of that scalp. It remains controversial as to whether the use of only 4 to 8 total scalp EEG channels is sufficient in this setting. Many groups have reported a lack of satisfaction with detection of embolic events and potential confusion regarding the nature of EEG changes when they do occur. The use of too few channels is a detriment to understanding the nature of ischemic changes. Since the use of a larger number of channels is generally straightforward, there seems no reason at this time to restrict the monitoring to an inordinately small number of recording channels and electrodes.

Traditional disk electrodes are commonly employed. These disks can be secured with collodion glue by an EEG technologist on the evening prior to the surgery, or in the preoperative room prior to induction of anesthesia. Preplacement allows for the careful measurement of electrode sites, thereby avoiding the various difficulties inherent in the amateur approach of placing electrodes just "by inspection." Once secured with collodion and filled with a conductive paste, the disk electrodes can continue to conduct EEG waves quite well for several days, if desired. The use of the collodion glue avoids dislodgment of electrodes when the patient is moved onto the operating table or repositioned.

As an alternative to disk electrodes, straight scalp needle electrodes or spiral needle electrodes can be used. Either can be applied rapidly. However, each has a relatively high level of electrical impedance. This high impedance can result in substantial electrical noise during monitoring in the operating room, which is an electrically hostile environment, with many pieces of equipment that generate 60 Hz of noise and other electrical interference. As such, needle electrodes, either straight or spiral, can produce EEG recordings subject to significant technical problems. The spiral needle electrodes are more secure than the straight ones, that is, less likely to be knocked loose by the anesthesiologist working around the head of the patient or during repositioning of the patient on the table. They are more expensive than straight needle electrodes and harder to clean and disinfect between patients. Some centers now consider needle electrodes to be disposable after one use, to avoid any danger of infection transmission.

An adequate ground electrode is also mandatory for good quality recordings without excessive contamination from 60 Hz noise. However, the ground to the EEG machine is generally an isoground rather than a true earth ground. In the operating room, the patient should be given only one true earth ground. This is generally the ground that is employed for the electrocautery device used by the surgeons. Placement of a second true ground would place the patient at risk for electrical burns in case of a loose ground or equipment malfunction. Further detrimental side effects of double grounding are also possible. The electroencephalography user should make sure that the ground lead used with his or her equipment is indeed optically isolated or otherwise prevented from creating a double ground situation. Most modern equipment does use isoground with optical isolation. Older equipment uses a true ground and therefore is disadvantageous for use in the operating room.

Filter band passes are usually set in traditional ways. A low-pass filter of 0.3 Hz is reasonable; it certainly should be no higher than 1.0 Hz. A high-pass filter of 70 Hz is preferable. The 60 Hz notch filter can be left on for EEG testing, as it is helpful for eliminating 60 Hz noise in the operating room and does not produce the same kind of artifact as is seen with somatosensory evoked potential (SEP) testing.

The electroencephalogram can be displayed on paper or can be reviewed on electronic video display alone. Often a combination of the two techniques is most advantageous (see Chapter 17). The review of the polygraph electroencephalogram on an electronic video display prevents the unnecessary accumulation of very large volumes of paper, while storage onto magnetic or optical disks provides necessary backup of the collected data. Printing of occasional pages onto paper in the operating room can provide a means for assessing for wave-shape changes over the course of the recording. Specifically, printing of the 1 minute's reading just prior to clamping of the carotid artery and the subsequent 1 or several minutes into the clamping episode is helpful for clarifying that there was no significant EEG change at the time of clamping. Likewise, printing out another several minutes' reading at the time of reclamping or unclamping is helpful for determining that no significant events occurred at that time, such as emboli at the time of unclamping or removal of a vascular shunt.

At many institutions, the entire record is made directly onto traditional EEG paper, without any electronic devices or storage. When paper recordings alone are used for the entire duration of the case, it is common to use a 10 mm/second or 15 mm/second paper speed. These slow paper speeds allow for considerable compression of the data, thereby reducing by 50 to 67 percent the amount of paper needed for the case. Much of the information needed can be still interpreted quite well at these slow paper speeds. Indeed, slow wave activity may be seen even better at such slow paper speeds, compared with the outpatient conventional speed of 30 mm/second. Some centers have now begun using 5 mm/second, and find the results to be satisfactory, while the need for paper is reduced by 83 percent. If EEG changes are difficult to interpret at a slow paper speed, the technologists or physician can always return to a 30 mm/second paper speed, to help in determining the cause or nature of significant changes.

Computer EEG analysis can now be used to produce frequency analysis and automated trending of the amount of EEG activity in fast and slow frequency bands. These automated trend displays can be helpful in supplementing the traditional visual analysis (Fig. 45–1). Visual reading of paper, or its electronic version displayed on a video screen, is hampered by the fact that changes over long periods of time may be missed because they have been so gradual. By using a supplemental frequency analysis trend, the gradual changes in the EEG recording can be observed over arbitrarily short or long time spans, including watching the changes over the entire course of the operative procedure. Such quantitative EEG analysis has been shown to be more sensitive than is routine electroencephalography for detecting changes occurring with ischemia.[2–4] When selective shunting is predicated on these more subtle degrees of EEG changes

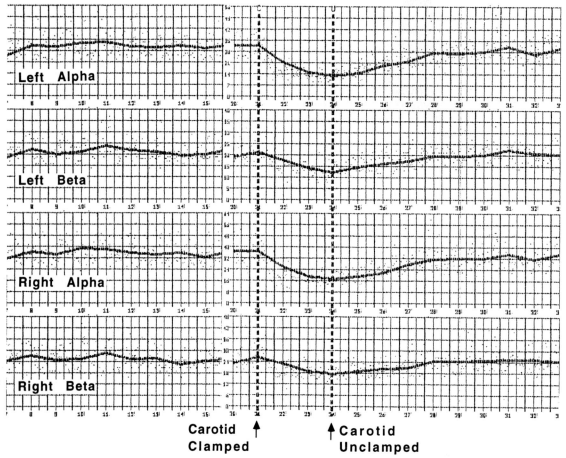

Trending EEG: Decreased Fast Activity Upon Carotid Clamping

Left Alpha

Left Beta

Right Alpha

Right Beta

Carotid ↑   ↑ Carotid
Clamped   Unclamped

FIGURE 45–1. Trends of electroencephalographic (EEG) features automatically plotted over 25 minutes of recording. These trends represent only the amount of fast activity seen, separated into the alpha and beta frequency bands. The data were recorded with a linked-ears reference and averaged across all eight channels on either side. Upon one carotid's being clamped, fast activity dropped more than 50 percent in both right and left alpha bands, compared with the preclamp average. The EEG changes generally occur over 15 to 30 seconds but appear slower here because this trend plots a moving average of 1 minute's EEG results. The EEG trend returns to baseline after a shunt is in place and functioning. Such a 50 percent or more loss of fast activity is considered sufficient to warrant placement of a shunt. (Courtesy of the University of California Los Angeles EEG Laboratory.)

detected by quantitative techniques, the incidence of shunting may increase from 25 percent of the population to 40 percent or more (see Chapter 17).

INTERPRETATION OF CHANGES

Interpretation of carotid endarterectomy EEG monitoring tests is based on changes from the patient's individual baseline reading. Each patient has a somewhat different EEG pattern under anesthesia, or at least there is a considerable variability among the general population. There is usually a mixture of fast and slow activity. Fast activity is 8 to 30 Hz, whereas slow activity is 7 Hz or less. Fast activity is considered good and is a measure of many normal brain functions. Fast activity includes the EEG bands alpha (8–13 Hz) and beta (14–30 Hz) in an awake subject. Slow activity is considered pathologic in many settings and includes the EEG bands delta (4 Hz or less) and theta (5–7 Hz) in an awake subject. Many anesthetic agents produce a moderate degree of slow activity themselves. Fast activity is also often caused by anesthetic agents. Isoflurane, a commonly used general anesthetic agent, generates considerable amounts of alpha-band activity, especially at the frontal regions.

At the time of clamping, the degree of decrease in fast activity, increase in background delta slow activity, or suppression of the entire EEG waveband should be assessed. The least degree of change is seen in a decrease of the background fast activity. This change is usually considered to be of clinical significance if it exceeds a 50 percent loss of fast activity (Fig. 45–2). The next greater degree of ischemic EEG change is that of an increase in slow activity, especially if the increase is greater than 50 percent compared with the reading before clamping. Sometimes a decrease in fast activity and an increase in slow activity are seen together. The worst degree of ischemic change and the most dire sign is when all EEG activity falls in amplitude or the pattern disappears entirely. When the EEG pattern becomes so suppressed, the degree of cortical ischemia is considered greatest, certainly much greater than the ischemia associated with an isolated decrease in fast activity.

Changes may be seen unilaterally or bilaterally. It is not uncommon for the changes to occur over both hemispheres, since the circle of Willis can share ischemia between the two hemispheres. Therefore, physicians who only look for interhemispheric asymmetries will miss some episodes of significant ischemia that affect both hemispheres.

At this author's institution, the practice is to discuss with the surgeon the degree of EEG changes occurring upon clamping. The surgeon makes the final determination about whether a shunt is indicated. In general, this indication corresponds to a greater than 50 percent decrease in overall EEG amplitude, a greater than 50 percent increase in slow activity, or a greater than 50 percent decrease in fast activity at the time of the clamping. In making this determination, the surgeon also needs to consider the confounding effects of any acute bolus of centrally active medication given at the time of clamping. Administration of such a bolus should be avoided if one wishes to avoid nonspecific medication-induced EEG changes.

RELEVANT RESEARCH REPORTS

Many studies in the electrodiagnostic and vascular surgery literature are pertinent to this issue. Among these, several deserve particular attention. Redekop and Ferguson,[5] in Ontario, studied 293 patients undergoing carotid endarterectomy. Shunts were not used in any of these cases, but EEG monitoring was used in all. Major EEG changes were seen in 11 of the 77 patients (14%) who had significant contralateral carotid stenosis or occlusion. Major EEG changes were seen in 11 of the 216 patients (5%) who did not have significant contralateral carotid stenosis or occlusion. In their study, the authors found that the risk of immediate postoperative deficit was significantly higher among the patients who showed major EEG changes intraoperatively (4 of 22, 18%) compared with those who showed no major EEG changes (5 of 271, 2%). They concluded that major EEG changes are infrequent, but that they identify a subgroup of patients at significantly higher risk for intraoperative stroke. There was no explanation of the five patients who suffered strokes despite stable EEG monitoring. Some EEG users have speculated that this morbidity had to do with complications occurring late in the case, such as emboli after unclamping.

Chiappa and colleagues[2] studied 367 patients who underwent carotid endarterectomy during which EEG monitoring was used. Significant EEG changes followed clamping of the carotid artery in 9.8% of cases. In half of these instances, the change was a decrease in background fast activity. In the same article, the authors discuss the various other kinds of changes that were seen with clamping. They compared visual analysis to quantitative EEG analysis and concluded that the latter was more useful than the former.

In classic work by Sundt and colleagues[6] at Mayo Clinic, later extended by McKay and colleagues[7] at the same institution, the relationship between EEG changes, cerebral blood flow, and carotid artery stump pressure was assessed. A high correlation was seen between cerebral blood flow and EEG waveform changes. To sustain a normal EEG pattern, the cerebral blood flow must be at least 18 mL/100 g of brain tissue/minute. The degree of EEG change below this level reflected the degree of severity of reduced blood flow. Regional cerebral blood flow also corresponds to stump pressure in the cross-clamped carotid artery. However, stump pressures do not reflect the effect of additional stenosis above the circle of Willis. Among 90 carotid endarterectomies, 28 percent of cases had stump pressures of less than 50 mm Hg despite cerebral blood flows above 24 mL/100 g/minute and normal EEG readings. In 8 percent of cases, stump pressures were more than 50 mm Hg, but regional blood flows were less than 18 mL/100 g/minute and EEG changes consistent with ischemia were observed. In 6 percent of cases, regional cerebral blood flow was marginally sufficient (18–24 mL/100 g/min), whereas stump pressure was more than 50 mm Hg and the EEG pattern remained unchanged. The impression is that electroencephalography is more readily related to cerebral function than is stump pressure, and that therefore it is a more reliable test for cerebral ischemia. The EEG pattern also can be monitored throughout the procedure, whereas stump pressure is only tested once.

An alternative neurophysiologic monitoring tool is somatosensory evoked potential (SEP). When used to monitor

BEFORE CLAMPING

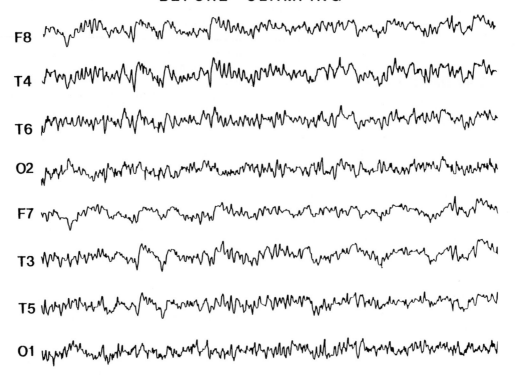

LEFT CAROTID CLAMPED

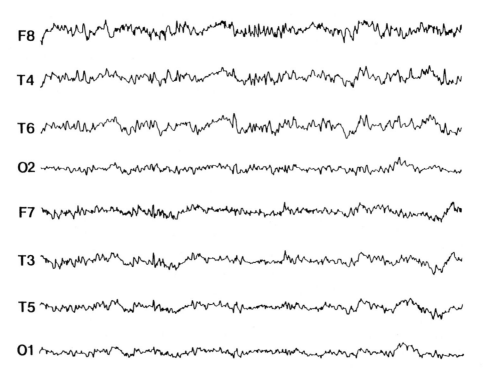

FIGURE 45–2. Electroencephalographic (EEG) changes during carotid endarterectomy recorded just before *(top)* and after *(bottom)* carotid clamping. Each record was made using a linked-ears reference. Only eight channels are shown here, even though more were recorded and observed on-line. In comparing the *bottom* record with the *top,* a relative suppression of the fast activity is seen over the left side after clamping. This change, considered a decrement of fast activity of greater than 50 percent, suggests ischemia due to clamping. The patient therefore received a vascular shunt as part of his endarterectomy procedure. (Courtesy of the University of California Los Angeles EEG Laboratory.)

hemispheric function, median nerve SEP is usually chosen. SEP monitoring in the operating room has become popular for a variety of situations.[8] For monitoring during carotid endarterectomies, SEP detects ischemia when blood flow falls below 18 mL/100 g/minute and disappears at 15 mL/100 g/minute.[9] SEP monitors only the somatosensory region. If an embolus occurs to any other region, SEP waves would likely remain unchanged. On the other hand, electroencephalography can monitor broadly across many cortical areas and is thus more likely to detect emboli. Both techniques are able to detect routine hypoperfusion from carotid clamping. Most institutions prefer to use EEG monitoring instead of SEP monitoring for carotid endarterectomies.

The SEP method has been compared with tests of neuropsychological changes in patients postoperatively. Neuropsychological test batteries were administered to 14 patients both before and after carotid endarterectomy.[10] Intraoperative ischemia was monitored with SEP in these patients. Patients whose cortical amplitudes decreased more than 50 percent performed worse on their postoperative neuropsychological tests than did those patients who had a lesser degree of or no evoked potential attenuation. The time elapsed since the first ischemic symptoms, the age and educational level of the patient, clamping time, occurrence of preoperative stroke, and time interval from surgery to assessment were not statistically related to the changes in neuropsychological abilities. These results suggested that intraoperative evoked potentials were indeed an index of risk for postoperative impairment. The worse the evoked potential attenuation was, the more likely the occurrence of postoperative neuropsychological deterioration. The 50 percent attenuation criteria can be considered tentative criteria for risk of such a postoperative deficit. Similar results were seen by the same investigators in a subsequent study of 34 patients.[11] These results show that even modest degrees of electrophysiologically detected cortical impairment, if left uncorrected intraoperatively, can lead to postoperative cognitive changes. Studies that only assess stroke and death as endpoints would miss detecting lesser degrees of postoperative cerebral impairment.

SUMMARY

Electroencephalographic monitoring during carotid endarterectomy is a valuable tool for detection of intraoperative cerebral ischemia. Although no monitoring technique has 100 percent sensitivity, EEG monitoring provides direct feedback about brain function moment by moment. It probably has a sensitivity better than 90 percent for ischemic events, and even higher for major ischemic events. Judiciously used, the technique can guide the surgeon about when to use a vascular shunt or when to search for other correctable problems.

REFERENCES

1. Jenkins GM, Chiappa KH, Young RR: Practical aspects of EEG monitoring during carotid endarterectomies. *Am J EEG Tech.* 1983;23:191.
2. Chiappa KH, Burke SR, Young RR: Results of electroencephalographic monitoring during 367 carotid endarterectomies: Use of a dedicated minicomputer. *Stroke.* 1979;10(4):381.
3. Ahn SS, Jordan SE, Nuwer MR, et al: Computerized EEG topographic brain mapping: A new and accurate monitor of cerebral circulation and function for patients undergoing carotid endarterectomy. *J Vasc Surg.* 1988;8:247.
4. Ahn SS, Jordan SE, Nuwer MR: Computerized EEG topographic brain mapping. In Moore W, ed. *Surgery for Cerebrovascular Disease.* New York: Churchill Livingstone; 1987;275.
5. Redekop G, Ferguson G: Correlation of contralateral stenosis and intraoperative electroencephalogram change with risk of stroke during carotid endarterectomy. *Neurosurgery.* 1992;30(2):191.
6. Sundt TM, Sharbrough FW, Anderson RE, Michenfelder JD: Cerebral blood flow measurements and electroencephalograms during carotid endarterectomy. *J Neurosurg.* 1974;41:310.
7. McKay RD, Sundt TM, Michenfelder JD, et al: Internal carotid artery stump pressure and cerebral blood flow during carotid endarterectomy: Modification by Halothane, Enflurane and Innovar. *Anesthesiology.* 1976;45(4):390.
8. Nuwer MR: *Evoked Potential Monitoring in the Operating Room.* New York: Raven Press; 1986.
9. Branston NM, Symon L: Cortical EP, blood flow and potassium changes in experimental ischemia. In Barber C, ed. *Evoked Potentials.* Baltimore: University Park Press; 1980;527.
10. Brinkman SD, Braun P, Ganji S, et al: Neuropsychological performance one week after carotid endarterectomy reflects intra-operative ischemia. *Stroke.* 1984;15:497.
11. Cushman L, Brinkman SD, Ganji S, Jacobs LA: Neuropsychological impairment after carotid endarterectomy correlates with intraoperative ischemia. *Cortex.* 1984;20:403.

CHAPTER 46

Technique of Carotid Endarterectomy

WESLEY S. MOORE

ADEQUACY OF CAROTID ARTERY MOBILIZATION

The principles of surgical exposure of the carotid artery are described in detail in Chapter 40. Following mobilization of the carotid bifurcation in preparation for endarterectomy (Fig. 46–1), it is quite important that the adequacy of mobilization be determined before the artery is clamped and an arteriotomy made. The common carotid artery, internal carotid artery, and external carotid artery must be mobilized for a sufficient length beyond the end of the plaque such that the application of a vascular clamp does not restrict total removal of the plaque and visualization of a clean endpoint. It is possible to assess the extent of the plaque both visually and by palpation. Visualization of the plaque through the arterial wall, in its most prolific portion, is easy. As the plaque begins to thin out, however, the surgeon may be misled as to the extent of the plaque if visualization alone is used. One technique that I find helpful is to place a right-angle clamp underneath the most distal extent of the artery being examined and to palpate the artery against the clamp in two planes in order to be assured that this is a soft and compliant segment of vessel that is disease free (Fig. 46–2).

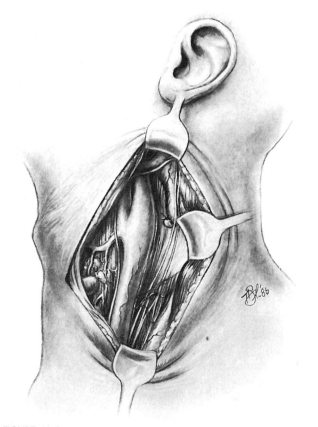

FIGURE 46–1. The dissected carotid bifurcation in relationship to the neck. Note that the common facial vein has been divided and ligated. This permits lateral retraction of the jugular vein and good exposure of the carotid bifurcation.

PLACEMENT OF ARTERIOTOMY

The location of the arteriotomy on the circumference of the carotid bifurcation is subject to considerable variation among surgeons. It is my preference to start the arteriotomy on the common carotid artery on the wall directly opposite, or 180 degrees away from the takeoff of the external carotid artery or directly opposite the flow divider. This permits the internal carotid artery to be opened in such a way that it will become bivalved, with the flow divider as its hinge. Prior to clamping the carotid artery, the patient is given 5000 U of heparin intravenously. In order to achieve proper rotation of the artery to permit placement of the arteriotomy as described, the arterial clamps must be placed on the common and internal carotid arteries in such a way that the opposing jaws are placed in an anterior-posterior position. This then permits counterclockwise rotation of the artery on its own axis such that the internal carotid artery will be positioned anterior to the exterior carotid artery (Fig. 46–3). A No. 11 blade is then inserted into the common carotid artery, and a preliminary incision is made. The arteriotomy is then enlarged with the use of Potts scissors. The arteriotomy is carried through the bulk of the atheromatous plaque. Particular care must be taken to ensure that the tip of the scissors lies within the lumen of the internal carotid artery. In the case of a bulky plaque, it is possible to place the tip of the scissors erroneously in the external carotid artery and to incise the flow divider as well as the wall of the artery itself. The arteriotomy is carried just beyond the extent of the plaque so as to enable the operator to visualize the endpoint when it is achieved (Fig. 46–4).

SELECTION OF ENDARTERECTOMY PLANE

The objective in selecting an endarterectomy plane is to encompass the atheromatous plaque while leaving behind as much of the normal, anatomic arterial wall as possible, in order to achieve a smooth transition between intimectomized surface and normal intima at the endpoints. A cross section of diseased arterial wall reveals the atheromatous plaque involving the arterial intima as the innermost layer. The next layer is an internal elastic lamina, separating the intima from a very thin layer composed of circular medial fibers. The next layer is the external elastic lamina, which separates the media from the durable adventitia.

Generally speaking, the easiest endarterectomy plane to achieve is that between the media and adventitia along the line of the external elastic lamina. Although some surgeons advocate this dissection plane as the best, in that it removes the circular medial fibers, it is my preference to establish a plane between the atheromatous plaque in the diseased intima and the media along the line of the internal elastic lamina. The reason for selecting this plane is that the transition between this plane and normal intima in the internal carotid artery will be much smoother, and a shelf or step-up

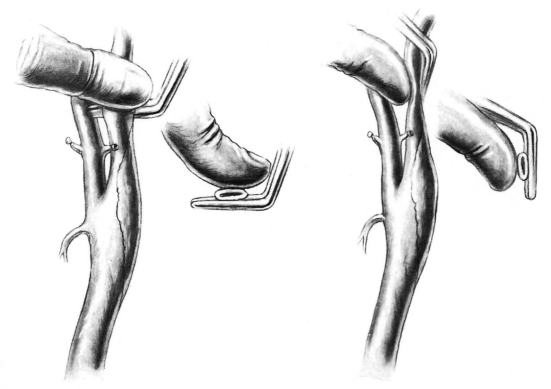

FIGURE 46–2. The bulky portion of the atheromatous plaque is usually visible on the adventitial surface of the carotid bifurcation. To be sure that a sufficient length of the internal carotid artery has been mobilized beyond the distal extent of the atheromatous plaque, the artery is carefully palpated against a right-angle clamp. This palpation is done in two planes to be sure that there is no residual atheromatous plaque at the distal end of the dissection.

effect can be avoided at the point of ending the intimectomy dissection (Fig. 46–5).

I prefer to start the endarterectomy plane in the bulkiest point of atheromatous plaque within the common carotid artery. The diseased intima is carefully separated from the circular medial fibers in a circumferential fashion with an endarterectomy dissector. As soon as this separation is carried as far as possible, the endarterectomy dissector is removed and a sharp right-angle clamp is inserted in the dissection plane; the remaining portion of the circumference is carefully separated with the use of the right-angle clamp. This technique is facilitated by having the assistant grasp the opposite wall with two pairs of thumb forceps, holding it in a flattened position, and allowing the right-angle clamp to emerge in the same dissection plane on the opposite wall as was started initially (Fig. 46–6). Once the right-angle clamp has totally encompassed the entire circumference of the atheromatous plaque, the proximal dissection of the plaque down to the proximal extent of the arteriotomy can be achieved by the gentle opening and closing of the clamp. As soon as the proximal extent of the intimectomy separation is achieved, it is my practice to incise the intima against the jaw of the right-angle clamp using a No. 15 blade (Fig. 46–7). This creates a sharp endpoint without residual proximal intimal flap. Even though there is a bit of a step at this level, it will not cause a problem, since it is in the direction of blood flow. However, if the step is rather prominent, this is easily controlled with two or three tacking sutures of 6-0 polypropylene. It is helpful to extend the arteriotomy more proximally on the common carotid artery so that, if a patch angioplasty is used for closure, the proximal endpoint site will be covered and widened with the pouch.

COMPLETION OF THE ENDARTERECTOMY

Once the proximal extent of the diseased intima has been divided, the intima can be elevated and separated from the medial fibers using an endarterectomy spatula. This is carried up toward the carotid artery bifurcation, at which point the orifice of the external carotid artery is encountered (Fig. 46–8). Generally, it is my practice to clear the external carotid artery and leave the internal carotid artery for last (Fig. 46–9). On occasion, however, it may be easier to do the internal carotid next and leave the external carotid artery for last. The orifice of the external carotid artery is gently separated away from the core of diseased intima in a circumferential fashion. This is done primarily with an endarterectomy spatula but may be facilitated using the tip of a mosquito clamp. As the core is gently drawn out, the assistant can evert the wall of the external carotid artery, using thumb forceps and gently applying traction toward the arterial clamp on the external carotid artery. In this combined effort, the intimal core may break free at the end of the plaque, leaving a sharp transitional endpoint in the external carotid artery. On occasion, it may be easier simply to mobilize the core of the intima with a mosquito clamp up to the point where the external carotid artery is clamped. The intimal core is then gently grasped with a mosquito clamp and avulsed at the point of arterial clamping. This usually results in a smooth clean endpoint. However, the lumen of the external carotid artery must be carefully inspected to ensure that no bits of residual atheromatous plaque are present. Once the core is delivered out of the external carotid artery, dissection is carried up the internal carotid artery in a careful

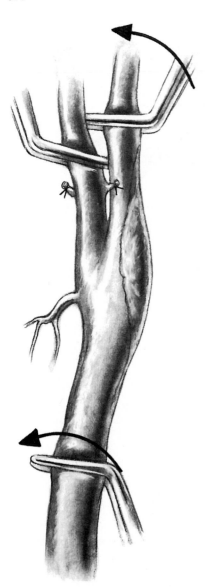

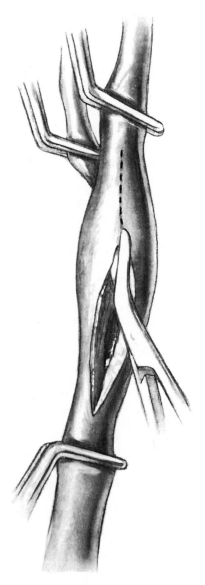

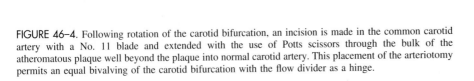

FIGURE 46–3. Vascular clamps are applied so as to permit a counterclockwise rotation, bringing the internal carotid artery anterior to the external carotid artery.

FIGURE 46–4. Following rotation of the carotid bifurcation, an incision is made in the common carotid artery with a No. 11 blade and extended with the use of Potts scissors through the bulk of the atheromatous plaque well beyond the plaque into normal carotid artery. This placement of the arteriotomy permits an equal bivalving of the carotid bifurcation with the flow divider as a hinge.

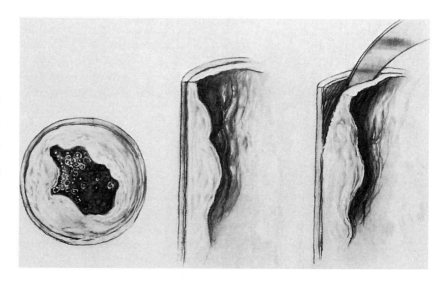

FIGURE 46–5. Cross section and longitudinal section showing the atheromatous plaque confined to the diseased intima, which is separated from the circular medial fibers by the internal elastic lamina. The circular medial fibers are separated from the adventitia by the external elastic lamina. The preferred endarterectomy plane removes the diseased intima, leaving the circular medial fibers behind and tightly attached to the adventitia.

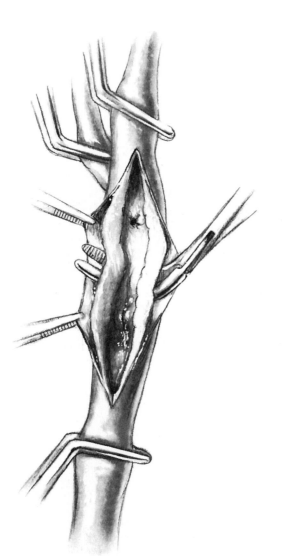

FIGURE 46–6. Following separation of the diseased intima on one side of the arteriotomy, a right-angle clamp is gently insinuated in the plane of dissection to emerge on the opposite side, which is being held flat by the first assistant with two pairs of forceps. This permits an intimectomy of equal depth on both sides of the arteriotomy.

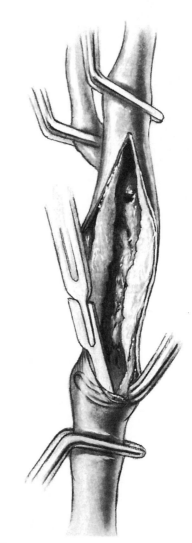

FIGURE 46–7. The right-angle clamp is brought down to the most proximal edge of the atheromatous plaque. The proximal endpoint is obtained sharply with a No. 15 blade.

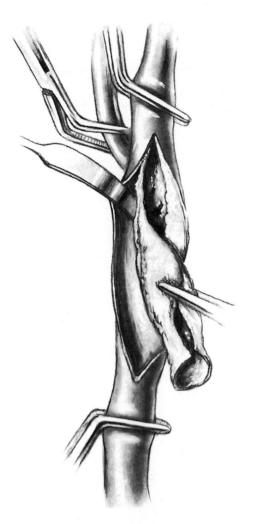

FIGURE 46–8. After the proximal extent of the atheromatous plaque has been divided, it can be reflected cephalad to complete the intimectomy up to the orifice of the external carotid artery.

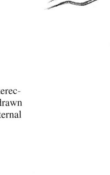

FIGURE 46–9. The orifice of the external carotid artery is cleared initially with an endarterectomy spatula and subsequently with the tip of a mosquito clamp. Once freed, it is withdrawn from the orifice of the external carotid artery at the same time that the clamp on the external carotid artery is released.

and circumferential fashion. The operating surgeon can usually visualize the point at which the diseased intima goes
into transition to normal intima. At this point, gentle traction
will result in a feathered separation of the distal extent of
the intimectomy, leaving behind a sharp endpoint with tight
adherence between the remaining intima and arterial wall
(Fig. 46–10). The intimectomized surface is then copiously
irrigated with a syringe filled with heparinized saline that is
forced through a flexible intracath in order to have a forcible
stream. The operating surgeon carefully looks for any bits
of floating debris on the intimectomized surface. If there are
elevated bits of circular medial fiber, these can be drawn out
at right angles to the arteriotomy. They can also be pulled
downward. Any remaining bits of material should never be
pulled cephalad for fear of elevating a new intimectomy
plane at the distal endpoint. A considerable amount of time
should be spent irrigating the distal endpoint to make sure
that it is tightly adherent and will not dissect when flow is
re-established. If there appears to be some residual elevation
of intima at the distal endpoint, this should be gently grasped
and pulled proximally, to free up any small circular segments
of nonadherent intima (Fig. 46–11).

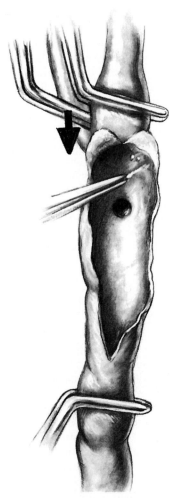

FIGURE 46–11. After the distal endpoint has been irrigated with heparinized saline, any small intimal flaps that remain should be gently grasped
with a pair of forceps and pulled downward until the residual intima is
firmly adherent to the media and adventitia.

PLACEMENT OF AN "OUTLYING" INTERNAL SHUNT

The technique of placement of an inlying internal shunt
has been described in detail in Chapter 41. An alternative to
the short, inlying shunt is the longer or outlying shunt. The
shunt I prefer is the Javid shunt, which is held in place with
Rumel tourniquets. When a decision has been made to use
a shunt either as a routine technique or because of inadequate
cerebral perfusion, the common and internal carotid arteries
are encircled with umbilical tapes. These are drawn through
short lengths of rubber tubing as a modified Rumel tourniquet. After the arteriotomy is made and extended well beyond the proximal and distal extent of the atheromatous
plaque, the Javid shunt, with a clamp across the tubing, is
inserted into the internal carotid artery. This is held in place
by pulling up on the umbilical tape. At the same time, the
rubber tubing is pushed down and clamped in place. The
artery is allowed to backbleed through the Javid shunt by

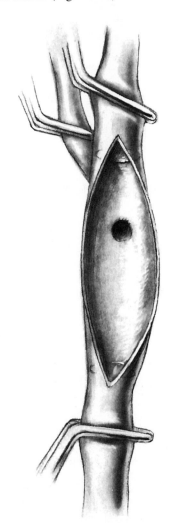

FIGURE 46–10. The completed intimectomized surface of the carotid
bifurcation. Note the clean, tapered endpoint at the internal carotid artery.
This should be visible directly through the arteriotomy. If necessary, the
arteriotomy should be extended further up the internal carotid artery in
order to visualize this endpoint directly.

temporary release of the clamp. The proximal portion of the shunt is then placed into the common carotid artery while the shunt is allowed to vigorously backbleed and displace air from the proximal cul-de-sac. The shunt is then clamped and the proximal Rumel tourniquet gently pulled up around the proximal portion of the Javid shunt. The proximal clamp on the carotid artery is removed, and the shunt is advanced retrograde into the common carotid artery. With the shunt firmly held in place with the proximal Rumel tourniquet, the clamp on the shunt is slowly opened so as to allow the operating surgeon careful visualization of the material that is entering the shunt. If the surgeon sees any air bubbles or any atheromatous debris, the shunt can be promptly clamped, removed from the proximal common carotid artery, and flushed, and the insertion procedure repeated. This is done until the material entering the shunt is completely clear; then the clamp is removed and flow is established through the internal shunt. With the shunt in place, endarterectomy can be carried out while the outlying loop of the shunt is moved from side to side to facilitate the endarterectomy maneuvers (Fig. 46–12).

PRIMARY CLOSURE OF THE ARTERIOTOMY

Most arteriotomy closures of the carotid artery can be made primarily without compromising available lumen, because the presence of an atheromatous plaque has actually dilated the carotid bifurcation, and, once the plaque is removed, the available tissue in both the common and the internal carotid arteries is somewhat larger than normal. I like to begin closure of the arteriotomy at the distalmost portion of the internal carotid artery using a 6-0 Prolene suture with a C-1 needle at each end. The initial knot is tied over the apex by placing one needle from within on one side of the apex and another needle on the opposite side. A similar maneuver is carried out at the proximal extent of the arteriotomy. Using a small purchase of tissue with stitches placed initially quite closely, a running suture is begun from the distal portion of the arteriotomy and carried down the internal carotid artery out onto the common carotid artery until approximately one half of the arteriotomy is closed. The proximal suture is then brought in a similar fashion toward the distal stitch. Before closure of the arteriotomy is completed, the internal carotid artery is vigorously backbled. This is followed by backbleeding of the external carotid artery. The arteriotomy closure is then completed and tied in its midportion.

PRIMARY CLOSURE WITH AN INTERNAL SHUNT

The presence of an internal shunt is somewhat cumbersome when proceeding with closure, but it has one advantage in that it provides a stent over which the internal carotid artery is closed. The closure is begun at the internal carotid artery, with suture placed as in primary closure. The suture is run down to the common carotid artery, and a second suture is begun on the common carotid artery and run distally to the point where both limbs of the internal shunt emerge

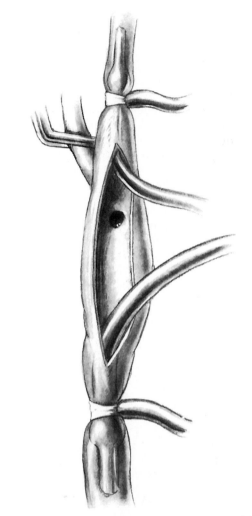

FIGURE 46–12. A Javid shunt in place following completion of the bifurcation endarterectomy.

and no further closure is permitted (Fig. 46–13). The internal shunt is then removed, and internal carotid, external carotid, and common carotid arteries are flushed out the open arteriotomy. A baby Satinsky clamp is then placed across the remaining open portion of the arteriotomy. This permits the restoration of blood flow beneath the clamp while the remaining portion of the arteriotomy is closed (Fig. 46–14).

ARTERIOTOMY CLOSURE WITH A PATCH

The use of a patch angioplasty is an attempt to minimize occurrent or recurrent stenosis of the internal carotid artery. Although the data in the literature are in conflict, it would appear that those who advocate a properly applied patch angioplasty now generally recommend that patch angioplasty be routinely used in female patients, patients with small internal carotid arteries, patients who require extension of the arteriotomy beyond the bulb of the internal carotid artery, and patients undergoing surgery for recurrent carotid stenosis. Patch material can consist of autogenous vein or prosthetic material of the surgeon's choice. I prefer to fashion

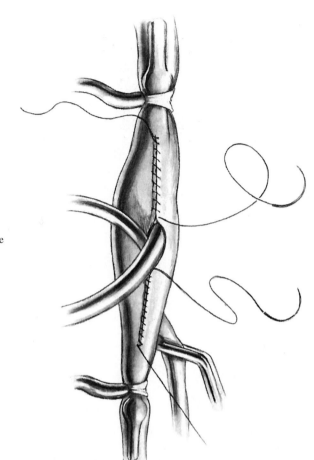

FIGURE 46–13. Closure of the arteriotomy is from both directions toward the midpoint of the arteriotomy where the shunt emerges.

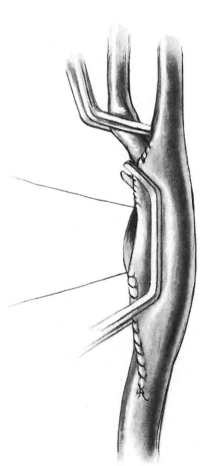

FIGURE 46–14. Following removal of the shunt, a partially occluding clamp is placed across the residual open portion of the arteriotomy to permit restoration of blood flow and completion of the arteriotomy closure over the clamp.

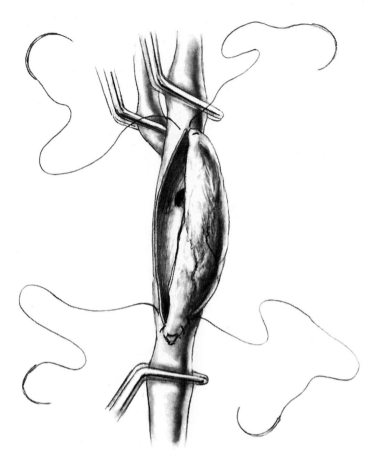

FIGURE 46–15. Placement of a patch and initiation of patch arteriotomy closure.

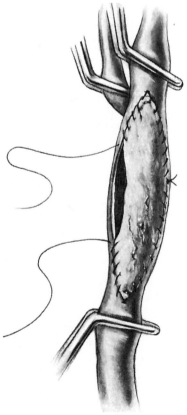

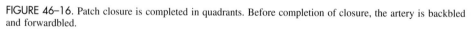

FIGURE 46–16. Patch closure is completed in quadrants. Before completion of closure, the artery is backbled and forwardbled.

the patch in appropriate length and diameter, presenting a somewhat elliptical shape. The distal suture can be placed first in the same manner as is used for primary closure, but with the stitch starting on one side of the apex of the patch, passing into the artery, and out the other side. The opposite limb of a double-armed suture is passed in the corresponding opposite portion of the apex of the arteriotomy. This is then tied in place (Fig. 46–15). One side of the patched closure of the arteriotomy is completed down to the midportion of the arteriotomy. The second or opposite side is completed to its opposite position. The proximal suture is then pulled up and tied, and a third quadrant is completed with the suture tied at the completed site of closure. As the fourth quadrant is being completed, but before complete closure of the arteriotomy, the internal carotid, external carotid, and common carotid arteries are backbled. The fourth quadrant is then completed and tied (Fig. 46–16).

An alternative method of endarterectomy has recently been described. Instead of making a longitudinal arteriotomy, the surgeon actually severs the internal carotid artery circumferentially at the bifurcation of the common carotid artery. The incision that severs the artery is placed obliquely, so that a relatively long opening remains on the common carotid artery. Endarterectomy of the internal carotid artery is done by everting the adventitia off the atheromatous plaque. This continues distally until the plaque ends and there is a clear intimal endpoint. Endarterectomy of the common and external carotid arteries is done through the open arteriotomy. The internal carotid artery is then reverted and circumferentially reanastomosed at the level of severance.

SEQUENCE OF FLOW RESTORATION

The sequence of restoration of blood flow is quite important to prevent embolization of air or debris into the internal carotid artery. While all three clamps are still in position, I prefer to open the internal carotid artery briefly to allow it to fill and distend the carotid bifurcation. I then clamp the origin of the internal carotid artery with a pair of arterial forceps. The external carotid and common carotid arteries are then opened, with flow restored between the common and external carotid arteries for several heartbeats. The forceps are then removed from the internal carotid artery and flow is established through that vessel. This represents the safest sequence for restoration of blood flow to the cerebral circulation.

WOUND CLOSURE

After meticulous hemostasis is achieved, I prefer to place a 7-mm Jackson Pratt drain in the depth of the wound next to the artery. The drain is brought out through a separate stab wound at the inferior margin of the neck incision. I close the platysma layer with a running suture of 3-0 Maxon and close the skin with 4-0 subcuticular sutures of Dexon. A clear Op-Site dressing is placed directly on the skin. The drain and dressing are removed the next morning. A bulky dressing can hide a hematoma for some time. A small, clear plastic dressing provides accurate visualization of the neck. If a hematoma occurs during the postoperative interval that is not evacuated by the Jackson Pratt drain, the patient should be returned to the operating room for drainage of the hematoma. Although it is a nuisance to have to return a patient to the operating room, evacuation of the hematoma markedly reduces wound morbidity. The frequency with which we have had to return patients to the operating room has dropped almost to zero since the utilization of the Jackson Pratt wound drain began.

SUMMARY

The carotid artery must be adequately mobilized so as to avoid clamp encroachment on the endpoints of endarterectomy. The arteriotomy is placed opposite the takeoff of the external carotid artery so as to split the common and internal carotid arteries on the flow divider.

An endarterectomy plane that encompasses the atheromatous plaque but that leaves the media and adventitia undisturbed is selected. An endarterectomy must be carried out in a slow, precise, and unhurried fashion in order to achieve a perfect result.

Although many arteriotomies can be closed primarily if care is taken, augmentation of circumference with patch closure is now used with increasing frequency. The sequence of restoring blood flow to the internal carotid artery is critical. Flow must be established first to the external carotid artery and then to the internal carotid artery in order to avoid embolization of air or atheromatous debris into the internal carotid artery. Meticulous hemostasis and careful wound closure minimize postoperative wound complications.

Acknowledgment

The author thanks Ted Bloodhart for his preparation of the illustrations.

CHAPTER 47

Arguments in Favor of Routine Patch Angioplasty of the Carotid Artery

RICHARD W. BOCK

In 1984, during an era of intense controversy regarding the appropriate use of carotid endarterectomy, vocal critics of the procedure conceded that its use might be warranted if its rates of major morbidity and mortality could be reduced to less than 5 percent.[1] A decade later, the important and effective role of carotid endarterectomy in stroke prevention has been solidly established,[2, 3] and little informed controversy remains regarding its use in symptomatic and, now, asymptomatic patients[4] with high-grade stenoses. Morbidity and mortality rates, even in multicenter trials with dozens of participating surgeons, have fallen dramatically. Yet never has the importance of a low complication rate and a durable procedure been so great as it is today.

Critical to the success of carotid endarterectomy within and outside of clinical trials have been significant refinements in selection of patients, the withdrawal from carotid surgery of many "occasional" practitioners, and major advances in surgical technique. Among these important intraoperative variables are anesthesia technique, cerebral monitoring, and appropriate use of carotid shunting. But perhaps most critical is the surgical procedure itself: a safe, durable result is almost completely dependent on the surgeon and his or her operation. The importance of careful dissection and thorough exposure of the internal carotid artery beyond the distal extent of disease is now widely accepted, as is adequate distal arteriotomy and the clear visualization of the endarterectomy endpoint itself. But although widespread agreement now exists on these topics, significant variation persists in the utilization of patch closure of the endarterectomized carotid artery.

Proponents of carotid patch angioplasty argue that the technique prevents narrowing of the internal carotid artery beyond the carotid bulb, that it allows a more anatomic reconstruction, and that it thereby prevents the most feared technical error associated with carotid endarterectomy: acute thrombosis and occlusion. They also argue that the incidence of recurrent carotid stenosis is significantly reduced with properly performed carotid patch closure. Opponents of patch angioplasty counter that the procedure adds time and complexity to the operation, that a new set of complications is associated with its use, and that endarterectomy can be safely performed with primary closure of the carotid artery.

This chapter reviews the technique of carotid patch angioplasty, theories underlying its use, histopathologic studies, and options for the patch material itself. Data regarding the effects of patch closure on acute complications and technical errors are carefully reviewed, studies on recurrent carotid stenosis are examined, and complications of patch closure are discussed. In the final section, important elements of operative strategy are summarized, together with the author's preference and rationale for the routine use of carotid patch angioplasty.

OPERATIVE TECHNIQUE OF CAROTID PATCH ANGIOPLASTY

Successful carotid endarterectomy begins with adequate distal dissection, arteriotomy beyond the distal extent of disease, and careful, thorough endarterectomy to the transition to normal internal carotid intima. Complete visualization of the distal endpoint is critical. Patch closure, utilizing either vein or prosthetic material, is then begun at the distal end of the arteriotomy.

Each needle of a double-armed monofilament suture is brought from inside to outside the vessel, passing less than 1 mm beyond the arteriotomy and equally close to its axis. Next, each needle is passed through the patch at corresponding points (some surgeons prefer a slightly wider placement of these two patch bites, a technique that produces a slight "opening" force on the vessel against the patch). The suture may then be tied, or a parachute closure may be begun. Continuous bites, always inside-out in the vessel, are then advanced down one side of the patch.

The width of both the arterial and the patch sutures is critical to proper patch angioplasty, as aneurysmal transformation must be avoided. As the suture line is advanced proximally, larger bites are taken of both artery and patch. When the distal extent of the endarterectomy is reached, usually after a few sutures, bites are deepened again. This widening is compensated for by the increased inner dimensions of the post-endarterectomized portion of the internal carotid artery. When the closure advances past the bifurcation into the common carotid artery, the patch and arterial wall bites are widened again. These stepwise but gradual changes in suture width are important in avoiding patch-induced aneurysmal transformation of the reconstructed carotid artery, an error that has been associated with turbulence throughout the cardiac cycle and persistent flow reversal[5] as well as thrombus formation, embolization, and recurrent carotid stenosis.[6] At a convenient juncture approximately halfway down the length of the patch, the first suture is tagged and the second side of the closure is begun with the remaining suture. Stepwise narrowing of the effective patch width is again accomplished by increasing the depth of the sutures as described.

After the second suture line reaches its approximate midpoint, each suture is tagged and a second double-armed suture is placed at the proximal (common carotid) end of the arteriotomy. The proximal end of the patch is trimmed. As the suture is advanced, the effective diameter of the reconstructed artery is again kept only slightly wider than its preoperative dimension by increasing the width of the suture bites. When the first proximal-based suture reaches its distal mate on the same side, the two are tied and tagged. The last side is then completed in the same fashion, and the vessels are sequentially backbled (internal carotid last) and the suture is tied. Flow is restored to the external and then the internal carotid arteries.

WHY DOES CAROTID PATCH ANGIOPLASTY WORK?

Patch closure after endarterectomy helps prevent acute thrombosis and occlusion by preventing narrowing of the critical distal end of the internal carotid artery closure. Simple logic dictates that primary closure *unavoidably* narrows the internal carotid artery; in fact, vessel diameter is reduced by approximately 15 percent,[5] and cross sectional area is diminished by a much greater factor. This may make no practical difference in the carotid bulb or in the common carotid artery, but at the distal end of the endarterectomy and of the arteriotomy itself, this narrowing may represent a technical defect sufficient for acute thrombosis, or it may amplify the effect of another, unseen defect in the endarterectomy endpoint soon after re-establishment of flow.[7]

Even if no immediate damage is done, the inescapable narrowing of the internal carotid artery produced by primary closure may interact with the normal postoperative histopathologic changes occurring in the vessel lumen to produce early postoperative thrombosis. After endarterectomy, the exposed deep arterial tunica media develops a layer of platelet aggregate that is soon followed by a thickened, edematous neointima.[7] This reduction in effective diameter of the vessel by either the platelet aggregate or the thickened neointima may be enough to cause thrombosis of a primarily closed artery, or it may worsen a previously noncritical technical defect and lead to postoperative occlusion. Patch closure, on the other hand, avoids narrowing of the critical distal endpoint of the endarterectomy. It may allow reconstruction of a more normal carotid bulb[8] or effectively move the bulb cephalad[9]; this reapproximation of normal anatomy may itself provide resistance to thrombosis. Saphenous vein patches may prevent early thrombosis by an additional mechanism: the neointimal edema and thickening seen in all endarterectomized vessels do not extend to the vein patch itself,[7] and effective vessel narrowing may thereby be lessened. Although vein patch angioplasty is believed by some surgeons to reduce initial platelet aggregation, this effect is not well documented in the literature.

The incidence of recurrent carotid stenosis, which may occur in the months and years following operation, is also reduced by carotid patch angioplasty, probably by extension of the mechanisms described. Since a thickened neointima overlying the endarterectomized vessel forms after each endarterectomy, primary closure of the vessel allows this layer to play a critical role in recurrent stenosis.[10] Preserving or slightly enlarging the reconstructed diameter of the internal carotid artery would prevent the neointima from precipitating a significant stenosis. When aggressive intimal thickening occurs in any postendarterectomy vessel in the first 2 years postoperatively, the recurrent stenosis is generally caused by this myointimal hyperplasia. When the recurrent lesion develops after 2 years, the pathology is usually recurrent (continuing) atherosclerosis. Hemodynamically significant effects of both processes may be significantly reduced by patch angioplasty.

MATERIALS USED FOR CAROTID PATCH ANGIOPLASTY

Saphenous Vein

Most surgeons who perform carotid patch closure after endarterectomy prefer to use saphenous vein. It has attractive theoretical benefits as an autologous tissue, it is almost always available at the necessary length, it rarely becomes infected, and it has favorable handling characteristics. For many years, the saphenous vein was customarily harvested at the ankle. However, reports of vein patch blowout[11–15] became more frequent, and the ankle saphenous vein was implicated as weaker and more susceptible to rupture than vein harvested from the groin (see section on Complications). A positive linear correlation exists between vein patch diameter and burst pressure, and saphenous veins measuring less than 4 mm in (preharvest) diameter pose a greater risk of rupture.[16] Saphenous vein from the groin is thicker, wider, and almost certainly safer for patch angioplasty, and today most autologous patches placed in the carotid position are fashioned from groin saphenous vein.

Many surgeons have been hesitant to use saphenous vein because of concern that the patient will later require autologous vein for lower extremity or coronary artery bypass. In a study of 134 patients undergoing carotid endarterectomy and patch closure with vein from the thigh, de Vries and associates[17] found only 13 patients who required secondary vascular procedures after a follow-up period averaging 45 months. Adequate saphenous vein was available in all but one patient.[17] In addition, it is doubtful whether removal of the limited length of vein required for carotid patch angioplasty makes a significant difference in the care of more than the rare vascular patient.

Cervical Vein

The use of common facial, external jugular, and internal jugular vein for carotid patch angioplasty has also been advocated.[18–20] One study of bursting pressures concluded that single-thickness cervical (facial or external jugular) vein has a bursting pressure of 10 pounds per square inch (psi) versus 83 psi for everted, double-thickness cervical vein and 94 psi for groin saphenous vein.[20] Therefore, cervical veins should always be everted and used double-thickness if they are employed as a carotid patch.

Polytetrafluoroethylene

Patches made of extended polytetraflouroethylene (PTFE) have been used in the carotid position for at least a decade.[21, 22] The disadvantages of autologous vein are avoided with the use of PTFE, and some feel that it is less thrombogenic and more infection-resistant than other prosthetic grafts; specific data to this effect are absent. In comparison with autologous vein patches, PTFE patches better resist subsequent aneurysm formation.[23] PTFE patches placed onto the carotid bifurcation do have a well-known propensity to bleed, often profusely.[24, 25] This bleeding is caused by leakage through needle holes at the periphery of the patch and is almost always controlled within a few minutes of unclamping by application of gentle pressure and topical thrombostatic agents. Nonetheless, this disadvantage, together with its suboptimal handling characteristics, has limited the appeal of PTFE for carotid patch angioplasty.

Dacron

Carotid closure with Dacron patch angioplasty has the advantages of availability, reduced operating time, and easy handling. Vein patch blowout, an unusual but devastating complication of vein patch angioplasty, is avoided, and no vein is taken that might later be required as a conduit. Collagen-coated Dacron obviates patch leakage and needle-hole bleeding after placement. Few data exist regarding the comparative thrombogenicity of Dacron and PTFE placed in the carotid position, but a major difference seems unlikely. Concerns regarding vein blowout, harvest time, and use of potential conduit, as well as PTFE-related bleeding, lead many surgeons to choose Dacron as the optimal patch material.[10, 24, 26, 27]

GEOMETRIC AND HISTOPATHOLOGIC CHANGES AFTER CAROTID PATCH ANGIOPLASTY

Canine studies have underscored the importance of carotid patch geometry in determining postoperative flow characteristics. Primary closure invariably decreases the diameter of the distal internal carotid vessel. Fietsam and coworkers[5] performed primary closure and patch angioplasty with 5 and 10 mm wide PTFE patches on normal dog carotid arteries. Primarily closed vessels displayed a significant increase in flow velocity across the arteriotomy, and a pressure gradient was consistently created. Large (10 mm) patches caused localized turbulence and significant spectral broadening that persisted throughout the cardiac cycle, clearly a pathologic state. Smaller (5 mm) patches produced arterial flow that was free of associated stenosis, pressure drops, turbulence, and flow disturbance. With the use of these moderate-sized patches, normal, preoperative flow characteristics were fully reapproximated.

Histopathologic changes after surgery begin with platelet aggregation on all endarterectomized surfaces within minutes after re-establishment of flow.[28] Platelet turnover and new aggregation continue for weeks, then give way to a thickened, edematous neointima. Smooth muscle cell migration into the developing neointima occurs concurrently.[29] Later, this neointima may recede or develop into chronic myointimal hyperplasia (to which women and patients who continue to smoke appear particularly susceptible). This layer develops on all endarterectomized surfaces but does not involve the luminal side of autologous vein grafts. Vein patching therefore increases the effective inner diameter, prevents circumferential deposition of the thicker, edematous intima, and may serve to mitigate recurrent stenosis.[7] The luminal surfaces of PTFE and Dacron patches undergo changes very similar to those that affect the endarterectomized arterial surface.[9, 22]

Histopathologic studies have shown that autologous vein patches develop fissuring and endothelial fragmentation soon after placement. The majority of the endothelium survives, but it appears not to influence the manner in which re-endothelialization takes place after endarterectomy[9]; in both patched and primarily closed vessels, regeneration of the endothelial monolayer proceeds from the endpoints of intact endothelium, not from the patch. The time until complete re-endothelialization occurs is also unaffected.[7] Biosynthetic function of the vein patch is initially abnormal, with increased thromboxane production relative to prostacyclin in the first 6 weeks, but thereafter prostacyclin formation predominates.[30]

PATCH ANGIOPLASTY AND PERIOPERATIVE COMPLICATIONS OF CAROTID ENDARTERECTOMY

Proponents of carotid patch angioplasty argue that the addition of a patch to carotid artery closure helps prevent acute thrombosis and occlusion, thereby reducing the incidence of perioperative stroke. Table 47–1 summarizes the effects of patch angioplasty versus primary closure reported in recent trials. No published study reports a significantly higher rate of acute thrombosis or perioperative stroke with patch angioplasty than with primary closure. Many trials show the reverse: rates of acute thrombosis or acute stroke or both are often significantly higher after primary closure.[8, 31–33] Because of the low incidence of serious perioperative neurologic complications and the resulting high numbers required to demonstrate statistical significance, several other studies show clear trends toward improvement with patch angioplasty but fail to reach appropriate P values.[13, 23, 34]

The large, prospective (but nonrandomized) study from Hertzer and associates[32] involved 917 patients undergoing carotid endarterectomy at the Cleveland Clinic. Among 483 patients receiving primary carotid artery closure, the perioperative stroke rate was 3.1 percent, whereas the 434 patients who underwent patch closure with ankle vein had a stroke rate of 0.7 percent. Unsuspected or symptomatic carotid thromboses numbered an additional 3.1 percent in the primary closure group versus 0.5 percent in the patched cohort. All differences were statistically significant. The nonrandomized series of Archie[31] and Little and colleagues[8] also demonstrated significant reductions in acute complications with patch angioplasty as compared with primary closure.

Two randomized, prospective studies have confirmed trends toward significant reductions in perioperative neurologic complications. Major complications occurred in 6.4 percent of the primary closure group studied by Eikelboom and associates,[34] whereas vein patch angioplasty resulted in a 4.5 percent rate. Lord and coworkers,[23] comparing primary closure with both autogenous vein and PTFE patch closure, reported a 10 percent rate of transient ischemic attack plus stroke with primary closure. The corresponding complication rate was 2.4 percent in the vein patch group and 2.1 percent among patients receiving PTFE patch angioplasty. Because of the low overall event rates, neither of these randomized studies attained statistical significance. More recently, a randomized, prospective, multicenter trial confirmed a statistically significant difference in perioperative carotid thrombosis between primary closure (6%) and saphenous vein patch angioplasty (0%).[33] Although other studies certainly exist that show no difference between patching and primary closure,[35, 36] no study shows an advantage for primary closure in preventing stroke or thrombosis.

In a recent editorial, Hertzer[37] discussed several surgeon-related factors that, in addition to the data presented here, also argue for routine patch angioplasty. He pointed out that as many as 64 percent of carotid endarterectomies are performed by surgeons who average two such operations per year, and that complication rates associated with carotid

TABLE 47–1. Effect of Patch Angioplasty on Acute Complication Rate

Study*	Patients, n	Study Design	Patch Type	Cerebral Protection	Endpoint	Patients Reaching Endpoint After Primary Closure, %	Patients Reaching Endpoint After Patch Closure, %
Little et al[8]	120	Consecutive Nonconcurrent	Ankle saphenous	Selective shunt (intraoperative EEG)	ICA/ECA/CCA Occlusion	8.6	0 (P = .04)
Archie and Green[16]	200	Consecutive Nonconcurrent	Ankle saphenous	Selective shunt (back pressure)	Stroke + death + occlusion + restenosis	10	0 (P < .01)
Hertzer et al[32]	917	Prospective Consecutive Concurrent	Ankle saphenous	Routine shunt	Ischemic stroke	3.1	0.7 (P < .1)
Katz et al[13]	89	Consecutive Nonconcurrent	Ankle saphenous	Routine shunt	Stroke	2.5	0 (ns)
Eikelboom et al[34]	129	Randomized Prospective	Ankle saphenous	Selective shunt (intraoperative EEG)	Stroke + death	6.4	4.5 (ns)
Lord et al[23]	140	Randomized Prospective	Groin saphenous and PTFE	Selective shunt (back pressure)	TIA + stroke	10	Saphenous 2.4 PTFE 2.1 (ns)
Clagett et al[29]	152	Randomized Prospective	Ankle saphenous	Routine shunt	TIA + stroke + death†	3.4	1.6 (ns)
Rosenthal et al[35]	1000	Multicenter Retrospective	Ankle saphenous and PTFE and Dacron	Varied	Stroke	1.6	Saphenous 0 PTFE 2.0 Dacron 1.6 (ns)
Ranaboldo et al[33]	213	Randomized Prospective Multicenter	Saphenous (unspecified) and Dacron	Routine shunt	Perioperative occlusion	6	0 (P < .05)

*For full bibliographic information, see reference list at end of chapter.
†Excludes "obligatory patch" group from analysis.
CCA, common carotid artery; ECA, external carotid artery; EEG, electroencephalogram; ICA, internal carotid artery; ns, not significant; PTFE, polytetrafluoroethylene; TIA, transient ischemic attack.

surgery are likely related to case volume. Patch angioplasty widens the margin of safety in carotid endarterectomy, mitigating the potentially devastating effects of small, subtle technical errors performed by occasional and seasoned carotid surgeons alike. Clearly, a preponderance of evidence supports carotid patch angioplasty as an effective means of reducing perioperative carotid thrombosis. Its routine use may prevent hundreds of perioperative strokes and deaths nationwide.

PATCH ANGIOPLASTY AND RECURRENT CAROTID STENOSIS

Recurrent stenosis following carotid endarterectomy was thought to be uncommon until postoperative surveillance with noninvasive imaging became commonplace. Depending on the criteria used to diagnose stenosis, recurrence rates measured with Doppler ultrasonography and duplex imaging ranged between 6.6 and 19 percent.[38–41] More recently, Gelabert and colleagues[42] emphasized the difference between residual stenosis, in which incomplete endarterectomy or other technical error has produced postoperative stenosis from the outset, and true recurrent stenosis. This latter process is caused either by myointimal hyperplasia, which is found in most restenoses diagnosed within the first 2 years, or by recurrent atherosclerosis, which is more common in recurrent stenosis arising after the second postoperative year.

The true significance of recurrent carotid stenosis is debated (see Chapter 71). Some surgeons argue that the long-term preservation of a widely patent carotid bifurcation with no significant narrowing is essential to the success of carotid endarterectomy. Others counter that, even when recurrent

hemodynamically significant stenosis is present, the majority of patients remain asymptomatic. They point to the very different histopathologic features seen in recurrent stenosis as compared with primary carotid lesions; the former lesions are generally smooth and fibrous and may be less likely to serve as an embolic source for stroke than primarily diseased vessels.[43] Finally, some surgeons believe that noninvasive diagnostic methods may be invalid following carotid endarterectomy. High-frequency and high-velocity areas seen on a duplex scan after endarterectomy could represent artifact from postoperative changes rather than true, hemodynamically significant stenoses. Certainly no study has fully validated duplex scanning for this purpose. Nonetheless, it seems logical that these postoperative duplex abnormalities probably document real lesions, and that avoidance of hemodynamically significant stenosis may improve the durability of carotid endarterectomy.

Pathogenesis of Recurrent Stenosis

The acute studies from Fietsam and associates[5] provide insight into mechanisms responsible for recurrent carotid stenosis. Primary closure produced immediate stenosis, but the dogs in this study were not endarterectomized and were therefore not observed chronically. Nonetheless, the postendarterectomy formation of a thickened neointima in humans is well known and could only worsen the initial stenosis caused by primary closure. Any degree of chronic myointimal hyperplasia would produce further stenosis. It seems likely that the mechanism of postendarterectomy recurrent stenosis is related to initial narrowing caused by technical factors at the distal arteriotomy and endarterectomy endpoint, subsequent intimal thickening occurring as a response to intimal obliteration, and chronic development of myointimal hyperplasia. Patch closure after endarterectomy may mitigate the effects of all three of these pathologic factors.

Just as primary closure may lead to restenosis, angioplasty with an overly wide patch may lead to thrombus formation and recurrent stenosis. The 10 mm patches in the study by Fietsam and colleagues[5] produced marked turbulence in the patched region. Thrombus may collect in these low-flow areas,[28] producing a risk of embolization and providing a substrate for atherogenesis (see the later discussion of Clagett and associates' series[36]). Preferential plaque formation is thought to occur in areas of low shear stress such as the outer carotid bulb,[44] a finding that could apply to vessels patched too widely after endarterectomy. Even after proper placement, vein patches have been reported to widen postoperatively.[23, 45] Synthetic patches composed of Dacron or PTFE appear to resist postoperative dilation, and the stenosis that follows patch angioplasty (rather than primary closure) appears more likely to remain hemodynamically insignificant.

Recurrent stenosis may be confused with persistent narrowing after inadequate endarterectomy; as many as one third of restenoses may actually represent this effect.[42] Sanders and coworkers[46] studied patients 1 year after endarterectomy and reviewed intravenous digital subtraction angiograms that had been obtained 1 week after surgery. They found that half of the patients with recurrent stenosis actually had lesions present immediately after surgery. These stenoses could have been caused by inadequate endarterectomy, other technical defects, or perhaps very early, aggressive myointimal hyperplasia. Regardless of pathogenesis, half of restenotic lesions measuring less than 50 percent (hemodynamically insignificant stenoses) undergo regression under continued follow-up,[46] and stenoses of even higher grade commonly regress over the course of long-term observation.[47]

Clinical Studies of Recurrent Stenosis and Patch Angioplasty

Studies of the relation between carotid patch angioplasty and carotid restenosis are detailed in Table 47–2. Seven series identified a significant decrease in recurrent stenosis among patients undergoing patch angioplasty compared with primary closure. The study by Hertzer and colleagues[32] was the largest, and although a threefold greater risk of restenosis was associated with primary closure, the study was criticized for its nonrandomized design, low threshold for the diagnosis of recurrent stenosis ($\geq$30% diameter reduction), and its use of continuous-wave Doppler rather than duplex studies. Nonetheless, their findings were confirmed by the randomized, prospective study of Eikelboom and associates[34] in which intravenous digital subtraction angioplasty and duplex findings of 50 percent or greater stenosis were used for the diagnosis of restenosis.[34] Primary closure was associated with a sixfold higher incidence of restenosis when compared with vein patch angioplasty. Two long-term follow-up studies of the same cohort reported a persistent advantage of patch angioplasty and found a particularly dramatic effect among women (70% 5-year restenosis rate with primary closure).

Two other randomized, prospective studies examined PTFE and Dacron patch angioplasty and reached the same statistically significant conclusion. Lord and associates[23] found no cases of restenosis in a group receiving either PTFE or groin saphenous vein patches, whereas 18 percent of the primarily closed group developed restenosis. Ranaboldo and associates[33] reported a 16 percent recurrence rate

TABLE 47–2. Effect of Patch Angioplasty on Recurrent Carotid Stenosis

Study*	Patients, n	Study Design	Patch Type	Postoperative Surveillance	Threshold for Diagnosis of Restenosis, %	Patients Experiencing Restenosis After Primary Closure, %	Patients Experiencing Restenosis After Patch Closure, %
Hertzer et al[32]	917	Consecutive Concurrent	Ankle saphenous	IVDSA + continuous-wave Doppler	$\geq$30	31	9 (P = .007)
Katz et al[13]	89	Consecutive Nonconcurrent	Ankle saphenous	Duplex	$\geq$50	19	2.4 (P < .05)
Eikelboom et al[34]	129	Randomized Prospective	Ankle saphenous	IVDSA + duplex	$\geq$50	21	3.5 (P < .01)
Ten Holter et al[50]	*1 year follow-up of Eikelboom series*			Duplex	$\geq$50	17	3.6 (P < .01)
De Letter et al[51]	*5 year follow-up of Eikelboom series*			Duplex	$\geq$50	Men: 11 Women: 70	Men: 14 (ns) Women: 5.5 (P = 0.07
Lord et al[23]	140	Randomized Prospective	Groin saphenous and PTFE	Duplex	$\geq$30	18	0 (P <.05)
Clagett et al[36]	152	Randomized Prospective	Ankle saphenous	B-mode ultrasonography	$\geq$25*	1.7	12.9 (P = .05)
Myers et al[52]	*5 year follow-up of Clagett series*			Duplex	$\geq$25	14.3	7.8 (ns)
Rosenthal et al[35]	1000	Multicenter Retrospective	Ankle saphenous and PTFE and Dacron	Duplex	$\geq$50	4	Saphenous 1 PTFE 5
Ranaboldo et al[33]	213	Randomized Prospective	Saphenous (unspecified) and Dacron	Duplex	$\geq$50	16	6 (P <.01)

*For full bioliographic information, see reference list at end of chapter.
†All but two of the recurrent stenoses measured less than 50%.
IVDSA, intravenous digital subtraction angiography; ns, not significant; PTFE, polytetrafluoroethylene.

after primary closure versus a 6 percent rate with Dacron patch angioplasty.

Only one series reports a higher carotid restenosis rate after patch angioplasty than after primary closure. Clagett and coworkers[36] randomly assigned patients to receive ankle saphenous vein angioplasty or primary closure and found a 12.9 percent restenosis rate among the 62 patients randomly assigned to receive patch angioplasty, which was significantly higher than the 1.7 percent rate in the primary closure group. Several factors may explain why this study runs counter to all other published reports: (1) Clagett and colleagues' series included only patients with large internal carotid arteries ($\geq$ 5 mm diameter) in their analysis, and all but one of the patients were men. A separate group of patients with smaller carotid vessels underwent ''obligatory'' vein patch angioplasty, and although not a single case of recurrent stenosis developed among these 30 patients, they were excluded from the analysis. This exclusion of patients who were most likely to benefit from patching limits the conclusions that can be drawn from this study. (2) B-mode ultrasonography without spectral analysis or duplex data was used to diagnose restenosis (spectral criteria were only used in the two patients whose stenosis reached 50%). (3) Although patients with B-mode ''stenoses'' of 25 percent or greater were counted as patch failures, all but two such stenoses measured less than 50 percent. (4) The participating surgeons may have fashioned overly wide patches. Increases in measured internal carotid artery diameter ranged from 1.8 to 2.9 mm, which corresponds to patch widths of 5.6 to 9.2 mm, respectively. Resulting increases in carotid artery cross sectional area therefore averaged between 43 and 83 percent with vein patching.

The mild, hemodynamically insignificant stenoses found in Clagett's vein patch group may have represented postoperative B-mode ultrasonographic artifact, or they may have been real. In the latter case, the clinical relevance of these mild stenoses is uncertain, as many such lesions subside.[46] And even if clinically relevant, these restenoses may have been produced by the overly wide patch angioplasties performed in this study; patch widths measuring 5.6 to 9.2 mm may have produced de facto carotid bulb aneurysms.[5]

Clearly, the weight of the evidence overwhelmingly supports the use of carotid patch angioplasty in reducing hemodynamically significant recurrent stenosis. Although selective patching may somewhat reduce the restenosis rate, it seems logical that a policy of routine patching will add significant benefit in reducing recurrent stenosis, as well as having the separate, significant advantage of reducing serious acute complications discussed in the preceding section.

COMPLICATIONS OF CAROTID PATCH ANGIOPLASTY

Potential complications of patch closure after carotid endarterectomy include vein patch blowout, postoperative hematoma, pseudoaneurysm formation, and infection. Advocates of primary closure also note the increased operating and carotid cross-clamp time required for patch placement and cite concern over loss of autologous graft when saphenous vein is used as the patch material. Although the reported incidence of most of these complications has been roughly equivalent between patched and primarily closed groups of endarterectomies, autologous vein patches placed in the carotid position carry an additional small but potentially devastating risk for acute rupture.

Vein Patch Blowout

The most feared complication of vein patch angioplasty is acute rupture of the patch in the perioperative period. The reported incidence of this complication ranges from 0.13 percent to 0.7 percent.[12] In about half of cases, major morbidity or death results from stroke, airway compromise, or other complications. A longitudinal split, presumably caused by central necrosis, is invariably found at reoperation. Almost without exception, reported cases of vein patch rupture have occurred in veins harvested from the lower leg and ankle.[12, 14, 15] Riles and colleagues[11] reported three patch ruptures among a subgroup of 75 patients in whom ankle vein was used as a patch, whereas none of their 600 patients in whom groin vein was used suffered blowout. Archie and Green[16] calculated mean rupture pressures in segments of fresh veins obtained in 157 patients undergoing bypass and found a positive linear correlation between vein graft diameter and the pressure required for vein rupture. Patch rupture pressures calculated from random application of a mathematical model were below 300 mm Hg in 5.7 percent of cases and below 200 mm Hg in 0.6 percent. Smaller veins were more frequent in women, who therefore had a higher theoretical rupture rate. Archie and Green found no vein measuring 4 mm or greater in diameter with a rupture strength of less than 300 mm Hg, and they therefore recommended that veins of small diameter not be used for carotid patch angioplasty. In response to these and other reports, most surgeons who perform vein patch angioplasty have shifted to the routine use of groin saphenous vein, a strategy that probably sharply reduces the risk of patch blowout.

Other Complications of Carotid Patch Angioplasty

Simple postoperative hematoma appears to occur with equal frequency after carotid patch closure with the use of vein or synthetic material as it does after primary closure.[8, 31–33] Carney and Lilly,[24] in a prospective evaluation of Dacron, PTFE, and autologous vein for patch angioplasty, found a significantly greater number of PTFE-patients with intraoperative blood losses exceeding 300 ml.[24] Because of this finding, and because PTFE patch placement was associated with increased operating time (presumably because of the additional time and efforts spent controlling the bleeding) and greater requirements for hemostatic agents, they concluded that PTFE was inferior to both Dacron and autologous vein. Others have reported similar bleeding problems with PTFE.[25]

Pseudoaneurysm formation is also occasionally seen after carotid endarterectomy,[18, 32] but its incidence seems to be less than 0.3 percent,[27, 48] and populations undergoing patched and primarily closed procedures appear to be at equivalent risk.[49] Prosthetic patch graft infections appear even more unusual,[32] with no such complications reported in many large series.

CONCLUSION

The literature and data supporting the use of carotid patch angioplasty are extensive, clear, and well established. Addition of patch closure to carotid endarterectomy reduces the incidence of perioperative stroke and acute thrombosis or occlusion of the carotid artery. It decreases the incidence of recurrent stenosis for years following surgery. Because very low rates of morbidity and mortality, as well as highly durable results, are critical to the effectiveness of the operation, a policy of routine patch angioplasty should be a key element in the surgeon's overall strategy for safe and effective carotid endarterectomy.

No definitive study has demonstrated a clear benefit of one class of patch material over another. Saphenous vein may be theoretically more attractive, but neither clinical series nor histopathologic studies have confirmed significant, concrete advantages over prosthetic materials. Patch blowout after angioplasty with ankle vein has a low but definite incidence; convincing data argue for abandoning the use of vein harvested from below the knee. Groin vein is a limited resource that may be needed later as a bypass conduit, and harvesting of the vein prolongs operating time. Finally, vein patches may undergo continuing postoperative widening and could theoretically compromise patch function by causing localized turbulence and thrombotic and atherogenic sequelae. PTFE patches are associated with bleeding problems which, while rarely serious, prolong operating time and may increase the incidence of simple postoperative hematoma. For these reasons, the author advocates routine carotid patch angioplasty with an albumin-impregnated, precut Dacron patch. Problems with harvest time, patch blowout, bleeding, and limited autologous conduit are all eliminated, and the concrete advantages in ensuring immediate and long-term success are preserved.

Patch angioplasty is only one part of an overall strategy for avoiding complications and ensuring a durable result. Most important is the careful, deliberate conduct of the operation: dissection and arteriotomy should *always* be performed distal to the atherosclerotic plaque. Direct visualization of the endarterectomy endpoint is critical. Cerebral protection with selective shunting, whether guided by measurement of backflow pressures, monitoring under local anesthesia, or intraoperative electroencephalography, is also important. Together, these technical details are as integral to the success of carotid endarterectomy as is a policy of routine carotid patch angioplasty.

REFERENCES

1. Chambers B, Norris J: The case against surgery for asymptomatic carotid artery stenosis. *Stroke.* 1984;15(6):964.
2. North American Symptomatic Carotid Endarterectomy Trial Collaborators: Beneficial effect of carotid endarterectomy in symptomatic patients with high-grade carotid stenosis. *N Engl J Med.* 1991;325(7):445. See comments.
3. European Carotid Surgery Trialists' Collaborative Group: MRC European Carotid Surgery Trial: Interim results for symptomatic patients with severe (70–99%) or with mild (0–29%) carotid stenosis. *Lancet.* 1991;337(8752):1235. See comments.
4. National Institute of Neurological Disorders and Stroke, National Institute of Health: Clinical advisory: Carotid endarterectomy for patients with asymptomatic internal carotid artery stenosis. *Stroke.* 1994;25(12):2523.
5. Fietsam R, Ranval T, Cohn S, et al: Hemodynamic effects of primary closure versus patch angioplasty of the carotid artery. *Ann Vasc Surg.* 1992;6(5):443.
6. Imparato AM: The role of patch angioplasty after carotid endarterectomy. *J Vasc Surg.* 1988;7(5):715. Editorial.
7. Stewart GW, Bandyk DF, Kaebnick HW, et al: Influence of vein-patch angioplasty on carotid endarterectomy healing. *Arch Surg.* 1987;122(3):364.
8. Little JR, Bryerton BS, Furlan AJ: Saphenous vein patch grafts in carotid endarterectomy. *J Neurosurg.* 1984;61(4):743.
9. Awad IA, Little JR: Patch angioplasty in carotid endarterectomy: Advantages, concerns, and controversies. *Stroke.* 1989;20(3):417. See comments.
10. Ouriel K, Green RM: Clinical and technical factors influencing recurrent carotid stenosis and occlusion after endarterectomy. *J Vasc Surg.* 1987;5(5):702.
11. Riles TS, Lamparello PJ, Giangola G, Imparato AM: Rupture of the vein patch: A rare complication of carotid endarterectomy. *Surgery.* 1990;107(1):10. See comments.
12. Tawes R Jr, Treiman RL: Vein patch rupture after carotid endarterectomy: A survey of the Western Vascular Society members. *Ann Vasc Surg.* 1991;5(1):71.
13. Katz MM, Jones GT, Degenhardt J, et al: The use of patch angioplasty to alter the incidence of carotid restenosis following thromboendarterectomy. *J Cardiovasc Surg.* 1987;28(1):2.
14. Scott EW, Dolson L, Day AL, Seeger JM: Carotid endarterectomy complicated by vein patch rupture. *Neurosurgery.* 1992;31(2):373. See comments.
15. O'Hara PJ, Hertzer NR, Krajewski LP, Beven EG: Saphenous vein patch rupture after carotid endarterectomy. *J Vasc Surg.* 1992;15(3):504.
16. Archie J Jr, Green J Jr: Saphenous vein rupture pressure, rupture stress, and carotid endarterectomy vein patch reconstruction. *Surgery.* 1990;107(4):389.
17. de Vries AC, Riles TS, Lamparello PJ, et al: Should proximal saphenous vein be used for carotid patch angioplasty: A clinical study of the need for vein in subsequent operations. *Eur J Vasc Surg.* 1990;4(3):301.
18. Whereatt N, Burke K, Littooy FN, Greisler HP, Baker WH: An evaluation of external jugular vein patch angioplasty after carotid endarterectomy. *Am Surg.* 1990;56(8):455.
19. Seabrook GR, Towne JB, Bandyk DF, et al: Use of the internal jugular vein for carotid patch angioplasty. *Surgery.* 1989;106(4):633.
20. Yu A, Dardik H, Wolodiger F, et al: Everted cervical vein for carotid patch angioplasty. *J Vasc Surg.* 1990;12(5):523.
21. Le Grand DR, Linehan RL: The suitability of expanded PTFE for carotid patch angioplasty. *Ann Vasc Surg.* 1990;4(3):209.
22. Deriu GP, Ballotta E, Bonavina L, et al: The rationale for patch-graft angioplasty after carotid endarterectomy: Early and long-term follow-up. *Stroke.* 1984;15(6):972.
23. Lord RS, Raj TB, Stary DL, et al: Comparison of saphenous vein patch, polytetrafluoroethylene patch, and direct arteriotomy closure after carotid endarterectomy. Part I. Perioperative results. *J Vasc Surg.* 1989;9(4):521.
24. Carney W Jr, Lilly MP: Intraoperative evaluation of PTFE, Dacron and autogenous vein as carotid patch materials. *Ann Vasc Surg.* 1987;1(5):583.
25. McCready RA, Siderys H, Pittman JN, et al: Delayed postoperative bleeding from polytetrafluoroethylene carotid artery patches. *J Vasc Surg.* 1992;15(4):661. See comments.
26. Treiman RL, Foran RF, Wagner WH, et al: Does routine patch angioplasty after carotid endarterectomy lessen the risk of perioperative stroke? *Ann Vasc Surg.* 1993;7(4):317.
27. Schultz GA, Zammit M, Sauvage LR, et al: Carotid artery Dacron patch graft angioplasty: A ten-year experience. *J Vasc Surg.* 1987;5(3):475.
28. Lusby R, Ferrell L, Englestad B, et al: Vessel wall and indium-111-labelled platelet response to carotid endarterectomy. *Surgery.* 1983;93(3):424.
29. Clagett G, Robinowitz M, Youkey J, et al: Morphogenesis and clinicopathologic characteristics of recurrent carotid disease. *J Vasc Surg.* 1986;3:10.
30. Govostis DM, Bandyk DF, Bergamini TM, Towne JB: Biochemical adaptation of venous patches placed in the carotid circulation. *Arch Surg.* 1989;124(4):490.
31. Archie J Jr: Prevention of early restenosis and thrombosis-occlusion after carotid endarterectomy by saphenous vein patch angioplasty. *Stroke.* 1986;17(5):901.
32. Hertzer NR, Beven EG, O'Hara PJ, Krajewski LP: A prospective study of vein patch angioplasty during carotid endarterectomy. Three-year results for 801 patients and 917 operations. *Ann Surg.* 1987;206(5):628.
33. Ranaboldo CJ, Barros D'Sa AA, Bell PR, et al: Randomized controlled trial of patch angioplasty for carotid endarterectomy. The Joint Vascular Research Group. *Br J Surg.* 1993;80(12):1528.
34. Eikelboom BC, Ackerstaff RG, Hoeneveld H, et al: Benefits of carotid patching: A randomized study. *J Vasc Surg.* 1988;7(2):240.
35. Rosenthal D, Archie J Jr, Garcia-Rinaldi R, et al: Carotid patch angioplasty: Immediate and long-term results. *J Vasc Surg.* 1990;12(3):326. See comments.
36. Clagett GP, Patterson CB, Fisher D Jr, et al: Vein patch versus primary closure for carotid endarterectomy. A randomized prospective study in a selected group of patients. *J Vasc Surg.* 1989;9(2):213.
37. Hertzer NR: The hidden statistics of carotid patch angioplasty. *J Vasc Surg.* 1994;19(3):555. Editorial.
38. Curley S, Edwards WS, Jacob TP: Recurrent carotid stenosis after autologous tissue patching. *J Vasc Surg.* 1987;6(4):350.
39. Barnes R, Nix M, Wingo J, Nichols B: Recurrent versus residual carotid stenosis. *Ann Surg.* 1985;203:652.
40. Thomas M, Otis S, Rush M, et al: Recurrent carotid stenosis following endarterectomy. *Ann Surg.* 1984;200:74.
41. Zierler R, Bandyk D, Thiele B, Strandness D: Carotid artery stenosis following endarterectomy. *Arch Surg.* 1982;117:1408.
42. Gelabert HA, el-Massry S, Moore WS: Carotid endarterectomy with primary closure does not adversely affect the rate of recurrent stenosis. *Arch Surg.* 1994;129(6):648.
43. O'Donnell TJ, Callow A, Scott G, et al: Ultrasound characteristics of recurrent

carotid disease: Hypothesis explaining the low incidence of symptomatic recurrence. *J Vasc Surg.* 1985;2:26.

44. Zarins C, Giddens D, Bharadvaj B, et al: Carotid bifurcation atherosclerosis: Quantitative correlation of plaque localization with flow velocity profiles and wall shear stress. *Circ Res.* 1983;53:502.

45. Archie J Jr: Early and late geometric changes after carotid endarterectomy patch reconstruction. *J Vasc Surg.* 1991;14(3):258.

46. Sanders EA, Hoeneveld H, Eikelboom BC, et al: Residual lesions and early recurrent stenosis after carotid endarterectomy. A serial follow-up study with duplex scanning and intravenous digital subtraction angiography. *J Vasc Surg.* 1987;5(5):731. See comments.

47. Healy D, Zierler R, Nicholls S, et al: Long-term follow-up and clinical outcome of carotid restenosis. *J Vasc Surg.* 1989;10:662.

48. Motte S, Wautrecht JC, Bellens B, et al: Infected false aneurysm following carotid endarterectomy with vein patch angioplasty. *J Cardiovasc Surg.* 1987;28(6):734.

49. Branch C Jr, Davis C Jr: False aneurysm complicating carotid endarterectomy. *Neurosurgery.* 1986;19(3):421.

50. Ten Holter JB, Ackerstaff RG, Thoe Schwartzenberg GW, et al: The impact of vein patch angioplasty on long-term surgical outcome after carotid endarterectomy. *J Cardiovasc Surg.* 1990;31(1):58.

51. De Letter JA, Moll FL, Welten RJ: Benefits of carotid patching: A prospective randomized study with long-term follow-up. *Ann Vasc Surg.* 1994;8(1):54.

52. Myers SI, Valentine RJ, Chervu A, et al: Saphenous vein patch versus primary closure for carotid endarterectomy: Long-term assessment of a randomized prospective study. *J Vasc Surg.* 1994;19(1):15.

CHAPTER 48

Arguments in Favor of the Routine Use of Primary Closure of the Carotid Artery

HUGH A. GELABERT

The recent publication of the results of the Asymptomatic Carotid Atherosclerosis Study (ACAS)[1] marks the completion of a remarkable period of prospective randomized study of the benefit of carotid endarterectomy. Several large multicenter studies have scientifically validated the results of endarterectomy,[1-6] demonstrating conclusively that carotid endarterectomy effectively reduces the risk of subsequent stroke. With the completion of these studies, concerns have begun to focus on several attendant problems, including the durability of the operation.

Recurrent stenosis has been cited as an important problem in limiting the benefit of carotid endarterectomy. Although there is some debate as to the impact of recurrent carotid stenosis, a significant number of clinicians believe that recurrent stenosis increases the risk of postoperative neurologic events. Advocates of routine patch closure for carotid endarterectomy hold that its use will reduce the incidence of restenosis. By extension, patch closure will reduce the number of postoperative neurologic events as well as reoperation for restenosis.

Central to this argument is an assessment of the significance of recurrent stenosis. Pathophysiologically, recurrent carotid lesions are vastly different from atherosclerotic plaques. The recurrent lesions are fibrous lesions commonly termed neointimal hyperplasia. They tend to be smooth and homogeneous, with high tensile strength and an intact endothelial surface. Thus, they present a very low potential for the development of thromboemboli and no risk of atheroemboli. Ultimately, the risk of recurrent stenosis lies in the possibility of progression to carotid occlusion. The consequence of a gradual carotid occlusion is thought to include an increased risk of stroke.

Several clinical studies have demonstrated that routine patch closure may reduce the incidence of recurrent stenosis.[7-13] It remains unclear whether this results in a reduction of significant restenosis. Several other studies have demonstrated that primary arterial closure may be accomplished with a very low incidence of restenosis.[14-16] Yet another group of investigators has noted increased restenosis in those patients undergoing patch closure of carotid endarterecotmy[17] (Table 48-1).

No study has clearly demonstrated that patch angioplasty reduces the incidence of reoperation for restenosis. This is in part because of disagreement as to the indications for such reoperations and in part because of the very low number of these events. If reoperation for recurrent stenosis is based on recurrence of symptoms or preocclusive stenosis (>90%), then the benefit of routine patch closure cannot be supported.

ROUTINE PRIMARY CLOSURE

Primary closure of a carotid arteriotomy is the technique in which a single suture line is used to approximate the adjacent walls of the artery following completion of the endarterectomy. This has long been the standard approach

to carotid artery repair. It has the advantages of simplicity, ease, and rapidity and does not expose the patient to the potential complications attendant on carotid patch closure. Routine primary closure implies that most carotid operations will be closed primarily, without an arterial patch. It should be noted, however, that the routine use of primary closure does not preclude the appropriate use of patch closure when warranted.

COMMON INDICATIONS FOR PATCH ANGIOPLASTY

As with most surgical innovations, patch closure may serve several purposes. The most common use of patch angioplasty is in anticipation of reducing the need for reoperation for recurrent stenosis. Patch closure allows stabilization of medial fibers of the arterial wall along the lateral margin of an arteriotomy. Thus, it may be employed as a remedy to prevent or repair small arterial dissections. Another use is to replace a portion of an arterial wall that has been inadvertently injured in the course of operation. An instance of such an event might be a tear occurring along the margin of the arteriotomy. Closure of such a defect may result in a stenosis, but use of a patch would repair the vessel.

The most evident and reasonable indication for the use of a patch closure is to avoid compromising the arterial lumen in the course of arteriotomy closure. Should the arterial lumen be inadvertently compromised, a stenotic lesion would result. This stenosis would then lead to several significant problems. In the early postoperative period, it may provide the nidus where platelets aggregate and thrombus

TABLE 48–1. Incidence of Recurrent Stenosis in Selected Series from 1985 to 1995

Author*	Year	Endarterectomies, n	Mean Follow-Up, mo	Recurrent Stenosis, %
Das et al.[30]	85	1726	42	1.8
Ricotta et al.[32]	92	449	60	3.9
Nitzberg et al.[45]	91	667	50	4
Green et al.[46]	91	686	36	5.2
Atnip et al.[39]	90	184	10	6
Sanders et al.[33]	87	109	24	8
Bertin et al.[47]	89	155	18	8.3
Mattos et al.[29]	93	409	42	10.8
Gelabert et al.[40]	94	268	36	11
Strepetti et al.[48]	89	210	72	12
O'Donnell et al.[49]	85	276	38	12.3
DeGroot et al.[50]	87	310	24	13
Salenius et al.[38]	89	257	77	13
Nicholls et al.[37]	85	145	18	17
Reilly et al.[36]	90	131	15	18
Healy et al.[43]	89	301	48	21
Bandyk et al.[34]	88	78	44	33

*For full bibliographic information see reference list at end of chapter.

may form, leading to embolic events, arterial thrombosis, or even stroke. In a later postoperative period, the narrowed closure may be mistakenly identified as a postoperative stenosis, possibly resulting in reoperation.

ADVANTAGES OF ROUTINE PATCH CLOSURE

Advocates of routine patch closure propose that problems such as recurrent stenosis, postoperative arterial occlusion, and postoperative embolic events would be eliminated by the incorporation of a patch in all arterial repairs. The use of a patch closure allows for a greater margin of error in the suturing of the endarterectomized arterial wall. Thus, where a primary closure might require close attention to the technical elements of suturing the artery, use of a patch allows a more liberal technique. Problems with the endarterectomy endpoint may be partially corrected by use of a patch. Small arteries will be less likely to be constricted in the course of repair. Thus, the incidence of early postoperative complications such as transient ischemic attack, stroke, arterial occlusion, and embolization might be reduced.

Proponents of routine patch closure also hold that the diagnosis of recurrent stenosis should be reduced by the use of patches. This results from the patch's providing a larger arterial lumen, which would then require a larger mass of hyperplastic tissue before a significant degree of stenosis is achieved. Presumably, this would ultimately lead to a reduction in late occlusions and late reoperations for significant restenosis.

DISADVANTAGES OF ROUTINE PATCH CLOSURE

Routine patch closure does present problems that may detract from its promise. Not all patients should be treated identically; to assume that patch closure is always required assumes that there is no difference in the size or shape of arteries. Additionally, it presumes that there is no difference in the arterial response to endarterectomy.

Large arteries that are patched inappropriately may be considered to have an iatrogenic pseudoaneurysm.[18] A larger than normal arterial circumference and cross sectional area may result from the incorrect use of a patch in a large artery. This, in turn, may predispose to complications of a pseudoaneurysm: expansion of the arterial lumen and accumulation of thrombus within the arterial lumen. Ultimately, these may lead to disruption of the arterial repair.[19–27] Another problem with the incorrect use of a patch is that it may lead to embolization and stroke. Although these complications are rare, they are avoidable by judicious and appropriate use of primary arterial repair. A second concern with patch closure is the incidence of prosthetic graft infection.[28] This is an episodic event, but it carries significant risk and necessitates a second operation for removal of the infected prosthesis and reconstruction with autologous tissue.[11]

An economic analysis of routine use of patch closure would certainly find fault with this approach.[29] In calculating the added expense associated with a patch closure, several elements must be considered: the cost of the patch, the added

cost of the longer operative time to close an artery with a patch, the cost of the antibiotic coverage that having a prosthesis may incur, and, in the case of saphenous vein patches, the cost of procuring the patch and closing the wounds. Although each of these elements is relatively small, on an aggregate scale they would represent a significant addition to the cost of care. If one considers the goal of patch closure—to reduce the incidence of recurrent stenosis—and one considers the small number of operations that are performed because of recurrent stenosis, then it is virtually impossible to justify the added cost imposed by a patch closure.

ADVANTAGES OF PRIMARY CLOSURE

The principal advantage of primary arterial closure is simplicity. This in turn yields secondary benefits such as shortened surgical time, lower potential for infectious complications, and elimination of aneurysmal complications following endarterectomy. Since primary closure requires one suture line, it is accomplished in at least half the time required to accomplish a patch closure. This in turn has secondary benefits. If the duration of surgery is shortened, the amount of anesthetic that is required is reduced. The total time during which the wound is open and exposed is also shortened, thus reducing the potential for wound contamination. The potential for wound sepsis is further reduced by avoidance of a foreign body within the wound. Finally, as mentioned previously, avoidance of patch closure on large arteries forestalls the possible problems associated with too large an arterial lumen: thromboembolism and arterial disruption.

DISADVANTAGES OF PRIMARY CLOSURE

Primary closure may itself give rise to several problems if it is done in an incorrect manner. The primary closure of a small artery results in a stenosis. This predisposes to the development of intimal hyperplasia and further compromise of the arterial lumen. Further, the possibility of an iatrogenic stenosis at the level of the endarterectomy endpoint leading to an intimal flap is not beyond reason. This could ultimately result in perioperative carotid thrombosis and stroke. The use of primary closure in patients who may be considered at increased risk of carotid restenosis may result in the development of intimal hyperplasia. Of particular concern would be patients with small arteries and patients whose risk factors include cigarette smoking, diabetes, or elevated cholesterol levels.

FACTORS AFFECTING IDENTIFICATION OF RECURRENT CAROTID STENOSIS

If the principal benefit of patch angioplasty is reducing the incidence of surgery for recurrent stenosis, then it is important to recognize that this event has not been well studied. In fact, the incidence of recurrent stenosis remains in dispute. Reports in recent years have placed the occurrence of restenosis between 1.8 and 70 percent.[13, 30] Furthermore, the rate of reoperation for recurrent stenosis varies from 0 to 4 percent.

Several factors account for these discrepancies. First is the lack of consensus as to what exactly a recurrent stenosis is. Some authors consider any evidence of a lesion, such as an abnormal B-mode image, sufficient evidence to proclaim a recurrent stenosis. Other authors consider any lesion that causes more than a 30 percent reduction of lumen diameter a recurrent stenosis.[7, 31] The most common criterion is a lesion causing more than a 50 percent reduction of the arterial lumen. This criterion has been widely adopted, since this degree of stenosis is associated with hemodynamic significance. Yet another criterion exists for defining a recurrent stenosis: lumen reduction greater than 80 percent.[32] This standard has been adopted by those who argue that a stenosis of any lesser degree does not pose embolic risk and is not preocclusive. The lack of consensus extends to the methods employed for identification of the lesions, the techniques used to confirm the adequacy of the original operation, the degree of stenosis that merits consideration as a recurrence of stenosis, and even the time frame during which a recurrent stenosis may appear.

A significant problem with most reports is the documentation of residual stenosis at the completion of the original carotid endarterectomy. Although many surgeons employ techniques such as routine completion arteriography, intraoperative duplex scanning, or immediate postoperative intravenous digital subtraction angiography, this is not a universal procedure. Current practices vary widely, from no formal assessment to the use of continuous wave Doppler probes.

Sanders and associates[33] noted that half of the postendarterectomy stenoses identified at 12 months were residual lesions. They concluded that technical errors that result in residual lesions may contribute significantly to the development of recurrent stenosis. Ricotta and associates[29] arrived at a similar conclusion, reporting that half of the severe (>80%) recurrent lesions identified in their study were in fact residual lesions that had progressed.

Bandyk and coworkers[34] observed the impact of residual stenosis on the outcome of carotid endarterectomy. Patients with no residual lesions had a 9 percent incidence of recurrent stenosis 24 months after surgery. Those who demonstrated hemodynamic evidence of a residual defect had a 21 percent incidence of restenosis at 24 months after surgery. Sawchuck and colleagues[35] noted that not all residual lesions result in recurrent stenosis. Reilly and colleagues[36] quantified the size of residual lesions and then correlated these with recurrent stenosis. They noted that the presence of residual defects increased the risk of recurrent stenosis. Furthermore, they observed that larger lesions seemed to be associated with more severe recurrent stenosis. This association was not arithmetic, however, and larger residual defects demonstrated a significantly increased propensity to develop severe recurrences.

INFLUENCE OF RISK FACTORS ON RECURRENT STENOSIS

If routine carotid patch closure is forsaken, then the question arises as to when it might be appropriate to employ a patch angioplasty in closing an arteriotomy. In answering this question, several authors have sought to correlate pre-existing risk factors with the risk of developing a recurrent stenosis. In a study of recurrent stenosis, Clagett and coworkers[17, 31] noted a disproportionate increase in recurrent stenosis among women and cigarette smokers. Similar findings were recorded by Nicholls and colleagues,[37] when they prospectively followed a cohort who had 145 endarterectomies over a period of 4 years. Again, they observed an increased risk of restenosis associated with female gender. These observations were again emphasized by Eikelboom and associates.[10] They observed recurrent stenosis in 55 percent of women who underwent primary closure, whereas it recurred in only 11 percent of men treated in the same manner. Interestingly, one report indicates that men may be at increased risk of restenosis. Salenius and colleagues[38] noted that 16 percent of men developed restenosis whereas only 8 percent of women in the study had a similar outcome.

Other risk factors that have been implicated in restenosis include diabetes and smoking.[17, 36] Atnip and colleagues[39] noted that diabetes was the only risk factor that appeared to be associated with an increased risk of restenosis in their report. They studied patients with 184 consecutive endarterectomies over a period of 5 years. During this time they observed recurrent stenosis in 11 arteries. Statistical analysis revealed that the only significant risk factor for recurrence among their patients was the presence of diabetes. This trend was also observed by Gelabert and colleagues,[40] when they reported a cohort study of 268 endarterectomies observed with serial duplex scans over a period of 2 years. They observed that cigarette smoking, gender, and diabetes appeared to be important factors in predisposing toward the development of recurrent stenosis.

Finally, the impact of lipid abnormalities has been noted by two groups. Salenius and associates[38] observed a statistically significant decrease in the occurrence of restenosis in patients with high levels of high-density lipoprotein and low levels of cholesterol and triglycerides. Those whose high-density lipoprotein was low and whose cholesterol and triglycerides were high appeared to be at increased risk of restenosis. Reilly and associates[36] observed a similar damaging effect of elevated cholesterol levels.

RESULTS OF ROUTINE USE OF PRIMARY CLOSURE

Several large studies have compared the results of patch angioplasty and primary closure with regard to posteruptive neurologic events as well as the occurrence of restenosis (Table 48–2). Archie[41] noted a benefit of patch angioplasty in reducing the incidence of recurrent stenosis. In a series of 200 consecutive, nonrandomized patients, recurrent stenosis occurred in 4 and occlusion in 1 patient who underwent primary closure. This contrasted with no such events in the patch closure group. The author concluded that the results of the study supported the use of vein patch angioplasty reconstruction of carotid endarterectomy to protect against restenosis and thrombotic occlusion.

Katz and associates[11] reported a series of 89 consecutive patients who underwent 47 primary closures and 42 patch closures following carotid endarterectomy. They were ob-

TABLE 48–2. Patch Angioplasty Compared to
Primary Closure in Nonrandomized Studies

Author*	Year	Endarter-ectomies, n	Mean Follow-Up, mo	Recurrent Stenosis, %		Statistical Significance
				No Patch	Patch	
Archie[41]	86	200	15	5	0	yes
Hertzer et al.[7]	87	917	21	31	9	yes
Katz et al.[11]	87	89	24	19	2.4	yes
Rosenthal et al.[42]	90	1000	33	4	4	no

*For full bibliographic information, see reference list at end of chapter.

served with repeated duplex scans for a period of 24 months. In the unpatched groups, 19 percent developed restenosis; in the patched group, 2.4 percent developed restenosis. Venous patch rupture occurred in three patients. There was a slightly increased (although not statistically significant) incidence of symptomatic restenosis in the unpatched group. The authors concluded that vein patch angioplasty reduced the incidence of restenosis. They did note the risk of vein patch rupture and suggested that saphenous vein from the thigh may be more durable than that obtained from the ankle.

Hertzer and colleagues[7] reported a series of 917 consecutive (nonrandomized) carotid endarterectomies performed at the Cleveland Clinic between 1983 and 1985. Primary closure was used in 483 cases, and patch closure was used in 434 cases. The mean follow-up period was 21 months. An increased incidence of perioperative carotid occlusion was observed among the non-patch group (total of 15 events), whereas the patch group suffered only two such events. Ipsilateral perioperative strokes occurred in both groups with equal frequency. The cumulative incidence of recurrent stenosis (>30% reduction in carotid diameter) was 31 percent for the primary closure and 9 percent for the patch closure. However, only 10 patients required reoperation for severe recurrent stenosis (3, vein patch; 7, nonpatched). The authors concluded that the results strongly suggest that vein patch enhances the durability and safety of carotid endarterectomy.

Finally, in 1990, Rosenthal and associates[42] conducted an ambitious review of 1000 consecutive carotid endarterectomies. They compared four groups: primary closure, polytetrafluoroethylene (PTFE) patch closure, Dacron patch closure, and vein patch closure. The incidence of early postoperative neurologic events was similar in all groups. Furthermore, they discovered no significant differences in the incidence of restenosis between any groups. They concluded that the method of carotid closure did not appear to affect the occurrence of ipsilateral stroke or restenosis.

PROSPECTIVE RANDOMIZED STUDIES

A survey of the medical literature indicates that there are nine prospective randomized studies that deal with the question of recurrent carotid stenosis. Of these, one is a pharmacologic study, one reports immediate postoperative results, and three report results with only 1 year of follow-up data. Given the natural history of recurrent stenosis, it is clear that a longer follow-up period is required. Thus, four prospective randomized studies are available for evaluation.

These studies compare patients undergoing carotid endarterectomy with and without patch closure (Table 48–3).

The first of these studies, by Clagett and associates,[31] randomly assigned patients to two arms: those receiving vein patches and those undergoing primary closure of the arteriotomy. The study was performed under the auspices of the Veterans Administration; accordingly, the population was all male. Additionally, the authors employed liberal criteria in defining recurrent stenosis: any recurrence was included. This is a significant difference from many other reports, in which recurrent stenosis is commonly defined as a lesion resulting in a greater than 50 percent reduction of the arterial lumen. Finally, the authors were careful to make a vital observation: they discriminated between residual lesions and recurrent lesions. With a mean follow-up period of 22 months, the authors found an increase in the incidence of recurrent stenosis in the vein patch group. The incidence of recurrent lesions in the primary closure group was 1.7 percent and in the vein patch group 12.9 percent. Although these differences are statistically significant, the authors note that most of the recurrent lesions resulted in a stenosis of less than 30 percent. The authors also noted that patch closure resulted in a significant increase in the operative time and did not result in a reduction of perioperative or late postoperative neurologic events.

The second prospective randomized study is by De Letter and colleagues.[13] In this study, patients undergoing 128 endarterectomies were divided into two groups: saphenous vein patch closure and primary closure. During the immediate postoperative period, the rates of stroke and death were similar in both groups (6.4%, primary closure; 4.5%, patch closure). One patient in the patch closure group suffered a patch rupture and hemorrhage. In one patient in the primary closure group, the internal carotid artery occluded, which resulted in a stroke. Long-term follow-up (5 years) indicated a 27 percent incidence of recurrent stenosis (>50%) in the primary closure group and a 12 percent incidence of restenosis in the patch closure group.

Subgroup analysis indicates no significant difference among men receiving primary closure or patch closure (11% vs. 14%). A similar analysis among the women in the study revealed a dramatic difference between the primary closure group and the patch group (70% vs. 5.5%). Unfortunately, the authors were not able to explain the reason for the dramatic incidence of restenosis among the women undergoing primary closure. Because they did not record the diameters of the arteries prior to endarterectomy, they were unable

TABLE 48–3. Prospective Randomized Studies
of Impact of Surgical Technique and Carotid
Restenosis: Primary Closure vs. Patch Closure

Author*	Year	Endarter-ectomies, n	Mean Follow-Up, mo	Recurrent Stenosis, %		Statistical Significance
				Primary	Patch	
Clagett et al.[31]	89	152	22	1.7	12.9	$P < 0.01$
De Letter et al.[13]	93	129	60	27	12	$P < 0.01$
Myers et al.[16]	94	163	59	7.8	14.3	$P = $ ns
Katz et al.[15]	94	100	36	3.9	0	$P = $ ns

*For full bibliographic information, see reference list at end of chapter.
ns, not significant.

to comment as to the likely impact of gender on arterial size and restenosis. It should be noted that no other study has ever identified such a remarkably high rate of restenosis. Additionally, the authors did assess the adequacy of arterial reconstruction with postoperative intravenous digital subtraction angiography, but they did not make note of the presence of residual stenosis in any of their patients. This implies that the incidence of restenosis may be over-reported in this study.

The last two prospective randomized studies appeared in 1994. Katz and associates[11] reported a series of 100 consecutive endarterectomies randomly assigned to primary and patch (PTFE) closure. The patients were followed closely using serial duplex scans over the 36-month follow-up period. The authors noted no significant difference between the groups with respect to perioperative neurologic events (4% primary vs. 2% patch) or recurrent stenosis (4% primary vs. 0% patch). They did note that one patient required reoperation for infection of the PTFE patch. The authors concluded that both primary closure and patch closure result in acceptably low rates of restenosis and that a significant difference between these groups could not be identified. It should be noted that because of the relatively small number of patients in this study, the power of the statistical analysis was limited. Additionally, the authors did not clearly separate residual stenosis from recurrence. Nonetheless, the study is well executed and represents a valuable contribution.

Myers and coworkers[16] reported a series of 163 endarterectomies randomly assigned over a 46-month period to either primary closure or vein patch. An additional group was formed of patients whose internal carotid arteries measured less than 5 mm in diameter and therefore underwent obligatory vein patching. Early postoperative results recorded three strokes: one in the primary closure group and two in the obligatory vein patch group. Long-term follow-up (59 months) identified 16 instances of recurrent stenosis: primary closure, 7.8%; vein patch, 14.3%; and obligatory patch, 5.3%. During the same period, two patients suffered strokes in the ipsilateral hemisphere (one primary, and one vein patch). The authors concluded that the use of a vein patch

did not yield a superior result and had no impact on the durability of carotid endarterectomy.

When examined as a group, the prospective randomized studies that have been published to date do not support the routine use of patch angioplasty in reconstruction of carotid endarterectomy. Although there may be some reason to use patch angioplasty in selected groups of high-risk patients, there appears to be no cogent reason to apply this technique in an indiscriminate manner. Careful attention to detail in performing the endarterectomy and closure appears to be as effective as patch closure both in perioperative and in long-term results.

CLINICAL SIGNIFICANCE OF RECURRENT STENOSIS

Ultimately, the impact of recurrent stenosis is related to the recurrence of symptoms and the need for reoperation. It has been argued that asymptomatic lesions are of little concern since they do not merit reoperation. Further, the actual frequency of recurrent symptoms or reoperation for recurrent stenosis is remarkably small (Table 48–4).

Atnip and coworkers[39] suggested that the indications for reoperation include recurrence of symptoms and the development of a preocclusive stenosis (>80%). In their report, they noted that only 6 percent of patients developed recurrent stenosis. Furthermore, ischemic symptoms developed in only 1.6 percent of all patients. They concluded that reoperation for recurrent stenosis was justified in the event of preocclusive stenosis or the development of ischemic symptoms.

Healy and associates[43] noted that the incidence of symptoms associated with recurrent stenosis was in the range of 14 percent. About 4 percent of their patients experienced recurrent symptoms along with the recurrent stenosis. Cook and coworkers[44] noted that lifetable analysis demonstrates no significant increased risk of transient ischemic attack, stroke, or death in patients with recurrent stenosis. Because of this benign course, the author suggests that routine surveillance may not be necessary.

TABLE 48–4. Reported Late Complications of Recurrent Stenosis

Author*	Year	Cases, n	Recurrent Stenosis, %	Late Occlusion, %	Occlusion Symptoms, %	
					CVA	TIA
Nicholls et al.[37]	85	145	22	0.68	0.68	—
Hertzer et al.[7]	87	917	31	0.43	—	—
Sanders et al.[33]	87	109	8	0.91	—	—
Eikelboom et al.[10]	88	129	11	2.40	—	—
Healy et al.[43]	89	301	21	0.66	0.33	—
Clagett et al.[31]	89	152	12.9	7.24	2.63	—
Salenius et al.[38]	89	257	13	1.94	—	—
Reilly et al.[36]	90	131	18	6.11	—	—
Mattos et al.[29]	93	409	10.8	1.71	0.24	0.24
Hansen et al.[14]	93	232	9.2	1.72	—	—
Myers et al.[16]	93	163	9.8	0	—	—
Gelabert et al.[40]	94	268	11	0	—	—
De Letter et al.[13]	93	129	27	0	—	—
Katz et al.[15]	94	100	3.9	0	—	—

*For full bibliographic information, see reference list at end of chapter.
CVA, cerebrovascular accident; TIA, transient ischemic attack.

Voicing a similar conclusion, Mattos and associates[29] noted that the incidence of symptoms with recurrent stenosis was virtually the same as that occurring in the absence of restenosis. They further note that the cost and effort involved in routine surveillance do not appear to translate into an improved clinical outcome. They concluded that a more cost-effective approach, such as investigating the occurrence of clinical symptoms rather than routine surveillance, may be appropriate.

CONCLUSION

Primary closure of carotid endarterectomy is a safe and simple technique that economizes time and resources. It results in a lower cost of surgery and a safer operation. Of particular importance is the appropriate application of this technique. When used in properly selected patients, primary closure is not associated with an increase in reoperation for recurrent stenosis and hyperplasia. It further avoids the possible complications that arise when a patch closure is used: infection, aneurysm, embolism, and arterial disruption.

Patch angioplasty closure of a carotid endarterectomy may be appropriate in selected instances. Patients who are at an increased risk of developing hemodynamically significant problems with primary closure may warrant patch angioplasty. Thus, patients with very small arteries, or those whose arterial closure appears to compromise the carotid lumen, may merit patch angioplasty. Use of patch angioplasty for patients with suspected risk factors is a debatable option. Of the several potential risk factors that have been identified, only gender has been correlated with recurrent stenosis in more than one or two reports. Still, in the absence of a prospective randomized report that correlates the occurrence of restenosis with a purported risk factor in a statistically significant manner, it is impossible to mandate patch closure.

Patch closure may reduce the incidence of recurrent stenosis for surgeons who have difficulty with primary arterial repair. Certainly, experienced surgeons with sound technique who routinely evaluate the adequacy of endarterectomy by intraoperative studies have no significant occurrence of restenosis among their patients. Patch angioplasty is certainly not necessary for any and all arterial closures. A policy of mandatory patch closure would be wasteful and dangerous. Finally, the use of patch angioplasty cannot guarantee the absence of postoperative symptoms or recurrent high-grade stenosis.

REFERENCES

1. Executive Committee for the Asymptomatic Carotid Atherosclerosis Study: Endarterectomy for Asymptomatic Carotid Artery Stenosis. *JAMA.* 1995;273:1421.
2. MRC European Carotid Surgery Trial: Interim results for symptomatic patients with severe (70–99%) or with mild (0–29%) carotid stenosis. *Lancet.* 1991;337:1235.
3. CASANOVA Study Group: Carotid surgery versus medical therapy in asymptomatic carotid stenosis. *Stroke.* 1991;22:1229.
4. North American Symptomatic Carotid Endarterectomy Trial Collaborators: Beneficial effect of carotid endarterectomy in symptomatic patients with high-grade carotid stenosis. *N Engl J Med.* 1991;325:445.
5. Hobson R, Weiss D, Fields W, et al: Efficacy of carotid endarterectomy for asymptomatic carotid stenosis. *N Engl J Med.* 1993;328:221.
6. Mayberg MR, Wilson SE, Yatsu F, et al: Carotid endarterectomy and prevention of cerebral ischemia in symptomatic carotid stenosis. *JAMA.* 1991;266:3289.
7. Hertzer NR, Beven EG, O'Hara PJ, Krajewski LP: A prospective study of vein patch angioplasty during carotid endarterectomy. Three-year results for 801 patients and 917 operations. *Ann Surg.* 1987;206:628.
8. Ranaboldo CJ, Barros D'Sa AA, Bell PR, et al: Randomized controlled trial of patch angioplasty for carotid endarterectomy. The Joint Vascular Research Group. *Br J Surg.* 1993;80:1528.
9. Lord RS, Raj TB, Stary DL, et al: Comparison of saphenous vein patch, polytetrafluoroethylene patch, and direct arteriotomy closure after carotid endarterectomy. Part I. Perioperative results. *J Vasc Surg.* 1989;9:521.
10. Eikelboom BC, Ackerstaff RG, Honeveld H, et al: Benefits of carotid patching: A randomized study. *J Vasc Surg.* 1988;7:240.
11. Katz MM, Jones GT, Degenhardt J, et al: The use of patch angioplasty to alter the incidence of carotid restenosis following thromboendarterectomy. *J. Cardiovasc Surg.* 1987;28:2.
12. Ten Holter JB, Ackerstaff RG, Thoe Schwartzenberg GW, et al: The impact of vein patch angioplasty on long-term surgical outcome after carotid endarterectomy. A prospective follow-up study with serial duplex scanning. *J Cardiovasc Surg.* 1990;31:58.
13. De Letter JA, Moll FL, Welten RJ, et al: Benefits of carotid patching: A prospective randomized study with long-term follow-up. *Ann Vasc Surg.* 1994;8:54.
14. Hansen F, Linbald B, Persson N, Berqvist D: Can recurrent stenosis after carotid endarterectomy be prevented by low-dose acetylsalicylic acid? A double-blind, randomised, and placebo-controlled study. *Eur J Vasc Surg.* 1993;7:380.
15. Katz D, Snyder SO, Gandhi RH, et al: Long-term follow-up for recurrent stenosis: A prospective randomized study of expanded polytetrafluoroethylene patch angioplasty versus primary closure after carotid endarterectomy. *J Vasc Surg.* 1994;19:198.
16. Myers SI, Valentine RJ, Chervu A, et al: Saphenous vein patch versus primary closure for carotid endarterectomy: Long-term assessment of a randomized prospective study. *J Vasc Surg.* 1994;19:15.
17. Clagett G, Rich N, McDonald P, et al: Etiologic factors for recurrent carotid artery stenosis. *Surgery.* 1983;93:313.
18. Archie J: The geometry and mechanics of saphenous vein patch angioplasty after carotid endarterectomy. *Texas Heart J.* 1987;14:395.
19. Archie J Jr, Green J Jr: Saphenous vein rupture pressure, rupture stress, and carotid endarterectomy vein patch reconstruction. *Surgery.* 1990;107:389.
20. Donovan D, Schmidt S, Townshend S, et al: Material and structural characterization of human saphenous vein. *J Vasc Surg.* 1990;12:531.
21. Smith JW: Delayed postoperative bleeding from polytetrafluoroethylene carotid artery patches. *J Vasc Surg.* 1992;16:663. Letter, comment.
22. O'Hara PJ, Hertzer NR, Krajewski LP, Beven EG: Saphenous vein patch rupture after carotid endarterectomy. *J Vasc Surg.* 1992;15:504.
23. Riles TS, Lamparello PJ, Giangola G, Imparato AM: Rupture of the vein patch: A rare complication of carotid endarterectomy. Surgery 1990;107:10. See comments.
24. Scott EW, Dolson L, Day AL, Seeger JM: Carotid endarterectomy complicated by vein patch rupture. *Neurosurgery.* 1992;31:373. See comments.
25. Spetzler RF: Carotid endarterectomy complicated by vein patch rupture. *Neurosurgery.* 1993;32:151. Letter, comment.
26. Tawes R Jr, Treiman RL: Vein patch rupture after carotid endarterectomy: A survey of the Western Vascular Society members. *Ann Vasc Surg.* 1991;5:71.
27. Van Damme H, Grenade T, Creemers E, Limet R: Blowout of carotid venous patch angioplasty. *Ann Vasc Surg.* 1991;5:542.
28. Motte S, Wautrecht JC, Bellens B, et al: Infected false aneurysm following carotid endarterectomy with vein patch angioplasty. *J Cardiovasc Surg.* 1987;28:734.
29. Mattos M, van Bemmelen P, Barkmeire L, et al: Routine surveillance after carotid endarterectomy: Does it affect clinical management? *J Vasc Surg.* 1993;17:819.
30. Das M, Hertzer N, Ratliff N, et al: Recurrent stenosis: A five year series of 65 reoperations. *Ann Surg.* 1985;202:28.
31. Clagett GP, Patterson CB, Fisher D Jr, et al: Vein patch versus primary closure for carotid endarterectomy. A randomized prospective study in a selected group of patients. *J Vasc Surg.* 1989;9:213.
32. Ricotta J, O'Brien M, DeWeese J: Natural history of recurrent and residual stenosis after carotid endarterectomy: Implications for postoperative surveillance and surgical management. *Surgery.* 1992;112:656.
33. Sanders EA, Honeveld H, Eikelboom BC, et al: Residual lesions and early recurrent stenosis after carotid endarterectomy: A serial follow-up study with duplex scanning and intravenous digital subtraction angiography. *J Vasc Surg.* 1987;5:731. See comments.
34. Bandyk D, Kabenick H, Adams M, Towne J: Turbulence occurring after carotid bifurcation endarterectomy: A harbinger of residual and recurrent carotid stenosis. *J Vasc Surg.* 1988;7:261.
35. Sawchuck A, Flanigan D, Machi J, et al: The fate of unrepaired minor technical defects detected by intraoperative ultrasonography during carotid endarterectomy. *J Vasc Surg.* 1989;9:671.
36. Reilly LM, Okuhn SP, Rapp JH, et al: Recurrent carotid stenosis: A consequence of local or systemic factors? The influence of unrepaired technical defects. *J Vasc Surg.* 1990;11:448.
37. Nicholls S, Phillips D, Bergelin R, et al: Carotid endarterectomy. Relationship of outcome to early restenosis. *J Vasc Surg.* 1985;2:375.
38. Salenius JP, Haapanen A, Harju E, et al: Late carotid restenosis: Aetiologic factors for recurrent carotid artery stenosis during long-term follow-up. *Eur J Vasc Surg.* 1989;3:271.

39. Atnip RG, Wengrovitz M, Gifford RR, et al: A rational approach to recurrent carotid stenosis. *J Vasc Surg.* 1990;11:511.

40. Gelabert HA, el-Massry S, Moore WS: Carotid endarterectomy with primary closure does not adversely affect the rate of recurrent stenosis. *Arch Surg.* 1994;129:648.

41. Archie J Jr: Prevention of early restenosis and thrombosis-occlusion after carotid endarterectomy by saphenous vein patch angioplasty. *Stroke.* 1986;17:901.

42. Rosenthal D, Archie J Jr, Garcia-Rinaldi R, et al: Carotid patch angioplasty: Immediate and long-term results. *J Vasc Surg.* 1990;12:326. See comments.

43. Healy D, Zierler R, Nicholls S, et al: Long-term follow-up and clinical outcome of carotid restenosis. *J Vasc Surg.* 1989;10:662.

44. Cook JM, Thompson BW, Barnes RW: Is routine duplex examination after carotid endarterectomy justified? *J Vasc Surg.* 1990;12:334.

45. Nitzberg R, Mackey W, Penderville W, et al: Long-term follow-up of patients operated for recurrent carotid stenosis. *J Vasc Surg.* 1991;13:121.

46. Green R, McNamara J, Ouriel K, DeWeese J: The clinical course of residual carotid arterial disease. *J Vasc Surg.* 1991;13:112.

47. Bertin V, Plecha F, Rodgers G, et al: Recurrent stenosis by duplex scan following carotid endarterectomy. *Arch Surg.* 1989;124:866.

48. Strepetti A, Schultz R, Feldhaus R, et al: Natural history of recurrent carotid artery stenosis. *Surg Gynecol Obstet.* 1989;168:217.

49. O'Donnell TJ, Callow A, Scott G, et al: Ultrasound characteristics of recurrent carotid disease: Hypothesis explaining the low incidence of symptomatic recurrence. *J Vasc Surg.* 1985;2:26.

50. DeGroot R, Lynch T, Jamil Z, Hobson R: Carotid restenosis: Long-term noninvasive follow-up after carotid endarterectomy. *Stroke.* 1987;18:1031.

CHAPTER 49

Intraoperative Assessment of the Technical Results of Carotid Endarterectomy: Angiography

MAX R. GASPAR and ALLEN W. AVERBOOK

It has been said that intraoperative carotid angiography is inconvenient, technically demanding, cumbersome, and time-consuming; that it does not show important details; and that it might be dangerous. It is none of those things: It is easy to perform, takes little time, shows significant details that might cause carotid endarterectomy to fail immediately or in the future, and in the experience of the authors and their associates, it has not contributed to morbidity or mortality.

EQUIPMENT, PERSONNEL, AND METHOD

Most operating tables have a slot capable of receiving an 11 by 14 inch x-ray cassette beneath the head of the patient. If the table is not equipped with such a slot, a simple wooden tunnel can be constructed for placement on the table beneath the head and shoulders of the patient (Fig. 49–1). It is not necessary to have a permanent overhead x-ray machine. A portable, battery-operated machine is satisfactory. Materials available in any operating room are all that are needed for injection of the dye (Fig. 49–2).

Upon completion of the arteriotomy closure, a $1\frac{1}{2}$ inch 21-gauge needle attached to connector tubing is introduced through the skin and musculature under direct vision into that portion of the common carotid artery that is not endarterectomized (Fig. 49–3). The long needle is needed when a transverse skin incision is made, but a butterfly needle can be used in the conventional incision when it is long enough. Prior to placement of the needle, a 20 mL syringe filled with saline solution is attached to the connector tubing, which

then is filled with the solution. There should be no bubbles in the tubing or the needle. The needle is always directed in a cephalad direction. Aspiration ensures proper placement of the needle in the lumen of the artery. The connector tubing is secured to a drape so that the needle will not be accidentally dislodged.

The surgeon is positioned behind a commercially available, portable, lead-shielded frame covered with sterile sheets (Fig. 49–4). With such a shield, it is not necessary to wear a lead apron. The portable x-ray unit is wheeled into position over the head and neck of the patient, so as to obtain not only a cervical carotid angiogram but also an intracerebral angiogram. The surgeon substitutes the 20 mL syringe with a 10 mL syringe filled with iothalamate meglumine (Conray-60), again checking that the needle is in place in the artery and that there are no air bubbles in the tubing. A 10 mL syringe provides more mechanical advantage than a 20 mL syringe for rapid injection. The x-ray technician starts the rotor of the machine and listens for the command to trigger the machine. This command is given as the plunger of the syringe passes through the 5 mL mark, while the dye is being injected as rapidly as possible. A tendency to stop injecting after giving the command "shoot" must be overcome so that the dye will not be swept out of the carotid artery during the split second between the surgeon's command and the technician's activation of the x-ray tube. The usual x-ray factors are 80 to 90 kilovolt peak at 30 to 40 milliampereseconds. This subjects the patient to a 130 millirad (mrad) dose to the thyroid, the most affected organ. The surgeon receives a dose of less than 1 mrad.

The key to successful intraoperative carotid angiography is the presence of an experienced technologist in the operating suite at all times during daytime operating hours. He or she is available for orthopedic, general surgical, and vascular surgical procedures. The technologist is fully acquainted with the apparatus and the procedures and develops

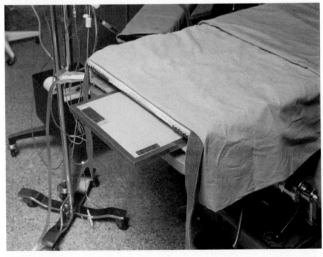

FIGURE 49–1. A simple wooden tunnel (note the upper side of the slot lined with brass tacks) used under the head of a patient when the operating table is not equipped with an x-ray slot. An 11 × 14 inch x-ray cassette is shown in the slot.

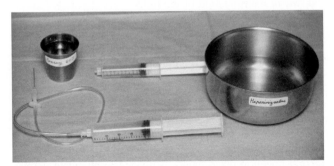

FIGURE 49–2. A 20 mL syringe filled with heparinized saline solution is attached with connector tubing to a $1\frac{1}{2}$ inch 21-gauge needle. After antegrade insertion of the needle into the common carotid artery proximal to the endarterectomized segment, the 10 mL syringe filled with Conray-60 is substituted for the saline-filled syringe.

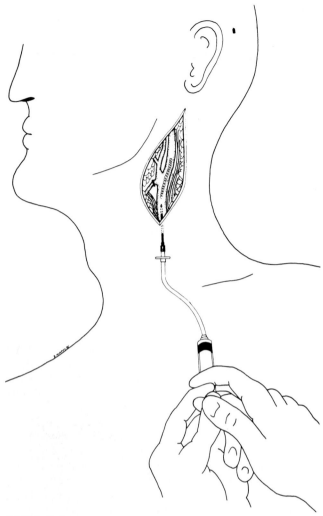

FIGURE 49–3. Placement of the needle through the skin and musculature in a cephalad direction. Two thumbs on the syringe supply power for rapid injection of the dye.

the x-ray films in an area adjacent to the operating room using a dry processor, which takes $2\frac{1}{2}$ minutes.

The time from placement of the needle to the return of the film to the operating room is between 5 and 7 minutes. The film is read by the surgeon and is later reviewed by the radiologist. There has been 99 percent agreement between the two in interpretation of the films.

Other investigators[1, 2] have used intra-arterial digital subtraction angiography with a C arm. This allows multiple views and playback, as well as permanent films, which may be an advantage for interpretation.

ARTERIOGRAPHIC FINDINGS

A satisfactory completion arteriogram is obtained with one injection of dye in 92 percent of cases (Fig. 49–5). A second injection occasionally is needed to elucidate details. Criteria for unacceptable arteriograms are the presence of (1) occlusion, (2) 30 percent stenosis, (3) intimal flap, (4) kink, and (5) clot (Figs. 49–6 through 49–11). Defects are corrected immediately. Defects in the common carotid artery

and the internal carotid artery have been repaired after the arteries are occluded and the arteriotomy is reopened. When the defect has been corrected, the straight in-line shunt (used routinely by our group) is replaced and the arteriotomy closed, occasionally with a patch. The mechanism producing the arteriographic defect is usually corrected within 5 to 7 minutes of occlusion time before replacement of the shunt. Defects seen in the external carotid artery are managed by placing an occluding clamp across the origin of the external carotid artery, thereby allowing continued blood flow to the brain through the internal carotid artery. A small transverse arteriotomy made in the external carotid artery provides enough exposure to extract plaque or intimal shreds with a small pituitary rongeur, after which the arteriotomy is closed with a continuous suture. A completion arteriogram is repeated. It has been necessary to reopen the artery for a second attempt at correction of the problem in less than 1 percent of cases.

In every case in which we have determined to reopen the artery based on the criteria we originally established, we have found a lesion to correct. On the other hand, tragedies have occurred on the few occasions on which the surgeon chose to ignore the indications or mistakenly judged that the demonstrated defect did not meet the criteria for reopening.

RESULTS

From 1967 to 1981, my colleagues and I used routine completion arteriography after carotid endarterectomy in 1105 consecutive operations.[3–5] It was the challenge from Blaisdell and colleagues[6] to assess our own results with intraoperative arteriography that prompted our adoption of this procedure in 1967. Arteriographic defects were noted in approximately 8 percent of cases, which compares favorably with the 26 percent of unsuspected intraluminal defects or thrombosis reported by Blaisdell and colleagues.[6]

There were internal carotid defects in approximately 4

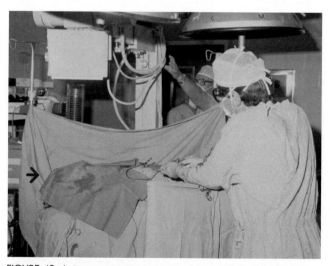

FIGURE 49–4. Surgeon standing in front of a portable lead-shielded frame while injecting dye as a portable x-ray unit is used. The patient's head is covered by a towel *(arrow)*. (From Larson SR, Gaspar MR, Movius HJ, et al: Intraoperative arteriography in cerebrovascular surgery. In Bergan JJ, Yao JST, eds: *Cerebrovascular Insufficiency.* New York: Grune & Stratton, 1982:353; with permission.)

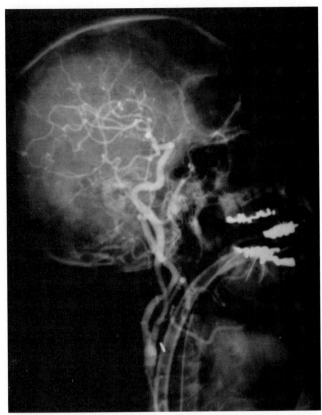

FIGURE 49–5. Satisfactory completion arteriogram of the carotid arteries, showing filling of cervical carotid vessels and intracerebral vessels. A temporary clip on the superior thyroid artery affords a reference point if there is a defect in the extracranial vessels that requires correction. (From Larson SR, Gaspar MR, Movius HJ, et al: Intraoperative arteriography in cerebrovascular surgery. In Bergan JJ, Yao JST, eds. *Cerebrovascular Insufficiency*. New York: Grune & Stratton; 1982:353; with permission.)

and mortality. In a recent survey of members of the Southern California Vascular Surgical Society, only 25 percent of the surgeons reported using completion angiography routinely, whereas 33 percent never use it, and 42 percent use it selectively (Gaspar MR, unpublished data). The procedure is not cumbersome and, if done routinely, can be technically perfected so that it is not time-consuming. Jernigan and colleagues[10] omitted completion angiography only once in 603 cases because of technical difficulties. The 5 to 10 minutes required is time well spent if the assessment protects the patient from a poor surgical outcome. As Lane and associates[11] noted, no operation is more important than carotid endarterectomy, in which a simple oversight can result in irreversible neurologic damage or death.

The possible dangers of intraoperative completion arteriography cannot be equated with those of preoperative diagnostic arteriography. The small amount of dye used is not harmful. Iothalamate meglumine does not pass the intact blood-brain barrier. Subintimal injection of the dye resulting in occlusion of the common carotid artery has been reported

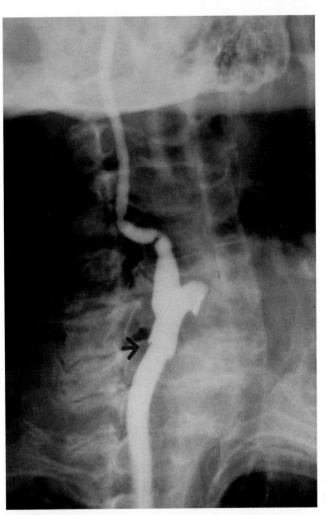

FIGURE 49–6. Completion arteriogram showing a kinked and stenotic internal carotid artery at the terminal point of the endarterectomy and occlusion of the external carotid artery. There was a pulse distal to the internal carotid stenosis, and on inspection the artery did not appear to be unduly kinked. The shelf in the common carotid artery at the proximal end of the endarterectomy is a common finding and is not considered significant if it is no more marked than in this example *(arrow)*.

percent of cases, external carotid defects in 3 percent of cases, and common carotid defects in 1 percent of cases. In our subsequent group of 308 cases, the internal carotid artery needed revision in six cases (1.94%), the external carotid in eight cases (2.6%), and the common carotid in one case (0.32%) for a total of 4.86 percent revision. In our most recently studied group of 120 cases, there were defects in the internal carotid artery in six cases (5%) and in the external carotid in three cases (2.5%).

Zierler and colleagues[7] and Courbier[8] noted 5 percent and 6 percent internal carotid defects, respectively, on completion arteriography. Andersen and colleagues[9] noted a 5.3 percent incidence of unacceptable arteriographic findings involving the common carotid, internal carotid, and external carotid arteries, and Jernigan and colleagues[10] needed to revise the endarterectomy in 2.4 percent of cases.

DISCUSSION

Vascular surgeons in general seem to accept completion arteriography for assessment of possible anastomotic or downstream intraluminal defects following femoral-popliteal and femoral-tibial bypass grafts. It is strange that they fail to do so for the internal carotid artery, which is an even more important run-off vessel in terms of risk of morbidity

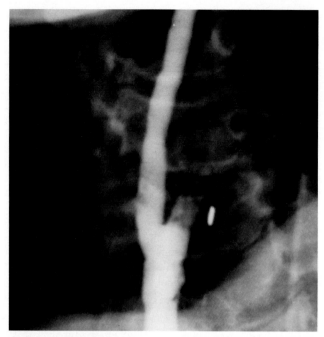

FIGURE 49–7. Occluded external carotid artery requiring transverse arteriotomy for correction.

when the needle has been directed caudad,[9] but we have had no such problem when the needle is directed cephalad. The cephalad direction of the needle is important because if dye is injected under the intima, it will flow into the area of the endarterectomy for decompression rather than flow caudad toward the aorta, possibly causing a dissection and occlusion. On withdrawal of the needle, the puncture site is under direct vision so that bleeding can be controlled with mild pressure or the use of Surgicel or, rarely, with a hemostatic stitch. It is not necessary to use a needle larger than 21

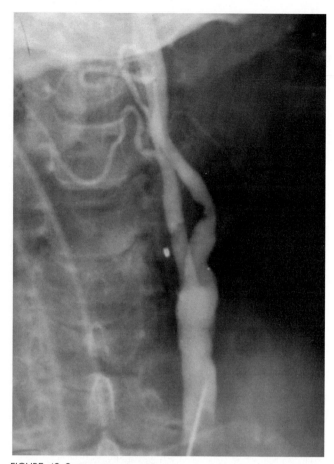

FIGURE 49–9. A greater than 30 percent stenosis of the internal carotid artery with a good pulse distal to the stenosis. Correction is required. There is an intimal flap in the external carotid artery.

gauge. In one case, an 18-gauge needle caused a hole from which fatal bleeding occurred postoperatively. The most vexing problem has been dislodgement of the needle before injection, but this problem can be avoided by careful placement of the needle and by securing of the needle to the drapes with a scratch pad (normally used for cleaning the blade of the electrocautery) or with a clamp that is removed during the actual injection.

The concentration of the dye column is important for interpretation of the film. We never use clamps on the arteries, nor do we occlude the common carotid arteries during injection, so blood continues to flow. If dye is injected when the common carotid artery is occluded, the dye column may be too concentrated and may obscure minimal defects. Forceful injection through a 21-gauge needle provides proper concentration when the x-ray machine is fired as the plunger passes the 5 to 3 mL mark on the syringe. This also provides an intracerebral angiogram.

The x-ray film is placed beneath the head of the patient so that an intracerebral angiogram is also obtained. On occasion, intracerebral arterial defects have been noted that have helped to explain postoperative neurologic deficits (see Fig. 49–11). Eleven (2.4%) intracerebral arterial defects not detected on the preoperative arteriogram were noted in a series of 457 cases intensively reviewed but not reported. Three of the 11 patients in whom an intracerebral defect was identified had a severe postoperative complication.

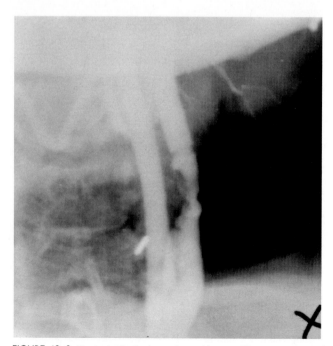

FIGURE 49–8. Fresh clot in the internal carotid artery. There was a normal pulse distal to the clot.

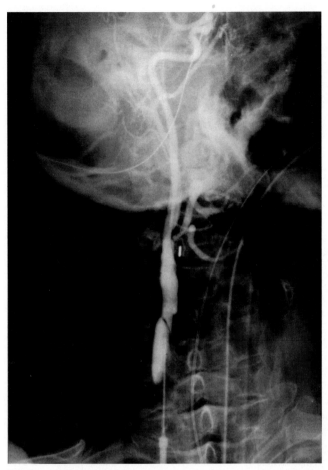

FIGURE 49–10. Intimal flap in the common carotid artery, an unusual finding.

Common carotid defects are not frequent. In the 457 cases mentioned earlier, common carotid defects were seen in only five patients, and only two of these were considered significant enough to be corrected. In one patient there was a fresh thrombus, and in the other there was a thick shelf with a moderate amount of fresh thrombus. During the operation, care is taken to fashion the proximal terminus of the endarterectomy in such a way that a thick shelf is not left. The completion angiogram usually shows a step off at the proximal point of termination of the endarterectomy (see Fig. 49–6).

The external carotid artery can supply up to 30 percent of the blood to the ipsilateral cerebral hemisphere.[12] A patent external carotid artery is essential if an extracranial-intracranial bypass is anticipated in the future,[13] and may be important for collateral blood supply if contralateral common or internal carotid occlusion develops. For these reasons, external carotid endarterectomy is a routine part of the operation, although removal of the terminal portion of the plaque is not under the surgeon's direct vision as it is in internal carotid endarterectomy. Careful attention is paid to the arteriograms, so any defects can be corrected (see Fig. 49–7). Moore and colleagues[14] showed the importance of overlooked external carotid artery intimal flaps by documenting three cases of stroke caused by thrombus in the external carotid artery protruding into the internal carotid artery.

The internal carotid artery is so important to the cerebral circulation that the surgeon performing carotid endarterectomy must be certain it is free of clot and debris and has no stenosis, intimal flaps, or kinks. Undoubtedly, after what appears to be a successful procedure, most surgeons believe they have performed a perfect operation. Surgeons who do not employ some sort of intraoperative imaging technique cannot know that they may have performed an imperfect operation. Perhaps they fall into the trap of feeling a pulse in the internal carotid artery and thinking this ensures patency, or perhaps they know most of their patients have no complications and therefore they are willing to risk submitting an occasional patient to a preventable hazard rather than learn how to master an imaging technique. Knowing that completion arteriography in femoral, popliteal, and tibial reconstructive operations often shows correctable defects should suggest that defects might also occur after carotid thromboendarterectomy.

Extension of the incision in the internal carotid artery to the end of the plaque and routine use of a shunt permit the terminal end of the plaque to be removed under direct vision; therefore tacking sutures or a patch is seldom necessary. We have rarely seen defects that could be attributed to the use of the shunt. Air bubbles, clots, and debris in the shunt are avoided by carefully placing the shunt first into the internal carotid artery above the plaque and noticing back-bleeding, and then by equally carefully placing the shunt into the common carotid artery. In only one of our early cases has "plowing" of the internal carotid intima been detected. Also, very few stenoses have been caused by suturing of the arteriotomy, because the straight in-line shunt acts as a stent during closure of the arteriotomy. Also, there have been no clamp marks on the internal carotid artery, because vessel loops are used to hold the shunt in position. Occasionally, a slight mark is observed on the internal carotid artery where the vessel loop has been located if it has been drawn up too tightly. Likewise, a faint transverse mark may be seen on the angiogram at the terminal point of the endarterectomy. Neither of these findings is considered sufficient indication for revision.

Technical defects probably account for a large percentage of postoperative morbidity and mortality after carotid endarterectomy. Scott and colleagues[15] were able to reduce their incidence of mortality from 4.8 to 1.5 percent and their incidence of perioperative stroke from 6.8 to 3.6 percent using intraoperative arteriography. We have had a similar experience. In our most recently studied series, the incidence of postoperative transient neurologic deficits was 0.65 percent, the stroke rate was 2.9 percent, and the mortality rate was 1 percent. One of the three deaths was due to stroke.

Small shreds of intima or intimal flaps that have not been removed might account for early recurrences caused by myointimal hyperplasia. In addition, they might be the nidus for later recurrence of atherosclerosis. Our known recurrence rate is less than 1%, which we attribute to very careful removal of all shreds of media, leaving a clean, shiny, endarterectomized surface.

REVIEW OF THE LITERATURE

Barnes and associates[16] reviewed the 18 publications from 1967 through 1985 on intraoperative monitoring of carotid

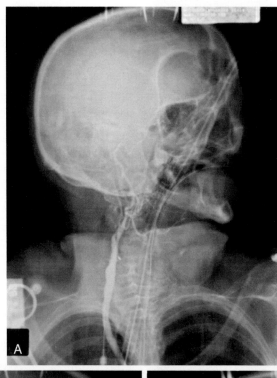

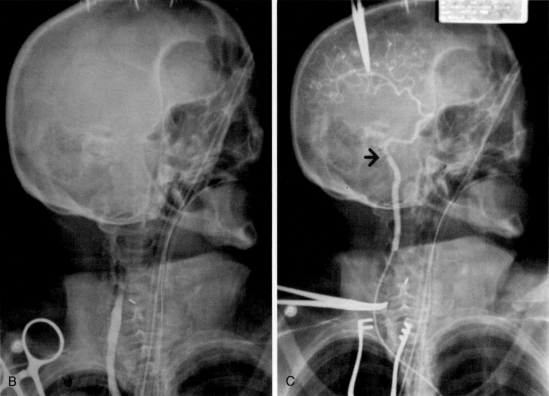

FIGURE 49–11. *A,* Completion arteriogram showing no flow in the internal carotid artery in spite of a good pulse. There is unusual filling of the common carotid artery below the site of needle insertion. *B,* A second arteriogram with the external carotid artery occluded by a vessel loop, showing blockage of the internal carotid artery and retrograde filling of the common carotid and subclavian arteries *(arrow),* indicating high resistance to forward flow. *C,* Arteriogram made with a feeding tube in the internal carotid artery, showing severe stenosis of the intracranial carotid artery *(arrow)* not appreciated on the preoperative arteriogram. (From Larson SR, Gaspar MR, Movius HJ, et al: Intraoperative arteriography in cerebrovascular surgery. In Bergan JJ, Yao JST, eds: *Cerebrovascular Insufficiency.* New York: Grune & Stratton; 1982:353; with permission.)

endarterectomy, approximately three fourths of which were done by arteriography and the remainder by noninvasive techniques. Of the 2274 reported cases, the overall incidence of residual carotid defects ranged from 5.3 to 42.9 percent, with an average of 11.9 percent. Common carotid and internal carotid artery defects were reported in 6.5 percent of cases, and external carotid artery defects in 4.4 percent. In 1494 cases in which carotid integrity was reported within 3 months of carotid endarterectomy, the incidence of defects ranged from 1.1 to 36 percent (average, 9.4%). The lowest incidence of early postoperative carotid defects was reported by Barnes and coworkers[16] (1.5%) and Blaisdell and coworkers[6] (1.1%), in the only two studies that used intraoperative monitoring techniques to identify and correct intraoperative defects. Barnes and colleagues opined that intraoperative detection and correction of defects reduced not only early residual defects but also recurrent carotid stenosis. Several authors have pointed out the relationship between defects found intraoperatively and residual lesions and also that between intraoperative defects and recurrent defects.[17–24] Teuween and associates[25] studied 33 percent of a group of patients by intravenous digital subtraction arteriography within 30 days after carotid endarterectomy. There were occlusions in 1.7 percent and more than 30 percent stenosis in 10 percent. Kinney and coworkers[24] found 5.9 percent of internal carotid arteries occluded at the first postoperative visit when intraoperative studies were omitted. It is logical to suspect that early residual lesions could result from uncorrected intraoperative defects. It is also logical to suspect that recurrent disease could result from a progression of events when minor stenoses, intimal flaps, kinks, and clots are left by failure to discover and correct them. Reilly and colleagues[20] noted a positive association between intraoperative defect size and the severity of later restenosis.

Courbier and associates[17] credit routine intraoperative carotid angiography with reducing the rate of operative mortality from 2.9 to 1 percent, that of stroke from 1.9 to 1 percent, and that of temporary neurologic deficit from 6.3 to 1 percent. The incidence of carotid restenosis was also reduced. Kinney and colleagues[24] also noted that patients with normal intraoperative flow studies had a significantly lower rate of late ipsilateral stroke.

Many investigators have employed ultrasonography,[11, 20, 26–28] angioscopy,[29] and Doppler spectral analysis[19] as well as arteriography intraoperatively to detect defects. Defects have been found by all modalities, ranging in incidence from 11 percent to 28 percent. Ultrasonography and angioscopy have tended to be too sensitive, identifying minor technical defects such as flaps only 1 to 3 mm in length.[28] It is often difficult to develop dependable criteria for determining whether the arteriotomy should be reopened, especially at the terminal end of the endarterectomy in the internal carotid artery. Investigators using ultrasonography have reopened the arteriotomy in 7 to 11 percent of cases. Using our original arteriographic criteria as a basis for determination, we have reopened the arteriotomy in approximately 8 percent of cases.

Dilley and Bernstein[30] compared B-mode ultrasonography with arteriography in 158 cases and found B-mode to be unsatisfactory in 8.2 percent because the probe did not allow examination of a high carotid bifurcation. They found the technique of B-mode scanning somewhat cumbersome, and

the number of artifacts in the image made the interpretation difficult. Their data suggested that neither intraoperative angiography nor B-mode imaging, when used alone, accurately depicted all intraoperative abnormalities.

COMMENT

Although technical defects are a preventable cause of postoperative stroke, they probably account for a large percentage of cases of postoperative morbidity and mortality after carotid endarterectomy in every surgeon's hands. Despite careful technique, residual defects are left. All investigators have reported intraoperative defects, ranging in incidence from 5 to 26 percent. Even a recent report from an experienced group noted the need to revise the endarterectomy in 13.9 percent of cases.[23] Surgeons who do not employ some type of imaging technique cannot know of the residual defects they leave, with possibly dire consequences for their patients.

We have favored intraoperative completion arteriography in nearly 2000 cases because it can be performed with equipment available in all operating rooms, it is easy to learn, x-ray films are more easily interpreted by surgeons than ultrasound images are, the entire internal carotid artery can be seen rather than just the bifurcation, and the technique affords an intracerebral study.

By using completion angiography as a means of quality control and having a heightened sensitivity to detail, we hoped to eliminate technical defects but have not been able to do so completely. We have reviewed our cases several times, and our percentage of necessary revisions has been surprisingly constant, ranging from 4.8 to 8 percent of cases. We agree with Bouchier-Hayes and colleagues[31] (emphasis is ours) that "clearly an operation which is undertaken to correct an angiographic defect should be shown to have achieved that objective *at the time of operation.*"

REFERENCES

1. Bredenberg CE, Iannettoni M, Rosenbloom M, et al: Operative angiography by intradigital subtraction angiography: A new technique for quality control of carotid endarterectomy. J Vasc Surg. 1989;9:530.
2. Roon AJ, Hoogerwerf D: Intraoperative angiography in carotid surgery. J Vasc Surg. 1992;16:239.
3. Rosental JJ, Gaspar MR, Movius HJ: Intraoperative arteriography in carotid thromboendarterectomy. Arch Surg. 1973;106:806.
4. Gaspar MR, Movius HJ, Rosental JJ: Routine intraoperative arteriography in carotid artery surgery. J Cardiovasc Surg. 1974(Spec Issue):477.
5. Larson SR, Gaspar MR, Movius HJ, et al: Intraoperative arteriography in cerebrovascular surgery. In Bergan JJ, Yao JST, eds. Cerebrovascular Insufficiency. New York: Grune & Stratton; 1982:353.
6. Blaisdell FW, Lim R Jr, Hall AD: Technical results of carotid endarterectomy: Arteriographic assessment. Am J Surg. 1967;114:239.
7. Zierler RE, Bandyk DF, Thiele BL: Intraoperative assessment of carotid endarterectomy. J Vasc Surg. 1984;1:73.
8. Courbier R: In discussion: Zierler RE, Bandyk DF, Thiele BL. Intraoperative assessment of carotid endarterectomy. J Vasc Surg. 1984;1:73.
9. Andersen CA, Collins GJ, Rich NM: Routine operative angiography during carotid endarterectomy: A reassessment. Surgery. 1978;83:67.
10. Jernigan WR, Fulton RL, Hamman JL, et al: The efficacy of routine completion operative angiography in reducing the incidence of perioperative stroke associated with carotid endarterectomy. Surgery. 1984;96:831.
11. Lane R, Ackroyd N, Appleberg M, Graham L: Application of ultrasound immediately following carotid endarterectomy. World J Surg. 1987;11:593.
12. Fields WS, Breutman ME, Weibel J: Collateral circulation of the brain. Monogr Surg Sci. 1965;2:183.
13. Connolly JE, Stemmer EA: Endarterectomy of the external carotid artery. Arch Surg. 1973;106:799.
14. Moore WS, Martello JY, Quinones-Baldrich WJ, Ahn SS: Etiologic importance

of the intimal flap of the external carotid artery in the development of post-carotid endarterectomy stroke. *Stroke.* 1990;21:1497.

15. Scott SM, Sethi GK, Bridgman AH: Perioperative stroke during carotid endarterectomy: The value of intraoperative angiography. *J Cardiovasc Surg.* 1982;23:363.

16. Barnes RW, Nix ML, Wingo JP, Nichols VT: Recurrent versus residual carotid stenosis: Incidence detected by Doppler ultrasound. *Ann Surg.* 1986;203:652.

17. Courbier R, Jausseran JM, Reggi M, et al: Routine intraoperative carotid angiography: Its impact on operative mortality and carotid restenosis. *J Vasc Surg.* 1986;2:343.

18. Sanders EACM, Hoeneveld H, Eikelboom BC, et al: Residual stenosis and early recurrent stenosis after carotid endarterectomy. *J Vasc Surg.* 1987;5:731.

19. Bandyk DB, Kaebnik HW, Adams MB, Towne JB: Turbulence occurring after carotid bifurcation endarterectomy. A harbinger of residual and recurrent carotid stenosis. *J Vasc Surg.* 1988;7:261.

20. Reilly LM, Okouhn SP, Rapp JH, et al: Recurrent carotid stenosis; A consequence of local or systemic factors? The influence of unrepaired technical defects. *J Vasc Surg.* 1990;11:448.

21. Green RN, McNamara J, Ouriel K, DeWeese JA: The clinical course of residual carotid arterial disease. *J Vasc Surg.* 1991;13:112.

22. Ricotta JJ, O'Brien MS, DeWeese JA: Natural history of recurrent residual stenosis after carotid endarterectomy: Implications for postoperative surveillance and surgical management. *Surgery.* 1992;112:656.

23. Donaldson MC, Ivarson BL, Mannick JA, Whittmore AD: Impact of completion angiography on operative conduct and results of carotid endarterectomy. *Ann Surg.* 1992;217:682.

24. Kinney EV, Seabrook GR, Kinney LY, et al: The importance of intraoperative detection of residual flow abnormalities after carotid artery endarterectomy. *J Vasc Surg.* 1993;17:912.

25. Teuween C, Eikelboom BC, Ludwig JW: Clinically unsuspected complications of arterial surgery shown by postoperative digital subtraction angiography. *Br J Radiol.* 1989;62:13.

26. Flanigan DP, Douglas DJ, Machi J, et al: Intraoperative ultrasonic imaging of the carotid artery during carotid endarterectomy. *Surgery.* 1986;100:893.

27. Schwartz RA, Peterson GA, Knowland KA, et al: Intraoperative duplex scanning after carotid artery reconstruction: A valuable tool. *J Vasc Surg.* 1988;7:620.

28. Sawchuk AP, Flanigan DP, Machi J, et al: The fate of unrepaired minor technical defects detected by intraoperative ultrasonography during carotid endarterectomy. *J Vasc Surg.* 1989;5:671.

29. Mehigan JT, Olcott C: Video angiography as an alternative to intraoperative arteriography. *Am J Surg.* 1986;152:139.

30. Dilley RB, Bernstein EF: A comparison of B-mode real time imaging and arteriography in the intraoperative assessment of carotid endarterectomy. *J Vasc Surg.* 1986;4:457.

31. Bouchier-Hayes D, DeCosta A, Macgowan WAL: The morbidity of carotid endarterectomy. *Br J Surg.* 1979;66:433.

Assessment of the Technical Results of Carotid Endarterectomy Using Real-Time Intraoperative Ultrasonography

D. PRESTON FLANIGAN

Carotid endarterectomy is the most common vascular operation performed in the United States. In 1985, approximately 107,000 carotid endarterectomies were performed, representing nearly a 10 percent increase over previous estimates.[1] Recently, the procedure has come under fire by those who believe that it may not be indicated in many patients who were previously considered candidates for the procedure. This criticism resulted in the formation of several randomized clinical trials to assess the role of carotid endarterectomy in both symptomatic and asymptomatic patients. The North American Symptomatic Carotid Endarterectomy Trial (NASCET) study was stopped prematurely because there were large differences in stroke rates in favor of surgically treated patients with greater than 70 percent stenoses. The group with lesser degrees of stenosis continues to be studied.[2] A European study showed similar preliminary results.[3] Other randomized studies are not yet completed. If these studies are to show a benefit for the surgical approach, the operative stroke rate must be minimized below currently accepted norms.

Although the incidence of stroke as a result of carotid endarterectomy is now less than 5 percent in most reported series, a considerable effort continues to be made to decrease this incidence further, thereby increasing the safety of the operation.[4–7] Although numerous factors may be implicated as causes of stroke during endarterectomy, many investigators have emphasized the importance of detecting technical errors that may occur during the operation.[5, 8–10]

Technical errors occurring during endarterectomy can result in stricture of the vessel, thrombosis, and the creation of intimal flaps. As early as 1967, Blaisdell and coworkers,[5] using intraoperative completion arteriography, showed that these defects occurred in 26 percent of carotid endarterectomies. Although it is not yet proved, it seems logical that detection and correction of these defects before the termination of a surgical procedure would be important in lessening morbidity from the operation. Other means of detection of technical defects such as inspection and palpation of the artery are highly subjective and are probably not reliable methods of detecting intraluminal defects.[5, 8] The combination of pulsed Doppler and spectrum analysis was reported by Zierler and associates,[9] and although the method was shown to be quite sensitive, subsequent intraoperative arteriography was required to provide an image of the defect. Thus, sound spectrum analysis can detect flow disturbances, but an image is much more valuable in the specific identification of the type of defect and in the decision process regarding repair of the defect.

Many investigators have suggested that intraoperative carotid arteriography be used routinely to detect intraoperative defects.[5, 8, 11–13] It is well known, however, that arteriography is an invasive procedure and may result in stroke,[14] new intraluminal defects,[15] radiation exposure to patient and surgeon alike, and adverse reactions to contrast.[16] A further shortcoming of arteriography is that it provides only a static image in a single plane at one point in time. The incidence of complication following routine intraoperative arteriography has been small, but a safer noninvasive method for the detection of defects would be preferable, particularly if such a method were even more accurate than arteriography. Intraoperative high-resolution real-time B-mode ultrasonography seems to meet these criteria.

LABORATORY INVESTIGATION

Before intraoperative ultrasonography was employed in the clinical arena, it was evaluated experimentally in the animal laboratory in a canine model. Defects consisting of intimal flaps, strictures, intraluminal thrombi, and subintimal hematomas were surgically created in a series of canine aortas and femoral arteries.[17] The accuracy of ultrasonography in correctly identifying these defects was then evaluated by several blinded observers. Ultrasonography correctly identified all strictures, intraluminal thrombi, and subintimal hematomas. All intimal flaps 2 mm or greater in size were also identified correctly; however, intimal flaps measuring 1 mm or less were correctly identified in only 68 percent of cases. In 90 percent of cases, measurement of the flap size was within 1 mm of the actual size of the flap. The correlation coefficient between actual flap size and ultrasonically measured flap size was 0.84.

Although ultrasonography was highly accurate in the correct identification of intraluminal defects, the experiment did not determine its accuracy in comparison with the standard of intraoperative arteriography. To assess this relationship, defects were once again created in canine aortas, but this time the defects were evaluated not only with intraoperative ultrasonography but also with both portable and serial biplane arteriography. Results of this experiment indicated that all three techniques were equally accurate in detecting strictures but that ultrasonography was more accurate and sensitive than both types of arteriography in detecting intimal flaps and intraluminal thrombi.[18]

With intraoperative ultrasonography established as more accurate than arteriography, it was decided to evaluate the technique clinically in the intraoperative evaluation of carotid endarterectomy sites.

CLINICAL EXPERIENCE

Over a 5-year period, 155 carotid endarterectomies were evaluated by intraoperative ultrasonic examination. The examination was performed at the completion of the endarterectomy, following closure of the arteriotomy and re-establishment of carotid artery flow. The wound was filled with

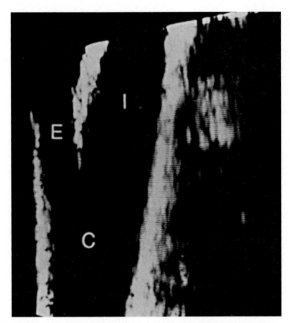

FIGURE 50–1. Intraoperative ultrasonography illustrating normal carotid bifurcation. C, common carotid; I, internal carotid; E, external carotid. (From Flanigan DP, Douglas DJ, Machi J: Intraoperative ultrasonic imaging of the carotid artery during carotid endarterectomy. *Surgery*. 1986;5:893; with permission.)

sterile saline to provide acoustic coupling between the ultrasound probe and the carotid artery. A variety of real-time B-mode instruments using either a 7.5- or 10-MHz probe (Biosound, Cooper, Diasonics, High Stoy, Technicare) were used.

Depending on the type of instrumentation, the probe was either gas sterilized or covered by a sterile disposable plastic sleeve filled with acoustic gel. A hand-held probe was used to perform multiple transverse and longitudinal scans of the common, external, and internal carotid arteries in each procedure. The entire endarterectomy site as well as areas of application of vascular clamps was examined for defects. Hard-copy data were kept on videocassette or Polaroid prints. An example of a normal postendarterectomy intraoperative carotid sonogram delineating the carotid bifurcation is shown in Figure 50–1.

During this series of operations, the decision to re-enter the carotid artery and correct the defect was based on the type, size, and location of the defect. Criteria were very subjective; defects were corrected if the operating surgeons considered them to pose a significant risk of stroke if left uncorrected. Two examples of such defects are shown in Figures 50–2 and 50–3.

The technical results of 155 endarterectomies were assessed in 143 patients with a mean age of 63 years. Intraluminal defects created as a result of surgery were detected by intraoperative ultrasonography in 43 of the 155 procedures (27.7%). More than one defect was present in six arteries. The types of defects and location of each are listed in Table 50–1. Intimal flaps accounted for 73 percent of the defects. Strictures accounted for 18 percent of the defects. Miscellaneous defects, such as arterial kinks, residual plaque, and intraluminal thrombi, accounted for the rest.

A decision not to re-enter the artery was made for 32 of the 43 arteries with ultrasonically detected defects (74%). Eleven of the 43 arteries (26%) that contained defects were re-entered for the purpose of correcting the defect. In 2 of these 11 arteries, more than one defect was present. Overall,

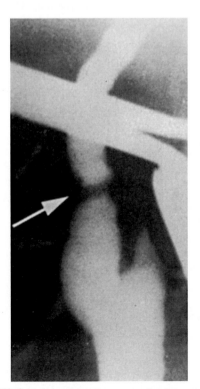
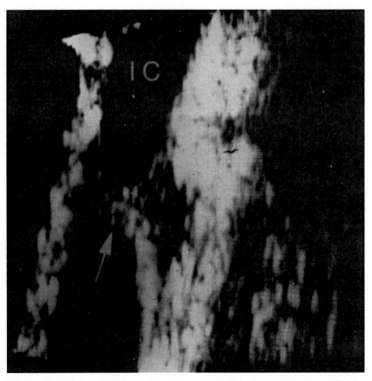

FIGURE 50–2. Arteriogram and corresponding intraoperative ultrasonography showing a clamp injury to the internal carotid artery. IC, internal carotid. (From Flanigan DP, Douglas DJ, Machi J: Intraoperative ultrasonic imaging of the carotid artery during carotid endarterectomy. *Surgery*. 1986;5:893; with permission.)

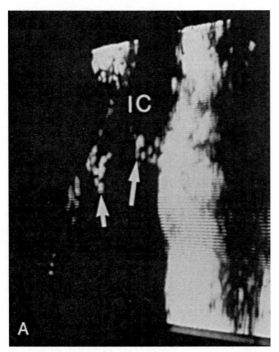
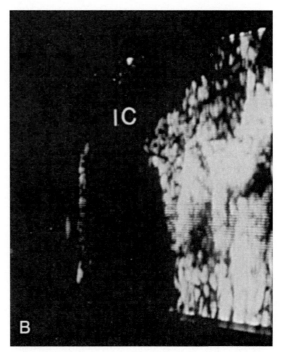

FIGURE 50–3. *A,* Intraoperative ultrasonography appearance of an intimal flap in the internal carotid (IC) artery. *B,* Ultrasonography of same segment of IC artery after correction of the defect. (From Flanigan DP, Douglas DJ, Machi J: Intraoperative ultrasonic imaging of the carotid artery during carotid endarterectomy. *Surgery.* 1986;5:893; with permission.)

7 percent (11 of 155) of the endarterectomy sites were re-entered on the basis of ultrasonic findings for the purpose of defect correction. In all cases, defects corresponding to those detected by ultrasonography were found upon reentry.

Patients were followed for the purpose of determining subsequent outcome. Follow-up was complete for 94 percent of the 155 endarterectomies. The mean length of follow-up was 13 months, with a range of 1 to 58 months. Permanent ipsilateral neurologic defects occurred in four patients within 30 days of operation, for an incidence of 2.8 percent. Three patients had a contralateral hemiparesis upon awakening from anesthesia, and one patient had an occlusion of the operated internal carotid artery 6 hours postoperatively. One additional patient had a transient contralateral hemiparesis that completely resolved within the first month postoperatively, for a temporary neurologic deficit rate of 0.7 percent. Cranial nerve injury occurred in 18 patients, for an incidence of 12.4 percent. Seventy-eight percent of these injuries had resolved at the time of last follow-up. Eight patients died during follow-up. Two of these deaths occurred within the first postoperative month, for an operative mortality of 1.5 percent.

Patients were divided into three groups for the purpose of comparing the incidence of postoperative stroke and cranial nerve injury. Group I had 104 endarterectomies available for follow-up in which no defect was found by ultrasonography.

TABLE 50–1. Distribution of Technical Defects Detected by Intraoperative Ultrasonography

Type of Defect	Total	ICA	ECA	CCA
Flap (mm)				
1	6	4	1	1
2	18	5	8	5
3	9	2 (1 corrected)	3 (2 corrected)	4
5	2	1 (corrected)	1	0
7	1	0	0	1 (corrected)
Total	36			
Stricture (%)				
20	4	0	4	0
30	1	1 (corrected)	0	0
40	1	1 (corrected)	0	0
50	3	3 (corrected)	0	0
Total	9			
Kink	2	1 (corrected)	1	0
Plaque	1	0	1 (corrected)	0
Thrombus	1	1 (corrected)	0	0

CCA, common carotid artery; ECA, external carotid artery; ICA, internal carotid artery.

TABLE 50–2. Incidence of Stroke and Cranial Nerve Injury

	Group I	Group II	Group III
Total endarterectomies, n	112	32	11
Available for follow-up, n	104	30	11
Mean follow-up, mo	13.5	12.6	13.2
Mean age, y	62.2	64.2	64.6
Perioperative stroke, n	4 (3.8%)	1 (3.3%)	0
Cranial nerve injury, n	10 (9.6%)	6 (20%)	2 (18%)

Group II had 30 endarterectomies available for follow-up in which technical defects were detected by ultrasonography but were not corrected. Group III had 11 endarterectomies available for follow-up in which defects were found by ultrasound and corrected (Table 50–2). The mean age and length of follow-up were not statistically different among the three groups (Student's t-test). Likewise, the incidence of stroke was not statistically different (χ^2 analysis). Cranial nerve injury occurred twice as frequently in groups II and III compared with group I; however, this difference was not statistically significant (χ^2 analysis). There was no complication in this series of endarterectomies, which could be attributable to the use of intraoperative ultrasonography.

This review suggests that the correction of defects judged to be a potential cause of stroke can be accomplished without additional neurologic complication. This is supported by the fact that the incidence of perioperative stroke was no different between the group of patients in whom the defect was corrected (group III) and the group of patients with a normal intraoperative ultrasonographic examination (group I). In addition, the retraction and manipulation involved with re-entering the artery and correcting the defect did not appear to lead to a higher incidence of cranial nerve injury, since the incidence was no different in group III as compared with groups I and II.

Defects judged by the operating surgeons as being significant enough to be a potential cause of stroke are illustrated in Table 50–3. Internal carotid artery defects represented 39 percent of all defects, but 70 percent of the defects were repaired. All strictures greater than 30 percent were repaired, as were most large intimal flaps. Kinks and thrombi were also considered significant enough for repair. External

carotid artery defects were corrected only when they coexisted with another defect thought to require repair.

A major problem with all types of intraoperative assessment for the detection of technical error is the determination of which defects are significant enough to warrant repair. The data presented suggest that intimal flaps less than or equal to 1 mm in the internal carotid artery, 1 to 3 mm intimal flaps in the common and external carotid arteries, and stenoses less than 30 percent can be left unrepaired without early sequelae. The data do not address, however, the subsequent fate of unrepaired defects. It is conceivable that such unrepaired defects might increase the incidence of recurrent carotid stenosis or carotid occlusion.

In order to assess this possibility, the author and colleagues[19] followed 80 carotid endarterectomies with serial postoperative duplex scans for 1 to 96 months (mean of 32 months). In this group, 21 arteries had shown minor defects on intraoperative ultrasonographic scans. Sixteen of the 19 intimal flaps had healed by the time of the first postoperative duplex scan (mean time after surgery, 27.5 months). Two of two stenoses were resolved by the first postoperative study as well. Of the remaining three intimal flaps, a 2 mm common carotid artery flap resolved by 52 months after surgery, a 1 mm internal carotid artery intimal flap was associated with a stable 30 percent stenosis at 37 months, and a 2 mm external carotid artery intimal flap was associated with occlusion of the external carotid artery at 45 months follow-up. These data suggest that minor technical defects as described earlier may be left unrepaired without long-term sequelae. Given the benign nature of these defects, it seems unwise to reclamp and reopen a carotid artery to repair these lesions and assume the potential risks inherent in that maneuver.

Duplex ultrasonography has also been used intraoperatively to assess the technical results of carotid endarterectomy. Schwartz and coworkers[20] studied 84 carotid endarterectomies and noted technical errors in 22 percent. Eleven percent of the defects were repaired. These numbers are similar to those presented for imaging ultrasound. No conclusion could be made regarding the superiority of one technique over the other, since the study was not designed for that purpose. The investigators did note a correlation between imaging and Doppler data, but large standard deviations in the Doppler data did not allow the determination of a velocity value that could be used to differentiate between normal and abnormal studies.

This author has used duplex scanning intraoperatively for the past 5 years with success equal to that achieved with imaging ultrasonography alone. The addition of pulsed Doppler is beneficial mainly in patients in whom the internal carotid ultrasonic image is suboptimal. No strict criteria have yet been developed for an abnormal intraoperative carotid artery velocity. Currently, I use 150 cm/second in the internal carotid artery as a cutoff value; values above this are considered abnormal. If the image demonstrates a benign lesion thought to be responsible for the abnormal velocity, re-exploration of the artery is not performed. If a normal sound spectrum is detected, arteriography is not performed. An abnormal Doppler spectrum, with or without a normal image, is considered an indication for arteriography to identify the lesion so that a decision can be made regarding the

TABLE 50–3. Type and Location of Technical Defects Corrected

Patient No.	Type of Defect	Location
1	3 mm flap	ICA
	3 mm flap	ECA
2	3 mm flap	ECA
	3 mm plaque	ECA
3	5 mm flap	ICA
4	7 mm flap	CCA
5	30% stenosis	ICA
6	40% stenosis	ICA
7	50% stenosis	ICA
8	50% stenosis	ICA
9	50% stenosis	ICA
10	Kink	ICA
11	Plaque	ICA

CCA, common carotid artery; ECA, external carotid artery; ICA, internal carotid artery.

need for repair. Further study will be required to determine whether these criteria are appropriate.

From a practical standpoint, intraoperative ultrasonography cannot always be employed in carotid endarterectomy. On occasion, very distal lesions may preclude adequate insonation of the distal internal carotid artery. If duplex scanning or stand-alone pulsed Doppler is available and can be used to obtain spectral data from the distal internal carotid artery, it should be employed. If the spectral data are abnormal or cannot be satisfactorily obtained, arteriography should be performed.

Regarding the practical application of the procedure, surgeons should not be concerned about the difficulty of learning the technical aspects of intraoperative ultrasonography. Several surgeons have been trained at our institution, and the learning curve has been quite short. Since intraoperative ultrasound has also been shown to be useful in many other surgical specialties, a single operative ultrasound machine with the appropriate number of specialty probes should get frequent use. Many companies have developed relatively inexpensive units for this purpose.

Since intraluminal defects will continue to occur after carotid endarterectomy, and because these defects represent a potential stroke risk, there will continue to be a need for intraoperative assessment of the technical results of carotid endarterectomy. Intraoperative ultrasonography appears to be a safe, highly accurate method of intraoperative assessment. Because of its safety and accuracy, it appears to be the best current method of intraoperative assessment in most patients. Regardless of the techniques employed, however, some type of objective intraoperative assessment of the technical results of carotid endarterectomy should be used if strokes from technical errors are to be prevented.

REFERENCES

1. Ernst CB, Rutkow IM, Cleveland RJ, et al: A report of the Joint Society for Vascular Surgery–International Society for Cardiovascular Surgery Committee on Vascular Surgical Manpower. *J Vasc Surg.* 1987;6:611.
2. NASCET collaborators: Beneficial effect of carotid endarterectomy in symptomatic patients with high grade carotid stenosis. *N Engl J Med.* 1991;325:445.
3. European carotid trialists' (ECST) collaborative group: MRC European carotid surgery interim results for symptomatic patients with severe (70–90%) or mild (0–29%) carotid stenosis. *Lancet.* 1991;337:1235.
4. Thompson JE, Talkington CM: Carotid endarterectomy. *Ann Surg.* 1976;184:1.
5. Blaisdell FW, Lim R, Hall AD: Technical result of carotid endarterectomy: Arteriographic assessment. *Am J Surg.* 1967;114:239.
6. Steed DL, Peitzman AB, Grundy BL, Webster MW: Causes of stroke in carotid endarterectomy. *Surgery.* 1982;92:634.
7. Collins GJ, Rich NM, Anderson CA, McDonald PT: Stroke associated with carotid endarterectomy. *Am J Surg.* 1978;135:221.
8. Rosental JJ, Gaspar MR, Movius HJ: Intraoperative angiography in carotid thromboendarterectomy. *Arch Surg.* 1973;106:806.
9. Zierler RE, Bandyk DF, Thiele BL: Intraoperative assessment of carotid endarterectomy. *J Vasc Surg.* 1984;1:73.
10. Lane SR, Appleberg M: Real-time intraoperative angiosonography after carotid endarterectomy. *Surgery.* 1982;1:5.
11. Plecha FR, Pories WJ: Intraoperative angiography in the immediate assessment of arterial reconstruction. *Arch Surg.* 1972;105:902.
12. Bowald S, Eriksson I, Fagerberg S: Intraoperative angiography in arterial surgery. *Acta Chir Scand.* 1978;114:463.
13. Dardik II, Ibrahim IM, Sprayregen S, et al: Routine intraoperative angiography. *Arch Surg.* 1975;110:184.
14. Anderson CA, Collins GJ, Rich NM: Routine operative arteriography during carotid endarterectomy: A reassessment. *Surgery.* 1978;83:67.
15. Pories WJ, Plecha FR, Castele TJ, Strain WH: Complications of arteriography and phlebography. In Beebe GH, ed. *Complications in Vascular Surgery.* Philadelphia: JB Lippincott; 1973:1.
16. Ansell G: Adverse reactions to contrast agents: Scope of problem. *Invest Radiol.* 1970;5:373.
17. Coelho JCU, Sigel B, Flanigan DP, et al: Detection of arterial defects by real-time ultrasound scanning during vascular surgery: An experimental study. *J Surg Res.* 1981;30:535.
18. Coelho JCU, Sigel B, Flanigan DP, et al: An experimental evaluation of arteriography and imaging ultrasonography in detecting arterial defects at operation. *J Surg Res.* 1982;32:130.
19. Sawchuk AP, Flanigan DP, Machi J, et al: The fate of unrepaired minor technical defects by intraoperative ultrasonography during carotid endarterectomy. *J Vasc Surg.* 1989;9:671.
20. Schwartz RA, Peterson GJ, Noland KA, et al: Intraoperative duplex scanning after carotid artery reconstruction: A valuable tool. *J Vasc Surg.* 1988;7:620.

CHAPTER 51

Surgery for Fibromuscular Dysplasia of the Carotid Artery: Indications, Technique, and Results

DAVID J. EFFENEY

Leadbetter and Burkland[1] described a young man in 1938 who had correctable hypertension as a result of unilateral renal artery dysplasia. Twenty years later, McCormack and coworkers[2] described four types of obstructive disease of the renal artery and called one of them fibromuscular hyperplasia. This disorder was thought to be confined to the renal arteries until 1964, when Palubinskas and Ripley[3] described fibromuscular disease in the internal carotid artery. A year later, Connett and Lansche[4] published the first histologic proof that the carotid artery is affected by fibromuscular dysplasia. Since then, fibromuscular disease has been shown to involve many of the medium-size arteries, including celiac, hepatic, superior mesenteric, and external iliac arteries.[5] In addition to the carotid arteries, the vertebral arteries may be involved with fibromuscular disease; the disorder has now been described in the intracranial arteries and is associated with intracranial aneurysms.[6, 7] This chapter deals with this curious disorder as it affects patients with extracranial carotid involvement.

PATHOLOGY

There are four distinct histologic types of fibromuscular dysplasia: intimal fibroplasia, medial fibroplasia, medial hyperplasia, and perimedial dysplasia.[8] The most common form affecting the carotid artery is medial fibroplasia. Fibromuscular dysplasia is not a generalized disorder. The disease affects segments of long arteries having few primary branches that serve as the origin of vasa vasorum to the parent vessel. The relationship of estrogens and other feminizing hormones to the development and progression of fibromuscular disease has been the subject of considerable speculation because of the marked female predominance in the reported series. There is no evidence to incriminate oral contraceptives or postmenopausal estrogen therapy as causative agents of the disease, but the feminizing hormones may have a facilitatory role in the development and progression of this disorder.

The reported pathologic observations in resected arteries, backed up by experimental work, have led to a concept of pathogenesis. The proposed model involves medium-size arteries that are somewhat longer than normal, the middle segments of which have a relatively poorer blood supply derived from vasa vasorum than that of vessels of normal length. In this situation, normal stresses on the arterial wall may lead to disruption of the internal elastic lamina and medial damage. The medial damage, in the presence of the continuing stresses, progresses to one or another of the histologic types of dysplasia, depending on which artery is involved, the depth of the medial injury, and the mechanisms of attempted repair. All these mechanisms may be modified by the hormonal environment.[9, 10]

ASSOCIATED CONDITIONS

Although the mean age of patients operated on for fibromuscular disease of the extracranial carotid artery is almost a decade younger than that of patients presenting with atherosclerotic disease, and despite the gender differences in the two cohorts, about 18 percent of patients have significant atherosclerosis of the carotid bulb as well as fibromuscular dysplasia of the middle segment of the carotid artery. Intracranial aneurysm is well recognized as being associated with extracranial fibromuscular disease. In a review of 101 patients at the University of California–San Francisco, Effeney and colleagues[11] reported that of the 35 patients with technically satisfactory intracranial views at the time of their initial arteriograms, five had intracranial aneurysms. The other major known association of extracranial fibromuscular disease is spontaneous dissection. Twelve percent of patients with a carotid dissection have evidence of fibromuscular disease in the contralateral internal carotid artery. The other arteries that were proved to be affected by fibromuscular disease in a cohort of 80 patients whose arteriograms were all reviewed by this author personally are shown in Table 51–1.

CLINICAL FEATURES

The largest reported series of patients with fibromuscular disease is from the University of California–San Francisco.[9, 11–15] The major symptoms and physical findings of 101 of these patients who have been previously reported are shown in Table 51–2. It must be remembered that all these patients underwent surgical correction of their fibromuscular dysplasia, and the table does not purport to show the total picture of the presentation of patients with fibromuscular disease. Stewart and associates[16] reported on 49 patients with fibromuscular dysplasia. That cohort was derived differently in that the investigators reviewed the records of patients with angiographically proven but mostly unoperated fibromuscular disease. In their group, only 22 percent were asymptomatic, and the largest number (29%) had transient ischemic attacks. Three patients (6%) had had completed strokes; the same number of patients had had

TABLE 51–1. Other Arteries Affected by Fibromuscular Disease in 80 Patients*

Artery	N
Renal	27
External iliac	8
Vertebral	6

*In addition, intracranial aneurysms were found in 5 of 35 patients.

TABLE 51–2. Major Symptoms and Physical Findings in 101
Patients With Fibromuscular Disease

Symptoms/Physical Findings	%
Symptoms	
Transient ischemic attack	41
Nonlocalizing neurologic	31
Bruit heard by patient	23
Amaurosis fugax	23
Completed stroke	22
Asymptomatic bruit	8
Prolonged ischemic attack	2
Other	6
Physical findings at presentation	
Carotid bruit	77
Hypertension	37
Electrocardiogram abnormality	17
Neurologic deficit	9

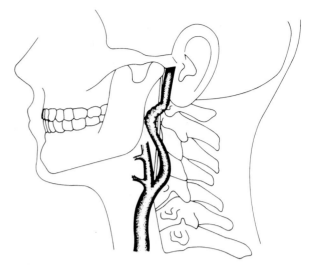

FIGURE 51–1. The internal carotid artery affected by fibromuscular dysplasia. Note that the artery is longer than normal, with the carotid bifurcation at the C4 disc. The artery is serpiginous. Fibromuscular dysplasia affects the midportion of the vessel, sparing the proximal and distal segments.

intracerebral hemorrhage at the time of presentation. Two other series reported symptoms at presentation remarkably similar to those reported in the San Francisco series.[10, 17] There is a disturbingly high incidence of completed stroke in this relatively young group of people, and a significant number of patients present with a residual neurologic deficit—in our experience, 9 percent. Kelly and Morris,[18] in their report of 25 patients undergoing operation, reported four patients who presented with stroke, for an incidence of 16 percent.

Fibromuscular disease causes a wide variety of symptoms. We do not know, however, what proportion of patients who have the disease anatomically will develop symptoms requiring operation.

ARTERIOGRAPHIC FINDINGS

The arteriograms of 80 patients with extracranial fibromuscular disease were personally reviewed; the comments in this section are based on that experience. Internal carotid arteries affected by fibromuscular disease are longer than those in normal patients and those who present with atherosclerosis (Fig. 51–1). The bifurcation of the carotid artery is usually at or below the C4 or C5 disc level. If the bifurcation is high, the internal carotid artery is frequently coiled or kinked. The lesions of fibromuscular disease are most commonly seen opposite the C1–C2 vertebral bodies, as fibromuscular disease affects the middle and extends into the distal third of the cervical portion of the carotid artery. The disease spares the proximal and most distal portions of the vessel.

Fibromuscular disease may be unilateral but much more commonly is bilateral. Frequently, one carotid artery displays signs of more advanced disease than the artery on the opposite side. There are three types of appearance of fibromuscular disease in the extracranial carotid artery. The classic string-of-beads sign is the most common, although a very localized lesion and the tubular form of fibromuscular disease are not uncommon.[6, 19, 20] The finding of a carotid dissection at the time of arteriography should lead to the examination of other vessels known to be at risk for fibromuscular disease.[9, 11] Because of the association of hypertension and carotid bifurcation atherosclerosis and the possibil-

ity of fibromuscular disease in other vascular beds, the arteriographic technique for all patients presenting with fibromuscular disease should be modified to define all the vessels involved. The intracranial vasculature must be included to enable us to define the true radiologic instance of simultaneously involved arteries and to better document asymptomatic aneurysms. Thus the angiographic technique should include an arch injection as well as selective carotid injections with intracranial views. In addition, a midstream aortogram should be performed to demonstrate the renal and external iliac arteries. The proximal visceral arteries are the only major vessels at risk that are not adequately demonstrated by this standard angiographic technique. The advances in digital subtraction imaging over the past few years suggest that these vessels should also be routinely imaged.

MECHANISM OF SYMPTOM PRODUCTION

Although it is true that extracranial fibromuscular disease often remains asymptomatic, the experience from San Francisco and other reported series confirms that once the patient develops symptoms related to fibromuscular disease, the course of the disease cannot be considered benign. Most patients develop neurologic symptoms and suffer transient ischemic attacks, amaurosis fugax, or completed strokes that are considered by many to be embolic phenomena.

Despite a substantial 18 percent incidence of associated atherosclerosis in our symptomatic cohort, corroborated by Stewart and coworkers'[16] incidence of about 20 percent, this cannot explain the majority of patients in whom focal neurologic symptoms and signs are their mode of presentation. The cause of symptoms in patients without associated atherosclerosis is still in question. Possibilities include thromboembolism of clot and platelet aggregates from the aneurysmal dilatations in the vessel, hypoperfusion due to a single critical stenosis or subcritical stenoses in series, or hypoperfusion on the basis of multiple-vessel involvement.

In some patients with fibromuscular disease, the symptoms may be caused by associated hypertension, extension of the disorder into the intracranial vessel, or intracranial aneurysm. Whatever the precise mechanism in individual patients, it is apparent that symptomatic patients must be evaluated carefully to determine some form of therapeutic intervention.

INDICATIONS FOR OPERATION

It was suggested by Patman and associates[21] that operation is unwarranted in all patients with fibromuscular disease until the natural history of the disease is "more clearly defined." This line of argument was further advanced by Stewart and colleagues[16] in their publication about the natural history of carotid fibromuscular dysplasia. This statement is so reasonable that it is difficult to dispute, as long as the patient remains asymptomatic. The dilemma remains, however, because the first symptom of carotid fibrodysplastic disease may be a completed stroke. Stewart and coworkers[16] argued that it may not be appropriate to apply criteria similar to those generally accepted for operations for atherosclerosis because the natural history of carotid fibromuscular dysplasia is different, but a study of their data leads to the conclusion that they have not proved their point.

Like Stewart and colleagues, I do not believe that asymptomatic patients with fibromuscular disease of the extracranial carotid artery should undergo surgery. These patients should be entered into a centralized register for systematic follow-up evaluation so that we can learn about the natural history of this disease. Fibromuscular disease is uncommon, and this, coupled with the lack of knowledge of the natural history, makes decision-making difficult when an individual physician is confronted with a patient with fibromuscular disease of the carotid artery. Studies of patients followed up at the University of California indicate that once carotid fibromuscular disease becomes symptomatic, serious neurologic sequelae commonly follow; in fact, 22 percent of patients have completed strokes. The wide variety and relative severity of the antecedent neurologic events point out the need for careful individual evaluation of these patients.

Most of these patients have been treated with aspirin and many with dipyridamole, yet their symptoms persisted at the time of presentation for surgical evaluation. There are no data to demonstrate the efficacy of any of these agents of medical treatment in patients whose symptoms are due to fibromuscular disease. Thus I believe that the symptoms that are valid indications for carotid reconstruction in atherosclerotic cohorts remain valid indications for patients with fibromuscular disease as well.

SURGICAL METHODS

The precise technique chosen in the management of patients with fibromuscular disease must be influenced by the location and extent of the disease process. If the lesion is in the accessible portion of the internal carotid artery, resection and primary anastomosis or autograft replacement may be feasible.[13, 14] Originally, standard surgical techniques were used in resection operations.[22] Primary anastomosis or saphenous vein or autologous artery interposition grafts were used to replace the diseased vessels. Carotid endarterectomy, without a shunt, was used in all patients who required this procedure for associated bifurcation atherosclerosis, and 4 percent of our patients underwent contralateral carotid endarterectomy. Since 1970, almost all patients have been treated by the graduated dilatation method described by Morris and coworkers.[23] No patients have been operated on for fibromuscular disease of the vertebral arteries.

INTRALUMINAL DILATATION

Intraluminal dilatation should be performed under general anesthesia. When bilateral carotid dilatations are undertaken, the procedures are staged a week apart. A transverse or slightly oblique skin crease incision is placed over the carotid bulb. The placement of this incision must be based on the findings of the preoperative arteriogram because of the high incidence of low carotid bifurcations in the patient cohort. The internal, external, and common carotid arteries are circumferentially cleaned from their investing fascia. Once these vessels have been mobilized, they are surrounded by soft rubber slings.

The key to this procedure is straightening the internal carotid artery. To achieve this, the vessel is mobilized high in the neck, at least to the level of the styloid process. The carotid sinus nerve can be divided, if necessary, to achieve further caudal movement of the bulb and enable the vessel to be straightened. The patient should be heparinized at the completion of the dissection, with sufficient time allowed for the heparin effect to be obtained before application of clamps to the external and common carotid arteries.

We have measured the stump or backflow pressure in all patients undergoing internal carotid artery dilatation and have not encountered any patient whose stump pressure was so low that shunting was required to preserve hemispheric blood flow. In those patients who do not require ipsilateral carotid endarterectomy, a 1 cm long arteriotomy is placed longitudinally in the carotid bulb. Two techniques are then available to ensure safe passage of the dilator. The first (Fig. 51–2A) involves caudal retraction on the internal carotid artery by means of a rubber sling during the passage of the dilators. Alternatively, the internal carotid artery may be supported by the fingers of the left hand and straightened while the dilator is passed cephalad (see Fig. 51–2B). A 1.5 mm dilator is used initially and passed into the carotid artery until resistance is encountered. Gentle pressure is applied with the artery completely straight, and the advance of the instrument is accompanied by loss of this resistance. Figure 51–3 shows the mechanisms involved in the disruption of the dysplastic membrane by passage of the dilator. Increasingly large dilators are then used to dilate the carotid progressively to the skull base. If the vessel is small, we use a maximum size of 3.5 mm; a larger dilator increases the risk of damage to the disease-free intima. For normal-size vessels, a maximum 4 mm dilator is used. When the final dilator has been removed, we allow a few seconds of vigorous backbleeding from the internal carotid artery to wash out any unattached intimal fragments or small thrombi. A clamp or forceps may be used to occlude the internal carotid artery. The short arteriotomy is closed with a continuous 6-0 suture. Using this technique, the entire occlusive phase of the proce-

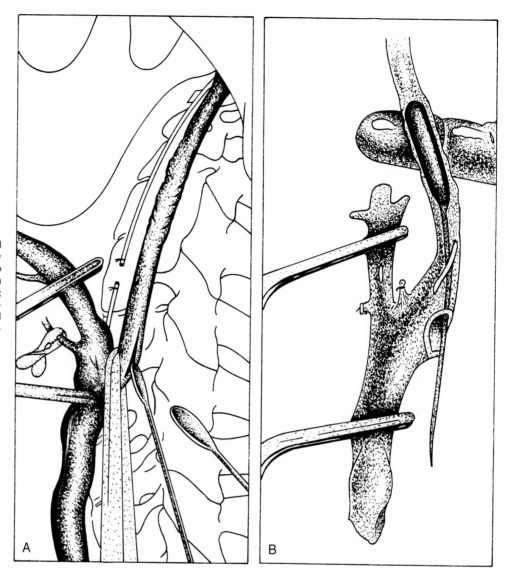

FIGURE 51–2. Two techniques used to control the internal carotid artery while the dilator is being passed into the artery. *A*, Caudal retraction on the sling straightens the artery during passage of the dilator. *B*, The fingers of the left hand control and straighten the artery during dilatation.

dure can be accomplished within 3 to 5 minutes. Since 1970, two patients have required resection of redundant carotid arteries combined with intraluminal dilatation.

An article by Lord and coworkers[24] described a technique of radiologic control of operative carotid dilatation. The technique involves interruption of carotid flow for up to 40 minutes. These workers argue that the method minimizes the risk of damaging the artery at the base of the skull while allowing immediate visualization of the result. I do not believe that intraoperative radiologic control offers any advantage over manually controlled rigid dilatation of the totally mobilized cervical carotid artery.

RESULTS OF THERAPY

To assess the outcome of patients managed surgically, we applied criteria previously published but generally accepted for other reconstructions of the extracranial carotid artery.[12] These criteria are as follows:

1. The lesion should be surgically accessible.

2. The operation must be performed with minimal risk to the patient.

3. The operative repair must be durable.

4. The benefits from the repair must be long lasting.

The results of treatment support the conclusion that the treatment of symptomatic fibromuscular disease is safe. In 150 operations in 101 patients, there were no deaths. The technique of intraluminal dilatation allows the accessibility requirement to be fulfilled. It obviates the need to attempt replacement of the carotid artery at the base of the skull, where exposure and control present great technical challenges. There was one instance of perforation in 150 dilatations. When this complication was reported,[9] the comment was made that it reinforced the absolute need for high mobilization and straightening of the carotid artery prior to passage of the rigid dilator.

The operation must be performed with meticulous attention to detail. If this is done, there can be an acceptably low morbidity accompanying the zero mortality figure. There were three early postoperative strokes in the 101 patients. Nine other patients had transient neurologic deficits or amau-

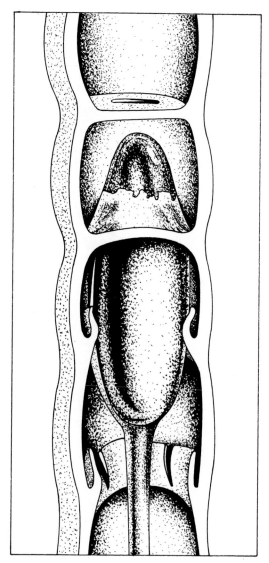

FIGURE 51–3. Radial rupture of dysplastic membranes during operative dilatation.

rosis fugax during the early postoperative period. The nonneurologic complications of the surgical management of symptomatic fibromuscular disease are the same as those seen with carotid endarterectomy and occur with the same frequency.

Early patency immediately after dilatation has been confirmed by arteriography routinely during the first few days after surgery, and some patients have been studied serially for up to 5 years. The durability of dilatation has been confirmed by these studies. In only one patient has a previously dilated artery been found to be occluded. Two patients underwent reoperation; one required redilatation 1 year after the first procedure for three episodes of transient ischemia due to a persistent band, and one had a subsequent carotid endarterectomy. In the long term, patients have been followed for up to 17 years. Three patients had strokes during this period, one of which was known to be caused by an embolus to the right middle cerebral artery 6 months after operation; in the other two cases, the cause of the stroke is unknown. Importantly, two patients had subarach-

noid hemorrhage from associated intracranial aneurysms, and neither of these patients had appropriate intracranial views prior to dilatation. Three patients represent inappropriate patient selection. They continue to have generalized neurologic symptoms with only minimal improvement since their initial presentation, despite a documented satisfactory anatomic repair.

DISCUSSION

Fibromuscular disease remains an enigma. Although reports give an incidence of 2.5 to 6.8 percent in patients undergoing carotid angiography,[6, 19] the real incidence in the community must be substantially lower. Thus it is a rare disease. It afflicts primarily women, and despite some recent contributions,[16, 25–28] the natural history of untreated lesions remains largely undefined.

The clinical conundrum remains that many patients remain asymptomatic, but the first symptom of fibromuscular disease may be a stroke. The true cause of symptom production in patients with this disorder remains unknown, although the usual clinical presentation of predominantly focal ischemia lends strong support to the thesis that the symptoms have a thromboembolic etiology.

Our lack of knowledge of the natural history makes patient selection for operative therapy difficult. The initial clinical and radiologic assessment of each patient must be complete. This is mandatory for two reasons: (1) to properly assess the individual patient for treatment recommendation, and (2) to document each case in a central register so that we may learn more about this unusual disease.

Following the history and detailed physical examination, radiologic assessment should be performed. With the rapid improvement in digital subtraction techniques, there can be no objection to a complete intra-arterial assessment to establish which vessels other than the carotid artery are affected by fibromuscular disease. However, the individual assessment of patients also requires standard intracranial views to look for aneurysms, and appropriate runs to document possible vertebral artery disease.

No data are available to confirm or deny the efficacy of any medical therapy for fibromuscular disease. We continue to use aspirin prophylactically in patients who are asymptomatic and to recommend surgery, most commonly graduated intraluminal dilatation, for patients who present with symptoms. In the cohort of patients followed after surgical therapy, the results of treatment have been gratifying in terms of the durability of the anatomic repair and the continued symptom relief afforded the patients. Others have reported the use of percutaneous transluminal angioplasty in the management of extracranial fibromuscular disease.[29–31] We have not used this technique and caution against its use, echoing the reluctance of Hodgins and Dutton[32] and Vitek and Morawetz[33] to use the percutaneous technique. A series of patients under control trial conditions would need to be presented, demonstrating an improved technical result over operative carotid dilatation, before percutaneous transluminal angioplasty could be recommended. Prophylactic surgery in asymptomatic patients is not recommended.

REFERENCES

1. Leadbetter WF, Burkland CE: Hypertension in unilateral renal disease. *J Urol.* 1938;39:611.
2. McCormack LJ, Hazard JB, Poutasse EF: Obstructive lesions of the renal artery associated with remedial hypertension (abstract). *Am J Pathol.* 1958;34:582.
3. Palubinskas AJ, Ripley HR: Fibromuscular hyperplasia in extrarenal arteries. *Radiology.* 1964;82:451.
4. Connett MC, Lansche JM: Fibromuscular hyperplasia of internal carotid artery: Report of a case. *Ann Surg.* 1965;162:59.
5. Nunn DB: Fibromuscular hyperplasia of the internal carotid artery. *Am Surg.* 1974;40:309.
6. Osborn AG, Anderson RE: Angiographic spectrum of cervical and intracranial fibromuscular dysplasia. *Stroke.* 1977;8:617.
7. Stanley JC, Fry WJ, Seeger JF, et al: Extracranial internal carotid and vertebral artery fibrodysplasia. *Arch Surg.* 1974;109:215.
8. Stanley JC, Gewertz BL, Bove EL, et al: Arterial fibrodysplasia: Histopathologic character and current etiologic concepts. *Arch Surg.* 1975;110:561.
9. Effeney DJ, Ehrenfeld WK, Stoney RJ, Wylie EJ: Fibromuscular dysplasia of the internal carotid artery. *World J Surg.* 1979;3:179.
10. Starr DS, Lawrie GM, Morris GC: Fibromuscular disease of carotid arteries: Long-term results of graduated internal dilatation. *Stroke.* 1981;12:196.
11. Effeney DJ, Krupski WC, Stoney RJ, Ehrenfeld WK: Fibromuscular dysplasia of the carotid artery. *Aust N Z J Surg.* 1983;53:527.
12. Effeney DJ, Ehrenfeld WK, Stoney RJ, Wylie EJ: Why operate on carotid fibromuscular dysplasia? *Arch Surg.* 1980;115:1261.
13. Ehrenfeld WK, Stoney RJ, Wylie EJ: Fibromuscular hyperplasia of the internal carotid artery. *Arch Surg.* 1967;95:284.
14. Ehrenfeld WK, Wylie EJ: Fibromuscular dysplasia of the internal carotid artery: Surgical management. *Arch Surg.* 1974;109:676.
15. Krupski WC, Effeney DJ, Ehrenfeld WK: Fibromuscular dysplasia, aneurysms, and spontaneous dissection of the carotid artery. In Bergan JJ, Yao JST, eds. *Cerebrovascular Insufficiency.* New York: Grune & Stratton; 1983:369.
16. Stewart MT, Moritz MW, Smith RB, et al: The natural history of carotid fibromuscular dysplasia. *J Vasc Surg.* 1986;3:305.
17. Collins GJ, Rich NM, Clagett GP, et al: Fibromuscular dysplasia of the internal carotid arteries: Clinical experience and follow-up. *Ann Surg.* 1981;194:89.
18. Kelly TF, Morris GC: Arterial fibromuscular disease. *Am J Surg.* 1982;143:232.
19. Houser OW, Baker HL: Fibrovascular dysplasia and other uncommon diseases of the cervical carotid artery: Angiographic aspects. *AJR Am J Roentgenol.* 1968;104:201.
20. Palubinskas AJ, Perloff D, Newton TH: Fibromuscular hyperplasia: An arterial dysplasia of increasing clinical importance. *AJR Am J Roentgenol.* 1966;98:907.
21. Patman RD, Thompson JE, Talkington CM, Garrett WV: Natural history of fibromuscular dysplasia of the carotid artery (abstract). *Stroke.* 1980;2:135.
22. Perry MO: Fibromuscular dysplasia. *Surg Gynecol Obstet.* 1974;139:97.
23. Morris GC Jr, Lechter A, DeBakey ME: Surgical treatment of fibromuscular disease of the carotid arteries. *Arch Surg.* 1968;96:636.
24. Lord RSA, Graham AR, Benn IV: Radiologic control of operative carotid dilatation: Aneurysm formation following balloon dilatation. *J Cardiovasc Surg.* 1986;27:158.
25. Corrin LS, Sandok BA, Houser OW: Cerebral ischemic events in patients with carotid artery fibromuscular dysplasia. *Arch Neurol.* 1981;38:616.
26. Harrington OB, Crosby VG, Nicholas L: Fibromuscular hyperplasia of the internal carotid artery. *Ann Thorac Surg.* 1971;9:516.
27. So EL, Toole JF, Dalal P, Moody DM: Cephalic fibromuscular dysplasia in 32 patients. *Arch Neurol.* 1981;38:619.
28. Wells RP, Smith RR: Fibromuscular dysplasia of the internal carotid artery: A long-term follow-up. *Neurosurgery.* 1982;10:39.
29. Belan A, Vesela M, Vanek I, et al: Percutaneous transluminal angioplasty of fibromuscular dysplasia of the internal carotid artery. *Cardiovasc Intervent Radiol.* 1982;5:79.
30. Garrido E, Montoya J: Transluminal dilatation of internal carotid artery in fibromuscular dysplasia: A preliminary report. *Surg Neurol.* 1980;16:469.
31. Hasso AN, Bird CR, Zinke DE, Thompson JR: Fibromuscular dysplasia of the internal carotid artery: Percutaneous transluminal angioplasty. *AJR Am J Roentgenol.* 1981;136:955.
32. Hodgins GW, Dutton JW: Subclavian and carotid angioplasties for Takayasu's arteritis. *J Can Assoc Radiol.* 1982;33:205.
33. Vitek JJ, Morawetz RB: Percutaneous transluminal angioplasty of the external carotid artery: Preliminary report. *AJNR.* 1982;3:541.

CHAPTER 52

Surgical Repair of Coils, Kinks, and Redundancy of the Carotid Artery: Indications, Techniques, and Results

LESLIE MEMSIC and RONALD W. BUSUTTIL

Carotid artery redundancy with kinking and coiling has long been recognized in both symptomatic and asymptomatic patients, but its clinical significance has been controversial. As experience with this anatomic variant has grown, it has become evident that under certain circumstances the condition can be responsible for ischemic cerebrovascular symptoms requiring thorough workup and often operative intervention.

PATHOLOGY

Carotid redundancy occurs with arterial elongation in a fixed space. Such tortuosity has been described in the coronal, sagittal, and transverse planes. Coiling is elongation and redundancy of the artery, resulting in an exaggerated S-shaped curvature or completed arterial loop (Fig. 52–1). Kinking is an acute angulation of one or more segments of the carotid artery associated with stenosis, atherosclerosis, or both in the affected segment (Figs. 52–2 and 52–3). Although carotid coils and kinks are undoubtedly manifestations of the same spectrum of pathology, they differ in configuration, symptomatology, and probable cause.[1]

HISTORICAL PERSPECTIVE

Tortuosity of the carotid artery was described as an incidental finding by anatomists in autopsy specimens as early as 1741.[2] Its clinical significance first became evident during the early 1900s, when Kelly, Fisher, and others[3–7] reported occasional hemorrhagic complications resulting from tonsillectomy in those patients with abnormal carotid artery configurations. It was not until the 1950s that redundant and kinked carotid arteries were proposed as possible sources of hemodynamic or embolic derangements leading to brain ischemia.[8] Agreement regarding the potential for these tortuous carotid arteries to produce cerebral symptoms, however, is not universal. Angiographic and autopsy studies indicate that carotid redundancy is not uncommon and that persons exhibiting such anatomy are, for the most part, asymptomatic and require no therapy.[9] However, a growing body of clinical experience suggests that although most carotid artery kinks are incidental findings with no clinical significance, a subset of patients manifest cerebral ischemic symptoms as a direct consequence of carotid angulation.

INCIDENCE

The incidence of angulated carotid arteries in the general population is unknown. Random anatomic studies in patients who have died of other causes suggest a 30 percent incidence.[7] Angiographic reviews indicate that redundant carotid arteries occur in 10 to 43 percent of patients studied, with kinking occurring in 4 to 16 percent.[10–12] Angulated carotid

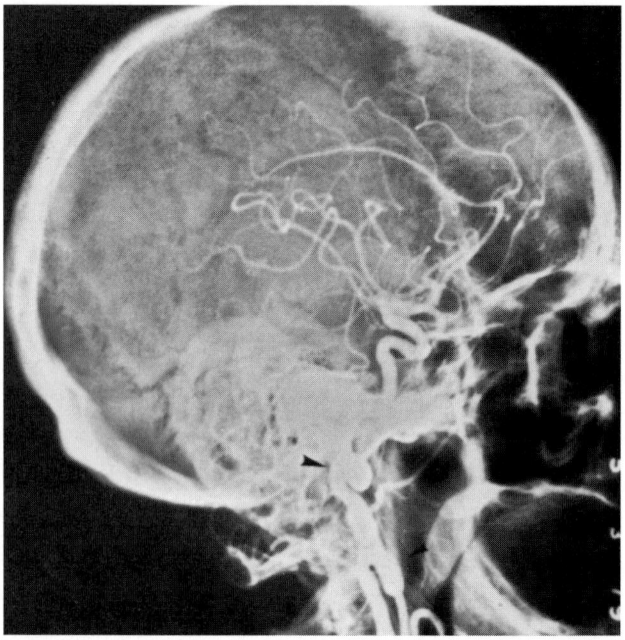

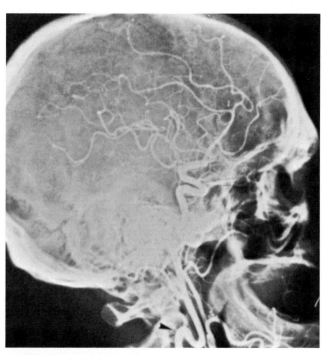

FIGURE 52–1. Angiogram showing two examples of carotid arterial coil *(arrowheads)*.

FIGURE 52–2. Angiogram showing a carotid kink with an angle of less than 60 degrees *(arrowhead)*.

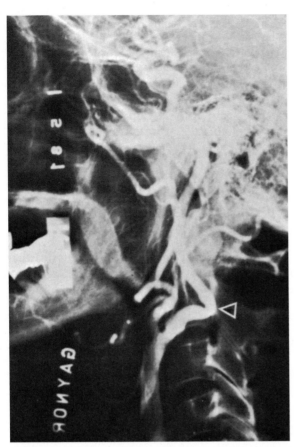

FIGURE 52–3. Angiogram showing a carotid kink with associated athero-sclerotic plaque distal to the kink *(arrowhead).*

arteries have been reported to occur in all ages, including fetuses, with the average age being 55 years. The numbers of males and females with angulated internal carotid arteries are equal, but women outnumber men 4:1 for common carotid artery kinking.

The incidence of symptomatic carotid elongation is even more difficult to estimate. It appears to be small but significant. In a series by Weibel and Fields,[1] 52 of 88 patients with unilateral or bilateral coiling of the internal carotid artery presented with cerebrovascular symptoms. Of these, only 11 percent (10 patients) were thought to be symptomatic as a result of the coiling itself. Since no stenosis of the coil was noted in nine patients, a direct correlation could be made between cerebrovascular ischemia and coiling in only 1 of 88 patients (1.1%). Other investigators conclude similarly that symptoms rarely occur when coiling is present unless atherosclerotic occlusive disease is also present in the carotid arteries or the vertebrobasilar system.

In a series of 65 patients in whom unilateral or bilateral kinking of the internal carotid artery was present, 51 percent (33 patients) experienced some degree of cerebrovascular insufficiency.[1] Workup revealed, however, that neurologic symptoms were not always related to the degree of angulation itself but to the presence of atheroma in the kinked segment. Symptoms of cerebrovascular insufficiency appeared to be directly related to the stenosis at the level of the kinking in only 10 of 33 patients, representing 18 percent of the total number of patients found to have kinking of the internal carotid artery.

Several other factors, such as variation in blood pressure, alterations in head and neck positions, and extracranial or intracranial occlusive diseases, contribute significantly to the production of cerebral symptoms. In 60 patients found to have severe carotid kinking (angle < 30 degrees) on angiogram in the study by Metz and coworkers,[12] 14 (23%) had had a significant cerebrovascular incident (stroke, eight; single transient ischemic attack, two; recurrent transient ischemic attack, four). In a series by Harrison and Davalos,[13] 46 of 424 patients (19%) evaluated by arteriography for cerebrovascular disease were found to have symptoms attributable to tortuosity of the carotid artery. All these studies are skewed by the fact that only patients who have had angiography are included in the statistical analysis.

Procedures to correct carotid kinks constitute a small portion of those operations performed for symptomatic carotid occlusive disease. Najafi and associates[14] reported a 5 percent incidence of kinking in a series of 308 patients undergoing carotid procedures. Vannix and colleagues[10] noted 15 instances of kinking in their series of 312 carotid reconstructions (4.8%); a review of the UCLA experience since 1977 reveals that only 10 of 670 carotid operations were performed for symptomatic carotid kinks, for an incidence of 1.4 percent.

ETIOLOGY

The etiology of carotid kinks and coils is multifactorial and involves both embryologic and developmental abnormalities as well as degenerative processes associated with atherosclerosis.

Embryologically, the carotid artery arises from the third aortic arch and the dorsal aorta. During fetal maturation, the carotid artery straightens as the fetal heart and large vessels recede into the thoracic cavity. If there is any discrepancy between the growth rate of the vascular system and that of the skeletal spine, the result is a redundancy of the carotid artery. This developmental disparity undoubtedly plays an important role in the pathogenesis of carotid elongation in children and perhaps in some adults as well. Approximately 50 percent of children with carotid angulation manifest it bilaterally, and they frequently have associated vascular anomalies such as aortic coarctation.

In adults there appears to be circumstantial evidence to support atherosclerosis as the responsible factor in the etiology of carotid angulation. Bilateral involvement is much less common in adults (<25%), and elongation is often accompanied by hypertension and peripheral vascular disease. The elongated carotid artery seen in adults has a weak inelastic wall, is quite friable, and is frequently associated with concomitant intimal ulceration and plaque deposition. Elongation of the aorta resulting from hypertension and age may be responsible for pushing up the origins of the innominate and carotid arteries, resulting in their redundancy. The issues of etiology and the role of atherosclerosis and age, however, remain controversial. In an extensive angiographic review by Metz and associates,[12] no association between severity of the kinking and either high blood pressure or increasing age was noted.

SYMPTOMS

Theoretically, carotid angulation can produce ischemic symptoms by either of two methods: by interfering with cerebral perfusion or by acting as a source of emboli to the brain. Impedance of cerebral blood flow can occur if the redundant carotid artery is severely angulated (<30–60 degrees) or if progressive sagging or sacculation occurs with advancing age. Arterial occlusion or embolization can result from coexisting atherosclerosis. This may occur more readily in an angulated artery than in a normal one owing to the dynamics of flow, just as it develops most frequently at regions of arterial bifurcation.

Although carotid coils not associated with atherosclerosis have been implicated as sources of cerebral ischemia on occasion, especially in children,[15] acutely angled carotid kinks are most commonly responsible for neurologic symptoms in patients with elongated carotid arteries. Neurologic ischemic symptoms produced by carotid kinks are the same as those seen in carotid ulceration or stenosis. Unilateral kinks may be manifested as amaurosis fugax, intermittent hemiparesis, aphasia, or stroke. Bilateral kinks can produce syncope, vertigo, global ischemia, and derangements of posterior circulation. Carotid angulation in children has been associated with learning disabilities as well as focal and grand mal seizures.

The development of symptoms may be related to position in patients with elongated arterial vessels. In these people, ipsilateral rotation usually results in the greatest reduction in carotid flow, but contralateral rotation, neck flexion, and neck extension can also exaggerate the kink and markedly reduce flow. In certain circumstances, head turning produces total occlusion of an otherwise patent but redundant artery. A history of either focal neurologic deficit or vertebrobasilar insufficiency triggered by head motion should arouse suspicion regarding the possibility of a carotid kink.

DIAGNOSIS

The initial patient workup is based on the presence of appropriate symptoms and on a high index of suspicion of a carotid kink. Physical examination is frequently unremarkable and usually reveals normal carotid pulses and absent bruits. An occasional patient may demonstrate a palpable thrill or prominent neck pulsation suggestive of an aneurysm.[16] Others may manifest bruits or thrills in the affected carotid artery only in particular head positions.

Noninvasive ocular plethysmography can be helpful in identifying hemodynamically significant carotid artery kinks and should be done in left, right, and neutral head positions owing to the positional nature of some kinked lesions (Fig. 52–4). In a study by Stanton and coworkers,[17] 14 of 16 patients taken to surgery for symptomatic carotid kinking were noted to have abnormal ocular plethysmography results preoperatively in the neutral or rotated head position or both.[5, 14] Operative flowmeter studies confirmed reduction in internal carotid artery blood flow of 30 to 80 percent during positional testing. All patients had normal postoperative ocular plethysmography test scores. Noninvasive studies are not useful in identifying non-flow-restrictive kinks associated with ulcerative plaques; therefore, arteriogram remains the definitive study for a symptomatic carotid lesion. In equivocal cases, complete angiographic evaluation of the carotid kink includes multiple views taken with the head in right and left rotation, flexion, and extension. It is also important to identify any associated atherosclerotic plaques that may be contributing to the patient's symptoms.

INDICATIONS FOR SURGERY

The natural history of carotid coils and kinks is unknown. It is likely that most patients who have these carotid configurations remain asymptomatic throughout life. Those who do experience cerebral symptoms generally undergo noninvasive studies and arteriography. Once a kink has been identified, it must be determined whether it is an incidental finding or, indeed, the pathology responsible for the patient's ischemic symptoms. Most surgeons would agree that any patient with focal hemispheric ischemic symptoms who has angiographic evidence of a kink with or without associated atherosclerosis should undergo surgical repair. In those patients who present with global or less specific complaints, a

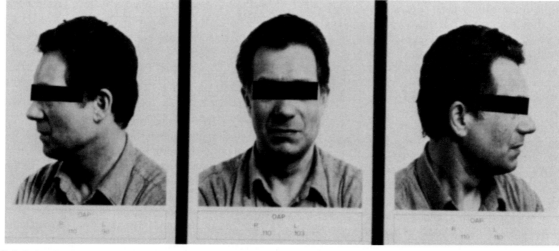

FIGURE 52–4. Patient head positions required for successful identification by oculoplethysmography of hemodynamically significant carotid artery kinks.

thorough workup is mandatory to exclude any other causes of neurologic dysfunction, including tumor, hypertension, or possible metabolic derangement. Furthermore, one should attempt to reproduce either symptoms or evidence of critical flow reduction on positional ocular plethysmography or arteriogram. In general, a kink associated with 70 percent luminal stenosis or an angle less than or equal to 60 degrees requires surgical repair.

Information is inadequate regarding management of an asymptomatic patient who has a kinked carotid artery demonstrated during angiography for an unrelated condition. In this situation, some physicians recommend prophylactic surgical repair if the kink is reducing the vessel diameter by 70 percent or consists of an acute angle of less than 60 degrees. Lesser degrees of narrowing should be treated expectantly, but because of the possibility of concomitant atherosclerotic plaque deposition or increasing redundancy with age or hypertension (unproven), these patients may warrant periodic ocular plethysmography and follow-up. If symptoms develop or ocular plethysmography suggests a hemodynamic stenosis, angiography is indicated.

In those patients who present with global or focal symptoms and who are found to have bilateral carotid kinks, a case can be made for repairing both lesions in a staged procedure if the lesions fit the aforementioned criteria. Some authorities, however, report resolution of symptoms with correction of only one side.[10]

SURGICAL THERAPY

The objectives of surgical therapy are elimination of the carotid kink and endarterectomy to remove all associated atherosclerotic plaque. The earliest surgical correction of a carotid kink, by Riser and colleagues[8] in 1951, involved tacking the redundant carotid artery to the fascia on the underside of the sternocleidomastoid muscle (Fig. 52–5). This procedure involved no resection and reduced the kink by realigning the vessel in a more vertical plane. Today this technique is rarely used and is reserved for high-risk patients with friable vessels in which no atherosclerotic plaque exists. Other nonresection techniques have also been advocated but are rarely, if ever, applied in practice. These methods include lysis of adhesions,[18] which may be helpful in the rare case in which carotid angulation occurs secondary to adhesions from an inflammatory source, and bypass.[19] In the bypass procedure, flow across the angulated segment is rerouted through a vein graft or fabric prosthesis. Such bypasses have a high rate of postoperative occlusion and have generally been abandoned.[20]

Preferred kink management involves partial resection of the common or internal carotid artery with reanastomosis to correct redundancy, with or without endarterectomy, depending on the coexistence of plaque. Both local and general anesthesia have been employed successfully.

One technique of kink correction is resection of the angulated area of the internal carotid artery with primary reanastomosis (Fig. 52–6). This procedure is often difficult, as many internal carotid arteries are small and friable and hold sutures poorly. An alternative means of kink repair is to remove a segment of normal proximal common carotid artery to straighten out the redundant portion of the internal

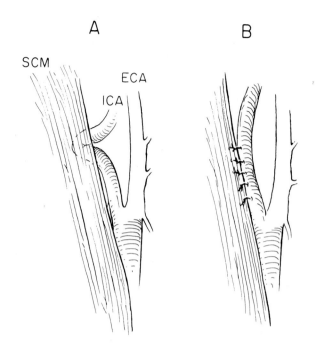

FIGURE 52–5. Drawing of the original operation of Riser in which the carotid kink *(A)* was eliminated by tacking of the redundant artery to the fascia on the underside of the sternocleidomastoid muscle *(SCM)* *(B)*. ECA, external carotid artery; ICA, internal carotid artery.

carotid artery with reanastomosis (Fig. 52–7). This procedure may necessitate ligation of the external carotid artery as in Figure 52–7A, unless it too is redundant, in which case it need only be stretched out as in Figure 52–7B. By performing resection and anastomosis of the common carotid artery, the surgeon can avoid suturing the more friable attenuated internal carotid artery.

A third method involves no resection but only transplantation of the origin of the internal carotid artery from the bifurcation, with reanastomosis more proximally to the anterior or lateral surface of the common carotid artery (Fig. 52–8).

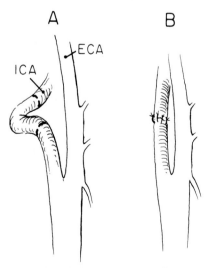

FIGURE 52–6. Surgical technique of kink repair in which the angulated area of the internal carotid artery *(A)* is resected with primary reanastomosis *(B)*.

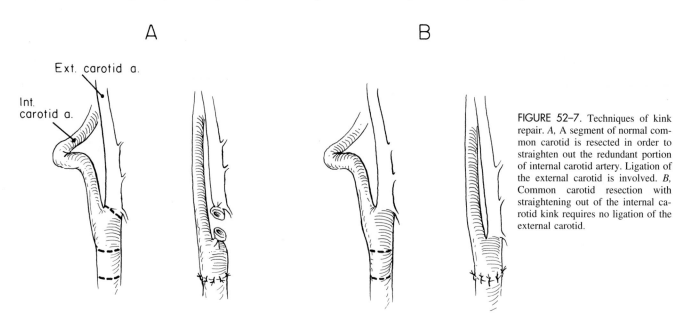

FIGURE 52–7. Techniques of kink repair. *A*, A segment of normal common carotid is resected in order to straighten out the redundant portion of internal carotid artery. Ligation of the external carotid is involved. *B*, Common carotid resection with straightening out of the internal carotid kink requires no ligation of the external carotid.

In all these operative procedures, it is imperative to mobilize the entire internal carotid artery from the base of the skull to the bifurcation to ensure that all kinks are eliminated. Endarterectomy is performed in all cases in which atherosclerosis accompanies kinking (Fig. 52–9). It is important to do this, because unless all kink-associated atheromas are removed at the time of operation, the patient may have persistent symptoms despite kink correction.

In the UCLA experience, kinks were associated with atherosclerotic plaque in 40 percent of patients and were symptomatic solely on the basis of angulation with diminished flow in 60 percent of patients. All patients who demonstrated hemodynamically significant stenoses had kinks with angles of less than 60 degrees.

The use of internal carotid shunts during repair should be selective. The principles governing the indications for shunting are the same as those used for general atherosclerotic lesions of the carotid artery. In operations for kink

correction, the internal shunt can be useful as a stent that facilitates repair. The redundancy of the vessel, however, poses a risk of intimal damage should the shunt be placed before full mobilization and straightening of the artery are done.

RESULTS OF SURGICAL CORRECTION

The results of the collective experience with surgical correction of symptomatic carotid kinks are excellent (Table 52–1).[10, 13, 14, 18, 20–27] Slightly less than 85 percent of patients reported alleviation or resolution of their symptoms, with a 5 percent death and stroke rate. On the basis of follow-up data from 5 months to 15 years, it appears that a good result manifested immediately after surgery is usually sustained.

Patients demonstrating the poorest results with surgical correction of carotid kinks include those with global, fairly nonspecific symptoms as well as those with significant neurologic deficits preoperatively. Patients exhibiting recurrent

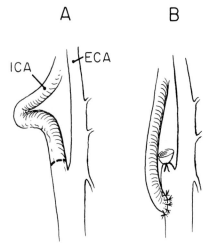

FIGURE 52–8. Technique of kink correction involving transplantation of the origin of the internal carotid artery from the bifurcation *(A)* and reanastomosing it more proximally to the common carotid artery *(B)*.

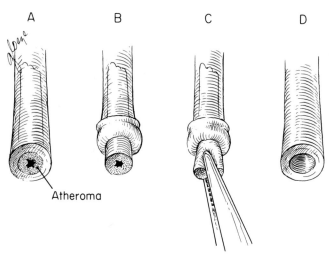

FIGURE 52–9. Eversion endarterectomy.

TABLE 52–1. Surgical Experience With Carotid Kinks

Study*	Patients, n	Surgical Therapy, n	Follow-up	Results	Percentage Improved
Goss[21]	6	1	3 months	U-1	0
Smathers and Smathers[22]	15	15	2 years 8 months	I-4, U-8, W-3 (thrombosis)	27
Freeman[23]	44	44	†	I-40, U-4	91
Hurwitt et al[20]	15	15	†	I-9, U-6	60
Henly et al[24]	7	7	†	I-6, U-1	86
Harrison and Davalos[13]	46	35	3 years	I-26, U-7, D-2 (stroke)	74
Najafi et al[14]	15	15	4 years 5 months	I-11, U-4	61
Sanger et al[25]	5	5	†	I-5	100
Derrick et al[18]	58	28	2–6 years	I-25, U-1	85
Rundles and Kimball[26]	8	5	13 months	I-3, U-2	60
Quattlebaum et al[27]	138	138	1–14 years	I-114 (E-39, G-61, F-14), U-24	83
Vannix et al[10]	15	5	1–24 months	I-13, U-I, W-1 (stroke)	87
UCLA	10	9	3 years 6 months	I-9	100
				Total	84.1

*For full bibliographic information, see reference list at end of chapter.
†Only immediate postoperative results given.
I, improved; U, unimproved; D, died; W, worse; E, excellent; G, good; F, fair.

focal transient ischemic attacks benefit the most from kink resection.

SUMMARY

Carotid coils and kinks result from both developmental and degenerative changes within the arterial system. Although coils are generally asymptomatic unless associated with atherosclerosis, carotid kinks with or without associated plaque may produce cerebral symptoms. Cerebral symptoms caused by carotid kinking may be triggered by positional changes. Ocular plethysmography may be helpful in the diagnosis, but arteriogram remains the definitive study. In general, asymptomatic patients may be followed expectantly. Symptomatic patients or patients with asymptomatic lesions exhibiting angles less than 60 degrees or causing greater than 70 percent luminal stenosis are candidates for surgical reconstruction.

REFERENCES

1. Weibel J, Fields WS: Tortuosity, coiling, and kinking of the internal carotid artery. II. Relationship of morphological variation to cerebrovascular insufficiency. Neurology (NY). 1965;15:462.
2. Schecter DC: Dolichocarotid syndrome. Cerebral ischemia related to cervical carotid artery redundancy with kinking. Parts I and II. N Y State J Med. 1979;79:1391.
3. Kelly AB: Tortuosity of the internal carotid in relation to the pharynx. J Laryngol Otol. 1925;40:15.
4. Fisher AGT: Sigmoid tortuosity of the internal carotid artery and its relation to tonsil and pharynx. Lancet. 1915;2:128.
5. Jackson JL: Tortuosity of the internal carotid artery and its relation to tonsillectomy. Can Med Assoc J. 1933;29:475.
6. McKensie W, Woolf GT: Carotid abnormalities and adenoid surgery. J Laryngol Otol. 1959;73:596.
7. Cairney J: Tortuosity of the cervical segment of the internal carotid artery. J Anat. 1924;59:87.
8. Riser MM, Geraud J, Ducoudray J, Ribaut L: Dolicho-carotide interne avec syndrome vertigneux. Neurology (Paris). 1951;85:145.
9. Hsu I, Kisten AD: Buckling of the great vessels: A clinical and angiographic study. Arch Intern Med. 1956;98:712.
10. Vannix RS, Joergenson FJ, Carter R: Kinking of the internal carotid artery: Clinical significance and surgical management. Am J Surg. 1977;134:82.
11. Bauer R, Sheehan S, Meyer JS: Arteriographic study of cerebrovascular disease. II. Cerebral symptoms due to kinking, tortuosity and compression of carotid and vertebral arteries in the neck. Arch Neurol. 1961;4:119.
12. Metz H, Murray-Leslie RM, Bannister RG, et al: Kinking of the internal carotid artery in relation to cerebrovascular disease. Lancet. 1961;1:424.
13. Harrison JH, Davalos PA: Cerebral ischemia: Surgical procedure in cases due to tortuosity and buckling of the cervical vessels. Arch Surg. 1962;84:85.
14. Najafi H, Javid H, Dye WS, et al: Kinked internal carotid artery. Arch Surg. 1964;89:135.
15. Sarkari NB, Holmes JM, Backerstaff ER: Neurologic manifestations associated with carotid loops in children. J Neurol Neurosurg Psychiatry. 1970;33:194.
16. Deterling RA Jr: Tortuous right common carotid artery simulating aneurysm. Angiology. 1952;3:483.
17. Stanton PE Jr, McCluskey DA Jr, James PA: Hemodynamic assessment and surgical correction of kinking of the internal carotid artery. Surgery. 1978;84:793.
18. Derrick JR, Kirksey TD, Estess M, Williams D: Kinking of the carotid arteries: Clinical considerations. Am Surg. 1966;32:503.
19. Derrick JR, Smith T: Carotid kinking as a cause of cerebral insufficiency. Circulation. 1962;25:849.
20. Hurwitt ES, Carton CA, Fell SC, et al: Critical evaluation and surgical correction of obstructions in the branches of the aortic arch. Ann Surg. 1960;152:472.
21. Goss HH: Kinks and coils of the cervical carotid artery. Surg Forum. 1959;9:721.
22. Smathers HM, Smathers WM: Carotid artery occlusion. Arch Surg. 1959;79:122.
23. Freeman TR: Surgery of carotid artery obstruction. J Med Assoc Ga. 1959;48:57.
24. Henly WS, Colley DA, Gordon WB Jr, DeBakey ME: Tortuosity of the internal carotid artery: Report of seven cases treated surgically. Postgrad Med. 1962;31:133.
25. Sanger PW, Robicsek F, Pritchard W, et al: Cerebral ischemia caused by kinking of the carotid artery. N C Med J. 1965;26:542.
26. Rundles WR, Kimball FD: The kinked carotid syndrome. Angiology. 1969;20:177.
27. Quattlebaum JH Jr, Wade JS, Whidden CM: Stroke associated with elongation and kinking of the carotid artery: Longterm follow up. Ann Surg. 1973;177:572.

External Carotid Endarterectomy: Indications, Techniques, and Results

E. JOHN HARRIS, JR. and CHRISTOPHER K. ZARINS

Naturally occurring collateral pathways connecting the external carotid artery branches and the intracranial cerebral circulation are well recognized and have been demonstrated anatomically, angiographically, and physiologically by various flow detection devices. Under normal circumstances, all internal carotid artery blood flow is directed intracranially, and flow through the collateral pathways is from intracranial vessels to the external carotid artery branches. Similarly, ocular blood supply is derived predominantly from the internal carotid artery via the ophthalmic artery. Thus, normally the external carotid arteries do not contribute significantly to intracranial or ocular blood flow. In the case of internal carotid artery occlusion, the direction of flow in the collateral pathways reverses, and flow courses from the external carotid branches to the intracranial branches of the internal carotid artery. Thus, with occlusion of the internal carotid artery, the external carotid artery may become an important source of blood flow to the brain.

Occlusive or atheromatous changes in the external carotid artery can lead to transient ischemic episodes or amaurosis fugax when they are ipsilateral to an occluded internal carotid artery. These symptoms arise by the same physiologic mechanisms observed with the internal carotid artery, that is, embolization or hypoperfusion. A number of investigators have demonstrated the potential for increasing cerebral blood flow in patients with ipsilateral internal carotid artery occlusion and external carotid artery stenosis by external carotid endarterectomy.[1–3] Embolization to the external carotid artery from the blind cul-de-sac of an occluded internal carotid artery can also be relieved by external carotid artery endarterectomy.

This chapter focuses on the indications, techniques, and results for external carotid endarterectomy performed alone for symptoms of cerebral or ocular ischemia with ipsilateral internal carotid artery occlusion.

INDICATIONS

The indications for external carotid endarterectomy include (1) ipsilateral transient ischemic attacks (hemispheric or ocular) or stroke in patients with occlusion of the ipsilateral internal carotid artery and severe external carotid artery stenosis;[4–6] (2) ipsilateral transient ischemic attacks (hemispheric or ocular) or stroke and occlusion of the ipsilateral internal carotid artery and moderate stenosis of the external carotid artery with ulceration;[7] (3) ipsilateral transient ischemic attacks (hemispheric or ocular) or stroke, with a nonstenotic ipsilateral external carotid artery and thrombus within the cul-de-sac of the occluded ipsilateral internal carotid artery (Table 53–1).[4, 8] The most clear-cut indication for external carotid artery endarterectomy is monocular amaurosis fugax in patients with ipsilateral internal carotid artery occlusion and a microembolic source in the origin of the external carotid artery or the occluded carotid sinus. Other, less clear indications for external carotid artery endarterec-

tomy include nonlateralizing hemispheric transient ischemic attacks, global ischemia, adjunctive procedure to extracranial-intracranial (EC-IC) bypass, and asymptomatic stroke prophylaxis.[5, 9, 10] Reports in the literature have not always clearly defined the indications for external carotid artery endarterectomy.

PATIENT SELECTION

Selection for external carotid artery endarterectomy among patients with clear indications has relied on diagnostic arteriography and duplex sonography for confirmation of appropriate lesions of the ipsilateral internal and external carotid arteries. In patients with less clear indications for external carotid artery endarterectomy, adjunctive studies, such as radiolabeled xenon (^{133}Xe) cerebral perfusion scans, have been utilized to aid the selection process. Patients with a severe reduction in total cerebral blood flow, as evidenced by the ^{133}Xe scan, and with bilateral internal carotid artery occlusion and external carotid artery stenosis can occasion-

TABLE 53–1. Indications for External Carotid Artery Endarterectomy

Symptoms	Anatomy
Ipsilateral transient ischemic attack Hemispheric Ocular	Ipsilateral ICA Occlusion Ipsilateral ECA High-grade stenosis
Ipsilateral stroke Hemispheric Ocular	Ipsilateral ICA Occlusion Ipsilateral ECA High-grade stenosis
Ipsilateral transient ischemic attack Hemispheric Ocular	Ipsilateral ICA Occlusion Ipsilateral ECA Moderate stenosis with ulceration
Ipsilateral stroke Hemispheric Ocular	Ipsilateral ICA Occlusion Ipsilateral ECA Moderate stenosis with ulceration
Ipsilateral transient ischemic attacks Hemispheric Ocular	Ipsilateral ICA Occlusion with thrombus in cul-de-sac Ipsilateral ECA No stenosis or lesion
Ipsilateral stroke Hemispheric Ocular	Ipsilateral ICA Occlusion with thrombus in cul-de-sac Ipsilateral ECA No stenosis or lesion
Global ischemia	Ipsilateral and contralateral ICA Occlusion Either ECA High-grade stenosis

ECA, external carotid artery; ICA, internal carotid artery.

ally benefit from external carotid artery endarterectomy to increase total cerebral blood flow. Successful external carotid artery revascularization can return blood flow, as measured by ^{133}Xe scan, to normal in 80 percent of these patients.[11] In spite of these findings, the role of external carotid artery reconstruction in relieving nonlateralizing symptoms, presumably secondary to hypoperfusion, is unclear and not an entirely proven indication. Nonetheless, blood flow measurement by ^{133}Xe scan may be helpful.

TECHNIQUES

External carotid endarterectomy, as with internal carotid artery endarterectomy, can be performed under general or local anesthesia, depending on surgeon preference. Continuous invasive blood pressure monitoring is preferred. The carotid artery bifurcation is exposed through one of two standard approaches: a transverse midcervical incision or a longitudinal incision along the anterior border of the sternocleidomastoid muscle. Systemic anticoagulation with intravenous heparin is recommended prior to initiation of arterial occlusion. Technical considerations of importance in external carotid endarterectomy include mobilization and control of the branches of the external carotid artery, sufficient to extend the arteriotomy up the external carotid artery beyond the distal edge of the plaque. Placement of the arteriotomy can be varied, with the understanding that the goals of the procedure are to exclude the cul-de-sac of the occluded internal carotid artery as an embolic source, to perform a standard thromboendarterectomy of the external carotid artery, and to close the arteriotomy without narrowing the external carotid artery. Since the external carotid artery becomes an important source of collateral cerebral blood flow with internal carotid artery occlusion, some surgeons have recommended selective use of an intraluminal shunt during external carotid artery revascularization.[6, 10, 12] Such shunting is technically difficult because of the many side branches, the small size, and the distal tapering of the external carotid artery. We have not found intraluminal shunting to be necessary based on continuous electroencephalographic (EEG) monitoring data.

Three general techniques of external carotid artery endarterectomy meet these goals. Our preferred technique begins primarily with amputation of the occluded internal carotid artery, whose distal end is ligated or oversewn. The arteriotomy is extended from the origin of the internal carotid artery along both the common carotid and external carotid arteries. Thromboendarterectomy is performed as previously described, with either primary closure or patch angioplasty (Fig. 53–1). Patch angioplasties with the use of prosthetic materials (Dacron and polytetrafluoroethylene), vein, and endarterectomized internal carotid artery have been described.[5] This technique of external carotid artery endarterectomy eliminates the internal carotid artery cul-de-sac, allows direct visualization of the endpoint of the endarterectomy, and allows the incision to be closed primarily or with patch angioplasty.

A second technique begins with a standard arteriotomy in the common carotid artery, which is then extended along the external carotid artery. Thromboendarterectomy is performed in standard fashion. The origin of the internal carotid artery

is then occluded intraluminally with interrupted sutures at its starting point. The arteriotomy is then closed primarily, or if necessary, with patch angioplasty with any of the materials described (Fig. 53–2).[6]

A third technique includes internal carotid artery angioplasty as an adjunct to closure of the endarterectomized external carotid artery. The internal carotid artery is mobilized beyond the bifurcation and ligated at the distal limit of the dissection. A Y-shaped arteriotomy is performed, with its base on the common carotid artery and the arms extending along both the internal and external carotid arteries. Standard thromboendarterectomy is performed to include all surfaces. The spatulated, transected internal carotid stump is then tapered to close the external carotid arteriotomy, facilitating a tapered transition from the common to the external carotid artery (Fig. 53–3).[5, 13]

RESULTS

The first report of external carotid endarterectomy ipsilateral to an internal carotid artery occlusion is credited to BB Jackson.[12] This article is interesting for its prose and its description of external carotid angioplasty using the stump of the internal carotid artery, but it describes a procedure performed for thrombosis of the common and external carotid arteries in the face of long-standing internal carotid artery occlusion, with excellent results, rather than discussing external carotid endarterectomy in regards to current indications. During this same period, the Baylor group was performing external carotid endarterectomy for hemispheric ischemic symptoms, both transient and fixed, in patients with ipsilateral internal carotid occlusion and stenosis of the origin of the external carotid artery.[2] Ten patients were reported, nine of whom had external carotid endarterectomy and Dacron patch angioplasty, and one of whom had thromboendarterectomy of both the common and external carotid arteries. Five of these patients had adjunctive vascular reconstruction of the contralateral carotid system. All patients were relieved of symptoms through 5 years of follow-up, although a 10 percent 30-day mortality was reported.

Subsequent experience with external carotid endarterectomy for symptomatic occlusion of the internal carotid artery, while uncommon compared with the experience with internal carotid endarterectomy, was notable for conflicting results provided by combining multiple small series of mixed patient populations.[3] The problem with these results is that they included multiple adjunctive surgical procedures with external carotid endarterectomy, performed on patients with variable preoperative neurologic deficits that increased the perioperative stroke and mortality rates. More acceptable results have been obtained when external carotid endarterectomy alone was performed to relieve specific hemispheric or retinal symptoms (Table 53–2).[7]

Connolly and Stemmer[14] reported an operative series of 45 patients with internal carotid artery occlusion, ipsilateral external carotid artery stenosis, and symptoms of ipsilateral hemispheric ischemia. All patients underwent external carotid endarterectomy, and half of the patients underwent attempts at ipsilateral internal carotid artery thromboendarterectomy. Unfortunately, the morbidity and mortality rates for the majority of these procedures were not reported. The

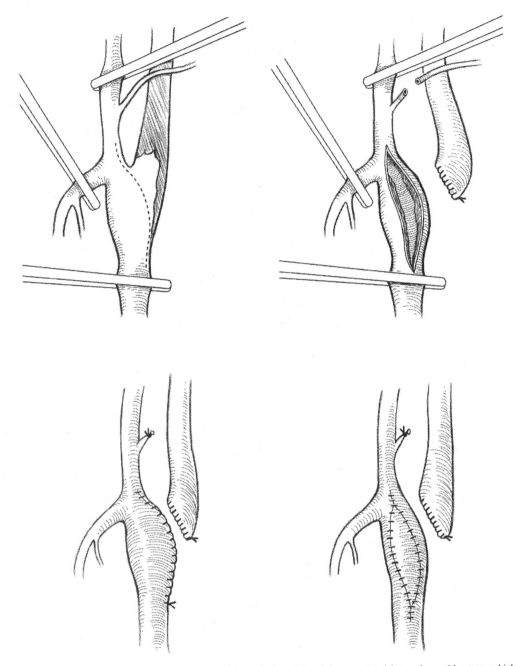

FIGURE 53–1. External carotid artery endarterectomy as performed through the origin of the amputated internal carotid artery, which is oversewn. The arteriotomy can be extended along the external carotid artery to enable visualization of the endpoint of the endarterectomy. The arteriotomy can be closed primarily or with a patch.

authors did observe improved symptoms and durability of the external carotid endarterectomy in nine of these patients, with a 2- to 5-year follow-up.

The remnant internal carotid artery "stump" observed following occlusion of this vessel was recognized as a potential source of embolic phenomena in 1978. Nine cases of ipsilateral hemispheric transient ischemia or ipsilateral amaurosis fugax or both were recognized in patients with remotely occluded internal carotid arteries and a remnant "stump" greater than 5 mm in length.[8] Seven of these patients underwent carotid bifurcation endarterectomy and either removal or obliteration of the internal carotid artery stump. Among those seven patients, there were no perioperative strokes, all

symptoms were improved or resolved, and one patient had a fatal myocardial infarction 2 weeks after the operation. The remaining two patients were observed; one underwent chronic anticoagulation and died from myocardial infarction 18 months later.

Correlation of successful external carotid artery revascularization ipsilateral to an internal carotid artery occlusion with improved regional cerebral blood flow was established in 1981.[11] Eight patients with internal carotid artery occlusion, ipsilateral external carotid artery stenosis, and ipsilateral hemispheric ischemic symptoms underwent external carotid endarterectomy with no postoperative strokes or mortality, all with improved or resolved symptoms. [133]Xe

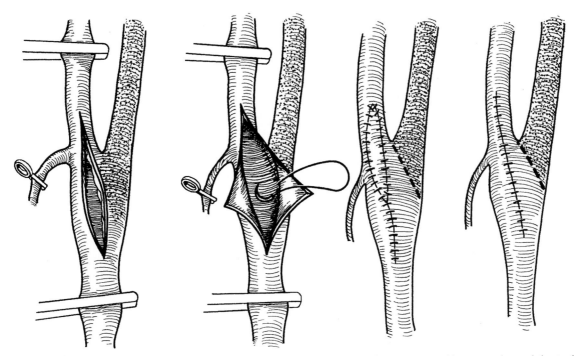

FIGURE 53–2. External carotid artery endarterectomy as performed through an arteriotomy on the common carotid artery, and extended onto the external carotid artery. After removal of the plaque, the internal carotid artery orifice is obliterated with suture, as illustrated. The arteriotomy can be closed primarily or with a patch.

inhalation cerebrography was obtained preoperatively and postoperatively in five of these patients, with improvement in the postoperative mean regional cerebral blood flow rate in all patients and normalization of the mean regional cerebral blood flow rate in 80 percent of these patients.

Enthusiasm for external carotid endarterectomy was tempered by the cautionary report of Halstuk and coworkers.[3] On the surface, they reported a 13.8 percent perioperative stroke rate and a 2.7 percent perioperative mortality rate in a series of 49 external carotid artery revascularizations. The authors concluded that although external carotid artery endarterectomy was technically easy, its use should be recommended with caution. Further review of these data identified several potential modifiers of the results. Only 29 patients had unilateral external carotid artery endarterectomy alone. The remaining 20 patients had additional procedures, including EC-IC artery bypass, inflow bypass from the supra-aortic trunks, and bilateral external carotid artery endarterectomies at the same operation. The majority of perioperative strokes and the only perioperative death occurred among these 20

FIGURE 53–3. External carotid artery endarterectomy is accomplished through a Y-shaped arteriotomy, extending from the common carotid artery onto the origins of both the external and internal carotid arteries. After removal of the plaque, the internal carotid artery is amputated and oversewn, and a segment of the endarterectomized internal carotid artery is used for patch angioplasty.

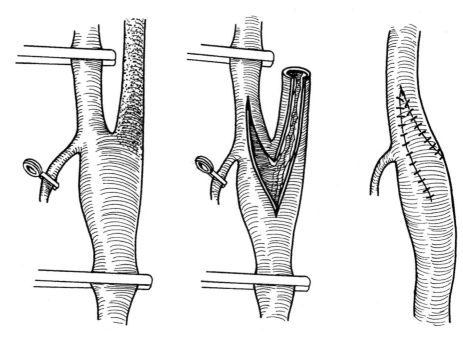

TABLE 53–2. Summary of Operative Results for External Carotid Artery Endarterectomy Performed Without Adjunctive Surgical Procedures

Study*	Patients, n	Mortality, n (%)†	Stroke, n (%)†
Fisher et al[13]	11	0	0
Floriani et al[15]	6	0	0
Satiani et al[16]	12	0	0
Sterpetti et al[5]	22	0	1 (4.5)
Street et al[17]	15	0	0
Rush et al[9]	19	0	0
Boontje et al[18]	11	0	0
Lamberth et al[4]	7	0	0
Halstuk et al[3]	29	0	2 (6.8)
McIntyre et al[6]	22	0	0
O'Hara et al[10]	30	0	0
Barnett et al[8]	7	1 (14.3)	0
Zarins et al[11]	8	0	0
Diethrich et al[2]	9	1 (11.1)	0
Totals	208	2 (0.9)	3 (1.4)

*For full bibliographic information, see reference list at end of chapter.
†30-day perioperative rate.

patients. Among the 29 patients undergoing external carotid artery endarterectomy alone, there were no perioperative deaths, and 2 perioperative strokes (6.8%). One of these strokes occurred 3 days postoperatively in a patient who was maintained perioperatively and postoperatively on an intra-aortic balloon pump.

Similar information was provided by the Cleveland Clinic with their report of 42 external carotid artery revascularizations performed in 36 symptomatic and 6 asymptomatic patients.[10] Among the 30 patients who had external carotid endarterectomy alone, the 30-day combined stroke and mortality rate was 0 percent. Among the 12 extended procedures requiring adjunctive EC-IC bypass, supra-aortic trunk inflow bypass, or external carotid artery reoperation, there were five perioperative neurologic events and one perioperative death, for a 30-day combined stroke and mortality rate of 50 percent.

A collective review published in 1987 attempted to further define the role of external carotid artery endarterectomy in patients with ipsilateral internal carotid artery occlusion and ipsilateral hemispheric or retinal ischemic symptoms.[7] Twenty-three series of external carotid artery revascularizations were reviewed, and all cases with procedures other than external carotid artery endarterectomy or bypass were excluded from further review. Analysis of 195 external carotid artery endarterectomies and 23 external carotid artery bypasses identified postoperative resolution of ischemic symptoms in 83 percent and marked symptomatic improvement in 7 percent of patients. The 30-day combined perioperative stroke and mortality rate was 7 percent, although several of these cases were from the Halstuk series,[3] and could be discounted for reasons cited earlier, lowering the combined stroke and mortality rate to 5 percent. The best results were identified in patients undergoing external carotid artery revascularization for indications of retinal ischemia or specific ipsilateral hemispheric ischemia. A separate retrospective review of 24 published series of external carotid artery reconstructions identified 192 operations in which external carotid endarterectomy was not associated with other procedures; the 30-day combined stroke and mortality rate was 1.6 percent.[5]

More recently, small series of patients have been retrospectively reviewed for outcome following external carotid artery endarterectomy for ipsilateral internal carotid artery occlusion and symptoms of ipsilateral hemispheric or retinal ischemia. In three compiled series, 28 patients underwent external carotid endarterectomy, all experienced resolution of preoperative symptoms, and the 30-day combined stroke and mortality rate was 0 percent.[13, 15, 16] Another series reviewed 16 patients with visual ischemic disturbances, ipsilateral internal carotid artery occlusion, and external carotid stenosis.[17] One patient underwent external carotid artery bypass and 15 patients underwent external carotid artery endarterectomy, with no perioperative deaths, strokes, or retinal ischemic episodes. All patients were relieved of ocular ischemia postoperatively, and two patients suffered recurrent amaurosis fugax when their repairs thrombosed, one at 24 and one at 53 months postoperatively.

External carotid artery endarterectomy performed in patients with ipsilateral internal carotid occlusion and nonlateralizing symptoms of hemispheric ischemia has been infrequent with poor results identified to date. Combining the series and review of Sterpetti and associates,[5] 18 of 36 patients (50%) undergoing external carotid artery endarterectomy for nonlateralizing symptoms were found to have relief from symptoms postoperatively.

Most recently, a series of 21 external carotid artery endarterectomies in patients with ipsilateral internal carotid artery occlusion and symptoms of either ipsilateral amaurosis fugax (14) or ipsilateral hemispheric ischemia (7) was reported.[9] The operations were performed safely, with no deaths or new strokes within 30 days of operation. Interestingly in this series, 14 percent of patients with amaurosis fugax and 71 percent of patients with hemispheric ischemia were not improved after external carotid endarterectomy. The patency and durability of external carotid endarterectomy were better when patch angioplasty was used than when primary closure was used.

CONCLUSION

Patients with internal carotid artery occlusion can develop ipsilateral amaurosis fugax and ipsilateral transient ischemic attacks. In this setting, the external carotid artery becomes an important source of collateral blood flow to the ipsilateral eye and cerebral hemisphere. Atherosclerotic occlusive disease of the external carotid artery can lead to the development of flow-limiting stenoses as well as ulcerating plaques. When these occlusive disease changes are associated with ipsilateral internal carotid artery occlusion, they can serve as a source of emboli to the ipsilateral eye and cerebral hemisphere. The occluded internal carotid artery stump can also serve as a source of emboli.

In patients with an occluded internal carotid artery, ipsilateral external carotid artery endarterectomy can improve cerebral and retinal perfusion or eliminate an embolic source. The successful endarterectomy should exclude the stump of the occluded internal carotid artery. Patch angioplasty of the endarterectomized external carotid artery is recommended.

External carotid artery endarterectomy is indicated for the treatment of ipsilateral amaurosis fugax or ipsilateral transient ischemic attacks in the presence of an ipsilateral internal carotid artery occlusion and either an ipsilateral significant external carotid artery stenosis or ulcerated plaque or in the presence of an internal carotid artery stump with thrombus. Morbidity and mortality rates for external carotid artery endarterectomy are acceptable and are improved by adjunctive bypass procedures and contralateral cerebral revascularization procedures performed in association with the external carotid artery endarterectomy. The role of external carotid artery endarterectomy in relieving nonlateralizing symptoms of cerebral ischemia is incompletely defined, and the procedure likely is of little benefit.

REFERENCES

1. DeBakey ME, Crawford ES, Cooley DA, et al: Cerebral arterial insufficiency: One to 11-year results following arterial reconstructive operation. *Ann Surg.* 1965;161:921.
2. Diethrich EB, Liddicoat JE, McCutchen JJ, et al: Surgical significance of the external carotid artery in the treatment of cerebrovascular insufficiency. *J Cardiovasc Surg.* 1968;15:213.
3. Halstuk KS, Baker WH, Littooy FN: External carotid endarterectomy. *J Vasc Surg.* 1984;1:398.
4. Lamberth WC: External carotid endarterectomy: Indications, operative technique, and results. *Surgery.* 1983;93:57.
5. Sterpetti AV, Schultz RD, Feldhaus RJ: External carotid endarterectomy: Indications, technique, and late results. *J Vasc Surg.* 1988;7:31.
6. McIntyre KE, Ely III RL, Malone JM, et al: External carotid artery reconstruction: Its role in the treatment of cerebral ischemia. *Am J Surg.* 1985;150:58.
7. Gertler JP, Cambria RP: The role of external carotid endarterectomy in the treatment of ipsilateral internal carotid occlusion: Collective review. *J Vasc Surg.* 1987;6:158.
8. Barnett HJM, Peerless SJ, Kaufmann JCE: "Stump" of the internal carotid artery. A source for further cerebral embolic ischemia. *Stroke.* 1978;9:448.
9. Rush DS, Holloway WO, Fogartie JE Jr, et al: The safety, efficacy, and durability of external carotid endarterectomy. *J Vasc Surg.* 1992;16:407.
10. O'Hara PJ, Hertzer NR, Beven EG: External carotid revascularization: Review of a ten-year experience. *J Vasc Surg.* 1985;2:709.
11. Zarins CK, DelBeccarro EJ, Johns L, et al: Increased cerebral blood flow after external carotid artery revascularization. *Surgery.* 1981;89:730.
12. Jackson BB: The external carotid as a brain collateral. *Am J Surg.* 1967;113:375.
13. Fisher DF, Valentine J, Patterson CB, et al: Is external carotid endarterectomy a durable procedure? *Am J Surg.* 1986;152:700.
14. Connolly JE, Stemmer EA: Endarterectomy of the external carotid artery. *Arch Surg.* 1973;106:799.
15. Floriani M, Giulini SM, Bonardelli S, et al: Surgical treatment of lesions obstructing the external carotid artery. *J Cardiovasc Surg.* 1989;30:414.
16. Satiani B, Das BM, Vasko JS: Reconstruction of the external carotid artery. *Surg Gynecol Obstet.* 1987;164:105.
17. Street DL, Ricotta JJ, Green RM: The role of external carotid revascularization in the treatment of ocular ischemia. *J Vasc Surg.* 1987;6:280.
18. Boontje AH: External carotid artery revascularization in the treatment of ocular ischemia. *J Cardiovasc Surg.* 1992;33:315.

CHAPTER 54

Accessible and Inaccessible Aneurysms of the Extracranial Carotid Artery

TAMMY K. RAMOS, EILEEN S. NATUZZI, and RONALD J. STONEY

Extracranial carotid artery aneurysms account for 1 to 4 percent of all peripheral artery aneurysms[1-3] and for only 2 percent of all extracranial carotid artery disease requiring surgery.[4] Current knowledge regarding these rare aneurysms is derived from isolated case reports[1, 5-11] and several small series.[2, 4, 12-16] The largest series was reported by McCollum and associates,[2] who treated 37 aneurysms occurring in 34 patients over a 21-year period at Baylor College of Medicine. At the University of California–San Francisco (UCSF), 34 patients with 35 extracranial carotid aneurysms have been treated surgically over the past 33 years, averaging one patient per year.

Only 2 percent of extracranial carotid artery aneurysms involve primarily the external carotid artery (Fig. 54–1); the remainder are distributed almost equally between the internal carotid and the common carotid arteries (Figs. 54–2 and 54–3).[7] Aneurysms that occur in the petrous portion of the internal carotid artery are usually considered along with intracranial aneurysms and are not covered in this chapter. Aneurysms demonstrated by conventional angiography to be located in the extracranial carotid arteries below a line drawn between the angle of the mandible and the top of the mastoid process are accessible by a standard cervical approach. In contrast, aneurysms located above this line have traditionally been considered inaccessible. However, over the past decade, several maneuvers have been described that extend the standard cervical approach cephalad, making some of these traditionally inaccessible aneurysms in the middle and distal extracranial internal carotid artery accessible for surgical therapy.

ETIOLOGY AND PATHOGENESIS

Atherosclerosis, previous carotid surgery, and trauma are the most common causes of extracranial carotid aneurysms (Table 54–1). In the UCSF series, only 29 percent of aneurysms were atherosclerotic, but in other series, atherosclerosis is responsible for nearly 50 percent of these aneurysms.[2, 4, 17] Hypertension, which is considered an important risk factor, is present in the majority of patients, and other clinical manifestations of extracarotid atherosclerosis are common, including aortic or peripheral artery aneurysms in 15 percent of patients.[2, 14, 17]

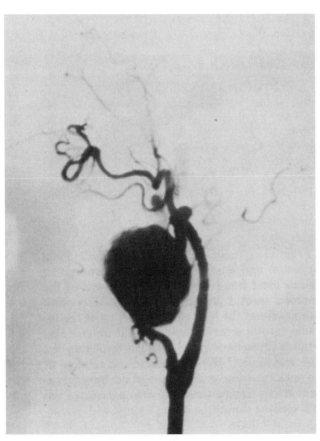

FIGURE 54–1. Saccular aneurysm of the proximal third of the external carotid artery.

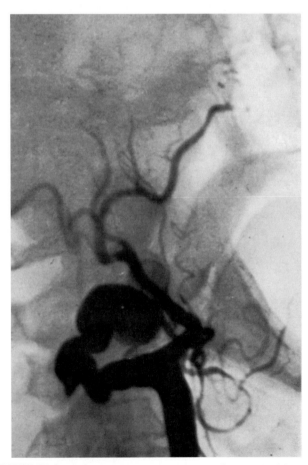

FIGURE 54–2. Fusiform multilobulated aneurysm of the proximal internal carotid artery.

424

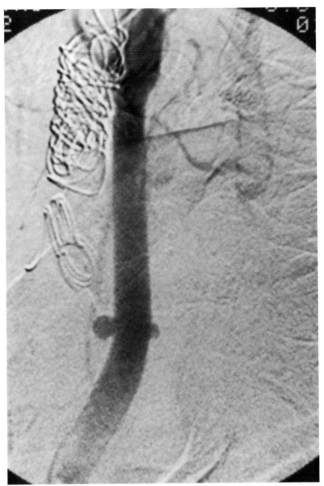

FIGURE 54–3. Saccular false aneurysms of the middle third of the right common carotid artery following penetrating neck trauma. Note the Gianturco coils in the right internal jugular vein that were placed percutaneously to close an associated arteriovenous fistula.

Although false aneurysm following carotid endarterectomy is an infrequent complication, it is the etiologic factor in 10 to 50 percent of all aneurysms in this location.[2, 12, 13, 16] False aneurysm occurs most often following endarterectomy with synthetic patch angioplasty, but it can also occur following vein patch angioplasty or primary arterial closure.[2, 13, 18, 19] Compared with larger veins, small-caliber veins, such as the greater saphenous vein harvested from the ankle, have a higher frequency of aseptic necrosis resulting in patch rupture.[20, 21] This usually occurs in the early postoperative period and presents with acute hemorrhage, but it may pre-

TABLE 54–1. Etiology of Extracranial Carotid Artery Aneurysms Treated at UCSF

Cause	Cases, n (%)
Previous carotid endarterectomy	13 (37.1)
Atherosclerosis	10 (28.6)
Trauma	5 (14.3)
Dissection	3 (8.6)
Congenital defect	3 (8.6)
Mycosis	1 (2.8)

sent later as a false aneurysm. This was thought to have occurred in at least one of the false aneurysms following carotid endarterectomy with vein patch angioplasty treated at UCSF. Of the 13 false aneurysms treated there, 5 occurred following patch closure of the carotid artery. In one case, Dacron was used; in the other four cases, greater saphenous vein was utilized. Rupture of silk sutures has been implicated as the most common cause of false aneurysm following primary arterial closure.[19] However, severe hypertension in the immediate postoperative period and infection, both of which were present in over half the patients in the UCSF series, are important contributing factors. *Staphylococcus aureus* (in four patients), *Pseudomonas aeruginosa* (in two patients), and *Streptococcus viridans* (in one patient) were the organisms responsible for mycotic pseudoaneurysms following carotid endarterectomy.

In the preantibiotic era, the most common causes of carotid aneurysms were syphilis, tuberculosis, and streptococcal pharyngitis,[22, 23] but today, mycotic aneurysms unrelated to carotid surgery are extremely rare. A recent review of the literature identified 22 reported cases.[24] In decreasing order, the arterial infections were the result of drug addiction (in four patients), dental infection (in three), septicemia (in three), endocarditis (in two), neck abscess (in one), trauma (in one), and arteriography (in one). In seven patients, the source was unknown. *Staphylococcus* was by far the most common organism involved, followed by *Streptococcus, Salmonella, Klebsiella,* and *Escherichia coli.* At UCSF, one patient was treated for a true mycotic aneurysm secondary to *Staphylococcus aureus* septicemia.

Ten to 30 percent of extracranial carotid artery aneurysms are the result of cervical trauma.[2, 4, 12, 13, 15] Disruption of continuity of the artery wall from penetrating trauma may lead to periarterial hematoma formation, with development of a pseudoaneurysm, arteriovenous fistula, or both (see Fig. 54–3). This injury may also result from iatrogenic puncture of the carotid artery as was seen in two patients treated at UCSF. It is more likely to occur during attempted central venous access with large-bore or stiff catheters, such as those required for pulmonary artery pressure monitoring or hemodialysis. One patient at UCSF was treated for an internal carotid artery pseudoaneurysm following an angiographic procedure. However, in most cases, penetrating trauma results in aneurysms of the common carotid artery, and blunt trauma more often leads to injury of the internal carotid artery. It is postulated that hyperextension and rotation of the neck lead to compression of the internal carotid artery against the transverse processes of the upper cervical vertebrae, causing fracture of the intima and resulting in thrombosis of the lumen or disruption of the artery wall, with pseudoaneurysm formation.[25, 26] An alternative explanation is based on the observation that most traumatic aneurysms occur at the distal extent of the mural dissection, opposite the styloid process.[15] The styloid process rotates with the skull on the dens, whereas the internal carotid artery lying within in the carotid sheath moves with the cervical spine. Therefore, it seems likely that a prominent styloid process may cause intimal disruption in certain instances of exaggerated neck rotation. One traumatic dissecting aneurysm following blunt cervical trauma was treated at UCSF.

Surgical treatment was required for three patients at UCSF with spontaneous carotid dissection associated with pseudoaneurysm formation (Fig. 54–4). Microscopic evaluation of the resected specimen revealed fibromuscular dysplasia as the etiology in one of these patients.[27, 28] Of interest, this patient was also treated for congenital berry aneurysms involving the intracranial carotid artery.[29, 30] Three patients treated at UCSF were thought to have true congenital aneurysms of the extracranial carotid artery. These aneurysms were similar in appearance to the berry type of intracranial aneurysm, and there were no other pathologic changes in the vessel wall. Hammon and coworkers[31] suggested that congenital aneurysms develop secondary to an as yet uncharacterized defect in the arterial media.

Rarely, extracranial carotid aneurysms are caused by arteriopathies other than fibromuscular dysplasia, including cystic medial necrosis,[32] Marfan syndrome,[33] Ehlers-Danlos syndrome,[34] Behçet disease,[35] idiopathic granulomatous arteritis,[36] and prior radiation therapy.[37] Approximately 10 percent of extracranial carotid artery aneurysms are bilateral,[2, 4, 12, 15] and occasionally they are associated with multiple systemic aneurysms.[38]

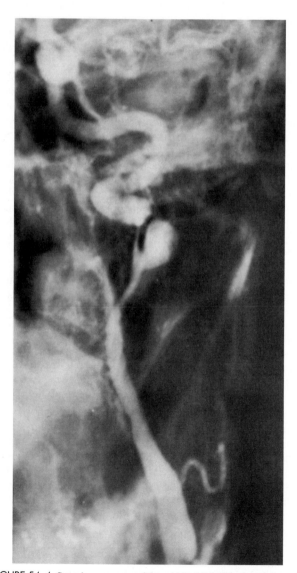

FIGURE 54–4. Saccular aneurysm of the middle third of the internal carotid artery associated with spontaneous dissection.

PRESENTATION

The most frequent presenting complaint is a pulsatile neck or pharyngeal mass (Table 54–2).[2, 4, 12, 16] Both pharyngeal masses and very large neck masses may be accompanied by dysphagia. Shipley and associates[23] pointed out that internal carotid aneurysms present in the pharynx, whereas common carotid aneurysms present in the neck. Although this was true in patients with atherosclerotic aneurysms presenting at UCSF, all patients with false aneurysms following carotid endarterectomy had pulsatile neck masses, presumably because of disruption of normal tissue planes and extension of the arteriotomy onto the common carotid artery.[14] When the pseudoaneurysms were infected, wound cellulitis and drainage were often present, and most patients complained of pain. Pain is also common with dissecting or expanding aneurysms, and it may be referred to the head, neck, and face.[39] In addition, facial pain may result from impingement of the facial and trigeminal nerves. Nerve encroachment with palsies of the fifth through twelfth cranial nerves has been reported.[40] Hoarseness due to compression of the vagus nerve and dysphagia related to involvement of both the vagus and the glossopharyngeal nerves are common symptoms of nerve encroachment. Involvement of postganglionic sympathetic fibers by aneurysms of the internal carotid artery may result in an incomplete Horner syndrome with ptosis and miosis. If there is no involvement of the external carotid artery, facial sweating remains normal because the postganglionic sympathetic fibers traveling with this vessel are spared.

Transient ischemic attacks and stroke account for the presenting symptoms and signs in 30 to 70 percent of patients with extracranial carotid artery aneurysms.[4, 12, 13, 15, 16] These central neurologic events are usually due to distal embolization of thrombotic or atheromatous material from the aneurysmal sac. Less frequently, they are related to hypoperfusion secondary to thrombosis, kinking, or compression of the arterial lumen by the aneurysm.[9, 14] Unlike abdominal aortic aneurysms, extracranial carotid artery aneurysms rarely rupture. When they do rupture, patients usually present with a rapidly enlarging neck mass that may quickly lead to airway compression. Unusual presentations of rupture, such as bleeding from the oropharynx and the ear canal, have also been described.[41, 42] Of the six patients treated at UCSF with acute hemorrhage, all had infected false aneurysms following carotid endarterectomy.

DIAGNOSIS

Physical examination may reveal a pulsatile submandibular neck mass in patients with aneurysms involving the

TABLE 54–2. Presentation of Extracranial Carotid Artery Aneurysms Treated at UCSF

Presentation	Cases, n (%)
Neck or pharyngeal mass	25 (71.4)
Pain	15 (42.9)
Transient ischemic attack	10 (28.6)
Hemorrhage	6 (17.1)
Dysphagia	3 (8.6)
Hoarseness	2 (5.7)
Stroke	2 (5.7)

common carotid artery or the proximal internal or external carotid artery. Overlying skin cellulitis or drainage may be present if the aneurysm is infected. When the middle or distal internal carotid artery is involved, a pulsatile pharyngeal mass may be present, but often aneurysms in this location are not palpable. On physical examination, the most frequently encountered lesion that must be distinguished from an aneurysm is a tortuous or kinked carotid artery. In this case, the pulsatile mass is palpated at the base of the neck, usually on the right side, and it typically occurs in overweight, hypertensive females. Other neck masses that may be confused with carotid artery aneurysms are carotid body tumors, brachial cleft cysts, cystic hygromas, and enlarged lymph nodes. Doppler ultrasonography with real-time imaging can accurately diagnose proximal aneurysms and differentiate them from other lesions. When distal aneurysms are suspected but not palpable by physical examination, duplex scanning is rarely helpful. A better noninvasive study in this situation is dynamic computed tomography. When computed tomographic scanning demonstrates prompt homogeneous enhancement of a parapharyngeal mass following intravenous contrast injection, the differential diagnosis is narrowed to aneurysm or paraganglioma.[43] Magnetic resonance imaging, which can accurately diagnose internal carotid artery dissecting aneurysms approximately 80 percent of the time, may be used as an alternative to computed tomography.[44] The advantage of magnetic resonance imaging is that it can be combined with magnetic resonance angiography. Although experience is limited, magnetic resonance angiography may confirm the diagnosis of an extracranial carotid artery aneurysm and provide additional information that is needed for preoperative planning. Currently, arteriography, using either conventional or digital subtraction techniques, remains the diagnostic study of choice. It provides essential information regarding the location and morphology of the aneurysm that helps determine resectability. In addition, arteriography can provide an accurate assessment of the contralateral carotid and intracranial circulations, which is helpful in planning the reconstruction. When very distal or large aneurysms are present, a balloon occlusion test may be performed at the time of arteriography to determine whether ligation without reconstruction is a therapeutic option.[45]

TREATMENT

It is thought that most extracranial carotid aneurysms enlarge and become symptomatic either from compression of adjacent structures or from distal embolization. However, knowledge of the natural history of these rare lesions is limited, as it is based on case reports and collected reviews that include few untreated patients. Winslow's[22] review of the literature in 1926 included 35 untreated patients with extracranial carotid aneurysms. He reported a long-term mortality of 71 percent for untreated patients compared with 30 percent for patients who underwent the only available surgical treatment, proximal carotid ligation. Many of the patients in Winslow's review had leutic aneurysms, so their outcome is probably not representative of more contemporary etiologies. Nevertheless, more recent reports continue to suggest a poor prognosis. In 1984, Zwolak and colleagues[17] reviewed

the outcome of conservative therapy in five patients with six atherosclerotic aneurysms and reported a 50 percent incidence of stroke ipsilateral to the aneurysm over a mean follow-up period of 6.3 years. As previously noted, a significant number of patients with extracranial carotid aneurysms present with central neurologic events, and when mycotic pseudoaneurysms are considered, the incidence of rupture is high. Therefore, with few exceptions, the presence of an extracranial carotid aneurysm is an indication for surgical treatment. One exception is spontaneous carotid dissecting aneurysms, which are best managed initially by anticoagulation. Healing with recanalization of the arterial lumen and resolution of the aneurysmal dilatation are the usual result. Surgical intervention is reserved for those few patients who have recurrent neurologic events despite adequate anticoagulation or in whom the aneurysmal dissection fails to resolve. In a minority of cases, small, asymptomatic, inaccessible true aneurysms may be best managed by expectant therapy.

Accessible Aneurysms

Resection of the aneurysm with restoration of arterial continuity is the procedure of choice for repair of an accessible carotid artery aneurysm (Table 54–3). Primary arteriorrhaphy and patch angioplasty can frequently be used to close the arterial defect following excision of a saccular aneurysm, whereas primary reanastomosis or interposition grafting is required to restore arterial continuity following removal of a fusiform aneurysm. An autogenous carotid reconstruction is preferred, and this is mandatory when replacing a potentially infected artery wall. If carotid artery elongation is not present, allowing for primary reanastomosis, internal or external iliac artery or greater saphenous vein can be harvested for the interposition graft. If the aneurysm involves the internal carotid artery without involvement of the external or common carotid arteries, an external carotid transposition can be performed by anastomosing the proximal external carotid artery to the distal internal carotid artery. When autogenous reconstruction is not required, a synthetic graft of polytetrafluoroethylene or Dacron is a satisfactory alternative. Similar to carotid endarterectomy, selective shunting is recommended for carotid aneurysm resection and reconstruction. Because the incidence of perioperative neurologic complications is generally higher following surgery for aneurysmal disease than for occlusive disease, more liberal criteria for shunting are used. In addition to a prior stroke and a low carotid backflow pressure,

TABLE 54–3. Treatment of Extracranial Carotid Artery Aneurysms at UCSF

Treatment	Cases, n (%)
Resection and reconstruction	26 (74.3)
Primary arteriorrhaphy	2
Patch angioplasty	8
Primary reanastomosis	6
Interposition grafting	8
Transposition external carotid artery	2
Resection and ligation	5 (14.3)
Exploration only	3 (8.6)
Extracranial-to-intracranial bypass only	1 (2.8)

poor collateral circulation on preoperative arteriography and an anticipated long cerebral ischemic time are indications for shunt placement. Special care must be taken in handling the aneurysm, and particularly when placing the shunt, to prevent distal embolization.

Inaccessible Aneurysms

Although once thought inaccessible, many carotid aneurysms located above a line drawn between the angle of the mandible and the top of the mastoid process on conventional cut-film angiography are now accessible for treatment (Fig. 54–5). Over the past decade, various techniques have been introduced to improve the exposure of the distal internal carotid artery. Several of these techniques have already been described in Chapter 43 and will be only briefly mentioned here. Purdue and associates[46] described a direct approach to distal internal carotid aneurysms through a proximal Y-shaped neck incision carried anterior and posterior to the pinna. The superficial parotid gland is elevated, and the mastoid process and styloid bone are resected, along with the posterior belly of the digastric and the stylohyoid muscles. Rather than resecting the mastoid process, Wylie and coworkers[47] showed that subperiosteal division of the vertical ramus of the mandible from its angle inferiorly to the mandibular notch superiorly can also provide access to this confined space at the base of the skull (Fig. 54–6). The narrow posterior fragment that remains attached to the temporomandibular joint can be rotated outward, and the mandible can be freely retracted anteriorly. At the end of the procedure, the mandible is reunited by wires at the angle

and across the teeth. An alternative to mandibular resection is anterior subluxation of the mandibular condyle onto the articular eminence of the temporal bone by wiring the ipsilateral angle to the nasal spine intraorally, as originally proposed by Fisher and colleagues.[48] More recently, Dossa and coworkers[49] described a modified technique for temporary mandibular subluxation that involves wiring the ipsilateral mandibular bicuspids or cuspids to the contralateral maxillary bicuspids or cuspids. Finally, Sundt and associates[15] claim that adequate anterior mobilization of the mandible can be accomplished by simply releasing the stylomandibular ligament after resection of the posterior belly of the digastric and the stylohyoid muscles. When an extended carotid exposure is anticipated, nasotracheal intubation allows closure of the mandible, which widens the retromandibular space and may be all that is necessary to expose aneurysms in the middle internal carotid artery. In addition, anterior displacement of the mandible by one of the previously described maneuvers is facilitated by nasotracheal intubation. When middle and distal internal carotid aneurysms can be exposed using one of the above techniques, resection of the aneurysm is the treatment of choice. If the aneurysm extends to the base of the skull, leaving no room for placement of a vascular clamp, backbleeding from the distal internal carotid artery can be controlled by either a balloon catheter or a tapered catheter used as an internal shunt placed into the artery within the bony foramen. Restoration of arterial continuity is accomplished using one of the methods of reconstruction already described for accessible aneurysms. When the aneurysm is large or associated with inflammation, the adjacent cranial nerves may be adherent

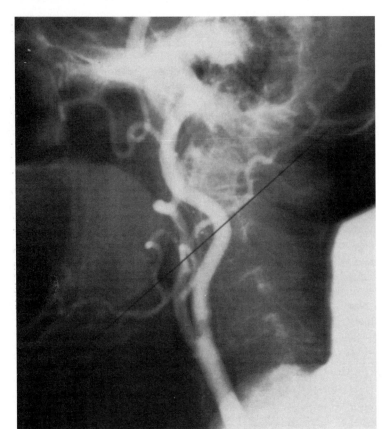

FIGURE 54–5. Lateral arteriogram of left carotid artery. The vascular segment above the black line drawn between the angle of the mandible and the top of the mastoid process may be "inaccessible" for treatment.

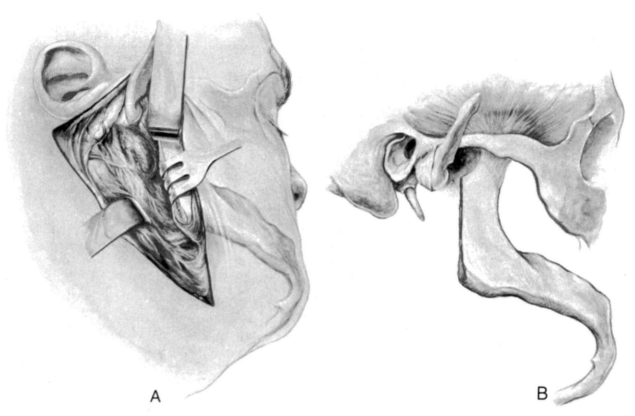

FIGURE 54–6. *A,* Operative drawing of the mandible split to extend accessibility to the distal internal carotid artery. *B,* Schematic view of the mandible split from mandibular angle to mandibular notch.

to it. In this situation, partial resection of the aneurysm or modified endoaneurysmorrhaphy, as described for the treatment of abdominal aortic aneurysms, may be the safest method of treatment, since each avoids complete mobilization of the aneurysm.[50]

Ligation

If there is adequate collateral blood supply to the ipsilateral cerebral hemisphere and the distal end of the involved internal carotid artery is truly inaccessible, ligation of the proximal internal carotid artery is appropriate (Fig. 54–7). Ligation results in thrombosis from the level of occlusion to the orifice of the ophthalmic artery. Postoperatively, these patients are given systemic heparin for 5 to 7 days to prevent extension of the thrombus beyond the ophthalmic artery into the intracranial branches of the internal carotid artery. The safety of ligating the internal carotid artery should be assessed preoperatively whenever possible. As previously suggested, this can be accomplished at the time of the arteriogram by performing a balloon occlusion test. Clinical monitoring with controlled reduction of the systemic blood pressure during the test occlusion improves the sensitivity, and actually obtaining a carotid backflow pressure reading is helpful.[45] The common carotid backflow pressure can be estimated noninvasively by means of ocular pneumoplethysmography, combined with digital common carotid artery compression. A close correlation exists between preoperative ocular pneumoplethysmography pressures and intraoperative preligation stump pressures.[51] Generally, intraoperative ca-

rotid backflow pressures of greater than 70 mm Hg indicate adequate collateral blood flow and permit safe ligation of the carotid artery. Carotid backflow pressures below 55 mm Hg constitute a significant risk of stroke.[52] In this situation, an extracranial-to-intracranial bypass between the superficial temporal artery and a cortical branch of the middle cerebral artery is performed prior to carotid ligation. Limited experience at UCSF with percutaneous balloon embolization of two inaccessible extracranial carotid artery aneurysms (results not included with surgically treated patients) suggests that this form of treatment may be an appropriate alternative, especially in patients who are poor surgical candidates.

RESULTS

Resection of the aneurysm with restoration of arterial continuity was possible in nearly 75 percent of the extracranial carotid artery aneurysms treated at UCSF. The methods of surgical reconstruction are listed in Table 54–3. Except for one reconstruction of the proximal right common carotid artery, all reconstructions were autogenous. Carotid ligation was performed in five patients, one of whom suffered a stroke and died. An extracranial-to-intracranial bypass was performed in one patient who had an internal carotid artery aneurysm extending to the base of the skull and a low preoperative carotid backflow pressure. Follow-up arteriogram revealed thrombosis of the involved internal carotid artery before operative ligation was performed. Surgical exploration was performed in three patients, one of whom was

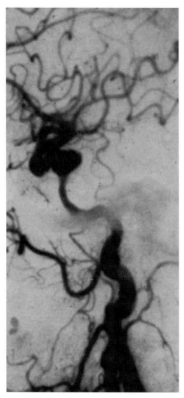 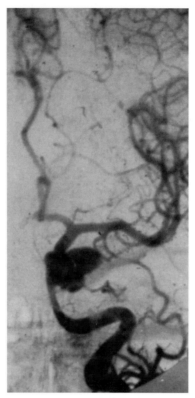 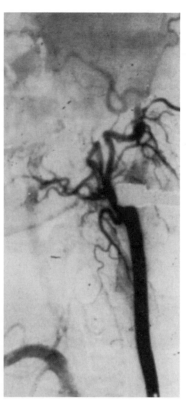

FIGURE 54–7. Distal internal carotid artery aneurysm at the base of the skull. The aneurysm was treated by ligation of the proximal internal carotid artery *(right)*.

found to have a small proximal internal carotid aneurysm associated with a spontaneous dissection that did not warrant resection. The other two patients were found to have unresectable aneurysms, and carotid ligation was not an option because of low carotid backflow pressures. Both patients elected to postpone further therapy. Perioperative cranial nerve deficits occurred in 14.3 percent of patients, but they were transient in all but one patient, who required a cricopharyngeal myotomy for achalasia. There was an 8.6 percent incidence of central neurologic events, with stroke occurring in three patients. The perioperative mortality rate was 5.7 percent. These results are similar to those reported in other contemporary series,[2, 4, 12, 13, 15, 16] in which both local cranial nerve deficits and central neurologic events have occurred in up to 25 percent of patients and perioperative mortality rates have ranged from 0 to 16 percent.

New techniques to improve exposure of the distal internal carotid artery have reduced the number of patients with extracranial carotid artery aneurysms that are truly inaccessible to surgical resection and reconstruction. Precise assessment of the aneurysm by magnetic resonance angiography or digital subtraction arteriography can identify most of these inaccessible aneurysms preoperatively. New techniques in interventional neuroradiology, including the balloon occlusion test, can provide accurate information for planning alternative treatment strategies such as percutaneous balloon embolization or operative ligation with or without extracranial-to-intracranial bypass. In summary, a small percentage of extracranial carotid artery aneurysms are inaccessible to surgical resection and reconstruction, but with the recent advances in radiologic and surgical techniques, all aneurysms are amenable to some form of treatment.

REFERENCES

1. Carrascal A, Mashiah A, Charlesworth D: Aneurysms of the extracranial carotid arteries. *Br J Surg.* 1978;65:590.
2. McCollum CH, Wheeler WG, Noon GP, DeBakey ME: Aneurysms of the extracranial carotid artery: Twenty-one years' experience. *Am J Surg.* 1979;137:196.
3. Welling RE, Taha A, Goel T, et al: Extracranial carotid artery aneurysms. *Surgery.* 1983;93:319.
4. Pratschke E, Schäfer K, Reimer J, et al: Extracranial aneurysms of the carotid artery. *Thorac Cardiovasc Surg.* 1980;28:354.
5. Boddie HG: Transient ischaemic attacks and stroke due to extracranial aneurysm of internal carotid artery. *Br Med J.* 1972;3:802.
6. Kaupp HA, Haid SP, Jurayj MN, et al: Aneurysms of the extracranial carotid artery. *Surgery.* 1972;72:946.
7. Schechter DC: Cervical carotid aneurysms. *N Y State J Med.* 1979;79:892.
8. Johnson JN, Helsby CR, Stell PM: Aneurysm of the external carotid artery. *J Cardiovasc Surg.* 1980;21:105.
9. Painter TA, Hertzer NR, Beven EG, O'Hara PJ: Extracranial carotid aneurysms: Report of six cases and review of the literature. *J Vasc Surg.* 1985;2:312.
10. Agrifoglio M, Rona P, Spirito R, et al: Extracranial carotid artery aneurysms. *J Cardiovasc Surg.* 1989;30:942.
11. Petrovic P, Avramov S, Pfau J, et al: Surgical management of extracranial carotid artery aneurysms. *Ann Vasc Surg.* 1991;5:506.
12. Rhodes LE, Stanley JC, Hoffman GL, et al: Aneurysms of extracranial carotid arteries. *Arch Surg.* 1976;111:339.
13. Busuttil RW, Davidson RK, Foley KT, et al: Selective management of extracranial carotid artery aneurysms. *Am J Surg.* 1980;140:85.
14. Krupski WC, Effeney DJ, Ehrenfeld WK, Stoney RJ: Aneurysms of the carotid arteries. *Aust N Z J Surg.* 1983;53:521.
15. Sundt TM, Pearson BW, Piepgras DG, et al: Surgical management of aneurysms of the distal extracranial internal carotid artery. *J Neurosurg.* 1986;64:169.
16. Sahlman A, Salo J, Kostiainen S, et al: Extracranial carotid artery aneurysms. *Vasa Band.* 1991;20:369.
17. Zwolak RM, Whitehouse WM Jr, Knake JE, et al: Atherosclerotic extracranial carotid artery aneurysms. *J Vasc Surg.* 1984;1:415.
18. Graver LM, Mulcare RJ: Pseudoaneurysm after carotid endarterectomy. *J Cardiovasc Surg.* 1986;27:294.
19. Bergamini TM, Seabrook GR, Bandyk DF, Towne JB: Symptomatic recurrent carotid stenosis and aneurysmal degeneration after endarterectomy. *Surgery.* 1993;113:580.
20. O'Hara PJ, Hertzer NR, Krajewski LP, Beven EG: Saphenous vein patch rupture after carotid endarterectomy. *J Vasc Surg.* 1992;15:504.
21. Scott EW, Dolson L, Day AL, Seeger JM: Carotid endarterectomy complicated by vein patch rupture. *Neurosurgery.* 1992;31:373.

22. Winslow N: Extracranial aneurysm of the internal carotid artery: History and analysis of the cases registered up to Aug. 1, 1925. *Arch Surg.* 1926;13:689.

23. Shipley AM, Winslow N, Walker WW: Aneurysm in the cervical portion of the internal carotid artery: An analytical study of the cases recorded in the literature between August, 1925 and July 31, 1936. *Ann Surg.* 1937;105:673.

24. Jebara VA, Acar C, Dervanian P, et al: Mycotic aneurysms of the carotid arteries—case report and review of the literature. *J Vasc Surg.* 1991;14:215.

25. Friedman WA, Day AL, Quisling RG, et al: Cervical carotid dissecting aneurysms. *Neurosurgery.* 1980;7:207.

26. Zelenoock GG, Dazmers A, Whitehouse WM Jr, et al: Extracranial internal carotid artery dissections. *Arch Surg.* 1982;117:425.

27. Miyauchi M, Shionoya S: Aneurysm of the extracranial internal carotid artery caused by fibromuscular dysplasia. *Eur J Vasc Surg.* 1991;5:587.

28. Bour P, Taghave I, Bracard S, et al: Aneurysms of the extracranial internal carotid artery due to fibromuscular dysplasia: Results of surgical management. *Ann Vasc Surg.* 1992;6:205.

29. Tokimura H, Todoroki K, Asakura T, et al: Coexistance of extracranial internal carotid artery aneurysm and multiple intracranial aneurysms. *Neurol Med Chir (Tokyo).* 1992;32:292.

30. Schievink WI, Mokri B, Peipgras DG: Angiographic frequency of saccular intracranial aneurysms in patients with spontaneous cervical artery dissection. *J Neurosurg.* 1992;76:62.

31. Hammon JW, Silver D, Young WG: Congenital aneurysm of the extracranial carotid arteries. *Ann Surg.* 1972;176:777.

32. Barnes WT, Jacoby GE: Aneurysm of the common carotid artery due to cystic medial necrosis treated by excision and graft. *Ann Surg.* 1962;155:82.

33. Hardin CA: Successful resection of carotid and abdominal aneurysm in two related patients with Marfan's syndrome. *N Engl J Med.* 1962;267:141.

34. Ruby ST, Kramer J, Cassidy SB, Tsipouras P: Internal carotid artery aneurysm: A vascular manifestation of type IV Ehlers-Danlos syndrome. *Conn Med.* 1989;53:142.

35. Tacal T, Cekirge S, Balkanci F, Besim A: Saccular extracranial carotid artery aneurysm secondary to Behcet's disease. Case report. *Acta Chir Scand.* 1993;17:70.

36. Adiseshiah M, Snait M, Fisher C: Carotid bifurcation aneurysm due to idiopathic granulomatous arteritis. *Br J Surg.* 1986;73:69.

37. Bole PV, Hintz G, Chander P, et al: Bilateral carotid aneurysms secondary to radiation therapy. *Ann Surg.* 1975;181:888.

38. Kubo S, Nakagawa H, Imaoka S: Systemic multiple aneurysms of the extracranial internal carotid artery, intracranial vertebral artery, and visceral arteries: Case report. *Neurosurgery.* 1992;30:600.

39. Fay T: Atypical facial neuralgia, a syndrome of vascular pain. *Ann Otol Rhinol Laryngol.* 1932;41:1030.

40. Lane RJ, Weisman RA: Carotid artery aneurysms: An otolaryngologic perspective. *Laryngoscope.* 1980;90:897.

41. Rittenhouse EA, Radke HM, Sumner DS: Carotid artery aneurysm: Review of the literature and report of a case with rupture into the oropharynx. *Arch Surg.* 1972;105:786.

42. Harrison DFN: Two cases of bleeding from the ear from carotid aneurysm. *Guys Hosp Rep.* 1954;103:207.

43. Duvall ER, Gupta KL, Vitek JJ, et al: CT demonstration of extracranial carotid artery aneurysms. *J Comput Assist Tomogr.* 1986;10:404.

44. Zuber M, Meary E, Meder J-F, Mas J-L: Magnetic resonance imaging and dynamic CT scan in cervical artery dissections. *Stroke.* 1994;25:576.

45. McIvor NP, Willinsky RA, TerBrugge KG, et al: Validity of test occlusion studies prior to internal carotid artery sacrifice. *Head Neck.* 1994;16:11.

46. Purdue GF, Pellegrini RV, Arena S: Aneurysms of the high internal carotid artery: A new approach. *Surgery.* 1981;89:268.

47. Wylie EJ, Stoney RJ, Ehrenfeld WK, Effeney DJ: Nonatherosclerotic diseases of the extracranial carotid artery. In *Manual of Vascular Surgery,* Vol. 2. New York: Springer-Verlag; 1986:187.

48. Fisher DR Jr, Clagett GP, Parker JI, et al: Mandibular subluxation for high carotid exposure. *J Vasc Surg.* 1984;1:727.

49. Dossa C, Shepard AD, Wolford DG, et al: Distal internal carotid exposure: A simplified technique for temporary mandibular subluxation. *J Vasc Surg.* 1990;12:319.

50. Creech O: Endo-aneurysmorrhaphy and treatment of aortic aneurysm. *Ann Surg.* 1966;164:935.

51. Gee W, Mehigan JT, Wylie EJ: Measurement of collateral cerebral hemispheric blood pressure by ocular pneumoplethysmography. *Am J Surg.* 1975;130:121.

52. Ehrenfeld WK, Stoney RJ, Wylie EJ: Relation of carotid stump pressure to safety of carotid artery ligation. *Surgery.* 1983;93:299.

CHAPTER 55

Carotid Body Paragangliomas: Diagnosis, Prognosis, and Surgical Management

JEFFREY L. BALLARD and LOUIS L. SMITH

The carotid body, derived from neural crest cells, is a minute oval structure of 0.1 to 0.5 cm located on the posterior aspect of the carotid bifurcation. The only known disease to affect the carotid body is neoplasm. The tumor, which arises from paraganglionic tissue, is appropriately termed ''paraganglioma.'' The surgical management of this interesting tumor is still controversial, despite new and more accurate diagnostic techniques and better operative management. The tumor is slow growing; it has a low but definite incidence of malignancy. Appropriate surgical therapy must be based on a knowledge of the pathogenetic behavior of the tumor as well as protection and preservation of the cerebral circulation.

The carotid body was first described by Von Haller in 1743.[1] More than a century elapsed before the first tumor of this structure was reported by Marchand[2] in 1891. Rieger was the first to excise a carotid body tumor in 1880 by ligation of the carotid vessels.[3] Unfortunately, his patient died. The first successful surgical removal of a carotid paraganglioma with preservation of the carotid vessels was reported by Albert in 1889.[4] Scudder[5] is credited with the first successful excision of a carotid body paraganglioma in the United States in 1903.

CLASSIFICATION

There has been confusion regarding the terminology used in reporting tumors arising from paraganglionic tissue. The carotid body paraganglioma has been referred to as ''chemodectoma'' or ''glomus carotica.'' These terms are misnomers. There is no relationship between glomus and paraganglionic tissue.[6, 7] True glomus tumors are highly organized arteriolovenular anastomoses that form a painful focus, usually in the nail bed, pads of the fingers and toes, ears, hands, and feet.[8] Further, no tumor at the carotid bifurcation has been demonstrated to arise from the nonchromaffin-reacting chemoreceptor cells of the carotid body. The term ''chemodectoma,'' originally introduced in 1950,[7] was used because the carotid body serves as a chemoreceptor organ that is responsive to excess carbon dioxide, lack of oxygen, and increased hydrogen concentration.

The carotid body is composed of cells derived from neural crest tissue that have migrated in close association with autonomic ganglion cells. Similar tissue is located along the vagus nerve, jugular venous system, aortic arch, visceral autonomic system, and adrenal medulla and forms an extensive multicentric paraganglia system. Some paragangliomas, particularly those that are adrenal derived, give a positive chromaffin reaction, and these functional tumors often produce catecholamines (eg, pheochromocytoma).[7] Glenner and Grimley[9] proposed a classification for paragangliomas according to anatomic site and functional activity, a modified version of which appears in Table 55–1. Thus, the precise nomenclature for a carotid body tumor is ''carotid body paraganglioma nonfunctional.'' Figure 55–1 shows the location of the different branchiomeric paragangliomas in relationship to the carotid bifurcation.

PATHOLOGY

The classic carotid body paraganglioma arises from the posteromedial aspect of the bifurcation of the common carotid artery. Hyperplasia of the carotid body has been noted in humans living at high altitudes and in patients with chronic obstructive pulmonary disease.[10, 11] In addition, Saldena and coworkers[12] reported a 10-fold increase in the incidence of paragangliomas in people living in the Peruvian Andes as compared with those living at sea level. Chronic hypoxemia seems to be a predisposing factor for the development of carotid body hyperplasia and may have a role in the development of paragangliomas.

Carotid body paragangliomas grow slowly but relentlessly. There has been no reported case of spontaneous regression of this neoplasm. A growth rate of approximately 2 cm every 5 years was noted by Farr.[13] Most tumors are 3 to 6 cm in diameter, but tumors as large as 15 cm have been reported.[14]

The tumor, which develops on the posterior aspect of the carotid bifurcation, adheres to the adventitia and spreads to the internal and external carotid arteries, thus producing the characteristic carotid bifurcation saddle deformity (Fig. 55–2). The tumor mass may be focal or may completely encase the carotid vessels. Upon gross examination, paragangliomas appear gray-pink with foci of hemorrhage; their consistency resembles liver tissue.

Microscopically, paragangliomas tend to reproduce the architecture of the normal gland. Although the tumors are occasionally circumscribed by surrounding connective tissue, a well-defined true capsule is not present. One of the hallmarks of a carotid body paraganglioma is its abundant vascularity. The blood supply may be so extensive as to suggest an angiomatous tumor at first evaluation. This rich blood supply can be visualized in later serial films taken during selective carotid injection. Figure 55–3 is a late radiograph of a carotid body tumor, demonstrating the characteristic rich blood supply. Typical nests of predominantly chief cells are organized into discrete islands within the alveolar reticular network and the dilated vascular sinusoids.

Cytoplasmic granules (100 to 300 μm) can be demonstrated within the chief cells by special silver stains and are thought to be the site for storage of catecholamines. Al-

---

TABLE 55–1. Classification of Paragangliomas

Branchiomeric
Jugulotympanic
Intercarotid
Intravagal
Laryngeal, coronary, pulmonary

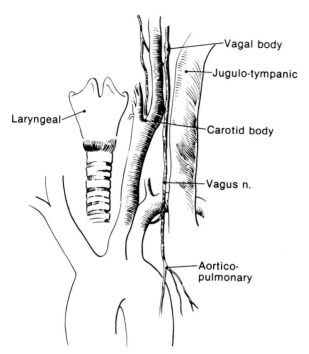

FIGURE 55–1. Sites of occurrence of the different paragangliomas in relation to the carotid bifurcation.

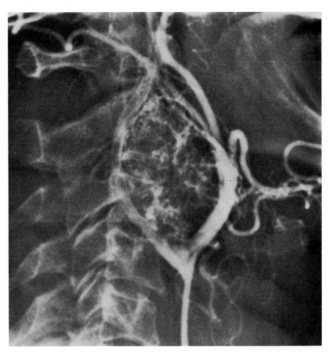

FIGURE 55–3. Marked vascularity in a carotid body tumor.

though the chromaffin reaction tends to be negative, most carotid paragangliomas contain catecholamines, which can usually be demonstrated by formalin-induced fluorescence. Most paragangliomas are nonfunctional, but a rare catecholamine-secreting carotid body tumor simulating a pheochromocytoma has been reported.[15]

Analysis of the DNA of resected paragangliomas suggests that aneuploid tumors with a high synthetic phase fraction may be more aggressive.[16, 17] Barnes and Taylor[18] observed

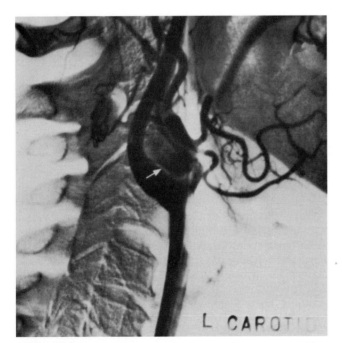

FIGURE 55–2. Saddle deformity of the carotid bifurcation produced by a carotid body tumor. Note the dense blush of the tumor (arrow).

perineural and vascular invasion only in tumors with abnormal DNA histograms. Although neither ploidy nor synthetic phase fraction has been correlated with survival, patients with aneuploid, high–synthetic phase fraction tumors may have a high propensity for recurrence.[17]

Malignant transformation is uncommon, occurring in 5 percent of our collected series (Table 55–2). There are no good histologic criteria by which malignancy can be diagnosed. Hyperchromatic nucleii, cellular pleomorphism, and mitotic figures are not reliable indicators of malignancy. The only reliable findings of malignancy are microscopic evidence of invasion of adjacent tissues and lymph nodes or distant metastasis. More than half of malignant tumors are metastatic to regional lymph nodes, and the remainder to distant viscera.

If one uses the criterion of lymph node involvement or distal metastasis, the incidence of malignancy in our collected series was 5 percent. Duration of follow-up is apparently important in this regard, since the longer these patients are followed, the higher the incidence of distant metastasis. Gaylis and Mieny[19] reported a 30 percent incidence of malignancy in 23 cases. Brown and associates reported intervals as long as 35 years between the discovery of the primary tumor and the appearance of metastatic disease. It seems prudent to exercise caution in discussing long-term "cure" with patients who have carotid body paragangliomas.

DIAGNOSIS

The usual presenting problem is a mass below the angle of the mandible. Other presenting signs and symptoms include cranial nerve dysfunction as well as nonspecific complaints such as headache, dizziness, tinnitus, hoarseness, dysphagia, and syncope. Examination will disclose a visible or palpable mass immediately below the angle of the mandible. Javid

TABLE 55–2. Carotid Body Paragangliomas: Selected Data From 575 Cases

Institution (Study Period)*	Total Cases, n	Bilateral, n	Familial, n	Arterial Reconstructions, n	Operative Stroke, n	Cranial Nerve Injury Site	Number	Deaths, n	Malignant Cases, n
Cleveland Clinic (1922–1978)[42]	39	4	2	6	1	Hypogl Vagus Facial	7 6 2	1	5
Cleveland Clinic (1979–1987)[41]	15	5	1	6	0	Vagus	4	0	0
Mayo Clinic (1931–1967)[43]	90	6	0	NA	16	Hypogl Vagus	17 15	4	2
Mayo Clinic (1965–1985)[52]	59	9	8	15	5	Hypogl Vagus Facial	6 11 6	1	1
Lahey Clinic (1982)[44]	36	3	0	NA	4	Hypogl Vagus Facial	5 3 1	4	NA
Sloan-Kettering (1937–1977)[13]	44	3	12	6	4	Cranial nerve palsy	7	5	4
Johns Hopkins University; Walter Reed (1946–1967)[45]	38	2	NA	5	0		0	0	2
University of Michigan (1945–1975)[46]	16	1	2	3	0	Hypogl	2	NA	NA
St. Luke's Hospital, Chicago (1954–1974)[21]	24	3	0	NA	0	Vagus	2	1	2
University of Toronto (1955–1980)[47]	27	3	2	8	1	Hypogl Vagus Facial	2 3 3	1	2
University of Leiden (1956–1988)[49,50]	91	5	20	4	1	Glosso Vagus	1 4	1	0
University of CA, San Francisco (1963–1981)[48]	19	1	1	4	3	Hypogl Vagus Facial	3 3 1	0	4
Massachusetts General Hospital (1982–1991)[51]	19	2	0	2	0	Vagus Facial	2 1	0	0
St. Joseph Hospital & Denver Presbyterian Hospital (1956–1990)[11]	33	3	1	NA	1	Cranial nerve palsy	4	1	3
St. Mary's Hospital, London (1975–1987)[22]	25	2	0	2	0	Cranial nerve palsy Cranial nerve injury	2 1	1	3
Totals	575	52 (9%)	49 (9%)	61 (11%)	36 (6%)		124 (22%)	20 (24%)	28 (5%)

*Superscript number refers to the number of the publication pertaining to these studies, as listed in the references at the end of the chapter.

Glosso, glossopharyngeal nerve; Hypogl, hypoglossal nerve; NA, not applicable.

and colleagues[21] noted bruits in 25 percent of their reported series. The mass is pulsatile but not expansile. This tumor has free mobility from side to side but not vertically. It is important to palpate both sides of the neck, since 9 percent of carotid body paragangliomas in our collected series were bilateral. A complete preoperative assessment should include careful pharyngoscopy, as there may be tumor extension into the pharynx or larynx.[22] Visualization of the vocal cords and a thorough neurologic examination may reveal subtle clues consistent with vagal nerve dysfunction or other cranial nerve involvement.

Diagnostic studies that are helpful in establishing an accurate diagnosis of a carotid paraganglioma include scintigraphy, duplex ultrasonography, computed tomography (CT), magnetic resonance imaging (MRI), and magnetic resonance angiography (MRA). Peters and coworkers[23] reported the use of intravenous ^{99}Tc-pertechnetate angioscan to diagnose a carotid body tumor. The specificity of this test is in question, since two additional patients thought to have carotid body paragangliomas were later found to have a venous malformation in one case and a nonvascular mass in the second case. This lesion was later demonstrated to be a tuberculous lymph node that resolved on chemotherapy. Duplex ultrasonography, which can accurately demonstrate location, structure, shape, and spatial relationships, can be a helpful study in young patients in whom neck cysts are common. Paragangliomas have been reported in patients as young as 6 months of age.[24] Doppler color-flow imaging has been shown to be accurate in the diagnosis of paragangliomas based on the classic widened contour of the bifurcation and the easily recognized tumor hypervascularity.[25, 26]

High-resolution CT scanning can accurately determine invasion of the soft tissues of the neck. It can also demonstrate intratympanic or intracranial extension of the tumor. It gives helpful information regarding the relationship of the carotid circulation and the jugular vein to the tumor. In addition, bony involvement of the base of the skull can be evaluated. The diffuse vascularity of paragangliomas differentiates them from other solid tumors of the head and neck. Their intense enhancement can be seen on dynamic CT scanning during the arterial phase.[27, 28]

Either conventional MRI (without and with gadolinium) or flow-sensitive MRI, including MRA, may supplant CT as the study of choice in the diagnosis of paragangliomas. Recent reports comparing MRI (with and without gadolinium) and MRA to CT have demonstrated that a carotid body paraganglioma as small as 5 mm in diameter can be accurately identified with either modality. The usual cutoff for detection of a carotid body paraganglioma with dynamic CT is 8 mm in diameter.[29] Additionally, MRI provides superb

soft-tissue contrast as well as soft tissue–bone differentiation.[29–31]

Despite the above-mentioned diagnostic studies, the most accurate and helpful invasive diagnostic study is the arch and cerebral angiogram. Obtaining cerebral runoff views will alert the surgeon to the presence of intracranial vascular abnormalities. Should hemodynamically significant carotid bifurcation disease exist, endarterectomy can be performed at the same operation. Selective external carotid and thyrocervical arterial injections are helpful in visualizing the blood supply to very large tumors. Precerebral angiography is also helpful in diagnosing paragangliomas in other locations. Figure 55–4 shows a vagal paraganglioma displacing the internal carotid artery forward. This is in contrast to the typical carotid body saddle deformity (see Fig. 55–2).

Selective embolization of the blood supply to paragangliomas may be employed preoperatively to aid in the removal of these vascular tumors. An expert angiographer, with a keen awareness of the variable vascular architecture associated with a paraganglioma, is key to the procedure. There can be collateral flow into the vertebral or internal carotid artery, with the possibility of reflux emboli and stroke. Ideally, the embolization procedure should be performed within hours of the proposed operation; otherwise, collateral arterial branches may form and contribute to blood loss during a delayed dissection.[32] When correctly performed, preoperative embolization of carotid paragangliomas has

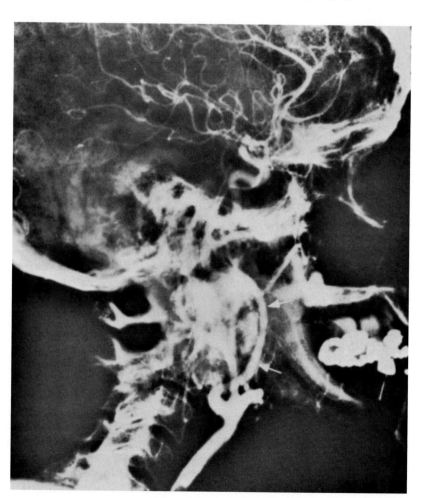

FIGURE 55–4. Vagal paraganglioma displacing the internal carotid artery forward *(arrows)*. Note the marked vascularity that is characteristic of this tumor.

proved to be a useful adjunct in the management of these highly vascular and complex lesions.[32, 33]

GENETIC CONSIDERATIONS

Chase[34] first reported a familial occurrence of carotid body paragangliomas in 1933. He also recognized the bilateral occurrence of this tumor. Sprong and Kirby[35] in 1949 reported 9 of 11 siblings in one family with carotid body paragangliomas.

Grufferman and colleagues[36] and Sobol and Dailey[7] have summarized the genetic origin of carotid body paragangliomas. Their observations indicate an autosomal dominant mechanism for transmission, with variable penetrance and expressivity. Carotid body paragangliomas are classified as dominant because of their average phenotypic expression of 40 percent. There is also a sex-equal ratio of occurrence. In Grufferman's study, bilateral tumors were noted in 31.8 percent of patients who are related genetically versus 4.4 percent in nonrelated individuals ($P = 7 \times 10^{-10}$). Other tumors derived from neural crest tissue, such as pheochromocytomas, thyroid medullary carcinomas, and tumors associated with von Recklinghausen neurofibromatosis syndrome, also demonstrate an autosomal dominant inheritance with variable penetrance and expressivity.[7]

Multiple carotid body paragangliomas have been reported in the same family; the presence of an associated pheochromocytoma in the same individual has also been reported.[22, 37, 38] Although the incidence of catecholamine-secreting carotid body paragangliomas is low, the possibility of an associated pheochromocytoma should include testing for urinary catechol metabolites in hypertensive patients.[39]

The association of carotid body paragangliomas and pheochromocytomas is one reason for the inclusion of this tumor with the amine precursor uptake and decarboxylation (APUD) group of neoplasms of familial origin.[40] Numerous authors have reported the finding of multiple paragangliomas in the same patient, further supporting the relationship of this neoplasm and the APUD tumors.[7, 11, 22, 41–43]

COLLECTED SERIES OF CAROTID BODY TUMORS

The authors have summarized 15 reports of carotid body paragangliomas from the literature (see Table 55–2).[11, 13, 21, 22, 41–52] This summary includes 575 pateints, 49 (9%) of whom had tumors of familial origin. There were 52 bilateral tumors (9%). Removal of the tumor required arterial reconstruction in 61 patients (11%), and 36 patients (6%) developed operative stroke. The operative mortality was 4 percent. Malignancy, as defined by the presence of lymph node involvement or distant metastasis, occurred in 5 percent of these patients.

It becomes evident from these data that carotid body paragangliomas have a high enough incidence of malignancy that removal should be encouraged unless age or associated illness is a contradication. Furthermore, the location of this tumor at the carotid bifurcation, immediately adjacent to the cerebral circulation and vital cranial nerve structures, makes it mandatory that surgeons managing these cases have experience in vascular surgical techniques. The operative stroke rate of 6 percent is high and reflects the disastrous management of early cases by tumor excision with acute ligation of the carotid circulation.

The tendency of paragangliomas to involve adjacent cranial nerves is evident by the frequent presence of hypoglossal or vagal nerve dysfunction. Vocal cord paralysis is seen occasionally in patients presenting with carotid body paragangliomas. It is important to obtain preoperative indirect laryngoscopy to determine vocal cord function. The incidence of operative cranial nerve injury in the 575 patients reported herein was 22 percent. Many of these nerve injuries were temporary, with subsequent complete recovery of function; however, the challenge of cranial nerve protection is apparent.

MANAGEMENT OF CAROTID BODY TUMORS

Surgical Removal

The surgical removal of a carotid body paraganglioma requires skill and keen judgment. Mathews[55] warned in 1915 that ''this rare tumor presents unusual difficulties to the surgeon, and should one encounter it without having suspected the diagnosis, the experience will not soon be forgotten.'' His statement is pertinent today. The problems associated with removal of carotid body paragangliomas led no less an authority than the father of American head and neck surgery, Hayes Martin,[56] to advocate a nonsurgical approach to most patients with carotid body paragangliomas.

Management of carotid body paragangliomas during the first half of this century included acute ligation of the internal carotid artery in difficult cases. Farr[13] reported a mortality rate of 50 percent with resection of the carotid bifurcation. Padberg and coworkers[46] reported a 30 percent stroke rate with sudden occlusion of the carotid vessels. An incredible report of the autopsy findings in a patient surgically treated for bilateral carotid body paragangliomas was reported by Rush.[57] The patient expired 16 hours postoperatively; at autopsy, both common carotid arteries were found to be ligated securely 2 or 3 cm below the bifurcations.

Resection of a carotid body paraganglioma can challenge a surgeon's skill, judgment, and endurance at every step. Despite the many unusual difficulties presented by this tumor, surgical resection remains the only curative therapy. The low but definite incidence of malignancy, its slow but relentless growth, and its propensity to incorporate adjacent structures make surgical excision advisable unless age, associated illness, or technical reasons preclude safe removal.

Shamblin and associates[45] at the Mayo Clinic classified carotid body tumors into three groups (Table 55–3). Groups 1 and 2 can usually be excised with preservation of the carotid circulation. Group 3 represents a very advanced lesion with encirclement of and extensive adherence to the carotid bifurcation. This type of tumor requires resection and autogenous vein reconstruction.

The carotid bifurcation is exposed through a standard anterior sternocleidomastoid incision or a modified T-radical neck incision for large tumors.[58] The common carotid, distal internal, and external carotid arteries are surrounded by vessel loops if possible. Management of the smaller group 1 lesions includes dissection on the posterolateral surface of the internal carotid artery, the area of least adherence. The basic principle of subadventitial resection, as first advocated by Gordon-Taylor,[59] involves cutting down to, but not into, the artery. The so-called white line that he described is basically the most superficial adventitial layer separating the tumor from the artery. Particular care must be taken to preserve the hypoglossal and vagus nerves, which may be involved at the superior and posterior aspects of the tumor.

A careful game plan is essential in managing certain group 2 and all group 3 carotid body paragangliomas. The surgeon must be prepared to resect the external carotid artery in certain group 2 lesions, as described by Krupski and associates,[50] for exposure and control of bleeding during tumor removal (Fig. 55–5). In a significant number of group 3 tumors, the dissection will include resection of the internal carotid artery as well. The decision to use a shunt during reconstruction in the latter case can be determined by measuring the internal carotid artery stump pressure prior to resection. It is wise to have one leg prepped and draped for harvest of the saphenous vein if necessary. The preferred reconstruction following resection of the internal carotid artery includes the use of a reverse saphenous vein segment. Arterial reconstruction was necessary in 11 percent of the 575 cases reviewed in Table 55–2.

In their reported series, Javid and colleagues[21] routinely employed an intraluminal shunt during resection of carotid body paragangliomas and noted a decrease in operative blood loss. The tumor blood supply from the external carotid artery is interrupted during resection by this maneuver.

The operative stroke rate following resection of carotid body paragangliomas was 6 percent, and the operative mortality rate was 4 percent in our selected series (see Table 55–2). Cranial nerve injuries were seen in 22 percent, again emphasizing the intimate relationship of these nerves to the superior and posterior aspects of this tumor. Recent series reporting operative results and employing modern vascular surgical techniques have reported no operative strokes and a mortality of less than 2.5 percent.[21, 22, 43, 53]

Preoperative Embolization

Preoperative embolization serves as a useful adjunct in the treatment of paragangliomas, particularly large bulky tumors, and has been reported by several authors.[30, 31, 53, 60] Hekster and coworkers[61] reported the treatment of five patients with large jugular paragangliomas by transfemoral

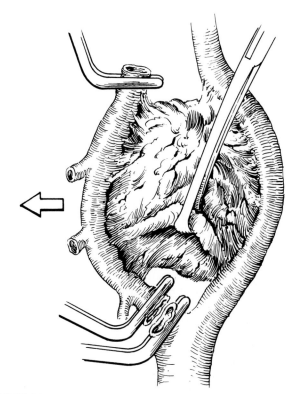

FIGURE 55–5. Resection of the external carotid artery to interrupt the rich blood supply to the tumor and to facilitate removal of large lesions. (From Krupski WC, Effeney DJ, Ehrenfeld WK, Stoney RJ: Cervical chemodectoma: Technical considerations and management options. *Am J Surg.* 1982;144:215; with permission.)

catheterization with the patients' own muscle tissue. Decrease in tumor size was noted in all five patients following embolization; however, a transient stroke occurred in one patient, and an allergic reaction to contrast material occurred in a second patient. These investigators cautioned that embolization alone is a temporary treatment, since the tumor can acquire a new blood supply and continue to enlarge, as occurred in several of their patients.

Using Ivalon sponge emboli via a transfemoral approach, Schick and associates[62] reported a 90 percent reduction in vascularity and a 30 percent reduction in size of a 12 cm carotid body tumor. Ward and colleagues[33] noted a significant decrease in operative blood loss and cranial nerve injury when six patients who were embolized were compared with 10 who were managed without preoperative embolization.

The technique of preoperative embolization, as described by Borges and coworkers,[63] involves careful mapping of the feeding vessels from the external carotid system. Selective catheterization of the large feeding branch from the ascending pharyngeal artery is the key to successful embolization. Avoidance of the posterior branch of this vessel is mandatory, as that branch is the blood supply to the ninth, tenth, and twelfth cranial nerves. In addition, occipital, vertebral, and ascending cervical arteries must be visualized to rule out collateral circulation from these sources. LaMuraglia and associates[53] used a microcatheter technique and angiography with opacified xylocaine to avoid inadvertent embolization of dangerous collateral anastomoses between tumor feeding vessels and the vertebral artery, internal carotid

TABLE 55–3. Classification of Carotid Body Tumors Based on Growth Characteristics

Group	Description
1	Tumor easily dissected from adjacent vessels (26% of cases)
2	Tumor partially surrounding the vessels and more adherent to the adventitia (46.4% of cases)
3	Tumor completely encircling the carotid bifurcation, making dissection impossible, even by experienced vascular surgeon (27.6% of cases)

Adapted from Shamblin WR, Remine WH, Sheps SG, et al: Carotid body tumor (chemodectoma): Clinicopathologic analysis of ninety cases. *Am J Surg.* 1971; 122:732; with permission.

artery, or cranial nerves. They recommend a neurologic examination before and after a test injection of opacified xylocaine to identify patients at high risk for cerebral injury or cranial nerve damage.[53] These techniques cause a marked reduction in the vascularity of the tumor and greatly facilitate the surgical excision.

Embolization is only an adjunct, and surgical excision should be undertaken soon after embolization because of the likelihood of recanalization and collateralization. Complications with this technique are unusual,[53] although stroke, allergic contrast reaction,[61] and even death have been reported with preoperative embolization of large head and neck paragangliomas.[64] The experience and judgment of the interventional radiologist are crucial to the success of the procedure, and embolizing material should not be used in equivocal situations.

Radiation Therapy

Radiation therapy is of little benefit as a primary treatment for carotid body paragangliomas.[45, 48, 65–67] Occasional reports of tumor regression can be found in the literature, but these are largely anecdotal.[44, 66, 67] Chambers and Mahoney[47] reported on a patient with an unresectable tumor who received a total of 8000 rads of radiation and survived 20 years with good palliation.

Postoperative radiation for partially resected or recurrent tumors may be of benefit.[13, 68] Extensive experience with radiation therapy in jugular paragangliomas was reported by Spector and Sobol.[69] These tumors are less accessible to surgical resection and are more likely to recur than carotid body paragangliomas. Radiation therapy therefore has a better-defined role in the treatment of these tumors. Twenty jugular paragangliomas were treated with 4000 to 6000 rads; 45 percent of the tumors showed a histologic response, 20 percent demonstrated complete regression, and 35 percent showed evidence of progressive enlargement. Moreover, although vascular sclerosis was prominent histologically in postirradiated specimens, the chief cells showed no significant response, indicating radioresistance.

One of the major difficulties in evaluating the effectiveness of radiation or even surgical therapy for malignant or recurrent paragangliomas is the remarkable chronicity of this neoplasm. Martin and associates[70] followed 28 patients with carotid body paragangliomas for an average of 11 years. Seven of these patients subsequently developed metastatic disease. One of these patients died 24 years after the onset of symptoms, and four others were alive 3, 15, 16, and 24 years after symptom onset with metastatic disease, at the time of their report.

Certainly, the remarkably slow growth rate of carotid body paragangliomas contraindicates surgical resection in elderly, poor-risk patients with limited life expectancy. However, Martin and coworkers[70] reported on the slow but unrelenting progress of this tumor. Two of the patients in their report died of their disease, and three others had painful and disabling involvement of the base of the skull and cranial nerves. This tendency toward inexorable infiltration of tissues in this critical neck location mandates an aggressive surgical approach in good-risk patients, including those with group 3 tumors. Recent reports advocate radiotherapy for advanced, recurrent, or partially resected paragangliomas.[66, 67] The recommended radiotherapy dose is 4500 cGy in 25 fractions, continuous course technique.[67] The long-term toxicity, particularly in previously nonirradiated patients, is minimal with the use of careful technique.[66, 67] Surgical resection is still possible should the need arise.[66, 67]

Presumably, the widespread availability of diagnostic procedures such as ultrasonography, CT scanning, angiography, MRI, and MRA will establish the diagnosis earlier in the course of this disease. An understanding of the anatomy of carotid body paragangliomas and the use of perioperative techniques, such as preoperative embolization, will reduce tumor size and operative blood loss, making surgical resection easier and more precise. The application of sound vascular surgical techniques—including resection of the internal carotid artery, where indicated, followed by vascular reconstruction—will reduce the operative stroke and mortality rates to a minimum.

REFERENCES

1. Gratist JH: Carotid tumors: Collective review. *Int Abst Surg.* 1943;7:117.
2. Marchand F: Carotid body tumor. *Int Beitr Wissen Med.* 1891;1:537.
3. Lahey FH, Warren KW: A long term appraisal of carotid body tumors with remarks on their removal. *Surg Gynecol Obstet.* 1951;92:481.
4. Staats EF, Brown RL, Smith RR: Carotid body tumors, benign and malignant. *Laryngoscope.* 1966;76:907.
5. Scudder CL, cited by Byrng JH: Carotid body and allied tumors. *Am J Surg.* 1958;95:371.
6. Bastsakis JG: *Tumors of the Head and Neck: Clinical and Pathologic Considerations,* 2nd ed. Baltimore: Williams & Wilkins; 1979:215.
7. Sobol SM, Dailey JC: Familial multiple cervical paragangliomas: Report of a kindred and review of the literature. *Otolaryngol Head Neck Surg.* 1990;120:382.
8. Robbins SL, Angell M, Kumas V: *Basic Pathology,* 3rd ed. Philadelphia: WB Saunders; 1981:282.
9. Glenner GG, Grimley PM: *Atlas of Tumor Pathology, 2nd ser.,* fascicle 9. Washington, DC: Armed Forces Institute of Pathology; 1974.
10. Arias-Stella J: Human carotid body at high altitudes. *Am J Pathol.* 1969;55:82a.
11. Williams MD, Phillips MJ, Nelson WR, Ranier WG: Carotid body tumor. *Arch Surg.* 1992;127:963.
12. Saldena MJ, Salem LE, Travezan R: High altitude hypoxia and chemodectomas. *Hum Pathol.* 1973;4:251.
13. Farr HW: Carotid body tumors: A 40 year study. *Cancer–Am J Clin.* 1980;30:260.
14. McCabe DP, Vaccaro PS, James AG: Treatment of carotid body tumors. *J Cardiovasc Surg.* 1990;31:356.
15. Glenner GG, Crout JR, Roberts WC: A functional carotid body-like tumor secreting lavarterenol. *Arch Pathol Lab Med.* 1962;73.
16. Sauter ER, Hollier LH, Farr GH Jr: The value of flow cytometric analysis in multicentric glomus tumors of the head and neck. *Cancer.* 1992;69:1452.
17. Sauter ER, Hollier LH, Bolton JS, et al: Prognostic value of DNA flow cytometry in paragangliomas of the carotid body. *J Surg Oncol.* 1991;46:151.
18. Barnes L, Taylor SR: Carotid body paragangliomas. *Arch Otolaryngol Head Neck Surg.* 1990;116:447.
19. Gaylis H, Mieny CJ: The incidence of malignancy in carotid body tumors. *Br J Surg.* 1977;64:885.
20. Brown JW, Burton RC, Dahlin DC: Chemodectoma with skeletal metastasis: Report of two cases. *Mayo Clin Proc.* 1967; 42:551.
21. Javid H, Chawla SK, Dye WS, et al: Carotid body tumor: Resection or reflection. *Arch Surg.* 1976;111:344.
22. McPherson GAD, Halliday AW, Mansfield AO: Carotid body tumors and other cervical paragangliomas: Diagnosis and management in 25 patients. *Br J Surg.* 1989;76:33.
23. Peters JL, Ward MW, Fisher C: Diagnosis of a carotid body chemodectoma with dynamic radionuclide perfusion scanning. *Am J Surg.* 1979;137:661.
24. Monro RS: The natural history of carotid body tumors and their diagnosis and treatment. *Br J Surg.* 1950;37:445.
25. Steinke W, Hennerici M, Aulich A: Doppler color flow imaging of carotid body tumors. *Stroke.* 1989;20:1574.
26. Derchi LE, Serafini G, Rabbi C, et al: Carotid body tumors: US evaluation. *Radiology.* 1992;182:457.
27. Shugas MA, Mafee MF: Diagnosis of carotid body tumors by dynamic computerized tomography. *Head Neck Surg.* 1982; 4:518.
28. Mafee MF, Valvassori GE, Shugar MA, et al: High resolution and dynamic sequential computed tomography. *Arch Otolaryngol.* 1983;109:691.
29. Vogl T, Bruning R, Schedel H, et al: Paragangliomas of the jugular bulb and carotid body: MR imaging with short sequences and Gd-DPTA enhancement. *AJR Am J Roentgenol.* 1989;153:583.
30. Rippe DJ, Grist TM, Uglietta JP, et al: Carotid body tumor: Flow sensitive pulse sequences and MR angiography. *J Comput Assist Tomogr.* 1989;13:874.

31. Arriaga MA, Lo WWM, Brackmann DE: Magnetic resonance angiography of synchronous bilateral carotid body paragangliomas and bilateral vagal paragangliomas. *Ann Otol Rhinol Laryngol.* 1992;101:955.
32. Smith RG, Shetty PC, Reddy DJ: Surgical treatment of carotid paragangliomas presenting unusual technical difficulties: The value of preoperative embolization. *J Vasc Surg.* 1988; 7:631.
33. Ward PH, Liu C, Vinuela F, Bentson JR: Embolization: An adjunctive measure for removal of carotid body tumors. *Laryngoscope.* 1988;98:1287.
34. Chase WH: Familial and bilateral tumors of the carotid body. *J Pathol Bacteriol.* 1933;36:1.
35. Sprong DH Jr, Kirby FG: Familial carotid body tumors: Report of nine cases in eleven siblings. *Ann West Med Surg.* 1949;3:241.
36. Grufferman S, Gillman MW, Pasternak LR, et al: Familial carotid body tumors: Case report and epidemiologic review. *Cancer.* 1980;46:2116.
37. Pritchett JW: Familial concurrence of carotid body tumor and pheochromocytoma. *Cancer.* 1982;49:2578.
38. Jensen JC, Choyke PL, Rosenfeld M, et al: A report of familial carotid body tumors and multiple extra-adrenal pheochromocytomas. *J Urol.* 1991;145:1040.
39. Levit SA, Sheps SG, Espinosa RE, et al: Catecholamine-secreting paraganglioma of the glomus jugulare region resembling pheochromocytoma. *N Engl J Med.* 1969;281:805.
40. Bolande RP: The neurocristopathies: A unifying concept of disease arising in neural crest maldevelopment. *Hum Pathol.* 1974;5:409.
41. Sundaram M, Cope V: Paragangliomas in the neck. *Br J Surg.* 1976;63:182.
42. Shedd DP, Arias JD, Glunk RP: Familial occurrence of carotid body tumors. *Head Neck.* 1990;12:496.
43. Kraus DH, Sterman BM, Hakaim AG, et al: Carotid body tumors. *Arch Otolaryngol Head Neck Surg.* 1990;116:1384.
44. Lees CD, Levine HL, Beven EG, et al: Tumors of the carotid body: Experience with 41 operative cases. *Am J Surg.* 1981;142:362.
45. Shamblin WR, Remine WH, Sheps SG, et al: Carotid body tumor (chemodectoma): Clinicopathologic analysis of ninety cases. *Am J Surg.* 1971;122:732.
46. Padberg FT, Cady B, Persson AV: Carotid body tumor: Lahey Clinic experience. *Am J Surg.* 1983;145:526.
47. Chambers RG, Mahoney WD: Carotid body tumors. *Am J Surg.* 1968;116:554.
48. Dent TL, Thompson NW, Fry WJ: Carotid body tumors. *Surgery.* 1976;80:365.
49. Rosen IB, Palmer JA, Goldberg M, et al: Vascular problems associated with carotid body tumors. *Am J Surg.* 1981; 142:459.
50. Krupski WC, Effeney DJ, Ehrenfeld WK, Stoney RJ: Cervical chemodectoma. Technical considerations and management options. *Am J Surg.* 1982;144:215.
51. VanAsperen DeBoer FRS, Terpstra JL, Vink M: Diagnosis, treatment and operative complications of carotid body tumors. *Br J Surg.* 1981;68:433.
52. Van Der Mey AGL, Fruns JHM, Cornelisse CJ, et al: Does intervention improve the natural course of glomus tumors? *Ann Otol Rhinol Laryngol.* 1992;101:635.
53. LaMuraglia GM, Fabian RL, Brewster DC, et al: The current surgical management of carotid body paragangliomas. *J Vasc Surg.* 1992;15:1038.
54. Nora JD, Hallett JW Jr, O'Brien PC, et al: Surgical resection of carotid body tumors: Long-term survival, recurrence, and metastasis. *Mayo Clin Proc.* 1988;63:348.
55. Mathews FS: Surgery of the neck. In Johnson AB, ed. *Operating Therapeusis,* Vol 3. New York: Appleton-Century-Crofts; 1915:315.
56. Martin HE: *Surgery of Head and Neck Tumors.* New York: Hoeber; 1957.
57. Rush BF: Familial bilateral carotid body tumors. *Ann Surg.* 1963;157:633.
58. Hallett JW Jr, Nora JD, Hollier LH, et al: Trends in neurovascular complications of surgical management for carotid body and cervical paragangliomas: A fifty-year experience with 153 tumors. *J Vasc Surg.* 1988;7:284.
59. Gordon-Taylor G: On carotid body tumors. *Br J Surg.* 1940;28:153.
60. Lasjaunias P, Menu Y, Bonnel D, et al: Non chromaffin paragangliomas of the head and neck: Diagnostic and therapeutic angiography in 9 cases explored from 1977 to 1980. *J Neuroradiol.* 1981;8:281.
61. Hekster REM, Luyendijk W, Matrical B: Transfemoral catheter embolization: A method of treatment of glomus jugulare tumor. *Neuroradiology.* 1973;5:208.
62. Schick PM, Hieshima GB, White RA, et al: Arterial catheter embolization followed by surgery for large chemodectoma. *Surgery.* 1980;87:459.
63. Borges LF, Heros RC, DeBrun G: Carotid body tumors managed with preoperative embolization: Report of two cases. *J Neurosurg.* 1983;59:867.
64. Pandya SK, Nagpal RD, Desai AP, et al: Death following external carotid artery embolization for a functioning glomus jugulare chemodectoma: Case report. *J Neurosurg.* 1978;48:1030.
65. Hewitt RI, Ichinose H, Weichert RF III, et al: Paragangliomas of the head and neck region: A clinical study of 69 patients. *Cancer.* 1977;39:397.
66. Schild SE, Foote RL, Buskirk SJ, et al: Results of radiotherapy for chemodectomas. *Mayo Clin Proc.* 1992;67:537.
67. Guedea F, Mendenhall WM, Parsons JT, Million RR: Radiotherapy for chemodectoma of the carotid body and ganglion nodosum. *Head Neck.* 1991;13:509.
68. Lack EE, Cubilla AL, Woodruff JM, et al: Paragangliomas of the head and neck region: A clinical study of 69 patients. *Cancer.* 1977;39:397.
69. Spector GJ, Sobol S: Surgery for glomus tumors at the skull base. *Otolaryngol Head Neck Surg.* 1980;88:524.
70. Martin C, Rosenfeld L, McSwain B: Carotid body tumors: A 16 year follow-up of seven malignant cases. *South Med J.* 1973;66:136.

CHAPTER 56

Preoperative and Postoperative Management of Patients Undergoing Carotid Endarterectomy

J. DENNIS BAKER

Most patients who undergo arterial reconstructions for cerebrovascular disease have other medical conditions that increase the chance of intraoperative and postoperative complications. Although the operation itself is short and involves only superficial dissection, the fluctuations in cardiopulmonary parameters that can occur during the operation represent a more serious threat of complications than is associated with other procedures that are carried out in older patients. Reducing the risk to a minimum requires not only expert surgical technique but also (1) optimal management of coexisting medical problems, (2) smooth anesthesia, and (3) careful attention to postoperative management, especially during the first 24 hours.

PREOPERATIVE ASSESSMENT

The presence of coronary artery disease is by far the greatest risk factor for complications, as it is present in more than one third of patients and causes up to one half of perioperative deaths. Other major risk factors include prior myocardial infarction, angina, congestive heart failure, and major dysrhythmias; a vigorous attempt should be made to achieve optimal medical management of these conditions preoperatively. Hertzer and colleagues[1] and Ennix and colleagues[2] proposed an aggressive approach by extending the cardiac examination to include coronary arteriography, with the aim of reducing the risk of carotid endarterectomy by performing staged or simultaneous coronary bypass for appropriate lesions. This approach has not become widely accepted because it exposes unnecessary numbers of patients to coronary artery studies while failing to decrease substantially the incidence of cardiac deaths after carotid operations. An alternative proposed by O'Donnell and associates[3] identified patients with advanced coronary disease by the use of Goldman's clinical classification.[4] (This method calculates a multifactorial index score that divides patients into four risk categories.) Only patients with the highest cardiac risk underwent coronary angiography. This selective approach found only 4 percent of patients to have combined carotid end arterectomy and coronary bypass grafting; the overall incidence of postoperative death from myocardial infarction was essentially the same as that achieved using the more aggressive cardiac examination. In recent years, there has been an increase in the use of stress thallium scanning to screen for significant coronary disease. Many cardiologists are using this test to select patients who may benefit from coronary angiography before carotid endarterectomy. To date there is no clear consensus as to the value of widespread preoperative nucleotide scanning to screen patients without symptoms of heart disease.

Hypertension is found in up to two thirds of patients undergoing carotid endarterectomy. Preoperative hypertension increases the risk of hypertensive episodes not only during endarterectomy but postoperatively as well. Studies have found that patients in whom an episode of hypertension develops during or early after operation are at increased risk of stroke.[5, 6] A multicenter study of 1160 patients undergoing carotid repair has found that severe preoperative hypertension (diastolic pressure > 110 mm Hg) is one of the clinical factors associated with postoperative stroke, myocardial infarction, and death.[7] In addition, an acute rise in blood pressure in persons with coronary disease may increase the chance of cardiac complications. As a result, it is important to reduce this risk by having full control of the blood pressure preoperatively. Uncontrolled hypertension is a contraindication to an elective carotid procedure. Patients who are taking major medications should be given their usual oral dose on the morning of surgery, as this has been found to make achievement of intraoperative blood pressure control easier.

Special attention is required in the preoperative evaluation of the patient who is to have an operation contralateral to a prior carotid endarterectomy. The most important concern is vocal cord function. The frequency of loss of vocal cord function is not fully appreciated by many surgeons, who often attribute postoperative hoarseness to irritation produced by the endotracheal tube. Many of the studies of cranial nerve complications only include patients with clearly symptomatic problems. In a study that included indirect laryngoscopy, Evans and coworkers[8] found vocal cord dysfunction in 25 percent of patients examined 2 days after operation. An earlier report on the initial part of this study reported that 36 percent of patients with vocal cord malfunctions were asymptomatic.[9] Many symptomatic patients fully recover their speech over a short period; however, in some cases this improvement is due to a compensatory shift of the normal cord rather than recovery of the affected side. In the study by Evans and associates,[8] follow-up examination revealed that almost half of the patients with deficits on the second day still had abnormalities at 6 weeks. In a long-term follow-up study of patients with postoperative vocal cord abnormalities, Sannella and associates[10] found that 42 percent had persisting dysfunction at 1 year or later. Since 64 percent of the patients with deficits had a normal-sounding voice, this characteristic does not exclude an occult problem. Some patients with persisting voice problems benefit from a Teflon injection to stabilize the paralyzed cord in a midline position.

Hypoglossal deficits are reported to occur in 2 to 11 percent of patients undergoing carotid operations.[8, 11] Patients with such lesions usually present with swallowing difficulties or tongue-biting, and in a few cases there may be interference with speech. Many of these problems resolve rapidly; however, Evans and associates[8] found that one third remained 6 weeks after surgery. A few patients have swallowing difficulties in spite of normal tongue function. These problems are thought to be caused by disturbance in the swallowing mechanism resulting from division of the ansa hypoglossi.

Vocal cord function should be assessed with laryngoscopic examination prior to contralateral carotid endarterectomy. Presence of a paralyzed cord is a serious problem because bilateral palsy can lead to a permanent tracheostomy. Likewise, hypoglossal function should be evaluated. Bilateral hypoglossal deficit can lead to speech impairment or upper airway obstruction, which, if sufficiently severe, may require tracheostomy.[12] Presence of vocal cord or hypoglossal palsy should be cause for a re-evaluation of recommendations for operation. If the first operation was performed recently, waiting a few months may result in a return to normal function. On the other hand, if the operation was performed more than a year before, the abnormality must be considered permanent. It may be appropriate not to perform the second endarterectomy, especially if the indication is an asymptomatic stenosis. If operation is to be performed in the presence of a permanent vocal cord or hypoglossal deficit, the surgeon must be sure to discuss with the patient the added risks that such an abnormality represents, especially the small possibility of the need for a permanent tracheostomy.

POSTOPERATIVE MANAGEMENT

All patients require close monitoring and observation after undergoing carotid endarterectomy, as even transient fluctuations in blood pressure or oxygenation can cause neurologic complications. After initial monitoring in the recovery room, it used to be the practice of most surgeons to keep the patient in an intensive care unit at least overnight. This provided continuous cardiac and arterial pressure monitoring and frequent evaluation of neurologic status. Pressures for cost containment are leading to reassessment of such policies. A number of hospitals now have step-down units that provide an intermediate level of observation combined with noninvasive monitoring, including electrocardiographic function, indirect blood pressure measurement, and pulse oximetry. For the patient who has been stable throughout the operation and in the recovery room, it is appropriate to use such a facility rather than insist that every patient requires the full service of the intensive care unit, including invasive monitoring.

When the patient first awakes, it is difficult to perform a detailed neurologic examination. The initial assessment should include facial and extremity motor function. Administration of postoperative narcotics should be kept to a minimum to avoid masking changes in mental status or other neurologic abnormalities. Most patients can be satisfactorily controlled with injections of 30 mg of codeine.

It is essential to maintain adequate ventilation and oxygenation and to check these functions with arterial blood gas determinations. Some patients experience respiratory depression after extubation, especially if a narcotic technique has been used, and may require reversal with naloxone (Narcan). Low initial doses should be used (<2 μg/kg body weight) to avoid the hypertension that can occur with higher levels.[13] This change in blood pressure probably results from a rapid release of the moderating effect of the narcotic. Any time that naloxone or similar drugs are used, the patient's respira-

tion must be followed closely to detect late depression, which can occur if the effect of the antagonist wears off while there is still a significant narcotic effect. This late respiratory depression, with its attendant hypoxia, has been identified as the cause of some postoperative complications.

An expanding neck hematoma is a potentially serious complication because if the condition progresses, there can be enough deviation and compression of the trachea to interfere with adequate ventilation. The initial physical examination of the patient in the recovery room should include evaluation of tracheal position and assessment of neck swelling. A drain in the operative site may provide a false sense of security, as it does not always prevent accumulation of a substantial hematoma. Any hematoma that produces tracheal deviation is an indication for returning the patient to the operating room for exploration and drainage of the hematoma. However, any degree of respiratory embarrassment requires either emergency tracheal intubation or immediate opening of the wound for decompression, since the patient's condition can deteriorate rapidly to the point of severe respiratory insufficiency and hypoxemia.

Blood pressure control is as important postoperatively as it is intraoperatively because of the increased risk of stroke and intracranial hemorrhage associated with hypertensive episodes.[5, 6, 14, 15] In addition, severe rises in pressure increase the risk of myocardial infarction. Postendarterectomy hypertension has been reported in 50 to 60 percent of patients, with most episodes occurring within the first 3 hours of recovery. Hypotheses for the mechanism of hypertension include modification in brain autoregulation and changes in baroreceptor function, either by trauma or by alterations in mechanical properties of the arterial wall with endarterectomy. Towne and Bernhard[6] demonstrated that preservation or division of the sinus nerve did not influence the incidence of postoperative hypertension; the influence of the carotid sinus must be questioned. Skydell and coworkers[16] found the use of halogenated inhalation anesthesia to be associated with an increased risk of hypertension, suggesting a change in autoregulation or some other effect on the brain. Recent studies have found increases in renin[17] and norepinephrine[18] in jugular vein samplings of patients with postoperative hypertension, implicating intracerebral production of these chemicals.

Intravenous medications prepared for intraoperative use should be moved with the patient to the recovery room, so that they are always available for immediate administration. Nitroprusside is the first choice for control of hypertension. The rate of the drip usually ranges from 0.5 to 5 μ/kg/min. When long periods of administration are required, an attempt should be made to reduce the dose to about 1 μ/kg/min to limit the risk of problems from accumulation of cyanide, an intermediate product in the metabolism of the drug. As the pressure is controlled, the dose of nitroprusside should be tapered because abrupt stopping can result in rebound hypertension, thought to be mediated by renin.[19] If the hypertension is prolonged, it is often helpful to give hydralazine and propranolol to permit tapering of the nitroprusside. Dopamine (Intropin), the choice for treatment of hypotension, is usually started at 5 μ/kg/min and adjusted for the desired effect. If the hypotension is associated with bradycardia, atropine should be the first agent tried. Hypotension of substantial severity or duration should trigger an evaluation of possible cardiac decompensation, such as acute failure, which may require additional treatment.

The fluid and electrolyte management in a patient after carotid endarterectomy is usually simple because there are usually few major shifts and limited intravenous replacement. In some cases, however, episodes of transient hypotension may have been treated with large volumes of fluid administration, sometimes including colloid. Intraoperative fluid volumes of more than 1500 mL require a formal evaluation, with measurement of electrolytes in the recovery room, as an occasional patient may require potassium or diuretic administration to correct an excess administration of 5 percent dextrose in water, especially a patient with severe cardiac disease.

Once the patient has been stable for 12 to 18 hours, the risk of acute changes is greatly reduced and the monitoring is stopped. This is the time for a full neurologic evaluation to check for small postoperative deficits. It is advisable to watch how well the patient can drink liquids before administering any medication or nutrition by mouth. Most patients have little trouble; they can return to their usual diet and be switched back to their usual oral medications. A small number have real problems with any swallowing and may be at risk of aspiration. The difficulty is often associated with a hypoglossal nerve palsy but may also occur in the presence of normal tongue function. In most cases, there is satisfactory recovery of swallowing function in 2 or 3 days, but an occasional patient may show very slow improvement. Such patients may handle solids and semisolids better than liquids, and fluids are best provided as sherbets or frozen ices. Hoarseness or inability to speak at a normal volume persisting beyond the second postoperative day should be evaluated with indirect laryngoscopic examination to check for vocal cord motion and edema. In a few patients, a troublesome degree of orthostatic hypotension develops, especially after a carotid endarterectomy on a second side. It is therefore wise to check lying and standing blood pressures before allowing the patient out of bed for the first time. Patients who have this complaint usually compensate gradually over a period of a few days and may benefit from frequent dangling of the legs over the side of the bed.

Overall, the critical management of the patient undergoing a carotid endarterectomy occurs intraoperatively and during the first hours of recovery. Careful observation and monitoring permit early identification and correction of problems. After initial stabilization on the night of operation, problems are uncommon, and most patients are ready for discharge within a few days.

REFERENCES

1. Hertzer NR, Rob CG, Satran R, et al: Fatal myocardial infarction following carotid endarterectomy. *Ann Surg.* 1981;194:212.
2. Ennix CL, Lawrie GM, Morris GC, et al: Improved result of carotid endarterectomy in patients with symptomatic coronary disease. *Stroke.* 1979;10:122.
3. O'Donnell TF, Callow AD, Willet C, et al: The impact of coronary artery disease on carotid endarterectomy. *Ann Surg.* 1983;198:705.
4. Goldman L: Cardiac risks and complications of noncardiac surgery. *Ann Surg.* 1983;198:780.
5. Lehv MS, Salzman EW, Silen W: Hypertension complicating carotid endarterectomy. *Stroke.* 1970;1:307.
6. Towne JB, Bernhard VM: The relationship of postoperative hypertension to complications following carotid endarterectomy. *Surgery.* 1980;88:575.
7. McCrory DC, Goldstein LB, Samsa GP, et al: Predicting complications of carotid endarterectomy. *Stroke.* 1993;24:1285.
8. Evans WE, Mendelowitz DS, Liapis C, et al: Motor speech deficit following carotid endarterectomy. *Ann Surg.* 1982;196:461.
9. Liapis CD, Satiani B, Florance CL, Evans WE: Motor speech malfunction following carotid endarterectomy. *Surgery.* 1981;89:56.
10. Sannella NA, Tober RL, Cipro RP, et al: Vocal cord paralysis following carotid endarterectomy: The paradox of return of function. *Ann Vasc Surg.* 1990;4:42.
11. Knoght FW, Yeager RM, Morris DM: Cranial nerve injuries during carotid endarterectomy. *Am J Surg.* 1987;154:529.
12. Gutrecht JA, Jones HR: Bilateral hypoglossal nerve injury after bilateral carotid endarterectomy. *Stroke.* 1988;19:261.
13. Cottrell JE, Newfield P: Anesthesia for neurovascular surgery. In Fein JM, Flamm ES, (eds). *Cerebrovascular Surgery.* New York: Springer-Verlag; 1985;213.
14. Caplan LR, Skillman J, Ojemann R, Fields WS: Intracerebral hemorrhage following carotid endarterectomy: A hypertensive complication? *Stroke.* 1978;9:457.
15. Hafner DH, Smith RB, King OW, et al: Massive intracerebral hemorrhage following carotid endarterectomy. *Arch Surg.* 1987;122:305.
16. Skydell JL, Machleder HI, Baker JD, et al: Incidence and mechanism of postcarotid endarterectomy hypertension. *Arch Surg.* 1987;122:1153.
17. Smith BL: Hypertension following carotid endarterectomy: The role of cerebral renin production. *J Vasc Surg.* 1984;1:623.
18. Ahn SS, Marcus DR, Moore WS: Post-carotid endarterectomy hypertension: Association with elevated cerebral norepinephrine. *J Vasc Surg.* 1989;9:351.
19. Cottrell JE, Illner P, Kittay J, et al: Rebound hypertension after sodium nitroprusside-induced hypotension. *Clin Pharmacol Ther.* 1980;27:32.

CHAPTER 57

Early Complications of Carotid Endarterectomy: Incidence, Diagnosis, and Management

NORMAN R. HERTZER

For nearly four decades, carotid endarterectomy has been arguably the most common and the most controversial operation performed on the atherosclerotic population. Although the surgical community has long accepted carotid endarterectomy as an appropriate means of durable stroke prevention in selected patients, reports such as those by Easton and Sherman,[1] Toole and associates[2] and Whisnant and associates[3] demonstrated that the late advantages of surgical management were seriously jeopardized by excessive operative morbidity. The validity of these earlier concerns has been confirmed by the results of subsequent prospective, randomized trials conducted in the United States and Europe.[4–8] Although each of these recent studies has shown that carotid endarterectomy is associated with statistically significant reductions in the subsequent incidence of stroke or transient ischemic attacks (TIAs) or both in patients who have at least 70 percent stenosis of the internal carotid artery, the superior results of surgical treatment are not so overwhelming that the procedure should continue to be performed in the presence of complication rates that exceed those found in the trials.

The incidence of permanent postoperative complications obviously must be reduced to an absolute minimum if carotid endarterectomy is to be considered as the preferred alternative for patients with a history of neurologic symptoms, and especially for those with asymptomatic carotid stenosis. Because of the frequency with which carotid endarterectomy currently is recommended and the irreparable consequences of some of its complications, there is no higher priority in the field of vascular surgery than establishing the safety of extracranial reconstruction. This chapter presents information concerning wound bleeding and infection, hypertension and hypotension, neurologic deficits, cranial nerve dysfunction, and other miscellaneous complications that may be associated with carotid bifurcation procedures.

WOUND COMPLICATIONS

Cervical Hematoma

By the nature of their selection, many patients who require carotid endarterectomy have previously received formal anticoagulation or antiplatelet management as adjunctive treatment of cerebrovascular disease. Preoperative intravenous heparin therapy is occasionally justified for patients scheduled for elective carotid endarterectomy after angiography has demonstrated symptomatic ulcerated lesions or high-grade carotid stenosis. But, since sodium heparin is easily and predictably controlled by protamine sulfate administered at the completion of the surgical procedure, heparin therapy is rarely associated with postoperative bleeding. Correction of the prothrombin time may take several days after the administration of coumadin derivatives has been discontinued. Therefore, chronic oral anticoagulation therapy

should be reversed with the use of parenteral vitamin K and fresh frozen plasma if sufficient time is not available to allow the prothrombin time to return spontaneously to the normal range. Antiplatelet agents, such as aspirin or dipyridamole, are so universally prescribed that they undoubtedly are the most common cause of troublesome surgical blood loss. In extreme circumstances, capillary bleeding caused by these agents is correctable by platelet transfusions, but patience and conventional hemostatic measures usually are sufficient to control bleeding.

The standard approach to the carotid bifurcation through an incision parallel to the anterior border of the sternocleidomastoid muscle provides a relatively avascular plane; postoperative bleeding that required reoperation occurred in only 0.7 to 2.5 percent of large series reported by Thompson,[9] Kunkel and colleagues,[10] and Welling and colleagues.[11] It is axiomatic that the best method to achieve hemostasis after an operation is to maintain it throughout the preliminary dissection. The common facial vein and other smaller vessels, such as the venous tributaries near the hypoglossal nerve and the artery to the sternocleidomastoid muscle, should be securely ligated with fine suture material to prevent delayed bleeding in the event that transient hypertension or straining occurs at the time the endotracheal tube is removed following general anesthesia. If an autogenous vein patch is applied to the arteriotomy, all branches should be ligated with sutures, or the venous segment should be filleted on an axis that enables most branches to be incorporated into the continuous suture that secures the patch to the artery. Although opinion may differ from one center to the next, a retrospective review of 697 carotid endarterectomies by Treiman and coworkers[12] has suggested that wound hematomas occur less frequently when the effects of heparin are reversed with protamine sulfate at the conclusion of the operation (1.8%) than when they are not (6.5%). Low-molecular-weight dextran occasionally is administered at the Cleveland Clinic to selected patients who require a deep endarterectomy plane because of ulcerated atheromatous disease, but this precautionary procedure has not appeared to cause any more bleeding than is caused by antiplatelet medication.

A large cervical hematoma can compromise the airway by shifting the trachea across the midline and can also compress the carotid bifurcation and the adjacent cranial nerves. Even if such problems do not occur, early reoperation should be seriously considered for any hematoma large enough to be obvious on physical examination, because the contained clot eventually liquefies and may drain through a chronic cutaneous sinus that is cosmetically unsatisfactory and could become infected (Fig. 57–1). The secondary procedure is limited to evacuation of the hematoma, hemostasis, irrigation, and reclosure over a temporary vacuum drain, so local anesthesia may be preferable to another general anesthetic.[10] A brief course of antibiotics is appropriate

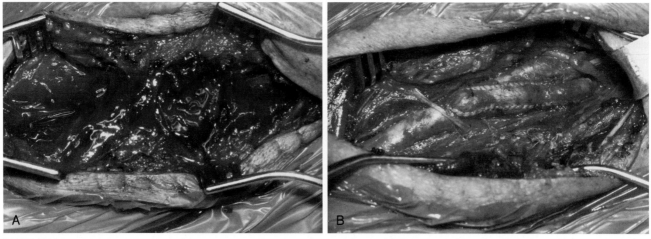

FIGURE 57–1. *A*, Operative photograph of a cervical hematoma that occurred during a hypertensive episode several hours after carotid endarterectomy. *B*, The same wound following evacuation of the hematoma, hemostasis, and irrigation with a dilute antibiotic solution.

whenever a hematoma has required an emergency reoperation.

Infection and False Aneurysm

Because of the rich arterial supply in the neck and the fact that most standard arterial procedures are completed within a reasonably short period of time, cervical infections and mycotic false aneurysms are very unusual complications of carotid endarterectomy. Thompson[9] encountered a wound infection after only one (0.09%) of 1140 operations, and each of the seven false aneurysms (0.6%) he encountered involved a prosthetic patch that had been applied with silk suture several years earlier. Even though many surgeons probably do not employ prophylactic antibiotic coverage during elective carotid reconstruction, infection is so rare as to be anecdotal in smaller series.

Infected false aneurysms occurred after only four (0.15%) of 2651 carotid endarterectomies performed at the Cleveland Clinic from 1977 through 1984[13] (Fig. 57–2). Because of suppuration and degeneration of the arterial wall, multiple ligation of the common, internal, and external carotid arteries was the only possible procedure in one patient who subsequently experienced TIAs in the ipsilateral cerebral hemisphere but who eventually became asymptomatic under oral anticoagulation therapy. The remaining three patients were managed initially by repair of the false aneurysms with the use of vein patch angioplasty in conjunction with systemic antibiotics. Each developed a recurrent false aneurysm that required carotid ligation, but none sustained a postoperative stroke. One other patient was transferred from another center because of chronic infection involving a prosthetic patch applied during endarterectomy several months previously. This patient was treated successfully by resection of the carotid bifurcation and saphenous vein bypass to the distal cervical segment of the internal carotid artery (Fig. 57–3); she remained asymptomatic following that reoperation.

Provided that significant contralateral carotid disease is not present, these limited examples suggest that infected false aneurysms usually require multiple ligation, unless it is feasible to excise the septic arterial wall completely and to replace it with an autogenous graft connected to an uncon-

taminated segment of the internal carotid artery. If there is severe contralateral carotid stenosis or occlusion, contralateral carotid endarterectomy or even middle cerebral artery bypass conceivably could be necessary as a preliminary procedure to provide adequate intracranial collateral circulation at the time that the infected carotid system is ligated. Fortunately, catastrophic infection almost never occurs.

HYPERTENSION AND HYPOTENSION

Etiology

Transient fluctuation in systemic blood pressure during the early postoperative period is not particularly unusual after any major vascular procedure involving atherosclerotic

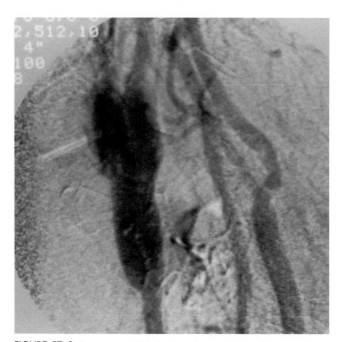

FIGURE 57–2. Intravenous digital subtraction angiogram demonstrating an infected false aneurysm discovered 8 weeks after previous carotid endarterectomy.

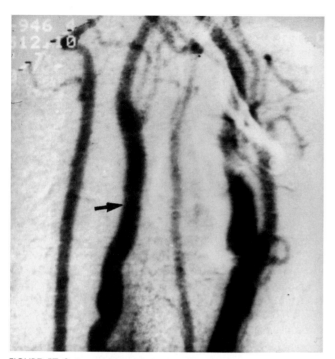

FIGURE 57–3. Intravenous digital subtraction angiogram obtained 2 years after the right carotid bifurcation and an infected Dacron patch were excised and replaced with a saphenous vein graft *(arrow)* extending to the distal cervical segment of the internal carotid artery.

patients; it is usually attributed to acute changes in intravascular volume, reduction in cardiac output, peripheral vasoconstriction, and preoperative dependency on antihypertensive medication or β-adrenergic blocking agents, such as propranolol. Despite the relatively limited surgical exposure, fluid replacement, and operative time necessary for extracranial procedures, however, hypertension and hypotension appear to be especially prevalent after carotid reconstruction and have been reported in 19 to 66 percent of patients requiring standard bifurcation endarterectomy.[14–18] Although Smith[19] introduced information suggesting that cerebral renin production may influence hypertension in a manner that was previously unrecognized, most research has traditionally been devoted to the possible contribution of the carotid sinus mechanism because of its perceived importance in blood pressure regulation, its proximity to the carotid bifurcation, and the fact that in several clinical studies, hypotensive episodes have been found to respond to local anesthetic blockade of the sinus nerve.[14, 17, 20]

As depicted in Figure 57–4, specialized neurons located in the adventitia of the carotid bulb monitor systemic blood pressure and respond to sustained pressure elevation by initiating a reflex arc to the upper brain stem mediated by the sinus nerve of Hering. Under normal circumstances, this negative feedback system produces compensatory bradycardia and reduction in blood pressure until baroreceptor stimulation has been relieved. Several investigations have presented evidence that interruption of the reflex arc by an injury to the carotid sinus nerve during endarterectomy can produce a hypertensive response because a sustained reduction in blood pressure is mistakenly perceived, particularly after staged bilateral carotid reconstruction has been performed.[14, 17, 21, 22] Angell-James and Lumley[20] have suggested

that, provided the sinus nerve is intact, patients may sustain transient postoperative hypotension because of excited baroreceptor activity caused by a relative increase in arterial diameter following the removal of a noncompliant bifurcation lesion.

It is important to appreciate the possible physiologic role of the sinus nerve, since sudden bradycardia and hypotension occurring either during manipulation of the carotid bifurcation or during the first few postoperative hours can often be controlled by infiltration of the sinus mechanism with a dilute solution of local anesthetic.[14, 17] Nevertheless, a consistent causal relationship between sinus nerve activity and extreme changes in postoperative blood pressure has not been established beyond speculation. Wade and coworkers[23] found that baroreceptor function is negligible in some older patients even prior to carotid reconstruction, and Towne and Bernhard[18] were unable to demonstrate that either routine preservation or transection of the sinus nerve had any measurable influence on systemic blood pressure after bifurcation endarterectomy. Considering that most patients who require extracranial procedures are older than 60 years of age and that many have associated cardiovascular disease, it seems reasonable to assume that blood pressure variance is often multifactorial. A number of reports have shown that compared with normotensive patients, patients with long-

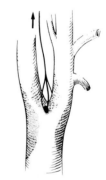

A. PREOPERATIVE

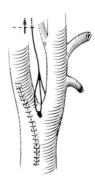

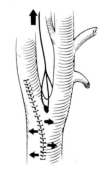

B. POSTOPERATIVE HYPERTENSION   **C. POSTOPERATIVE HYPOTENSION**

FIGURE 57–4. *A,* Schematic illustration of normal sinus nerve activity preceding carotid endarterectomy. *B,* Postoperative hypertension may be associated with interruption of the baroreceptor reflex caused by sinus nerve injury. *C,* Postoperative hypotension may be a compensatory response to an increase in arterial diameter in the presence of an intact sinus nerve. (From Hertzer NR: Non-stroke complications of carotid endarterectomy. In Bernhard VM, Towne J, eds. *Complications in Vascular Surgery,* 2nd ed. Orlando: Grune & Stratton; 1985; 744; with permission.)

standing hypertension are at significant risk for sustained hypertension after carotid endarterectomy, especially if preoperative medical control is inadequate.[18, 21, 22] By the same token, Ranson and colleagues[24] found that an uncorrected deficit in intravascular volume was the principal factor responsible for postoperative hypotension in their experience, and that reflex bradycardia was a serious complication only in the presence of hypovolemia. Moreover, Tarlov and associates[25] were able to reduce the incidence of postoperative hypotension from 54 percent to only 18 percent by employing colloid infusions to maintain central venous pressure at normal levels. Irrespective of the possible contribution of the carotid sinus, adequate preoperative preparation is obviously a critical consideration, and elective extracranial reconstruction should not be performed until recognized hypertension or volume deficits have been resolved.

Complications and Management

Few physicians would disagree that profound hypotension has potentially dangerous consequences to any patient after carotid endarterectomy. Reduction in cerebral perfusion could encourage platelet aggregation within the carotid bifurcation that was operated on and seems especially undesirable for those patients who have had previous strokes or severe contralateral carotid stenosis. Considering that advanced coronary disease is prevalent among patients requiring extracranial procedures, hypotensive episodes in this particular group could also lead to subendocardial ischemia or myocardial infarction. Conversely, injudicious pharmacologic attempts to reverse hypotension in hypovolemic patients with associated coronary atherosclerosis may also be hazardous. In a group of 135 patients suspected to have ischemic heart disease, Riles and associates[26] reported that the incidence of postoperative myocardial infarction rose from 2.0 to 8.1 percent when vasopressors were used to manipulate blood pressure after carotid reconstruction.

Even if it occurs in conjunction with a neurologic deficit, however, the specifically deleterious effect of transient postoperative hypertension is more controversial. Wallace and Levy[27] found that hypertension commonly is the result, rather than the cause, of cortical deficits in more than 80 percent of patients who present with spontaneous strokes; they suggested that autonomic blood pressure elevation may be a normal reflex to protect the ischemic brain. Satiani and coworkers[22] have advised against pharmacologic treatment of transient postoperative hypertension, concluding from their experience that neurologic complications were more likely to be caused by sudden, excessive blood pressure reduction than by mild to moderate hypertension itself.

Nevertheless, several studies have demonstrated that stroke and mortality are substantially greater risks among patients who experience any wide variance from their usual range of blood pressure immediately after extracranial procedures.[18, 21, 24, 28, 29] Bove and colleagues[21] encountered neurologic deficits in 9 percent of patients who became either hypertensive or hypotensive, whereas no complications occurred among those with stable blood pressure. Towne and Bernhard[18] reported postoperative strokes in 10 percent of patients who had hypertensive episodes as compared with 3.4 percent of those who remained normotensive. Although intracranial hemorrhage is a rare complication of sustained

postoperative hypertension after carotid endarterectomy, Caplan and associates[28] have described case reports that imply that this catastrophe is most likely to occur in chronically hypertensive patients who have a history of previous strokes and experience an abrupt, overwhelming improvement in cerebral perfusion after correction of high-grade carotid stenosis. Isolated examples at the Cleveland Clinic of this irreversible and invariably fatal complication have involved precisely this subset of factors and generally have occurred after a delay of several days following an apparently successful operation (Fig. 57–5).

Judging from these accumulated data, postoperative hypertension and hypotension should be prevented whenever possible and warrant prompt but cautious management when they do occur. Chronic hypertension should be brought under optimal medical control preceding elective endarterectomy, even if postponement of the surgery is necessary to accomplish this objective. A relative contraction of intravascular volume should be anticipated in patients who receive long-term diuretic or antihypertensive treatment, in the elderly, and in those with unexpectedly high hematocrit values. Selected patients may require at least central venous pressure measurement and sometimes Swan-Ganz pulmonary artery catheterization to monitor rapid expansion of circulating blood volume if postoperative hypotension fails to respond to conventional treatments.

Although definitions are arbitrary, blood pressure should generally be maintained at preoperative levels, and at the Cleveland Clinic, pharmacologic management is begun if postoperative values exceed 180 mm Hg systolic or fall below 100 mm Hg in patients who were previously normotensive. Sodium nitroprusside is a peripheral vasodilator that provides prompt and responsive blood pressure control when titrated intravenously as 50 mg in 250 to 500 mL of 5 percent dextrose in water (D_5W). Hypotension associated with bradycardia may respond to parenteral atropine sulfate (0.5 to 1.0 mg), but both Cafferata and colleagues[14] and Pine and colleagues[17] are convinced that this situation is ideally managed by infiltration of local anesthetic into the carotid sinus through a percutaneous catheter. Provided that hypovolemia has already been corrected, dopamine hydrochloride (200 to 400 mg in 250 mL D_5W) can be used to reverse transient hypotension, which is otherwise refractory to management.

Extreme fluctuations in blood pressure following carotid reconstruction nearly always are self-limited.[22, 30] Although some patients require pharmacologic manipulation for as long as a full day after staged bilateral carotid endarterectomy, most who experience postoperative hypertension or hypotension can be withdrawn from intravenous medication within a few hours of operation. Although it is temporary, widely labile blood pressure should be recognized and controlled before it can lead to further, more serious consequences.

ISCHEMIC STROKE

Although other complications may occur, operative stroke and mortality rates are the critical criteria for determining the early success or failure of carotid endarterectomy. At most centers, remarkable progress has been made in both

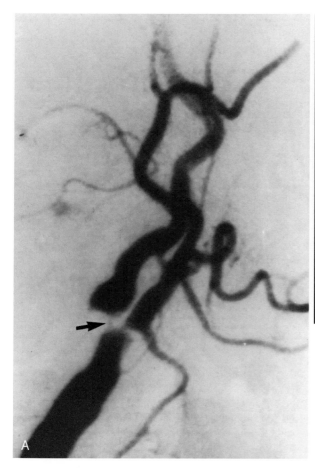
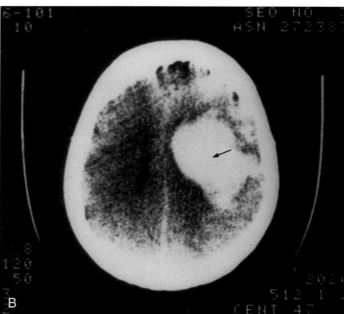

FIGURE 57–5. *A,* Intra-arterial digital subtraction angiogram demonstrating severe, subtotal stenosis *(arrow)* of the right internal carotid artery in a hypertensive patient. *B,* Computed tomogram of a hemorrhagic infarction *(arrow)* in the right cerebral hemisphere that occurred on the fifth postoperative day after elective carotid endarterectomy.

respects since the Joint Study of Extracranial Arterial Occlusion assessed the results of the first decade of carotid reconstruction. According to this multicenter investigation, prior to 1969, 8.4 percent of patients died within 30 days of their extracranial operations, and fatal complications occurred in 42 percent of patients in whom the indication for surgical intervention was an acute stroke within the previous 2 weeks.[31, 32] Subsequent reports, such as those by Thompson and associates[33] and DeWeese and associates[34] were encouraging because they confirmed the safety and durable protection from late stroke offered by carotid endarterectomy in appropriate patients, namely those with TIA or stable completed strokes with good functional recovery. Because of such classic studies, the importance of careful patient selection received the emphasis it deserved, and the composite stroke and mortality risk rates of elective carotid endarterectomy steadily declined as fewer patients underwent operations in the presence of acute, unstable neurologic deficits or complete occlusion of the internal carotid artery. After 1970, the overall incidence of grave complications fell to 3 percent or less in many series.[30] As testimony to this progress, a subcommittee of the American Heart Association stated in 1989 that the 30-day mortality rate for all carotid endarterectomies should not exceed 2 percent and defined the acceptable risks for perioperative stroke according to specific surgical indications (asymptomatic stenosis, <3 percent; previous TIA, <5 percent; prior ischemic infarction, <7 percent; recurrent carotid stenosis, <10 percent).[35]

There is no assurance, however, that the personal experi-

ence or institutional specialty interest represented by large published series accurately reflects the results of carotid reconstruction throughout the countless hospitals in the United States at which an escalating number of extracranial procedures have been performed. Pooled data comprising the collective efforts of surgeons who, as individuals, are infrequently responsible for the management of patients with cerebrovascular disease occasionally have demonstrated iatrogenic stroke rates that fail to meet even reasonable expectations.[36] Although controversial, such studies inevitably provoke speculation concerning the unreported results of carotid endarterectomy in those hospitals at which a formal survey of complications may never have been attempted. Unless the safety of extracranial reconstruction has specifically been determined within the hospital in which it is to be performed, carotid endarterectomy is likely to be recommended on the basis of published results from centers hundreds or thousands of miles away. With their report of an unexpected stroke and mortality rate of 21 percent in southern Illinois nearly 20 years ago, Easton and Sherman[1] shattered any illusion that the success of carotid endarterectomy was universal.

Incidence

Table 57–1 summarizes the results of carotid endarterectomy reported in large series of patients at academic vascular centers since 1980. Virtually all contemporary methods for operative monitoring and cerebral protection are represented

TABLE 57-1. Reported Complication Rates for Carotid Endarterectomy: Studies from Academic Medical Centers

Study*	Patients, n	Anesthesia	Cerebral Monitoring	Carotid Shunt, %	Neurologic Complications, %			Mortality Rate, %
					TIA	Stroke	Total	
Ott et al[37]	309	General	NA	0	1.9	1.3	3.2	0.6
Bardin et al[38]	456	General	Back pressure	75	4.2	2.6	6.8	0.9
Hertzer et al[39]	314	General	NA	100	NA	1.9	NA	1.0
Peitzman et al[40]	314	Regional (80%)	Test clamp	8	0.6	3.2	3.8	1.9
Towne and Bernhard[41]	312	General	NA	83	2.2	2.9	5.1	0.6
Whittemore et al[42]	219	General	EEG	16	1.4	0.9	2.2	2.2
Baker et al[43]	940	General	Back pressure	0	2.2	2.4	4.7	0.6
Ouriel et al[44]	402	General	EEG (35%)	17	3.2	3.2	6.5	NA
Sachs et al[45]	557	General	NA	100	2.2	2.3	4.5	0.7
Hertzer et al[46]	917	General	NA	100	0.8	2.0	2.8	0.4
Corson et al[47]	399	Mixed	NA	32	1.0	1.7	2.8	1.0
Till et al[48]	389	Mixed	NA	5	NA	2.6	NA	2.3
Mackey et al[49]	598	General	NA	17	NA	2.8	NA	1.0
Pinkerton and Gholkar[50]	685	Mixed	EEG	10	NA	1.8	NA	0.9
Mattos et al[51]	544	General	NA	NA	NA	2.9	NA	1.3
McCrory et al[52]	1160	NA	NA	42	NA	3.4	NA	1.4
Riles et al[53]	3062	Regional (89%)	NA	19	NA	2.2	NA	NA
Total	11,577					2.4		1.0 (n = 8113)

*For full bibliographic information, see reference list at end of chapter.
EEG, operative electroencephalography; NA, data not available; TIA, transient ischemic attack.

in this composite group of nearly 12,000 operations, including general anesthesia with either internal carotid backflow pressure measurements or continuous electroencephalography (EEG), as well as local or regional anesthesia with test carotid clamping. Among 16 studies for which adequate information is available, carotid shunting was consistently employed in 5 and was entirely avoided in 2. Selective shunting was performed in the remaining 9 studies but, since objective indications were observed only in 5 of these, shunts clearly appeared to be necessary in a limited subset of approximately 8 to 20 percent of patients who were assessed by backflow pressure values, EEG changes, or the clinical response to temporary carotid occlusion.[40, 42, 44, 50, 53] Operative mortality ranged from 0.4 to 2.3 percent and, despite substantial differences in intraoperative monitoring and formal cerebral protection, the incidence of neurologic complications was remarkably similar in all these series. At most, 4.2 percent of patients experienced temporary deficits; more importantly, a maximum of only 3.4 percent sustained permanent ischemic strokes.

In a previous summary of data published from 1977 through 1984 (Table 57-2), surgical indications were described in detail for 9496 procedures.[54] Iatrogenic strokes occurred in 1.6 percent of patients with asymptomatic carotid stenosis and in 2.5 percent of those with previous neurologic symptoms. Serious neurologic complications occurred in more than twice as many patients with a history of previous strokes (3.9 percent) than in those whose preoperative symptoms had been restricted to TIAs (1.8 percent). Although the angiographic severity of contralateral carotid stenosis usually was omitted from the reports, patency of the internal carotid artery opposite to endarterectomy was designated for 2589 patients in the composite series. Operative strokes occurred in 6.1 percent of those with documented contralateral carotid occlusion, compared with 1.1 percent of all other patients. Conclusions regarding anesthetic management and the use

of carotid shunts were less convincing. Permanent deficits occurred in conjunction with general anesthesia in 2.2 percent, with local or regional anesthesia in 1.3 percent, and with shunting or nonshunting in 1.9 percent and 1.8 percent, respectively.

It must be noted, however, that a critical comparison of results in the shunted and nonshunted groups is difficult because shunts were employed in most of the referenced studies for selected patients who appeared to require cerebral

TABLE 57-2. Specific Considerations Concerning Incidence of Permanent Stroke After Carotid Endarterectomy

Specific Considerations	Composite Results of Representative Series*	
	Patients, n	Permanent Operative Strokes, n (%)
Surgical indications		
Asymptomatic carotid stenosis	1784	29 (1.6)
Neurologic symptoms	7712	194 (2.5)
Transient ischemia	3288	58 (1.8)
Previous strokes	933	36 (3.9)
Contralateral carotid status		
Patent	2276	26 (1.1)
Occluded	313	19 (6.1)
Anesthetic management		
General	7494	163 (2.2)
Local or regional	447	6 (1.3)
Cerebral protection		
Shunt	1973	37 (1.9)
No shunt	4479	80 (1.8)
Total	14606	323 (2.2)

*From available data.
From Hertzer NR: Early complications of carotid endarterectomy: Incidence, diagnosis and management. In Moore W, ed. Surgery for Cerebrovascular Disease. New York: Churchill Livingstone; 1987;634; with permission.

protection. In one study in which no patient selection was practiced, Baker and colleagues[43] found operative strokes significantly more common among patients with low back-flow pressure associated with contralateral carotid occlusion (11%) than in those with only one (2.8%) or neither of these features (0.9%). Since even the advocates of routine operative shunting concede that cerebral protection appears to be necessary in only a small group of patients who require carotid endarterectomy, it is unlikely that the perpetual controversy associated with this topic will be resolved within the foreseeable future unless substantive data are available to correlate the incidence of postoperative complications with the preoperative neurologic status as well as the angiographic appearance of the contralateral carotid system. As demonstrated in Table 57–2, each of these parameters seems to influence the perioperative stroke rate in selected patients, irrespective of the overall excellence of early results. Intraoperative microembolization, postoperative platelet aggregation, and internal carotid thrombosis almost certainly cause as many, if not more, iatrogenic strokes than does cerebral ischemia during temporary clamp occlusion. Although technical perfection clearly is more relevant than carotid shunting in most operations, the critical issue simply is whether at least some patients require both.

The Community Hospital Experience

Most publications concerning carotid endarterectomy originate from academic surgical centers, but far more operations are performed in community hospitals. Table 57–3 contains a summary of the scant information regarding the results of carotid reconstruction in this largely unreported sector since 1980. A total of 10 series comprising 9361 patients collected from individual practices yielded a mortality rate of only 1.1 percent and an incidence of permanent perioperative stroke of just 1.5 percent. These exemplary results were closely comparable to those from major vascular centers and undoubtedly represent the extensive individual experience of a limited number of surgeons who dominated the field of extracranial reconstruction in their community hospitals during each study.

In comparison, Table 57–3 also presents a summary of nine community surveys representing a total of 19,464 patients. Seven of these surveys were conducted retrospectively, the only exceptions being two reports from the prospective computer registry maintained by the Cleveland Vascular Society.[65–70] The composite perioperative stroke and mortality rates for all nine of these surveys were 3.1 percent and 1.7 percent, respectively. If the data from the Cleveland Vascular Society were excluded on the arguable grounds that they had been submitted by the responsible surgeons without impartial review, the stroke and mortality rates would be slightly higher for the remaining seven retrospective surveys comprising 8861 patients (4.1% and 1.8%). Although these figures still appear to be quite acceptable, it must be noted that these community data reflect a broad range of perioperative risk, the highest of which is excessive by contemporary standards.

TABLE 57–3. Reported Complication Rates for Carotid Endarterectomy: Studies and Surveys from Community Practices

Study*	Patients, n	Anesthesia and Cerebral Monitoring	Carotid Shunt, %	Neurologic Complications, %			Mortality, %
				TIA	Stroke	Total	
Individual Practices							
Whitney et al[55]	1197	General	0	1.2	2.3	3.5	1.8
Carmichael[56]	445	General	1	0.9	1.6	2.5	0.2
Cranley[57]	882	NA	NA	2.1	1.0	3.1	1.1
Hafner and Evans[58]	1200	Local	9	0.8	0.9	1.7	0.7
Nunn[59]	651	General	100	NA	1.5	NA	0.8
Edwards et al[60]	3028	General	97	1.3	1.0	2.3	1.5
Gibbs and Guzzetta[61]	566	General	10	1.6	1.6	3.2	0.5
McKittrick et al[62]	370	General	2	3.2	2.4	5.7	1.4
Hoyne[63]	272	General; EEG, back pressure	18	2.2	2.9	5.1	0.4
Hans[64]	750	NA	NA	0.5	2.6	3.1	0.5
Total	9361				1.5		1.1
Community Surveys							
Hertzer et al[65]	2646	Mixed	NA	NA	2.5	NA	1.2
Moore et al[66]	510	General; EEG, back pressure (33%)	75	2.0	5.3	7.3	1.6
Fode et al[67]	3328	Mixed	44	2.5	4.2	6.7	2.0
Kempczinski et al[68]	750	NA	34	NA	5.1	NA	2.3
Toronto Cerebrovascular Study Group[69]	358	NA	NA	5.0	4.5	9.5	1.5
Rubin et al[70]	8535	Mixed	NA	NA	2.1	NA	1.6
Kirshner et al[71]	1035	Mixed	25	2.4	4.3	6.8	1.4
Brook et al[72]	1302	NA	NA	NA	6.6	NA	3.0
Rosenthal et al[73]	1000	General	54	1.5	1.3	2.8	0.9
Total	19,464				3.1		1.7

*For full bibliographic information, see reference list at end of chapter.
EEG, operative electroencephalography; NA, data not available; TIA, transient ischemic attack.

An early study by Easton and Sherman[1] also employed pooled data to calculate community stroke and mortality rates of 21 percent in southern Illinois. This series included a substantial number of patients with preoperative strokes and was collected retrospectively from many surgeons whose training in cerebrovascular surgery was undesignated and whose practical experience was confined to fewer than four carotid procedures annually. Although the results of this investigation were unacceptable by any reasonable criteria even at the time of their publication, the lingering question concerning whether they accurately reflect the unreported standards at many other community hospitals has yet to be resolved. Nevertheless, additional data from the same two hospitals participating in the southern Illinois survey are now available and clearly demonstrate that unsatisfactory results are amenable to impressive improvement, provided that they are discovered in the first place.

In another study from Springfield that reached the conclusion that contralateral carotid disease did not influence the incidence of ischemic stroke at the time of unilateral reconstruction, Moore and associates[66] incidentally reported the results of the 510 carotid endarterectomies that consecutively followed the 228 operations described by Easton and Sherman in 1977. Although fewer surgeons contributed to the original investigation than to this follow-up report, the frequency with which previous strokes served as the indication for endarterectomy declined from 43 percent in the initial series to 19 percent thereafter. During the second of these consecutive study periods, there were striking reductions in the incidence of postoperative stroke from 14 percent to 4.1 percent and in operative mortality from 6.6 percent to 1.6 percent. Further information from the same hospitals also has confirmed that nearly all patients have benefited from the enhanced safety of carotid endarterectomy.[74] The rate of nonfatal neurologic complications was reduced from 18 percent to 2.6 percent in patients with asymptomatic carotid stenosis, from 18 percent to 5.2 percent in those with preoperative TIA, and from 6.7 percent to 3.2 percent in those with nonhemispheric symptoms. In comparison, the frequency of neurologic complications among patients with a history of previous strokes declined from 15 percent to only 12 percent. The series of reports from the Springfield area is especially important because it illustrates so unmistakably that unsatisfactory results must first be discovered before they can be corrected.

Prospective Randomized Trials

Finally, Table 57–4 summarizes information concerning perioperative complications for the surgical treatment groups containing a total of 1318 patients in five prospective, randomized trials of carotid endarterectomy and best medical management for high-grade symptomatic or asymptomatic carotid stenosis. Several elements of these data appear to be noteworthy. First, the composite stroke and mortality rates for all five trials (4.7% and 1.2%, respectively) not only exceed the comparable figures at academic medical centers (see Table 57–1) and in private community practices (see Table 57–3) but also fail to meet the expectations of even retrospective community surveys (see Table 57–3), which previously had widely been considered inappropriate. Despite this finding, however, three of the randomized trials demonstrated significant reductions in stroke risk among symptomatic patients who were randomly assigned to receive surgical treatment.[4–6] The results of the two remaining trials devoted to asymptomatic carotid stenosis are less conclusive, but the larger of these did determine that surgical management was advantageous in reducing the combined endpoints of subsequent stroke or TIA.[7] Therefore, there is reason to believe that the benefits of carotid endarterectomy that either have been proved or strongly suggested by the results of randomized trials are transferable to all practice settings, provided that appropriate indications are clearly defined and complication rates are kept within reasonable limits.

Etiology and Management of Operative Stroke

Although there may be other contributing factors, cerebral embolization and cortical ischemia caused by internal carotid occlusion are the two basic mechanisms for intraoperative or delayed strokes following carotid endarterectomy. Clinical attention has generally been devoted to atheromatous embolization and clamp ischemia occurring at the time of operation, but Whitney and coworkers[55] found that more than one half of all neurologic complications among patients in their large series presented as isolated events within the first few days after an apparently successful procedure. Although delayed postoperative deficits often are undesignated in other reports, they undoubtedly occur with similar frequency at all centers; they are probably related to the aggregation of platelets and fibrin at the endarterectomy site with subsequent intracranial embolization (Fig. 57–6) or spontaneous thrombosis of the internal carotid artery.

In an effort to prevent platelet thrombi, aspirin therapy (5 grains twice daily) is administered empirically on the preoperative evening and for the first month after carotid

---

TABLE 57–4. Reported Complication Rates for Carotid Endarterectomy: Prospective Randomized Trials

Study*	Patients, n	Anesthesia and Cerebral Monitoring	Carotid Shunt, %	Neurologic Complications, %			Mortality, %
				TIA	Stroke	Total	
Towne et al[7]	211	General	NA	NA	2.4	NA	1.9
NASCET[4]	328	NA	NA	NA	5.2	NA	0.6
ECST[5]	657	NA	NA	NA	5.6	NA	1.1
Mayberg et al[6]	90	Mixed	44	NA	2.2	NA	3.3
Total	1286				4.7		1.2

*For full bibliographic information, see reference list at end of chapter.
ECST, European Carotid Surgery Trial; NA, data not available; NASCET, North American Symptomatic Carotid Endarterectomy Trial; TIA, transient ischemic attack.

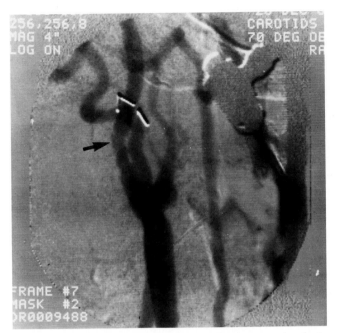

FIGURE 57–6. Intravenous digital subtraction angiogram suggesting platelet aggregation *(arrow)* near the origin of the internal carotid artery in a patient who experienced a dense contralateral hemiplegia several hours after right carotid endarterectomy.

reconstruction at the Cleveland Clinic. And, in those patients with extensive atheromatous ulceration that requires a deep endarterectomy extending into the subadventitial plane of the arterial wall, an infusion of low-molecular-weight dextran (35 to 50 mL/hr) is begun prior to the arteriotomy closure and is continued until the following day. Neither of these precautions is beyond speculation, but both are predicated on the accepted principle that platelet inhibition must precede the first pass of blood across the endarterectomy surface to be effective against the accumulation of gray platelet thrombus that is commonly found in patients who require urgent reoperations because of early neurologic complications.

The precise onset of intraoperative deficits is impossible to determine when the patient is under general anesthesia, but studies of cases in which regional anesthesia is used seem to confirm that most intraoperative ischemic events are embolic, as they become evident in awake patients either during preliminary carotid manipulation or at the time that flow is restored after a period of clamp ischemia which itself was well tolerated.[75, 76] Recent information derived from computed tomographic (CT) studies also may implicate embolization as the predominant source of intraoperative neurologic complications. Zukowski and coworkers[77] obtained preoperative CT scans in 65 patients scheduled for carotid endarterectomy, only 6 of whom had a recognized history of prior strokes. Of the ulcerated surgical specimens, 62 percent were associated with CT-documented cerebral infarcts, compared with only 8 percent of lesions without ulcers. In another series of 107 consecutive patients who underwent CT scans before elective carotid reconstruction, Graber and associates[78] found that postoperative neurologic complications occurred in 22 percent of with those preoperative CT infarcts, compared with 4.5 percent of those with normal scans. The composite results of these two studies

suggest that ulcerated bifurcation lesions produce more microemboli than are clinically evident and that additional intraoperative embolization may be responsible for the traditionally greater risk of carotid endarterectomy among patients known to have had previous strokes.

Although Ortega and associates[79] discovered asymptomatic internal carotid occlusion postoperatively in 5 percent of patients who had early noninvasive carotid testing, data from other centers suggest that when the operation is performed by an experienced surgeon, technical complications are exceedingly unusual. Although previous strokes or contralateral carotid occlusion substantially increased the risk of operative stroke in their series of 3062 operations, Riles and coworkers[53] determined that technical problems occurred after only 0.8 percent of standard procedures. In a series of 262 endarterectomies performed at the Cleveland Clinic that were assessed by postoperative digital subtraction angiography, internal carotid occlusion was identified in only five patients (1.9%), three of whom (1.1%) were asymptomatic.[39] Two of these three patients had extensive atherosclerosis involving diminutive internal carotid arteries that had nearly escaped detection at the time of preoperative angiography (Fig. 57–7), leaving only one patient in the entire study group (0.4%) who sustained asymptomatic internal carotid occlusion that was entirely unanticipated.

The relative merits of intraoperative angiographic and ultrasonographic scanning are presented in Chapters 52 and 53, but it should be noted that Lye and associates[80] encountered unexplained vasospasm involving the distal cervical segment of the internal carotid artery in 9.8 percent of immediate angiograms, a finding that may represent another potential source for postoperative occlusion that is not directly related to the endarterectomy site. Provided that vasospasm occurs with comparable frequency in other series, however, the results reported by Riles and colleagues and from the Cleveland Clinic imply that it is probably transient and has limited practical significance.

Management Options

When a patient awakens with a neurologic deficit after carotid endarterectomy under general anesthesia, a prompt decision is required concerning whether a reoperation should be performed. If thrombosis of the internal carotid artery has occurred, time is critically important because a zone of ischemic brain tissue may be converted to a hemorrhagic infarct if thrombectomy is delayed for more than even an hour.[81] Reoperation cannot be advised as a universal approach to all early complications, however, since an immediate deficit may also have been caused by atheromatous embolization at the time of the initial procedure. Under these circumstances, reopening of the endarterectomy segment has no therapeutic value and may be detrimental because of the additional clamp ischemia that then is imposed on what otherwise might be only a transient neurologic event.

Difficult decisions regarding the management of immediate complications are inevitably influenced by such considerations as preoperative neurologic status, gross appearance of the original lesion, satisfaction of the surgeon with the primary procedure, and, perhaps most importantly, the severity of the postoperative deficit. An emergency reoperation clearly would be appropriate for a patient found to have a

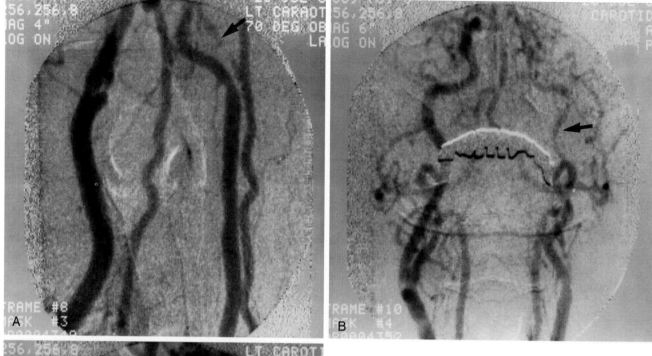

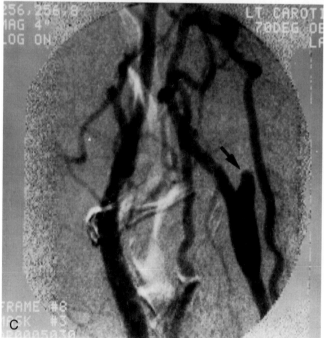

FIGURE 57–7. *A,* Preoperative intravenous digital subtraction angiogram demonstrating a ''string sign'' *(arrow)* representing the internal carotid artery. *B,* Frontal view confirmed that the distal internal carotid segment *(arrow)* was patent but diminutive. *C,* Postoperative intravenous study demonstrated internal carotid occlusion *(arrow)* despite the use of vein patch angioplasty at the time of bifurcation endarterectomy.

dense contralateral hemiplegia in the recovery room after correction of a smooth asymptomatic stenosis involving a small internal artery and a difficult arteriotomy closure. Conversely, noninvasive studies or a diagnostic angiogram might instead be warranted for another patient who awakens with mild to moderate clumsiness in the opposite hand following endarterectomy and patch angioplasty of a symptomatic ulcerated lesion in a carotid bifurcation of normal diameter (Fig. 57–8). Rosenthal and associates[75] and Perdue[82] found that reoperations were indicated in only 19 to 21 percent of patients who experienced cerebral ischemia related to carotid endarterectomy, but both of these reports concluded that urgent exploration was worthwhile in the

presence of an acute, profound deficit. An aggressive approach also may be justified in yet a smaller group of patients who recover from anesthesia without complications, only to sustain obvious deficits within the next several hours. Since intraoperative embolization is not a plausible explanation for such delayed ischemia, internal carotid thrombosis must be a serious consideration in this setting even though fibrin microemboli from the endarterectomy segment have been known to occur.

The priority objective during a remedial procedure is to re-establish cerebral perfusion by the expeditious insertion of a temporary shunt. General anesthesia may be necessary if the patient is too confused to be cooperative, but simple

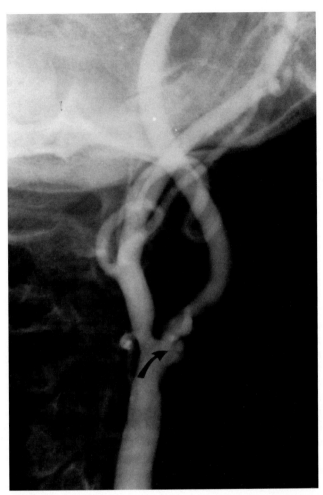

FIGURE 57–8. Seldinger angiogram of an ulcerated stenosis *(arrow)* associated with previous transient ischemic attacks in the ipsilateral cerebral hemisphere. Postoperative digital subtraction angiography was performed when the patient awakened from general anesthesia with clumsiness of the contralateral hand following carotid endarterectomy and vein patch angioplasty. The endarterectomy site was normal, and the mild deficit resolved entirely within a matter of hours.

local anesthesia may conserve additional time.[81] After the arteriotomy has been reopened, removal of the platelet thrombus, which is often found within the bifurcation, may be sufficient to restore retrograde bleeding from the internal carotid artery. Propagated clot extending into the ipsilateral siphon may require the use of a small balloon embolectomy catheter, but the catheter must not be advanced beyond even minimal resistance, and it should be inflated cautiously to avoid precipitating a carotid–cavernous sinus fistula.[83, 84] Once a shunt has been inserted, all adherent thrombus is removed from the endarterectomy segment, and technical defects, such as intimal flaps, are corrected. In fact, such problems are rarely identified, possibly because the architecture of the carotid bifurcation is no longer amenable to critical inspection once the arteriotomy has been reopened. At the conclusion of any reoperation, the arteriotomy should be closed with an autogenous vein patch in order to make every reasonable effort to prevent recurrent thrombosis.

From 1977 through 1984, 11 (0.4%) of the 2651 patients who underwent carotid endarterectomy at the Cleveland Clinic required urgent reoperations because of early, symp-

tomatic thrombosis of the internal carotid artery.[85] Because men made up approximately 70 percent of those scheduled for carotid reconstruction during the study period,[39] the composition of this small subset (six women and five men) suggests that women may be more likely to experience early thrombosis because of the small diameter of their arteries. Only two patients had obvious neurologic symptoms at the time they recovered from general anesthesia. The remaining deficits occurred within the next 8 hours in three patients, within 8 to 24 hours in five, and on the second postoperative day in one patient. Features that could have contributed to thrombosis were identified in five patients, including postoperative hypotension in two, an uncorrected internal carotid kink or loop each in one, and a small internal carotid artery in another. Diagnostic angiograms were obtained for two patients, while nine others underwent reoperations simply on the basis of their clinical deterioration. Eight (73%) of the 11 patients demonstrated substantial neurologic improvement after thrombectomy and patch angioplasty, five of whom either became asymptomatic or had only mild residual impairment. One patient (9%) died with a hemorrhagic cerebral infarction 3 days after early thrombosis of the operated artery in conjunction with contralateral internal carotid occlusion. These limited data tend to support the concept that prompt thrombectomy and patch angioplasty can be performed and that neurologic improvement can be realistically expected.

Focal Motor Seizures

Focal seizure activity occurring within the ipsilateral cerebral hemisphere several days after carotid endarterectomy has been reported in at least three series and may be related either to fibrin emboli from the surgical site or to cortical hyperperfusion associated with a fragile capillary bed. Youkey and colleagues[86] added four examples of this unusual complication to those already described by Sundt and associates[87] and Wilkinson and associates[88] and made several observations concerning the composite group of 18 patients. All required correction of high-grade carotid stenosis and experienced jacksonian seizures from 3 to 11 days later, despite subsequent confirmation of carotid patency on the basis of angiography or noninvasive hemodynamic testing. Eight patients (44%) had a history of preoperative ipsilateral strokes, but none apparently was neurologically unstable at the time of carotid reconstruction. Although postoperative hypertension did not occur, severe unilateral headache seemed to be a harbinger of seizure activity in several patients, and three (17%) sustained fatal intracerebral hemorrhage as a consequence of their complications.

While fibrin emboli have been suggested as the etiology of such focal seizures,[88] 9 of the 18 patients in the collected series were receiving prophylactic heparin, aspirin, or dipyridamole at the time their symptoms began. In fact, anticoagulation may have been a contributing risk factor. In retrospect, the recipient capillary network appeared to be especially sensitive to an abrupt improvement in flow because of prior subtotal stenosis or previous strokes, and at least one patient was found to have pericapillary hemorrhages during postmortem examination.[86] It is difficult to draw absolute conclusions concerning such a rare syndrome, but the available data suggest that patients who demonstrate signs and symptoms of cerebral edema should be kept under close observation even if seizure activity has not yet occurred. Bed rest, fluid restriction, and maintenance of the blood pressure at a level slightly lower than normal probably are appropriate, and any form of anticoagulation seems to be contraindicated. Like the swollen limb after extremity revascularization, the morbidity of cerebral edema undoubtedly declines as the integrity of the capillary bed is restored.

CRANIAL NERVE DYSFUNCTION

Incidence

The etiology and prevention of major ischemic stroke have been universal sources of concern for 40 years but, until the 1980s, even the incidence of cranial nerve dysfunction caused by direct manipulation during carotid endarterectomy has been a matter of conjecture. Surprisingly few reports concerning extracranial reconstruction have addressed cranial nerve complications, but such problems have been estimated to occur in 7.9 to 17 percent of patients assessed on the basis of retrospective clinical features.[24, 34, 89] Although their consequences may seem to be incidental in comparison with those of cerebral infarction, cranial nerve injuries often impose serious inconvenience or disability on the patient and may have medicolegal implications. Most importantly, a number of studies have suggested that trauma to the vagus, the hypoglossal, and other cervical nerves is usually avoidable, provided reasonable precautions are observed during preliminary exposure of the carotid bifurcation and subsequent application of vascular clamps.[90-92]

Several investigations indicate that carotid reconstruction is associated with at least transient cranial nerve dysfunction more frequently than has traditionally been suspected. In a series comprising a total of 116 patients and 128 operations, Liapis and colleagues[93] and Evans and colleagues[94] discovered early postoperative dysfunction involving the vagus and the recurrent laryngeal nerves in 15 percent and the hypoglossal nerve in 5.6 percent; they also found that as many as 35 percent of patients had integrated motor deficits that could only be detected by speech pathologists. Previous

experience employing direct otolaryngologic examinations after 450 consecutive carotid procedures at the Cleveland Clinic is presented in Table 57–5.[13, 30, 95] In this study there was evidence of surgical injury to the vagus or the recurrent laryngeal nerve in 6.7 percent, to the hypoglossal nerve in 5.8 percent, and to the marginal mandibular branch of the facial nerve and the superior laryngeal nerve, each in 1.8 percent.

Probably the most salient feature of this prospective study was the fact that a substantial number of iatrogenic cranial nerve injuries were overtly asymptomatic and might have escaped detection without formal evaluation. Twenty-four (38%) of 64 injuries to the vagus, the recurrent laryngeal, and the superior laryngeal nerves were not obvious during cursory clinical inspection. Considering the transient nature of cranial nerve dysfunction in most patients, this distinction has little importance among those requiring only unilateral carotid endarterectomy. Simultaneous dysfunction of both recurrent laryngeal or hypoglossal nerves, however, may seriously compromise the upper airway and impair respiration as well as oral nutrition.[92, 96] Accordingly, laryngoscopic examination to confirm the integrity of the recurrent laryngeal and hypoglossal nerves appears to be warranted during the interval between staged bilateral operations in order to avoid the possibility of injuries on both sides, which could require an extended period of assisted ventilation. If an important cranial nerve palsy is noted, it is prudent to postpone an elective contralateral procedure until the dysfunction has resolved, especially in patients having asymptomatic carotid stenosis on the opposite side.

As indicated in Table 57–5, most iatrogenic injuries are temporary and are probably caused by blunt traction. Follow-up examinations were performed to reassess 55 (76%) of the 72 injuries documented at the Cleveland Clinic, and 45 (82%) of these deficits resolved spontaneously during mean intervals of 2 to 3 postoperative months. Mild stretch injuries may be unavoidable during difficult operations involving either high bifurcations or lesions extending into the distal cervical segment of the internal carotid artery, but such patients at least may be reassured that their dysfunction probably represents a temporary inconvenience rather than a permanent disability.

TABLE 57–5. Early Incidence and Late Results of Cranial Nerve Dysfunction Following 450 Carotid Endarterectomies at the Cleveland Clinic

Postoperative Dysfunction	Cranial Nerves			
	Recurrent Laryngeal, n (%)	Hypoglossal, n (%)	Marginal Mandibular, n (%)	Superior Laryngeal, n (%)
Early incidence				
Symptomatic	21 (4.7)	16 (3.6)	8 (1.8)	3 (0.7)
Asymptomatic	9 (2.0)	10 (2.2)	0 (—)	5 (1.1)
Total	30 (6.7)	26 (5.8)	8 (1.8)	8 (1.8)
Late results				
Follow-up examinations	24 (80)	20 (77)	7 (88)	4 (50)
Recovery				
Complete	20 (83)	17 (85)	6 (86)	2 (50)
Mean interval, mo	3	2	3	2
Incomplete	4 (17)	3 (15)	2 (14)	2 (50)
Maximum interval, mo	14	12	9	2

Data from Hertzer,[13] Hertzer,[30] and Hertzer et al.[46] (See reference list for full bibliographic information).

Surgical Considerations

An example of the normal anatomy of several cranial nerves adjacent to the carotid bifurcation is depicted in Figure 57–9.

The Vagus Nerve

The vagus nerve (tenth cranial nerve) usually lies within the carotid sheath posterior to the artery and medial to the internal jugular vein, but it occasionally requires mobilization from an anomalous position lateral, or even anterior, to the distal common carotid artery at the time of bifurcation endarterectomy. The recurrent laryngeal nerve branches from the vagus in the mediastinum, loops around the subclavian artery on the right side and the aortic arch on the left, and then enters the tracheoesophageal groove posterior to the thyroid gland. Very rarely, the recurrent laryngeal nerve originates from the vagus near the carotid bifurcation and crosses behind the common carotid artery to enter the larynx.

Although concealed by the strap muscles and never demonstrated during carotid reconstruction, the recurrent laryngeal nerve conceivably may be injured by the sharp blades of self-retaining retractors that are placed too deeply and engage the nerve behind the trachea. Since recurrent laryngeal dysfunction is the most obvious manifestation of unilateral vagal injury, however, it is likely that most postoperative complications attributed to the recurrent laryngeal nerve are instead the result of trauma to the vagus itself. The vagus may be injured by electrocautery, by application of the proximal carotid clamp, or by dissection of the nerve from the distal internal carotid artery during the correction of high lesions. In any event, the ipsilateral vocal cord is paralyzed in the paramedian position, producing hoarseness and loss of an effective cough mechanism. Although vocal cord palsy customarily resolves within several weeks, Teflon injection to return the cord to the midline position may be necessary to improve phonation if the deficit persists beyond 6 to 12 months.

The Hypoglossal Nerve

The hypoglossal nerve (twelfth cranial nerve) descends from the hypoglossal canal in a relatively constant position medial to the internal carotid artery and the internal jugular vein before passing diagonally to enter the base of the tongue anterior to the external carotid artery. Hypoglossal injury produces ipsilateral deviation on protrusion of the tongue as well as the annoyance of inarticulate speech and clumsiness during mastication.

Transection of the hypoglossal nerve is an improbable event because it is a well-recognized landmark during carotid endarterectomy. Nevertheless, the twelfth nerve often interferes with surgical exposure of the internal carotid artery because it is tethered in position by the descending hypoglossal nerve, by the artery and vein to the sternocleidomastoid muscle, and, in many patients, by the occipital branch of the external carotid artery. Elective division of any or all of these structures may be necessary, since the hypoglossal nerve is more likely to be injured by excessive retraction than by appropriate steps to mobilize it. Forceful elevation of the posterior belly of the digastric muscle also impinges on the hypoglossal nerve, and both this muscle and its tendon can be divided without functional loss.

The Superior Laryngeal Nerve

The superior laryngeal nerve originates from the vagus immediately below the jugular foramen and passes obliquely behind the internal and external carotid arteries to supply an external branch to the cricothyroid muscle and the inferior pharyngeal constrictor, as well as a sensory internal branch to the mucosa of the larynx. Injury to the superior laryngeal nerve principally results in mild relaxation of the ipsilateral vocal cord as manifested by early fatiguability of the voice and impairment of high pitch, both of which may be of substantial concern to vocalists or public speakers. This comparatively small nerve is usually shrouded by the carotid sinus (see Fig. 57–9) and is susceptible to trauma by the distal internal carotid clamp. In addition, either the motor or

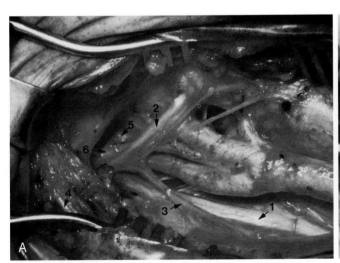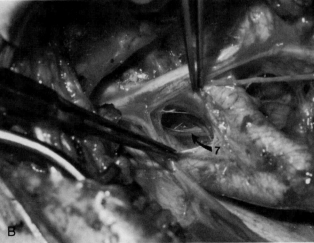

FIGURE 57–9. A, Operative photograph demonstrating the vagus nerve *(1)*, the hypoglossal nerve *(2)*, the ansa hypoglossi *(3)*, and the greater auricular nerve *(4)*. The artery and vein to the sternocleidomastoid muscle *(5)* have been divided, but the hypoglossal nerve remains tethered by the occipital artery *(6)*. B, The superior laryngeal nerve *(7)* lies posterior to the internal carotid artery and crosses medial to the carotid sinus and the external carotid artery to enter the larynx.

the sensory branch may be injured by dissection near the external carotid artery and its superior thyroid branch.

The Marginal Mandibular Nerve

The marginal mandibular branch of the facial nerve emerges from the anterior border of the parotid gland, courses forward across the masseter muscle and the ramus of the mandible, and innervates the muscles at the angle of the mouth and the lower lip. Although the nerve lies between the platysma and the deep cervical fascia and does not directly enter the surgical field, it is drawn inferiorly by rotation of the head to the opposite side and may be compressed by a retractor blade employed to elevate the mandible during the exposure of a high bifurcation, particularly if the incision has not been extended on a line posterior to the earlobe. Although marginal mandibular nerve injury imposes little functional disability, it does cause obvious drooping at the corner of the mouth, which is cosmetically unsatisfactory to many patients.

The Glossopharyngeal Nerve

Motor filaments of the glossopharyngeal nerve (ninth cranial nerve) cross the distal internal carotid artery before entering the middle pharyngeal constrictor and the tensor muscle of the soft palate. Trauma to these branches is a consideration only when an exceedingly long internal carotid lesion requires endarterectomy but, when such an injury does occur, it is one of the most troublesome of all cranial nerve deficits. Patients who experience ninth nerve dysfunction find it difficult to ingest solid food because of middle constrictor paralysis, and they are even less tolerant of oral fluids because nasopharyngeal reflux is not prevented by the flaccid soft palate. At least a brief period of parenteral or nasogastric tube nutrition may be necessary under these circumstances.

Fortunately, both the middle pharyngeal constrictor and the palate receive multiple motor fibers from the ipsilateral nerve as well as from the glossopharyngeal nerve on the opposite side, and serious disability usually is restricted to the first 2 postoperative weeks, with complete resolution within a month thereafter. Identification and preservation of the ninth cranial nerve may be one of the most important ancillary advantages to extended maneuvers that have been described to facilitate exposure of the internal carotid artery near the base of the skull, such as mandibular subluxation and detachment of the styloid process.[97, 98]

The Greater Auricular Nerve

Although it is a cervical rather than a cranial nerve, the greater auricular nerve passes posterolaterally to the sternocleidomastoid muscle to enter the surgical field during carotid endarterectomy. It is susceptible to either transection or stretch injury, particularly if sharp retractor blades are permitted to slide anterior to the muscle. Greater auricular trauma may produce either sensory loss or painful paresthesia involving the scalp and the external ear, both of which appear to be remarkably uncomfortable to patients who experience them.

REFERENCES

1. Easton JD, Sherman DG: Stroke and mortality rate in carotid endarterectomy: 228 consecutive operations. *Stroke.* 1977;8:565.
2. Toole JF, Yusoon CP, Janeway R, et al: Transient ischemic attacks: A prospective study of 225 patients. *Neurology (NY).* 1978;28:746.
3. Whisnant JP, Sandok BA, Sundt TM Jr: Carotid endarterectomy for unilateral carotid system transient cerebral ischemia. *Mayo Clin Proc.* 1983;58:171.
4. North American Symptomatic Carotid Endarterectomy Trial Collaborators: Beneficial effect of carotid endarterectomy in symptomatic patients with high-grade carotid stenosis. *N Engl J Med.* 1991;325:445.
5. European Carotid Surgery Trialists' Collaborative Group: MRC European carotid surgery trial: Interim results for symptomatic patients with severe (70–99%) or with mild (0–29%) carotid stenosis. *Lancet.* 1991;337:1235.
6. Mayberg MR, Wilson SE, Yatsu F, et al: Carotid endarterectomy and prevention of cerebral ischemia in symptomatic carotid stenosis. *JAMA.* 1991;266:3289.
7. Towne JB, Weiss GD, Hobson RW II: First phase report of cooperative Veterans Administration asymptomatic carotid stenosis study—operative morbidity and mortality. *J Vasc Surg.* 1990;11:252.
8. Hobson RW II, Weiss DG, Fields WS, et al: Efficacy of carotid endarterectomy for asymptomatic carotid stenosis. *N Engl J Med.* 1993;328:221.
9. Thompson JE: Complications of carotid endarterectomy and their prevention. *World J Surg.* 1979;3:155.
10. Kunkel JM, Gomez ER, Spebar MJ, et al: Wound hematomas after carotid endarterectomy. *Am J Surg.* 1984;148:844.
11. Welling RE, Ramadas HS, Gansmuller KJ: Cervical wound hematoma after carotid endarterectomy. *Ann Vasc Surg.* 1989;3:229.
12. Treiman RL, Cossman DV, Foran RF, et al: The influence of neutralizing heparin after carotid endarterectomy on postoperative stroke and wound hematoma. *J Vasc Surg.* 1990;12:440.
13. Hertzer NR: Non-stroke complications of carotid endarterectomy. In Bernhard VM, Towne J, eds. *Complications in Vascular Surgery,* 2nd ed. Orlando: Grune & Stratton; 1985;740.
14. Cafferata HT, Merchant R, DePalma RG: Avoidance of postcarotid endarterectomy hypertension. *Ann Surg.* 1982;196:465.
15. Davies MJ, Cronin KD: Post carotid endarterectomy hypertension. *Anaesth Intens Care.* 1980;8:190.
16. Ownes ML, Wilson SE: Prevention of neurologic complications of carotid endarterectomy. *Arch Surg.* 1982;117:551.
17. Pine R, Avellone JC, Hoffman M, et al: Control of postcarotid endarterectomy hypotension with baroreceptor blockade. *Am J Surg.* 1984;147:763.
18. Towne JB, Bernhard VM: The relationship of postoperative hypertension to complications following carotid endarterectomy. *Surgery.* 1980;88:575.
19. Smith BL: Hypertension following carotid endarterectomy: The role of cerebral renin production. *J Vasc Surg.* 1984;1:623.
20. Angell-James JE, Lumley SP: The effects of carotid endarterectomy on the mechanical properties of the carotid sinus and carotid sinus nerve activity in atherosclerotic patients. *Br J Surg.* 1974;61:805.
21. Bove EL, Fry WJ, Gross WS, Stanley JC: Hypotension and hypertension as consequences of baroreceptor dysfunction following carotid endarterectomy. *Surgery.* 1979;85:633.
22. Satiani B, Vasko JC, Evans WE: Hypertension following carotid endarterectomy. *Surg Neurol.* 1979;11:357.
23. Wade JG, Larson CP Jr, Hickey RF, et al: Effect of carotid endarterectomy on carotid chemoreceptor and baroreceptor function in man. *N Engl J Med.* 1970;282:823.
24. Ranson JHC, Imparato AM, Clauss RH, et al: Factors in the mortality and morbidity associated with surgical treatment of cerebrovascular insufficiency. *Circulation.* 1969;39(suppl I):I-269.
25. Tarlov E, Schmidek H, Scott RM, et al: Reflex hypotension following carotid endarterectomy: Mechanism and management. *J Neurosurg.* 1973;39:323.
26. Riles TS, Kopelman I, Imparato AM: Myocardial infarction following carotid endarterectomy: A review of 683 operations. *Surgery.* 1979;85:249.
27. Wallace JD, Levy LL: Blood pressure after stroke. *JAMA.* 1981;246:2177.
28. Caplan LR, Skillman J, Ojemann R, Fields WS: Intracerebral hemorrhage following carotid endarterectomy: A hypertensive complication? *Stroke.* 1978;9:457.
29. White JS, Sirinek KR, Root HD, Rogers W: Morbidity and mortality of carotid endarterectomy. *Arch Surg.* 1981;116:409.
30. Hertzer NR: Postoperative management and complications of extracranial carotid reconstruction. In Rutherford RB, ed. *Vascular Surgery.* Philadelphia: WB Saunders; 1984;1304.
31. Bauer RB, Meyer JS, Fields WS, et al: Joint study of extracranial arterial occlusion. *JAMA.* 1969;208:509.
32. Blaisdell WG, Clauss RH, Galbraith JC, et al: Joint study of extracranial arterial occlusion. *JAMA.* 1969;209:1889.
33. Thompson JE, Austin DJ, Patman RD: Carotid endarterectomy for cerebrovascular insufficiency: Long-term results in 592 patients followed up to thirteen years. *Ann Surg.* 1970;172:663.
34. DeWeese JA, Rob CG, Satran R, et al: Results of carotid endarterectomies for transient ischemic attacks: Five years later. *Ann Surg.* 1973;178:258.
35. Beebe HG, Clagett GP, DeWeese JA, et al: Assessing risk associated with carotid endarterectomy. *Circulation.* 1989;79:472.
36. Hertzer NR: Presidential address. Outcome assessment in vascular surgery: Results mean everything. *J Vasc Surg.* 1995;21:6.

37. Ott DA, Cooley DA, Chapa L, Coelho A: Carotid endarterectomy without temporary intraluminal shunt. Study of 309 consecutive operations. *Ann Surg.* 1980;191:708.

38. Bardin JA, Bernstein EF, Humber PB, et al: Is carotid endarterectomy beneficial in prevention of recurrent stroke? *Arch Surg.* 1982;117:1401.

39. Hertzer NR, Beven EG, Modic MT, et al: Early patency of the carotid artery after endarterectomy: Digital subtraction angiography after two hundred sixty-two operations. *Surgery.* 1982;92:1059.

40. Peitzman AB, Webster NW, Loubeau JM, et al: Carotid endarterectomy under regional (conductive) anesthesia. *Ann Surg.* 1982;196:59.

41. Towne JB, Bernhard VM: Neurologic deficit following carotid endarterectomy. *Surg Gynecol Obstet.* 1982;154:849.

42. Whittemore AD, Kauffman JL, Kohler TR, Mannick JA: Routine electroencephalographic (EEG) monitoring during carotid endarterectomy. *Ann Surg.* 1983;197:707.

43. Baker WH, Littooy FN, Hayes AC, et al: Carotid endarterectomy without a shunt: The control series. *J Vasc Surg.* 1984;1:50.

44. Ouriel K, May AG, Ricotta JJ, et al: Carotid endarterectomy for nonhemispheric symptoms: Predictors of success. *J Vasc Surg.* 1984;1:339.

45. Sachs SM, Fulenwider JT, Smith RB III, et al: Does contralateral carotid occlusion influence neurologic fate of carotid endarterectomy? *Surgery.* 1984;96:839.

46. Hertzer NR, Beven EG, O'Hara PJ, Krajewski LP: A prospective study of vein patch angioplasty during carotid endarterectomy. *Ann Surg.* 1987;206:628.

47. Corson JD, Chang BB, Shah DM, et al: The influence of anesthetic choice on carotid endarterectomy outcome. *Arch Surg.* 1987;122:807.

48. Till JS, Toole JF, Howard VJ, et al: Declining morbidity and mortality of carotid endarterectomy. The Wake Forest University Medical Center Experience. *Stroke.* 1987;18:823.

49. Mackey WC, O'Donnel TF Jr, Callow AD: Carotid endarterectomy contralateral to an occluded carotid artery: Perioperative risk and late results. *J Vasc Surg.* 1990;11:778.

50. Pinkerton JA Jr, Gholkar VR: Should patient age be a consideration in carotid endarterectomy? *J Vasc Surg.* 1990;11:650.

51. Mattos MA, Hodgson KJ, Londrey GL, et al: Carotid endarterectomy: Operative risks, recurrent stenosis, and long-term stroke rates in a modern series. *J Cardiovasc Surg.* 1992;33:387.

52. McCrory DC, Goldstein LB, Samsa GP, et al: Predicting complications of carotid endarterectomy. *Stroke.* 1993;24:1285.

53. Riles TS, Imparato AM, Jacobowitz GR, et al: The cause of perioperative stroke after carotid endarterectomy. *J Vasc Surg.* 1994;19:206.

54. Hertzer NR: Early complications of carotid endarterectomy: Incidence, diagnosis and management. In Moore, ed. *Surgery for Cerebrovascular Disease.* New York: Churchill Livingstone; 1987;634.

55. Whitney DG, Kahn EM, Estes JW, Jones DE: Carotid artery surgery without a temporary indwelling shunt: 1917 consecutive procedures. *Arch Surg.* 1980;115:1393.

56. Carmichael JD: Carotid surgery in the community hospital: 467 consecutive operations. *Arch Surg.* 1980;115:937.

57. Cranley JJ: Presidential address. Stroke: A perspective. *Surgery.* 1982;91:537.

58. Hafner CD, Evans WE: Carotid endarterectomy with local anesthesia: Results and advantages. *J Vasc Surg.* 1988;7:232.

59. Nunn DB: Carotid endarterectomy in patients with territorial transient ischemic attacks. *J Vasc Surg.* 1988;8:447.

60. Edwards WH, Edwards WH Jr, Jenkins JM, Mulherin JL Jr: Analysis of a decade of carotid reconstructive operations. *J Cardiovasc Surg.* 1989;30:424.

61. Gibbs BF, Guzzetta VJ: Carotid endarterectomy in community practice: Surgeon-specific versus institutional results. *Ann Vasc Surg.* 1989;3:307.

62. McKittrick JE, MacLean WB, Lim RA: Carotid endarterectomy in patients with contralateral carotid occlusion: Is the risk increased? *Ann Vasc Surg.* 1989;3:324.

63. Hoyne RF: Review of 272 consecutive carotid endarterectomies in a small community. *Surg Gynecol Obstet.* 1990;170:522.

64. Hans SS: Concurrent audit of early outcome for 1617 consecutive arterial reconstructions. *Surg Gynecol Obstet.* 1993;176:382.

65. Hertzer NR, Avellone JC, Farrell CJ, et al: The risk of vascular surgery in a metropolitan community. With observations on surgeon experience and hospital size. *J Vasc Surg.* 1984;1:13.

66. Moore DJ, Modi JR, Finch WT, Sumner DS: Influence of the contralateral carotid artery on neurologic complications following carotid endarterectomy. *J Vasc Surg.* 1984;1:409.

67. Fode NC, Sundt TM Jr, Robertson JT, et al: Multicenter retrospective review of results and complications of carotid endarterectomy, 1981. *Stroke.* 1986;17:370.

68. Kempczinski RF, Brott TG, Labutta RJ: The influence of surgical specialty and caseload on the results of carotid endarterectomy. *J Vasc Surg.* 1986;3:911.

69. Toronto Cerebrovascular Study Group: Risks of carotid endarterectomy. *Stroke.* 1986;17:848.

70. Rubin JR, Pitluk HC, King TA, et al: Carotid endarterectomy in a metropolitan community: The early results after 8535 operations. *J Vasc Surg.* 1988;7:256.

71. Kirshner DL, O'Brien MS, Ricotta JJ: Risk factors in a community experience with carotid endarterectomy. *J Vasc Surg.* 1989;10:278.

72. Brook RH, Park ED, Chassin MR, et al: Carotid endarterectomy for elderly patients: Predicting complications. *Ann Intern Med.* 1990;113:747.

73. Rosenthal D, Archie JP, Garcia-Rinaldi R, et al: Carotid patch angioplasty: Immediate and long-term results. *J Vasc Surg.* 1990;12:326.

74. Modi JR, Finch WT, Sumner DS: Update of carotid endarterectomy in two community hospitals: Springfield revisited. *Stroke.* 1983;14:128. Abstract 30.

75. Rosenthal D, Zeichner WD, Lamis PA, Stanton PE Jr: Neurologic deficit after carotid endarterectomy: Pathogenesis and management. *Surgery.* 1983;94:776.

76. Jernigan WR, Fulton RL, Hamman JL, et al: The efficacy of routine completion operative angiography in reducing the incidence of perioperative stroke associated with carotid endarterectomy. *Surgery.* 1984;96:831.

77. Zukowski AJ, Nicolaides AN, Lewis RT, et al: The correlation between carotid plaque ulceration and cerebral infarction seen on CT scan. *J Vasc Surg.* 1984;1:782.

78. Graber JN, Vollman RW, Johnson WC, et al: Stroke after carotid endarterectomy: Risk as predicted by preoperative computerized tomography. *Am J Surg.* 1984;147:492.

79. Ortega G, Gee W, Kaupp HA, McDonald KM: Postendarterectomy carotid occlusion. *Surgery.* 1981;90:1093.

80. Lye CR, Morrow IM, Downs AR: Carotid artery spasm. A cause of postendarterectomy thrombosis? *Arch Surg.* 1982;117:1531.

81. Kwaan JHM, Connolly JE, Sharefkin JB: Successful management of early stroke after carotid endarterectomy. *Ann Surg.* 1979;190:676.

82. Perdue GD: Management of postendarterectomy neurologic deficits. *Arch Surg.* 1982;117:1079.

83. Eggers F, Lukin R, Chambers AA, et al: Iatrogenic carotid-cavernous fistula following Fogarty catheter thromboendarterectomy: Case report. *J Neurosurg.* 1979;51:543.

84. Kakkasseril JS, Tomsick TA, Arbaugh JA, Cranley JJ: Carotid cavernous fistula following Fogarty catheter thrombectomy. *Arch Surg.* 1984;119:1095.

85. Painter TA, Hertzer NR, O'Hara PJ, et al: Symptomatic internal carotid thrombosis after carotid endarterectomy. *J Vasc Surg.* 1987;5:445.

86. Youkey JR, Clagett GP, Jaffin JH, et al: Focal motor seizures complicating carotid endarterectomy. *Arch Surg.* 1984;119:1080.

87. Sundt TM, Sharbourgh FW, Piepgras DG, et al: Correlation of cerebral blood flow and electroencephalographic changes during carotid endarterectomy with results of surgery and hemodynamics of cerebral ischemia. *Mayo Clin Proc.* 1981;56:533.

88. Wilkinson JT, Adams HP, Wright CB: Convulsions after carotid endarterectomy. *JAMA.* 1980;244:1827.

89. Matsumoto GH, Cossman D, Callow AD: Hazards and safeguards during carotid endarterectomy: Technical considerations. *Am J Surg.* 1977;133:458.

90. Imparato AM, Bracco A, Kim GE, Bergmann L: The hypoglossal nerve in carotid arterial reconstructions. *Stroke.* 1972;3:576.

91. DePalma RG: Optimal exposure of the internal carotid artery for endarterectomy. *Surg Gynecol Obstet.* 1977;144:249.

92. Verta MJ, Applebaum EL, McClusky DA, et al: Cranial nerve injury during carotid endarterectomy. *Ann Surg.* 1977;185:192.

93. Liapis CD, Satiani B, Florance CL, Evans WE: Motor speech malfunction following carotid endarterectomy. *Surgery.* 1981;89:56.

94. Evans WE, Mendelowitz DS, Liapis C, et al: Motor speech deficit following carotid endarterectomy. *Ann Surg.* 1982;196:461.

95. Hertzer NR, Feldman BJ, Beven EG, Tucker HM: A prospective study of the incidence of injury to the cranial nerves during carotid endarterectomy. *Surg Gynecol Obstet.* 1980;151:781.

96. Bageant TE, Tondini D, Lysons D: Bilateral hypoglossal-nerve palsy following a second carotid endarterectomy. *Anesthesiology.* 1975;43:595.

97. Fisher DF Jr, Clagett GP, Parker JI, et al: Mandibular subluxation for high carotid exposure. *J Vasc Surg.* 1984;1:727.

98. Sandmann W, Hennerici M, Aulich A, et al: Progress in carotid artery surgery at the base of the skull. *J Vasc Surg.* 1984;1:734.

X

Results of Carotid Endarterectomy: Retrospective Data

CHAPTER
58

The Importance of Establishing Uniform Reporting Standards in Evaluating the Results of Carotid Endarterectomy

ROBERT B. RUTHERFORD

In the late 1960s and early 1970s, a large cooperative, multicenter study of extracranial arterial occlusive disease was carried out in North America, the central feature of which was a prospective randomized trial of carotid endarterectomy (CEA) versus medical therapy. Much valuable information was contained in the many reports that emanated from this major cooperative effort, including the distribution of arteriosclerotic lesions in extracranial and intracranial arteries in symptomatic patients,[1] the high risk of operating in the face of profound acute stroke,[2] and the natural history of patients after complete carotid occlusion.[3] However, the only "take away" message from the randomized trial was that statistically significant superiority of CEA over nonoperative therapy could be shown only for patients with transient ischemic attacks (TIAs) originating ipsilateral to an "appropriate" carotid lesion, ostensibly a unilateral carotid stenosis.[3, 4] Benefit to patients with asymptomatic carotid stenosis or with completed stroke could not be shown. Two decades later, we are emerging from an "epidemic" of prospective randomized CEA trials designed to settle the same issues. At this point, the results of two trials of symptomatic carotid stenosis are incomplete for carotid stenosis in the 30 to 70 percent range,[5, 6] and potentially the best trial of CEA for asymptomatic carotid stenosis is still unreported.[7]* Little progress has been made, judging from continuing debates on many of the same issues. Consensus conferences are still being held, searching for just what surgeons and neurologists can agree on (Moore WS, unpublished information; Nicolaides A, et al, unpublished information). In the roughly 20-year interval between CEA trials, the literature was filled with innumerable retrospective reports on the results of CEA, with multiple prospective randomized trials of the efficacy of antiplatelet therapy and a

large number of "natural history" studies of asymptomatic carotid stenosis, spawned by Doppler ultrasonography imaging techniques and the opportunity for serial noninvasive surveillance, all yielding conflicting impressions. Elsewhere in this book (see Chapter 4), Mitchell and I present an analysis of the literature on the degree of carotid stenosis as an independent predictor of stroke. Because of a number of irregularities, the majority of studies on the subject had to be excluded from the analysis, obscuring the true dimensions and shape of the plot relating degree of carotid stenosis to stroke risk. Among other things, there were varying definitions of stroke, questionable accuracy and inconsistency in the methods used to estimate carotid stenosis, broad and differing ranges used in stratifying the degree of carotid stenosis, lack of separation of ipsilateral stroke from stroke in other territories, different ways of dealing with outcome in patients with bilateral carotid stenosis, and differing endpoints used in outcome analysis. It is likely that if standardized reporting practices had been developed and adopted at the outset and, as a result, more uniform clinical trial protocols and outcome criteria had been used, many if not most of the central issues still being debated in this field might have been settled. Until they are, uncertainty or dispute will continue to mar everyday life-and-death clinical decisions, and reporting bias, conscious or unconscious, will continue to infect the literature. It is no coincidence that papers written by surgeons are generally the most supportive of CEA and those written by neurologists tend to downplay its claimed efficacy.

However, the task of producing universally accepted standards for reports on cerebrovascular disease is not an easy one, or it might have been accomplished long ago. An acceptable clinical classification system has eluded us for over three decades, being either too simple to encompass all the complexities of cerebrovascular insufficiency or too complex for widespread adoption.[8, 9] Well-intentioned and well-organized attempts to overcome this impasse, such as the Marseilles Consensus Conference on Stroke,[10] could not resolve the many differences, although it served as an impetus for more focused efforts. It stimulated the CHAT classification system (so called because it is based on *Current*

---

*A clinical alert from this last trial was recently sent out that announced the trial's closure because of the finding of significant advantage of CEA over medical therapy (55% relative stroke risk reduction). The results were published in *Stroke* (1994;25:2523) and showed a 66% relative stroke risk reduction in males, but only a 17% reduction in females. The data have been the subject of varied interpretations and cautious warnings against universal application of CEA to *all* symptomatic patients with over 60% stenosis (Hertzer NR: *J Vasc Surg.* 1996;23:167).

458

status and *History*, the responsible *Arterial* lesion as demonstrated arteriographically, and the pathologic status of the *Target* organ), described elsewhere in this book (see Chapter 59), and suggested standards for reports dealing with cerebrovascular disease produced under the joint aegis of the Society for Vascular Surgery and the North American chapter of the International Society for Cardiovascular Surgery (SVS/ISCVS).[11, 12] To date, these suggested standards have not elicited an official response from neurologists. The task of developing standardized reporting practices for evaluating the results of CEA is made doubly difficult because it has all the complexities of evaluating arterial reconstructive surgery performed on patients with atherosclerotic occlusive disease as well as the already mentioned generic problems of dealing with cerebrovascular disease.

At the very least, we need to adopt uniform standards that stratify patients by clinical (neurologic function) status, by associated risk factors, and by the important characteristics of the carotid lesion itself (e.g., stenosis, ulceration), as well as by the modifying effect of significant lesions—in series or in parallel—on the cerebrovascular blood supply and by the status of the affected end organs—namely, the brain or eye—so that meaningful changes can be reliably gauged and the outcome of CEA objectively appraised. This task also requires that certain technical aspects of the operation itself be documented and that specific complications be properly reported.

Carotid endarterectomy cannot be evaluated in isolation. Comparison is the key to proper evaluation. CEA can be compared with nonoperative treatment (with "best medical therapy" applied to both groups), with some form of percutaneous endovascular intervention, or with itself, with some significant difference (eg, patient's neurologic status, timing of operation, technique, or adjunctive procedure) being isolated for comparison. For some comparisons, initial outcome criteria will suffice, but for most, long-term results must be weighed. Either way, the essential outcome criteria by which to gauge success or failure must be identified.

There has already been much discussion, if not debate, over many, if not most, of these key aspects. To recount all the options used in the past or proposed for the future, with their pros and cons, is beyond the scope of this chapter. Rather, I present a perspective gleaned from almost 9 years as the chairman of the SVS/ISCVS ad hoc committee on reporting standards, as a primary coauthor of its suggested standards for reports dealing with cerebrovascular disease,[12] and as one who has proposed standards for evaluating the long-term results and grading the complications of vascular surgery.[13, 14] Recommendations derived from these efforts are presented and discussed.

CLINICAL CLASSIFICATION

In 1960, Whisnant and coworkers[8] proposed a classification for focal cerebral ischemia with the following categories: incipient stroke (transient symptoms, arbitrarily defined as lasting less than 24 hours), advancing stroke (progressing or evolving symptoms), and completed stroke. The incipient strokes soon became known as TIAs. This classification system became widely used, and additional categories such as crescendo TIA and reversible ischemic neurologic deficit (RIND) were eventually added. The major limitation of such

clinically based classifications is that they do not provide for stratification of patients according to underlying disease. In an effort to overcome this problem, in 1975, the National Institute of Neurological and Communicative Disorders and Stroke (NINCDS) proposed a comprehensive classification covering six areas: timing, mechanism, anatomy, pathology, clinical status, and neurologic status.[9] Although the NINCDS classification was comprehensive, its complexity made it impractical for most clinical reports.

After an international symposium on this subject in Marseilles in 1984, Courbier[10] proposed a two-level system consisting of a primary clinical classification with a secondary description of arterial and intracerebral lesions. Subsequently, Hye and associates[11] further elaborated on this approach and developed the CHAT scheme, analogous to the TNM (primary *Tumor*, regional *Nodes*, and *Metastasis*) staging system used for tumor classification. The SVS/ISCVS ad hoc committee adopted a modified version of the CHAT system as the best approach to a broad-based clinical classification rather than a more restrictive classification specific to the needs of vascular surgeons.[12] The committee recommended that clinical status be reported much as the CH part of the CHAT classification system. The major categories for current clinical presentation include asymptomatic, brief stroke (less than 24 hours); temporary stroke (full recovery between 24 hours and 3 weeks); and permanent stroke (signs or symptoms lasting longer than 3 weeks), with separation into major and minor deficits. In addition, a category of changing stroke was included to identify those patients in whom the outcome of the current clinical episode is unknown before treatment. Patients with acute stroke, stroke in evolution, or crescendo TIA would fit in this category, subgrouped under improving stroke, fluctuating stroke, and deteriorating stroke to further stratify patients with an indeterminate natural history who are subjected to CEA. The category of nonspecific dysfunction was created for those patients who do not fit any of the more precise classifications (eg, syncope or other nonlateralizing symptoms of global ischemia). The past history section has the same categories as clinical presentation, except that there is no need for the changing stroke categories.

GRADING NEUROLOGIC DEFICITS AND DISABILITY

Grading the severity of residual neurologic deficit after stroke, either before or after CEA, has a practical value in assessing the risks and benefits of that operation. For many purposes, strokes can be classified as major or minor, based simply on whether patient independence is maintained. If a more refined gauging of neurologic complications is required, use of a neurologic event severity scale (Table 58–1) is recommended, adapted from the randomized trial of extracranial–intracranial bypass.[15] This scale is graded from 1 (brief stroke or TIA) to 11 (death), based on the presence or absence of impairment in any one or more of five domains (swallowing, self-care, ambulation, communication, and comprehension).

RISK FACTORS

The underlying disease process here is primarily atherosclerosis. The same risk factors contributing to its severity

TABLE 58–1. Neurologic Event Severity Scale

Severity Grade	Impairment*	Neurologic Symptoms	Neurologic Signs
1	None	Present	Absent
2	None	Absent	Present
3	None	Present	Present
4	Minor, in one or more domains	Present	Present
5	Major, in only one domain	NA†	NA
6	Major, in any two domains	NA	NA
7	Major, in any three domains	NA	NA
8	Major, in any four domains	NA	NA
9	Major, in all five domains	NA	NA
10	Reduced level of consciousness	NA	NA
11	Death	NA	NA

*Impairment in the domains of swallowing, self-care, ambulation, communication, and comprehension. If independence is maintained despite the impairment, the stroke is classified as minor; if independence is lost, it is classified as major.
†NA (not applicable) indicates that neurologic signs and symptoms have been integrated into the higher grades of impairment.
Adapted from the EC/IC Bypass Study Group: The international cooperative study of extracranial/intracranial arterial anastomosis (EC/IC bypass study): Methodology and entry characteristics. *Stroke.* 1985;16:397. Copyright © 1985 The American Heart Association. Used with permission.

contribute to outcome (survival, recurrent stroke, restenosis) and, primarily through coronary disease, affect operative risk. If valid differences are to be claimed in these outcome criteria, treatment groups should be comparable with regard to major risk factors. Operative risk may be gauged by a number of standard schemes such as Goldman's scale,[16] but noninvasive cardiac screening tests may serve an adjunctive role in evaluating patients prior to CEA.[17] For example, Eagle and colleagues'[18] approach of combining "clinical markers" with dipyridamole thallium scanning, as indicated, can be used to identify patients as having low, intermediate, or high risk for cardiac events. Since coronary disease is a contributing factor in the majority of deaths after CEA, intergroup comparisons of operative mortality should be backed by objective assessment of cardiac risk, if valid differences are to be claimed. Similarly, neurologic status (clinical class) affects the risk of postoperative neurologic deficit and deserves stratification for valid intergroup comparisons.

Finally, a simple grading of arteriosclerotic risk factors (eg, 0, none; 1, mild; 2, moderate; 3, severe) such as that recommended by the SVS/ISCVS[19] for diabetes, tobacco use, hypertension, hyperlipidemia, and cardiac status is proposed to ensure valid intergroup comparisons of many early and late outcome criteria.

The carotid bifurcation lesion should be stratified according to degree of stenosis and, where possible, ulceration. Arteriographic and duplex scan strata for degree of stenosis should be identical and convertible, to facilitate longitudinal follow-up studies (eg, in pentiles of 20%). Degree of stenosis should be reported in *diameter* reduction, with the smallest internal carotid artery diameter being related to its normal diameter above the stenosis.[12] This recommendation also applies to standardizing duplex scan findings. In this regard,

quality control of accuracy should be based on reasonably current internal comparisons with arteriograms. Other investigators' criteria should not be used without internal quality control. Ulceration should be graded minimal, moderate, or severe (ie, deep—>4 mm—multiple, or complex), with 2 mm depth separating the first two grades.[12]

The problem of dealing with bilateral carotid disease—or worse yet, multiple tandem or parallel lesions within the blood supply to the brain—is a difficult one. Significant contralateral carotid disease (eg, internal carotid artery occlusion) can affect the severity of an ipsilateral stroke as well as the accuracy of duplex scan surveillance, causing overestimation of the severity of ipsilateral stenosis using standard velocity criteria. Occlusive lesions and congenital variations in collateral pathways between hemispheres and between the anterior and posterior circulations can also affect outcome. Although this potential may be functionally assessed by a transcranial Doppler study, this is not universally available or used, and it is not technically feasible in a significant proportion of patients. Until a better approach is devised, the following simple grading scale is offered: 0, no hemodynamically significant lesion in any major collateral artery (ie, neither of the conditions described by the next grade); 1, greater than 60 percent narrowing in the contralateral carotid pathway (from aortic arch to siphon) or greater than 80 percent narrowing in the vertebrobasilar pathway (bilateral vertebral involvement required); 2, both of the conditions described by the previous grade; and 3, a complete occlusion in both contralateral carotid and vertebrobasilar pathways.

Ocular findings can be graded on clinical and ophthalmologic grounds as 0, absent; 1, transient; 2, permanent partial impairment (includes all forms of chronic ocular ischemia); and 3, blind. Brain computed tomographic and magnetic resonance imaging findings should characterize infarcts as ischemic or other, new or old (based on enhancement), small (less than 2 cm diameter) or large or multiple, and in the ipsilateral carotid territory or elsewhere. Ipsilateral focal atrophy may deserve inclusion.

Carotid endarterectomy data should include essential technical details such as type of anesthesia, method of monitoring for cerebral protection (stump pressure, electroencephalogram, transcranial Doppler), use of shunt, total crossclamping time and time without shunt (if used), use of patch angioplasty, and method of assessing technical adequacy.

RESULTS OF CAROTID ENDARTERECTOMY

Table 58–2 lists reportable complications following operations for cerebrovascular disease. Postoperative central neurologic complications should be reported using the C part of the CHAT clinical classification scheme, as previously suggested (eg, brief, temporary, or permanent stroke). Similarly, permanent strokes should be either stratified as major or minor or graded according to the neurologic event severity scale (see Table 58–1). The latter has particular value for clinical trials and operations for acute stroke or permanent stroke with partial deficit. Postoperative strokes should be separated further into the following categories: intraoperative stroke, when the deficit is detected at the first opportunity to

---

TABLE 58-2. Reportable Complications of Operations to Treat Extracranial Cerebrovascular Disease

---

Mortality
    Nonstroke related
    Stroke related
Permanent neurologic morbidity
    Stroke, major
    Stroke, minor
    Cranial nerve injury
Transient neurologic morbidity
    Brief stroke
    Temporary stroke
    Cranial nerve injury
Asymptomatic occlusive events
    Occlusion
    Residual stenosis (technical)
    Recurrent stenosis

---

examine the patient after operation; early postoperative stroke, with worsening detected after the initial evaluation and up to 30 days; and late postoperative stroke, occurring after 30 days. As usual, death from any cause during this same 30-day period must be counted as an operative death; deaths from stroke must be separated from those from other causes. Cranial nerve injuries should be identified separately and be listed by nerve and whether the deficit is temporary or permanent.

Permanent cranial nerve injuries should be included with stroke when reporting permanent neurologic deficit. The latter, along with perioperative death (up to 30 days), is ordinarily combined in the permanent morbidity and mortality rate as a major yardstick of the risk of CEA. In that regard, fatal postoperative strokes should not be counted twice.

Unlike other arterial reconstructions, the long-term success of CEA cannot be gauged by patency because, with few exceptions, the carotid artery is patent preoperatively. Nor can it be gauged by continued symptomatic or functional improvement, because many patients will have had either transient or no ischemic symptoms to start with. Freedom from stroke or symptoms of cerebral ischemia is the most valid index of success.[13, 20] Cerebral ischemic events caused by disease outside the carotid territory should be recorded but *not* counted against CEA, except in clinical trials in which it is pitted against systemic (eg, antiplatelet) therapy for stroke prevention. Nonlateralizing symptoms should also be counted in the event there is carotid restenosis. The rate of significant carotid restenosis (arbitrarily 60% or more) should be recorded separately. Obviously, symptomatic restenoses will also be counted in the late ischemic event or stroke rate, so duplication must be avoided if these failure criteria are combined. In summary, the primary measure of

the long-term efficacy of CEA should be a stroke- or ischemic event–free interval specific for that carotid artery distribution, with treatment group data presented and analyzed using either the Kaplan-Meier[21] or the classic life table method.[22, 23]

REFERENCES

1. Hass WK, Fields WS, North RR, et al: Joint study of extracranial arterial occlusion. II. Arteriography, techniques, sites and complications. *JAMA.* 1968;203:159.
2. Fields WS, Lemak NA: Joint study of extracranial arterial occlusion. X. Internal carotid artery occlusion. *JAMA.* 1976;235:2734.
3. Blaisdell WF, Claus RH, Galbraith JG, et al: Joint study of extracranial arterial occlusion. IV. A review of surgical considerations. *JAMA.* 1969;209:1889.
4. Fields WS, Maslenikov V, Meyer JS, et al: Joint study of extracranial arterial occlusion. V. Progress report of prognosis following surgery or nonsurgical treatment for transient cerebral ischemic attacks and cervical carotid artery lesions. *JAMA.* 1970;211:1993.
5. North American Symptomatic Carotid Endarterectomy Trial (NASCET): Beneficial effect of carotid endarterectomy in symptomatic patients with high-grade carotid stenosis. *N Engl J Med.* 1991;325:445.
6. European Carotid Surgery Trialists' Collaborative Group (ECSTCG): MRC European carotid surgery trial: Interim results for symptomatic patients with severe (70–99%) or with mild (0–29%) carotid stenosis. *Lancet.* 1991;337:1235.
7. Asymptomatic Carotid Atherosclerosis Study Group: Study design for randomized prospective trial of carotid endarterectomy for asymptomatic atherosclerosis. *Stroke.* 1989;20:844.
8. Whisnant JP, Sickert RG, Millikan CH: Appraisal of the current trend toward surgical treatment of occlusive cerebral vascular disease. *Med Clin North Am.* 1960;44:857.
9. National Institute of Neurological and Communicative Disorders and Stroke: A classification and outline of cerebrovascular disease. *Stroke.* 1975;6:564.
10. Courbier R, ed.: *Basis for a Classification of Cerebral Arterial Diseases.* Amsterdam: Exerpta Medica; 1985.
11. Hye RJ, Dilley RB, Browse NL, Bernstein EF: Evaluation of a new classification of cerebrovascular disease (CHAT). *Am J Surg.* 1987;154:104.
12. Baker JD, Rutherford RB, Bernstein EF, et al: Suggested standards for reports dealing with cerebrovascular disease. *J Vasc Surg.* 1988;8:721.
13. Rutherford RB: Reporting standards for long-term results of vascular surgery. In Yao JST, Pearce WH, eds. *Vascular Surgery: Long-Term Results.* Philadelphia: WB Saunders; 1993:1.
14. Rutherford RB: Suggested standards for reporting complications in vascular surgery. In Towne JB, Bernhard WM, eds. *Complications in Vascular Surgery*, 3rd ed. St. Louis: Quality Medical Publishing; 1991:1.
15. The EC/IC Bypass Study Group: The international cooperative study of extracranial/intracranial arterial anastomosis (EC/IC bypass study): Methodology and entry characteristics. *Stroke.* 1985;16:397.
16. Goldman L: Assessment of the patient with known suspected ischaemic heart disease for non-cardiac surgery. *Br J Anaesth.* 1988;61:38.
17. Rutherford RB: Assessment of cardiac risk for carotid surgery. In Bernstein E, Callow A, Nicolaides A, Shiffrin E, eds. *Cerebral Revascularisation.* London: Med-Orion Publishing; in press.
18. Eagle KA, Coley CM, Newell JB, et al: Continuing clinical and thallium data optimizes preoperative assessment of cardiac risk before major vascular surgery. *Ann Intern Med.* 1989;110:859.
19. Rutherford RB, Flanigan DP, Gupta SK, et al: Suggested standards for reports dealing with lower extremity ischemia. *J Vasc Surg.* 1986;4:80.
20. Rutherford RB: Recommended standards for reports on vascular disease and its management. In Callow A, Ernst CB, eds. *Vascular Surgery: Theory and Practice.* Norwalk, CT: Appleton & Lange, 1995.
21. Lee ET: *Statistical Methods for Survival Data Analysis.* Belmont, CA: Wadsworth; 1980:75.
22. Peto R, Pike MC, Armitage P, et al: Design and analysis of randomized trials required prolonged observations of each patient. I. Introduction and design. *Br J Cancer.* 1976;34:585.
23. Peto R, Pike MC, Armitage P, et al: Design and analysis of randomized trials required prolonged observations of each patient. II. Analysis and examples. *Br J Cancer.* 1977;35:1.

CHAPTER 59

The CHAT Classification

EUGENE F. BERNSTEIN

The CHAT classification of vascular disease was designed to separate various current (C) and historical (H) presentations of disease and their separate angiographic (A) and target (T) organ manifestations from one another, with the aim of identifying specific factors or groups of factors that would be important in determining appropriate management approaches or prognosis. Initially, asymptomatic patients with prior contralateral symptoms were shown to have a different prognosis from those with a completely negative contralateral history of cerebrovascular disease.[1, 2] In addition, the system provided information about the improved prognosis of patients with amaurosis fugax compared with patients with cortical transient ischemic attacks (TIAs), both of which had previously been grouped within the overall classification of TIAs.[1, 2] The CHAT classification system was adopted by the subcommittee on reporting standards for cerebrovascular disease of the Society for Vascular Surgery and the International Society for Cardiovascular Surgery in 1988.[3] In addition, that committee advocated the use of a risk factor severity scale for the cerebrovascular area that had been proposed by the subcommittee on reporting standards for lower-extremity ischemia. The availability of these two schemes—a classification of the presentation of cerebrovascular disease and a risk factor classification—suggested that specific risk factors, and a total risk factor score, could be related to the long-term outlook after successful carotid endarterectomy. This approach seemed particularly appropriate because of the growing number of reports emphasizing the importance of such risk factors in determining the likelihood of future stroke and early death.[4–8] In addition, a larger database with longer follow-up was available to provide long-term data in our patients. Special attention was paid to those patients who were operated on for asymptomatic carotid lesions but were subclassified under the CHAT classification.

METHODS

To evaluate the relation of known risk factors with late stroke and early death after carotid endarterectomy, we analyzed the indications for surgery according to CHAT in 633 patients who had undergone 714 carotid operations and had been followed in the Vascular Registry of the Scripps Clinic and Research Foundation. All operations were performed by two surgeons who have used the same operative indications and technical surgical methods since 1978. All patients undergoing carotid surgery also had complete angiographic studies to document the technical status of the repair after their operative procedures. Other details of operative technique have been published previously.[9]

The chart of each patient in the registry was re-evaluated, and a CHAT classification (Table 59–1) and risk factor grading (Table 59–2) were performed at the time of initial clinical presentation. Risk factors studied included diabetes, tobacco use, hypertension, cholesterol, and cardiac, renal, and pulmonary function. The grading scale was the one recommended by the subcommittee and ranged from 0 to 3

462

for each factor. A total risk factor score was determined by adding the grade score for each of the seven risk factors. In addition, analyses of the effects of age (by decade) and gender were performed. A breakdown of the subgroups analyzed within the group of patients operated on for asymptomatic lesions is detailed in Table 59–3. All analyses were based on the endpoints of ipsilateral stroke (after hospital discharge following carotid surgery), death, and stroke-free survival.

All data concerning the original presentations of the patients, details of the operative procedures, early morbidity and late follow-up were entered in a VAX Model 11/750 computer (Digital Equipment Corp., Maynard, MA) of the General Clinical Research Center of the Scripps Clinic using CLINFO (BBN Software Products Corp., Cambridge, MA) software for clinical data management and analysis. Life table analyses were performed according to the product limit method of Kaplan and Meier,[10] and comparisons between groups were made with Gehan's modification of the Wilcoxon test.[11] Categorical data in contingency tables were analyzed using Pearson's χ^2 test.

Logistic regression analyses were performed to assess the relative significance of the various risk factors as predictors of outcome events, ipsilateral stroke, and death.[12] For these analyses, all graded risk factors were dichotomized into 0–1 (negative-positive) variables. In particular, this facilitates reporting odds ratios and the associated 95 percent confidence intervals for these variables. The estimated odds ratio approximates how much more likely it was that the particular outcome (stroke or death) would occur among those with the factor present (ie, positive) than among those with the factor absent (ie, negative).

RESULTS

Risk Factor Incidence

In the 633 patients who were operated on and studied for an average of 44 months thereafter, late ipsilateral stroke was observed in 16, and late contralateral stroke was noted in 33. Four of these contralateral strokes occurred in the 81 patients in whom the contralateral side had also been subjected to endarterectomy, and 29 were seen in hemispheres that had not been operated on. In the total patient group, the incidence of hypertension was 59.7 percent; tobacco use, 52.9 percent; cardiac disease, 47.3 percent; hyperlipidemia, 38.8 percent; pulmonary disease, 30.6 percent; diabetes, 15.0 percent; and renal disease, 14.2 percent.

Univariate CHAT Analysis

An initial assessment of the Kaplan-Meier life table analyses according to the major clinical symptom presentation is summarized in Table 59–4, in which the 5-year probability of remaining stroke free, of surviving, and of surviving stroke free is documented. The table also separates the patients according to the CHAT scheme. The asymptomatic

TABLE 59–1. The CHAT Classification of Stroke

C — Current Status (<1 yr)		H — History (>1 yr)	A — Artery		T — Target	
Symptoms	Vascular Territory	Symptoms/ Vascular Territory	Site	Pathology	Site	Pathology
0—asymptomatic	a—carotid ocular (amaurosis fugax)	Same categories as current status	0—no lesion	a—arteriosclerosis	0—no lesion	h—hemorrhage
1—brief stroke, TIA (<24 hr)	b—carotid cortical	Current clinical	1—appropriate lesion	c—cardiogenic embolus	1—appropriate lesion	i—infarct
2 — temporary stroke with full recovery (24 hr to 3 wk)	c—vertebrobasilar	1–5/a–e	2—lesion in another vascular pathway	d—dissection	2—lesion in another vascular territory	j—lacunar
3—permanent stroke, minor (>3 wk)	d—other focal		3—combined appropriate lesion and lesion in another vascular pathway	e—aneurysm	3—combined appropriate lesion and lesion in another vascular territory	m—AVM
4—permanent stroke, major (>3 wk)	e—diffuse	Subscript s is used to indicate prior operation		f—fibromuscular		n—neoplasm
5—nonspecific dysfunction				r—arteritis		q—other
6—improving stroke				t—trauma		r—retinal embolism
7—fluctuating stroke						
8—deteriorating stroke						

AVM, arteriovenous malformation—significant, 50% stenosis or disease thought to be the source of symptoms; TIA, transient ischemic attack.
From Baker JD, Rutherford RB, Bernstein EF, et al: Suggested standards for reports dealing with cerebrovascular disease. *J Vasc Surg.* 1988; 8:721; with permission.

TABLE 59–2. Risk Factor Categories

Risk Factor	0	1	2	3
Diabetes	None	Adult onset, no insulin	Adult onset, insulin controlled	Juvenile onset
Tobacco use	None (or abstinence >10 yr)	None currently, abstinence 1–10 yr	Current, <1 pack/day (or abstinence <1 yr)	Current ≥1 pack/day
Hypertension	Diastolic <90 mm Hg	Easily controlled, single drug	Requires 2 drugs	>2 drugs or uncontrolled
Hyperlipidemia	Cholesterol and triglycerides within normal limits for age	Mild elevation, diet controlled	Type II, III, or IV, requiring strict diet control	Requires drug control
Cardiac	Asymptomatic, normal ECG	Asymptomatic, remote MI (>6 mo), occult MI by ECG	Stable angina, controlled ectopy, asymptomatic arrhythmia, drug-compensated congestive failure	Unstable angina, symptomatic or poorly controlled ectopy or dysrhythmia, poorly compensated failure, MI <6 mo
Renal	No renal disease, creatinine <1.5 mg/dL, clearance >50 mL/min	Creatinine 1.5–3.0 mg/dL clearance 30–49 mL/min	Creatinine 3.1–5.9 mg/dL, clearance 15–30 mL/min	Creatinine >6.0 mg/dL, clearance <15 mL/min, dialysis or transplant
Pulmonary	Asymptomatic, normal chest radiograph film, PFT >80% of predicted	Asymptomatic or mild dyspnea on exertion, mild radiographic parenchymal changes, PFTs 65–80% of predicted	Levels between those in category 1 and those in category 3	Vital capacity <1.85 L, FEV_1 <1.2 L or <35% of predicted, maximal voluntary ventilation <28 L/min or <50% of predicted, Pco_2, >45 mm Hg, supplemental O_2 required, pulmonary hypertension

ECG, electrocardiogram; FEV_1, 1-second forced expiratory volume; MI, myocardial infarction; PFT, pulmonary function test.
From Baker JD, Rutherford RB, Bernstein EF, et al: Suggested standards for reports dealing with cerebrovascular disease. *J Vasc Surg.* 1988; 8:721; with permission.

TABLE 59–3. Subdivisions of Asymptomatic Carotid Stenosis Patients by CHAT Analysis

Indication	CHAT Code
Asymptomatic carotid stenosis	C_0
History of no prior cerebrovascular symptoms either hemisphere	C_0H_0
History of contralateral brief stroke (TIA)—amaurosis fugax	C_0H_{1a}
History of contralateral brief stroke (TIA)—cortical	C_0H_{1b}
History of contralateral brief stroke (TIA)—vertebrobasilar	C_0H_{1c}
History of contralateral temporary stroke	C_0H_2
History of contralateral permanent stroke, minor	C_0H_{3a}
History of contralateral permanent stroke, major	C_0H_{3b}
History of prior carotid surgery, ipsilateral	C_{0s}
History of prior carotid surgery, contralateral	$C_0H_{0-3,\,s}$
Artery, appropriate lesion only	C_0HA_1
Artery, bilateral or tandem lesions	C_0HA_3
Target, no CT/MRI lesions, bilateral	C_0HAT_0
Target, positive CT/MRI, ipsilateral only	C_0HAT_1
Target, positive CT/MRI, contralateral only	C_0HAT_2
Target, positive CT/MRI, bilateral	C_0HAT_3

CT, computed tomography; MRI, magnetic resonance imaging; TIA, transient ischemic attack.

TABLE 59–5. Probability of Stroke-Free Survival 5 Years After Carotid Endarterectomy in All Patients

Risk Factor Score	Patients, n	Stroke Free	Survival	Stroke-Free Survival
0–3	253	0.94	0.86	0.81
4–5	172	0.94	0.75	0.73
6	87	0.91	0.68	0.66
7–9	94	0.94	0.66	0.63
10–14	24	0.83	0.35	0.28

Braces, $P < 0.01$.

patient group is first presented as a single entity and then subdivided based on the patient's past history of contralateral symptoms. The small group with a prior history of contralateral permanent stroke has a higher likelihood of late stroke when compared with those with no history of contralateral disease (Fig. 59–1).

Patients presenting with TIAs are subdivided by CHAT into those with amaurosis fugax, anterior cortical lesions, and vertebrobasilar symptoms. Varying grades of preoperative stroke are also separated. The most striking finding of this analysis is the relative absence of ipsilateral stroke in all groups, with a 97 percent probability of all patients remaining stroke free at 5 years after carotid endarterectomy.

The worst outlook for recurrent stroke was after surgery for an asymptomatic lesion in patients with a history of contralateral cortical stroke with permanent deficit, and in patients in whom cortical stroke with minor residual deficit was the indication for ipsilateral carotid surgery. Survival data document a mortality rate of approximately 5 percent per year in patients with all indications for carotid surgery, except for those with minor ocular deficits, in which no deaths occurred ($P < 0.001$).

Total Risk Factor Score

The likelihood of stroke or death by 5 years after carotid endarterectomy as a function of the total risk factor score was examined. In Table 59–5, these results are summarized for all patients, indicating that there is no effect on late stroke with a total score from 0 to 9 and no statistically significant effect with any score. But each increment of the

TABLE 59–4. Probability of Stroke-Free Survival 5 Years After Carotid Endarterectomy

Indication	CHAT Class	Conventional Class	Patients, n	Stroke Free	Survival	Stroke-Free Survival
Asymptomatic, all cases	C_0	Asymptomatic	180	0.95	0.79	0.75
Asymptomatic, no prior history	C_0H_0	Asymptomatic	144	0.95	0.83	0.80
Asymptomatic, contralateral amaurosis fugax	C_0H_1	Asymptomatic	6	1.00	0.83	0.83
Asymptomatic, contralateral TIA	C_0H_2	Asymptomatic	8	1.00	0.54	0.54
Asymptomatic, contralateral permanent stroke	C_0H_3	Asymptomatic	15	0.80	0.66	0.53
Amaurosis fugax	C_{1a}	TIA	125	0.97	0.79	0.81
Cortical TIA	C_{1b}	TIA	155	0.96	0.70	0.70
Vertebrobasilar TIA	C_{1c}	TIA	29	1.00	0.69	0.68
Temporary stroke with full recovery	C_{2a-e}	Stroke, RIND	27	1.00	0.66	0.66
Stroke, minor deficit, ocular	C_{3a}	Stroke	16	1.00	1.00	1.00
Stroke, minor deficit, cortical	C_{3b}	Stroke	47	0.89	0.67	0.59
Miscellaneous indications in smaller groups			43			
All indications			615	0.97	0.76	0.75

*Excludes 9 permanent operative strokes out of 714 operations (1.3%).
RIND, reversible ischemic neurologic deficit; TIA, transient ischemic attack.

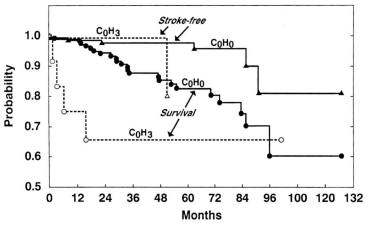

FIGURE 59–1. Kaplan-Meier survival curves depict the probability of stroke and of survival in patients presenting with asymptomatic stenoses who had no history of any prior contralateral neurologic symptoms (C_0H_0) and in those presenting with asymptomatic stenoses with a history of contralateral stroke (C_0H_3).

total risk factor score did have a significant effect on the likelihood of early death ($P < 0.01$) and, consequently, on stroke-free survival ($P < 0.01$).

When all those patients operated on for asymptomatic lesions were grouped together (Table 59–6), the total risk factor score had no effect on stroke. When limited to patients with global (eg, both hemispheres) asymptomatic states (C_0H_0), however, the patients with scores of 4–5 and 10–14 were significantly more likely to experience late stroke ($P < 0.01$). In contrast to the relative absence of any effect on late stroke, in each of these analyses, the total score had a highly significant effect on the probability of early death.

Univariate Risk Factor Analysis

The effect of each of the specific risk factors was then analyzed for each clinical presentation by CHAT. In Table 59–7, the effects of varying risk grades for tobacco use, hypertension, and cardiac disease are presented for asymptomatic patients. None of these individual factors had any obvious or statistically significant effect on the likelihood of stroke, survival, or stroke-free survival.

In Table 59–8, CHAT analyses of the data related to arterial (A) and target (T) organ risk factors are summarized. None of the comparisons indicates any significant risk factor

predictive for stroke following carotid endarterectomy. However, more advanced degrees of arterial disease (A_3) and a positive computed tomography or magnetic resonance imaging scan for infarction (T_{li}) were correlated with an increased probability of early death.

MULTIVARIATE LOGISTIC ANALYSIS

Results of logistic regression analysis are presented for two outcomes and for different CHAT classifications in Table 59–9 (stroke) and Table 59–10 (survival). Data are presented as a standardized coefficient (ie, a coefficient divided by the standard deviation) for each variable in the relevant logistic regression equation. Positive coefficients denote increased risk of stroke or death. A standardized coefficient of less than -2 or greater than $+2$ is "significant" at approximately the $P = 0.05$ level. Gender was coded 0, female and 1, male; negative coefficients indicate that males have a decreased risk relative to females for either stroke or death. Data are also presented as P values and odds ratios.

In the asymptomatic group, only diabetes had a significant effect on the likelihood of late stroke (odds ratio, 18.8). Hypertension approached this level as a negative predictive

TABLE 59–6. Probability of Stroke-Free Survival 5 Years After Carotid Endarterectomy in Asymptomatic Patients

Indication	Risk Factor Score	Patients, n	Probability at 5 Years		
			Stroke Free	Survival	Stroke-Free Survival
Asymptomatic (C_0)	0–3	63	0.96	0.95 ⌝	0.91 ⌝
	4–5	53	0.86	0.85 ⌟	0.88 ⌟
	6	27	0.95	0.75 ⌝	⌐0.69
	7–9	23	1.00	0.54 ⌟	0.54 ⌟
	10–14	16	0.88	0.43	⌊0.36
	Total	182			
Asymptomatic (C_0H_0)	0–3	45	1.00 ⌝	⌐0.97 ⌝	⌐0.97 ⌝
	4–5	47	0.86 ⌟	0.83 ⌟	0.79 ⌟
	6	24	0.94	0.64 ⌟	0.71 ⌟
	7–9	16	1.00	⌊0.70	⌊0.70
	10–14	11	0.82 ⌟	⌊0.58	⌊0.49
	Total	143			

Braces, $P < 0.01$.

TABLE 59–7. Effect of Risk Factors on Probability of Stroke-Free Survival
5 Years After Carotid Endarterectomy in Asymptomatic Patients

Risk Factor	Degree of Risk	Patients, n	Probability at 5 Years		
			Stroke Free	Survival	Stroke-Free Survival
Tobacco use	0	77	0.91	0.82	0.78
	1	30	0.95	0.84	0.79
	2	23	0.91	0.79	0.75
	3	54	0.95	0.70	0.68
Hypertension	0	66	0.89	0.90	0.81
	1	59	0.98	0.85	0.83
	2	37	0.94	0.63	0.60
	3	21	1.00	0.58	0.58
Cardiac disease	0	95	0.98	0.89	0.88
	1	28	0.96	0.91	0.87
	2	39	0.82	0.61	0.48
	3	23	0.96	0.60	0.58

TABLE 59–8. CHAT Analysis of Arterial (A) and Target (T) Organ Factors on Late Stroke and Death Following Carotid Endarterectomy

Groups at Risk	Patients, n	Probability of Difference at 5 Years		
		Stroke Free	Survival	Stroke-Free Survival
All patients	372/219	0.42	0.02	0.03
A_1 vs. A_3	127/37	0.97	0.11	0.05
T_0 vs. T_2				
CHAT analysis				
C_0A_1 vs. C_0A_3	104/714	0.60	0.02	0.09
C_0A_1 vs. C_2A_1	104/93	0.76	0.02	0.09
C_1A_1 vs. C_1A_3	91/34	*	0.08	0.04
C_2A_1 vs. C_2A_3	93/52	0.84	0.94	0.90
C_1T_0 vs. C_1T_{1i}	21/2	*	*	*
C_2T_0 vs. C_2T_{1i}	43/6	*	0.23	0.26
C_1T_{1i} vs. C_2T_{1i}	21/43	*	0.96	0.98

*Inadequate number of events to permit statistical evaluation.

CT, computed tomography; MRI magnetic resonance imaging; TIA, transient ischemic attack.

A_1, appropriate unilateral arterial lesion; A_3, bilateral arterial lesion; C_0, asymptomatic stenosis; C_1, ocular TIA (amaurosis fugax); C_2, cortical TIA; T_0, negative CT/MRI; T_{1i}, positive and appropriate CT/MRI—infarction.

TABLE 59–9. Logistic Analysis of the Influence of Specific Risk
Factors on the Probability of Late Stroke After Carotid
Endarterectomy in Asymptomatic Patients

Risk Factor	Coefficient/SD	P Value	Odds Ratio
Gender	−0.245	0.81	0.9
Age	0.979	0.33	1.9
CHAT positive history	−0.823	0.41	0.5
Diabetes	2.180	0.03	18.8
Tobacco use	0.039	0.97	1.0
Hypertension	−1.730	0.08	0.4
Cholesterol	0.964	0.34	1.8
Cardiac	1.360	0.17	2.3
Renal	−0.408	0.68	0.7
Pulmonary	0.417	0.68	1.9

TABLE 59–10. Logistic Analysis of the Influence of Specific Risk
Factors on the Probability of Survival After Carotid
Endarterectomy in Asymptomatic Patients

Risk Factor	Coefficient/SD	P Value	Odds Ratio
Gender	−1.200	0.23	0.6
Age	0.566	0.57	1.4
CHAT positive history	0.909	0.36	1.6
Diabetes	−0.357	0.72	0.6
Tobacco use	0.539	0.59	1.4
Hypertension	1.350	0.18	2.0
Cholesterol	−0.240	0.81	0.9
Cardiac	1.420	0.16	2.0
Renal	1.960	0.05	3.0
Pulmonary	0.792	0.43	1.5

factor for stroke ($P = 0.08$). None of the risk factors predicted early death in asymptomatic patients, but renal disease approached significance (see Table 59–10).

DISCUSSION

The value of the CHAT analysis in this study is to separate patients within the traditional groups of asymptomatic stenosis, TIA, and stroke into several subgroups based on other details of their current and past histories. This analysis has confirmed the value of such an approach, since important and statistically significant differences have been shown between such subgroups, which may weigh heavily in the decision to advise surgery as well as in determining the prognosis for a patient. For example, those asymptomatic patients with no prior history of contralateral neurologic symptoms had a much lower probability of late stroke (96% stroke free at 5 years) than those who were operated on for a contralateral lesion opposite a prior stroke resulting in a permanent residual deficit (80% stroke free at 5 years). In addition, the likelihood of survival of the two groups was markedly different. Similar differences have been shown in the past between patients with amaurosis fugax and those with cortical TIAs.[1, 2] The differing patterns of risk factor importance brought out by the current data re-emphasize the separateness of these clinical entities, which have been grouped together in the past. In addition, there are potentially many other important distinctions that remain to be discovered within the CHAT classification, if one could analyze a much larger database with longer follow-up. The value of the arterial and target organ subclassifications within each clinical and historical group cannot be evaluated adequately until a vastly larger database is available, probably requiring pooling of data from a number of institutions. It is hoped that reports such as this will stimulate the cooperative reviews required to provide a detailed analysis of the value of all the CHAT factors and combinations.

CONCLUSIONS

CHAT analysis and risk factor grading of patients following carotid endarterectomy have permitted an evaluation of the importance of standard risk factors in determining the probability of late stroke and survival following such surgery. The incidence of late stroke in the entire patient group, regardless of clinical presentation, was 3 percent at 5 years, by life table analysis. There were no significant differences related to clinical preoperative presentation. In asymptomatic patients with carotid stenosis, a previous history of contralateral stroke predicted a higher likelihood of late ipsilateral stroke. Higher risk factor states in asymptomatic patients predicted a greater likelihood of late stroke.

Specific risk factors and the total risk factor score did not predict late stroke after carotid endarterectomy, although they were powerful predictors of early death in every clinical subgroup analyzed. Logistic analysis indicated that few risk factors were important predictors of late stroke or early death and that these predictors were different for each clinical presentation subgroup. For asymptomatic patients, only diabetes predicted the likelihood of late stroke with a very high odds ratio (18:8). None of the risk factors predicted early death in asymptomatic patients.

REFERENCES

1. Bernstein EF, Browse NL: The CHAT classification of stroke. *Ann Surg.* 1989;209:242.
2. Hye RJ, Dilley RB, Browse NL, Bernstein EF: Evaluation of a new classification of cerebrovascular disease (CHAT). *Am J Surg.* 1987;154:104.
3. Baker JD, Rutherford RB, Bernstein EF, et al: Suggested standards for reports dealing with cerebrovascular disease. *J Vasc Surg.* 1988;8:721.
4. Wolf PA, Kannel WB, Verter J: Current status of risk factors for stroke. *Neurol Clin.* 1983;1:317.
5. Dyken ML, Wolf PA, Barnett HJM, et al: Risk factors in stroke. *Stroke.* 1984;15:1105.
6. Whisnant JP: Classification of cerebrovascular diseases. III. *Stroke.* 1990;21:637.
7. Whisnant JP, Wiebers DO: Clinical epidemiology of transient cerebral attacks (TIA) in the anterior and posterior cerebral circulation. In Sundt T, ed. *Occlusive Cerebrovascular Disease: Diagnosis and Surgical Management.* Philadelphia: WB Saunders; 1987:60.
8. Sacco RL, Foulkes MA, Mohr JP, et al: Determinants of early recurrence of cerebral infarction: The stroke data bank. *Stroke.* 1989;20:983.
9. Thomas M, Otis SW, Rush M, et al: Recurrent carotid artery stenosis following endarterectomy. *Ann Surg.* 1984;200:74.
10. Kaplan EC, Meier P: Non-parametric estimation from incomplete observations. *JASA.* 1958;55:457.
11. Gehan EA: A generalized Wilcoxon test for comparing arbitrary singly censored samples. *Biometrika.* 1965;52:203.
12. Dixon WJ, et al: Stepwise logistic regression. In *BMDP Statistical Software Manual,* Vol. 2. Berkeley: University of California Press; 1990.

CHAPTER 60

Risk of Operation as a Function of Indication: Retrospective Institution and Individual Surgeon Reviews

RICHARD F. KEMPCZINSKI

Carotid endarterectomy (CEA) is the most commonly performed, major, noncardiac, vascular operation in the United States. Despite a significant decline in the mid-1980s following the publication of several studies that were critical of the procedure and suggested that it was being overutilized and was associated with unacceptably high morbidity and mortality, there has been a resurgence of interest following publication of the results of the North American Symptomatic Carotid Endarterectomy Trial.[1] It has been estimated that more than 80,000 CEAs are now performed annually in the United States.[2] Widely divergent morbidity and mortality rates for the procedure have been published, ranging from a combined stroke and death rate under 5 percent to one in excess of 20 percent.[3] This chapter analyzes the results of recent large, retrospective reviews of CEA in an effort to establish the current risks of operation and to relate those risks to the indications for operation.

SELECTION OF REPORTS

The apparent morbidity of CEA can vary greatly, depending on which series from the medical literature one chooses to cite. As a broad generalization, articles from individual surgeons or institutions summarizing their own experience have usually reported the most favorable results; broad, multi-institutional studies in which there has been an independent, external review of the data have usually been more pessimistic. In order to try to arrive at the most balanced summary of current risks for CEA, we applied several benchmarks to the papers being considered for inclusion in this review. Since there have been significant improvements in anesthetic and perioperative medical management in the 40 years following the introduction of CEA, we limited our search to papers published within the last 10 years in the hope that these would more accurately represent the current state of the art. Furthermore, although it remains unproved that individual surgeons or referral centers with a lot of experience in CEA generally achieve superior results, this argument seems logical, so we tried to select papers reporting a large number of cases. But because the experience of individual surgeons or institutions can be subject to significant selection bias, reflecting referral patterns, the nature of local patient populations, or distinctly superior surgical skills, we tried to include large multi-institutional or regional experiences in the hope that these would be more broadly representative. Finally, whenever possible, we tried to focus on reports in which there was an external review of the actual medical records by individuals other than members of the operating team, in the belief that these were less likely to present a biased view of the outcome. None of the papers we chose satisfied all these requirements.

In 1984, Dyken and Pokras[4] used the National Hospital Discharge Survey to examine the results of CEA in patients admitted to short-stay, nonmilitary, non-Veterans Administration hospitals. They collected data on 82,000 CEAs performed in 1982. Although they did not review individual medical records and focused only on the risk of perioperative death, this report is the most broadly based analysis of the risk of mortality following CEA. Two years later, Fode and colleagues[5] published a retrospective, multicenter audit of CEAs performed in 46 different institutions. Although participation was initially solicited from members of the cerebrovascular section of the American Association of Neurologic Surgeons, participation was not limited to members of this group. Case material was included from vascular surgeons and general surgeons, but all correspondence was through neurosurgeons and neurologists. There was no preselection process, and the goal of this study was to achieve a broad-based view of the spectrum of CEA in North America. In general terms, this study found that the risk of stroke or death was statistically lower in larger institutions (greater than 700 beds) and for patients who were operated on for amaurosis fugax or for unspecified reasons. Patients who were monitored with electroencephalography during surgery had lower overall morbidity. Endarterectomy combined with coronary artery bypass or simultaneous bilateral endarterectomies also had a statistically higher incidence of stroke or death than unilateral procedures.

In 1986, Brott and associates[6] reported their findings following a review of all CEAs (750) performed in the Greater Cincinnati area from July 1983 through June 1984. The records of all patients undergoing this procedure in the 16 general medical surgical hospitals serving the area were personally reviewed by one of the authors. These records included physicians' notes, nurses' notes, anesthesia records, operative notes, angiograms, and other radiographic reports. This detailed, albeit retrospective, review of an entire community's annual experience with CEA is unique in the medical literature.

In 1988, Winslow and coworkers[7] performed a retrospective review of the complete medical records of 1302 Medicare patients at three geographically distinct sites to determine the results of and appropriateness of indications for CEA. Based on a list of 864 possible indications for CEA previously developed from a review of the medical literature, their panel of nine "nationally known experts in vascular surgery" determined that only 35 percent of the patients in this sample had undergone CEA for "appropriate" reasons. They also concluded that CEA appeared to be substantially overused in the areas they surveyed. Furthermore, in situations in which the complication rate was equal to or above the study's aggregate complication rate (9.8%), CEA was judged not to be warranted even in cases in which there was an appropriate indication, because the risk would almost certainly outweigh the benefits.

In order to determine whether CEA is indicated in the management of asymptomatic, hemodynamically significant carotid artery stenosis, the National Institutes of Health funded a prospective, randomized, multicenter clinical trial of surgical versus best medical therapy. In selecting surgeons for participation in this asymptomatic carotid atherosclerosis study, the executive committee agreed that the results of CEA depend on the competence of the surgeon as well as the quality of the institution in which he or she practices. Accordingly, in order to select individuals qualified to participate in this study, 48 centers around the country were asked to submit a one-page data sheet on the last 100 CEAs (total, 5641) they had performed.[8] It detailed patient history, indications for surgery, the degree of stenosis, and the associated morbidity and mortality rates. Once a center was accepted for participation in the study, each potential participating surgeon (total, 164) was asked to submit the details of his or her last 50 consecutive endarterectomies. On-site audits to verify these data were not performed. The database resulting from these submissions represents one of the largest series of CEAs reported to date.

In June 1993, Riles and colleagues[9] reported their 30-year experience with patients undergoing cerebrovascular surgery in the Division of Vascular Surgery at New York University Medical Center. The records of 3062 primary CEAs performed on 2365 patients from 1965 to 1991 were reviewed. This represents one of the largest, most carefully analyzed single-institution series in which morbidity and mortality are related to both indication for operation and the surgical technique employed. (Although perioperative mortality was not specified in the original report, this information was graciously provided by Dr. Riles in a personal communication.)

The studies represent a combined database representing more than 96,000 CEAs (Table 60–1). With one exception,[4] complications were segregated by indication, and the data satisfied most of the criteria we had established.

RESULTS

Overall Results

Table 60–1 summarizes the overall results for CEA, irrespective of indication. Analysis of more than 96,000 CEAs demonstrates an average perioperative mortality of 2.6 percent and a stroke rate of 2.9 percent. Since several of the studies did not distinguish between death from all causes and death due to stroke, the risk of ''death or stroke'' could not be computed. A modified meta-analysis of the data was used to combine the individual reports.

The risk of death ranged from 0.8 to 3.4 percent, and the

TABLE 60–2. Carotid Endarterectomy for Prior Stroke

Study*	CEA, n	Death, %	Stroke, %
McCullough et al[11]	533	5.8	4.7
Fode et al[5]	477	3.6	5.5
Brott et al[6]	370	2.4	6.5
Moore et al[8]	1096	1.6	1.9
Riles et al[9]	677	2.7	4.3
Meta-analysis	3153	2.9	4.0

*For full bibliographic information, see reference list at end of chapter.
CEA, carotid endarterectomy.

perioperative stroke rate was 1.5 to 6.4 percent. The best results were generally seen in reports from individual surgeons analyzing their own data. The worse results occurred in those series in which there was external review of the actual medical records.[7]

In all the studies, the diagnosis of postoperative stroke was based on clinical findings. However, in 1986, Berguer and associates[10] reported their experience with 100 consecutive carotid reconstructions in 91 patients who were prospectively studied with preoperative and postoperative computed tomographic (CT) brain scans. Following operation, 96 of those procedures appeared to be free of neurologic complications, but CT scans revealed new deficits in 8 of these patients. Furthermore, two patients experienced transient episodes of cerebral ischemia that quickly resolved, and both of these patients had new deficits on CT scan. Thus, 10 percent of patients who would have been judged clinically to have undergone complication-free carotid reconstructions had silent infarcts, as documented on CT scan. There is no reason to believe that a similar incidence of clinically unrecognized stroke did not occur in the retrospective series. Thus, one must assume that there is some additional, undetermined incidence of silent infarction that occurs during CEA and goes unrecognized.

Carotid Endarterectomy for Prior Stroke

In 1985, McCullough and coworkers[11] reviewed the reported experience with CEA after completed stroke. They also included their own personal experience with 59 additional operative cases. They concluded that patients with fixed, mild to moderate neurologic deficits due to carotid artery lesions were protected from recurring neurologic complications by CEA. Table 60–2 summarizes their data and compares it with similar subgroups of patients in the previously described retrospective series. Perioperative mortality for this indication did not differ significantly from the overall results of CEA (average, 2.9%). The risk of stroke, however, was significantly higher, averaging 4.0 percent (range, 1.9–6.5%).

Carotid Endarterectomy for Transient Ischemic Attack or Amaurosis Fugax

Table 60–3 reports the results of approximately 18,000 CEAs performed on symptomatic patients without clinical evidence of a fixed neurologic deficit. One of the largest retrospective reviews of CEA in such patients was reported

TABLE 60–1. Overall Results for Carotid Endarterectomy

Study*	CEA, n	Death, %	Stroke, %
Dyken & Pokras[4]	82,000	2.8	NA
Fode et al[5]	3328	2.0	4.0
Brott et al[6]	750	2.3	5.1
Winslow et al[7]	1302	3.4	6.4
Moore et al[8]	5641	0.8	1.5
Riles et al[9]	3062	1.3	2.2
Meta-analysis	96,083	2.6	2.9

*For full bibliographic information, see list of references at end of chapter.
CEA, carotid endarterectomy; NA, information not available.

TABLE 60–3. Carotid Endarterectomy for Transient Ischemic Attacks or Amaurosis Fugax

Study*	CEA, n	Death, %	Stroke, %
Fode et al[5]	1283	1.6	4.8
Nunn[12]	12,307	1.0	1.8
Moore et al[8]	3034	0.5	1.8
Riles et al[9]	1320	1.1	2.4
Meta-analysis	17,944	1.0	2.0

*For full bibliographic information, see reference list at end of chapter.
CEA, carotid endarterectomy.

by Nunn in 1988.[12] That author personally performed 651 CEAs in 605 patients in a community hospital over a 23-year period. In addition, the author summarized the morbidity and mortality rates previously reported in five large retrospective series comprising more than 12,000 CEAs performed for this indication. Overall, morbidity and mortality rates for the series reviewed were surprisingly low, especially considering the report of the patients who underwent routine CT scans prior to CEA.[10] Seventeen percent of "asymptomatic" patients and 19 percent of those with "transient" neurologic deficits were found to have ipsilateral infarcts on their preoperative CT scans. Thus, even if we assume that nearly 20 percent of the patients who underwent CEA for "transient cerebral ischemia" had cerebral infarcts, perioperative neurologic morbidity averaged only 2 percent, and the combined morbidity and mortality was only 3 percent.

Carotid Endarterectomy for Asymptomatic Stenosis or Ulcer

Asymptomatic stenosis or ulcer remains the most controversial indication for CEA. Norris and Zhu[13] compared CT scans and carotid duplex findings in 115 patients with asymptomatic carotid stenosis, 203 patients with transient ischemic attacks and carotid stenosis, and 63 patients with transient ischemic attacks without carotid stenosis. Cerebral infarcts ipsilateral to the carotid stenosis were found in 10 percent of patients with mild (35–50%) stenosis, 17 percent of those with moderate (50–75%) stenosis, and 30 percent of those with severe (>75%) stenosis. This difference was highly significant.

In 1992, Freischlag and colleagues[14] reviewed their experience with 141 CEAs performed on 123 asymptomatic patients with high-grade (>75%) carotid stenosis. Remarkably, there were no perioperative deaths and only two postoperative strokes. During a mean follow-up of 56.6 months, no patient suffered a stroke in the hemisphere ipsilateral to endarterectomy. This paper confirmed that in competent hands, well-selected patients can undergo prophylactic CEA with negligible morbidity and with significant reduction in late neurologic complications, especially when compared with the previous natural history data.[13] Table 60–4 summarizes the results of 2757 CEAs performed for asymptomatic stenosis. Average mortality was 1.4 percent, and neurologic morbidity was 1.6 percent, for a combined complication rate of 3.0 percent.

The issue of prophylactic endarterectomy for asymptomatic ulcerative lesions remains even less clear. In 1982,

Dixon and associates[15] reviewed the natural history of 153 asymptomatic, nonstenosing ulcerative lesions of the carotid bifurcation in 141 patients. Ulcers were classified as small (type A), large (type B), or compound (type C). During the course of study, which extended up to 10 years, 3 percent of patients with type A ulcers, 21 percent with type B, and 19 percent with type C had hemispheric strokes without antecedent transient ischemic attacks on the side appropriate to the lesion. The interval annual stroke rate was 4.5 percent for type B ulcers and 7.5 percent for type C ulcers. Based on their findings, the authors recommended prophylactic operation for such lesions in good-risk surgical candidates.

In contrast, Harward and colleagues[16] reported on 91 angiographically documented asymptomatic carotid artery ulcers in 79 patients. Mean follow-up was 54 months. Of the 90 ulcerative lesions for which follow-up was available, 64 were categorized as type A and 26 were categorized as type B. There were no patients in the series with compound type C ulcers, since it was the authors' policy to perform prophylactic CEA on such lesions. They confirmed a low 0.5 percent annual stroke rate for patients with type A ulcers, a finding that was essentially identical to the 0.9 percent annual stroke rate for similar lesions in the series by Dixon and coworkers.[15] However, in contrast to the 4.5 percent annual stroke rate for type B ulcers reported by those authors, Harward and associates found only a 0.5 percent annual stroke rate for type B ulcers—identical to the rate for type A ulcers. The authors concluded that asymptomatic type A and B ulcers carried an insignificant risk of stroke and did not warrant prophylactic endarterectomy. Thus, both groups agreed that patients with type C ulcers represented a high risk for ipsilateral stroke and should undergo prophylactic endarterectomy and that those with type A ulcers had a low risk and did not warrant surgical intervention. They differed on their management recommendations for type B, or moderate, ulcers.

Based on an earlier retrospective review of the medical literature, an ad hoc committee of the American Heart Association published recommendations for maximum allowable perioperative morbidity and mortality following CEA.[17] They stipulated that perioperative mortality, from all causes and for all indications, should not exceed 2 percent. When endarterectomy is performed for asymptomatic patients, a maximum complication rate of 3 percent is acceptable. For patients undergoing operation for transient cerebral ischemia, a complication rate of less than 5 percent is desirable. In the highest risk group of patients with previous mild to moderate

TABLE 60–4. Carotid Endarterectomy for Asymptomatic Carotid Artery Stenosis

Study*	CEA, n	Death, %	Stroke, %
Fode et al[5]	396	2.8	2.5
Brott et al[6]	380	2.1	3.7
Moore et al[8]	1511	0.8	0.9
Freischlag et al[14]	141	0.0	1.4
Riles et al[9]	329	2.1	1.5
Meta-analysis	2757	1.4	1.6

*For full bibliographic information, see reference list at end of chapter.
CEA, carotid endarterectomy.

cerebral infarction, a perioperative complication rate of 7 percent or less is permissible. Although these results do not represent the best that have been reported in the medical literature, they are realistic targets for the medical community at large.

CONCLUSIONS

Retrospective studies are of only limited value in determining the results of a specific surgical procedure because they often reflect significant bias in the selection of patients for surgery and the indications for treatment. Community-based studies, especially those in which there has been an objective, external review of the actual medical records, generally show results inferior to those from surgeons reviewing their own data. In general, the more serious the indications for surgery, the higher the neurologic morbidity. Surgical mortality, since it is dictated by the patient's general medical condition, remains relatively constant, ranging from 1.7 to 2.9 percent, and appears to be unaffected by indication. Accurate comparison of alternative forms of therapy for specific conditions generally comes from prospective, randomized, multicenter studies, several of which are currently under way for CEA.

REFERENCES

1. North American symptomatic carotid endarterectomy trial collaborators: Beneficial effect of carotid endarterectomy in symptomatic patients with high-grade stenosis. *N Engl J Med.* 1991;325:445.
2. Pokras R, Dyken ML: Dramatic changes in the performance of endarterectomy for disease of the extracranial arteries of the head. *Stroke.* 1988;19:1289.
3. Easton JD, Sherman DG: Stroke and mortality rate in carotid endarterectomy: 228 consecutive operations. *Stroke.* 1977;8:565.
4. Dyken ML, Pokras R: The performance of endarterectomy for disease of the extracranial arteries of the head. *Stroke.* 1984;15:948.
5. Fode NC, Sundt TM, Robertson JT, et al: Multicenter retrospective review of results and complications of carotid endarterectomy in 1981. *Stroke.* 1986;17:370.
6. Brott TG, Labutta RJ, Kempczinski RF: Changing patterns in the practice of carotid endarterectomy in a large metropolitan area. *JAMA.* 1986;255:2609.
7. Winslow CM, Solomon DH, Chassin MR, et al: The appropriateness of carotid endarterectomy. *N Engl J Med.* 1988;318:721.
8. Moore WS, Vescera CL, Robertson JT, et al: Selection process for surgeons in the asymptomatic carotid atherosclerosis study. *Stroke.* 1991;22:1353.
9. Riles TS, Imparato AM, Jacobowitz GR, et al: The cause of perioperative stroke after carotid endarterectomy. *J Vasc Surg.* 1994;19:206.
10. Berguer R, Sieggreen MY, Lazo A, et al: The silent brain infarct in carotid surgery. *J Vasc Surg.* 1986;3:442.
11. McCullough JL, Mentzer RM, Harman PK, et al: Carotid endarterectomy after a completed stroke: Reduction in long-term neurologic deterioration. *J Vasc Surg.* 1985;2:7.
12. Nunn DB: Carotid endarterectomy in patients with territorial transient ischemic attacks. *J Vasc Surg.* 1988;8:447.
13. Norris JW, Zhu CZ: Silent stroke and carotid stenosis. *Stroke.* 1992;23:483.
14. Freischlag JA, Hanna D, Moore WS: Improved prognosis for asymptomatic carotid stenosis with prophylactic carotid endarterectomy. *Stroke.* 1992;23:479.
15. Dixon S, Pais O, Raviola C, et al: Natural history of nonstenotic, asymptomatic ulcerative lesions of the carotid artery. *Arch Surg.* 1982;117:1493.
16. Harward TRS, Kroener JM, Wickbom IG, et al: Natural history of asymptomatic ulcerative plaques of the carotid bifurcation. *Am J Surg.* 1983;146:208.
17. Beebe HG, Clagett GP, DeWeese JA, et al: Assessing risk associated with carotid endarterectomy: A statement for health professionals by an ad hoc committee on carotid surgery standards of the Stroke Council, American Heart Association. *Stroke.* 1988;20:314.

CHAPTER 61

Risk of Carotid Endarterectomy Based on Community Audit

MARGARET O'DONOGHUE, JOSEPH P. BRODERICK, and THOMAS BROTT

For years, the appropriateness of surgery for carotid artery stenosis has been debated. Central to this debate are estimates of the risk of operative complications. Numerous community-based studies have been performed in an effort to quantify the risk of carotid endarterectomy (CEA). This chapter reviews selected population-based, referral-based, and institutional studies of carotid surgery.

POPULATION-BASED STUDIES

Population-based studies of surgery have the advantage of being free from the performance bias of more selective series. Consequently, they may give the most accurate assessment of overall risk. Table 61–1 lists the complication rates for CEA from several population-based studies.

Brott and Thalinger[1] reviewed all the CEAs performed at the 16 general hospitals in Greater Cincinnati during 1980. The combined perioperative morbidity and mortality rate in their series was 9 percent. The study was repeated by Brott and coworkers[2] for all CEAs performed from July 1983 through June 1984. There was a 74 percent increase in the total number of CEAs performed in metropolitan Cincinnati and a decrease in the morbidity and mortality rate to 6 percent. Kirshner and associates[3] did a similar retrospective review of all CEAs in the six acute-care hospitals of Rochester, New York, in 1984 and 1985. Their stroke rate was comparable to that reported by Brott, but their combined morbidity and mortality rate was slightly lower at 4.8 percent. Over a 20-month period in 1986–1987, Burns and Willoughby[4] prospectively studied all CEAs performed in public and private hospitals in south Australia. Their mortality rate of 1.3 percent was also lower than that in the Cincinnati studies, but their higher stroke rate resulted in an almost identical perioperative morbidity and mortality rate of 5.9 percent.

Two studies used Medicare records to calculate complication rates of carotid surgery. Richardson and Main[5] investigated all CEAs performed on Medicare patients in the commonwealth of Kentucky in 1983. They found a lower stroke rate (3.8%) but a higher mortality rate (3.1%); the combined rate of permanent neurologic deficit or death was 5.1 percent. They also performed a concurrent study for the first 6 months of 1984. The stroke and death rates both fell, giving a combined morbidity and mortality rate of 4.3 percent. The authors believed that knowledge of the ongoing study may have altered practice patterns, contributing to the improved outcome. Fisher and colleagues[6] also did a retrospective review of Medicare files. Their study looked only at mortality rates for Medicare patients undergoing CEA in New England from April 1984 through June 1985. They found a perioperative death rate of 2.5 percent, nearly the same as that found in the Cincinnati studies.

Finally, Dyken and Pokras[7] attempted to collect data for a study of CEAs in the entire United States between 1971 and 1982. They used the National Hospital Discharge Survey to sample nonfederal hospitals and subsets of those hospitals' discharge records. Data from military and Veterans Administration hospitals were added. The number of procedures performed increased by more than fivefold between 1971 and 1982. The average mortality rate over the 12-year period was 2.8 percent, consistent with the rates in the aforementioned studies.

Several of these population-based studies sought to relate risk to the indication for surgery. Table 61–2 shows that among the four studies with data separated by indication, the proportion of patients in each group is relatively similar. The risk of nonfatal stroke for each study is illustrated in Figure 61–1. In general, the risk of stroke appears to be greater for patients with symptoms referable to the stenosed carotid artery than for those without symptoms. In some studies, the difference in stroke rates between symptomatic and asymptomatic patients was greater than in others. Differences among the studies also exist with respect to estimates of mortality rate by indication (Fig. 61–2). Kirshner and coworkers[3] found no difference in risk between asymptomatic and symptomatic patients; Burns and Willoughby[4] and Richardson and Main[5] reported increased mortality in the symptomatic group.

TABLE 61–1. Complication Rates for Carotid Endarterectomy: Population-Based Studies

Study*	Year	Population	Patients, n	CEAs, n	TIA, %	Nonfatal Stroke, %	Fatal Stroke, %	Death, %	Disabled or Dead, %
Brott & Thalinger[1]	1930	Cincinnati, OH	371	431	4.0	7.0	1.6	2.8	9.0
Brott et al[2]	1983–1984	Cincinnati, OH	656	750	2.9	4.3	0.8	2.3	6.0
Kirshner et al[3]	1984–1985	Rochester, NY	1035	1035	NA	5.8	0.9	1.4	4.8
Burns & Willoughby[4]	1986–1987	S. Australia	223	239	3.8	6.3	1.3	1.3	5.9
Richardson & Main[5]	1983	Kentucky†	705	738	2.8	3.8	1.2	3.1	5.1
Fisher et al[6]	1984–1985	New England†	2089	NA	NA	NA	NA	2.5	NA
Dyken & Pokras[7]	1971–1982	USA	>500,000	>500,000	NA	NA	NA	2.8	NA

*For full bibliographic information, see reference list at end of chapter.
†Medicare patients only.
CEA, carotid endarterectomy; NA, data not available; TIA, transient ischemic attack.

TABLE 61-2. Indications for Carotid Endarterectomy: Population-Based Studies

Study*	TIA, %	Stroke, %†	Asymptomatic, %‡	Nonipsilateral Symptoms, %§
Brott and Thalinger[1]	32.7	17.2	30.1	20.0
Brott et al[2]	32.5	16.5	30.1	20.8
Kirshner et al[3]	46.3	13.7	21.4	18.6
Burns and Willoughby[4]	36.8	17.6	24.3	19.2

*For full bibliographic information, see reference list at end of chapter.
†Includes events classified as reversible ischemic neurologic deficits.
‡Includes patients with and without bruits.
§Includes patients with contralateral symptoms, posterior circulation symptoms, and generalized complaints.
TIA, transient ischemic attack.

REFERRAL-BASED STUDIES

There are numerous non-population-based series of CEAs in the literature. Table 61–3 lists selected recent series involving two or more hospitals. Series from single institutions will be considered separately.

As might be expected, there is considerably more variation in complication rates among the referral-based studies than among the population-based studies. Easton and Sherman's study[8] was a retrospective review of CEAs at two community hospitals in Springfield, Illinois. The study by Modi and associates[9] analyzed CEAs performed at the same two hospitals for the 6 years following the period covered by Easton and Sherman. There is a striking difference between the two studies with regard to morbidity and mortality rates. Modi attributed this difference to possible improvements in "patient selection, radiologic service, and peri-operative management." Modi's group reported only "major" strokes. Even so, when only those strokes causing permanent deficits are considered in Easton and Sherman's study, this still results in a morbidity rate of 9.6 percent.

The university-based studies of the Toronto Cerebrovascular Study Group[10] and Healy and coworkers[11] of the University of Washington reported complication rates fairly similar to those of Modi and associates. The mortality rate in Healy's series, however, was particularly low. Both Hertzer and coworkers[12] and Rubin and colleagues[13] reviewed the computer registry of the Cleveland Vascular Society to compile data on CEAs performed by its members at a variety of hospitals. Fode and associates'[14] study involved the recruitment of many medical centers of different types. The individual centers contributed data by providing retrospectively collected information about their cases on statistical forms. There are similarities between this study and that of Hertzer. Both studies involved voluntary participation by surgeons: the Cleveland studies focused on vascular surgeons voluntarily enrolled in the Cleveland Vascular Society, and the study by Fode involved voluntary participation, predominantly by neurosurgeons.

In general, these more selective studies have lower morbidity and mortality figures than the population-based studies. Like the population-based studies, several of the referral-based studies separated complication rates by the indication for surgery (Figs. 61–3 and 61–4). Unlike the population-based studies (see Fig. 61–1), the referral-based studies fail to show any consistent trend toward higher stroke rates in symptomatic patients than in asymptomatic patients. The same can be said for mortality rates (see Figs. 61–2 and 61–4).

The CASANOVA study,[15] which is included in Figures 61–3 and 61–4, differs from the other studies in several ways. First, it consists of *only* asymptomatic patients. Second, it excluded any patient with less than 50 percent or greater than 90 percent stenosis. Finally, it was a randomized, prospective study of surgery performed at 10 medical centers in Europe. Of the 204 patients assigned to no surgery or unilateral surgery for bilateral disease, 118 underwent CEA. The morbidity and mortality figures for the surgical group in this series are similar to the rates for asymptomatic patients in most of the other referral-based studies.

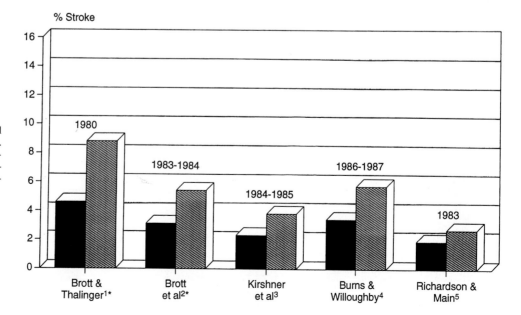

FIGURE 61–1. Risk of nonfatal stroke: population-based studies. Solid block, asymptomatic presentation; shaded block, symptomatic presentation. *Asymptomatic group includes nonhemispheric strokes.

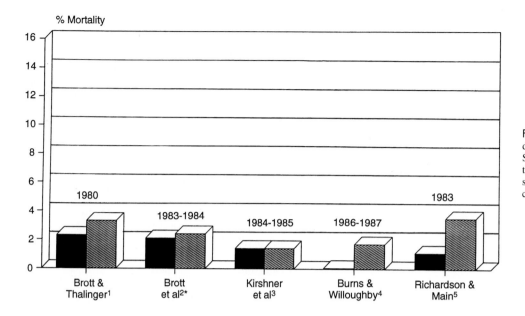

FIGURE 61–2. Mortality rate by indication: population-based studies. Solid block, asymptomatic presentation; shaded block, symptomatic presentation. *Asymptomatic group includes nonhemispheric strokes.

TABLE 61–3. Complication Rates for Carotid Endarterectomy: Referral-Based Studies

Study*	Year	Hospitals, n	Setting	Nonfatal Stroke (%)	Death (%)	Disability or Death (%)
Easton and Sherman[8]	1970–1976	2	Community	14.5	6.6	16.2
Modi et al[9]	1976–1982	2	Same as Easton	2.5†	1.9	4.2
Toronto[10]	1982	5	University affiliated	3.6	1.4	5.0
Healy et al[11]	1980–1987	2	University affiliated	3.0	0.5	3.0
Hertzer et al[12]	1978–1981	20 +	Mixed	2.5	1.2	3.8
Rubin et al[13]	1973–1985	44	Same as Hertzer	1.3	1.6	2.7
Fode et al[14]	1981	46	Multicenter	4.2	1.2	3.9

*For full bibliographic information, see reference list at end of chapter.
†Major strokes only.

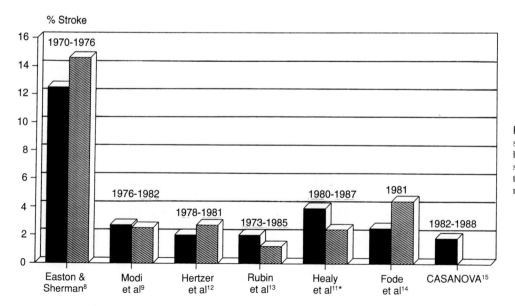

FIGURE 61–3. Risk of nonfatal stroke: referral-based studies. Solid block, asymptomatic presentation; shaded block, symptomatic presentation. *Asymptomatic group includes nonhemispheric strokes.

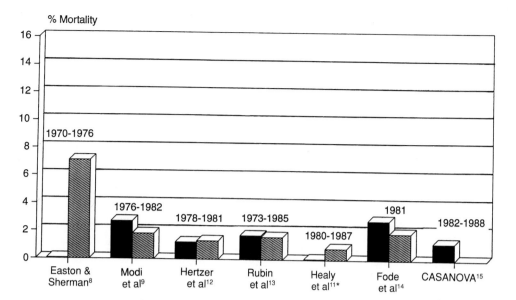

FIGURE 61–4. Mortality rate by indication: referral-based studies. Solid block, asymptomatic presentation; shaded block, symptomatic presentation. *Asymptomatic group includes nonhemispheric strokes.

INSTITUTION-BASED STUDIES

Table 61–4 lists examples of studies of CEA performed at a single hospital.[16–26] Except for three studies,[17, 21, 22] all the institution-based studies report a lower incidence of nonfatal stroke than in the population-based studies. Three of the studies from single hospitals had no deaths,[18, 22, 26] but the mortality rates otherwise overlapped those from the population-based studies. It is possible that the smaller number of cases in institutional series accounts for the zero mortality rate in the aforementioned reports. Comparing the single hospital studies with the referral-based studies demonstrates significant overlap in both morbidity and mortality rates (excluding the study by Easton and Sherman,[8] which has much higher rates than any other study in either group).

Figures 61–5 and 61–6 illustrate those studies with stroke and death rates broken down by indication. Deruty and colleagues[23] and Mattos and associates[25] showed the same increase in risk for those with symptomatic disease as in the population-based studies, but the DeBord study[24] did not. Analyses of the risk of death by indication are variable, as in both the population- and referral-based studies. The studies by the Friedmann,[19] Thompson,[16] and Mattos[25] groups found higher risks in symptomatic patients than in asymptomatic patients, but the Ruvolo,[18] Deruty,[23] and DeBord[24] groups found the rates to be exactly the same for both groups. Turner and coworkers[27] studied only symptomatic patients at a Veterans Administration hospital and found a stroke rate of 4.9 percent and a mortality rate of 2.1 percent—higher than in any of the other hospital-based studies.

OTHER RISK FACTORS

Many of the studies discussed in the preceding sections have looked at factors other than the indication for surgery as potential markers or causes of increased risk in patients

TABLE 61–4. Complication Rates for Carotid Endarterectomy: Institutional Studies

Study*	Year	Hospital Type	CEAs, n	Nonfatal Stroke, %	Death, %	Disability or Death, %
Thompson et al[16]	1957–1977	University	1022	NA	2.1	NA
Slavish et al[17]	1977–1982	Community	743	5.2	2.7	4.4
Ruvolo et al[18]	1977–1985	Community	100	1.0	0.0	0.0
Friedmann et al[19]	1971–1988	Community	688	3.8	1.0	3.2
Maxwell et al[20]	1979–1988	Community	810	1.5	2.7	4.2
Salenius et al[21]	1965–1984	University	331	5.7	3.9	9.7
Asaph et al[22]	1986–1987	Community	243	4.9	2.5	7.4
	1988–1990	Community	148	4.0	0.0	4.0
Deruty et al[23]†	1978–1989	University	260	2.0	3.0	5.0
DeBord et al[24]	1985–1989	Community	324	1.5	1.5	2.8
Mattos et al[25]	1976–1991	University	544	2.9	1.3	4.2
Krupski et al[26]	1980–1983	University	100	2.0	0.0	2.0
		Community	100	2.0	1.0	2.0
			100	1.0	1.0	2.0

*For full bibliographic information, see reference list at end of chapter.
†Operative complications were assessed at 6 months.
CEA, carotid endarterectomy; NA, data not available.

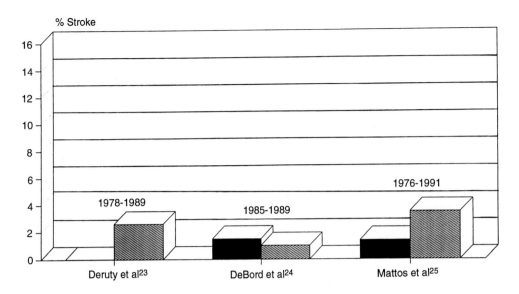

% Stroke

FIGURE 61–5. Risk of nonfatal stroke: institutional studies. Solid block, asymptomatic presentation; shaded block, symptomatic presentation.

undergoing CEA. Patient characteristics were analyzed in several studies. Brott and Thalinger,[1] Kirshner and associates,[3] Easton and Sherman,[8] and Maxwell and colleagues[20] found no significant increase in complications with age. Fisher and coworkers[6] and Salenius and associates,[21] however, reported worse outcomes in the elderly. In the Fisher group's series,[6] there was a progressive increase in the operative mortality with age: from a rate of 1.1 percent in patients aged 65 to 69 to 4.7 percent in those over 80 years old. Salenius and coworkers[21] found that the mean age of patients with complications was significantly higher than the age of those without complications (62.1 vs. 57.8 years old). They also noted that none of the 52 patients under 50 years of age had any complications. Kirshner and associates[3] found that women had a higher stroke rate, and Maxwell and colleagues[20] stated that in patients under age 75, women had an increased risk of stroke or death. The Salenius group[21] found that pre-existing adult-onset diabetes mellitus or hypertension had no effect on outcome, whereas the Kirshner study[3] reported a higher stroke rate for patients with hypertension;

it also found that a history of prior myocardial infarction was associated with a worse outcome. Rihal and coworkers[28] found that overt coronary artery disease did not affect perioperative outcome but was associated with late morbidity and mortality. Both Kirshner[3] and Salenius[21] found that patients with contralateral carotid artery stenosis or occlusion suffered more strokes, whereas Mattos[25] and Mackey and colleagues[29] saw no effect on contralateral occlusion on perioperative outcome. The study by Mackey's group also found no late effects. Perhaps confounding these results is the fact that the group with contralateral occlusions contained more asymptomatic patients.

Many studies have assessed risk in terms of characteristics of the surgeon or hospital involved. Most studies found no relationship between the number of CEAs performed by a given surgeon and that surgeon's complication rate.[1, 3, 4, 8, 12, 17, 19, 20, 22] Richardson and Main[5] reported a "nonlinear" increase in complication rates for surgeons performing few CEAs per year. The study by Rubin and colleagues[13] of CEAs performed by members of the Cleveland Vascular

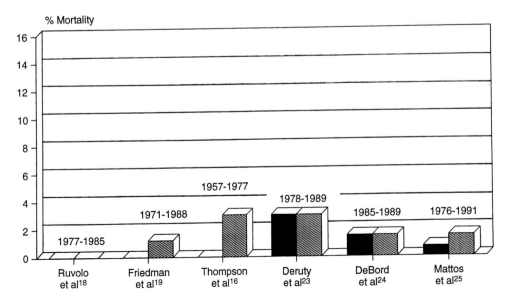

% Mortality

FIGURE 61–6. Mortality rates by indication: institutional studies. Solid block, asymptomatic presentation; shaded block, symptomatic presentation.

Society, unlike the prior report by Hertzer and colleagues,[12] describes an increased incidence of perioperative stroke for surgeons who perform fewer than 15 CEAs per year as compared with those performing the surgery more often (3.4% vs. 1.5–1.9%). Another potential outcome variable—the specialty of the surgeon—also seems to have little identifiable effect on outcome. Kempczinski and associates[30] found no significant difference in complication rates between vascular, general, cardiac, or neurosurgeons. Friedmann and coworkers[19] found no difference between vascular and neurosurgeons; similar results were noted by Asaph and colleagues.[22] In terms of the influence of specialty training and experience, Rubin's group[13] found that having done a fellowship in vascular surgery did not alter a surgeon's complication rate. In the study by Brott and Thalinger,[1] 29 CEAs were performed by surgical house officers; there were no major strokes and no deaths.

Krupski and coworkers[26] compared 100 surgeries at each of three hospital settings: a university hospital, private community hospitals, and a Veterans Administration (VA) hospital (see Table 61–3). The complication rates were equally low in all three. CEAs at the VA hospital were performed by residents in surgery, with the supervision of senior staff. Although CEAs took an average of 1 hour longer overall, and resulted in 10 minutes' longer ischemia time at the VA hospital, there was no increase in the rate of morbidity or mortality. Other groups have looked at risk as a function of the hospital size. Results of these analyses have been variable: no effect based on hospital size,[3, 12] a higher mortality rate in hospitals performing fewer surgeries per year,[6] and a decreased morbidity and mortality rate for hospitals with more than 700 beds.[14]

Perhaps there is something about the surgical procedure itself that influences the outcome. Some studies have found that whether a shunt is used as part of the procedure has no bearing on the risk for surgical complications.[1, 8] Maxwell and colleagues[20] found that those patients who were selectively shunted because they developed neurologic deficits when the carotid artery was clamped had an increased risk of stroke or death. This, however, is likely a reflection of the importance of collateral circulation rather than an effect of the surgical technique. Some have suggested that a second CEA carries more risk than the first,[21] but others have not found this to be the case.[20] Fode and associates[14] found that combining CEA with coronary artery bypass surgery or performing simultaneous bilateral CEAs resulted in a higher complication rate, a finding consistent with that of Brott and Thalinger.[1] In their study, combined CEA–coronary artery bypass graft surgery resulted in death in 4 of 17 patients.

The use of aspirin seems to be one factor in reducing the risk of perioperative complications. Salenius and coworkers[21] associated both aspirin and intraoperative heparin with reduced risk of complication. The Mayo Asymptomatic Carotid Endarterectomy Study[31] had to be terminated early because of the high prevalence of myocardial infarction in the surgical group. The use of aspirin had been discouraged in the surgical group, and the nonuse of aspirin correlated significantly with the perioperative occurrence of myocardial infarction.

Finally, Ruvolo and colleagues[18] suggest that the rate of complications reported in a series of CEAs may be higher if a neurologist, rather than a surgeon, is the author.

COMMUNITY-BASED STUDIES OF CEA IN PERSPECTIVE

The operative risk estimates from community-based studies of CEA can be clinically applied only in light of the estimated benefit of the surgery. Some authors have attempted to define the natural history of asymptomatic disease and found an annual ipsilateral stroke rate of 1.2 to 2.5 percent.[32, 33] This relatively low rate of stroke has caused these authors to be skeptical about the benefit of CEA in asymptomatic patients. A high mortality rate was noted but was related mostly to cardiovascular rather than cerebrovascular disease. Turner and coworkers[27] followed patients with symptomatic carotid stenosis who had undergone CEA at a VA hospital and found that after 8 years, less than 50% of the patients were alive and stroke free.

Fortunately, several prospective trials have become available to settle the question of risk versus benefit for CEA. The North American Symptomatic Carotid Endarterectomy Trial (NASCET),[34] the European Carotid Surgery Trial,[35] and the Veterans Affairs Cooperative Study[36] all demonstrate that, at least for symptomatic carotid stenoses of 70 percent or greater, the benefits of CEA outweigh the risks. For stenoses of 0 to 29 percent, the European trial showed that surgery is not beneficial. The Veterans Affairs study group also published a prospective study of CEA in asymptomatic patients.[37] The high cardiovascular mortality rate in patients randomized to either medical treatment or medical treatment

TABLE 61–5. Complication Rates for Carotid Endarterectomy: Community-Based vs. Prospective Studies

Study*	CEAs, n	Nonfatal Stroke (%)	Death (%)	Death or Disability (%)
NASCET[34]	328	5.2	0.6	2.1
European[35]	657	5.6	1.1	3.2
Veterans (symptomatic)[36]	92	3.3	3.3	4.3
Veterans (asymptomatic)[37]	211	3.8	1.9	4.7
Population-based*	3193	5.2	2.2	5.9
Referral-based†	13,123	2.7	1.8	3.9
Institutional‡	5513	2.6	1.6	3.8

*For full bibliographic information, see reference list at end of chapter.
†Average of results from all population-based studies in Table 61–1 with pertinent data available.[1–5]
‡Average of results from all referral-based studies in Table 61–3.[8–11, 13, 14] Hertzer et al[12] is excluded to prevent overlap with Rubin et al.[13]
§Average of results from all institutional studies in Table 61–4 with pertinent data available.[17–26]

plus surgery resulted in a similar combined stroke and death rate for both groups. There was a lower incidence of neurologic events (transient ischemic attack, amaurosis fugax, and stroke) in the surgical group, but it was estimated that a much larger study population would have been required to demonstrate a significant benefit from surgery. It is hoped that more information on the benefit of surgery in asymptomatic patients will become available shortly as the results of other prospective trials are published.

Table 61–5 compares the operative risks of four prospective trials with the risks found in community-based studies. The death and disability rates in the prospective studies are lower than in the population-based studies but comparable to the referral-based and institutional studies. These differences are significant when attempting to extrapolate the results of prospective trials, conducted at selected medical centers, to the much wider range of community medical centers. Accordingly, it may be appropriate to design additional population-based studies of CEA to examine the practical application of the favorable surgical results from the NASCET, European, and VA studies.

REFERENCES

1. Brott T, Thalinger K: The practice of carotid endarterectomy in a large metropolitan area. Stroke. 1984;15:950.
2. Brott TG, Labutta RJ, Kempczinski RF: Changing patterns in the practice of carotid endarterectomy in a large metropolitan area. JAMA. 1986;255:2609.
3. Kirshner DL, O'Brien MS, Ricotta JJ: Risk factors in a community experience with carotid endarterectomy. J Vasc Surg. 1989;10:178.
4. Burns RJ, Willoughby JO: South Australian carotid endarterectomy study. Med J Aust. 1991;154:650.
5. Richardson JD, Main KA: Carotid endarterectomy in the elderly population: A statewide experience. J Vasc Surg. 1989;9:65.
6. Fisher ES, Malenka DJ, Solomon NA, et al: Risk of carotid endarterectomy in the elderly. Am J Public Health. 1989;79:1617.
7. Dyken ML, Pokras R: The performance of endarterectomy for disease of the extracranial arteries of the head. Stroke. 1984;15:948.
8. Easton JD, Sherman DG: Stroke and mortality rate in carotid endarterectomy: 228 consecutive operations. Stroke. 1977;8:565.
9. Modi JR, Finch WT, Sumner DS: Update of carotid endarterectomy in two community hospitals: Springfield revisited. Stroke. 1983;14:128. Abstract.
10. Toronto cerebrovascular study group: Risks of carotid endarterectomy. Stroke. 1986;17:848.
11. Healy DA, Clowes AW, Zerler RE, et al: Immediate and long-term results of carotid endarterectomy. Stroke. 1989;20:1138.
12. Hertzer NR, Avellone JC, Farrell CJ, et al: The risk of vascular surgery in a metropolitan community. J Vasc Surg. 1984;1:13.
13. Rubin JR, Pitluk HC, King TA, et al: Carotid endarterectomy in a metropolitan community: The early results after 8535 operations. J Vasc Surg. 1988;7:256.
14. Fode NC, Sundt TM, Robertson JT, et al: Multicenter retrospective review of results and complications of carotid endarterectomy in 1981. Stroke. 1986;17:370.
15. CASANOVA study group: Carotid surgery versus medical therapy in asymptomatic carotid stenosis. Stroke. 1991;22:1229.
16. Thompson JE, Patman RD, Talkington CM: Asymptomatic carotid bruit: Long term outcome of patients having endarterectomy compared with unoperated controls. Ann Surg. 1978;188:308.
17. Slavish LG, Nicholas GG, Gee W: Review of a community hospital experience with carotid endarterectomy. Stroke. 1984;15:956.
18. Ruvolo L, Holada W, Brait K: Carotid endarterectomy in a nonteaching community hospital. N J Med. 1987;84:431.
19. Friedmann P, Garb JL, Berman J, et al: Carotid endarterectomy: Clinical results in a community-based teaching hospital. Stroke. 1988;19:1323.
20. Maxwell JG, Rutherford EJ, Covington DL, et al: Community hospital carotid endarterectomy in patients over age 75. Am J Surg. 1990;160:598.
21. Salenius J-P, Harju E, Riekkinen H: Early cerebral complications in carotid endarterectomy: Risk factors. J Cardiovasc Surg. 1990;31:162.
22. Asaph JW, Janoff K, Wayson K, et al: Carotid endarterectomy in a community hospital: A change in physicians' practice patterns. Am J Surg. 1991;161:616.
23. Deruty R, Mottolese C, Pelissou-Guyotat I, Lapras C: The carotid endarterectomy: Experience with 260 cases and discussion of the indications. Acta Neurochir (Wien). 1991;112:1.
24. DeBord JR, Marshall WH, Wyffels PL, et al: Carotid endarterectomy in a community hospital surgery practice. Am Surg. 1991;57:627.
25. Mattos MA, Barkmeier LD, Hodgson KJ, et al: Internal carotid artery occlusion: Operative risks and long-term stroke rates after contralateral carotid endarterectomy. Surgery. 1992;112:670.
26. Krupski WC, Effeney DJ, Goldstone J, et al: Carotid endarterectomy in a metropolitan community: Comparison of results from three institutions. Surgery. 1985;98:492.
27. Turner DA, Tracy J, Haines SJ: Risk of late stroke and survival following carotid endarterectomy procedures for symptomatic patients. J Neurosurg. 1990;73:193.
28. Rihal CS, Gersh BJ, Whisnant JP, et al: Influence of coronary heart disease on morbidity and mortality after carotid endarterectomy: A population-based study in Olmsted County, Minnesota (1970–1988). J Am Coll Cardiol. 1992;19:1254.
29. Mackey WC, O'Donnell TF, Callow AD: Carotid endarterectomy contralateral to an occluded carotid artery: Peri-operative risk and late results. J Vasc Surg. 1990;11:778.
30. Kempczinski RF, Brott TG, Labutta RJ: The influence of surgical specialty and caseload on the results of carotid endarterectomy. J Vasc Surg. 1986;3:911.
31. Mayo asymptomatic carotid endarterectomy study group: Results of a randomized controlled trial of carotid endarterectomy for asymptomatic carotid stenosis. Mayo Clin Proc. 1992;67:513.
32. Hennerici M, Hülsbömer H-B, Hefter H, et al: Natural history of asymptomatic extracranial arterial disease. Brain. 1987;110:777.
33. Norris JW, Zhu CZ, Bornstein NM, Chambers BR: Vascular risks of asymptomatic carotid stenosis. Stroke. 1991;22:1485.
34. North American symptomatic carotid endarterectomy trial collaborators: Beneficial effect of carotid endarterectomy in symptomatic patients with high-grade carotid stenosis. N Engl J Med. 1991;325:445.
35. European carotid surgery trialists' collaborative group: MRC European carotid surgery trial: Interim results for symptomatic patients with severe (70–99%) or with mild (0–29%) carotid stenosis. Lancet. 1991;337:1235.
36. Mayberg MR, Wilson SE, Yatsu F, et al: Carotid endarterectomy and prevention of cerebral ischemia in symptomatic carotid stenosis. JAMA. 1991;266:3289.
37. Hobson RW II, Weiss DG, Fields WS, et al: Efficacy of carotid endarterectomy for asymptomatic carotid stenosis. N Engl J Med. 1993;328:221.

CHAPTER
62

Upper Limit of Risk for Performance of Carotid Endarterectomy: Position Statement of the Stroke Council of the American Heart Association

HUGH G. BEEBE

In 1989, an Ad Hoc Committee of the Stroke Council of The American Heart Association (AHA) published a position paper on morbidity and mortality limits for carotid endarterectomy. This chapter examines briefly the rationale, major difficulties encountered, and results of the process that led to that publication.

The contextual background of the development of these guidelines deserves some mention because it influenced the publication, and because our perception of carotid endarterectomy is already different from that held only 6 years ago.

RATIONALE

In 1986, the need for a dialogue between the neurology and surgical communities was expressed from a grassroots level to the Chairman of the Stroke Council, AHA. The concern emanated from widely disparate reports of short-term results of carotid surgery published separately by neurologic and surgical groups and the expression of concern that surgical prophylaxis of stroke was unproved and too widely applied, and inflicted stroke as an operative complication in too many cases.[1]

Surgeons working in centers with institutional commitment to cerebrovascular disease and low morbidity from carotid endarterectomy were concerned that the reputation of an effective treatment to prevent stroke in properly selected cases would be damaged through misapplication of the procedure.

Thus, from the outset, the intent of a position paper on morbidity and mortality limits was to protect carotid endarterectomy during the interval when the randomized trials, subsequently reported or nearing completion, were underway. Furthermore, as an adjunct to expressing an opinion about morbidity and mortality limits, a stimulus could be provided to audit the results of carotid surgery for comparison with such limits.

In preparing the statement, something that appears to be unique was also being attempted: an interdisciplinary multispecialty group with the imprimatur of an authoritative body was to establish a boundary beyond which results were declared unacceptable. The goal, distinct from that of many reports already in the literature describing excellent results, was to show which results required remedial action.

AREAS OF CONTROVERSY

The principal issues that required resolution were the following:

1. A definition of morbidity. It was initially expanded to include cardiac events, cranial nerve injury, and postopera-

tive transient ischemia symptoms, but during draft revisions was condensed finally to include only stroke.

2. What to do with many unusual and smaller categories of patients who cannot be classified as being asymptomatic or having TIAs or prior stroke. Symptoms and characteristics of these patients include progressive stroke, unstable neurologic symptoms, vertebrobasilar insufficiency, global ischemia, and diseases such as fibromuscular dysplasia or aneurysm. Eventually simplicity prevailed, and focus was limited to the large majority of patients who fit common clinical categories.

3. The actual percentage values of the limits. This issue required a continuing dialogue among participants over several months before consensus was achieved.

4. Whether a position statement had the appearance of an endorsement of carotid endarterectomy when not all authorities agreed that convincing data were available to support the use of the procedure. A disclaimer was incorporated into the statement.

5. The language describing morbidity and mortality levels as "acceptable limits" or "unacceptable limits." The issue appeared subtle but was in fact of major importance. Eventually, language was adopted that suggested that data were insufficient to be able to define "acceptable" limits. The emphasis was turned to stating a limit beyond which results clearly were not acceptable.

Other concerns surfaced during the ongoing discussion, one of which was the legal implication of declaring unacceptable limits. This was resolved by legal review and by placing emphasis on the individual hospital's responsibility to take action in the case of a deviation from standards.

One of the most vexing difficulties was how to establish audit criteria that would apply with equal fairness to established surgeons with a large, long-term experience and to those with a much smaller caseload volume, such as a surgeon beginning practice. Biostatistical consultation revealed the problem (Table 62–1).

TABLE 62–1. Difference Between Long-Term and Short-Term Experience as It Affects Statistical Analysis

Morbidity Event Incidence, %	Cases Required for Statistical Significance, n	
	$\alpha = 0.5$ $\beta = 0.1$	$\alpha = 0.5$ $\beta = 0.2$
1.5 vs 10	153	115
1 vs 4	564	424
2.5 vs 5	1208	909
3 vs 5	2010	1513
5 vs 8	1413	1063

479

Based on the average practicing surgeon's volume of carotid endarterectomy cases, too many years of experience would be required for the analysis to be meaningful. Instead, a moving average of results of the last 100 cases was adopted. Adding morbidity-free cases to any surgeon's experience to bring the total up to 100 allows all volumes of individual experience to be evaluated and compared. Hypothetical calculations reveal that morbidity and mortality rates in excess of the limits will be shown promptly enough to protect patients and still allow enough experience to be both statistically valid and fair.

RESULTS

The simultaneous publication of the Special Report in the journals *Stroke*[2] and *Circulation*[3] in 1989 provided a guide to the procedure for physicians and surgeons, quality assurances for hospitals, and assistance for credentialing bodies in evaluating the results of carotid surgery. The Ad Hoc Committee on Carotid Surgery Standards of the Stroke Council of the AHA included Hugh G. Beebe, MD, Chairman; G. Patrick Clagett, MD; James A. DeWeese, MD; Wesley S. Moore, MD; James T. Robertson, MD; Burton Sandok, MD; and Philip A. Wolf, MD. The statement follows.*

Carotid endarterectomy for arteriosclerotic occlusive disease of the carotid artery bifurcation and the internal carotid artery has been widely used as a method of reducing stroke risk. There is a variable risk that surgery may induce the condition it is designed to prevent, stroke due to cerebral infarction. Incidence of this complication varies among surgeons and medical institutions.

The risk of carotid endarterectomy should properly influence the indication for surgery. If the risk of operating on a patient is low in relation to the risk of not operating, then the benefit of carotid endarterectomy as a least-risk strategy may be proportionately great and worthwhile. The converse is also true. If morbidity and mortality of carotid endarterectomy are excessive in proportion to the natural history of the untreated or nonoperatively treated lesion, surgery should be avoided.

The ad hoc committee recognizes there are insufficient data to define acceptable morbidity and mortality limits for carotid endarterectomy for various indications. Nevertheless, the committee believes the *upper limits of morbidity and mortality that should prompt individual peer review can be defined. These recommendations are based on current data and are likely to change.*

CATEGORIES OF INDICATIONS FOR OPERATION

Morbidity and mortality limits are categorized by clinical indications for operation, which are defined as follows:

• *Absence of symptoms:* No symptoms, either transient or per-

manent, referable to the carotid artery lesion. Thus, surgery for nonhemispheric, nonclassic symptoms such as dizziness falls in this category.

• *Transient ischemic attack:* An episode (1) that produces a distinct neurological deficit such as paresis, paresthesia, or dysphasia that clears in less than 24 hours, and after which the patient's clinical status returns to what it was before the attack, and that is referable to the carotid artery; or an episode (2) in which the patient has transient loss of vision in one eye.

• *Ischemic stroke:* A focal ischemic neurological deficit that does not clear in 24 hours.

• *Recurrent carotid disease:* Recurrence of disease in an artery after carotid endarterectomy.

UPPER LIMITS OF MORBIDITY AND MORTALITY

In this position statement, morbidity refers specifically to stroke that occurs during or after endarterectomy. It does not include other nonspecific complications or adverse effects that may be associated with surgical procedures.

The 30-day mortality rate from all causes for all carotid endarterectomies should not exceed 2%.

Combined morbidity and mortality due to stroke during or after carotid endarterectomy is categorized by indication for surgery and listed below:

Indication	Limit
Absence of symptoms	< 3%
Transient ischemic attack	< 5%
Ischemic stroke	< 7%
Recurrent carotid disease in the same artery after endarterectomy	< 10%

A small minority of patients will have indications for surgery outside these categories and should be evaluated individually.

The lowest expected morbidity and mortality levels for each category are not known; a more direct comparison of surgical and nonsurgical treatment may be needed, requiring further revision of these limits. The scientific councils of the American Heart Association will continue to monitor these levels and make appropriate revisions as necessary.

MONITORING SURGERY RESULTS

The Ad Hoc Committee on Carotid Surgery Standards recommends that all medical institutions that treat extracranial arterial occlusive disease continually monitor results of surgery through a formal, ongoing audit, which should be made in comparison with these limits and definitions.

For the purposes of the audit, either of the two following methods for establishing an adequate data base are recommended:

1. For experienced surgeons, 100 consecutive cases should be reviewed retrospectively, and afterward a consecutive moving average of 100 total cases categorized by indication for operation evaluated as an ongoing audit.

2. For less experienced surgeons whose smaller caseload does not permit such analysis, available cases should be brought to 100 of total cases without morbidity. Thus, a beginning surgeon would be assigned 100 trouble-free cases as a theoretical statistical basis. For example, 75 cases without morbidity or mortality would be added proportionately by indication categories to a beginning surgeon's 25 cases to form a statistical basis of 100 total cases. From that point on, a consecutive moving average of all additional

*Originally published in Beebe HG, Clagett PG, DeWeese JA, et al: Special Report: A statement for health professionals by the committee on carotid surgery standards of the Stroke Council, American Heart Association. *Stroke.* 1989;20:314 and in Beebe HG, Clagett PG, DeWeese JA, et al: Assessing risk associated with carotid endarterectomy. *Circulation.* 1989;79:472, both © 1989 by the American Heart Association. Reprinted here with permission of the publisher.

cases belonging to that surgeon, categorized by indication for operation, would constitute the data base.

If the morbidity and mortality limits suggested in this position statement are exceeded in any category, the Ad Hoc Committee on Carotid Surgery Standards recommends that individual hospital quality of care procedures be used to determine the appropriate action.

REFERENCES

1. Barnett HJM, Plum F, Walton JN: Carotid endarterectomy: An expression of concern. *Stroke.* 1984;15:941.
2. Beebe HG, Clagett PG, DeWeese JA, Moore WS, Robertson JT, Sandok B, Wolf PA: Special Report: A statement for health professionals by committee on carotid surgery standards of the Stroke Council, American Heart Association. *Stroke.* 1989;20:314.
3. Beebe HG, Clagett PG, DeWeese JA, Moore WS, Robertson JT, Sandok B, Wolf PA: Assessing risk associated with carotid endarterectomy. *Circulation.* 1989;79:472.

Rationale and Method for Auditing Individual Surgeons: Relationship to Hospital Privileges

RICHARD F. KEMPCZINSKI

RATIONALE

Differences in outcome between medical and surgical therapy for some of the clinical manifestations of extracranial carotid artery disease are quite small. If surgical morbidity and mortality were excessive in such cases, it might be impossible to demonstrate a benefit for carotid endarterectomy (CEA). In order to properly compare alternative forms of therapy, one must know how long the patient is likely to survive, that is, the natural history of the disease; the immediate, perioperative risks of surgery; and the clinical course of patients after surgical therapy. Figure 63–1 demonstrates that a surgeon who performs CEA for a specific indication with a perioperative complication rate of 5 percent (line A) would begin to show a benefit to his or her patients after 2 years; an individual with a perioperative complication rate of 20 percent (line C) could not document any real benefit within the 5-year follow-up period typical of most studies.[1] Once the operative risks for CEA are known and the natural history of medically treated patients is documented (information that should be available from well-conducted, randomized trials), each surgeon should be able to determine whether endarterectomy, in his or her hands, is appropriate for a specific indication. Certainly, without an external audit of results, an individual surgeon's undocumented recollections of his or her own surgical morbidity and mortality rates is highly suspect. In one communitywide study of CEA, only 40 percent of the strokes that were identified in a detailed review of the medical records were, in fact, coded or reported on the patient's medical record face sheet.[2] Additional support for this assumption can be drawn from the observation that objective, external reviews of CEA have consistently shown higher morbidity and mortality rates compared with reports based on a surgeon's review of his or her own personal experience.

Following a series of highly critical reports suggesting that CEA was overutilized in the United States and carried excessive morbidity and mortality,[3] there were numerous articles in the lay press urging patients to familiarize themselves with local results before submitting to this procedure. However, without an up-to-date surgical registry based on audited reviews of actual medical records, it is virtually impossible, even for referring physicians, to obtain objective data on individual surgeons in their community. Therefore, in order to reassure referring physicians and their patients that particular surgeons can perform the procedure with acceptable morbidity and mortality, regular, objective auditing of results is essential. Furthermore, the information provided by such audits would be invaluable to hospital credentialing committees not only to ensure that only qualified surgeons were permitted to perform this procedure in the first place but also to guarantee that their ongoing results conformed to local community standards. Finally, in this era of cost-conscious medical practice, it is reasonable to assume that surgeons will be included on specific reimbursement panels based on such considerations as length of stay and documented surgical morbidity.

THE SURGICAL REGISTRY

Since the outcome of CEA should be continuously monitored, a computerized registry must be established to track each surgeon's results.[4] In order to ensure maximum compliance and avoid concerns about breach of confidentiality, it should be an institutional or communitywide resource. Depending on the technology and expertise available in a given community, such a registry could be created on a hospital mainframe computer or on one of the more powerful microcomputers readily available from a number of vendors. The registry should include sufficient data on patient demographics and risk factors to permit stratification of results by risk. The indications for the procedure should be well documented, and all perioperative complications, as well as long-term follow-up, should be included. In order to preserve both patient and surgeon confidentiality, patients can be entered by their hospital identification numbers or social

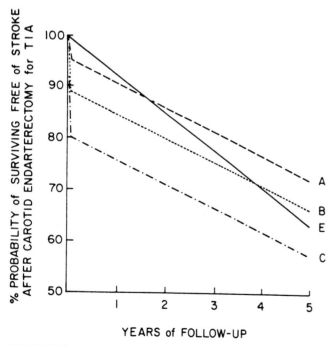

FIGURE 63–1. Approximate life table comparison of best medical therapy *(E)* versus carotid endarterectomy performed with three different rates of perioperative morbidity. *A*, Low (5%) risk; *B*, medium (10%) risk; *C*, high (20%) risk. (From Warlow C: Carotid endarterectomy: Does it work? *Stroke.* 1984;15:1073. Copyright 1994 The American Heart Association. Reproduced with permission.)

security numbers. In the same way, each surgeon should be assigned a unique identification number, and all reports based on the registry should be coded using this number.

A simple data-entry form to collect all the required information should be made available in the operating room or surgeons' lounge of all participating hospitals. This form should be completed by the operating surgeon and returned promptly to a central registry office. To ensure that all operations and complications are being accurately reported, a peer review nurse should be hired to monitor the operating room log of each of the participating institutions. Furthermore, each patient's chart should be audited regularly to confirm that all complications have been noted and recorded. Gathering follow-up data can be much more difficult. However, if most patients in the registry are being followed in their respective hospital's vascular diagnostic laboratory, each laboratory could be regularly provided with a list of all active patients in the registry, and the results of follow-up carotid duplex scans could be used to update each patient's record.

AUDITING THE RESULTS OF CAROTID ENDARTERECTOMY

Once the registry is established and a decision to implement a surgical audit program is made, an organizing committee, composed of representatives from each of the specialties involved in the care of patients with extracranial carotid vascular disease, should be formed. This committee should define the mechanism for data collection and entry into the registry and should resolve appropriate confidentiality issues. In addition, after a thorough review of the medical literature, community performance standards should be established. These should be reviewed and approved by all participating surgeons. A critical issue that must be addressed by the organizing committee is the method and frequency of objective, external audits. Depending on the volume of carotid surgery in any given institution, audits should be conducted at least every 3 years. In busy institutions, annual audits may be appropriate.

New surgeons joining a hospital staff or those just entering practice may have an insufficient number of CEAs in the registry to accurately determine their surgical morbidity rates. The concept of the "moving 100 cases" is one method for dealing with this problem.[5] New surgeons joining a hospital staff would automatically be assigned 100 hypothetical complication-free CEAs. As a surgeon performs actual operations, each one is added to his or her list and a hypothetical case is eliminated. This process continues until all 100 hypothetical cases are replaced by real ones. For example, if a new surgeon performed only three CEAs during his first year on staff and each of these was complicated by a stroke, that surgeon's perioperative stroke rate would be 3 percent rather than 100 percent.

At regular intervals established by the organizing committee, the registry would be audited and the results of each surgeon's performance would be reported to it in confidence, along with the results for the community at large. If a surgeon disagreed with the nurse's assessment on one or more cases, an appeals mechanism should be invoked to permit review of the charts in question by a committee of peers to resolve the disagreement. Surgeons falling below the predetermined performance standards would then have all their cases for the period in question examined by a peer review committee within each institution. These detailed chart reviews would try to determine whether there were any unusual risk factors or extenuating circumstances that might have contributed to the adverse outcome.

HOSPITAL PRIVILEGES

Annual renewal of hospital privileges for specific vascular procedures such as CEA should be based on regular audits of individual surgical performance. Once the data from a computerized vascular registry, as outlined above, were regularly available, renewal of hospital privileges could be linked to performance. Surgeons applying for privileges to perform CEA generally fall into two broad categories. Established surgeons should be required to submit operative notes and discharge summaries from their last 50 consecutive CEAs for review by the credentialing or peer review committee. Based on this material, the committee should determine whether that surgeon's results fall within acceptable community standards. For new surgeons who do not have a sufficient number of cases that can be reviewed, the committee should determine whether the individual's training qualifies him or her for temporary privileges to perform this procedure. The committee should also solicit the recommendations of the directors of the programs where these individuals trained and review the results of any CEAs performed by them during their training. The "moving 100 concept," as described earlier, could be used to ensure that every complication during their early experience would not immediately trigger a performance standard violation. Before permanent privileges are conferred, an audit of a sufficient number of real cases should be performed to ensure that actual results meet community standards.

Surgeons whose results fall outside of the published performance standards would face potential action by the credentialing committee if a review of their patients' hospital records failed to disclose any mitigating circumstances.[6] Depending on how far their results fell outside the norm, committee action might include imposition of a 1-year probationary period, during which the medical records of all patients being considered for CEA would be reviewed by the committee for appropriateness of indications and during which the physician might be required to arrange for an accredited surgeon to assist him or her during such procedures. For particularly egregious outliers or for repeat offenders, additional training might be required before recertifying such individuals to perform CEA. Finally, persistent and recurrent unacceptable performance could result in permanent suspension of hospital privileges. At every step in this process, individual surgeon's confidentiality must be protected, and access to due process must be ensured.

CONCLUSIONS

An institutional or communitywide registry should be established to monitor the results of several index vascular procedures, such as CEA. Regular audits of the registry should be made available to participating surgeons and used to identify individuals whose results fall outside of predetermined performance standards. Such a registry would not only help maintain public confidence but could also reassure referring physicians that all surgeons credentialed to perform this procedure were, in fact, qualified. Continuation of operating privileges should be tied to maintenance of acceptable performance standards and should be monitored by a committee of peers established at each institution. Provided that the ''rules of the game'' are determined in advance and approved by all participating surgeons prior to implementation, and provided that patient and surgeon confidentiality is protected, such a system can provide an invaluable safeguard to both patients and referring physicians without exposing the institution or the individual members of the committee to undue legal liability.

REFERENCES

1. Warlow C: Carotid endarterectomy: Does it work? *Stroke.* 1984;15:1068.
2. Brott T, Thalinger K: The practice of carotid endarterectomy in a large metropolitan community. *Stroke.* 1984;15:950.
3. Barnett HJM, Plum F, Walton JN: Carotid endarterectomy—an expression of concern. *Stroke.* 1984;15:941.
4. Kempczinski RF: Monitoring vascular surgical performance. *J Vasc Surg.* 1991;13:532.
5. Beebe HG, Clagett GP, DeWeese JA, et al: Assessing risk associated with carotid endarterectomy: A statement for health professionals by an ad hoc committee on carotid surgery standards of the Stroke Council, American Heart Association. *Stroke.* 1988;20:314.
6. Moore WS: Guidelines for hospital privileges in vascular surgery. *J Vasc Surg.* 1991;13:527.

Immediate and Long-Term Outcome of Surgery for Asymptomatic Carotid Stenosis

JOHN J. RICOTTA

Carotid endarterectomy is advocated as a prophylactic measure to prevent clinical neurologic events. The following assumptions are inherent in this approach: (1) A high-risk group can be identified in which the stroke risk is sufficient to warrant therapeutic intervention; (2) carotid endarterectomy can be performed with a complication rate low enough to make it a feasible therapeutic alternative; and (3) as an intervention, carotid endarterectomy is significantly more efficacious than current optimal medical therapy in reducing long-term stroke risk. In the case of patients with lateralizing symptoms and an ipsilateral severe stenosis, these three assumptions have been fulfilled, and the benefit of endarterectomy is clearly established.[1, 2] Two multicenter trials have been reported[3, 4] and a third has recently been concluded[5] to address this issue in asymptomatic patients. Details of these trials are presented elsewhere in this volume (Section XI). This chapter focuses on the published results in patients with asymptomatic stenosis who have been subjected to carotid endarterectomy, with special attention to perioperative morbidity and mortality as well as late results. Although these data do not address the question of whether a high-risk group of asymptomatic patients can be identified, they should help define whether endarterectomy is a safe and efficacious procedure for stroke prevention.

CAVEATS

Before proceeding further, three controversial issues need to be identified. It is beyond the scope of this chapter to discuss these in detail, but it is important to mention them at the outset in order to place the problem in perspective. Each of these questions remains the subject of active debate, and all have an impact on the interpretation of results. The different positions taken on these three topics cause some of the confusion surrounding the proper indications for carotid endarterectomy in asymptomatic patients.

The first issue is the difference between an asymptomatic patient and an asymptomatic stenosis. In many studies, 30 percent or more of patients with asymptomatic stenosis have had contralateral neurologic symptoms or carotid endarterectomy[3–7] or bilateral endarterectomy for asymptomatic stenosis.[8–12] These patients have been included in trials along with patients who have no symptoms referable to the contralateral carotid artery. Although it is easy to accept that the risk for these patient groups might be different, few data are available on which to base a definitive conclusion. A retrospective analysis by Kirshner and colleagues[6] indicated that perioperative complications after endarterectomy for asymptomatic stenosis were limited to patients with evidence of contralateral carotid disease. Further complicating this issue are data that suggest that approximately 20 percent of patients with clinically asymptomatic carotid stenosis have evidence of intracranial infarctions on computed tomography (CT);[13, 14]

whether these patients are a high-risk group remains unknown. In general, studies reported to date have relied on clinical rather than imaging criteria to classify patients.

A second major issue involves the definition of appropriate clinical endpoints—stroke, transient ischemic attack (TIA), carotid occlusion, and death. Should stroke alone be used to determine efficacy, or is the measure of all neurologic endpoints (stroke and TIA) more appropriate? Should only ipsilateral events be considered, or is it more appropriate to evaluate all neurologic events? Is asymptomatic carotid occlusion an important event and a potential endpoint? Inclusion of TIA as an endpoint can be justified by the importance of TIA in the face of severe stenosis seen by the North American[1] and European[2] trials and the high incidence of CT-demonstrated infarctions in patients with TIA alone.[13, 14] Reports of increased stroke risk (6% per year) associated with carotid occlusion support its inclusion as an important clinical endpoint,[15–17] although this has not been done in prospective trials. These arguments assume great significance, since the Veterans Administration trial in asymptomatic stenosis,[3] for example, showed a benefit for surgery in the reduction of all ipsilateral neurologic events but not of ipsilateral stroke alone. Hertzer[18] and others have argued that it is unfair to expect carotid endarterectomy to influence late mortality (most of which is cardiac) and that perioperative mortality and overall neurologic morbidity (early and late) are more appropriate criteria for evaluating the efficacy of endarterectomy. The repeated failure of carotid endarterectomy to influence the late death rate emphasizes the importance of this argument.

The final major issue of concern is the determination of the degree of stenosis. Although most studies have now adopted a standard method of reporting the percentage of diameter reduction using the distal normal internal carotid artery,[5] this has not been uniform practice in past reports. Various methods have been used to report the percentage of stenosis,[1, 2] and it has not always been specified whether diameter or area was measured. It is well established that there is an inherent measurement variability of plus or minus 10 percent in measurements of diameter, even angiographically.[19] In addition, in many reports, severity of stenosis is often quantitated primarily by noninvasive studies, including spectral analysis or ocular pneumoplethysmography, and then confirmed by angiography in the operative group of patients. Although this is clinically appropriate in asymptomatic patients (indeed, angiography is restricted to the surgical arm of the asymptomatic carotid atherosclerosis study),[5] these differences must be kept in mind when comparing the severity of stenosis reported in the various studies in the literature as well as when making recommendations based on calculated degrees of stenosis, which seem deceptively absolute.

With these reservations in mind, I proceed to review

the results of surgical series of patients with asymptomatic stenosis (in contrast to asymptomatic patients).

PERIOPERATIVE MORBIDITY AND MORTALITY

Major perioperative morbidity and mortality are related to stroke and myocardial infarction. These occur with about equal frequency as a cause of early morbidity and postoperative mortality. The majority of neurologic deficits are the result of technical error, and most myocardial infarctions reflect underlying myocardial disease or are related to perioperative control of blood pressure. Complication rates are generally related to neurologic status prior to surgery and are lowest in asymptomatic patients.[9, 20–22]

Perioperative neurologic morbidity in asymptomatic patients has generally been reported as less than 4 percent (Table 64–1).[3, 4, 6–12, 21–34] In the late 1970s[35] and early 1980s,[24, 27] several series were presented in which perioperative stroke rates were unacceptably high, but more recent reports have clearly established that endarterectomy can be done safely in the majority of patients with asymptomatic stenosis. Although some of the series in Table 64–1 include individual[7, 8, 12, 21] or institutional[22, 29] experiences, others present the experience of multiple institutions[26] or community-wide surveys.[6, 24, 27, 28, 30] Data from the three major randomized trials,[3–5] all involving multiple centers and multiple surgeons, indicate stroke rates from 1.5 to 3.3 percent. A meta-analysis of the 7360 operations constituting these data yields a stroke rate of 2.1 percent.

Perioperative mortality is relatively evenly divided between stroke and myocardial infarction. Data from Love and coworkers,[36] which identified abnormal thallium scans in 7 of 15 patients with asymptomatic severe carotid stenosis, underline the high prevalence of coronary artery disease in this patient group. Perioperative nonfatal myocardial infarction occurs in 0 to 2 percent of patients after carotid endarterectomy for asymptomatic stenosis.[3, 4, 6] Mortality after carotid endarterectomy for asymptomatic stenosis is low, averaging 1.4 percent in the 7360 cases collected from the literature since 1984 (Table 64–2). The more important figure, including both perioperative stroke and death (see Table 64–2), is also low for the entire group—3.2 percent—although there are a number of series in which this number appears to be unacceptably high for operations on asymptomatic patients.[24, 26–28] The stroke council of the American Heart Association has suggested that the combined neurologic morbidity and mortality for patients with asymptomatic stenosis should not exceed 3 percent.[37] In contrast, Chambers and Norris[38] suggested that surgery for asymptomatic stenosis might benefit a select group if the combined perioperative incidence of stroke and death was less than 5 percent. Whether this more liberal criterion should be applied is yet to be decided.

Review of the two published randomized studies[3, 4] and one large multi-institutional review[26] indicates that overall death and complication rates sometimes exceed the American Heart Association standards. In the Veterans Administration trial,[3] endarterectomy was found effective in reducing overall ipsilateral neurologic events. In the CASANOVA study,[4] no benefit was found, but in this study, complications from angiography approached those of surgical intervention. These data emphasize the need to carefully select patients for operation and the need for meticulous angiographic evaluation. It is important to restrict intervention to patients in whom the risks of stroke or myocardial infarction are minimal if carotid endarterectomy is to be truly effective as a method of stroke prevention.

Long-term data on stroke risk are available from several series of patients operated on for asymptomatic carotid stenosis (Table 64–3).[3, 4, 7, 8, 10–12, 21, 22, 29, 32, 33, 39] These data have been variously presented in terms of total stroke risk, ipsilateral stroke risk, and survival. Although all three are important, endarterectomy is likely to affect only ipsilateral stroke risk. Some authors used life table methods, and others reported mean follow-up and cumulative stroke and mortality. For purposes of comparison and analysis, stroke rate has been presented in Table 64–3 when possible. The available data indicate that late stroke risk after carotid endarterectomy is low (generally 1 to 1.5% per year). Not all strokes occur in the ipsilateral hemisphere, and a number of patients in these series had subsequent contralateral endarterectomy.

Late mortality remains high in this group of patients (see Table 64–3). In the Veterans Administration study reported by Hobson and associates,[3] no difference was seen between the medical and surgical group when rates of late stroke and death were combined for analysis. The late incidence of death was very high in this veteran population (40%), with the majority of deaths resulting from myocardial infarction. Similar results have been reported in most other series, with no difference in late mortality between medical and surgical groups. These data should not serve as an indictment of the

TABLE 64–1. Perioperative Stroke After Asymptomatic Stenosis, Abstracted from Reports Since 1984

Study*	Year	Procedures, n	Strokes, n (%)
Slavish et al[23]	1984	190	5 (2.6)
Brott & Thalinger[24]†	1984	130	10 (7.7)
White et al[25]	1984	32	0 (0.0)
Hertzer & Aronson[22]	1985	655	12 (1.8)
Moore et al[11]	1985	81	2 (2.5)
Fode et al[26]†	1986	572	20 (3.5)
Cafferata & Gainey[27]†	1986	92	12‡ (13.0)
Kempczinski et al[28]	1986	381	14 (3.7)
Hertzer et al[29]	1986	116	4 (3.4)
Moneta et al[10]	1987	56	1 (1.8)
Rosenthal et al[8]	1987	42	0 (0.0)
Rubin et al[30]†	1988	1055	19 (1.8)
Callow & Mackey[21]	1989	179	2 (1.1)
Caracci et al[9]	1989	100	2 (2.0)
Kirshner et al[6]†	1989	222	6 (2.7)
Edwards et al[7]	1989	411	2 (0.5)
Treiman et al[31]	1990	377	7 (1.8)
Mattos et al[32]	1992	146	2 (1.4)
Freischlag et al[12]	1992	141	2 (1.4)
Thompson[33]	1993	326	4 (1.2)
Moore et al[34]§	1991	1511	13 (0.9)
CASANOVA[4]§	1991	334	10 (3.0)
Hobson et al (VA)[3]§	1993	211	5 (2.4)
Total		7360	154 (2.1)

*For full bibliographic information, see reference list at end of chapter.
†Multi-institutional experience.
‡Includes stroke and death.
§Randomized studies.

TABLE 64-2. Perioperative Mortality and Total Stroke and Mortality After Asymptomatic Stenosis, Abstracted from Reports Since 1984

Study*	Year	Procedures, n	Death, n (%)	Stroke and Death, n (%)
Slavish et al[23]	1984	190	5‡ (2.6)	5 (2.6)
Brott & Thalinger[24]†	1984	130	4 (3.1)	14 (10.8)
White et al[25]	1984	32	0 (0.0)	0 (0.0)
Hertzer & Aronson[22]	1985	655	8 (1.2)	21 (3.2)
Moore et al[11]	1985	81	0 (0.0)	2 (2.5)
Fode et al[26]†	1986	572	17 (3.0)	37 (6.5)
Cafferata & Gainey[27]†	1986	92	12‡ (13.0)	12 (13.0)
Kempczinski et al[28]	1986	381	8 (2.1)	22 (5.7)
Hertzer et al[29]	1986	116	1 (0.9)	5 (4.3)
Moneta et al[10]	1987	56	0 (0.0)	1 (1.8)
Rosenthal et al[8]	1987	42	0 (0.0)	0 (0.0)
Rubin et al[30]†	1988	1055	18 (1.7)	37 (3.5)
Callow & Mackey[21]	1989	179	1 (0.6)	3 (1.7)
Caracci et al[9]	1989	100	1 (1.0)	3 (3.0)
Kirshner et al[6]†	1989	222	1 (0.4)	7 (3.1)
Edwards et al[7]	1989	411	1 (0.2)	3 (0.7)
Treiman et al[31]	1990	377	1 (0.3)	8 (2.1)
Mattos et al[32]	1992	146	1 (0.7)	3 (2.1)
Freischlag et al[12]	1992	141	0 (0.0)	2 (1.4)
Thompson[33]	1993	326	1 (0.3)	5 (1.5)
Moore et al[34]§	1991	1511	12 (0.8)	25 (1.7)
CASANOVA[4]§	1991	334	4 (1.2)	9 (4.2)
Hobson et al (VA)[3]§	1993	211	4 (1.9)	9 (4.3)
Total		7360	100 (1.4)	238 (3.2)

*For full bibliographic information, see reference list at end of chapter.
†Multi-institutional reports.
‡Includes death and stroke.
§Randomized studies.

operation, which can be performed with minimal risk, but rather as a reminder of the high incidence of coronary atherosclerosis in this patient population and the need for careful follow-up and management of coronary disease after

TABLE 64-3. Long-Term Follow-Up After Carotid Endarterectomy for Asymptomatic Stenosis

Study*	Patients, n	Follow-Up	Stroke Rate, %	Survival Rate, %
Thompson[33]	67	55 mo†	1/yr	68
Moore et al[11]	81	5 yr	1.6/yr	78
Moneta et al[10]	56	24 mo	2/yr	85
Rosenthal et al[8]	42	10 yr	1/yr	57
Hertzer and Aronson[22]	126	5 yr	1.6/yr	72§
				43¶
Callow and Mackey[21]	179	56 mo†	1.1/yr	75§
				46¶
Edwards et al[7]	411	1–104 mo	13	86
Mattos et al[32]	146	64 mo†	0.8/yr	80§
				60¶
CASANOVA[4]‡	331	42 mo†	11	84
Hobson et al (VA)[3]	221	41 mo†	1.6	59
Hertzer et al[29]	95	35 mo†	1.6	86
Bernstein et al[39]	87	4 yr	1.2	69
Freischlag et al[12]	123	56 mo†	1.1	76§
				66¶

*For full bibliographic information, see reference list at end of chapter.
†Mean follow-up time.
‡Includes 6.7% perioperative stroke.
§At 5 years.
¶At 10 years.

carotid surgery. Appropriate measures to reduce this late cardiac mortality remain to be defined.

CONCLUSIONS

Review of retrospective as well as prospective surgical series indicates that carotid endarterectomy can be performed safely in patients with asymptomatic stenosis. A significant number of these patients will have some evidence of contralateral cerebral ischemia or carotid stenosis, and there are isolated data to suggest that risks may be increased in this subgroup. Patient selection by clinical or noninvasive criteria should aim to minimize perioperative coronary ischemic events.

Endarterectomy is effective in minimizing the long-term incidence of ipsilateral neurologic events. However, these patients remain at increased risk for contralateral neurologic problems and late death, particularly from myocardial infarction. Optimal treatment of these patients requires recognition of these long-term risks and development of appropriate treatment strategies to reduce them.

REFERENCES

1. North American symptomatic carotid endarterectomy trial collaborators: Beneficial effect of carotid endarterectomy in symptomatic patients with high grade carotid stenosis. *N Engl J Med.* 1991;325:445.
2. European carotid surgery trialist's collaborative group/MRC European carotid surgery trial: Interim results for symptomatic patients with severe (70–99%) or with mild (0–29%) carotid stenosis. *Lancet.* 1991;337:1235.

3. Hobson RW II, Weiss DG, Fields WS, et al: Efficacy of carotid endarterectomy for asymptomatic carotid stenosis. *N Engl J Med.* 1993;328:221.

4. CASANOVA study group: Carotid surgery versus medical therapy in asymptomatic carotid stenosis. *Stroke.* 1991;22:1229.

5. Asymptomatic carotid atherosclerosis study group: Study design for a randomized prospective trial of carotid endarterectomy for asymptomatic atherosclerosis. *Stroke.* 1989;20:844.

6. Kirshner DL, O'Brien MS, Ricotta JJ: Risk factors in a community experience with carotid endarterectomy. *J Vasc Surg.* 1989;10:178.

7. Edwards WH, Edwards WH Jr, Jenkins JM, Mulherin JL Jr: Analysis of a decade of carotid reconstructive operations. *J Cardiovasc Surg.* 1989;30:424.

8. Rosenthal D, Rudderman R, Borrero E, et al: Carotid endarterectomy to correct asymptomatic carotid stenosis: Ten years later. *J Vasc Surg.* 1987;6:226.

9. Caracci BF, Zukowski AJ, Hurley JJ, et al: Asymptomatic severe carotid stenosis. *J Vasc Surg.* 1989;9:361.

10. Moneta GL, Taylor DC, Nicholls SC, et al: Operative vs. non operative management of asymptomatic high grade internal carotid artery stenosis: Improved results with endarterectomy. *Stroke.* 1987;18:1005.

11. Moore DJ, Miles RD, Gooley NA, Sumner DS: Noninvasive assessment of stroke risk in asymptomatic and nonhemispheric patients with suspected carotid disease. *Ann Surg.* 1985;202:491.

12. Freischlag JA, Hanna D, Moore WS: Improved prognosis for asymptomatic carotid stenosis with prophylactic carotid endarterectomy. *Stroke.* 1992;23:479.

13. Street DL, O'Brien MS, Ricotta JJ, et al: Observations on computerized cerebral tomography in carotid endarterectomy patients. *J Vasc Surg.* 1988;7:798.

14. Norris JW, Zhu CZ: Silent stroke and carotid stenosis. *Stroke.* 1992;23:483.

15. Barnett HJM: Delayed cerebral ischemic episodes distal to occlusion of major cerebral arteries. *Neurology.* 1980;28:764.

16. Cote R, Barnett HJM, Taylor DW: Internal carotid occlusion: A prospective study. *Stroke.* 1983;14:898.

17. Nicholls SC, Kohler TR, Beregelin RO, et al: Carotid artery occlusion: Natural history. *J Vasc Surg.* 1986;4:479.

18. Hertzer NR: Carotid endarterectomy—a crisis in confidence. *J Vasc Surg.* 1988;7:611.

19. Oleary TH, Byran FA, Goodison MW, et al: Measurement variability of carotid atherosclerosis: Real time (B mode) ultrasonography and angiography. *Stroke.* 1987;18:1011.

20. Thompson JE, Patman RD, Talkington CM: Asymptomatic carotid bruits—long term outcome of patients having endarterectomy compared to unoperated controls. *Ann Surg.* 1978;188:308.

21. Callow AD, Mackey WC: Long term follow up of surgically managed carotid bifurcation atherosclerosis. *Ann Surg.* 1989;210:308.

22. Hertzer NR, Aronson R: Cumulative stroke and survival 10 years after carotid endarterectomy. *J Vasc Surg.* 1985;2:93.

23. Slavish LG, Nicholas GG, Gee W: Review of a community experience with carotid endarterectomy. *Stroke.* 1984;15:957.

24. Brott T, Thalinger K: The practice of CEA in a large metropolitan area. *Stroke.* 1989;15:950.

25. White JS, Sirinek KP, Root HD, Rogers W: Morbidity and mortality of CEA: Rates of occurrence in asymptomatic patients. *Arch Surg.* 1981;116:409.

26. Fode NC, Sundt TM, Robertson JJ, et al: Multicenter retrospective review of results and complications of carotid endarterectomy in 1981. *Stroke.* 1986;17:370.

27. Cafferata HT, Gainey MD: CEA in the community hospital: A continuing controversy. *J Cardiovasc Surg.* 1986;27:557.

28. Kempczinski RF, Brott TG, LaButta RJ: The influence of surgical specialty and caseload on the results of carotid endarterectomy. *J Surg.* 1986;3:911.

29. Hertzer NR, Flanagan RA, O'Hara PJ, Beveu EG: Surgical vs. non operative treatment of asymptomatic carotid stenosis. *Ann Surg.* 1986;204:163.

30. Rubin JR, Pitluk HC, King TA, et al: Carotid endarterectomy in a metropolitan community: Early results after 8535 operations. *J Vasc Surg.* 1988;7:256.

31. Treiman RL, Cassman DV, Foran RF, et al: The risk of carotid endarterectomy for the asymptomatic patient: An argument for prophylactic operation. *Ann Vasc Surg.* 1990;4:29.

32. Mattos MA, Hodgson KJ, Londrey GL, et al: Carotid endarterectomy: Operative risks, recurrent stenosis, and long term stroke rates in a modern series. *J Cardiovasc Surg.* 1992;33:387.

33. Thompson JE: Carotid endarterectomy for asymptomatic carotid stenosis: An update. *J Vasc Surg.* 1991;13:669.

34. Moore WS, Vescera CL, Robertson JT, et al: Selection process for surgeons in the asymptomatic carotid atherosclerosis study. *Stroke.* 1991;22:1353.

35. Easton JD, Shermann DG: Stroke and mortality rate in carotid endarterectomy: 228 consecutive operations. *Stroke.* 1977;8:565.

36. Love BB, Groover-McKay M, Pailler J, et al: Coronary artery disease and cardiac events with asymptomatic and symptomatic cerebrovascular disease. *Stroke.* 1992;23:939.

37. Beebe HG, Clagett GP, DeWeese JA, et al: Assessing risk associated with carotid endarterectomy. *AHA Stroke Council Special Report.* Oct. 20, 1988:472.

38. Chambers B, Norris JW: The case against surgery for asymptomatic carotid stenosis. *Stroke.* 1984;15:964.

39. Bernstein EF, Humber PB, Collins GM, et al: Life expectancy and late stroke following carotid endarterectomy. *Ann Surg.* 1983;198:80.

The Effect of Risk Factor Modification and Antiplatelet Treatment in Reducing Stroke Risk in Patients with Transient Cerebral Ischemic Attack or Prior Stroke

D. J. THOMAS

It is common practice to consider all the main vascular risk factors together as if their effects on different parts of the circulation were the same. Stroke and myocardial infarction are quite different diseases with different pathophysiologies. Although there are some advantages in discussing overall risk factors for vascular disease, it is important to appreciate that they have different effects in different parts of the circulation. Furthermore, within cerebrovascular disease, the inter-relationships between risk factors differ for cerebral hemorrhage, cerebral thrombosis, and cerebral embolism.

The more risk factors a patient has, the more likely that patient is to have vascular events, and the poorer the prognosis. There is an unfortunate tendency to give a blanket risk of, say, 7 percent per year of having a major vascular event in patients presenting with transient ischemic attack (TIA), but this is just an average value for patients who have been included in clinical trials. A relatively young patient with amaurosis fugax may well have an annual risk of 2 percent or less. An elderly patient with a history of smoking, hypertension, ischemic heart disease, peripheral vascular disease, and bilateral carotid disease may have an annual risk of almost 30 percent. Patients with tight carotid stenoses but no previous history of TIA may be only slightly less at risk from a stroke than patients who have already had TIAs.

Risk factor modification and other possible vascular treatments in patients with TIA are likely to have different impacts on the chance of myocardial infarction and on the chance of stroke. Furthermore, drugs may be required at different dosages to prevent stroke compared with myocardial infarction. It should be emphasized that TIA and carotid stenosis are important markers for the presence of coronary atheroma. Indeed, the most common cause of death in TIA patients is myocardial infarction.

RISK FACTORS

A list of the important risk factors to consider in patients presenting with TIAs is given in Table 65–1.

Age

Age is by far the most important risk factor for stroke.[1] This is often ignored because it is impossible to modify age. But since the effect of risk factors tends to be cumulative, it is probably more important to treat elderly patients than patients presenting similarly but at a younger age. Patient compliance is also important. It is not everlasting and needs reinforcement. Compliance may be better in elderly patients, who are more frightened of stroke than younger individuals,

often because they have seen contemporaries succumb. They may continue to take antiplatelet medication long after young patients have abandoned it.

Hypertension

Hypertension is usually cited as being the most important risk factor for stroke that is amenable to treatment. There is now incontrovertible evidence that raised blood pressure is associated with both cerebral thrombosis and cerebral hemorrhage. There is also excellent evidence that reducing blood pressure significantly reduces the risk of stroke, not only in middle-aged individuals but also in the elderly.[2, 3] Hypertension should also be treated after a patient has had a stroke, to reduce the chance of recurrence. It is important to resume treatment of hypertension after carotid endarterectomy. This needs emphasis, because patients often believe that surgery has cured their cerebrovascular problems and they stop taking medication for hypertension.

The presence of hypertension, particularly untreated hypertension, increases the risk of carotid endarterectomy and other vascular surgery.[4] One reason for this increased risk is a shift of the cerebral blood flow autoregulatory curve so that hypertensive patients are more vulnerable to perioperative hypotension.[5] This does not have to be absolute hypotension, just a relative drop in perfusion pressure compared with the preoperative state.

There is as yet no clear evidence as to which hypotensive agent has the advantage in preventing cerebrovascular complications. It seems to be the reduction in blood pressure that is important, not necessarily how it is achieved. It is important, however, to avoid symptoms suggestive of hemodynamic insufficiency in patients receiving antihypertensive or antianginal treatment, particularly in those with impaired circulation to the brain stem (producing vertebrobasilar TIAs on treatment) and those with known carotid occlusion or severe bilateral stenoses. Blood pressure treat-

TABLE 65–1. Risk Factors for Stroke

Increasing age
Hypertension
Transient ischemic attacks
Cardiac disease
Peripheral vascular disease
Polycythemia
Diabetes
Hyperlipidemia
Oral contraceptive use
Cigarette smoking
Alcohol use
Elevated plasma fibrinogen

ment is less effective in preventing myocardial infarction than in preventing stroke, but the exact reasons for this are still obscure.[2] After a cerebrovascular event, it is advisable to avoid treating the surge of hypertension that often occurs as a reaction to the event,[6] because so doing may impair blood flow through the necessary collateral vessels and exacerbate the resulting disability.

Transient Ischemic Attack

The occurrence of an episode of transient monocular blindness or TIA is associated with an increased risk of stroke. It appears that the number of TIAs that a patient suffers is related to the risk of eventual stroke.[4] Therefore, even very transient attacks should not be ignored, and every attempt should be made to control them.

Patients who are thought to have had transient cerebral ischemia but who are found on examination to have minor residual neurologic signs or are found to have evidence on brain scan of cerebral infarction are at increased risk of developing cerebral infarct, particularly during surgery.[4] Patients who have actually had a minor stroke rather than a TIA also appear to be at higher risk.[4]

Associated Cardiac Disease

The presence of cardiac disease increases the risk of stroke in patients presenting with TIA. Every effort should be made to optimize cardiac function.[7]

It has been appreciated for decades that rheumatic heart disease with atrial fibrillation is a harbinger of thromboembolic stroke. More recently, it has been shown that atrial fibrillation without obvious structural cardiac disease is also linked with an increased chance of embolic cerebral infarction.[8] Anticoagulant therapy in such patients is indicated and effective.

Cardiac failure is also associated with an increased risk of stroke and should be corrected promptly. Evidence of cardiomegaly on chest radiograph is associated with an adverse risk, even in patients without any history of cardiac symptoms or disease.[9] Its presence reinforces the need for careful management of hypertension.

Peripheral Vascular Disease

The presence of substantial peripheral vascular disease in TIA patients appears to be associated with an increased cerebral risk.[4] Obviously, patients with aortic aneurysms requiring surgical repair are at risk from perioperative cerebrovascular events. Poorly controlled peripheral vascular disease may be associated with an increase in plasma fibrinogen and other clotting factors, resulting in increased risk of cerebral thrombosis. Efforts should be made to improve the control of peripheral vascular disease whenever possible.

Polycythemia and High Hematocrit

Polycythemia rubra vera increases the risk of stroke by 20-fold. Interestingly, it has much less of an impact on the chance of myocardial infarction.

Treating polycythemia by therapeutic venesection has been shown to reduce the risk of occlusive vascular disease.[10]

However, it is important to emphasize that venesection may result in a reactive thrombocytosis,[11] so these patients should receive antiplatelet treatment to prevent a thrombotic event from occurring during hemodilution.

High normal or elevated hematocrit, without polycythemia rubra vera, is also associated with an increased risk of cerebrovascular disease. There is no evidence as yet that reducing hematocrit by venesection in these groups results in a reduced risk of stroke. However, many of these patients without polycythemia rubra vera have high hematocrit levels as a result of cigarette smoking, alcohol use, or diuretic therapy, and an improved prognosis may be achieved by modifying these factors.[11]

Diabetes

Diabetes mellitus is associated with increased risk of atheroma and of both myocardial infarction and cerebrovascular disease.[12] There is good animal experimental evidence that uncontrolled blood sugar results in larger cerebral infarction and that adequate reduction of blood sugar leads to smaller cerebral infarcts.[13] This has yet to be proved in humans, but based on experimental evidence from the laboratory, it seems prudent to optimize the treatment of diabetes, particularly in the early phase after a TIA or stroke.

Hyperlipidemia

The impact of hyperlipidemia on the occurrence of cerebrovascular events is much less striking than its impact on ischemic heart disease. Treatment of hyperlipidemia goes through cycles of popularity. At the moment, it is recommended only for high-risk individuals with a possible familial hyperlipidemia or for those with multiple associated risk factors.[14] It is one of the risk factors that is probably not worth treating in very elderly patients.

There is some evidence that a drastic reduction in blood lipids leads to a regression of atheroma. There are some anecdotal accounts in humans, but as yet, there is no convincing evidence that the modest reduction in cholesterol that can be achieved in most patients results in regression of atheroma.

Oral Contraceptive Use

When the oral contraceptive pill was first introduced, it undoubtedly resulted in a number of strokes in young women.[15] The improved formulation of oral contraceptives, particularly the reduction in the estrogen content, has led to a definite decrease in the risk of stroke. However, it is essential that oral contraceptive use be stopped if a woman develops cerebrovascular symptoms, even if her focal symptoms occur during migrainous phenomena. It is good policy that no woman who smokes should take oral contraceptives, particularly if she is over 30. When a woman has a TIA while on hormone replacement therapy, the therapy should be stopped.

Cigarette Smoking

Cigarette smoking seems to be much more important in myocardial infarction and peripheral vascular disease than in cerebrovascular disease. Indeed, it is only recently that smoking has been shown to be an independent risk factor for stroke.[16] The reason for this is that most patients who suffer stroke are elderly, and many of them have never smoked. They tend to obscure the important group of young stroke patients in whom smoking is an important risk factor. It is probably worthwhile to attempt to get all patients presenting with vascular symptoms to stop smoking.

Cigarette smoking may also be associated with underlying carcinoma. It should be appreciated that patients with an underlying carcinoma may have a hyperthrombotic tendency and actually present with TIA or minor stroke. It is prudent to look clinically and perform some simple investigations to rule out the possibility of an underlying neoplasm.

Alcohol Use

There is some early evidence suggesting that one or two units of alcohol per day may be associated with a reduced risk of occlusive vascular disease. (One unit is approximately 100 mL wine, 300 mL beer, or 35 mL spirits.) Heavy alcohol intake in young and middle-aged individuals, however, is associated with an increased risk of stroke. This increased risk is largely due to cerebral hemorrhage, although there is a slight increase in cerebral infarction.[17] Cerebral hemorrhage may be associated not only with cerebral trauma but also with the clotting disturbances that occur as a result of hepatic disease associated with alcohol use.

Obesity

Obesity does not appear to be an independent risk factor for stroke. However, if obesity is reduced, blood pressure tends to fall, and the chance of developing diabetic complications is reduced, as is their severity if they do occur.

Reduced Physical Activity

Lack of exercise seems to be bad for the heart and peripheral vascular system but apparently is not associated with an increased risk of stroke. Nevertheless, it seems sensible to suggest increased physical activity in order to improve cardiac and peripheral vascular function and to help reduce blood pressure.

Following Carotid Endarterectomy

After the efforts and risks involved in carotid endarterectomy, the opportunity to improve patients' lifestyles should be taken in the hope that a carotid restenosis will be prevented or delayed. Although in some centers in the United Kingdom surgeons will not operate unless patients agree to give up smoking, there is no definite evidence that continuing to smoke causes restenosis. There is also no definite evidence that reducing lipids substantially delays restenosis. The author's view is that both should be advised until further information is available.

Because of the tendency for patients to believe that they are cured after surgery, they must be cautioned to continue with hypotensive and antiplatelet treatment.

ANTIPLATELET THERAPY

Medical therapy is crucial in the prevention of cerebrovascular complications in at-risk individuals. Only a small percentage of patients at risk from stroke have a relevant carotid stenosis that is amenable to endarterectomy. Also, all the clinical trials that have shown benefits of surgery have involved medical treatment plus surgery versus medical treatment alone. We do not know what effect surgery alone would have against best medical treatment.

The treatment choices available for antiplatelet therapy are aspirin, ticlopidine, dipyridamole, sulfinpyrazone, and fish oil.

Contraindications

Antiplatelet therapy is contraindicated in patients with a past history of cerebral hemorrhage or subarachnoid hemorrhage. It is also potentially dangerous to use in patients with peptic ulcers or with a past history of gastrointestinal hemorrhage. Patients with bleeding diathesis, including thrombocytopenia, should not be so treated. Severely hypertensive patients not responding to medical treatment may have larger cerebral hemorrhages if they are on aspirin than if they are not. Diabetic patients with poorly controlled retinopathy may have catastrophic intraocular bleeding as a result of antiplatelet treatment. Allergies and side effects are not uncommon with antiplatelet drugs.

Up to 20 percent of the population may be unable to tolerate aspirin, however low the dose. A slightly higher proportion find dipyridamole an unacceptable drug. Probably less than 10 percent of patients have difficulty tolerating ticlopidine.

Aspirin Therapy

Antiplatelet trials have been carried out in three main groups: TIA and stroke, ischemic heart disease, and primary prevention. Data from over 100,000 patients treated in clinical trials with antiplatelet therapy are now available.[18] Most patients have been treated with aspirin, but the dosage has varied from as low as 30 mg up to 1200 mg a day. Some patients have been treated with ticlopidine alone. Some trials have included patients treated with a combination of dipyridamole and aspirin. Relatively few patients have been treated with sulfinpyrazone.

The results of these trials indicate that antiplatelet treatment confers approximately a 25 percent reduction in risk of stroke, myocardial infarction, or vascular death. It is therefore to be recommended in at-risk individuals, such as those who present with TIA.

There is a minor reluctance to operate on patients who are currently taking aspirin therapy because of the increased risk of oozing at the time of surgery and postoperative cervical hematomas, sometimes requiring re-exploration. However, the benefits of aspirin treatment probably outweigh the disadvantages by reducing the risk of deep vein thrombosis and pulmonary embolism.[19]

The 25 percent reduction in risk is relatively modest and should not cause complacency. A similar efficacy for an antibiotic in treating an infection would not be acceptable.

More efficient alternative medical treatments for the prevention of occlusive vascular disease need to be developed.

Particularly in the primary prevention studies, the occurrence of cerebral hemorrhage in subjects treated with aspirin is a cause of some concern. The current recommendation is that since the benefits of treatment are low in low-risk individuals, and since there is a recognized albeit small risk of hemorrhage, it is preferable to delay the use of antiplatelet therapy.[18] Interestingly, antiplatelet treatment seems to be more cardio- than cerebroprotective.

Debate continues about the optimum dose of aspirin. There is still insufficient information about which dose to use in which patient. It is not yet clear, for example, whether a higher dose of aspirin is required for cerebral protection than for cardiac protection. A medium dose (160 to 325 mg/day) has been the most widely used and has the most extensive evidence of benefit.[18]

Most patients taking 300 mg of aspirin a day will have some evidence of an antiplatelet effect, as evidenced by bleeding time or other tests of platelet function. A significant proportion of patients taking less than 100 mg a day will demonstrate no such antiplatelet activity. This does not necessarily mean that the lower doses are ineffective.

The author's current practice is to start patients on 300 mg of aspirin daily. In patients who have a history of indigestion, it is justified to use enteric-coated aspirin. If patients develop indigestion on 300 mg of ordinary aspirin a day, they can be switched to 300 mg of enteric-coated aspirin daily. Alternatively, the dose of aspirin can be reduced to 150 mg and, if necessary, to 75 mg.

Some patients cannot tolerate even tiny doses of aspirin, either because of allergy or because of the resulting indigestion or constipation. In these patients, an alternative antiplatelet agent should be considered.

The main worrying side effect of aspirin therapy is gastrointestinal bleeding. The United Kingdom TIA aspirin trial[9] suggested that gastrointestinal bleeding was much more common in patients treated with 1200 mg daily than in those on 300 mg. However, in some other studies, this dose-related risk of bleeding was not confirmed.

The tendency of aspirin to produce bleeding can be beneficial. It sometimes leads to bleeding from, for example, a bladder or gastrointestinal tumor. This may lead to earlier diagnosis and earlier treatment of such tumors, and possibly improved prognosis. Therefore, when bleeding occurs in patients on aspirin therapy, the existence of an underlying problem revealed by the aspirin should be considered. The bleeding should not automatically be attributed solely to aspirin.

Ticlopidine

Ticlopidine has been shown to be an effective antiplatelet agent.[20, 21] It is certainly as powerful as aspirin—possibly more so—but the evidence is not sufficiently convincing at this stage for it to be recommended as the first-line drug.[22] One problem is that in a small percentage of patients, a reversible leukopenia can occur. It can also have gastrointestinal side effects; in a small proportion of patients, diarrhea can be troublesome.

Dipyridamole

Although dipyridamole has been shown to be an effective antiplatelet agent in the laboratory, the clinical trials have suggested that when used in combination with aspirin (which acts in a different way as an antiplatelet agent), dipyridamole does not confer any extra protection. There are insufficient data on the use of dipyridamole alone to justify recommending its widespread use, but that does not mean that it is ineffective.[18] For the moment, its use is restricted to patients with artificial heart valves who require a combination of an anticoagulant and an antiplatelet agent to reduce the risk of cerebral and systemic emboli. Further evidence is required on the use of dipyridamole alone.

Other Agents

There are insufficient data on sulfinpyrazone and fish oils as antiplatelet agents to justify recommending their use at this time.

CONCLUSIONS

Aspirin can be recommended as a first-line antiplatelet agent in patients presenting with TIAs. It appears to confer a 25 percent risk reduction for stroke, myocardial infarction, and vascular death. In people without significant vascular risk factors and without a history of amaurosis fugax or TIA, the benefits are less, and it may be preferable to delay aspirin treatment because of the risk of cerebral hemorrhage. Aspirin also seems to reduce the risk of deep venous thrombosis and pulmonary embolism in patients undergoing surgery.

Based on the present evidence, the choice of 300 mg of aspirin a day seems reasonable. In the presence of indigestion, enteric-coated aspirin may be used or a lower dose of aspirin may be considered—for example, 150 or 75 mg daily, or possibly on alternate days.

Other antiplatelet agents have not been demonstrated to be significantly better than aspirin in treating TIA patients. In patients unable to take or tolerate aspirin, ticlopidine should be used.

If TIAs continue despite antiplatelet therapy, alternative treatment with anticoagulation should be considered.

REFERENCES

1. Wolf PA, Kannel WB, McGee DL: Prevention of ischaemic stroke: Risk factors. In Barnett HJM, Stein BM, Mohr JP, et al, eds. *Stroke: Pathophysiology, Diagnosis and Management*, Vol 2. New York: Churchill Livingstone; 1986:971.
2. Collins R, Peto R, MacMahon S, et al: Blood pressure, stroke and coronary heart disease. Part 2. Short-term reductions in blood pressure: Overview of randomised drug trials in their epidemiological context. *Lancet*. 1990;335:827.
3. MRC working party: Medical Research Council trial of treatment of hypertension in older adults: Principal results. *BMJ*. 1992;304:405.
4. European carotid surgery trialists' collaborative group: MRC European carotid surgery trial: Interim results for symptomatic patients with severe (70–99%) or with mild (0–29%) carotid stenosis. *Lancet*. 1991;337:1235.
5. Strandgaard S, Olesen J, Skinhoj E, Lassen NA: Autoregulation of brain circulation in severe arterial hypertension. *BMJ*. 1973;1:507.
6. Wallace JD, Levy LL: Blood pressure after stroke. *JAMA*. 1981;246:2177.
7. Wolf PA, Kannel WB, McNamara PM, Gordon T: The role of impaired cardiac function in atherothrombotic brain infarction: The Framingham study. *Am J Public Health*. 1973;63:52.
8. Wolf PA, Dawber TR, Thomas HE Jr, Kannel WB: Epidemiologic assessment of

chronic atrial fibrillation and risk of stroke: The Framingham study. *Neurology (NY)*. 1978;28:973.

9. UK TIA study group: The United Kingdom transient ischaemic attack (UKTIA) aspirin trial: Final results. *J Neurol Neurosurg Psychiatry*. 1991;54:1044.

10. Pearson TC, Wetherley-Mein G: Vascular occlusive episodes and venous haematocrit in primary proliferative polycythaemia. *Lancet*. 1978;2:1219.

11. Challoner T, Briggs C, Rampling MW, Thomas DJ: A study of the haematological and haemorrheological consequences of venesection. *Br J Haematol*. 1986;62:671.

12. Fuller JH, Shipley MJ, Rose G, et al: Mortality from coronary heart disease and stroke in relation to degree of glycaemia: The Whitehall study. *BMJ*. 1983; 287:867.

13. Kushner M, Nencini P, Reivich M, et al: Relation of hyperglycaemia early in ischaemic brain infarction to cerebral anatomy, metabolism and clinical outcome. *Ann Neurol*. 1990;28:129.

14. Smith GD, Song F, Sheldon TA: Cholesterol lowering and mortality: The importance of considering initial level of risk. *BMJ*. 1993;306:1367.

15. Collaborative group for the study of stroke in young women: Oral contraception and increased risk of cerebral ischemia or thrombosis. *N Engl J Med*. 1973; 288:871.

16. Wolf PA, Kannel WB, Verter J: Current status of risk factors for stroke. *Neurol Clin*. 1983;1:317.

17. Kannel WB, Wolf PA: Epidemiology of cerebrovascular disease. In Ross Russell RW, ed. *Vascular Disease of the Central Nervous System*. London: Churchill Livingstone; 1983:1.

18. Antiplatelet trialists' collaboration: Collaborative overview of randomised trials of antiplatelet treatment. Part 1. Prevention of death, myocardial infarction and stroke by prolonged antiplatelet therapy in various categories of patients. *BMJ*. 1994;308:81.

19. Antiplatelet trialists' collaboration: Collaborative overview of randomised trials of antiplatelet treatment. Part 3. Reduction in pulmonary embolism and venous thrombosis by antiplatelet prophylaxis among surgical and medical patients. *BMJ*. 1994;308:235.

20. Hass WK, Easton JD, Adams HP: A randomised trial comparing ticlopidine hydrochloride with aspirin for the prevention of stroke in high risk patients. *N Engl J Med*. 1989;321:501.

21. Gent M, Blakely JA, Easton JD, et al: The Canadian American ticlopidine study (CATS) in thrombo-embolic stroke. *Lancet*. 1989;1:1215.

22. Warlow CP: Ticlopidine, a new antithrombotic drug, but is it better than aspirin for long term use? *J Neurol Neurosurg Psychiatry*. 1990;53:185.

Immediate and Long-Term Results of Carotid Endarterectomy in Reducing Stroke Risk in Patients with Hemispheric and Monocular Transient Ischemic Attack

JAMES T. ROBERTSON

Carotid endarterectomy for significant carotid stenosis or ulceration is a logical operation for the prevention of transient monocular blindness, transient cerebral ischemia, and small strokes.[1, 2] Use of the procedure has been severely criticized regarding its efficacy and appropriateness.[3–6] In 1984, it was the most commonly performed peripheral vascular procedure.[4, 7] Approximately 107,000 cases were done in 1985 but, subsequent to criticism concerning the indications for surgery and the associated morbidity and mortality rates, the number of cases was reduced to approximately 70,000 in 1990. Currently, approximately 70,000 carotid endarterectomies are performed annually. Whisnant and colleagues[8] estimate that 35,000 new patients with carotid ischemic events become candidates for carotid endarterectomy annually. If one half of the 70,000 procedures are performed in asymptomatic patients, then their estimate is accurate.

Several authors prior to 1991 opined that the risk of morbidity, stroke, and death from the procedure was conservatively in the 10 percent range.[3] Medical guidelines indicated that surgical mortality rates of less than 1 percent and stroke-related morbidity of less than 3 percent in patients with transient ischemic attacks and stroke were acceptable risks. An American Heart Association Consensus recommended that the combined morbidity and mortality of carotid endarterectomy should not exceed 3 percent for asymptomatic lesions, 5 percent for transient ischemic episodes, 7 percent for ischemic stroke, and 10 percent for recurrent carotid stenosis. In addition, the 30-day mortality rate from all causes related to endarterectomy should not exceed 2 percent. At the same time, institutional audits were recommended to ensure surgical adherence to these recommendations.

BENEFIT OF SURGERY OVER MEDICAL THERAPY

In 1987, the North American Symptomatic Carotid Endarterectomy Trial (NASCET) was begun.[9, 10] At the International Stroke Conference of the American Heart Association in February of 1991, H. J. M. Barnett, the principal investigator, reported on an interim analysis of approximately 600 patients who had been randomly assigned to receive either medical or surgical therapy for transient ischemic attack or a mild nondisabling stroke, ipsilateral to a 70 to 90 percent narrowing of the internal carotid artery.[10] After carotid endarterectomy, this group of symptomatic patients with high-grade carotid stenosis demonstrated a major reduction in fatal and nonfatal ipsilateral carotid stroke, despite perioperative risk of any stroke or death from any cause. When data concerning perioperative morbidity and mortality rates or

their 32-day equivalent in the medical group were included in the analysis, over 26 percent of the medical group but only 9 percent of the surgical patients were shown to have experienced fatal or nonfatal ipsilateral stroke at 24 months. This represented an absolute reduction in risk for stroke of 17 percent and a relative risk reduction of 65 percent in favor of surgical treatment.[9] Carotid endarterectomy was beneficial in the prevention of any stroke of any severity in any territory. The European study headed by Charles Warlow produced similar results.[11] It can therefore be stated without equivocation that the only proven indication for carotid endarterectomy in a patient with transient cerebral ischemic attacks or a small stroke is 70 percent or greater stenosis ipsilateral to the site of the event.

Generally, most vascular surgeons and many neurologic surgeons are convinced that carotid endarterectomy has now been proved to be beneficial and that no further studies are indicated to selectively determine the role of the procedure in patients with symptoms of transient ischemia or small cerebral infarction. In addition, carotid endarterectomy may be indicated in patients with a 50 percent carotid stenosis or a large ulcerated plaque in conjunction with ipsilateral transient ischemic attacks, a reversible ischemic neurologic deficit, small stroke, or selected recurrent symptomatic carotid stenosis.[12–16] Occasionally, patients may require surgery for progressive stroke, progressive retinal ischemia, acute carotid occlusion, symptomatic carotid stump syndrome, global cerebral ischemia due to multiple large-vessel occlusive disease, selected tandem lesions in which the proximal stenosis is greater than the distal, and certain cases of symptomatic carotid dissection and carotid aneurysm.

The Veterans Administration (VA) Carotid Endarterectomy and Prevention of Cerebral Ischemia and Symptomatic Carotid Stenosis Trial[2] was terminated prematurely after the publication of the NASCET and European Carotid Surgery Trial results. The VA study demonstrated that a selected cohort of men with symptoms of cerebral or retinal ischemia in the distribution of the high-grade internal carotid artery stenosis (50% or greater) was best treated by carotid endarterectomy. Statistical rates for primary endpoints in the nonsurgical group exceeded those previously reported from prior prospective and retrospective studies. In this trial, stroke or crescendo transient ischemic attacks were noted in 6 percent of nonsurgical patients at 1 month and 19 percent at a mean of 1 year after initial presentation. In comparison, symptomatic patients who received aspirin in prior prospective multicenter trials had annual stroke rates ranging from 3 to 7 percent. Nonsurgical patients in the original carotid endarterectomy trial had an approximate annual stroke rate of 6.7 percent. The stroke risk in the VA group was greatest in temporal proximity to the presenting event. The NASCET and the European Carotid Surgery Trial demonstrated high rates of cerebral ischemia in nonsurgical patients similar to the rates observed in the VA trial. These results negated previous opinions about the risk of symptomatic carotid stenosis.

PATIENT SELECTION

Two major multicenter retrospective reviews from 1981 emphasize that surgical and medical skills have improved. Particularly, the surgical selection criteria used in NASCET have considerably reduced the risk of negative effects from carotid endarterectomy. Fode, Sundt, Robertson, Peerless and Shields reported a multicenter retrospective audit of 3328 carotid endarterectomies performed during 1981 in 46 institutions. Overall, there was a 2.5 percent risk of transient neurologic dysfunction following surgery and a 6 percent risk of stroke or death. The intrainstitutional combined major morbidity and mortality rate varied from 0 to 21 percent. Institutions with more than 700 beds had a statistically lower incidence of stroke or death. The incidence of stroke or death postoperatively was significantly lower for patients who were operated on for amaurosis fugax or for unspecified reasons. Patients who were operated on for a progressive stroke had a high incidence of stroke, but patients who did not undergo surgery were at greatest risk for stroke. The incidence of postoperative stroke or death was related to the type of arterial repair; vein patch grafting was associated with statistically better results than both fabric patch grafting and primary closure. When all patients who were not monitored during surgery were compared with all patients who had electroencephalographic (EEG) monitoring, a significant statistical difference was found in favor of the EEG group. Among patients who had endarterectomy combined with coronary artery bypass or simultaneous bilateral endarterectomies, there was a statistically significant higher incidence of stroke or death than among those who had unilateral carotid endarterectomy. Since neurosurgeons were the correspondents in this study, the question of bias can be raised. However, this retrospective study based on the cases done in 1981 probably represented a cross section of carotid endarterectomy procedures performed in North America.

In 1988 Winslow and coworkers, from the Rand Corporation, reported on the appropriateness of carotid endarterectomy after developing a list of 864 possible reasons for performing the procedure and asking a panel of nationally known experts to rate the appropriateness of each indication with the use of a modified Delphi technique. Subsequently, on the basis of these ratings, the appropriateness of carotid endarterectomy in a random sample of 1302 Medicare patients in three geographic areas who underwent the procedure in 1981 was determined. This controversial report indicated that 35 percent of the patients had carotid endarterectomy for appropriate reasons, 32 percent for equivocal reasons, and 32 percent for inappropriate reasons. Of the patients who underwent inappropriate surgery, 48 percent had less than 50 percent stenosis of the operated carotid artery. Of all the procedures, 54 percent were performed in patients who did not have transient ischemic attacks in the carotid distribution. Of these procedures, 18 percent were judged appropriate, as compared with 55 percent in patients with

transient ischemic attacks in the carotid distribution. After carotid endarterectomy, 9.8 percent of patients had a major complication (stroke with residual deficit at the time of hospital discharge or death within 30 days of surgery). This high complication rate indicated that the risk would almost certainly outweigh the benefits of surgery as opposed to medical therapy.

LARGE MULTICENTER TRIALS

Salient comments about the European Carotid Surgery Trial,[11] NASCET,[9] and the Symptomatic Trial in the VA Hospitals[2] are warranted. In these multicenter trials, the 30-day combined incidence of stroke and death was 7.5 percent in the European trial, 5.8 percent in NASCET, and 5.5 percent in the VA trial (which excluded one preoperative stroke). In NASCET, if the analysis is restricted to the most serious events for major stroke and death, the rates were 2.1 percent and 0.6 percent, respectively. The perioperative death rate was 3.3 percent in the VA studies and 0.9 percent in the European trial. The benefits from surgery were apparent in both trials from 2 to 4 months postoperatively. This raises the serious question about whether beneficial results in the symptomatic high-grade group could have been reported earlier. Nevertheless, the beneficial surgical results clearly persisted for nearly 3 years of reported observation. Atherogenic risk factors were observed to have a definite effect on stroke occurrence ipsilaterally in the medically treated patient. The proportion of the medical group who experienced an ipsilateral stroke within 2 years was 17 percent in the low-risk group (up to five risk factors), 23 percent in the moderate-risk group (six risk factors), and 39 percent in the high-risk group (more than seven risk factors). The prognosis of the surgical patients did not vary significantly among risk groups and averaged 9 percent at 2 years. The degree of high-grade carotid stenosis, for example 70 to 79 percent, 80 to 89 percent, and 90 to 99 percent, correlated with the degree of risk reduction after surgery. The absolute risk reduction for all ipsilateral stroke at 2 years was 26 percent among patients with stenosis of 90 to 99 percent at entry, 18 percent among those with stenosis of 80 to 89 percent, and 12 percent among those with stenosis of 70 to 79 percent. Similar results were reported from the European Carotid Surgery Trial. Among 778 symptomatic patients with severe stenosis (70 to 99 percent) who were randomly assigned to treatment with carotid endarterectomy or medical care alone, 7.5 percent of the surgical patients had an ipsilateral stroke or died within 30 days of surgery. An analysis of the risks of ipsilateral stroke during the next 3 years yielded an additional risk rate of 2.8 percent for surgical patients, as compared with 16.8 percent for medical patients. The European study concluded that the immediate risk of surgery outweighed any potential long-term benefit in the 374 symptomatic patients with mild stenosis (0–29%). The degree of benefit that individual patients received from carotid endarterectomy was directly proportional to the risk they faced without surgery, and those with the highest risk at entry benefited the most. The original estimates of 4 to 7 percent per year risk of stroke, based on results in placebo trials, substantially underestimated the risk of stroke among symptomatic patients with high-grade stenosis. The risk of stroke at 2 years among medically treated patients was 26 percent for ipsilateral stroke, 28 percent for stroke in any territory, and 32 percent for any stroke or death.

Although these immediate and long-term results from studies of carotid endarterectomy in patients with 70 percent or greater stenosis clearly confirmed the benefit of surgery, the surgeons were selected only after audits of their endarterectomy results confirmed their expertise.[9, 17] If this quality control had not been applied, the perioperative risk for major stroke and death would have been more than 2.1 percent, and the benefit of endarterectomy would be shown to be less.[9] If the rate of major complications had approached 10 percent, the benefits associated with surgical treatment would be in doubt.

EMERGENCY CAROTID SURGERY

A few comments about the value of emergency carotid endarterectomy in the acute treatment of ischemic stroke should be made. Reported studies have not proved the benefit of emergency surgery. Early reports condemned the practice because of the high incidence of death and worsening deficits from either intracerebral hemorrhage or the exacerbation of cerebral edema; however, emergency carotid endarterectomy continues to be performed. Emergency endarterectomy for the obtunded or comatose patient or the patient with a major hemiplegia is contraindicated. As early as 1965, Hunter and colleagues,[18] based on their experience with 21 patients, insisted that emergency endarterectomies be confined to patients who have less than a severe deficit. Such patients improved over the expected natural course of the disease. Patients with severe deficits were not helped by surgery, and frequently their conditions worsened. Clinically, the development of intracerebral hemorrhage was caused by revascularization of an acute stroke and the lack of careful control of blood pressure during the postoperative period.[19–22] Several additional reports have indicated that emergency carotid endarterectomy may be of value in selected patients with acute stroke. Walters and coworkers[23] reported on 64 emergency carotid endarterectomies that were performed either because of clinical indications (acute stroke or crescendo transient ischemic attacks) or because of angiographic indications (presumed acute carotid occlusion, presence of intraluminal thrombosis, or extremely high-grade stenosis usually with a "string sign"). Of the 36 patients who preoperatively were neurologically intact or had mild deficits, 33 patients (92%) were the same or improved postoperatively, and 3 (8%) were worse. There was no mortality. Among the 15 patients presenting with moderate deficits, 12 (80%) were the same or improved after the procedure, but 2 (13.3%) were worse and 1 (6.6%) died of a myocardial infarction. Of the 13 patients presenting with severe deficits, 10 (77%) were the same or improved, and none was made neurologically worse by the operation; however, 3 (23%) of the patients died, and 2 of the 10 who survived had medical complications. Eight of the 13 with severe deficits developed their sudden deficit while in the hospital, and emergency evaluation and operation could be performed. Emergency carotid endarterectomy was safely performed on neurologically intact patients or on patients with only a mild to moderate deficit with either clinical or angiographic indica-

tions. Emergency endarterectomy should only be considered after the onset of a severe deficit when there is hope of completing the procedure within the first few hours of the onset of the deficit. Meyer and colleagues,[24] Goldstone and Effeney,[25] and McCormick and colleagues[26] have reported additional patients.

CONCLUSIONS

The literature fails to render proven indications for emergency carotid endarterectomy. The following conclusions regarding efficacy are proposed:

1. The completely occluded carotid artery can usually be reopened successfully during the first 48 hours after occlusion. If there is retrograde flow in the intracranial portion of the internal carotid artery down to the petrous portion of the carotid artery, the vessel can frequently be reopened regardless of the presumed time of occlusion.

2. Patients with mild or mild to moderate neurologic deficits of recent onset can undergo surgery early after the onset of the deficit with safety, provided that they have a normal level of consciousness, that the computed tomographic scan does not show a large stroke with significant mass effect, and that there is no evidence of disruption of the blood-brain barrier on the enhanced computed tomographic scan. However, it is unlikely that operating on these patients early is better or safer than waiting and operating 4 to 6 weeks later.

3. Patients with crescendo transient ischemic attacks or with a stroke-in-evolution who have only a mild or at most a mild to moderate deficit can be operated on safely and with efficacy.

4. Patients with moderately severe to severe neurologic deficits of abrupt onset should be considered for emergency endarterectomy only when the procedure can be completed within the first few hours after the onset of the deficit; whether these patients fare better with surgery is not known at present but is considered unlikely.

In summary, providing that complications can be minimized, the indications and results of emergency endarterectomy will demand better definition when the concept of "brain attack" and more immediate stroke evaluation become commonplace. Transluminal angioplasty and thrombolysis of acutely occluded arteries are feasible as adjunct treatments in acute stroke care; their efficacy remains to be proved.[27]

REFERENCES

1. Eastcott HHG, Pickering GW, Rob CG: Reconstruction of internal carotid artery in a patient with intermittent attacks of hemiplegia. *Lancet.* 1954;2:299.
2. Mayberg MR, Wilson SE, Yatsu F, et al, for the Veterans Administration Cooperative Studies Program 309 Trialist Group: Carotid endarterectomy and prevention of cerebral ischemia in symptomatic carotid stenosis. *JAMA.* 1991;266:3289.
3. Barnett HJM, Plum F, Walton JN: Carotid endarterectomy: An expression of concern. *Stroke.* 1984;15:941.
4. Dyken ML, Pokras R: The performance of endarterectomy for disease of the extracranial arteries of the head. *Stroke.* 1984;15:948.
5. Warlow CP: Carotid endarterectomy: Does it work? *Stroke.* 1984;15:1068.
6. Whisnant JP, Fisher L, Robertson JT, Scheinberg P: Does carotid endarterectomy decrease stroke and death in patients with transient ischemic attacks? *Ann Neurol.* 1987;22:72.
7. Pokras R, Dyken ML: Dramatic changes in the performance of endarterectomy for diseases of the extracranial arteries of the head. *Stroke.* 1988;19:1289.

8. Whisnant JP, Matsomoto N, Elveback LR: Transient cerebral ischemic attacks in a community. *Mayo Clin Proc.* 1973;48:194.

9. North American Symptomatic Carotid Endarterectomy Trial Collaborators: Beneficial effect of carotid endarterectomy in symptomatic patients with high-grade carotid stenosis. *N Engl J Med.* 1991;325:445.

10. Clinical Alert: Benefit of Carotid Endarterectomy for Patients with High-Grade Stenosis of the Internal Carotid Artery. National Institute of Neurological Disorders and Stroke. February, 1991.

11. European Carotid Surgery Trial (ECST) Collaborative Group: MRC European carotid surgery interim results for symptomatic patients with severe (70–99%) or mild (0–29%) carotid stenosis. *Lancet.* 1991;337:1235.

12. The Asymptomatic Carotid Atherosclerosis Study Group: Study design for randomized prospective trial of carotid endarterectomy for asymptomatic atherosclerosis. *Stroke.* 1989;20:844.

13. Ojemann RG, Heros RC, Crowell RM: Atherosclerosis of the carotid circulation: Evaluation and management. In Ojemann RG, ed. *Surgical Management of Cerebrovascular Disease*, 2nd ed. Baltimore: Williams & Wilkins; 1988;25.

14. Sekhar LN, Heros RC, Lotz PR, et al: Atheromatous pseudo-occlusion of the internal carotid artery. *J Neurosurg.* 1980;52:782.

15. Sundt TM Jr, Whisnant JP, Houser OW, Fode NC: Prospective study of the effectiveness and durability of carotid endarterectomy. *Mayo Clin Proc.* 1990;65:625.

16. Thompson JE, Austin DJ, Patman RD: Endarterectomy of the totally occluded carotid artery for stroke. *Arch Surg.* 1967;95:791.

17. Moore WS, Vescera CL, Robertson JT, Baker WH, Howard VJ, Toole JF: Selection process for surgeons in the Asymptomatic Carotid Atherosclerosis Study. *Stroke.* 1991;1353.

18. Hunter JA, Julian OC, Dye WS, et al: Emergency operation for acute cerebral ischemia due to carotid artery obstruction: Review of 26 cases. *Ann Surg.* 1965;162:901.

19. Bruetman ME, Fields WS, Crawford ES, DeBakey ME: Cerebral hemorrhage as a complication of surgery in carotid artery occlusion. *Trans Am Neurol Assoc.* 1963;88:52.

20. Caplan LR, Skillman J, Ojemann R, et al: Intracerebral hemorrhage following carotid endarterectomy: A hypertensive complication? *Stroke.* 1978;9:457.

21. Gonzalez LL, Lewis CM: Cerebral hemorrhage following successful endarterectomy of the internal carotid artery. *Surg Gynecol Obstet.* 1966;122:773.

22. Heros RC, Nelson PB: Intracerebral hemorrhage after microsurgical cerebral revascularization. *Neurosurgery.* 1980;6:371.

23. Walters BB, Ojemann RG, Heros RC: Emergency carotid endarterectomy. *J Neurosurg.* 1987;66:817.

24. Meyer FB, Sundt TM Jr, Piepgras DG, et al: Emergency carotid endarterectomy for patients with acute carotid occlusion and profound neurological deficits. *Ann Surg.* 1986;203:82.

25. Goldstone J, Effeney DJ: The role of carotid endarterectomy in the treatment of acute neurologic deficits. *Prog Cardiovas Dis.* 1980;22:415.

26. McCormick PW, Spetzler RF, Bailes JE, et al: Thromboendarterectomy of the symptomatic occluded internal carotid artery. *J Neurosurg.* 1992;76:752.

27. Brown MM, Butler P, Gibbs J, et al: Feasibility of percutaneous transluminal angioplasty for carotid artery stenosis. *J Neurol Neurosurg Psychiatry.*

SUGGESTED READING

Donaldson MC, Drezner AD: Surgery for acute carotid occlusion: Therapy in search of predictability. *Arch Surg.* 1983;118:1266.

Mentzer RM Jr, Finkelmeier BA, Crosby IK, et al: Emergency carotid endarterectomy for fluctuating neurologic deficits. *Surgery.* 1981;89:60.

Rob CG: Operation for acute completed stroke due to thrombosis of the internal carotid artery. *Surgery.* 1969;65:862.

Shueart WA, Garrido E: Reopening some occluded carotid arteries. Report of four cases. *J Neurosurg.* 1976;45:442.

Immediate and Long-Term Results of Carotid Endarterectomy in Reducing Recurrent Stroke Risk in Patients with Prior Hemispheric Stroke

RICHARD L. FEINBERG and HUGH H. TROUT III

In the 40 years since the first report of successful surgical reconstruction of the carotid bifurcation for symptomatic atherosclerotic occlusive disease,[1] carotid endarterectomy (CEA) has been the subject of much scrutiny and continuing controversy. Large, multi-institutional, prospective, randomized clinical trials have now eliminated any remaining questions regarding the efficacy of CEA in reducing stroke risk among patients suffering from transient ischemic attacks (TIAs) who have documented high-grade (ie, greater than 70%) stenosis of the ipsilateral internal carotid artery.[2, 3] Similarly, prospective randomized clinical trials are currently under way to determine the efficacy of CEA in reducing the risk of stroke among patients with asymptomatic occlusive disease of the carotid bifurcation.[4, 5]

Although the efficacy of CEA in reducing future stroke risk among patients with significant bifurcation occlusive disease and prior hemispheric stroke who have made a good recovery is commonly accepted, it has not, to date, been specifically addressed in any prospective controlled trial. Furthermore, given current practical considerations, it is unlikely that any such randomized comparison between CEA and best medical therapy for this group of patients will occur in the near future. Consequently, the rationale for the continued use of CEA to reduce the incidence of recurrent stroke in selected patients with prior stroke and hemodynamically significant carotid bifurcation atherosclerosis must rely on a reasoned appraisal of the most reliable data from applicable contemporary series and comparison with the best available data regarding the natural history of ischemic stroke. Recognizing the methodologic and analytic shortcomings inherent in this type of analysis, we endeavor in this chapter to establish whether the use of CEA in selected patients with prior ischemic stroke is supported by the best available data.

The appropriateness of the performance of CEA in patients who have had prior cerebral infarction was initially questioned as a result of several early reports that described prohibitive rates of early postoperative hemorrhagic infarction and death in patients subjected to operation.[6–8] It is important to note, however, that most of the patients reported in these series had experienced acute, severe neurologic deficits in the period shortly before surgery, and many had poorly controlled hypertension as a complicating factor. These reports are of primarily historical interest and account for the early discrediting of CEA as an operation for patients with established stroke. Although the past 3 decades have witnessed an evolution in the understanding of the pathophysiology of the microvascular changes occurring within the cerebral bed following acute ischemic infarction, the use of CEA in the setting of acute cerebral infarction is still highly controversial and will not be considered further in this discussion. The remainder of this chapter concerns the role of CEA in patients with prior stable infarction who have subsequently recovered satisfactorily, with only mild to moderate residual deficit.

The initial questions to be considered in assessing the appropriateness of CEA in patients with prior fixed stroke with good recovery are whether the procedure can be performed with acceptable perioperative morbidity and mortality, and whether these rates are comparable to those for patients undergoing surgery with TIA as an indication. Table 67–1 summarizes several recent series from various centers reporting experience with CEA performed in patients with prior fixed stroke.[9–16] These series have been chosen for analysis because of their relative currency (with one exception, they have been performed or reported in the 1980s or 1990s) and because they specifically address the subgroup of patients operated on for prior ischemic stroke. For historical perspective, and because of the large number of cases accumulated, the 1970 report by Thompson and coworkers[9] is included. Perioperative morbidity, defined for the purposes of this analysis as the occurrence of a new minor or major permanent neurologic deficit in either the ipsilateral or contralateral hemisphere within 30 days of the procedure, ranges from 0 to 4.8 percent among these series. Combined morbidity and mortality rates from these same series, totaling 830 CEAs, range from 2.8 to 10.3 percent. These results generally fall well within the range recommended by the ad hoc committee on carotid surgery standards of the Stroke Council of the American Heart Association for CEA performed for prior stroke (ie, less than or equal to 7%).[17] Most of these series, in fact, report combined morbidity and mortality rates within the range considered acceptable (less than 5%) for CEA performed for the indication of prior TIA.

Thompson and colleagues,[9] as part of their larger retrospective review of 748 CEAs performed between 1957 and 1970, reported a perioperative stroke incidence of 4.2 percent among 262 patients undergoing CEA for prior ischemic stroke. Several of the perioperative strokes were fatal, resulting in a 6.1 percent perioperative mortality rate—excessive by current standards. These authors noted, however, that 11 of the 16 operative deaths in this group occurred early in their experience and were among patients operated on emergently for acute profound strokes. They concluded that CEA should not be performed on patients with acute profound strokes and adopted this policy during the latter portion of their reported experience. Eliminating these early errors in patient selection results in an adjusted perioperative mortality rate of 1.9 percent for these authors in patients with prior stable ischemic strokes, and a combined operative morbidity and mortality rate of 6.1 percent in such patients.

As part of their series of 456 consecutive CEAs performed

TABLE 67–1. Thirty-Day Morbidity and Mortality of Carotid Endarterectomy Performed for Prior Fixed Hemispheric Infarction

Study*	Year	Patients, n	Stroke, n (%)	Death, n (%)	Morbidity and Mortality, n (%)
Thompson et al[9]	1970	262	11 (4.2)	16 (6.1)	27 (10.3)
Bardin et al[10]	1982	127	5 (3.9)	4 (3.1)	9 (7.0)
Whittemore et al[11]	1984	28	0 (0)	1 (3.5)	1 (3.5)
McCullough et al[12]	1985	59	2 (3.4)	1 (1.7)	3 (5.1)
Rosenthal et al[13]	1988	104	5 (4.8)	2 (1.9)	7 (6.7)
Healy et al[14]	1989	36	1 (2.8)	0 (0)	1 (2.8)
Piotrowski et al[15]	1990	129	3 (2.3)	2 (1.6)	5 (3.9)
Makhoul et al[16]	1993	85	4 (4.7)	0 (0)	4 (4.7)
Total		830	31 (3.7)	26 (3.1)	57 (6.8)
Total (1984–93)		441	15 (3.4)	6 (1.4)	21 (4.8)

*For full bibliographic information, see reference list at end of chapter.

between 1970 and 1979, Bardin and associates[10] reported perioperative strokes in five (3.9%) and mortality in four (3.1%) of 127 patients operated on after a previous completed stroke. After assessing the subsequent course of these patients on long-term follow-up, these authors questioned the efficacy of CEA for stroke risk reduction in this category of patients. Yet their combined perioperative morbidity and mortality rate of 7.0 percent must be considered to be within the range generally held to be acceptable for this subgroup of patients. In a retrospective review of 28 patients undergoing CEA at the Brigham and Women's Hospital at a mean of 11 days following the occurrence of a small fixed hemispheric stroke, Whittemore and coworkers[11] reported no new neurologic deficits and one death in the perioperative period, for a combined morbidity and mortality rate of 3.5 percent. McCullough and colleagues[12] documented two perioperative strokes and one death (5.1% combined morbidity and mortality) among 59 patients undergoing CEA with prior stable stroke as the indication. Eighteen of their patients had continuing evidence of transient cerebral ischemia in the ipsilateral distribution during the period immediately preceding operation.

Rosenthal and associates,[13] in a 10-year review of 253 patients suffering either stroke or reversible ischemic neurologic deficit, demonstrated a 4.8 percent incidence of perioperative stroke and a combined morbidity and mortality rate of 6.7 percent among the subgroup of 104 patients with documented stroke who underwent CEA. The reports of Healy, Piotrowski, and Makhoul and their coworkers provide additional data suggesting that CEA can be performed safely in patients with prior stable stroke (see Table 67–1).[14–16]

The collated results from these eight series demonstrate a 30-day perioperative stroke incidence of 3.7 percent and a perioperative mortality rate of 3.1 percent for a combined morbidity and mortality of 6.8 percent. Furthermore, if one considers only the six most recent reports (ie, those published within the past 10 years), thus eliminating the excessive mortality figures included in the earliest series, the net result is a total of 441 CEAs with cumulative perioperative stroke and death rates of 3.4 percent and 1.4 percent, respectively.

Having established that CEA can be performed safely in patients with stable prior hemispheric stroke with acceptable short-term morbidity and mortality risk, we must now inquire as to the durability of cerebral protection afforded by

successful CEA in this cohort of patients. Before undertaking this analysis, however, two points must be emphasized: First, it is of primary importance in the assessment of the long-term results of CEA that a distinction be made between central neurologic ischemic events occurring *ipsilateral* to the operated carotid artery during the follow-up period and those occurring in other distributions. Although CEA, when performed successfully, may confer some partial protective effect on the contralateral cerebral hemisphere, it should primarily be expected to reduce the incidence of subsequent *ipsilateral* ischemic stroke. Second, the calculation of subsequent long-term ipsilateral stroke rates ideally should be tabulated by the life table method, in accordance with the recommendations of the ad hoc committee on reporting standards of the Society for Vascular Surgery and the North American chapter of the International Society for Cardiovascular Surgery.[18] This method affords the most reliable means of accounting for the large proportion of patients in such series who, because of intercurrent death from extracerebral cardiovascular causes, are eventually lost to analysis before complete follow-up can be obtained. Unfortunately, there is great variability—among even the more recent series cited earlier—in the reporting methods employed for assessing the efficacy of CEA in reducing the long-term risk of recurrent stroke. Table 67–2 summarizes the long-term results of CEA with regard to recurrent stroke risk among these selected series reporting patients operated upon for prior stroke.[9–16, 19] It should be noted that the incidences of subsequent stroke reported by the Thompson and Bardin groups (1.5 and 2.9% per year, respectively) represent overall stroke occurrence rates; there was no distinction in either of these reports between ipsilateral and contralateral neurologic endpoints. And although the reports by the Whittemore and McCullough groups are specific in detailing the incidence of ipsilateral strokes during the follow-up period, the admirably low stroke recurrence rates reported (3.8% at 2 years and 3.4% at 4 years, respectively) are tabulated as crude stroke rates rather than by the life table method. As a result, a slight underestimation of recurrent stroke incidence is likely in these reports, and comparison with other contemporary series is rendered more difficult.

The five most recent of the series summarized in Table 67–2 all employ the life table method in analyzing the long-term risk of recurrent stroke, and each specifically assesses ipsilateral stroke as a distinct endpoint. For the 434 patients

TABLE 67–2. Long-Term Results of Carotid Endarterectomy Performed for Prior Fixed Hemispheric Infarction

Study*	Year	Patients, n	Follow-Up, mo	Method	Subsequent Stroke Rate, %/yr	Ipsilateral Stroke Rate, %/yr
Thompson et al[9]	1970	262	6–156	crude	1.5 (20 @ 13)	NA
Bardin et al[10]	1982	127	56†	life table	2.9 (14.5 @ 5)	NA
Whittemore et al[11]	1984	28	6–108	crude	NA	1.9 (3.8 @ 2)
McCullough et al[12]	1985	59	42†	crude	NA	0.9 (3.4 @ 4)
Hertzer and Arison[19]	1985	80	120–168	life table	3.1 (31 @ 10)	1.1 (11 @ 10)
Rosenthal et al[13]	1988	104	12–120	life table	NA	3.2 (16 @ 5)
Healy et al[14]	1989	36	NA	life table	NA	6.2 (24.8 @ 4)
Piotrowski et al[15]	1990	129	0–99	life table	1.8 (9 @ 5)	1.3 (6.5 @ 5)
Makhoul et al[16]	1993	85	1–130	life table	NA	1.6 (14 @ 9)

*For full bibliographic information, see reference list at end of chapter.
†Mean.
NA, information not available.

undergoing CEA for prior fixed stroke in these five series, long-term cumulative ipsilateral recurrent stroke rates range from 1.1 percent per year in the report by Hertzer and Arison[19] (which contains the longest follow-up reported to date) to 6.2 percent per year reported by Healy and coworkers,[14] whose 36 patients constitute the smallest cohort among these series. Presumably, the actual incidence of recurrent stroke following CEA for prior hemispheric infarction lies somewhere within this range, perhaps closer to 2.7 percent per year, the arithmetic mean of the cumulative long-term annual ipsilateral stroke rates reported in these five series.

In order to determine whether the above-mentioned perioperative stroke and death rates and the long-term cumulative ipsilateral stroke incidence following CEA in patients with prior fixed hemispheric neurologic deficits represent an improvement over the natural course of the disease, it is essential to attempt to estimate the incidence and severity of recurrence in patients who have not had surgery. Unfortunately, a direct comparison between natural history studies and the results of contemporary series of CEA for prior stroke is made difficult by the fact that few, if any, natural history studies employ actuarial analysis of subsequent cerebral ischemic events; the territory of subsequent strokes is often not documented; and the presence or degree of atherosclerotic occlusive disease in the carotid arteries is seldom described. Thus, at best, these reports offer a crude estimation of the incidence of subsequent stroke (from all causes), in any or all territories, following an initial stroke that may or may not have resulted from a hemodynamically significant ipsilateral carotid bifurcation lesion.

As a result, it is difficult to extrapolate from the available natural history data to the population of patients with which we are concerned (ie, patients sustaining discrete, stable hemispheric strokes with arteriographically proven, ipsilateral, hemodynamically significant carotid artery stenosis). Table 67–3 depicts the rates of recurrent stroke from several series reporting on the results of medical therapy in patients following ischemic stroke. A review of the data from these and other studies[20–31] reveals two important points: (1) patients surviving an ischemic stroke have a high rate of recurrent stroke (5–20% per year), and (2) recurrent stroke carries a higher rate of significant morbidity and mortality in this group of patients than would be expected based on the severity of the initial stroke. Even if we consider only the data from the more recent series—assuming that they

reflect the results of the best medical therapy currently available—it is apparent that the incidence of recurrent stroke remains roughly 7 to 9 percent per year with nonoperative treatment following an initial ischemic stroke. In the Swedish cooperative study,[31] the only prospective, randomized, double-blind trial of the comparative efficacy of aspirin versus placebo in reducing the incidence of recurrent stroke among survivors of a prior ischemic cerebral infarction, 253 patients were randomly assigned to receive aspirin and 252 were randomly assigned to receive placebo. Of the 176 patients who remained in the aspirin group for the full 2-year follow-up period of this study, 32 developed recurrent cerebral infarction, for an annual stroke recurrence rate of 9.1 percent per year. This was statistically indistinguishable from the 171 patients remaining in the placebo group, for whom the annual stroke recurrence rate was 9.4 percent per year. Furthermore, the authors of this study conceded that patients at some of the participating centers underwent angiography and were treated outside of the study (either with CEA or with formal anticoagulation) if hemodynamically significant stenosis of the extracranial carotid arteries was identified. Consequently, the stroke recurrence rates from this study are likely to reflect a population with lesser degrees of carotid stenosis and, as such, probably underestimate the actual incidence of recurrent stroke in the patients under consideration here: those with prior cerebral infarction

TABLE 67–3. Recurrence Rates for Ischemic Stroke Based on Studies of Natural History with Best Medical Therapy

Study*	Year	Stroke Recurrence Rate, %/yr
Baker et al[20]	1968	7
Robinson et al[21]	1968	21
Acheson and Hutchinson[22]	1971	13
Matsumoto et al[23]	1973	4
Beevers et al[24]	1973	4–14
HSCSG[25]	1974	6
Sacco et al[26]	1982	5–8
Swedish Cooperative[31]	1987	9
CATS[30]	1989	8–11
NASCET[3]	1991	13†
Tass[29]	1992	5

*For full bibliographic information, see reference list at end of chapter.
†Includes patients with transient ischemic attacks without prior stroke.

and high-grade ipsilateral carotid occlusive disease. In the Canadian American Ticlopidine Study (CATS),[30] a randomized, double-blind, placebo-controlled trial of the antiplatelet agent ticlopidine among 1053 patients with recent ischemic cerebral infarction, the annual event rate for fatal and nonfatal recurrent stroke was 7.8 percent per year for the treatment group and 11.4 percent per year for the control group. A recent postcompletion analysis of the subgroup of 927 patients with previous ischemic infarction from the Ticlopidine Aspirin Stroke Study (TASS)[29] revealed a cumulative 14.2 percent incidence of recurrent fatal or nonfatal stroke at 3 years among patients treated with ticlopidine (4.7% per year); the 3-year cumulative recurrent stroke rate among patients in the aspirin group was 16.0 percent (5.3% per year). Absent from both the CATS and the TASS reports is any information regarding the presence or severity of occlusive disease of the carotid bifurcation ipsilateral to the qualifying stroke in the patients studied; thus, the suitability of using the stroke recurrence rates reported in these studies as controls against which to judge the results of CEA is questionable at best.

Although, to date, no prospective randomized study has been designed and conducted specifically to address the comparative efficacy of CEA plus best medical therapy versus medical therapy alone for the subset of patients with prior fixed hemispheric stroke and carotid bifurcation stenosis, data reported from the North American Symptomatic Carotid Endarterectomy Trial (NASCET)[3] and the European Carotid Surgery Trial (ECST)[2] offer additional, albeit indirect, support for the effectiveness of CEA in this patient cohort.

Among the 659 patients with high-grade carotid stenosis reported in the NASCET in 1991, 31 percent of the medically treated patients and 33 percent of those undergoing CEA had documented prior hemispheric infarction. Although data from these two groups were not specifically enumerated, the authors stated that, upon analysis of the influence of multiple individual risk factors (including prior stroke) on outcome, there was "no significant difference in event rates among patients with different numbers of base-line risk factors." These authors went on to state that "our original estimates of the risk of stroke (4–7% per year), based on results in placebo groups in trials of antithrombotic drugs, substantially *underestimated* the risk of stroke among symptomatic patients with high grade stenosis." The risk of ipsilateral stroke among medically treated patients in this study (calculated using actuarial methods) was 26 percent at 2 years. Although specific data for the subset of patients with prior hemispheric stroke were not given, it seems reasonable to assume that the actuarial, annualized ipsilateral stroke rate for the 103 such patients in this study would be at least this great.

In a similar vein, a full 50 percent of the 778 patients with severe carotid stenosis reported in the ECST had previous hemispheric stroke as their indication for randomization into the trial. Although the authors of this report found that a history of prior stroke had no adverse effect on the outcome for patients undergoing CEA (compared with patients undergoing CEA for prior TIA), there was a significantly worse outcome among the subgroup of patients with prior stroke who received best medical treatment alone: "In patients allocated no-surgery a logrank analysis of time to ipsilateral

ischaemic stroke revealed three interrelated adverse prognostic factors, other than the degree of carotid stenosis—a history of stroke, residual neurologic signs, and infarction on the pre-randomisation [computed tomographic] scan." Again, although individual data for the surgically and medically treated groups of patients with prior stroke were not specifically given in this report, an interpolation of the analysis follows a logical symmetry with the results from the NASCET study and strongly suggests a beneficial effect of CEA on the course of patients with prior hemispheric infarction and hemodynamically significant ipsilateral carotid stenosis.

In conclusion, a review of the retrospective data from several recent series demonstrates that CEA can be performed safely in patients who have previously sustained a stable, fixed hemispheric stroke and made a good recovery. The subsequent long-term incidence of recurrent stroke in the ipsilateral carotid territory following successful CEA in such patients is acceptably low, approximates that for patients operated on for transient cerebral ischemia, and appears to be superior to the long-term incidence of recurrent stroke for similar patients treated nonoperatively. These conclusions, based on retrospective review and comparison with historical control series, appear to be confirmed by data from the recent prospective randomized trials of CEA, an analysis of which indicates that, among the specific subgroups with antecedent stroke, the beneficial role of CEA over nonoperative therapy in this patient population is real and statistically verifiable.

REFERENCES

1. Eastcott HHG, Pickering GW, Rob CG: Reconstruction of the internal carotid artery in patient with intermittent attacks of hemiplegia. *Lancet.* 1954;2:994.
2. European carotid surgery trialists' collaborative group: MRC European carotid surgery trial: Interim results for symptomatic patients with severe (70–99%) or with mild (0–29%) carotid stenosis. *Lancet.* 1991;337:1235.
3. North American symptomatic carotid endarterectomy trial collaborators: Beneficial effect of carotid endarterectomy in symptomatic patients with high-grade carotid stenosis. *N Engl J Med.* 1991;325:445.
4. Hobson RW, Weiss DG, Fields WS, et al: Efficacy of carotid endarterectomy for asymptomatic carotid stenosis. *N Engl J Med.* 1993;328:221.
5. Asymptomatic carotid atherosclerosis study group: Study design for randomized prospective trial of carotid endarterectomy for asymptomatic atherosclerosis. *Stroke.* 1989;20:844.
6. Rob CG: Operation for acute completed stroke due to thrombosis of the internal carotid artery. *Surgery.* 1969;65:862.
7. Wylie EJ, Hein MF, Adams JE: Intracranial hemorrhage following surgical revascularization for treatment of acute strokes. *J Neurosurg.* 1964;21:212.
8. Bruetman ME, Fields WS, Crawford ES, DeBakey ME: Cerebral hemorrhage in carotid artery surgery. *Arch Neurol.* 1963;9:458.
9. Thompson JE, Austin DJ, Patman RD: Carotid endarterectomy for cerebrovascular insufficiency: Long-term results in 592 patients followed up to thirteen years. *Ann Surg.* 1970;172:663.
10. Bardin JA, Bernstein EF, Humber PB, et al: Is carotid endarterectomy beneficial in prevention of recurrent stroke? *Arch Surg.* 1982;117:1401.
11. Whittemore AD, Ruby ST, Couch NP, Mannick JA: Early carotid endarterectomy in patients with small, fixed neurologic deficits. *J Vasc Surg.* 1984;1:795.
12. McCullough JL, Mentzer RM Jr, Harman PK, et al: Carotid endarterectomy after a completed stroke: Reduction in long-term neurologic deterioration. *J Vasc Surg.* 1985;2:7.
13. Rosenthal D, Borrero E, Clark MD, et al: Carotid endarterectomy after reversible ischemic neurologic deficit or stroke: Is it of value? *J Vasc Surg.* 1988;8:527.
14. Healy DA, Clowes AW, Zierler RE, et al: Immediate and long-term results of carotid endarterectomy. *Stroke.* 1989;20:1138.
15. Piotrowski JJ, Bernhard VM, Rubin JR, et al: Timing of carotid endarterectomy after acute stroke. *J Vasc Surg.* 1990;11:45.
16. Makhoul RG, Moore WS, Colburn MD, et al: Benefit of carotid endarterectomy following prior stroke. *J Vasc Surg.* 1993;18:666.
17. Beebe HG, Clagett GP, DeWeese JA, et al: Assessing risk associated with carotid endarterectomy: A statement for health professionals by an ad hoc committee on carotid surgery standards of the Stroke Council, American Heart Association. *Circulation.* 1989;79:472.

18. Baker JD, Rutherford RB, Bernstein EF, et al: Suggested standards for reports dealing with cerebrovascular disease. *J Vasc Surg*. 1988;8:721.

19. Hertzer NR, Arison R: Cumulative stroke and survival ten years after carotid endarterectomy. *J Vasc Surg*. 1985;2:661.

20. Baker RN, Schwartz WS, Ramseyer JC: Prognosis among survivors of ischemic stroke. *Neurology*. 1968;18:933.

21. Robinson RW, Demirel M, LeBeau RJ: Natural history of cerebral thrombosis: Nine to nineteen year follow-up. *J Chron Dis*. 1968;21:221.

22. Acheson J, Hutchinson EC: The natural history of focal cerebral vascular disease. *Q J Med*. 1971;40:15.

23. Matsumoto N, Whisnant JP, Kurland LT, Okazaki H: Natural history of stroke in Rochester, Minnesota, 1955 through 1969: An extension of a previous study, 1945 through 1954. *Stroke*. 1973;4:20.

24. Beevers DG, Fairman MJ, Hamilton M, Harpur JE: Antihypertensive treatment and the course of established cerebral vascular disease. *Lancet*. 1973;1:1407.

25. Hypertension-stroke cooperative study group: Effect of antihypertensive treatment on stroke recurrence. *JAMA*. 1974;229:409.

26. Sacco RL, Wolf PA, Kennel WB, McNamara PM: Survival and recurrence following stroke: The Framingham study. *Stroke*. 1982;13:290.

27. Sobel E, Alter M, Davanipour Z, et al: Stroke in the Lehigh Valley: Combined risk factors for recurrent ischemic stroke. *Neurology*. 1989;39:669.

28. Homer D, Whisnant JP, Schoenberg BS: Trends in the incidence rates of stroke in Rochester, Minnesota, since 1935. *Ann Neurol*. 1987;22:245.

29. Harbison JW: Ticlopidine versus aspirin for the prevention of recurrent stroke: Analysis of patients with minor stroke from the ticlopidine aspirin stroke study. *Stroke*. 1992;23:1723.

30. Gent M, Blakely JA, Easton JD, et al: The Canadian American ticlopidine study (CATS) in thromboembolic stroke. *Lancet*. 1989;1:1215.

31. Britton M, Helmers C, Samuelsson K: High-dose acetylsalicylic acid after cerebral infarction: A Swedish cooperative study. *Stroke*. 1987;18:325.

CHAPTER 68

Intellectual Function Following Carotid Endarterectomy

STANLEY N. COHEN

For many years, it was believed that dementia was caused by "hardening of the arteries" to the brain. In 1951, Fisher[1] reported a patient with dementia who was found to have a bilateral carotid occlusion. It was suggested that impaired cerebral blood flow might be the underlying cause of the dementia. Other reports published in the 1950s supported this proposal.[2, 3] With the knowledge that the degree of atherosclerotic changes in the brain did not correlate with the degree of dementia of the Alzheimer's type, this concept of dementia had fallen by the wayside. Nonetheless, it had been the experience of many neurosurgeons and vascular surgeons that, following carotid endarterectomy (CEA), patients noted improvement in their subjective ability to think. During the past 2 decades, numerous studies have been performed to investigate and attempt to validate this observation. Many of the data are conflicting and controversial.

In order to understand the problem, several questions must be addressed through clinical studies. What is the effect of normal aging on cerebral blood flow? Do "flow-restrictive" lesions cause sufficient reduction in flow to cause clinically significant decreases in mentation? If they do, does correction of the lesion with CEA restore function to a more normal state? Does CEA prevent further deterioration?

CEREBRAL BLOOD FLOW AND MENTATION

Zemcov and coworkers[4] studied cerebral blood flow (CBF) in cognitively intact normal subjects and cognitively intact subjects with evidence of atherosclerosis using the xenon[133] inhalation technique. These workers found significant decreases in both hemispheres in both the gray and white matter compartments. The areas of decreased flow were primarily in the temporal, parietal, and occipital regions. Although subjects with atherosclerosis demonstrated a trend toward less flow than the age-matched normals, the difference was not significant.

MacInnes and colleagues[5] studied 79 elderly patients, 59 healthy nondemented volunteers, and 20 patients with dementia of the Alzheimer's type (DAT). They compared CBF as measured by the xenon[133] inhalation technique with the results on the Luria-Nebraska Neuropsychological Battery (LNNB). The decrements in the gray matter flow paralleled the decrements in test battery performance. There was a trend toward decreased white matter flow with poorer LNNB results, but this did not reach statistical significance.

Hachinski and associates[6] studied CBF using intracarotid xenon[133] in patients clinically diagnosed as having DAT and multi-infarct dementia (MID). These investigators found that the proportion of fast-clearing tissue was decreased in both groups. The fast-clearing compartment is believed to be a reflection of gray matter activity. The CBF per 100 grams of brain tissue was normal in the DAT group but was decreased in the MID group. The decrease in CBF in the MID group correlated with the degree of dementia. Hachin-

ski and his colleagues stated: "This suggests a close relationship between decrease in CBF and mental deterioration when cerebrovascular disease is the cause." However, the data in these three studies were not sufficient to differentiate whether the decrease in blood flow was the cause of the decreased mental functioning or an epiphenomenon resulting from the decreased brain tissue due to the neuronal loss in normal aging or the multiple infarctions in the MID patients.

Rogers and coworkers[7] went one step further by prospectively studying 181 healthy volunteers over a 7-year period with neurologic examinations, a formal cognitive test battery, Hachinski's ischemic index, and regional CBF with the xenon[133] inhalation technique. Six volunteers developed DAT and 10 developed MID. Subjects who developed MID were found to have had a drop in their CBF 2 years prior to developing symptoms. The DAT subjects had decreases in CBF only after symptoms developed. This supports the idea that the CBF decrease in DAT is secondary to the decreased metabolic demand rather than the cause of it.

Our understanding of CBF and its relationship to cerebral metabolism and brain function has expanded with the use of positron emission tomography (PET). In normal cerebral circulation, the amount of oxygen provided to the brain exceeds the metabolic needs of the brain. Under normal conditions, the brain uses only 35 to 40 percent of the oxygen provided. This leaves 60 to 65 percent to act as a reserve in case of decreased CBF. The relationship between CBF and oxygen consumption ($CMRO_2$) can be measured by the PET scan. This measure is called the oxygen extraction fraction (OEF). In the face of decreasing CBF, the OEF can increase from its normal rate of about 40 percent to about 80 percent before there will be alterations in $CMRO_2$.[8] Only after the OEF reserve is depleted will decreased flow cause ischemic metabolic alterations. Frackowiack and associates[9] used the PET scan technique to study regional cerebral oxygen supply and utilization in dementia. Like the Hachinski and Rogers groups,[6, 7] Frackowiack and coworkers studied both DAT and MID. They found decreased CBF and decreased oxygen utilization in both groups, but the OEF was normal. Since there was no evidence of increased oxygen extraction, the oxygen supply to the brain was adequate for the metabolic needs of the tissue. They concluded that chronic ischemia was not the cause of the dementia in either clinical setting.

Most studies indicate that CBF is decreased in all types of dementia.[10] The thrust of the data is that chronic ischemia due to flow-restrictive lesions does not cause DAT or MID. Can we generalize from that and infer that flow-restrictive lesions do not alter normal cerebral metabolism to cause diminished mental functioning prior to causing traditional ischemic symptoms? Baron and coworkers[11] studied a patient suffering from left hemispheric transient ischemic attacks (TIAs) with a PET scan. The patient showed a decreased CBF and an increased OEF—the misery perfusion syndrome. After an extracranial-to-intracranial (EC–IC) middle cerebral artery bypass, the CBF and OEF returned to normal and the

TIAs disappeared. In a subsequent report by the same group,[12] 12 patients were studied, 11 of whom had ischemic cerebral symptoms and all of whom had at least one carotid artery occluded. As a group, the patients had a significant decrease in CBF and CMRO$_2$ on the side of the planned operation. After EC–IC bypass, the CBF and CMRO$_2$ returned to normal values in both hemispheres. OEF values in the patients as a group were normal both before and after the operation. Some patients had traditional responses in that, postoperatively, the CMRO$_2$ rose with an increase in CBF and a reduction in the OEF. In six patients, the CMRO$_2$ rose with the CBF, without alteration in the OEF. This finding contradicts traditional ideas that, in the face of decreased CBF, the OEF should increase prior to the decrease in CMRO$_2$. This indicates that some patients can have decreased cerebral metabolism due to decreased CBF without increased oxygen extraction. The postoperative improvement indicates that this impaired metabolism is reversible. A third group of patients had a postoperative increase in CMRO$_2$ that was greater than the change in CBF, indicating a paradoxical rise in the OEF.

The data reviewed thus far indicate that the decreased blood flow found in the traditional dementing illnesses does not play a primary role in the etiology of decreased mental functioning. However, other studies in nondemented patients indicate that decreased CBF of a chronic nature can cause impaired metabolic cerebral function as reflected by the CMRO$_2$. This decrease in metabolic function has a complex relationship with CBF and oxygen extraction and is potentially reversible with revascularization. It is unknown whether this potential decrease in metabolic activity has a clinical correlate in level of mental function. The questions that must now be addressed are whether decreased CBF in nondemented patients can cause abnormal mental function and whether a decrease in mental function is reversible with CEA.

CLINICAL STUDIES WITH NO CONTROL GROUP

Williams and McGee[13] prospectively studied 11 patients with symptomatic cerebrovascular disease and documented carotid artery stenosis or occlusion or both. Of the six patients on whom clinical details were available, three presented in coma and two had hemiparesis. Neuropsychological testing included the Wechsler Bellevue Intelligence Scale Form I, Wechsler Memory Scale (WMS) Form I, trail making A and B, and the Rorschach test. The patient group was compared with published results for approximately age-matched subjects. Although no statistical analysis was presented in the article, the authors stated that the preoperative occlusive group "stand[s] up fairly well on intellectual and memorial functions" when compared with published results in normal subjects. The psychological test results from the Rorschach test revealed that the "over-all current psychological functioning of this carotid occlusive group tended toward deficit on the low side of average in most areas." Nine patients underwent CEA. No mention was made of the time elapsed between the neurologic ictus and the surgery. Six of these patients were available for retest at 1 month following the operation. Neurologically, all six had "marked diminu-

tion" of symptoms. Formal postoperative testing on intellectual, memorial, and psychological tests showed slight or no change for better or worse.

Goldstein and colleagues[14] tested six patients pre- and postoperatively. Testing was performed 3 to 4 days before the operation and about 3 months postoperatively. The patients were all suffering from TIAs. Three of the six also had "mild" to "moderate" fixed strokes. The mean duration of cerebrovascular symptoms had been 12 months. Testing included the Wechsler Adult Intelligence Scale (WAIS) and the Halstead-Reitan battery, including a category test, finger tapping, tactual performance test, speech sounds perception test, trail making, and aphasia screening. The WAIS scores were slightly better in the postoperative patients, but the authors thought that the difference could be attributed to a practice effect. The authors found the most outstanding improvement in the category test. Several of the other Halstead-Reitan subtests showed improvement, some of which reached statistical significance.

Perry and associates[15] tested 20 patients preoperatively and 3 months postoperatively using eight subtests of the Halstead-Reitan battery. They also measured blood flow using an electromagnetic flowmeter. In comparison with published results for normal subjects, 13 of the 20 showed "impairment" on the preoperative testing. Postoperatively, the patients showed significant improvement. The preoperative flow impairment did not correlate with the neuropsychological impairment index.

After observing dramatic subjective change in two patients who had bilateral CEA, Horne and Royle[16] studied 16 symptomatic patients before and after CEA using the WMS, six subtests from the WAIS, and the Benton visual retention test. They found that after CEA, their patients showed significant improvement in the object assembly subtest and the WAIS performance scale IQ. The other tests showed no significant change.

Owens and coworkers[17] examined 28 patients undergoing unilateral endarterectomies. Eleven of the 28 had fixed neurologic deficits prior to surgery. Each of the patients was tested preoperatively, 3 days postoperatively, and again 3 months postoperatively. The test battery included Raven's progressive matrices, finger tapping, spatial orientation, arithmetic, vocabulary, short-term memory, and short-interval perception. On each test date, a computed tomographic scan of the brain and a radionuclide brain scan were performed. Two patients suffered clinically and radiographically apparent strokes. Five others were found to have 2 to 4 cm cortically located infarcts in the distribution of the middle cerebral artery without clinically apparent deficit. On analyzing the data, Owens and colleagues found that there were only two groups of patients large enough for statistical analysis: those with significant preoperative stenosis and no postoperative infarct and those with postoperative infarction. Preoperatively, there were no significant differences between the groups. On the 3-day postoperative test, the hand contralateral to the operated side showed improvement in the stenosis group and deterioration in the infarction group. Comparing the two groups, there were significant differences in spatial orientation, short-term memory, arithmetic, and vocabulary. On the 3-month postoperative test, the stenosis group showed no change from the 3-day test. The infarction group showed improvement on seven of the eight tests, with significant improvement on three of the tests. Owens and colleagues concluded that "endarterectomy improves certain aspects of intellectual performance."

Hemmingsen and coworkers[18] studied 14 patients with TIA and 11 patients with "minor stroke." The stroke patients had suffered their ischemic events 4 to 6 weeks before the initial testing. Each of the patients was studied before the CEA, 1 to 2 weeks after the surgery, and again 8 months postoperatively. Four patients suffered postoperative strokes. Testing included word pairs, story recall, visual gestalts, trail making, facial recognition, word fluency, digit span, similarities, and block design. The preoperative testing showed results below normal. The testing performed in the immediate postoperative period showed significantly worse test performance. The delayed retest, however, showed improved test scores. These investigators noted that when the analysis was based on the side of the surgery, the test results that improved were appropriate to the side of the surgery. Right-sided CEA improved scores on visual gestalt and block design. Patients with left CEA showed significant improvement in word pairs, story recall, and trail making. The authors felt that because of the relationship between the side of the surgery and the improvement in lateralized function, the improvement could not be attributed to retest learning effect.

Brinkman and associates[19] studied 14 patients with bilateral carotid disease with greater than 75 percent occlusion. All the patients had been symptomatic with either TIAs or small stable strokes. Each of the fixed deficits had occurred at least 6 weeks prior to surgery. Five patients had TIAs within 1 week of the surgery. Two of the patients suffered postoperative infarction. Neuropsychologic testing was performed 2 days prior to surgery and in the first postoperative week. The test battery included the WAIS, Russell's revised WMS, trail making, and the Reitan sensory-perceptual examination. No significant changes were found in test results when the group data were considered. Patients showing somatosensory evoked potential changes during surgery had significant deterioration in postoperative test scores. These investigators also found that the timing of the ischemic event (ie, a more recent event) was significantly associated with greater postoperative improvement.

Diener and coworkers[20] tested 23 patients before surgery and 10 months after surgery. These workers found intellectual functions slightly improved, mnemonic functions worse, and psychomotor functions and dimension of personality unchanged. They concluded that CEA "on the average does not cause a significant improvement."

Bennion and colleagues[21] prospectively studied 53 patients undergoing unilateral CEA. Eighteen of the patients had prior strokes. Neuropsychological tests included Raven's matrices, finger tapping, spatial orientation, arithmetic, vocabulary, and short-term memory. Testing was performed preoperatively, 3 to 7 days postoperatively, and 3 months postoperatively. There were no significant differences between test periods on finger tapping, arithmetic, vocabulary, and Raven's matrices. There was an early nonsignificant improvement followed by a significant deterioration in spatial orientation and short-term memory. Using a composite score for the entire test battery, there was a significant improvement at 3 days followed by a significant worsening at 3 months. There was very little difference between the baseline studies and the 3-month testing. When the authors looked at the subgroup of patients with greater than 50 percent stenosis preoperatively, there was no difference in the outcome when compared with the group as a whole. Their 3-month postoperative scores showed no significant improvement as compared with baseline scores.

Nine prospective studies have been reviewed. Each assessed the cognitive effects of CEA by comparing the patients' preoperative test scores with the test results obtained in the same patients a period of time following the surgery. The results are summarized in Table 68–1. Three studies examined neuropsychological test results in the first 2 weeks after surgery. One showed a nonsignificant trend toward improvement in those patients who did not have an operative infarction,[17] one showed significant improvement,[21] and one showed worsening.[18] Four studies tested the patients 3 months postoperatively. One demonstrated improvement,[15] two showed mild improvement,[14, 17] and one showed no change.[21] One study with an 8-month follow-up found improvement on tests lateralized to the side of the CEA.[18] On a 10-month follow-up, another study found no significant improvement.[20] There is no consistent pattern to the test results from study to study.

Each of these studies attempted to use the individual patient as his or her own control, comparing the preoperative test scores with the postoperative results. There are obvious problems with this. A patient faced with impending surgery in 1 to 2 days will have a certain amount of apprehension that may interfere with test performance. This preoperative anxiety will not be present at the time of retest months later. There is also a potential retest learning effect. One way examiners could avoid this learning effect is to use different versions of the standardized tests being given. Another method of avoiding a retest learning effect is to get at least three baseline neuropsychological test batteries in order to establish a range of variation for the patient's scores. Unfortunately, some of these studies did not use measures to avoid the learning effect. The combination of changing test conditions, learning effect, and lack of consistency of findings between studies makes it clear that more carefully controlled studies are needed to get a better understanding of this issue.

CONTROLLED STUDIES

In commenting on another study,[22] Blaisdell[22a] documented that the National Cooperative Study of Extracranial Cerebral Vascular Disease had performed "extensive psychological testing" on 1500 patients with cerebrovascular disease. No significant difference was found between surgically treated and nonsurgically treated groups. That study found that "for every patient who improved following operation there appeared to be an equivalent number of medically managed patients who improved spontaneously" (Table 68–2).

In 1968, Duke and coworkers[23] studied 47 patients with symptomatic cerebrovascular disease who were divided into three groups based on their angiographic findings. Patients with no evidence of large-vessel disease were considered to have small-vessel disease (SVD). Patients with large-vessel disease were divided into two groups: those who underwent

TABLE 68–1. Neuropsychologic Testing After Carotid Endarterectomy: Studies Without Separate Control Group

Study*	Patients, n	Timing of Testing	Tests with Improved Results	Tests with Unchanged Results	Tests with Worse Results	Overall
Williams and McGee[13]	6	1 mo	—	WAIS, WMS, trails A & B, Rorschach	—	No change
Goldstein et al[14]	6	3 mo	Halstead-Reitan, category test, finger tap, seashore rhythm	WAIS, speed sounds	—	Mild improvement
Perry et al[15]	20	3 mo	Halstead-Reitan	—	—	Improvement
Horne and Royle[16]	16	Unknown	WAIS performance IQ, object assembly	WMS, WAIS verbal, Benton visual retention	—	Mild improvement
Owens et al[17]	28	3 mo	FT contralateral, spatial perception, SIT perception, STM	FT ipsilateral, Raven's vocal	—	Mild improvement
Hemmingsen et al[18]	25	1–2 wk	—	—	Whole battery	Lateralized improvement
		8 mo	—	—	—	
Brinkman et al[19]	14	1 wk	—	WAIS, WMS, trails, Reitan sensory-perceptual	—	No change
Diener et al[20]	23	10 mo	—	Intellectual, psychomotor, personality	Mnemonic functions	No change
Bennion et al[21]	53	3–7 days	—	Spatial, STM, finger tap, arithmetic, vocal, Raven's	—	Improvement
		3 mo	—	Finger tap, arithmetic, vocabulary, Raven's, spatial, STM	—	No change

*For full bibliographic information, see reference list at end of chapter.

FT, finger tapping; SIT, short-interval perception; STM, short-term memory; WAIS, Wechsler Adult Intelligence Scale; WMS, Wechsler Memory Scale.

endarterectomy (LVD-O) and those who did not have an operation (LVD-N). Dividing the patients between surgical and nonsurgical groups was not done on a randomized basis. Testing included the WAIS, trail making, and finger tapping. The interval between test sessions averaged between 10 and 19 months for the three groups. There was no change in test results for trail making and finger tapping in any of the groups between the two test periods. On the WAIS, the patients with SVD showed significant improvement on retest in all three scales: verbal, performance, and full-scale IQ. The LVD-O patients showed significant improvement on the performance and full-scale IQ. The LVD-N patients did not show significant gain on the retest. It was believed that the improvement seen in the SVD and LVD-O groups could be due to a retest learning effect, which was not found in the LVD-N group. The authors interpreted this as indicating that "surgery did not restore the skills that were in existence before the onset of the disease process, but it did stop the deterioration accompanying the vascular disease."

Haynes and coworkers[22] and King and associates[24] studied 17 patients with symptomatic carotid artery disease. They also chose nine patients about to undergo non-neurologic surgical procedures who had no evidence of carotid stenosis to serve as controls. Presurgical to postsurgical changes in intellectual and cognitive functions were assessed by means of the verbal-comprehension and perceptual-organization Cohen factors from the WAIS. Some patients were also tested with trail making and assessed with the Minnesota Multiphasic Personality Index (MMPI) and State-Trait Anxiety Inventory. The testing was performed 24 hours before the surgery and 4 to 8 weeks after the operation. The patients undergoing endarterectomy showed significant improvement in verbal intelligence, perceptual organization abilities, and trail making. Of interest, the control group showed deterioration in test scores in all parameters. The authors concluded

"that this operative procedure improves cognitive functioning and perceptual motor abilities, lessens the predisposition to experience anxiety, and serves to reduce the severity of some personality changes generally associated with senility."

Matarazzo and colleagues[25] studied 17 patients with symptomatic carotid disease who underwent CEA. They had three "control" groups, including 29 healthy police officers, 35 chronic schizophrenics, and 16 patients with cerebrovascular disease who did not undergo CEA. CEA patients were analyzed both as a group and individually. These authors found that "the changes in neuropsychological functioning following carotid endarterectomy were (1) nonexistent in these 17 patients 20 weeks after their surgery and (2) equally importantly, little different from the changes due to measurement error and other random influences from test to retest which are shown in our 3 reference comparison groups receiving no surgery." They found that most individuals improved on the retest due to the practice effect alone. Although some individuals in the surgical group had a marked improvement from test to retest, the authors found that there were comparable individuals in the other reference groups.

Kelly and associates[26] studied 35 patients who were to have CEA following a TIA. None of their patients had suffered stroke, and none was operated on for asymptomatic stenosis. As a control group, 17 patients with peripheral vascular disease with no evidence of carotid stenosis were studied. The neuropsychological test battery included WMS, Wells-Ruesch Memory for Objects Test, Minitest for Differential Diagnosis of Aphasia–Sentence Production Subtest, Benton Controlled Word Association Test, Peabody Picture Vocabulary Test, Rush-Presbyterian–St. Lukes Test of Stereognosis and Praxis, Spreen-Benton Right-Left Discrimination Test, Stanford-Benet Intelligence Test–Picture Absurdities Subtest, Educational Testing Service Hidden Patterns Test, Gorham Proverbs Test, State-Trait Anxiety Scale, and the Mini-Mult Test. Their operative morbidity and mortality included two strokes and two stroke deaths (test results not included in the data analysis). The preoperative test results showed no group differences between the CEA and control groups. Postoperatively, both groups displayed significant improvement on the Hidden Patterns Test and the Spreen-Benton Right-Left Discrimination Test. These results were believed to be due to a retest practice effect. Only the CEA group was found to have significant improvement of the WMS and the Benton Controlled Word Association Test. On further analysis, the most improvement was found in the younger and better educated patients who had a lower admitting blood pressure and less evidence of other vascular disease.

Bornstein and coworkers[27] studied three groups of pa-

tients: 55 patients about to undergo CEA, 13 having a non-neurosurgical procedure, and 14 with symptomatic cerebrovascular disease who were not having CEA. The CEA patients showed a greater postoperative improvement. All the patients undergoing a right CEA who had a history of stroke showed improvement. The authors stated, ''As expected, stroke patients improve more than TIA patients.''

Boeke[28] compared a group of 14 patients suffering from TIA who had CEA with a control group undergoing cholecystectomy. The patients were tested 24 hours before surgery and 4 weeks after surgery. Five patients were retested 4.5 months postoperatively. The neuropsychological testing included reaction time, 15-word test, recurring faces test, finger tapping, and word fluency. The authors found that both study groups improved on the 15-word test and the recurring faces test. This was attributed to the practice effect. Further analysis revealed no difference between the right and left

TABLE 68–2. Neuropsychological Testing After Carotid Endarterectomy: Controlled Studies

Study*	Patients (Controls), n	Timing of Testing, mo	Tests with Improved Results	Tests with Unchanged Results	Tests with Worse Results	Overall
National Cooperative Study[22a]	1500	—	—	—	—	No change
Duke et al[23]	47	10–19	WAIS-performance and full scale IQ	Trail making, finger tapping	—	No improvement, but prevents deterioration
Haynes et al[22] and King et al[24]	17 (9)	1–2	WAIS-verbal intelligence, perceptual organization, trail making	—	—	Improvement
Matarazzo et al[25]	17 (29, 35, 16)	5	—	—	—	No change
Kelly et al[26]	35	1–2	WMS, Benton controlled word association	Hidden patterns, Spreen-Benton right-left discrimination	—	No change
Bornstein et al[27]	69 (13)	—	—	—	—	Improvement
Boeke[28]	14	1	—	Reaction time, 15-word test, recurring faces, finger tapping, word fluency	—	No change
Parker et al[29]	53	6	—	WAIS, WMS, Halstead-Reitan, sickness impact profile, profile mood states	—	No change
Jacobs et al[30]	12 (12)	—	Buschke's selective reminding, TWR, CLTR, trail making	—	—	Improvement
Van den Burg et al[31]	20 (40)	—	—	Raven's progressive matrices, 15-word test, recurring faces, finger tapping, Minn. manipulating test	—	No change
Greiffenstein et al[32]	30 (15)	2–3	WAIS-performance time-dependent neuropsychological test (right CEA only)	WAIS-R verbal IQ, WAIS-R performance IQ (left CEA)	—	Right CEA: selective improvement; left CEA: no improvement
Meyer et al[33]	8 (18)	36	—	Cognitive capacity screening examination	—	No change

*For full bibliographic information, see reference list at end of chapter.
CEA, carotid endarterectomy; CLTR, consistent long-term retrieval; TWR, total words retrieved; WAIS, Wechsler Adult Intelligence Scale; WMS, Wechsler Memory Scale.

CEA patients. Age was not a factor in test performance. Overall, mental functioning in the CEA group did not improve.

Parker and associates[29] divided 53 patients into three clinical groups: those with symptomatic carotid disease undergoing CEA, those with symptomatic carotid disease not undergoing CEA, and those cerebrally asymptomatic about to undergo unrelated surgical procedures. Patients undergoing CEA were not assigned to their groups by random selection. They were studied with WAIS, WMS, Halstead-Reitan neuropsychological battery, Sickness Impact Profile, and Profile of Mood States. Testing was performed preoperatively and 6 months postoperatively. They found that "the results did not support the conclusion of improved mental status or increased psychosocial well-being in patients who received carotid endarterectomies."

Jacobs and colleagues[30] studied 24 patients with cerebrovascular symptomatology, either TIA or small stable stroke. Twelve had carotid stenosis, which they labeled low flow–endangered brain (LFEB), and 12 had nonstenotic ulcers. Neuropsychological testing included the Buschke selective reminding procedure, including long-term storage, long-term retrieval, consistent long-term retrieval, and total words retrieved. Also tested were trail making, digit symbol substitution, sensory perceptual examination, and finger tapping. The surgical morbidity included one postoperative stroke. The LFEB patients improved significantly on all subtests of memory. On total words retrieved and consistent long-term retrieval, the LFEB patients scored significantly better than did the nonstenotic ulcer patients. On trail making, both groups showed improvement, but the LFEB group showed significantly more improvement.

Van den Burg and coworkers[31] studied 60 patients with the Groningen Intelligence Test, Raven's progressive matrices, 15-word test (immediate and delayed), recurring faces, four-choice reaction time, verbal fluency, finger tapping, and Minnesota Manipulation Test. Twenty patients had symptomatic cerebrovascular disease and underwent CEA; 20 had peripheral vascular disease, with no evidence of carotid disease; and the remaining 20 were asymptomatic normal subjects. The preoperative testing showed motor slowing in patients who had prior stroke. When the effects of prior stroke and education were partialed out, there was no difference among groups in either cognitive or motor testing. The authors believed that this indicated that stenosis by itself does not cause cognitive impairment. There was no difference among groups in the amount of postoperative change. Van den Burg and associates did find that the CEA patients had more subjective improvement than the other groups. They thought that this may be the reason for some surgeons having the subjective impression that CEA causes cognitive improvement.

Greiffenstein and associates[32] studied 45 symptomatic patients who were candidates for CEA. Fifteen underwent left CEA, 15 underwent right CEA, and 15 did not have the surgery. Each was studied with WAIS-R, trails A and B, finger oscillation, symbol digit, and the Buschke selective reminding procedure. In the surgical groups, the patients were tested 1 month to 1 week before the operation and 2 to 3 months after the operation. In the nonsurgical group, the patients were tested 1 week before the scheduled surgery and 1 week after the operation was postponed. Patients in

the right CEA group showed significant improvement in the performance IQ test but not the verbal. This was thought to be due to reduced problem-solving time rather than increased accuracy. The right CEA group also had improved time-dependent neuropsychological testing. The left CEA group and the nonsurgical group did not show significant improvement in any area.

Meyer and coworkers[33] prospectively studied three groups of patients with symptomatic cerebrovascular disease and MID. Eighteen patients received antiplatelet medication and risk factor modification (medical management), 10 received medical management plus EC–IC bypass, and 8 received medical management plus CEA. A cognitive test battery, CBF studies, and neurologic examinations were performed over a 3-year period. If left untreated, each group would be expected to have deterioration in both CBF and cognitive testing, but there was no such decline. Nor did any of the groups show improvement in cognitive scores or sustained improvement in CBF. There was no difference among treatment groups.

Twelve prospective controlled studies have been reviewed. Only the National Cooperative Study was a randomized study in which comparable patients were assigned to each treatment group. Unfortunately, detailed results of the neuropsychological testing in this study were not published, and the data are available only in a sketchy form.[22] However, this study showed no significant improvement in the operative group as compared with the nonoperative group. In each of the other studies, there was nonrandom selection of the control group. Most of the studies chose groups of patients who had no evidence of cerebrovascular disease as their control, and the operative group was selected based on the presence of symptomatic cerebrovascular disease. This can lead to potential problems in the interpretation of results. This is best exemplified by the study of Matarazzo and coworkers,[25] in which the "controls" were younger, healthier, and in other ways very different from the patient group. They found that both patient and control groups had retest improvement, indicating an important practice effect. The studies of Duke and colleagues[23] and Jacobs and associates[30] also documented a practice effect in the surgical groups. However, in their "control" populations of nonoperated cerebrovascular patients, significantly less practice effect was seen. Thus, it may be specious to conclude that the lack of a significant difference between a surgical group and a noncerebrovascular nonsurgical control indicates a negative study.

The comparison of symptomatic cerebrovascular patients with patients with no evidence of cerebrovascular disease raises other problems. As noted in the section on uncontrolled studies, emotional factors may play a significant role. This was emphasized by the results of the study of van den Burg and coworkers.[31] They found that CEA patients had greater subjective improvement than noncerebrovascular patients in the absence of objective evidence of improvement. Another important factor is the role of acute or subacute cerebrovascular symptoms on the initial test results. Does a TIA or a small stable stroke have any negative effect on neuropsychological test results? If it does, then one should expect improvement on retest even in the absence of practice effect. Patients with no cerebrovascular disease undergoing non-neurologic surgery would not have this type of retest improvement. There is evidence that acute and subacute cerebral ischemia does affect neuropsychological testing. Brinkman and colleagues[19] found that patients with more recent cerebral symptoms showed the greatest improvement on retest scores. They also found that patients with intraoperative somatosensory evoked potential changes, indicating possible intraoperative ischemia, showed significant postoperative deterioration in their test scores. Perhaps the strongest evidence that recent cerebral ischemia causes subacute and temporary deterioration in neuropsychological test scores is the study by Owens and associates.[17] They found evidence of postoperative infarction in seven patients (asymptomatic in five). This study affords the rare opportunity of having prestroke neuropsychological test data on carefully evaluated patients. These patients showed dramatic deterioration in their immediate postischemic test results as compared with their baseline testing. More importantly, 3 months after their ischemia, they showed significant improvement in testing, with no intervening surgical procedure. Therefore, studies doing "baseline" testing in a patient who has had subacute symptomatic cerebrovascular disease and repeat testing 2 to 3 months later may be demonstrating improvement as part of the natural history of the disease rather than as the product of any therapeutic intervention.

The data are conflicting and flawed. In an excellent review on the same subject almost two decades ago, Asken and Hobson[34] found that "due to inconsistent results and methodological shortcomings, no satisfactory conclusions can be reached at this point." Although much work has been done in the intervening years, it is clear that there is no final answer on the effect of CEA on intellectual functioning. The ideal study would be prospective and randomized. In addition to using traditional neuropsychological testing, newer objective physiologic tests such as PET scanning and brain mapping should be incorporated. Preoperative neuropsychological testing should be repeated three times in order to establish a true baseline and avoid a retest learning effect. In order to avoid the variable effects of the postischemic period, the patients should be either asymptomatic or cerebrally stable for several months. In order to avoid the effect of age on neuropsychological and physiologic tests, the patients should be from a relatively small, homogeneous age group. With such a study, we will have a more definitive answer on the effect of CEA on intellectual functioning. Until such a study is done, performing CEA to improve intellectual function or to prevent intellectual deterioration cannot be justified.

REFERENCES

1. Fisher M: Senile dementia: A new explanation of its cause. *Can Med Assoc J.* 1951;65:1.
2. Williams C, Bruetsch W: Mental deterioration and occlusion of the internal carotid arteries in the neck. *Am J Psychiatry.* 1958;115:256.
3. Hurwitz JJ, Groch S, Wright I, et al: Carotid artery occlusive syndrome. *AMA Arch Neurol.* 1959;1:491.
4. Zemcov A, Barclay L, Blass JP: Regional decline of cerebral blood flow with age in cognitively intact subjects. *Neurobiol Aging.* 1984;5:1.
5. MacInnes WD, Golden CJ, Gillen RW, et al: Aging, regional cerebral blood flow, and neuropsychological functioning. *J Am Geriatr.* 1984;32:712.
6. Hachinski VC, Iliff LD, Zilhka E, et al: Cerebral blood flow in dementia. *Arch Neurol.* 1975;32:632.
7. Rogers RL, Meyer JS, Mortel KF, et al: Decreased cerebral blood flow precedes multi-infarct dementia, but follows senile dementia of Alzheimer's type. *Neurology.* 1986;36:1.
8. Frackowiak RSJ, Wise RJS: Positron tomography in ischemic cerebrovascular disease. *Neurol Clin.* 1983;1:183.
9. Frackowiak RSJ, Pozzilli C, Legg NJ, et al: Regional cerebral oxygen supply and utilization in dementia. *Brain.* 1981;104:753.
10. Hastak SM, Hachinski VC: Multi-infarct dementia: An expanding concept. In Barnett HJM, Mohr JP, Stein BM, Yatsu FM, eds. *Stroke.* New York: Churchill Livingstone; 1992:799.
11. Baron JC, Bousser MG, Rey A, et al: Reversal of focal "misery perfusion syndrome" by extra-intracranial arterial bypass in hemodynamic cerebral ischemia. *Stroke.* 1981;12:454.
12. Samson Y, Baron JC, Bousser MG, et al: Effects of extra-intracranial arterial bypass on cerebral blood flow and oxygen metabolism in humans. *Stroke.* 1985;16:609.
13. Williams M, McGee TF: Psychological study of carotid occlusion and endarterectomy. *Arch Neurol.* 1964;10:293.
14. Goldstein SG, Kleinknecht RA, Gallo AE: Neuropsychological changes associated with carotid endarterectomy. *Cortex.* 1970;6:308.
15. Perry PM, Drinkwater J, Tayler GW: Neuropsychological tests and carotid arterial disease. *Br J Surg.* 1974;61:922.
16. Horne DJ, Royle JP: Cognitive changes after carotid endarterectomy. *Med J Aust.* 1974;1:316.
17. Owens M, Pressman M, Edwards AE, et al: The effect of small infarcts and carotid endarterectomy on postoperative psychological test performance. *J Surg Res.* 1980;28:209.
18. Hemmingsen R, Mejsholm B, Boysen G, et al: Intellectual function in patients with transient ischemic attacks (TIA) or minor stroke. *Acta Neurol Scand.* 1982;66:145.
19. Brinkman SD, Braun P, Ganji S, et al: Neuropsychological performance one week after carotid endarterectomy reflects intra-operative ischemia. *Stroke.* 1984;15:497.
20. Diener HC, Hamster W, Seboldt H: Neuropsychological functions after carotid endarterectomy. *Eur Arch Psychiatry Neurol Sci.* 1984;234:74.
21. Bennion RS, Owens ML, Wilson SE: The effect of unilateral carotid endarterectomy on neuropsychological test performance in 53 patients. *J Cardiovasc Surg.* 1985;26:21.
22. Haynes CD, Gideon DA, King GD, et al: The improvement of cognition and personality after carotid endarterectomy. *Surgery.* 1976;80:699.
22a. Blaisdell FW: Discussion. *Surgery.* 1976;80:704.
23. Duke R, Bloor B, Nugent G, et al: Changes in performance on WAIS, trailmaking test, and finger tapping associated with carotid artery surgery. *Percept Mot Skills.* 1968;26:399.
24. King GD, Gideon DA, Haynes CD, et al: Intellectual and personality changes associated with carotid endarterectomy. *J Clin Psychol.* 1977;33:215.
25. Matarazzo RG, Matarazzo JD, Gallo AE: IQ and neuropsychological changes following carotid endarterectomy. *J Clin Neuropsychol.* 1979;1:97.
26. Kelly MP, Garron DC, Javid H: Carotid artery disease, carotid endarterectomy and behavior. *Arch Neurol.* 1980;37:743.
27. Bornstein RA, Benoit BG, Trites RL: Neuropsychological changes following endarterectomy. *Can J Neurol Sci.* 1981;8:127.
28. Boeke S: The effect of carotid endarterectomy on mental functioning. *Clin Neurol Neurosurg.* 1981;83:209.
29. Parker JC, Granberg BW, Nichols WK, et al: Mental status outcomes following endarterectomy: A six month analysis. *J Clin Neuropsychol.* 1983;5:345.
30. Jacobs LA, Ganji S, Shirley JG, et al: Cognitive improvement after extracranial reconstruction for the low flow-endangered brain. *Surgery.* 1983;93:683.
31. Van den Burg W, Saan RJ, Van Zomeren AH, et al: Carotid endarterectomy: Does it improve cognitive or motor functioning? *Psychol Med.* 1985;15:341.
32. Greiffenstein MF, Brinkman S, Jacobs L, Braun P: Neuropsychological improvement following endarterectomy as a function of outcome measure and reconstructed vessel. *Cortex.* 1988;24:223.
33. Meyer JS, Lotfi J, Martinez G, et al: Effects of medical and surgical treatment on cerebral perfusion and cognition in patients with chronic cerebral ischemia. *Surg Neurol.* 1990;34:301.
34. Asken M, Hobson RW: Intellectual change and carotid endarterectomy, subjective speculation or objective reality: A review. *J Surg Res.* 1977;23:367.

CHAPTER 69

Carotid Endarterectomy for Global or Nonfocal Symptoms: Indications and Results

WILLIAM H. BAKER

Patients with nonhemispheric cerebrovascular symptoms remain an enigma to physicians. The patient's symptoms are often difficult to evaluate, ranging from specific cranial nerve disorders to giddiness. The vertebral arteries cannot be palpated as can carotid arteries, and vertebral bruits are either hidden or confused with arch lesions or carotid lesions. Carotid emboli may be observed during an ophthalmoscopic examination, but no such window exists in the vertebrobasilar system. Noninvasive evaluation of the vertebral arteries is limited during the usual cerebrovascular examination. Angiography of the carotid system produces sharp contrast images, whereas the vertebral system is often ignored.

Yet despite these obstacles and frustrations, physicians have surmised that posterior circulation symptoms are caused by low flow. Furthermore, isolated series have suggested that carotid endarterectomy, an operation that improves flow globally but not specifically in the posterior circulation, will relieve symptoms in a significant portion of patients. This latter statement is controversial. Thus the purpose of this chapter is to review the setting in which carotid endarterectomy may be of value in patients with global or nonfocal symptoms.

PATIENT EVALUATION

Proper patient evaluation is paramount in obtaining satisfactory results in the treatment of vertebrobasilar insufficiency. In a study by Baker and Barnes,[1] dizziness was present in 60 percent of patients (Fig. 69–1). Other symptoms included specific cranial nerve dysfunctions that are easier to pinpoint. Because there are multiple causes of dizziness as well as these other more specific syndromes, a precise history must be obtained and a physical examination performed. Is the feeling of faintness associated with changes in position, or is a true vertigo present? If the patient has a sensation of faintness or giddiness, the investigator must exclude postural hypotension on physical examination. The patient may be taking vasoactive drugs to counteract hypertension that predispose to this condition. An extensive cardiac evaluation might disclose the presence of dysrhythmias (evident on Holter monitoring) or other causes of reduced cardiac output, such as aortic valvular stenosis (found on echocardiogram) or coronary artery disease (discovered by exercise testing). A hypertensive patient often gives a history of intermittent episodes of dizziness. In addition, the physician must rule out metabolic causes, dizziness secondary to medication, and psychiatric disorders. In patients who appear to have vestibular or auditory pathology on a physical examination, a thorough ear, nose, and throat evaluation is indicated. Perhaps the most important aspect of the evaluation is a complete neurologic examination. Surgery on any artery cannot be expected to reverse permanent neurologic dysfunction, such as an unremitting ataxia.

(A discussion of specific syndromes such as the dysarthria–clumsy-hand syndrome, pure motor hemiplegia, pure sensory stroke, homolateral ataxia, and crural paresis syndrome is beyond the scope of this chapter. The reader is referred to standard neurologic texts for a more complete review of these syndromes.)

The vascular examination emphasizes palpation of the head and neck pulses as well as auscultation over these arteries. The blood pressure should be obtained in each arm in an effort to identify subclavian artery lesions. The pitfalls of the vascular examination are well known and have been clearly elucidated by Barnes and colleagues.[2] In essence, a normal physical examination may miss a severe stenosis or total occlusion. Conversely, a carotid bruit does not necessarily indicate the presence of severe carotid stenosis. For these reasons, most patients with significant symptoms are evaluated noninvasively.

Noninvasive evaluation has evolved so that in most laboratories, duplex scanning is employed routinely. Indirect examination such as the supraorbital Doppler examination or ocular plethysmography is rarely performed. Excellent laboratories are able to identify 90 percent of patients who have significant carotid artery stenosis.

The presence of an abnormal noninvasive examination does not guarantee that a patient with global symptoms will improve if a carotid lesion is found and corrected. In an older review of 53 patients undergoing cerebrovascular Doppler studies for nonhemispheric symptoms, Baker and Barnes[1] found the supraorbital Doppler examination to have no pre-

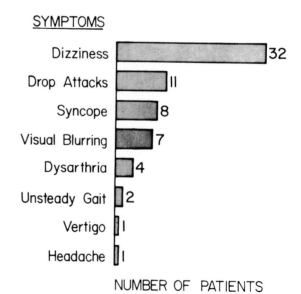

SYMPTOMS

Dizziness 32
Drop Attacks 11
Syncope 8
Visual Blurring 7
Dysarthria 4
Unsteady Gait 2
Vertigo 1
Headache 1

NUMBER OF PATIENTS

FIGURE 69–1. Incidence of nonhemispheric symptoms. (From Baker WH, Barnes RW: The cerebrovascular Doppler examination in patients with nonhemispheric symptoms. *Ann Surg.* 1977;186(2):190; with permission.)

dictive value for therapeutic success or failure. Ouriel and associates[3] reported in 1986 that 72 percent of patients with abnormal ocular plethysmographic studies were relieved of symptoms, compared with 32 percent with normal studies. Not surprisingly, an earlier study by these authors reported increased success in patients with more severe carotid stenosis.[4] The value of isotope brain scanning, computed tomography, positron emission tomography, and transcranial Doppler to predict alleviation of nonhemispheric symptoms following carotid endarterectomy has yet to be established.

A "normal" noninvasive carotid examination effectively eliminates carotid endarterectomy as a therapeutic choice. Yet vertebral, nonocclusive subclavian, and intracranial lesions may still be present. An arteriogram may be required to ferret out these latter lesions.

PATHOGENESIS

Nonhemispheric transient ischemic attacks are generally considered secondary to decreased blood flow in the vertebrobasilar arterial system. In general, the surgical approach to correct this abnormality is aimed at increasing global cerebral perfusion. This can be done by a direct approach to stenotic vertebral arteries, by extracranial-to-intracranial anastomosis to bypass occluded vessels, or by carotid endarterectomy.

The rationale for improving the posterior circulation by carotid endarterectomy is dependent on an intact circle of Willis. In a series of 350 autopsy studies of normal brains, the circle of Willis was normal in 183 (52.3%).[5] The most common anomaly was a stringlike vessel (less than 1 mm outer diameter). This occurred alone or in combination with other anomalies in 96 specimens (27.4%). The most frequent stringlike vessel was the posterior communicating artery. As a single anomaly, this occurred in 28 (8%) of the autopsy specimens. An additional 21 (6%) had bilaterally symmetrical stringlike posterior communicating arteries. In all, stringlike anomalies involved the posterior communicating artery in 22 percent of normal brains. It is also interesting to note that the embryonic origin of the posterior communicating artery from the internal carotid artery persisted in 14.6 percent of the circles of Willis in normal brains. Similar findings were noted by Fisher.[6] In another study, Alpers and Berry[7] looked at the anatomic configuration of the circle of Willis in the presence of cerebrovascular disorders and noted a 38 percent incidence of stringlike posterior communicating arteries in brains with cerebral softness, as compared with 22 percent in normal brains. In this study, it was also noted that the embryonic origin of the posterior communicating artery from the internal carotid artery persisted in 29 percent of cases, as compared with 14.6 percent in normal brains. Absent posterior communicating arteries were rarely encountered in normal brains (0.6%), but there was a 1.5 percent incidence in brains with cerebral softening. Stringlike anterior communicating arteries occurred in 1 to 2 percent of normal brains and in 4 percent of brains with cerebral softening.

Harward and coworkers[8] attempted to correlate these anatomic variables to clinical results in performing carotid endarterectomy for vertebrobasilar insufficiency. They believed that clinical improvement was more predictable when at least one posterior communicating artery was visualized angiographically (92% of patients asymptomatic or improved). Of note is that two-thirds of the patients with nonvisualized posterior communicating arteries also became asymptomatic or improved after carotid endarterectomy. In general, the combination of significant vertebral artery disease and nonvisualized posterior communicating arteries predicted a poor result after carotid endarterectomy. Of interest, a report by Archie[9] demonstrated vertebrobasilar-to-carotid flow despite visualization of the posterior communicating arteries in only 4 of his 12 patients.

Naritomi and colleagues[10] postulate that posterior circulation symptoms occur on the basis of cerebral or brainstem emboli and result in cerebral dysautoregulation. Their conclusions are based on regional cerebral blood flow measurements in patients with symptoms of vertebrobasilar insufficiency. They suggest that vertebrobasilar insufficiency may be initiated by cerebral thromboembolism from the vertebrobasilar system, but thereafter, cerebral dysautoregulation and postural hypotension may be the predominant factors in the subsequent occurrence of transient symptoms. It is postulated that the central neurogenic control mechanisms are injured by the initial thromboembolic event, predisposing the patient to repeated episodes of ischemia due to alterations in perfusion pressure. As time progresses and repeated ischemic episodes occur, the dysautoregulation appears to become more progressive and diffuse. Thus, vertebrobasilar insufficiency may occur purely on the basis of a flow-limiting lesion and subsequent global hypoperfusion, or from an initial thromboembolic event with cerebral dysautoregulation and symptomatic hypoperfusion.

TREATMENT

Once the patient has been thoroughly evaluated and a significant carotid stenosis identified, carotid endarterectomy should be considered. The validity of this approach is debatable. In a review of 18 patients undergoing carotid endarterectomy for nonhemispheric symptoms, McNamara and coworkers[11] noted that 8 of 18 patients (44%) continued to have transient ischemic attacks with patterns identical to those identified preoperatively. They also noted that three of these eight patients developed hemispheric cerebral infarctions during follow-up evaluation. All 52 patients with pure hemispheric symptoms who underwent carotid endarterectomy were free of stroke during a comparable period of time. Recurrent transient ischemic attacks occurred in 15 percent of the patients with hemispheric symptoms. A particularly high-risk group consisted of eight patients with both hemispheric and nonhemispheric symptoms. Only three were free of symptoms at the end of follow-up, which averaged 40 months.

Other authorities, however, report much better results. Rosenthal and associates[12] reported an overall 80 percent improvement rate with a mean follow-up of 59 months in 114 patients undergoing carotid endarterectomy for vertebrobasilar insufficiency alone, vertebrobasilar insufficiency plus transient ischemic attacks, or vertebrobasilar insufficiency coupled with completed stroke. DeWeese and colleagues[13] noted total improvement in only 13 percent of patients undergoing carotid endarterectomy for posterior circulation symptoms. Harward and coworkers[8] reported an improved outcome in those patients undergoing carotid endarterectomy for posterior circulation symptoms, particularly if an angiographically intact posterior communicating artery was demonstrated. They also noted a greater likelihood of vertebral stenosis in those patients who underwent carotid endarterectomy but did not obtain relief of their symptoms. Ford and associates[14] reported complete relief of symptoms in 71 percent of 46 patients undergoing carotid endarterectomy for posterior circulation symptoms without vertebral or subclavian stenosis, compared with symptom relief in 61 percent of patients with concomitant vertebral or subclavian stenosis. Their study made no reference to the integrity of the circle of Willis. Jacobs and coworkers[15] evaluated cognitive function with neuropsychiatric testing in 12 patients with low-flow endangered brains undergoing carotid endarterectomy. When these patients were compared with a matched group undergoing carotid endarterectomy for nonhemodynamically significant lesions, a marked improvement in mental function was noted. The issue of improving mental capabilities by increasing cerebral perfusion is, however, a controversial one.

Vascular surgeons should not have tunnel vision for a "favorite" carotid bifurcation lesion but should consider other arterial lesions as well. Patients with ipsilateral carotid and vertebral lesions may have both lesions fixed during the same operation.[16] A routine carotid endarterectomy is performed; later, through the same or a different incision, the vertebral artery is endarterectomized, bypassed, or reimplanted into the side of the common carotid artery. In patients with multiple lesions, carotid endarterectomy may be combined with extra-anatomic bypass. Finally, in carefully selected healthy patients in whom extra-anatomic bypass is not possible, direct arch reconstruction may be undertaken safely.

Carotid endarterectomy in patients with posterior circulation symptoms is a controversial issue with a wide diversity of clinical results. Careful patient selection is necessary to obtain an acceptable rate of clinical improvement. Evaluation of the integrity of the circle of Willis would logically improve the predictability of operative success. Likewise, if total cerebral blood flow reduction is demonstrated, alleviation of a flow-limiting stenosis should improve low-flow-related symptoms.

CONCLUSIONS

A patient with nonspecific neurologic symptoms should undergo a thorough history and physical examination as well as routine and specialized laboratory procedures in an effort to identify significant carotid lesions. Complete angiography is obtained to clearly delineate carotid stenosis, arch lesions, and vertebral artery lesions. Intracranial views are necessary to identify intracranial arterial pathology. In patients with severe carotid stenosis, carotid endarterectomy can be expected to afford relief to a significant number of them. Operation should be undertaken only by surgeons with proven good operative results, because the indication for surgery is controversial.

REFERENCES

1. Baker WH, Barnes RW: The cerebrovascular Doppler examination in patients with nonhemispheric symptoms. *Ann Surg.* 1977;186:190.
2. Barnes RW, Liebman PR, Marszalek PB, et al: The natural history of symptomatic carotid disease in patients undergoing cardiovascular surgery. *Surgery.* 1981;90:1075.
3. Ouriel K, Rocotta JJ, Green RM, DeWeese JA: Carotid endarterectomy for nonhemispheric cerebral symptoms: Patient selection with ocular pneumoplethysmography. *J Vasc Surg.* 1986;4:115.
4. Ouriel K, May AG, Ricotta JJ, et al: Carotid endarterectomy for nonhemispheric symptoms: Predictors of success. *J Vasc Surg.* 1984;1:339.
5. Alpers BJ, Berry RG, Paddison RM: Anatomical studies of the circle of Willis in normal brain. *Arch Neurol Psychiatr.* 1959;81:409.
6. Fisher CM: The circle of Willis: Anatomical variations. *Vasc Dis.* 1965;2:99.
7. Alpers BJ, Berry RG: Circle of Willis in cerebral vascular disorder. *Arch Neurol.* 1963;8:68.
8. Harward TRS, Wickbom IG, Otis SM, et al: Posterior communicating artery visualization in predicting results of carotid endarterectomy for vertebrobasilar insufficiency. *Am J Surg.* 1984;148:43.
9. Archie JP: Improved carotid hemodynamics with vertebral reconstruction. *Ann Vasc Surg.* 1992;6:138.
10. Naritomi H, Sakai F, Meyer JS: Pathogenesis of transient attacks within the vertebrobasilar arterial system. *Arch Neurol.* 1979;36:121.
11. McNamara JO, Heyman A, Silver D, Mandel ME: The value of carotid endarterectomy in treating transient cerebral ischemia of the posterior circulation. *Neurology (NY).* 1977;27:682.
12. Rosenthal D, Cossman D, Ledig CB, Callow AD: Results of carotid endarterectomy for vertebrobasilar insufficiency. *Arch Surg.* 1978;113:1361.
13. DeWeese JA, Rob CG, Satran R, et al: Results of carotid endarterectomies for transient ischemic attacks—five years later. *Ann Surg.* 1972;178:285.
14. Ford JJ Jr, Baker WH, Ehrenhaft JL: Carotid endarterectomy for nonhemispheric transient ischemic attacks. *Arch Surg.* 1975;110:1314.
15. Jacobs LA, Ganji S, Shirley JG, et al: Cognitive improvement after extracranial reconstructions for the low flow-endangered brain. *Surgery.* 1983;93:683.
16. Malone JM, Moore WS, Hamilton R, Smith M: Combined carotid-vertebral vascular disease. *Arch Surg.* 1980;115:783.

CHAPTER 70

Tandem Lesions of the Extracranial and Intracranial Carotid Artery: Management and Results

JAMES J. SCHULER and D. PRESTON FLANIGAN

The predilection for atherosclerosis to involve certain arteries or portions of arteries preferentially while leaving other areas unaffected has been frequently observed. In the carotid arterial system, both angiographic and pathologic studies have demonstrated that the carotid bifurcation is more frequently involved with atherosclerosis than any other portion of the extracranial carotid artery, and that the intracerebral portion of the carotid artery, especially the carotid siphon, is the most frequent site of intracerebral atherosclerosis.[1–9] The occurrence of carotid siphon stenosis in conjunction with ipsilateral carotid bifurcation stenosis has been termed a tandem carotid lesion.[10–12]

Lesions at the carotid bifurcation are considered surgically accessible; numerous authorities have documented the causal relationship between strokes or transient ischemic attacks (TIAs) and hemodynamically significant stenoses or embolic events, or both, arising from atherosclerotic plaques at the carotid bifurcation. They have likewise demonstrated both the immediate and long-term benefits of carotid bifurcation endarterectomy.[13–21] Lesions in the carotid siphon, however, are considered surgically inaccessible; therefore, until quite recently, very little was known about their clinical significance or natural history. In spite of this lack of information numerous investigators have suggested that carotid bifurcation endarterectomy may be contraindicated in the presence of ipsilateral carotid siphon stenosis because of an increased risk of perioperative stroke.[19, 23–24] Another factor contraindicating the procedure is the possible failure of carotid bifurcation endarterectomy alone to relieve symptoms of TIAs or decrease the chances of stroke.[10, 25–27] The siphon stenosis would remain as a possible cause of either a hemodynamically significant stenosis or a continuing source of emboli to the brain. It is quite probable that these suggestions concerning siphon stenosis were formulated on the basis of clinical impressions or theoretic considerations, or both, since a thorough review of the relevant literature that existed at the time they were made has failed to reveal any studies comparing the results of carotid bifurcation endarterectomy in patients with and without siphon stenosis. In the mid 1980s, two independent studies[11, 12] and, more recently, three additional confirmatory studies[28–30] specifically addressed the question of whether patients with carotid tandem lesions are at an increased risk of stroke or will fail to experience short- or long-term relief of symptoms following carotid bifurcation endarterectomy alone. The results of these studies are discussed in detail later in this chapter and will serve as the basis for a rational plan of management for patients with carotid tandem lesions.

TANDEM LESIONS: ANATOMY AND PATHOLOGY

The internal carotid artery is divided into four segments: (1) the cervical or extracranial portion, which is approximately 8 cm long, extending from the bifurcation of the common carotid artery to the carotid canal, where it enters the skull and becomes intracranial; (2) the petrous portion, which averages 4.5 cm in length and lies in the carotid canal within the petrous portion of the temporal bone; (3) the cavernous portion, which also averages 4.5 cm in length, extending throughout the length of the cavernous sinus to the medial border of the anterior clinoid process; and (4) the cerebral or intradural portion, which averages 1 cm in length, extending from the point at which the internal carotid artery pierces the dura mater to its division into anterior and middle cerebral arteries.[7] The distal portion of the internal carotid artery in the petrous bone and the entire portion within the cavernous sinus and the intradural portion make two S-shaped turns, commonly referred to as the carotid siphon.[7] The most common sites for atherosclerosis in the carotid artery system are at the carotid bifurcation (including the carotid sinus) and in the carotid siphon.

Solberg and Eggen[1] subjected the entire carotid arterial systems of 961 autopsied patients who had died from all causes to detailed pathologic analysis. These atherosclerotic plaques were shown to begin as fatty streaks and to progress to fibrous and eventually calcified plaques. Solberg and Eggen showed that this process of plaque ''growth'' is progressive, is identifiable in one third to one half of patients as early as the third decade of life in both the carotid bifurcation area and the siphon, is present in 80 to 100 percent of autopsied patients by the sixth decade, and has a characteristic pattern for each arterial segment regardless of age, sex, or geographic location in which the patient lived. They also demonstrated that ''complicated lesions,'' that is, plaques showing evidence of intraplaque hemorrhage, ulceration, or plaque necrosis, are present in up to 42 percent of carotid bifurcations and 68 percent of carotid siphons examined from patients in their sixth decade. These investigators as well as others[3–5, 7] documented the relative absence of atherosclerotic involvement of that segment of the carotid artery between the distal extent of the carotid sinus and the middle to distal portion of the carotid artery within the petrous bone. It is postulated that because this portion of the vessel is relatively straight, it is subjected to classic laminar flow patterns, unlike the area of the carotid sinus and the multiple S curves of the carotid siphon, where turbulence and ''eddy currents'' are known to occur.[1, 3–5] The carotid bifurcation and carotid sinus area are thin-walled and elastic, whereas the internal carotid artery in its distal cervical and sinus portions is relatively thick-walled and muscular, as is the carotid siphon; yet the distal cervical portion is almost uniformly found to be free from atherosclerosis. Therefore, it is likely that the hemodynamic factors just discussed, rather than arterial wall composition, play a dominant role in the development of tandem lesions.

Numerous investigators[1, 5, 31–35] have pointed out the great propensity for calcification in carotid siphon plaques and have noted that this calcification tends to occur predominantly in the muscle of the media and especially in the elastic lamina underlying the plaque, whereas the calcification seen in plaques that occur at the carotid bifurcation seems to be more diffuse and involves more completely the substance of the plaque itself. The tendency for the carotid siphon to undergo diffuse calcification in its elastica and media without any other evidence of true atherosclerosis has likewise been pointed out by various authorities.[31–35] Fisher and associates[35] examined most carefully the degree of carotid calcification and showed that the process of siphon calcification is progressive, begins in the third decade, and is more pronounced in females and patients with hypertension, and that the degree of siphon calcification does not correlate with the degree of atherosclerosis found elsewhere, such as the carotid bifurcation, the aorta, and the coronary arteries. These workers also point out that since the carotid siphon wall is so susceptible to diffuse calcification, which turns it into a brittle tube that shatters easily when opened with scissors during autopsy and thus makes accurate calculation of the percentage of siphon stenosis very difficult, earlier studies that assessed the degree of siphon stenosis without first decalcifying the artery may have overestimated the true incidence and especially the degree of siphon stenosis.

These investigators also point out that atherosclerosis affecting the carotid siphon tends to assume one of two morphologic patterns. In areas in which the subintima, elastica, and media of the siphon are heavily calcified, the atherosclerotic plaques are thin and usually fibrous and tend not to form deep or irregular ulcerations, to protrude into the lumen, or to pile up, which causes significant stenosis. By contrast, plaques in noncalcified or lightly calcified areas more closely resemble plaques seen elsewhere in the carotid bifurcation, in that they are more apt to form irregular ulcerated lesions and to cause luminal stenosis. Because of this, Fisher and associates[35] postulated that diffuse calcification of the carotid siphon may actually hinder the formation or retard the growth of typical obstructive atherosclerosis in the siphon.

The findings of DiChiro and Libow[34] tend to support this view. These investigators failed to show any differences in the cerebral blood flow or cerebrovascular resistance between two groups of healthy elderly men, one with carotid siphon calcification and the other without. This tends to support the findings of other authorities, who showed that the degree of carotid siphon calcification does not correlate with the degree of occlusive atherosclerosis at the carotid bifurcation or elsewhere in the body, that the degree of calcification in the siphon is not an accurate predictor of the degree of luminal stenosis caused by obstructing atherosclerotic plaques, and that the degree of siphon calcification does not accurately correlate with the occurrence of previous stroke or TIAs.[31–33, 35] In light of this, it is likely, as pointed out by Fisher and colleagues,[35] that earlier studies based on either the degree of calcification in the siphon, as assessed by plain radiographs of the skull, or autopsy examination of the carotid siphon without its first having been decalcified may have overemphasized the importance of siphon calcification as a ''marker'' for cerebrovascular disease and overestimated the degree of stenosis in the lumen of the carotid siphon.

INCIDENCE OF CAROTID SIPHON STENOSIS AND TANDEM LESIONS

The true incidence of carotid siphon stenosis and, therefore, carotid tandem lesions is difficult to glean from the literature. This is because reports containing this information are based on such diverse types of studies as random autopsy series, autopsy series of patients who previously had cerebrovascular symptoms, autopsy series correlating radiographic evidence of carotid siphon calcification as assessed by plain skull films with subsequent autopsy results, contrast arteriographic studies in patients with cerebrovascular symptoms, long-term follow-up studies of patients with a variety of radiographically demonstrable intracerebral carotid artery lesions, and the results of carotid bifurcation endarterectomy in patients with and without tandem lesions. In view of the great diversity of the methods used to define the incidence and severity of siphon disease and tandem lesions, it is not surprising that the reported incidence is quite variable.

In a random autopsy series, Solberg and Eggen[1] examined both carotid arteries from 961 patients aged 25 to 69 years from their origins to their branching to anterior and middle cerebral arteries. These workers found that the incidence of fibrous atherosclerotic plaque occurring at both the carotid bifurcation and the carotid siphon increased from 10 to 20 percent for those patients in their third decade, to 80 to 100 percent for those patients in their sixth decade. The incidence of so-called complicated lesions, that is, atherosclerotic plaques showing evidence of intraplaque hemorrhage, plaque ulceration, necrosis, superimposed thrombosis, or calcification, occurred at the carotid bifurcation in 20 to 40 percent of patients and at the siphon in 60 to 70 percent of patients. The overall incidence of tandem lesions in this series was 40 to 50 percent; however, since the percentage of siphon stenosis and the percentage of bifurcation stenosis are not addressed in this study, it is impossible to discern what percentage of these tandem lesions would be detectable on angiography. It is thus impossible to correlate this autopsy study with angiographic studies of patients with symptoms.

In another autopsy series, 50 to 58 percent of men and 26 to 38 percent of women over the age of 35 examined by Schwartz and Mitchell[3] had moderate to severe degrees of carotid siphon stenosis, whereas 54 to 80 percent of men and 63 to 68 percent of women had carotid bifurcation stenosis. Although this study is well done and fairly accurately defines the incidence of siphon stenosis, it does not provide data to define the incidence of tandem lesions. Hass and coworkers,[8] in Report II of the Joint Study of Extracranial Arterial Occlusion, showed that 17.1 percent of patients had angiographically demonstrable carotid siphon stenosis and 67.9 percent had carotid bifurcation stenosis. In the same report, an additional 17 percent of patients had carotid bifurcation occlusion and 17.3 percent had carotid siphon occlusion. From the data presented in the report, it is impossible to determine what percentage of patients had true carotid tandem lesions and what percentage of patients had carotid siphon occlusion caused by propagation of clot from occlusion of the proximal internal carotid artery at the level of the bifurcation.

In an angiographic study, Eisenberg and colleagues[36] showed that 11 percent of patients with amaurosis fugax and 3 percent of patients with hemispheric TIAs had isolated carotid siphon stenosis, an overall incidence of 5 percent isolated siphon stenosis. This study also presents the data in such a manner that it is impossible to derive the incidence of tandem lesions. In a natural history study of patients with angiographic evidence of 33 percent or greater siphon stenosis, Craig and associates[37] reported that only 10 percent had tandem lesions. This figure is quite low and is probably explained by the fact that this series of patients was preselected such that only those with significant carotid siphon stenosis were analyzed. In a similar natural history study, Marzewski and coworkers[38] reported a series of 66 patients with greater than 50 percent stenoses of the carotid siphon. Of the 85 carotid siphon stenoses identified (19 patients had bilateral siphon stenosis), 53 lesions had associated carotid bifurcation stenosis. Thus, the incidence of tandem lesions in this series was 62 percent. Roederer and associates[12] reported 141 patients (282 carotid arterial systems) in whom the angiographic findings were correlated with both the presenting symptoms and outcome following carotid endarterectomy. Siphon stenosis was found in 84 percent of the carotid arterial systems. Most of these siphon stenoses caused a 20 to 29 percent reduction in diameter. Nine percent caused a greater than 50 percent diameter reduction, and 10 percent of siphons showed total occlusion. Since only one of 282 carotid bifurcations examined was normal, it can be determined that the incidence of tandem lesions in this study is 84 percent. In a previous report, our group described a 48 percent incidence of carotid tandem lesions.[11] The most likely explanation for the discrepancy in the incidence of tandem lesions in the last two reports cited is that in the report by Roederer and coworkers,[12] carotid siphon stenoses of 1 to 20 percent were included in the calculations of the incidence of tandem lesions, whereas in the report by Schuler and colleagues[11] only those patients with siphon stenosis greater than 20 percent diameter reduction were considered. It can be seen that the reported incidence of siphon stenosis varies from 5 percent[36] to almost 100 percent,[1] and that the incidence of tandem lesions varies from 10 percent[37] to 84 percent.[12] Some portion of these great differences is obviously attributable to differences in (1) patient population, (2) the definition of siphon disease (ie, calcification with minimal or no diameter reduction versus strictly diameter reduction), (3) the method of determining siphon disease (ie, angiography versus autopsy), and (4) what degree of siphon stenosis is clinically meaningful (ie, any degree of siphon stenosis[12, 29] versus 20 percent or more siphon stenosis).[11, 28, 30, 37, 38] If only those reported patients are considered who have siphon stenosis of 20 percent or greater in conjunction with carotid bifurcation stenosis, the incidence of tandem lesions falls somewhere in the range of 30 to 60 percent. It must be remembered, however, that most of these figures are derived from angiographic studies of series of patients presenting with symptoms of cerebrovascular disease that are of sufficient severity to prompt angiographic evaluation. The real incidence in the general population is therefore probably lower.

In assessing the relationship between tandem lesions and symptoms, it is logical to ask which lesion—either the one at the carotid bifurcation or the one in the carotid siphon, or possibly both—is responsible for the symptoms, since rational therapy necessarily depends on which lesion is the cause of symptoms. The study by Schuler and colleagues[11] compared two groups of patients—those with and without tandem lesions. Both groups underwent elective carotid endarterectomy. The primary indication for endarterectomy in the group without tandem lesions was hemispheric TIAs and or amaurosis fugax or both in 66 percent, previous resolved strokes in 19 percent, vertebrobasilar insufficiency in 4 percent, and asymptomatic lesions in 11 percent. In the group with tandem lesions, the primary indication for endarterectomy was TIAs or amaurosis fugax in 61 percent, previous resolved stroke in 18 percent, vertebrobasilar insufficiency in 2 percent, and asymptomatic bifurcation lesions in 18 percent. None of these differences between the two groups as regards the presenting symptoms or primary indication for bifurcation endarterectomy was statistically significant. There were likewise no discernible trends that would be expected to become statistically significant if larger numbers of patients were involved in the analysis. In addition, there was no discernible relationship between the nature of the presenting symptoms and the degree of siphon stenosis. It follows that most symptoms are attributable to the carotid bifurcation lesion rather than to the carotid siphon lesion.

Roederer and colleagues[12] also evaluated the relationship between siphon disease and preoperative symptoms. In their series, there was a 40 percent probability that a patient would have hemispheric symptoms on the side of a completely normal carotid siphon, a 41 percent probability of hemispheric symptoms if the siphon stenosis was 1 to 49 percent, a 40 percent probability if the siphon stenosis was 50 to 99 percent, and a 43 percent probability of symptoms if the siphon was completely occluded. These data obviously do not support any correlation between the severity of carotid siphon stenosis and the occurrence of cerebral ischemic events and again suggest that most hemispheric events originate in lesions at the carotid bifurcation.

THE RESULTS OF CAROTID ENDARTERECTOMY IN PATIENTS WITH TANDEM LESIONS

The two major concerns expressed in the literature regarding tandem lesions are that carotid bifurcation endarterectomy in the presence of ipsilateral siphon stenosis either will fail to relieve symptoms[10, 25–27] or will lead to an increased risk of stroke.[19, 22–24] Five independent studies have recently provided data regarding the safety and efficacy of carotid bifurcation endarterectomy in patients with tandem lesions.

Schuler and colleagues[11] compared the results of carotid endarterectomy in two groups of patients; one group (44 patients who underwent 47 carotid endarterectomies) had carotid bifurcation stenosis only and the other group (35 patients who underwent 44 carotid endarterectomies) had carotid siphon stenosis of greater than 20 percent in conjunction with carotid bifurcation stenosis. The two groups were equally matched as regards age, sex distribution, incidence of diabetes and hypertension, type of presenting symptoms, and length of follow-up. All patients in both groups who were symptomatic before surgery experienced immediate relief of symptoms following carotid bifurcation endarterectomy (Table 70–1). In the 44 patients with carotid bifurcation disease only, there were no intraoperative strokes, no strokes within 30 days of operation, and four late

TABLE 70–1. Results of Carotid Endarterectomy in Patients with and Without Tandem Lesions

Condition	Bifurcation Disease Only, n(%)	Tandem Lesions, n(%)
Operative stroke	0/47(0)	5/44(11.4)
Intraoperative stroke	0/47(0)	2/44(4.5)
Stroke within 30 days of operation	0/47(0)	3/44(6.8)
Immediate relief of symptoms	41/41*(100)	29/29†(100)
Late stroke referable to operated side	4/46(8.7)	2/39(5.1)
Late development of symptoms referable to operated side	3/46(6.5)	2/39(5.1)

*Excludes five carotid bifurcation lesions that were asymptomatic prior to surgery and one nonstroke death.

†Excludes eight carotid bifurcation lesions that were asymptomatic prior to surgery, five operative strokes, and two nonstroke-related operative deaths.

From Schuler JJ, Flanigan DP, Lim LT, et al: The effect of carotid siphon stenosis on stroke rate, death, and relief of symptoms following elective carotid endarterectomy. *Surgery.* 1982; 92:1058.

strokes (8.7%) referable to the cerebral hemisphere on the operated side. In the 35 patients with tandem lesions who underwent 44 carotid endarterectomies, there were two intraoperative strokes (4.5%) three strokes occurring within 30 days of operation (6.8%), and two late strokes (5.1%) referable to the operated side. None of the differences between the group with tandem lesions and the group with bifurcation stenosis only were statistically significant.

The major concern regarding tandem lesions has dealt with the subgroup of patients who have a greater degree of siphon stenosis than of bifurcation stenosis. Therefore, the 18 patients with, more severe siphon stenosis than bifurcation stenosis were compared with the 17 patients with less severe siphon stenosis than bifurcation stenosis plus the patients with no siphon stenosis. Again, there were no statistically significant differences in operative, perioperative, or late stroke rates, nor was there any difference in immediate and long-term relief of symptoms between those patients with more severe siphon stenosis than bifurcation stenosis and the remainder of the patients (Table 70–2).

To evaluate whether differences in stroke rate or mortality rate are related to the absolute degree of siphon stenosis rather than the degree of siphon stenosis relative to bifurcation stenosis, those patients with tandem lesions were divided into two groups: those with siphon stenosis greater than or equal to 50 percent and those with siphon stenosis less than 50 percent. Again, as shown in Table 70–3, none of these differences between the group with siphon stenosis greater than 50 percent and the group with siphon stenosis less than 50 percent were statistically significant.

In this study, the only significant difference between patients with tandem lesions and those with bifurcation disease only was that the patients with tandem lesions required bilateral carotid endarterectomy more frequently (26%) than did those with bifurcation disease only (7%). Although the patients with tandem lesions tended, in general, to fare more poorly than did the patients with bifurcation disease only, there were no statistically significant differences between the two groups in any parameters examined. It is possible that a larger number of patients in both groups or a longer period of follow-up would show significant differences; however,

TABLE 70–2. Results of Carotid Endarterectomy in Patients with Siphon Stenosis More Severe than Bifurcation Stenosis (Group A) Compared with Those with Siphon Stenosis Less Severe than Bifurcation Stenosis Plus Those Patients with Bifurcation Stenosis Only (Group B)

Condition	Group A, n(%)	Group B, n(%)
Operative stroke	2/18(11.1)	3/73(4.1)
Intraoperative stroke	1/18(5.6)	1/73(1.4)
Stroke within 30 days of operation referable to operated side	1/18(5.6)	2/73(2.7)
Immediate relief of symptoms	12/12*(100)	58/58†(100)
Late stroke referable to operated side	1/17(5.9)	5/68(7.4)
Late development of symptoms referable to operated side	1/17(5.9)	4/68(5.9)

*Excludes four carotid bifurcation lesions that were asymptomatic prior to surgery plus two operative strokes.

†Excludes nine carotid bifurcation lesions that were asymptomatic prior to surgery, three operative strokes, two nonstroke-related deaths, and one death 6 weeks after operation resulting from unknown causes.

From Schuler JJ, Flanigan DP, Lim LT, et al: The effect of carotid siphon stenosis on stroke rate, death, and relief of symptoms following elective carotid endarterectomy. *Surgery.* 1982; 92:1058.

this is speculative, since the patients without tandem lesions would likewise remain at risk.

In a similar study, Roederer and colleagues[12] reported the results of carotid endarterectomy in 141 patients who underwent 149 carotid endarterectomies. In this series, 82 percent of the endarterectomized sides had carotid siphon stenosis of some degree and 62 percent had siphon stenosis greater than 20 percent. There were no perioperative strokes in this series. During follow-up evaluation extending to 56 months, 18 patients experienced recurrent symptoms on the endarterectomized side. Thirteen patients experienced TIAs, and five patients had strokes. Severe (greater than 50%) siphon stenosis was present in 11 percent of cerebral hemispheres of patients who experienced recurrent symptoms and also in 11 percent of hemispheres of patients who remained completely asymptomatic. The proportion of cerebral hemispheres in which focal recurrent symptoms were found was

TABLE 70–3. Results of Carotid Endarterectomy in Patients with Carotid Siphon Stenosis of Greater than 50 Percent Compared with Those with Siphon Stenosis of Less than 50 Percent

Condition	<50 Percent Stenosis, n(%)	>50 Percent Stenosis, n(%)
Operative stroke	4/30(13.3)	1/14(7.1)
Intraoperative stroke	2/30(6.7)	0/14(0.0)
Stroke within 30 days of operation	2/30(6.7)	1/14(7.1)
Immediate relief of symptoms	17/17*(100.0)	12/12†(100.0)
Late stroke referable to operated side	1/26(3.8)	1/13(7.7)
Late development of symptoms referable to operated side	1/26(3.8)	1/13(7.7)

*Excludes seven carotid bifurcation lesions that were asymptomatic prior to surgery, four operative strokes, and two nonstroke-related operative deaths.

†Excludes one carotid bifurcation lesion that was asymptomatic prior to surgery and one operative stroke.

From Schuler JJ, Flanigan DP, Lim LT, et al: The effect of carotid siphon stenosis on stroke rate, death, and relief of symptoms following elective carotid endarterectomy. *Surgery.* 1982; 92:1058.

12 percent when the siphon was mildly diseased and 22 percent when the carotid siphon was completely normal. It can be seen that the patients in Roederer's series,[12] 82 percent of whom had tandem lesions, are not at increased risk of stroke following carotid endarterectomy (no perioperative strokes) or at increased risk of recurrence of symptoms, since those patients without siphon stenosis had essentially the same rate of recurrence of symptoms as those with siphon stenosis. Furthermore, there was no relationship between the degree of siphon stenosis and the risk of developing recurrent symptoms.

More recently, Mattos and coworkers[30] analyzed the results of carotid endarterectomy relative to early and late stroke and death in 354 patients who underwent 393 carotid endarterectomies over a 16-year period. Siphon stenosis of greater than 20 percent was present in 84 arteries. In this series, there were no statistically significant differences in perioperative mortality rates, perioperative stroke rates, or late ipsilateral stroke-free rates in those patients with tandem lesions as compared with those patients with carotid bifurcation stenosis alone. The only significant difference in the two groups of patients was an increased incidence of late death caused primarily by cardiac disease in the group with siphon stenosis.

Lord and colleagues[28] likewise reported no significant difference in the perioperative stroke rate following carotid endarterectomy between patients with 50 to 80 percent siphon stenosis and those patients with no siphon stenosis or "insignificant" siphon stenosis. All three of the strokes in this series of 169 carotid endarterectomies occurred in patients with no radiographic evidence of significant siphon stenosis. These authors also concluded that moderate siphon stenosis (50–80%) does not increase the risk of perioperative cerebral infarction.

Mackey and colleagues[29] compared the results of carotid endarterectomy in a series of 597 patients, 134 of whom had both intracranial stenosis and carotid bifurcation stenosis and 463 of whom had only carotid bifurcation stenosis. In 66 percent of the 134 patients, the intracranial stenosis involved the carotid siphon. These authors likewise showed no statistically significant differences in perioperative stroke morbidity, perioperative mortality, or late stroke-free rates between those patients with combined intracranial stenosis and carotid bifurcation stenosis and those patients with carotid bifurcation stenosis only.

The data presented in these five studies do not support the previous suggestions in the literature that patients with tandem lesions are at a greater risk of stroke[19, 22–24] or recurrence of symptoms.[10, 35–37]

The relatively benign natural history of siphon stenosis is more clearly defined in a report by Borozan and associates.[39] Ninety-three patients with isolated carotid siphon stenosis of greater than 20 percent were followed for 1 to 62 months (mean, 27.6 months). None of these patients had ipsilateral carotid bifurcation disease or intracranial stenosis in any area other than the carotid siphon. Of these 93 patients, 71 had unilateral siphon stenosis and 22 had bilateral siphon stenosis, yielding 115 cerebral hemispheres at risk. At the time of arteriography, 93 cerebral hemispheres were in asymptomatic patients and 22 were in patients who had preceding focal neurologic events (TIAs or resolved stroke). Among asymptomatic patients during follow-up, 64.5 per-

cent of hemispheres were found in patients who remained asymptomatic, 6.5 percent in patients who experienced TIAs, and 4.3 percent in patients who had a stroke. Among initially symptomatic patients during the same follow-up period, 63.6 percent of hemispheres were found in patients who became asymptomatic, 9.1 percent in patients who experienced recurrent TIAs, and 9.1 percent in patients who had a stroke. In the initially asymptomatic group of patients, 22.5 percent died during follow-up, whereas in the initially symptomatic group, 22.7 percent died during the same period of follow-up. The overall incidence of nonfatal stroke and TIAs was 6.5 and 8.6 percent, respectively, at a mean follow-up of 27.6 months. There was no significant difference in the incidence of stroke or TIA between those patients who were asymptomatic at the time of presentation and those who were symptomatic at presentation. Likewise, the percentage of siphon stenosis in all patients who experienced TIAs or stroke (35.4%) was not significantly different from that in patients who remained asymptomatic (32.3%). Borozan and coworkers[39] conclude that although patients with carotid siphon stenosis are at an increased risk for stroke or TIA compared with the population at large, they are at much less risk for stroke than are patients with TIAs caused by carotid bifurcation disease.[21]

THE RATIONALE FOR CAROTID BIFURCATION ENDARTERECTOMY IN PATIENTS WITH TANDEM LESIONS

Several reports have indicated that approximately 30 to 40 percent of untreated patients who have TIAs will experience a frank stroke within 5 years of the onset of TIAs, and most of these strokes will occur during the first 1 to 2 years after the onset of TIAs.[21, 40–44] The combined intraoperative, perioperative, and late stroke rate of 15.9 percent in those patients with tandem lesions, as reported by Schuler and colleagues,[11] the 0 percent perioperative stroke rate and 3.4 percent late stroke rate in patients reported by Roederer and colleagues,[12] the 0 percent stroke rate reported by Lord and colleagues,[28] the 1.9 percent stroke rate reported by Mackey and colleagues,[29] and the 3.6 percent perioperative stroke rate reported by Mattos and colleagues[30] are all obviously much lower than the 30 to 40 percent stroke rate that would be expected based on previously reported natural history studies.[21, 40–44] The combined results of carotid endarterectomy in patients with tandem lesions in the five series mentioned are also superior to the total stroke rates reported for aspirin-treated patients in the Canadian cooperative study,[45] the American aspirin trial,[46] the AICLA aspirin trial,[47] and the aspirin trial in the prevention of stroke reported by Sorensen and associates.[48] Furthermore, none of these aspirin trials in the prevention of stroke clearly defines the incidence of carotid siphon stenosis or tandem lesions in the treated group. The combined results of carotid endarterectomy in patients with tandem lesions[11, 12, 28–30] are likewise superior to the results of treating patients who present with TIAs with systemic anticoagulants such as coumadin, as reported by Whisnant and associates,[49] and Siekert and associates.[50]

More recently, two separate prospective randomized studies[51, 52] compared the results of carotid endarterectomy

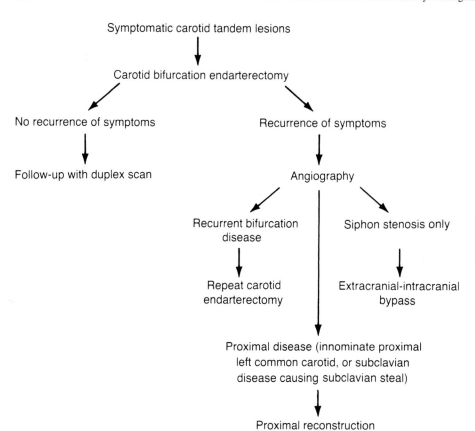

FIGURE 70–1. Clinical algorithm useful in making decisions regarding the diagnostic evaluation and the short-term and long-term management of patients with symptomatic carotid tandem lesions.

with those of best medical management in symptomatic patients with carotid bifurcation stenosis of 70 to 99 percent. In the NASCET trial,[51] the incidence of any ipsilateral stroke at the 2-year follow-up examination in the medically treated group was 26 percent, and in the European Carotid Surgery trial,[52] the incidence of ipsilateral stroke in the medically treated group was 16.8 percent at the 3-year follow-up examination. The results of carotid endarterectomy in patients with tandem lesions in the five series previously mentioned[11, 12, 28–30] are obviously far superior to those reported in patients receiving best medical management.

Although none of the patients with tandem lesions reported by Schuler and colleagues[11] or Roederer and colleagues[12] required extracranial to intracranial bypass, it seems reasonable that in those patients with carotid tandem lesions who, following carotid bifurcation endarterectomy, present with recurrence of TIAs or stroke and who are found to have no disease other than siphon stenosis, extracranial to intracranial bypass[48] or a short trial of aspirin therapy should be considered.

Based on the results of carotid endarterectomy in patients with tandem lesions,[11, 12] we have derived and follow the clinical management algorithm depicted in Figure 70–1. In summary, (1) approximately one half of all patients with symptoms of cerebrovascular disease have carotid tandem lesions; (2) the severity of the siphon stenosis bears no relationship to the severity of the bifurcation stenosis and is unrelated to the type or severity of presenting symptoms; (3) patients with tandem lesions do not have a significantly higher rate of operative stroke, late stroke, or operative mortality following carotid bifurcation endarterectomy, as compared with those without tandem lesions; (4) patients

with tandem lesions who are subjected to carotid endarterectomy have the same immediate uniform relief of presenting symptoms following carotid bifurcation endarterectomy as do those patients with bifurcation disease only, thus indicating that the vast majority of patients are experiencing symptoms secondary to either embolic or hemodynamic events originating in the carotid bifurcation; and (5) patients with tandem lesions subjected to carotid endarterectomy have a stroke rate less than would be expected if they received no therapy, were treated with aspirin, or were treated with systemic anticoagulation. We conclude that carotid endarterectomy is indicated in symptomatic patients with tandem lesions for relief of symptoms and prevention of stroke.

REFERENCES

1. Solberg LA, Eggen DA: Localization and sequence of development of atherosclerotic lesions in the carotid and vertebral arteries. *Circulation.* 1971;43:711.
2. Janeway R, Toole JF: Vascular anatomic status of patients with transient ischemic attacks. *Trans Am Neurol Assoc.* 1972;97:137.
3. Schwartz CJ, Mitchell JRA: Atheroma of the carotid and vertebral arterial systems. *Br Med J.* 1961;2:1057.
4. Schwartz CJ, Mitchell JRA: Observations on localization of arterial plaques. *Circ Res.* 1962;11:63.
5. Fisher CM, Gore I, Okabe N, White PD: Atherosclerosis of the carotid and vertebral arteries. Extracranial and intracranial. *J Neuropath Exp Neuro.* 1965;24:455.
6. Luessenhop AJ: Occlusive disease of the carotid artery: Observations on the prognosis and surgical treatment. *J Neurosurg.* 1959;16:705.
7. Samuel KC: Atherosclerosis and occlusion of the internal carotid artery. *J Pathol Bacteriol.* 1956;71:391.
8. Hass WK, Fields WS, North RR, et al: Joint study of extracranial arterial occlusion. II. Arteriography, techniques, sites and complications. *JAMA.* 1968;203:159.
9. Martin MJ, Whisnant JP, Sayre GP: Occlusive vascular disease in the extracranial cerebral circulation. *Arch Neurol.* 1961;5:64.
10. Wylie EJ, Ehrenfeld WK: Extracranial Occlusive Cerebrovascular Disease: Diagnosis and Management. Philadelphia; WB Saunders, 1970.
11. Schuler JJ, Flanigan DP, Lim LT, et al: The effect of carotid siphon stenosis on

stroke rate, death, and relief of symptoms following elective carotid endarterectomy. *Surgery.* 1982;92:1058.

12. Roederer GO, Langlois YE, Chan ARW, et al: Is siphon disease important in predicting outcome of carotid endarterectomy? *Arch Surg.* 1983;118:1177.

13. Imparato AM, Riles TS, Gorstein F: The carotid bifurcation plaque: Pathologic findings associated with cerebral ischemia. *Stroke.* 1979;10:238.

14. Gomensoro JB, Maslenikov V, Azambuja N, et al: Joint study of extracranial arterial occlusion. VIII. Clinical-radiographic correlation of carotid bifurcation lesions in 177 patients with transient cerebral ischemic attacks. *JAMA.* 1973;224:985.

15. Millikan CH: The pathogenesis of transient focal cerebral ischemia: The Lewis A. Conner memorial lecture. *Circulation.* 1965;32:438.

16. Thompson JE, Austin DJ, Patman RD: Carotid endarterectomy for cerebrovascular insufficiency: Long-term results in 592 patients followed up to 13 years. *Ann Surg.* 1970;4:663.

17. DeWeese JA, Rob CG, Satran R, et al: Surgical treatment for occlusive disease of the carotid artery. *Ann Surg.* 1968;168:85.

18. Nunn DB: Carotid endarterectomy: An analysis of 234 operative cases. *Ann Surg.* 1973;182:733.

19. Bauer RB, Meyer JS, Fields WS, et al: Joint study of extracranial arterial occlusion. III. Progress report of controlled study of long-term survival in patients with and without operation. *JAMA.* 1969;208:509.

20. DeWeese JA, Rob CG, Satran R, et al: Results of carotid endarterectomies for transient ischemic attack. Five years later. *Ann Surg.* 1973;178:258.

21. Thompson JE, Patman RD, Talkington CM: Carotid surgery for cerebrovascular insufficiency. *Curr Prob Surg.* 1978;15:6.

22. Day AL, Rhoton Al, Quisling RG: Resolving siphon stenosis following endarterectomy. *Stroke.* 1980;2:278.

23. Hugenholtz H, Elgie RG: Carotid thromboendarterectomy: A reappraisal: Criteria for patient selection. *J Neurosurg.* 1980;53:776.

24. Sundt TM, Sandok BA, Whisnant JP: Carotid endarterectomy: Complications and preoperative assessment of risk. *Mayo Clin Proc.* 1975;50:301.

25. Fields WS: Selection of stroke patients for arterial reconstructive surgery. *Am J Surg.* 1973;125:527.

26. Fields WS: Selection of patients with ischemic cerebrovascular disease for arterial surgery. *World J Surg.* 1979;3:147.

27. Blaisdell WF, Clauss RH, Galbraith IG, et al: Joint study of extracranial arterial occlusion. IV. A review of surgical considerations. *JAMA.* 1969;209:1889.

28. Lord RSA, Raj TB, Graham AR: Carotid endarterectomy, siphon stenosis, collateral hemispheric pressure, and perioperative cerebral infarction. *J Vasc Surg.* 1987;6:391.

29. Mackey WC, O'Donnell TF, Callow AD: Carotid endarterectomy in patients with intracranial vascular disease: Short-term risk and long-term outcome. *J Vasc Surg.* 1989;10:432.

30. Mattos MA, van Bemmelen PS, Hodgson KM, et al: The influence of carotid siphon stenosis on short- and long-term outcome after carotid endarterectomy. *J Vasc Surg.* 1993;17:902.

31. Ratinov G: Extradural intracranial portion of carotid artery: A clinicopathologic study. *Arch Neurol.* 1964;10:66.

32. Bostrom K, Hassler O: Radiological study of arterial calcification: Intracranial arteries. *Neurology (NY).* 1965;15:1168.

33. Scotti G, DeGrandi C: Intimal and medial calcifications of the carotid siphon and cerebrovascular disease. *Radiology.* 1975;116:667.

34. DiChiro G, Libow LS: Carotid siphon calcification and cerebral blood flow in the healthy aged male. *Radiology.* 1971;99:103.

35. Fisher CM, Gore I, Okabe N, White PD: Calcification of the carotid siphon. *Circulation.* 1965;32:538.

36. Eisenberg RL, Nemzek WR, Moore WS, Mani RL: Relationship of transient ischemic attacks and angiographically demonstrable lesions of carotid artery. *Stroke.* 1977;8:483.

37. Craig DR, Meguro K, Watridge C, et al: Intracranial internal carotid artery stenosis. *Stroke.* 1982;13:825.

38. Marzewski DJ, Furlan AJ, St. Louis P, et al: Intracranial internal carotid artery stenosis: Long-term prognosis. *Stroke.* 1982;13:821.

39. Borozan PG, Schuler JJ, LaRosa MP, et al: The natural history of isolated carotid siphon stenosis. *J Vasc Surg.* 1984;1:744.

40. Acheson J, Hutchinson EC: The natural history of focal cerebral vascular disease. *Q J Med.* 1971;40:15.

41. Goldner JC, Whisnant JP, Taylor WF: Long-term prognosis of transient cerebral ischemic attacks. *Stroke.* 1971;2:160.

42. Millikan CH: Reassessment of anticoagulant therapy in various types of occlusive cerebrovascular disease. *Stroke.* 1971;2:201.

43. Millikan CH, McDowell FH: Progress in cerebrovascular disease: Treatment of transient ischemic attacks. *Stroke.* 1978;9:299.

44. Toole JF, Janeway R, Choi K, et al: Transient ischemic attacks due to atherosclerosis. *Arch Neurol.* 1975;32:5.

45. Barnett HJM, Gent M, Sackett DL, et al: A randomized trial of aspirin and sulfinpyrazone in threatened stroke. *N Engl J Med.* 1978;299:53.

46. Fields WS, Lemak NA, Frankowski RF, Hardy RJ: Controlled trial of aspirin in cerebral ischemia *Stroke.* 1977;8:301.

47. Bousser MG, Eschwege E, Haguenau M, et al: AICLA controlled trial of aspirin and dipyridamole in the secondary prevention of atherothrombotic cerebral ischemia. *Stroke.* 1983;14:5.

48. Sorensen PS, Pedersen H, Marquardsen J, et al: Acetylsalicylic acid in the prevention of stroke in patients with reversible cerebral ischemic attacks: A Danish cooperative study. *Stroke.* 1983;14:15.

49. Whisnant JP, Matsumoto N, Elveback LR: The effect of anticoagulant therapy on the prognosis of patients with transient cerebral ischemic attacks in a community: Rochester, Minnesota, 1955 through 1969. *Mayo Clin Proc.* 1973;48:844.

50. Siekert RG, Whisnant JP, Millikan CH: Surgical and anticoagulant therapy of occlusive cerebrovascular disease. *Ann Intern Med.* 1963;58:637.

51. North American Symptomatic Carotid Endarterectomy Trial Collaborators: Beneficial effect of carotid endarterectomy in symptomatic patients with high-grade carotid stenosis. *N Engl J Med.* 1991;325:445.

52. European Carotid Surgery Trialists' Collaborative Group: MRC European Carotid Surgery Trial: Interim results for symptomatic patients with severe (70–99%) or with mild (0–29%) carotid stenosis. *Lancet.* 1991;337:1235.

53. Sherman RL, Reichman OH: Superficial temporal artery to middle cerebral artery (STA-MCA) bypass. *Bruit.* 1983;7:50.

CHAPTER 71

Recurrent Stenosis of the Carotid Artery: Incidence, Diagnosis, Prognosis, and Management

J. DENNIS BAKER

From the early days of arterial reconstruction, surgeons had better long-term results with endarterectomy of the carotid bifurcation than with other sites. Whereas endarterectomy for leg ischemia was frequently followed by restenosis or occlusion, the carotid artery seemed to be free of these problems. Not until 1968, almost 15 years after the first carotid operations, was there a formal assessment of this impression. Edwards and coworkers[1] evaluated long-term results in 75 patients followed from 5 to 9 years. Thirty surviving patients underwent follow-up angiography 5 years or more after operation. Only 3 of the 43 operated arteries (7%) had restenosis with 50 percent or greater reduction of lumen diameter, leading to the conclusion that ''carotid endarterectomy is a worthwhile and durable procedure.''

The rapid expansion in the volume of carotid surgery in the 1970s, together with the growing proportion of operations performed for asymptomatic lesions, demanded a more complete understanding of the long-term results. During the past 15 years, a number of studies have evaluated both symptomatic and asymptomatic postoperative stenosis, together with the pathology and risk factors associated with the problem.

INCIDENCE

In 1976, Stoney and String[2] reviewed the results of 1654 operations over a 22-year span and found 24 cases of symptomatic restenosis (1.5%). This low incidence of recurrence was echoed by several others, but Kartchner[3] found a 4 percent recurrence rate when he included asymptomatic lesions identified by noninvasive tests. He suggested that this total restenosis rate was a more accurate reflection of the magnitude of the problem. Kremen and associates[4] further focused the emphasis on asymptomatic restenosis when they reported an incidence of 8.1 percent identified by ocular pneumoplethysmography.

Table 71–1 summarizes some of the studies of carotid restenosis reported during the past 17 years. In this group, the incidence of symptomatic restenosis ranged from 1 to 8 percent (mean, 2%). The groups that carried out postoperative noninvasive surveillance had a somewhat higher incidence of symptomatic restenosis, possibly resulting from closer follow-up evaluation. Asymptomatic restenosis was found in 7 to 23 percent of operated arteries (mean, 13%). Some of the variation in this incidence may have resulted from differences in noninvasive methodology used. Pierce and colleagues[5] found a 7 percent incidence of asymptomatic restenosis using intravenous digital subtraction angiography for follow-up evaluation. All the recent studies used duplex scanning for surveillance.

PATHOLOGY

In 1968, Edwards and coworkers[1] pointed out that all three patients operated on for restenosis had a fibrous thickening of the arterial wall rather than typical atherosclerosis. These investigators commented that it was not possible to develop a cleavage plane for endarterectomy, and patch angioplasty was required. Stoney and String[2] found that the character of the lesion was related to the time from the original operation. Intimal fibrosis similar to that described by Edwards and coworkers was seen with recurrences that developed within the first 2 years, whereas atherosclerotic plaques were found in the later lesions. Subsequent studies have reported the same pattern of pathology; however, in some cases, early lesions may show atherosclerosis, and late lesions may be fibrous. In addition, it is not unusual for mixed lesions to be made up of both fibrous and atherosclerotic components.

Most restenoses occur within the region of the previous endarterectomy, suggesting that recurrence is the result of postoperative alterations of the healing process (Fig. 71–1). (The remainder of the lesions are found above or below the extent of the arteriotomy, reflecting technical problems, including clamp injuries, endpoint problems, and incomplete or inadequate extent of endarterectomy.) Most of the studies of the healing process after carotid operations have focused on the thrombus, which covers the exposed media. As soon as flow is re-established, platelets adhere to the subendothelial structures. There is platelet degranulation with release of adenosine diphosphate and thromboxane, triggering further aggregation. The platelet mass is stabilized by fibrin with formation of a thrombus composed of red blood cells, platelets, and fibrin. Lusby and colleagues[6] studied the dynamics of the interaction of platelets with the endarterectomy site using a ^{111}In radiotracer technique. Their animal experiments showed that the concentration of labeled platelets reached a peak at 1 hour, and 8 of 14 arteries still showed platelet activity at 1 week. Once the endarterectomy site was completely covered by endothelium, platelet activity could not be detected.

In normal blood, an extensive mass of thrombus may develop; experimental studies by Dirrenberger and Sundt[7] showed that systemic anticoagulation with heparin reduces the extent of the thrombus but does not prevent its formation. They also demonstrated that the maximum size of the luminal thrombus occurs within the first few hours and that there is reduction in thickness by the second to third day. During the following weeks, there is a further decrease in the thrombus, with gradual covering by endothelium. Autopsy studies by French and Rewcastle[8] showed that full endothelial covering can occur within 1 month in humans. Using serial angiograms, Schultz and coworkers[9] demonstrated that local irregularities at the endarterectomy site remodeled and became smooth over several months.

TABLE 71–1. Incidence of Carotid Restenosis

Study*	Operations, N	Screening Method	Symptomatic Restenosis, %	Asymptomatic Restenosis, %	Follow-Up	Comments
Stoney and String[2]	1654	None	1	—	5 mo–13 yr	—
Cossman et al[26]	301	None	3	—	1–24 mo mean 12 mo	The study was limited to restenosis within 24 months.
Kremen et al[4]	173	Noninvasive	2	8	1–12 yr mean 43 mo	All symptomatic patients had contralateral occlusions.
Hertzer et al[10]	1250	None	1	—	1–20 yr mean 45 mo	Most patients had contralateral tight stenosis or occlusion; most restenoses occurred at site of previous endarterectomy.
Cossman et al[15]	468	None	3	—	—	No occlusions were found.
Catelmo et al[27]	199	Noninvasive	5	8	1–8 yr	—
Thompson et al[41]	1286	None	1	—	Mean 9.4 yr	—
Baker et al[12]	133	Noninvasive	2	11	1 mo–5 yr mean 20 mo	Two arteries with abnormal noninvasive tests reverted to normal on follow-up.
Salvian et al[16]	105	Noninvasive	5	7	6 mo–6 yr mean 28 mo	In 75% of cases there were endpoint problems.
Pierce et al[5]	75	IV DSA	3	7	1–13 yr	—
O'Donnell et al[21]	276	Noninvasive	2	11	1–15 yr mean 38 mo	Restenosis appeared earlier in common carotid than in internal carotid.
Healy et al[11]	301	Noninvasive	4	23	Mean 48 mo	Regression of some high-grade lesions.
Salenius et al[42]	133	Noninvasive	8	14	Mean 81 mo	—
Atnip et al[17]	184	Noninvasive	2	4	Mean 35 mo	Three regressions.
Reilly et al[18]	108	Noninvasive	—	18	Mean 15 mo	Regression of some high-grade lesions.
Mattos et al[23]	409	Noninvasive	2	11	11 y mean 42 mo	—

*For full bibliographic information, see reference list at end of chapter.
IV DSA, intravenous digital subtraction angiography.

Most of the emphasis has been on the platelet interaction with the exposed media and the resulting luminal thrombus, but changes in the remaining vessel wall may also be related to restenosis. French and Rewcastle[8] described focal necrosis of the media with an inflammatory reaction within the first week. The severity of the process was quite variable within any given specimen, and the overall extent was unrelated to the time from operation. Polymorphonuclear leukocyte infiltration was centered around the sites of medial necrosis. Dirrenberger and Sundt[7] found nuclear swelling and cyto-

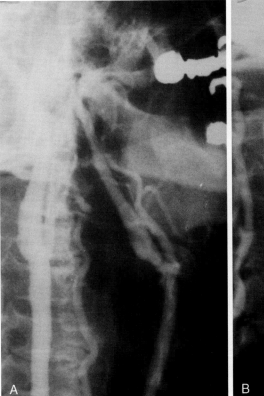
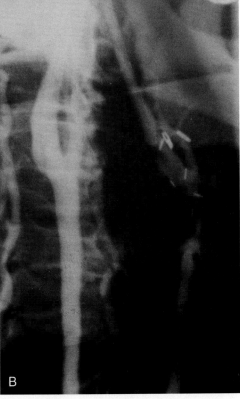

FIGURE 71–1. *A*, Angiogram showing the location of the original atherosclerotic plaque. *B*, Recurrent lesion in the area of endarterectomy.

plasmic vacuolation in smooth muscle cells of the media. In addition, there were areas of hemorrhage into the media.

Intimal fibrosis, also termed myointimal hyperplasia or fibroplasia, is the lesion most often found with restenosis in the first 2 years. At operation, there is a smooth narrowing with a white, glistening appearance and a firm or rubbery consistency. The process may extend through the thickness of the media, so that it is not possible to establish a dissection plane for endarterectomy. Microscopic examination reveals a homogeneous field of densely packed spindle-shaped cells, but no lipid, hemosiderin, or calcium is found (Fig. 71–2). Electron microscopic examination shows the cells to have features of both fibroblasts and smooth muscle cells.[10] It is likely that these cells are normally involved in the healing process of any endarterectomy but that in some situations there is excessive cell proliferation and collagen production, resulting in stenosis. It is not known whether the cells themselves are abnormal or whether there is some external factor responsible for the abnormal growth pattern.

Late restenoses usually result from recurrence of atherosclerosis and have the same gross and microscopic features found in the original lesion, including lipid collections, foam cells, and calcification (Fig. 71–3). The luminal surface may be irregular or ulcerated. Some plaques can be easily removed by endarterectomy, whereas others have a more fibrous reaction, making it difficult to create a suitable plane for dissection. The fact that some restenoses have elements of both intimal fibrosis and atherosclerotic changes leads to speculation over whether these pathologic findings represent two different entities or early and late manifestations of the same process. It is difficult to accumulate evidence to answer the question, since many of the reoperations do not remove the recurrent lesion and there are few autopsies on patients with recurrences.

Healy and associates[11] found that 78 of 301 patients followed developed evidence of more than 50 percent diameter reduction by duplex scan; however, subsequent examinations in 20 of these patients were interpreted as showing less

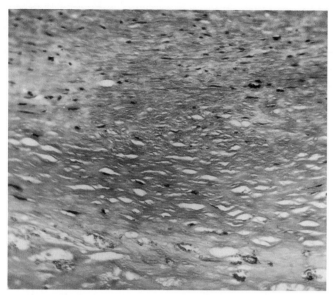

FIGURE 71–3. Atheromatous plaque typically found in late restenosis. (Hematoxylin and eosin stain; original magnification ×200.)

than 50 percent stenosis. These findings were interpreted as evidence that some advanced myointimal lesions undergo regression. Other studies have reported similar cases of abnormal noninvasive tests converting back to normal, but the incidence has been much lower: Baker and coworkers[12] had 2 of 133 patients; and Thomas and colleagues[13] had 3 of 257. An argument could be made that these cases may have represented errors in noninvasive testing rather than extensive restenosis with regression; however, in a study employing early and late intravenous digital subtraction angiography, Eikelboom and associates[14] demonstrated decrease or disappearance of 10 stenoses. Although the specific changes accounting for reduction in the extent of the recurrent lesion are not known, it appears that a remodeling process can occur, at least in some patients.

RISK FACTORS

A number of studies have tried to identify factors associated with recurrence after carotid endarterectomy, but the results are contradictory in many cases. Table 71–2 summarizes the findings of different groups and shows the areas of agreement and disagreement. Many of the factors are those normally associated with advanced atherosclerosis, but it may be that early restenosis is related to other factors entirely. Thus, series with a large proportion of early lesions would not identify hypertension, lipid disorders, and diabetes as predictors of recurrence. Two studies found a preponderance of women but offered different explanations for sex as a risk factor. Cossman and colleagues[15] suggested that restenosis might occur more frequently because of the smaller size of the internal carotid artery in women. Thomas and coworkers[13] postulated that the sex-related incidence resulted from differences in platelet reactivity. The Salvian,[16] Atnip,[17] and Reilly[18] groups specifically did not find female gender to be a predictive factor. To date there is no agreement on which risk factors have clinical relevance. The

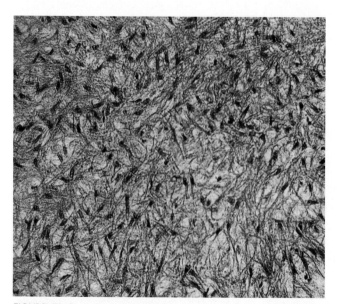

FIGURE 71–2. Microscopic appearance of fibrotic lesion. (Hematoxylin and eosin stain; original magnification ×200.)

TABLE 71–2. Risk Factors Identified in Different Series

Study*	Age	Sex	Hyperlipidemia	Hypertension	Diabetes	Other Vascular Disease	Postop Smoking	Other
Cossman et al[26]	+		+	+	+			
Hertzer et al[10]			+	+				
Cossman et al[15]		+						
Catelmo et al[27]			+	+	+			Bilateral endarterectomy
Clagett et al[43]	+		−	−	−	−	+	
Salvian et al[16]	−	−		−	−	−		Endpoint problem
Thomas et al[13]		+		−	−		−	
O'Donnell et al[21]			+			+		
Salenius et al[42]			+	−		−	−	
Atnip et al[17]	−			−	+		−	
Reilly et al[18]	−		+	+			+	Technical problem

*For full bibliographic information, see reference list at end of chapter.
+, Factor associated with restenosis; −, factor studied but not associated.

greatest problem in this area is the fact that most of the series have small numbers of patients with restenosis, making statistical identification of risk factors difficult if not impossible.

DETECTION AND MANAGEMENT

In many settings, recurrent stenoses are identified when they become symptomatic. Patients who have had surgery for the treatment of symptoms are very sensitive to even minor symptoms, which in most cases are the same as those that occurred preoperatively. Even patients who were originally asymptomatic are also sensitive to symptoms, because they have usually been instructed about transient ischemic attacks (TIAs). Asymptomatic restenosis also may be detected when the patient has angiography for evaluation of symptoms related to the contralateral carotid artery.

In contrast to this passive approach to detection, Kremen and associates[4] and subsequent investigators advocate an active search using noninvasive diagnostic techniques in order to find asymptomatic recurrences. In the past, noninvasive surveillance usually consisted of testing at the time of the annual checkup, but recognition of the fact that many restenoses occur earlier has led to earlier examinations. An advantage of using noninvasive tests is that one can check the patient during the early postoperative period to distinguish technical errors or residual disease from new lesions. A survey showed that most vascular surgeons used noninvasive testing for checkups after carotid endarterectomy.[19] On average, the first examination was 3 to 4 months after the operation, with subsequent checkups at 8- to 12-month intervals.

The management algorithm for symptomatic restenosis is simple, as most surgeons consider this an indication for angiography and reoperation unless the patient has developed a major medical contraindication. (It is important to distinguish patients who have remained symptomatic after endarterectomy from those who had a definite symptom-free period before the return of symptoms.) Most often, the initial presentation is a TIA; in the series summarized in Table 71–1, TIAs occurred almost six times as often as strokes. Although there are no data regarding the actual incidence of thromboembolic stroke from recurrent stenosis, the argument

for treating a symptomatic lesion in order to reduce the risk of stroke applies for a recurrent lesion, as it did for the original one.

The management of an asymptomatic restenosis is neither simple nor clear-cut, primarily because there are few data on the risk of stroke if the lesion is left untreated. Overall, the generalization that appears in the current literature is that asymptomatic restenosis is well tolerated by most, since less than one fifth of these patients become symptomatic. Multiple studies have shown that the new lesion may be quite different from the original one, so that it is not appropriate to presume the same prognosis or risk of stroke. The risk is likely to be related to the pathology of the new lesion: fibrous or atheromatous. It is also probable that the prognosis depends on the status of the opposite carotid artery. Cossman and coworkers[15] found that the only patients who became symptomatic in follow-up were those with contralateral occlusions. Hertzer and colleagues[10] reported that 10 of the 13 symptomatic recurrences had tight stenosis or occlusion of the other carotid artery. These data suggest that the status of the remainder of the cerebral circulation should be considered in the treatment algorithm.

There are three general approaches to the management of asymptomatic restenosis. The most conservative attitude is to operate only when the patient develops symptoms, since most lesions remain silent and only rarely present with stroke as the first symptom.[5] Proponents of this method emphasize the importance of educating patients regarding the different presentations of TIAs and of not delaying follow-up should any symptoms appear.

A second approach is to operate on those patients with asymptomatic restenosis who are considered at high risk for the development of symptoms. In the past, many surgeons considered a hemodynamically significant stenosis (one that reduces the lumen diameter more than 50 or 60%) an indication for repeat operation. Recently the group at increased risk has been reduced to include only those with "preocclusive" lesions (greater than 75 or 80% stenosis). Presence of a contralateral occlusion is considered to increase the risk of a recurrent lesion and may prompt operating on less severe degrees of stenosis.

A third, more selective, approach is advocated by Gee,[20] who measures the carotid collateral pressure to determine the relative risk of a given recurrent lesion. This technique involves indirect measurement of the ophthalmic artery pressure during carotid artery compression using ocular pneumoplethysmography and correlates well with internal carotid artery backpressure (stump pressure) measured intraoperatively. A collateral pressure below 60 mm Hg shows that the hemisphere is at high risk of stroke should the stenosis progress to occlusion and is an indication for reoperation. By contrast, higher pressures predict that the patient will tolerate occlusion of the involved artery, so prophylactic operation is not necessary. Some investigators have found that the hemisphere with an occluded carotid artery is at an increased risk for stroke, but these studies did not examine subsets determined by collateral pressure measurements.

A more recent approach to functional evaluation employs transcranial Doppler to evaluate the vascular reserve. The hypothesis is that patients with impaired autoregulation distal to a tight stenosis are at increased risk of stroke, especially if the lesion progresses to occlusion. The testing is performed by comparing the baseline velocity in the middle cerebral artery with velocities recorded in response to hypo- or hypercapnea or to the administration of acetazolamide. Several centers are conducting studies to evaluate the prognostic value of intracranial vasoreactivity. In the future, this parameter may be important in clinical decision making.

It is possible that further experience with B-mode ultrasonography of the carotid bifurcation will provide additional criteria for operation on recurrences. O'Donnell and coworkers[21] demonstrated that most new lesions are homogeneous by ultrasonography examination, indicating a fibrous lesion with a benign prognosis. Heterogeneous lesions, suggestive of complex atheromas, were found one-eighth as often in recurrences as in primary lesions. If identification of complex plaques can be achieved with suitable accuracy in other vascular laboratories, the presence of such a lesion may come to be accepted as an additional indication for prophylactic reoperation.

During the past 10 years, there has been a swing toward more extensive use of noninvasive testing to monitor the results of carotid endarterectomies, with an increase in the use of more complex (thus more time-consuming and expensive) tests, such as duplex scanning. However, the different approaches to the management of postendarterectomy stenoses may require a re-evaluation of the follow-up routines. Pierce and colleagues[5] stated that periodic noninvasive tests may not be necessary for routine clinical follow-up, although they recognize the value of such testing in the study of the natural history of carotid endarterectomy. In a study of 78 carotid endarterectomies followed with duplex scanning, Cook and coworkers[22] found no increase in TIA or stroke in patients who developed greater than 50 percent restenosis. They concluded that routine postoperative surveillance is not necessary and should be reserved to follow contralateral lesions or to evaluate recurrent symptoms. The emphasis should be placed on educating patients about the symptoms of TIAs so that any new episodes will result in early re-evaluation. Mattos and associates[23] followed 380 consecutive patients with 409 endarterectomies for up to 177 months (mean, 42 months). Only one patient with recurrent stenosis greater than 50 percent developed a stroke, and this was in relation to occlusion of an internal carotid artery. The authors concluded that early restenosis is a relatively benign lesion and that patients may be as well served with careful clinical

follow-up for symptoms as with frequent noninvasive tests. Duplex scanning becomes appropriate after the first 3 years to detect degenerative lesions, which may carry a higher risk of stroke than early fibrotic stenosis. The main reason for earlier testing is to evaluate contralateral, asymptomatic stenoses.

OPERATION

Repeat carotid endarterectomy is usually more difficult than the original operation due to the scarring and the loss of normal dissection planes. Special care must be taken with the identification and mobilization of the cranial nerves. The hypoglossal nerve usually presents the greatest problem, for it can be pulled down over the bifurcation by the fibrosis and can be difficult to free up as much as needed. Rapp and Stoney[24] reported a 16 percent incidence of cranial nerve injuries, with 10 of 17 involving the hypoglossal nerve. Most surgeons treat the intraoperative period of carotid occlusion in the same way as for primary operations—shunting or not shunting according to their normal practice. There is no evidence to suggest that any different approach is required for restenosis.

The management of the stenotic lesion depends to a great extent on the pathology. A regular atheroma can be treated by simple endarterectomy and primary closure. When the stenosis consists of intimal fibrosis or atheroma combined with fibrosis, it is usually difficult to establish a satisfactory plane of dissection, so these recurrences are treated with patch angioplasty or a combination of endarterectomy plus patching. The consistency of the plaque may be so hard as to require sharp dissection with a scalpel to remove any part of it. The survey on recurrent carotid stenosis conducted by McBride and Callow[25] found that approximately 75 percent of operations included patch angioplasty. It is not possible to predict from the postoperative interval which patients can be managed by simple repeat endarterectomy; some lesions within the first 2 years are simple atheroma, and some late lesions are heavily fibrotic. One must therefore always be prepared for a patch. Reports in the literature show that saphenous vein is used most frequently for reconstruction; however, some surgeons use prosthetic graft material as their first choice. Experience has shown that segments taken from neck veins are too thin and should be avoided. A few lesions have such advanced scarring as to preclude reconstruction with patch angioplasty, thereby requiring the use of an interposition graft.

The outcome of operation for restenosis is comparable to that obtained with primary procedures, except for an increased incidence of cranial nerve problems. Management problems during the operation and in the early recovery period can usually be anticipated, for they often duplicate what occurred at the initial operation. Although there have been cases of a second episode of restenosis, there are no published data to permit estimates of incidence and possible risk factors for this problem.

PREVENTION OF RESTENOSIS

Although the incidence of recurrent stenosis is low, there are continuing efforts to reduce the problem further. The most common approach is the postoperative use of antiplatelet agents, usually a combination of aspirin and dipyridamole, to modify platelet activity. Two reasons proposed for this drug therapy are (1) reduction of the amount of mural thrombus on the endarterectomy surface as a result of decreased platelet aggregation and adhesiveness; and (2) possible reduction of the release of platelet mitogenic factor, which stimulates the migration of myofibroblasts into the area of repair. Most of the experimental work on the value of antiplatelet therapy has been done in relationship to the modification of myointimal proliferation at graft anastomoses, but the conclusions from this work are not necessarily applicable to the reduction of postendarterectomy stenosis. A number of the clinical studies to date have used aspirin with or without dipyridamole and have failed to show any benefit. In three of the studies listed in Table 71–1, 60 to 84 percent of patients with recurrences had been treated.[5, 26, 27] Experimental studies by Bomberger and coworkers[28] as well as others have shown that aspirin and dipyridamole interfere with arterial healing. Of particular importance is the finding of Lusby and associates that patients taking antiplatelet drugs showed no difference in platelet activity at the endarterectomy site compared with controls.[6]

It is important to note that most surgeons start the drugs postoperatively. It may be that an increased benefit can be achieved by treating before operation, so that the effect is present at the time the vessel is unclamped, which is when the majority of the thrombus is formed. Experience with coronary artery bypass with vein grafts shows a benefit from antiplatelet therapy when the drug is given before operation.[29] Two recent randomized studies have addressed this issue by starting the medication preoperatively. Harker and colleagues[30] treated 163 patients undergoing endarterectomy with aspirin (325 mg) and dipyridamole. Comparison of the treatment group with the placebo group showed no difference in the incidence of restenosis. Likewise, Hansen and associates[31] found that low-dose aspirin (75 mg daily) had no effect on restenosis in a study of 232 patients. For the present, one can only conclude that the use of antiplatelet therapy to prevent restenosis remains unproved.

Attempts to reduce the incidence of restenosis should not overlook other drugs, such as heparin or dextran. Using a hypercholesterolemic rabbit model, Barker and associates[32, 33] demonstrated that prolonged administration of either of these agents brought about a reduction in the size of the thrombus formed at an endarterectomy and a significant increase in patency rates. The original explanation proposed for the resulting benefit was based on reduction of lipid levels. A more likely explanation is that the drugs interfere with or modify the platelet activity or the nature of the resulting thrombus in a beneficial way. Supporting the postoperative use of heparin is Lusby's observation that one patient on continuous heparin had no evidence of platelet activity at the endarterectomy site in contrast to patients both with and without antiplatelet therapy.[6]

A different approach to the prevention of restenosis is the routine use of patch angioplasty for all carotid endarterectomies. Some surgeons have used this technique for many years, but there are few data to prove its superiority. Imparato[34] stated that his restenosis rate with this method is lower than that achieved with primary closure. In 1987, Hertzer and coworkers[35] reported a large experience from the Cleve-

land Clinic with patients undergoing carotid surgery with and without vein patch angioplasty. During the 3-year follow-up period, 332 patients were studied with digital angiography or noninvasive studies. Only 3 percent of the arteries that were patched developed greater than 50 percent stenosis, compared with 11 percent of those that were closed primarily. In a randomized study of carotid patching, Eikelboom and associates[36] found that restenosis greater than 50 percent was found in 4 percent of the angioplasty patients compared with 21 percent of those with primary closure. Other studies have had opposite results. A multicenter study of 1000 carotid endarterectomies reported by Rosenthal and colleagues[37] found that patching had no influence on restenosis rates during a median follow-up of 26 months. Similarly, a study by Myers and associates[38] of 163 operations randomizing vein patch versus simple closure found no significant difference in restenosis over a mean follow-up of 5 years. Although there is no clear consensus regarding routine use of a patch, many surgeons appear to be using the technique more frequently. It must be remembered that use of a vein patch is not without potential problems, for there is a small risk of disruption of the vein in the early postoperative period, often with serious morbidity or death.[35, 39, 40]

A third approach to prevention is the proposal by Callow that a deeper endarterectomy be performed in order to avoid leaving behind lipid-laden smooth muscle cells. The technique is based on the assumption that the deeper cells of the media contribute to abnormal myofibroblast proliferation to a greater extent than the media cells adjacent to the endarterectomy site. The work of French and Rewcastle[8] suggests that the deeper dissection plane may increase the chance of recurrence. These workers found thicker deposition of mural thrombus at sites where the residual media was thin or where adventitia was exposed. Callow and colleagues are currently evaluating the merits of deep endarterectomy.[44]

DISCUSSION

In view of the increasing number of carotid operations for asymptomatic lesions, it is necessary to reassess patient selection in regard to risk of restenosis. Operations on asymptomatic patients carry a risk of converting them to symptomatic patients who will require a second operation, but this risk is low. Hertzer and coworkers[10] found that all their patients who had undergone prophylactic endarterectomy became symptomatic when they developed restenosis. In a review of a 16-year experience with 380 patients, Mattos and associates[23] concluded that patients with restenosis were at no higher risk of stroke than those free of restenosis. Although prognostic factors for recurrence are not clearly established, the patient's risks need to be considered in the management algorithm for asymptomatic carotid stenosis. For example, Thomas and colleagues[13] questioned the appropriateness of prophylactic operation for women in view of the increased risk of restenosis they found in their review.

Other questions requiring further study include the role of prophylactic drug therapy, with special emphasis on new approaches to modulating the hyperplastic response. The low frequency of carotid restenosis and the even lower rate of operations for this condition create difficulties in studying this complication. This low incidence requires a large number of patients in prospective studies in order to achieve statistical significance; it is possible that the only way to answer some of the questions is through multicenter cooperative projects. Another problem is the lack of a good experimental model from which to obtain a better understanding of the pathology of the normal and abnormal healing processes. Much of the experimental work to date has involved evaluation of response to injury by normal arteries when what may be needed are further experiments on hypercholesterolemic animals in order to approach the situation of the postendarterectomy patient.

REFERENCES

1. Edwards WS, Wilson TAS, Bennett A: The long-term effectiveness of carotid endarterectomy in the prevention of strokes. *Ann Surg.* 1968;168:765.
2. Stoney RJ, String ST: Recurrent carotid stenosis. *Surgery.* 1976;80:705.
3. Kartchner MM: Discussion. *Surgery.* 1976;80:710.
4. Kremen JE, Gee W, Kaupp HA, McDonald KM: Restenosis or occlusion after carotid endarterectomy. *Arch Surg.* 1979;114:608.
5. Pierce GE, Iliopoulus JI, Holcomb MA: Incidence of recurrent stenosis after carotid endarterectomy determined by digital subtraction angiography. *Am J Surg.* 1984;148:848.
6. Lusby RJ, Ferrell LD, Englestad BL, et al: Vessel wall and indium-III labeled platelet response to carotid endarterectomy. *Surgery.* 1983;93:424.
7. Dirrenberger RA, Sundt TM: Carotid endarterectomy: Temporal profile of the healing process and effects of anticoagulation therapy. *J Neurosurg.* 1978;48:201.
8. French BN, Rewcastle NB: Sequential morphological changes at the site of carotid endarterectomy. *J Neurosurg.* 1974;41:745.
9. Schultz H, Fleming JFR, Awerbuck B: Arteriographic assessment of carotid endarterectomy. *Ann Surg.* 1970;171:509.
10. Hertzer NR, Martinez BD, Benjamin SP, Beven EG: Recurrent stenosis after carotid endarterectomy. *Surg Gynecol Obstet.* 1979;149:300.
11. Healy DA, Zierler RE, Nicholls SC, et al: Long-term follow-up and clinical outcome of carotid restenosis. *J Vasc Surg.* 1989;10:662.
12. Baker WH, Hayes AC, Mahler D, Littooy FN: Durability of carotid endarterectomy. *Surgery.* 1983;94:112.
13. Thomas M, Otis SM, Rush M, et al: Recurrent carotid artery stenosis following endarterectomy. *Ann Surg.* 1984;200:79.
14. Eikelboom BC, Ackerstaff RGA, Ludwig JW, et al: Residual lesions after carotid endarterectomy and the development of restenosis: A prospective DSA and duplex study. In Proceedings of the San Diego Symposium on Noninvasive Diagnostic Techniques in Vascular Disease;1985 (abstract):90.
15. Cossman DV, Treiman RL, Foran RF, et al: Surgical approach to recurrent carotid stenosis. *Am J Surg.* 1980;140:209.
16. Salvian A, Baker JD, Machleder HI, et al: Cause and noninvasive detection of restenosis after carotid endarterectomy. *Am J Surg.* 1983;146:29.
17. Atnip RG, Wengrovitz M, Gifford RM, et al: A rational approach to recurrent carotid stenosis. *J Vasc Surg.* 1990;11:511.
18. Reilly LM, Okuhn SP, Rapp JH, et al: Recurrent carotid stenosis: A consequence of local or systemic factors? The influence of unrepaired technical defects. *J Vasc Surg.* 1990;11:448.
19. Baker JD: How vascular surgeons use noninvasive testing. *J Vasc Surg.* 1986;4:272.
20. Gee W: Ocular pneumoplethysmography. In Bernstein EF, ed. *Noninvasive Diagnostic Techniques in Vascular Disease*, 2nd ed. St. Louis: CV Mosby; 1982:220.
21. O'Donnell TF, Callow AD, Scott G, et al: Ultrasound characteristics of recurrent carotid disease: Hypothesis explaining the low incidence of symptomatic recurrence. *J Vasc Surg.* 1985;2:26.
22. Cook JM, Thompson BW, Barnes RW: Is routine duplex examination after carotid endarterectomy justified? *J Vasc Surg.* 1990;12:334.
23. Mattos MA, van Bemmelen PS, Barkmeier LD, et al: Routine surveillance after carotid endarterectomy: Does it affect clinical management? *J Vasc Surg.* 1993;17:819.
24. Rapp J, Stoney RJ: Recurrent carotid stenosis. In Bernhard VM, Towne JB, eds. *Complications in Vascular Surgery*, 2nd ed. Orlando: Grune & Stratton; 1985:763.
25. McBride K, Callow AD: Recurrent stenosis after carotid endarterectomy. In Bernhard VM, Towne JB, eds. *Complications in Vascular Surgery.* New York: Grune & Stratton; 1980:259.
26. Cossman D, Callow AD, Stein A, Matsumoto G: Early restenosis after carotid endarterectomy. *Arch Surg.* 1978;113:275.
27. Catelmo NL, Cutler BS, Wheeler HB, et al: Noninvasive detection of carotid stenosis following endarterectomy. *Arch Surg.* 1981;116:1005.
28. Bomberger RA, DePalma RG, Ambrose TA, Manalo P: Aspirin and dipyridamole inhibit endothelial healing. *Arch Surg.* 1982;117:1459.
29. Cheseboro JH, Clements IP, Fuster V: A platelet inhibitor drug trial in coronary artery bypass operations. *N Engl J Med.* 1982;307:73.
30. Harker LA, Bernstein EF, Dilley RB, et al: Failure of aspirin plus dipyridamole to prevent restenosis after carotid endarterectomy. *Ann Intern Med.* 1992;116:731.
31. Hansen F, Lindblad B, Persson NH, Bergqvist D: Can recurrent stenosis after carotid endarterectomy be prevented by low-dose acetylsalicylic acid? A double-blind, randomized and placebo controlled study. *Eur J Vasc Surg.* 1993;7:380.
32. Barker WF, Barokonski A: The use of heparin and dextran in arterial reconstruction. *Acta Chir Scand.* 1967;387(suppl):97.
33. Pilcher DB, Barker WF: Retardation of experimental atherosclerosis in endarterectomized arteries by the administration of heparin and dextran. *Am J Surg.* 1970;120:270.
34. Imparato AM: Discussion. *J Vasc Surg.* 1985;2:40.
35. Hertzer NR, Beven EG, O'Hara PJ, Krajewski LP: A prospective study of vein patch angioplasty during carotid endarterectomy. *Ann Surg.* 1987;206:628.
36. Eikelboom BC, Ackerstaff RGA, Hoeneveld H, et al: Benefits of carotid patching: A randomized study. *J Vasc Surg.* 1988;7:240.
37. Rosenthal D, Archie JP, Garcia-Rinaldi R, et al: Carotid patch angioplasty: Immediate and long-term results. *J Vasc Surg.* 1990;12:326.
38. Myers SI, Valentine RJ, Chervu A, et al: Saphenous vein patch versus primary closure for carotid endarterectomy: Long-term assessment of a randomized prospective study. *J Vasc Surg.* 1994;19:15.
39. Riles TS, Lamparello PJ, Giangola G, Imparato AM: Rupture of the vein patch: A rare complication of carotid endarterectomy. *Surgery.* 1990;107:10.
40. Tawes RL, Treiman RL: Vein patch rupture after carotid endarterectomy: A survey of the Western Vascular Society members. *Ann Vasc Surg.* 1991;5:71.
41. Thompson JE, Patman RD, Talkington CM, Garrett WV: Restenosis following carotid endarterectomy. In Vieth FJ, ed. *Critical Problems in Vascular Surgery.* E. Norwalk, CT: Appleton-Century-Crofts; 1982:361.
42. Salenius JP, Haapanen A, Harju E, et al: Late carotid restenosis: Aetiologic factors for recurrent carotid artery stenosis during long-term follow-up. *Eur J Vasc Surg.* 1989;3:271.
43. Clagett GP, Rich NM, McDonald PT, et al: Etiologic factors for recurrent carotid artery stenosis. *Surgery.* 1983;93:313.
44. Callow AD, O'Donnell TF: Recurrent carotid stenosis: Frequency, clinical implications and some suggestions concerning etiology. In Bergan JJ, Yao JST, eds. *Reoperative Arterial Surgery,* Orlando: Grune & Stratton; 1986:513.

XI

Results of Carotid Endarterectomy: The Prospective Randomized Trials

CHAPTER

72

Carotid Endarterectomy for Asymptomatic Carotid Stenosis: Review of the Veterans Administration Cooperative Clinical Trial

ROBERT W. HOBSON II and THE VA COOPERATIVE ASYMPTOMATIC CAROTID ARTERY STENOSIS STUDY GROUP

Performance of carotid endarterectomy in patients with asymptomatic carotid stenosis continues to be a controversial aspect of the surgical management of extracranial carotid occlusive disease. Data from a recently published clinical trial on the efficacy of operative intervention in asymptomatic carotid stenosis form the basis for this chapter.[1, 2] Conducted by the Department of Veterans Affairs, this prospective randomized trial adds information on the topic among male patients. However, final judgment will await publication of data from the National Institutes of Health–sponsored Asymptomatic Carotid Atherosclerosis Study (ACAS).[3]

METHODS

This clinical trial was conducted at 11 Department of Veterans Affairs medical centers (see Appendix) to define the influence of carotid endarterectomy on the combined incidence of neurologic outcome events, including transient ischemic attack, transient monocular blindness, and stroke, in patients with asymptomatic carotid stenosis. Data on 444 adult male patients with asymptomatic carotid stenosis, shown arteriographically to reduce the diameter of the arterial lumen by 50 percent or more (in the presence of positive ocular pneumoplethysmography[4] or duplex scan[5]), were studied. All patients underwent arteriographic confirmation of significant stenosis. The threshold lesion for randomization was a stenosis of 50 percent or more—comparing the least transverse diameter at the point of maximal stenosis with the measured diameter of the postbulbar internal carotid artery once its diameter had become uniform, which, in the presence of positive noninvasive studies,[4, 5] was considered to be an area reduction of 75 percent. Patients were randomly assigned to optimal medical management, including aspirin therapy, plus carotid endarterectomy (211 patients), versus optimal medical management alone (233 patients). All patients were followed independently by a vascular surgeon and a neurologist at each participating center during a mean follow-up of 47.9 months. The mean age of the clinical population was 64.5 years, and clinical characteristics of

randomized patients at entry are summarized in Table 72–1. Thirty-two percent of the trial's patients had a history of ischemic events due to contralateral stenosis, and 80 percent of these events were reported as transient ischemic attacks. Two-thirds of the sample involved patients with bilaterally asymptomatic cerebral hemispheres. Patients randomized to carotid endarterectomy underwent operation within 10 days of randomization.

Medical exclusionary criteria included previous cerebral infarction, previous endarterectomy with restenosis, previous extracranial-to-intracranial bypass, high surgical risk due to associated medical illness, chronic anticoagulant therapy, aspirin intolerance or chronic high-dose aspirin therapy, life expectancy less than 5 years, surgically inaccessible lesions, and noncompliance with or refusal to participate in the protocol.

PATIENT FOLLOW-UP

The study initiated enrollment of patients on April 1, 1983, and patient acquisition was completed in October 1987. Clinical follow-up ended on March 31, 1991. Mean follow-up as measured from the time of entry to the first neurologic event, death, or loss to follow-up was 47.9 months.

All patients initially received 650 mg of aspirin twice daily. This was modified to a lower-dose regimen (325 mg daily) for patients with aspirin intolerance during the subsequent clinical follow-up.[6, 7] Patients who experienced clinically defined neurologic outcome events were evaluated independently by the vascular surgeon and the neurologist at each center, and their conclusions were submitted for blinded review and adjudication to the endpoints committee.

NEUROLOGIC OUTCOME EVENTS

The results for all neurologic events, contralateral and ipsilateral, are summarized in Table 72–2. Eighty-four events

TABLE 72–1. Patient Characteristics at Study Entry*

Characteristics	Surgical Group (n = 211)	Medical Group (n = 233)
Mean age (SD)		
Race, %	64.1 (6.8)	64.7 (6.7)
Caucasian	88	86
African American	6	8
Hispanic	1	3
Native American	2	3
Asian American	2	0
Previous contralateral symptoms, %	32	33
Daily smoker, %	52	49
Previous smoker, %	43	42
History of, %		
Diabetes	30	27
Myocardial infarct	28	25
Angina pectoris	30	25
Congestive heart failure	5	7
Hypertension	63	64
Arrhythmia	17	14
Peripheral vascular disease	61	59

*There were no significant differences between treatment groups.

From Hobson RW, Weiss DG, Fields WS, et al: Efficacy of carotid endarterectomy for asymptomatic carotid stenosis. N Engl J Med. 1993;328:221. Reprinted by permission of the New England Journal of Medicine. Copyright 1993 Massachusetts Medical Society.

were observed, 27 (12.9%) in the surgical group and 57 (24.5%) in the medical group, which represented an absolute risk reduction of 11.6 percent ($P < 0.002$; relative risk 0.51; 95% confidence interval: 0.32, 0.81). Results for ipsilateral events only are presented in Table 72–3. There were 65 ipsilateral events, 17 (8.0%) in the surgical group and 48 (20.6%) in the medical group. The absolute risk reduction was 12.6 percent ($P < 0.001$; relative risk 0.38; 95% CI: 0.22, 0.67). Analysis of the ipsilateral neurologic events in the medical group demonstrated an incidence of 24 events (19.2%; 12 strokes, 7 transient ischemic attacks, 5 episodes of transient monocular blindness) for stenoses of 50 to 75 percent and 24 events (22.4%; 10 strokes, 8 transient ischemic attacks, 6 episodes of transient monocular blindness) for stenoses of 76 to 99 percent, which did not represent a significant difference.

The temporal distribution of neurologic outcome events over the duration of follow-up was determined by construction of Kaplan-Meier survival curves, with survival defined as the time until the first neurologic event. Data for ipsilateral events are summarized in Figure 72–1. The numbers of

patients remaining event free and enrolled in the study at the beginning of each 12-month interval are provided under the graph. Treatment group comparisons by the log-rank test demonstrated significant differences in favor of the surgical group ($P < 0.001$).

STROKE AND DEATH ANALYSIS

The incidence of stroke and death for this high-risk group of patients is presented in Table 72–4. No significant differences were observed between treatment groups.

SURGICAL MORBIDITY AND MORTALITY

Morbidity and mortality data for carotid endarterectomy have been published previously.[8] The 30-day operative mortality was 1.9 percent (4 of 211); three deaths occurred as a

TABLE 72–2. Combined Neurologic Endpoints for Ipsilateral and Contralateral Events

Endpoint	Surgical Group (n = 211)		Medical Group (n = 233)	
	n	%	n	%
Transient ischemic attack	9	4.3	17	7.3
Transient monocular blindness	1	0.5	12	5.2
Stroke (nonfatal and fatal)	17	8.1	28	12.0
Total*	27	12.9	57	24.5

*$P < .002$; relative risk 0.51; 95% confidence interval: 0.32, 0.81.

From Hobson RW, Weiss DG, Fields WS, et al: Efficacy of carotid endarterectomy for asymptomatic carotid stenosis. N Engl J Med.1993;328:221. Reprinted by permission of the New England Journal of Medicine. Copyright 1993 Massachusetts Medical Society.

TABLE 72–3. Combined Neurologic Endpoints for Ipsilateral Events Only

Endpoint	Surgical Group (n = 211)		Medical Group (n = 233)	
	n	%	n	%
Transient ischemic attack	6	2.8	15	6.4
Transient monocular blindness	1	0.5	11	4.7
Stroke* (nonfatal and fatal)	10	4.7	22	9.4
Total†	17	8.0	48	20.6

*$P = 0.056$.

†$P < .001$; relative risk, 0.38; 95% confidence interval: 0.22, 0.67.

From Hobson RW, Weiss DG, Fields WS, et al: Efficacy of carotid endarterectomy for asymptomatic carotid stenosis. N Engl J Med. 1993;328:221. Reprinted by permission of the New England Journal of Medicine. Copyright 1993 Massachusetts Medical Society.

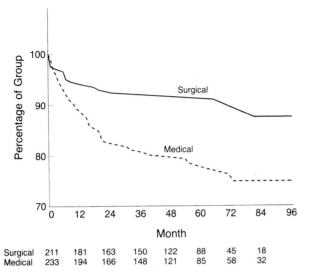

| Surgical | 211 | 181 | 163 | 150 | 122 | 88 | 45 | 18 |
| Medical | 233 | 194 | 166 | 148 | 121 | 85 | 58 | 32 |

FIGURE 72–1. Kaplan-Meier curves of an analysis of event-free rates for first ipsilateral stroke and transient ischemic attack, including transient monocular blindness. The time until the first event for surgical and medical groups is presented. The numbers of patients remaining event free and enrolled in the study at the beginning of each 12-month period are provided under the graph. Comparisons by the log-rank test between treatment groups demonstrated significant differences in favor of the surgical group ($P <$ 0.001). The relative risk (surgical versus medical) was 0.38 (95% confidence interval: 0.22, 0.67). (From Hobson RW II, Weiss DG, Fields WS, et al: Efficacy of carotid endarterectomy for asymptomatic carotid stenosis. *N Engl J Med.* 1993;328:221. Reprinted by permission of the *New England Journal of Medicine.* Copyright 1993 Massachusetts Medical Society.)

result of myocardial infarction, and one was caused by myocardial infarction followed by stroke. Five postoperative strokes (nonfatal) occurred, for an incidence of 2.4 percent. Three nonfatal strokes (0.4%; 3 of 714) occurred as a result of arteriography; one was associated with significant hemiparesis (0.15%), and two were associated with minimal neurologic deficits. The 30-day postrandomization permanent stroke and death rate was 4.7 percent for the surgical group, assigning all complications of arteriography for this trial to the surgical group. In contrast, during the first 30 days after assignment of patients to the medical group, one death due to suicide (0.4%) and two neurologic events (0.9%)

occurred—one permanent stroke and one transient ischemic event.

DISCUSSION

The results of the VA clinical trial indicate that carotid endarterectomy when combined with optimal medical management reduces the incidence of ipsilateral neurologic outcome events in high-risk male patients with arteriographically confirmed asymptomatic carotid stenosis. In addition, the incidence of ipsilateral stroke alone (see Table 72–3) was significantly ($P = 0.056$) reduced in the surgically managed group. However, when the four perioperative deaths (1.9%) were added to this analysis, the 30-day perioperative stroke and death rates between groups were not significantly different. Besides emphasizing the importance of maintaining low perioperative complication rates among patients, our current clinical protocol also includes a rigorous evaluation of the coronary circulation using stress thallium scans as indicated.[9] Carotid endarterectomy is indicated in patients with high-grade asymptomatic stenosis who have been cleared for the risks of coronary artery disease and are expected to live 5 or more years. Although this trial was unable to confirm the influence of carotid endarterectomy on the combined incidence of stroke and death, a modest effect could not be excluded because of the trial's sample size. Data from the ACAS trial,[3] with an anticipated sample size of over 1600 patients, may be able to address this important question.

Surgical complications included an operative mortality of 1.9 percent, a permanent stroke rate of 2.4 percent, and an associated stroke rate due to arteriography of 0.4 percent. Although the combined perioperative stroke and death rate of 4.7 percent was higher than the 3.0 percent cited by Callow and colleagues,[10] multiple individual institutional reports have demonstrated performance well within the 3 percent combined stroke and death rate.[11–15] As a more rigorous clinical review of patients' coronary risk factors is exercised, many institutions will achieve extremely low or no mortality. These institutional reports further emphasize the potential value of carotid endarterectomy in selected patients with high-grade asymptomatic carotid stenosis.

This trial combined transient ischemic attack and stroke alone in the analysis of neurologic outcome. The investigators determined that this was justified because of the importance of transient ischemic attack as an indicator or predictor of stroke. Furthermore, defining differences between transient ischemic attack and stroke with minimal disability may constitute an unnecessarily rigid distinction in view of their similarity in clinical definition,[16] the subsequent risk of stroke after transient events,[17] and the acknowledged 30 to 40 percent incidence of abnormal computed tomography and magnetic resonance scans in patients with transient ischemic attack alone.[18, 19] Results of the North American Symptomatic Carotid Endarterectomy Trial[17] confirmed that transient ischemic attack in the presence of high-grade stenosis is an important factor for predicting stroke. Patients with transient ischemic attack or nondisabling stroke, ipsilateral to a 70 percent or greater carotid stenosis, were reported to have a 26 percent incidence of stroke on life-table analysis during the first 2 years of follow-up. An analysis of relevant data

TABLE 72–4. Stroke, Stroke Death, and All Other Deaths*

Event	Surgical Group (n = 211)		Medical Group (n = 233)	
	n	%	n	%
Nonfatal stroke	17	8.0	25	10.7
Stroke death	1	0.5	4	1.7
MI, cardiac, sudden†	44	20.9	47	20.2
Other medical	19	9.0	17	7.3
Unknown	6	2.8	10	4.3
Total*	87	41.2	103	44.2

*No significant difference (relative risk 0.92; 95% confidence interval: 0.69, 1.22).
†Includes four perioperative deaths.
MI, myocardial infarction.
From Hobson RW, Weiss DG, Fields WS, et al: Efficacy of carotid endarterectomy for asymptomatic carotid stenosis. *N Engl J Med.* 1993;328:221. Reprinted by permission of the *New England Journal of Medicine.* Copyright 1993 Massachusetts Medical Society.

(see Fig. 72–1) from our trial demonstrated that 26 of the 32 ipsilateral strokes also occurred during the first 2 years of the clinical trial. Furthermore, as observed in our studies of the medical treatment group, half of the neurologic outcome events were strokes that were not preceded by transient ischemic attack.

One approach to the performance of carotid endarterectomy for asymptomatic stenosis has been the identification of a subset of high-risk patients who might benefit from operative intervention. Degree of stenosis has emerged as an important risk factor. Chambers and Norris[20] prospectively followed 500 asymptomatic patients with carotid bruits and observed ischemic cerebrovascular events in 18 percent (5.5% strokes) of patients during the first year and in 22 percent during the first 2 years among those with stenoses of more than 75 percent reduction in cross-sectional area. In patients with stenoses of less than 75 percent, the rates were less than 3 and 6 percent for the first 1 and 2 years, respectively. Although the threshold lesion in the VA trial was a 50 percent reduction in diameter on arteriography, the added requirement of a positive noninvasive study resulted in a comparably significant stenosis approximating a 75 percent area reduction in most patients. This probably accounts for the comparability of ipsilateral neurologic event rates between the Toronto data[20] and this clinical trial.[2] Exclusion of patients with high-grade stenosis or rapid progression in the severity of stenosis from a recently reported clinical trial,[21]

allocating them to surgical management, probably neutralized any potentially significant differences between the surgical and medical groups.

In summary, we conclude that carotid endarterectomy in combination with optimal medical management, including antiplatelet therapy, can reduce the incidence of ipsilateral neurologic outcome events in high-risk male patients with arteriographically confirmed asymptomatic carotid stenosis. Although we supported randomization of identified patients to the ACAS protocol,[3] patients who are geographically remote from such centers or who are unwilling to participate in a randomized study should be considered for operative intervention. Nevertheless, caution must be observed, because not all patients are operative candidates. The primary cause of death in these patients remains coronary atherosclerosis, and this must be carefully evaluated before considering operation in an asymptomatic patient. Each surgeon also has the responsibility of defining by local clinical audit the institutional complication rate for carotid endarterectomy. Without thorough clinical evaluation and knowledge of the morbidity and mortality of carotid endarterectomy, operative intervention cannot be recommended routinely. Although carotid endarterectomy did not appear to have a significant effect on the combined incidence of stroke and death in this study, a firm conclusion on this important aspect of treatment must await publication of data from clinical trials involving larger numbers of patients.

Appendix: Study Organization

PLANNING COMMITTEE

Robert W. Hobson II, M.D., chairman; William S. Fields, M.D.; Andrew Gage, M. D.; Jerry Goldstone, M.D.; Clair Haakenson, R.Ph., M.S.; Wesley S. Moore, M.D.; Jonathan B. Towne, M.D.; David G. Weiss, Ph.D.; Creighton B. Wright, M.D.

EXECUTIVE COMMITTEE

Robert W. Hobson II, M.D., chairman; Cindy Colling, R.Ph., M.S., pharmacist; William S. Fields, M.D., consultant in neurology; Jerry Goldstone, M.D., consultant in vascular surgery; Wesley S. Moore, M.D., consultant in vascular surgery; Jonathan B. Towne, M.D., consultant in vascular surgery; David G. Weiss, Ph.D., assistant chief, Cooperative Studies Program Coordinating Center, Perry Point; Creighton B. Wright, M.D., consultant in vascular surgery

STUDY ADMINISTRATIVE COORDINATORS

Sandy Rossos, M.S.; Adele George, R.N.

DATA MONITORING BOARD

Allan D. Callow, M.D., Ph.D., chairman; Roger E. Flora, Ph.D.; James C. Grotta, M.D.; Anthony Imparato, M.D.

CENTRAL NEURORADIOLOGIST

In Sook Song, M.D.

ENDPOINT COMMITTEE

Louis R. Caplan, M.D.; William S. Fields, M.D.; Jerry Goldstone, M.D.; Wesley S. Moore, M.D.; Creighton B. Wright, M.D.

VA COOPERATIVE STUDIES PROGRAM COORDINATING CENTER

C. James Klett, Ph.D.; Joseph F. Collins, Sc.D.; David G. Weiss, Ph.D.; Peggy Jackson; Dorothy Morson; Bertha D. Carter; Barbara McMullen; Robert Kuhn, Ph.D.; Barbara Miller, M.S.; Mike Lee, M.S.; Diana Preston; Debra Davis; Linda Linzy; Cathy Lucas

VA COOPERATIVE STUDIES PROGRAM

Daniel Deykin, M.D.; Janet Gold; Ping Huang, Ph.D.

PARTICIPATING VA MEDICAL CENTERS

Atlanta, GA. Robert B. Smith, M.D.; John Ammons, M.D.; Rita Giannetti, R.N.
Boston, MA. Rudolph W. Vollman, M.D.; Willard John-

son, M.D.; Russell Butler, M.D.; Carlos Kase, M.D.; Janis Hamilton, R.N.; Nancy Walker, R.N.

Buffalo, NY. Andrew A. Gage, M.D.; C. Steven Powell, M.D.; Emilio Soria, M.D.; Walter A. Olszewski, M.D.; Ireneo Gutierrez, M.D.; Delores E. Young, R.N.; Karen Burch, R.N.

East Orange, NJ. Thomas G. Lynch, M.D.; Frank Padberg, M.D.; Said Shanawani, M.D.; Dolores A. Johnson, R.N.; Carolyn Rogers, R.N.

Iowa City, IA. Loren F. Hiratzka, M.D.; John Corson, M.D.; William T. Talman, M.D.; Cheryl Martin, R.N.; Vickie B. Griffith, R.N.; John Yutzy, R.N.; Brenda Lutes, R.N.

Little Rock, AR. Bernard W. Thompson, M.D.; Diane Morgan, R.N.; Colette McDonald, R.N.

Los Angeles (Sepulveda), CA. J. Dennis Baker, M.D.; E. Jeffrey Metter, M.D.; Nadine Rabey, A.S.; DeEtte Dix, P.A.

Milwaukee (Wood), WI. Jonathan B. Towne, M.D.; Dennis Bandyk, M.D.; Varun K. Saxena, M.D.; John Navine, R.N.; Kathy Catarozoli, R.N.; Debra Lanza, R.N.; Pat Parson, R.N.

San Francisco, CA. William C. Krupski, M.D.; Joseph Rapp, M.D.; Frank Sharp, M.D.; Sande Perez, R.N.

Tucson, AZ. Jerry Goldstone, M.D.; Victor Bernhard, M.D.; Enrique Labadie, M.D.; Martha Nash, R.N.; Barbara Phelps, R.N.; Jennifer Vance, R.N.; Gary Anderson, V.S.

West Los Angeles (Wadsworth), CA. R. Eugene Zierler, M.D.; Bruce Stabile, M.D.; Samuel E. Wilson, M.D.; Stanley Cohen, M.D.; Lynne Emma, R.N.; Cathy Hubbert, R.N.

COOPERATIVE STUDIES PROGRAM CLINICAL RESEARCH PHARMACY COORDINATING CENTER

Clair Haakenson, R.Ph., M.S.; Dennis Toussaint, R.Ph., M.S.; Larry Young, R.Ph., M.S.; Cindy Colling, R.Ph., M.S.

REFERENCES

1. Veterans Administration cooperative study group: Role of carotid endarterectomy in asymptomatic carotid stenosis. *Stroke.* 1986;17:534.
2. Hobson RW, Weiss DG, Fields WS, et al: Efficacy of carotid endarterectomy for asymptomatic carotid stenosis. *N Engl J Med.* 1993;328:221.
3. Asymptomatic carotid atherosclerosis study group: Study design for randomized prospective trial of carotid endarterectomy for asymptomatic atherosclerosis. *Stroke.* 1989;20:844.
4. Gee W, Mehigan JT, Wylie EJ: Measurement of collateral cerebral hemispheric blood pressure by ocular pneumoplethysmography. *Am J Surg.* 1975;130:121.
5. Blackshear WM Jr, Phillips DJ, Thiele BL, et al: Detection of carotid occlusive disease by ultrasonic imaging and pulsed Doppler spectrum analysis. *Surgery.* 1979;86:698.
6. Krupski WC, Weiss DG, Rapp JH, et al: Adverse effects of aspirin in the treatment of asymptomatic carotid artery stenosis: Complications related to high and low dose protocols. *J Vasc Surg.* 1992;16:588.
7. Hobson RW, Krupski WC, Weiss DG, et al: Influence of aspirin in the management of asymptomatic carotid stenosis. *J Vasc Surg.* 1993;17:257.
8. Towne JB, Weiss DG, Hobson RW II: First phase report of Veterans Administration asymptomatic carotid stenosis study—operative morbidity and mortality. *J Vasc Surg.* 1990;11:252.
9. Eagle KA, Coley CM, Newell JB, et al: Continuing clinical and thallium data optimizes preoperative assessment of cardiac risk before major vascular surgery. *Ann Intern Med.* 1989;110:859.
10. Callow AD, Caplan LR, Correll JW, et al: Carotid endarterectomy: What is its current status? *Am J Med.* 1988;85:835.
11. Thompson JE, Patman RD, Talkington CM: Asymptomatic carotid bruits—long-term outcome of patients having endarterectomy compared to unoperated controls. *Ann Surg.* 1978;188:308.
12. Wylie EJ: Is an asymptomatic carotid stenosis a surgical lesion? In Courbier R, Jausseran JM, Reggi M, eds. *Arteriopathies Cerebrales Extra-craniennes Asymptomatiques.* Lyon, France: Medicale Observal; 1980:231.
13. Moore DJ, Miles RD, Gooley NA, Sumner DS: Noninvasive assessment of stroke risk in asymptomatic and nonhemispheric patients with suspected carotid disease. Five-year follow-up of 294 unoperated and 81 operated patients. *Ann Surg.* 1985;202:491.
14. Treiman RL, Cossman DV, Foran RF, et al: The risk of carotid endarterectomy for the asymptomatic patient: An argument for prophylactic operation. *Ann Vasc Surg.* 1990;4:29.
15. Anderson R, Hobson RW, Padberg FT, et al: Carotid endarterectomy for asymptomatic carotid stenosis: A ten year experience with 120 procedures in a fellowship program. *Ann Vasc Surg.* 1991;5:111.
16. Toole JF: The Willis lecture: Transient ischemic attacks, scientific method, and new realities. *Stroke.* 1991;22:99.
17. North American symptomatic carotid endarterectomy trial collaborators: Beneficial effect of carotid endarterectomy in symptomatic patients with high-grade carotid stenosis. *N Engl J Med.* 1991;325:445.
18. Perrone P, Candelise L, Scott G, et al: CT evaluation in patients with transient ischemic attack: Correlation between clinical and angiographic findings. *Eur Neurol.* 1979;18:217.
19. Awad I, Modic M, Little JR, et al: Focal parenchymal lesions in transient ischemic attacks: Correlation of computed tomography and magnetic resonance imaging. *Stroke.* 1985;17:399.
20. Chambers BR, Norris JW: Outcome in patients with asymptomatic neck bruits. *N Engl J Med.* 1986;315:860.
21. CASANOVA study group: Carotid surgery versus medical therapy in asymptomatic carotid stenosis. *Stroke.* 1991;22:1229.

CHAPTER 73

Design and Current Status of the Asymptomatic Carotid Atherosclerosis Study

VIRGINIA J. HOWARD

DESIGN

The Asymptomatic Carotid Atherosclerosis Study (ACAS) is a prospective, multicenter, randomized clinical trial designed to determine whether the addition of carotid endarterectomy to aspirin therapy and risk-factor modification reduces the incidence of ipsilateral transient ischemic attack (TIA) and retinal or cerebral infarction in patients with asymptomatic carotid stenosis. Eligibility criteria require that patients have unilateral or bilateral surgically accessible stenosis of the common or internal artery of at least 60 percent diameter, that they be asymptomatic in the artery to be randomly assigned to treatment, and that symptoms in the distribution contralateral to the stenosis have not occurred within 45 days prior to randomization. All patients receive intensive counseling and interventions for reduction of risk factors, including hypertension, obesity, tobacco abuse, and other recognized risk factors for strokes. All patients also receive one tablet (325 mg) of aspirin daily. One half of patients are randomly assigned to undergo a carotid endarterectomy within 2 weeks of randomization. Postrandomization physical and neurologic examinations, cognitive function, event detection, drug counts, and carotid Doppler ultrasonographic studies are performed. Computed tomographic scans and Folstein Mini-Mental Status examinations are performed at the time of entry and of exit and also at the time of verified endpoint occurrence.

Based on data from other endarterectomy trials, ACAS investigators have recently had the opportunity to re-evaluate the original endpoints of the study. Even during the initial planning phase, the investigators understood that the combined events of TIA and stroke may not be as relevant clinically as stroke alone but chose combined ipsilateral TIA and stroke as the primary endpoint because of statistical power considerations.[1] However, if the ACAS has the same stroke rate and the same treatment effect as the recently reported asymptomatic Veterans Affairs trial,[2] and if 4 or more years' worth of follow-up data are accrued, there will be excellent statistical power in ACAS for an analysis of stroke alone. Therefore, the ACAS investigators proposed, and the National Institute of Neurological Disorders and Stroke and the Monitoring Committee have approved, a change in the ACAS primary endpoint, removing TIA and leaving ipsilateral retinal or cerebral infarction or any perioperative stroke or death as the primary endpoint. No change has been made in the clinical conduct of the study. An ACAS patient with a verified TIA endpoint is still considered for post-TIA endarterectomy if he or she is a surgical candidate. The effect is a change in the interim stopping rules; specifically, the Monitoring Committee will *not* notify the investigators if a significant treatment effect is found for the combined ipsilateral stroke *and* TIA endpoint.

Consideration is also being given to extending recruitment beyond the original goal of 1500 patients to 1800, possibly providing a more rapid answer to the question of whether "stoke only" is a significant endpoint. Furthermore, continuing recruitment increases the chance of obtaining a sufficient sample size for subset analyses for gender and for categories of 60 to 80 percent and 81 to 99 percent stenosis.

DETERMINATION OF HEMODYNAMICALLY SIGNIFICANT STENOSIS

A major criterion for a patient's inclusion in the ACAS is the demonstration of a hemodynamically significant stenosis of the internal or common carotid artery by noninvasive or invasive techniques. The presence of such a stenosis can be established using one or more of the following criteria: (1) arteriographic evidence of a 60 percent (diameter) stenosis, (2) a "highly significant" peak systolic flow on Doppler, or (3) a "significant" peak systolic flow on Doppler and a positive ocular pneumoplethysmographic (OPG-Gee) examination. Patients who are randomly assigned to surgery on the basis of Doppler alone or Doppler and OPG-Gee examinations are required to have an arteriogram prior to undergoing endarterectomy.

To ensure consistent interpretation of arteriograms across centers, the ACAS group has developed a standard protocol for arteriographic measurements and has implemented a training and certification program for an ACAS investigator and study coordinator at each center. Study-wide standards for determining hemodynamic significance by noninvasive testing have also been developed to ensure that the measurements (1) are consistent across all participating clinical centers; (2) provide a positive predictive value (PPV) greater than 90 percent for a stenosis of 60 percent or more as measured by arteriography (PPV is the probability of finding a high-grade stenosis by arteriography given a Doppler value that is above the cutoff point); and (3) provide a PPV greater than 95 percent for a stenosis of 60 percent or more, as measured by arteriography. Doppler cutoff points are established for each Doppler device by comparing data collected on a set of approximately 50 consecutive patients from both Doppler examinations and arteriograms performed within 42 days of each other. Regression techniques are employed to model the relationship between the Doppler peak systolic value and the degree of stenosis measured by arteriography. When a Doppler machine is changed during the recruitment phase, a validation study on the new machine is conducted prospectively. Centers are encouraged to keep both the old and the new machines until the new one is validated with a cutoff point.

DETERMINATION OF ASYMPTOMATIC STATUS

In addition to the eligibility requirement of a hemodynamically significant stenosis, patients must never have had a stroke or ischemic attack in the distribution of the artery to be randomized and never have had a vertebrobasilar attack. With respect to the contralateral artery, potential candidates must not have had a stroke or transient ischemic attack within the previous 45 days.

A diagnosis and classification of previous TIA or stroke can be made by an ACAS physician at the clinical center based on symptoms reported by the patient, findings on the neurologic examination, and information contained in the patient's medical records. A diagnosis of previous TIA or stroke can also be made by a computerized TIA/stroke algorithm developed as part of the ACAS trial. A diagnosis by the algorithm is derived from symptoms reported by the patient on the TIA/stroke questionnaire developed by the ACAS.[3] The TIA/stroke questionnaire is a standardized instrument that increases the consistency of diagnosis across the clinical centers. Prior to randomization, personnel from each clinical center are trained, evaluated, and certified on the use of the questionnaire and the algorithm.

FOLLOW-UP SCHEDULE

Completeness of follow-up is vital to achieving the objectives of the study. Patients in the surgical group are scheduled for a follow-up visit 30 days after endarterectomy; patients in the medical group are seen 42 days after randomization. The discrepancy in times for the initial posttreatment follow-up reflects a projected average 12-day delay between randomization and surgery.

Three months after randomization, patients in both treatment arms return for a clinical visit. Following this visit, scheduled telephone interviews and visits to the clinic are alternated every 3 months for the duration of the 5-year study. The scheduled date of the visit or phone interview is determined by the date of randomization, not by the date of the previous contact. All interviews and examinations in the clinic should be made within 10 days of the scheduled date. If the follow-up schedule must be changed because of illness, geographic relocation, or extended vacation, procedures are followed to document the change in schedule. Evaluations performed at these visits are

1. Thirty days after treatment: visit to the clinic for brief medical history; physical, neurologic, and mini-mental status examinations; TIA/stroke questionnaire; event detection; and determination of adherence to prescribed drug regimen. Doppler and postoperative examinations given to the surgical group only.

2. At the third month and every 6 months thereafter: visit to the clinic for brief medical history; physical, neurologic, and mini-mental status examinations; TIA/stroke questionnaire; event detection; and determination of adherence to prescribed drug regimen. For the first 2 years, follow-up includes a repeat Doppler examination at 3 months and every 6 months thereafter. For the remaining 3 years, repeat Doppler is performed annually.

3. At the sixth month and every 6 months thereafter: telephone contact for brief medical history, TIA/stroke questionnaire, event detection, and determination of adherence to prescribed drug regimen.

4. At exit, ie, the last visit to the clinic (for most patients, at follow-up month 57), all patients are to have a repeat computed tomographic scan unless the patient had one within the 6-month period prior to the exit visit.

Patients who notify the coordinators about symptoms of a possible TIA or stroke and patients who report possible events during the regularly scheduled telephone interviews are scheduled for a evaluation at the clinic by both a participating ACAS neurologist and a surgeon as soon as possible. The endpoint verification system is then invoked.

ENDPOINT VERIFICATION SYSTEM

When a patient responds positively to any of the six major symptoms on the TIA/stroke questionnaire, separate neurologic examinations by a participating neurologist and a surgeon are immediately scheduled. Visits are scheduled for any symptoms except positional numbness or positional dizziness alone or symptoms lasting less than 30 seconds. Similarly, if, during one of the regularly scheduled follow-up visits, signs are detected that may be indicative of a cerebral or vertebrobasilar stroke with or without reported symptoms, a second neurologic examination is immediately scheduled. Both the neurologist and the surgeon record the results of their evaluation on the Primary Endpoint Diagnosis form. The diagnoses from the TIA/stroke algorithm are recorded on the TIA/Stroke Follow-Up form. If the local physicians disagree on a diagnosis, the patient coordinator notifies the physicians and gives them the opportunity to review their findings together.

A packet containing the TIA/Stroke Follow-Up form, the two Neurological Examination forms, and the two Primary Endpoint Diagnosis forms are sent by facsimile transmission to the Statistical Coordinating Center (SCC). The SCC removes clinic-identifying information and any comments regarding treatment, diagnosis, or degree of stenosis. The SCC selects one of the six external endpoint reviewers and sends him or her, by facsimile transmission, the endpoint review packet, consisting of the edited Neurological Exam forms and the TIA/Stroke Form.

The external endpoint reviewer completes the review of the case as soon as possible and phones the diagnosis to the SCC. The SCC immediately reviews the diagnoses from the two clinical physicians, the external reviewer, and the TIA/stroke algorithm. If the three physicians agree in their diagnoses, the endpoint is considered to be verified. In cases in which the three physicians are in agreement but disagree with the TIA/stroke algorithm, each physician is asked to document on the Primary Endpoint Diagnosis Form the reason for disagreement with the algorithm.

If there is any variance in diagnoses among the three physicians, the SCC immediately schedules an adjudication conference call among the three physicians, the patient coordinator, and the SCC. In coordinating the discussion of each case, at the beginning of the call, the SCC reminds all parties that no mention of the patient's treatment is to be made during the call to ensure blinded assessment by the endpoint reviewer. After discussion, if a consensus is reached, the physician revising his initial diagnosis completes a Revised Primary Endpoint Diagnosis form and sends the form to the SCC, who forwards it to the patient coordinator at the clinical center for entry into the computerized data base.

In cases in which consensus cannot be reached during the adjudication conference call, the SCC sends the endpoint packet by facsimile transmission to a second external endpoint reviewer. If, after consultation between the reviewers, both reviewers determine that an ischemic event in the distribution of the randomized artery has occurred, a primary endpoint is declared and the patient is released from his or her treatment protocol. If the two reviewers do not agree that an endpoint has been reached, the patient continues under his or her assigned treatment protocol with increased surveillance to quickly detect any repeat of symptoms.

This entire process is to be completed within 3 days of the first reporting of the symptoms or signs that initiated the review. This 3-day period was determined by the Surgical Management and Executive Committees to be an acceptable period to delay surgical treatment for medical protocol patients who began experiencing symptoms, if surgery is determined to be indicated by the patient's physician. Given this time limitation, the responsibilities of the persons involved in the review process are fourfold. First, all data collection and transfer must be accomplished within 2 days of the first report of signs or symptoms. Second, all persons involved in the review process must be available for an adjudication conference call, if necessary, within 3 days of the first report of signs or symptoms. Third, physicians at the clinical centers are committed, by their agreement to participate in this study, to maintain the assigned treatment modality until after completion of the endpoint review process. Fourth, the review process must be completed as quickly as possible, without regard for treatment assignment. In particular, an unhurried attitude on the part of the clinic's physicians may be interpreted by the endpoint reviewer to mean that the patient is in the surgical arm, which in turn may subtly bias the reviewer in his or her diagnosis.

As an added procedure to decrease differential bias and to increase reliability, all potential endpoints (excluding positional numbness and positional dizziness without accompanying symptoms and cases in which none of the symptoms lasts at least 30 seconds) are reviewed again by the full Endpoints Review Committee, composed of all six external reviewers. This full review determines the final diagnosis used in all analyses.

SURGICAL QUALITY CONTROL

The skill of the surgeons participating in the ACAS has a direct and major impact on the recovery of those patients treated by carotid endarterectomy. Because this is a prophylactic operation, it is clear that the lower the mortality and neurologic morbidity rates associated with the operation, the greater the opportunity that the surgically treated group may fare better than the medically treated group. For this reason, the Executive Committee established a Surgical Management Committee, whose responsibility it is to screen credentials

of potential participating surgeons from the centers involved in the study.

The last 50 carotid endarterectomies performed by each individual surgeon are reviewed, with focus on the average patient length of stay; the percentage of patients with surgical indications for amaurosis fugax, TIA, stroke, or other conditions, and the percentage of patients with postoperative results of TIA, stroke, all other morbidities, death, and no complications. The criteria established for safety include an operative morbidity and mortality rate of 5 percent for patients undergoing surgery for TIA, and an operative morbidity and mortality rate of less than 3 percent for patients undergoing surgery for asymptomatic carotid stenosis. Surgeons for whom few data were available were reviewed by the committee as a whole, and, in some cases, acceptance was deferred until additional data could be collected (ie, another 50 cases), in order to get a better profile of the surgeon.[4]

In addition to certification criteria for surgeons participating in the ACAS, there is also a continuing audit of results at individual institutions. The SCC monitors each surgeon's in-study complication rate. If an ACAS patient suffers a postoperative TIA or stroke or dies, that institution is automatically placed on watch. If a second incident occurs, a formal institutional audit is carried out by the Surgical Management Committee. Factors surrounding the postoperative complications, such as whether or not it was the same surgeon or a different surgeon, and possibly further review of the surgical results from individual surgeons at that institution are part of the institutional audit.

CURRENT STATUS

As of June 1, 1993, 1517 patients were enrolled in this study from 39 clinical centers in the United States and Canada. The accrual rate is now about 24 patients per month. The baseline characteristics of the first 1498 patients indicate that there is a male to female ratio of 2:1; approximately 85 percent of the patients are 60 and older and half are between the ages of 60 and 69. About one fourth have had a previous hemispheric event contralateral to the artery being studied.

TABLE 73–1. Results of Doppler and Arteriogram Validation Study*

Status of Doppler Analysis	Number of Machines
Lower cutoff point determined, sensitivity ≥ 70%†	25
Lower cutoff point determined, sensitivity 50–70%†	21
Cutoff point determined, sensitivity < 50%†	7‡
Sensitivity not determined	2**
No cutoff point determined	9††
Total	64

*As of June 1, 1993.
†Refers to sensitivity of lower cutoff point.
‡Four of these are at centers that also have a more sensitive machine.
**Cutoff points determined by comparison of patient data from Doppler machine and from previously analyzed machine.
††Eight of these are at centers with at least one Doppler machine with an established cutoff point.

Seventy-five percent of the patients were found to have a bruit associated with the artery being studied. Patients with recognized risk factors for stroke, such as hypertension, diabetes, or smoking, are balanced between the two treatment groups.

At the time of this report, data from the Doppler/Angiogram Validation Study have been analyzed on 64 instruments from 37 clinical centers (Table 73–1). At their individual cutoff points, 21 devices (33%) had a sensitivity above 50 percent, and 46 devices (72%) had a sensitivity above 70 percent. However, for nine instruments (14%), the relationship between the Doppler reading and the angiogram was too weak to establish any cutoff point, and for seven instruments (11%), a cutoff point could be established but the sensitivity was less than 50 percent. For two machines, the sensitivity could not be determined because the cutoff points were derived from comparison of patient data from the new machine with data from the previously analyzed machine.

In the ACAS, the cutoff points are set to keep the percentage of false-positive findings small, or equivalently, the PPV large. A false-positive is a case in which the Doppler result is above the established cutoff point but the degree of stenosis, as measured by arteriography, is less than 60 percent. The study utilizes an upper cutoff point that can be used without an OPG-Gee examination for confirmation for which there must be confidence that the PPV is at least 95 percent, ie, that the percentage of false-positives is no more than 5 percent. The study utilizes a lower cutoff point for which there is confidence that the percentage of false-positives is no more than 10 percent. (This confidence is related both to the quality and to the quantity of the data.) With the lower cutoff point, an OPG-Gee examination must be performed to confirm high-grade stenosis.

The criteria for determining hemodynamically significant stenosis for the 1498 randomized patients is shown in Table 73–2. Approximately half of the patients were randomly assigned on the basis of a "highly significant" Doppler reading, ie, at or above the 95 percent PPV cutoff point, and 40 percent were randomly assigned on the basis of arteriographic evidence of a 60 percent diameter stenosis. Only 13 centers utilize ocular pneumoplethysmography in eligibility determination (6% of total randomizations), but at one center with 135 randomizations, 52 percent of the cases were randomly assigned based on positive results from an OPG-Gee examination and a Doppler reading at the 90 percent PPV cutoff point.

The results of this method of determining the cutoff point are as follows. Out of the current 364 ACAS patients ran-

TABLE 73–2. Source of Determination of Significant Stenosis

	Patients, n (%)
Doppler cutoff point at 95% PPV*	813 (54)
Arteriogram positive†	586 (39)
Doppler cutoff point at 90% PPV and positive OPG-Gee‡	94 (6)
Total	1498

*Doppler sonography showing a peak systolic frequency greater than the machine-specific 95 percent (PPV) cutoff point determined by correlation of Doppler flow velocities with arteriography in 50 consecutive cases *and* no negative arteriogram within preceding 2 months.

†Conventional or arterial digital subtraction arteriogram indicating diameter stenosis of 60 percent or greater, using minimal residual lumen (MRL) and the distal lumen (DL) in the equation $\{1 - (MRL/DL)\} \times 100$.

‡Doppler ultrasonography showing a peak systolic frequency greater than the machine-specific 90 percent PPV cutoff point *and* positive OPG-Gee (a difference in ophthalmic artery systolic pressures $\geq$ 5 mm Hg or with an ophthalmic-brachial ratio {(ophthalmic artery systolic pressure minus 39) divided by (brachial artery systolic pressure)} less than 0.43) *and* no negative arteriogram within preceding 2 months.

OPG, ocular pneumoplethysmographic examination; PPV, positive predictive value.

domly assigned to surgery who then had to have a postrandomization arteriogram (ie, they had no prior arteriogram), 29 (8.0%) were found by arteriography to have less than 60 percent stenosis. Thus, the method performed substantially as designed, as the percentage of false-positive results is approximately 10 percent. Additionally, four patients (1% of those with postrandomization arteriograms) were excluded from the study surgery because of intracranial arterial disease detected by the postrandomization arteriogram.

ADDENDUM

On September 14, 1994, the external Monitoring Committee advised the National Institutes of Health to stop the study based on an analysis from a median follow-up of 2.7 years: utilizing Kaplan-Meier estimates in an intention-to-treat analysis, a 55 percent reduction was found in the 5-year relative risk for primary endpoints among patients who underwent surgery. A copy of the complete Clinical Advisory can be found published in *Stroke.*[6] The ACAS investigators are now completing the follow-up examinations, expanding the database, performing additional statistical analyses, and seeking expeditious publication of results.

Acknowledgment

This work was supported by USPHS National Institute of Neurological Disorders and Stroke Grant #NS22611.

Appendix

Asymptomatic Carotid Atherosclerosis Study (ACAS)

Principal Investigator: James F. Toole, M.D.

Operations Center:
Department of Neurology
Bowman Gray School of Medicine
Medical Center Boulevard
Winston-Salem, NC 27157-1078

Statistical Coordinating Center:
Collaborative Studies Coordinating Center
Department of Biostatistics
School of Public Health
University of North Carolina
Chapel Hill, NC 27514

Funding Agency: National Institute of Neurological Disorders and Stroke

Participating Clinical Centers: University of Arizona Health Science Center, University of Arkansas for Medical Sciences, Barrow Neurological Institute, Bowman Gray School of Medicine of Wake Forest University, University of California at Los Angeles School of Medicine, University of California at San Diego, California Pacific Medical Center, University of Cincinnati, Columbia University, Francis Scott Key Medical Center, Harbin Clinic, Henry Ford Hospital, Milton S. Hershey Medical Center, Hopital de L'Enfant Jesus, University of Iowa Hospitals and Clinics, University of Kentucky Chandler Medical Center, Lehigh Valley Hospital Center, Loyola University Medical Center, Marshfield Clinic, Medical College of Virginia, University of Medicine and Dentistry of New Jersey, University of Mississippi, New England Medical Center, University of New Mexico School of Medicine, Northwestern University Medical School, Ochsner Clinic, Oregon Health Sciences University, Roanoke Neurological Associates, St. John's Mercy Medical Center, Singing River Hospital, Sunnybrook Medical Centre, University of Tennessee, University of Texas Southwestern Medical Center, Victoria Hospital, Virginia Mason Clinic, University of Western Ontario, Yale University.

REFERENCES

1. The Asymptomatic Carotid Atherosclerosis Study Group: Study design for randomized prospective trial of carotid endarterectomy for asymptomatic atherosclerosis. *Stroke.* 1989;20:844.
2. Hobson R, Weiss D, Fields W, et al and the Veterans Affairs Cooperative Study Group: Efficacy of carotid endarterectomy for asymptomatic carotid stenosis. *N Engl J Med.* 1993;328:21.
3. Lefkowitz DS, Brust JCM, Goldman L, et al: A pilot study of the endpoint verification system in the Asymptomatic Carotid Atherosclerosis Study. *J Stroke Cerebrovasc Dis.* 1992;2:92.
4. Moore WS, Vescera CL, Robertson JT, et al: Selection process for surgeons in the Asymptomatic Carotid Atherosclerosis Study. *Stroke.* 1991;22:1353.
5. Howard G, Chambless LE, Baker WH, et al: A multicenter validation study of Doppler ultrasound versus angiography. *J Stroke Cerebrovasc Dis.* 1991;1:166.
6. National Institute of Neurological Disorders and Stroke—Clinical Advisory: Carotid endarterectomy for patients with asymptomatic internal carotid artery stenosis. *Stroke.* 1994;25:2523.

ADDITIONAL ACAS PUBLICATIONS

1. Howard VJ, Johnson J, Chambless LE, et al: Training and certification of personnel in the Asymptomatic Carotid Atherosclerosis Study. *Controlled Clin Trials.* 1989;10:344. Abstract.
2. Bealer J, Reed JF, Castaldo JE: The influence of a NIH funded study in a community hospital. *Controlled Clin Trials.* 1989;10:352. Abstract.
3. Chambless LE, Smith M: Estimating positive predictive value from a regression model: Screening with a noninvasive test. *Controlled Clin Trials.* 1989;10:325. Abstract.
4. Schenk EA, Baker W, Kuehner ME, et al: Pathology of carotid endarterectomy specimens from patients in the Asymptomatic Carotid Atherosclerosis Study (ACAS). *Stroke.* 1991;22:148. Abstract.
5. Brott T, for the Asymptomatic Carotid Atherosclerosis Study Group: Silent cerebral infarction in the Asymptomatic Carotid Atherosclerosis Study (ACAS). *Stroke.* 1991;22:147. Abstract.
6. Fisher M, for NASCET and ACAS Study Groups: Morphometric analysis of carotid artery plaques. *Stroke.* 1992;23:160. Abstract.
7. Howard VJ, Grizzle J, Diener HC, et al: Comparison of multicenter study designs for investigation of the efficacy of carotid endarterectomy. *Stroke.* 1992;23:583.
8. Wilcox M: Asymptomatic Carotid Atherosclerosis Study: Role of the clinical coordinator. *J Vasc Nurs.* 1992;10:10.
9. Fisher M, Martin A, Cosgrove M, et al: Carotid artery plaques in the NASCET and ACAS projects. *Neurology.* 1992;42(suppl):III-204. Abstract.
10. Howard VJ: Recruitment of clinical centers in an investigator-initiated multicenter clinical trial. *Controlled Clin Trials.* 1992;13:394. Abstract.
11. Toole JF, Hobson RW, Howard VJ, Chambless LE: Nearing the finish line? The Asymptomatic Carotid Atherosclerosis Study. Stroke 1992;23:1054. Editorial.
12. Toole JF, Howard VJ, Chambless LE, et al, for the ACAS Study Group: Results of a Doppler/angiogram validation study applied to eligibility criteria in the Asymptomatic Carotid Atherosclerosis Study (ACAS). *J Stroke Cerebrovasc Dis.* 1992;2(suppl):S14. Abstract.
13. Adams HP, Castaldo J, Chambless LE, et al, for the ACAS Investigators: Identification and management of risk factors for atherosclerosis: Experience in a multicenter trial of carotid endarterectomy. *J Stroke Cerebrovasc Dis.* 1992;2(suppl):S19. Abstract.
14. Fisher M, Martin A, Cosgrove M, et al: Morphologic features of asymptomatic carotid plaques. *Neurology.* 1993;43(suppl):754S. Abstract.

CHAPTER 74

Prospective Randomized Trial of Symptomatic Patients: Results from the NASCET Study

H. J. M. BARNETT

The North American Symptomatic Carotid Endarterectomy Trial (NASCET) was designed to evaluate, by randomized trial, the benefit of carotid endarterectomy in patients with symptoms due to arteriosclerotic disease of the carotid artery. Symptoms had to have occurred or recurred as recently as 120 days (since modified to 180 days) prior to entry into the trial and had to have been clearly focal in the appropriate retina or hemisphere, expressed as transient or persisting ischemic events, but not resulting in major disabling permanent stroke. Patients were not eligible if there was coincidental serious disease or organ failure that would prohibit surgery or appeared likely to restrict survival to less than 5 years. A cardiac condition likely to produce thromboembolism was a cause for exclusion, as was intracranial or inaccessible cerebral artery disease of more significance than the disease at the bifurcation. Patients had to be able and willing to sign informed consent to randomization. Selective catheterization to visualize the four major vessels, including intracranial views, was required as a prelude to randomization.

Fifty American and Canadian centers were recruited to randomize patients. Between January 1988 and February 1991, 659 patients who had symptoms accompanying carotid stenosis of between 70 and 99 percent were entered into the trial; 331 were randomized to receive best medical care alone, and 328 to receive best medical care with the addition of carotid endarterectomy. During this same period, 705 patients with symptoms related to stenosis of between 30 and 69 percent were randomized—349 to receive medical care and 356 to receive medical care plus endarterectomy.

To comply with a set of predetermined "stopping rules," confidential analyses were begun in 1989. In February 1991, these analyses disclosed to the investigators and to the monitoring committee that patients in the surgical arm with 70 percent stenosis or greater were surviving free of stroke significantly better than those in the medical group. The analyses disclosed no benefit for patients with less than 70 percent stenosis. The entry of patients into the trial continues for this moderate group, but entry to the "severe" group was closed in February 1991. The participating physicians and surgeons were advised of these results, and the patients in the medical arm of the severe group were advised to have endarterectomy if no contraindications had arisen since randomization.

The results for patients with this degree of severe stenosis can be summarized directly from the results paper: "Life-table estimates of the cumulative risk of any ipsilateral stroke at two years were 26% in the 331 medical patients and 9% in the 328 surgical patients—an absolute risk reduction ($\pm$ SE) of 17 $\pm$ 3.5% ($P < 0.001$). For a major or fatal ipsilateral stroke, the corresponding estimates were 13.1% and 2.5%—an absolute risk reduction of 10.6 $\pm$ 2.6% ($P < 0.001$). Carotid endarterectomy was still found to be beneficial when all strokes and deaths were included in the analysis ($P < 0.001$)."[1]

In order to generalize these results and assume this degree of benefit, two conditions must be present. First, the surgical skill must be no less than that of the NASCET surgeons. There was an overall 30-day stroke morbidity and mortality of 5.8 percent, reduced to 2.1 percent when minor transient strokes were not included. Second, there must be strict measurement of the stenosis by arteriography (not ultrasonography), with the numerator being the narrowest linear diameter carefully measured (as opposed to estimated by eyeballing) and the denominator being the artery beyond the bulb and the disease. An indication of the importance of this measurement comes from a recent notation from the European Carotid Surgery Trial (ECST), which reported that only 48 percent of its severe stenosis patients would have been classified as such by NASCET.[2] Measurement is critical, and arteriography is the only measurement against which benefit has been evaluated.

The durability of the benefit of endarterectomy for this group of patients is reflected in the survival curves projected out to 60 months (Fig. 74–1). Only 9 percent of the patients in the surgical group had experienced an ipsilateral stroke at 24 months, and this rose to only 11 percent at 48 months. Although the occurrence of strokes in other territories and of death was not affected by the procedure, the stroke-free survival at 60 months was substantially and significantly better after endarterectomy than after medical care alone.

Functional status was measured in all patients on an 11-point scale that had been developed by the investigators for the EC/IC Bypass Study.[3] The surgical patients had a persistently superior functional status than did the medical patients (Fig. 74–2).

Investigators for NASCET were of the opinion that stroke-free survival was the compelling benefit to be sought from endarterectomy. The mere reduction or elimination of transient ischemic attacks (TIAs) was not considered a goal by itself, nor could the addition of TIA to the outcome event of stroke or stroke and death be claimed as evidence of a worthwhile benefit if stroke reduction alone or stroke-free survival were not attainable. We recorded TIA at every follow-up visit and can attest to the surgery's ability to reduce the recurrence of TIA in this group of patients. Adding ipsilateral TIA to ipsilateral stroke as a combined outcome event increases the absolute difference between medical and surgical results at 2 years to 42 percent, compared with an absolute difference of 17 percent when TIA is not attributed equal importance as stroke (Fig. 74–3).

SECONDARY OBSERVATIONS FROM NASCET

Data generated during NASCET have allowed us to examine a number of important issues relevant to the application

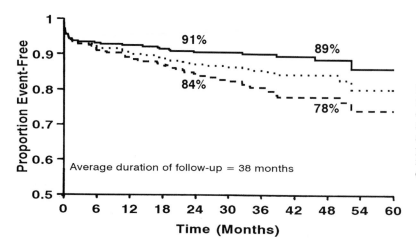

FIGURE 74-1. Kaplan-Meier survival curves demonstrating the durability of endarterectomy for patients with 70 percent or greater linear diameter stenosis (by arteriogram). The average length of follow-up was 38 months, and the percentage of patients with ipsilateral stroke at 24 months was 91 percent; this figure decreased only to 89 percent at 48 months. Solid line, ipsilateral strokes; dotted line, all strokes; dashed line, all strokes and death.

FIGURE 74-2. Functional status over time averaged for medical and surgical patients with severe stenosis. The functional status is the sum of the first ten domains, range = 10–70. Dead patients are censored at death. (From Barnett HJM, The North American Symptomatic Carotid Endarterectomy Trial chapter. In Greenhalgh RM, Hollier LH, eds. *Surgery for Stroke*. London: WB Saunders Co, Ltd; 1993;383–391; with permission.)

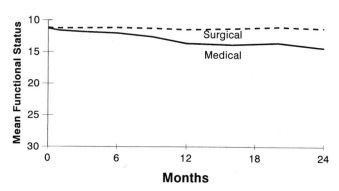

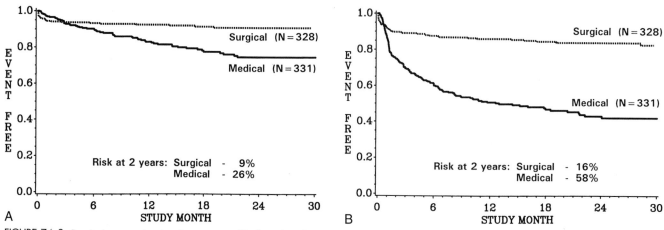

FIGURE 74-3. Survival curves showing the outcome of ipsilateral stroke (A) and the outcome for ipsilateral stroke or transient ischemic attack (TIA) (B) in the medical and surgical groups. There is substantial evidence that endarterectomy reduces TIA occurrences in addition to stroke and death. (From Barnett HJM, The North American Symptomatic Carotid Endarterectomy Trial. In Greenhalgh RM, Hollier LH, eds. *Surgery for Stroke*. London: WB Saunders Co, Ltd; 1993;383–391; with permission.)

TABLE 74–1. Cumulative Risk at 2 Years of Ipsilateral Stroke

% Stenosis	Medical Group, %	Surgical Group, %	Difference, %
70–99	26.0	9.0	17.0
90–99	34.6	8.5	26.1 (±8)
80–89	28.5	10.6	17.9 (±6)
70–79	19.9	7.4	12.5 (±5)

of endarterectomy to this group of patients with symptomatic severe stenosis. These observations are incidental and come from small numbers of patients in some instances. Although caution is recommended in interpreting the generalizability of these observations, this cautionary note is modified somewhat because the observations were made during a 5-year period of prospective follow-up using a protocol and source documents designed to acquire these data.

Deciles of Stenosis. Benefit from surgery and, conversely, the gravity of outlook for medically treated patients declined from the 10th to the 8th decile (Table 74–1). This decline has been verified by observations made in the ECST and recently disclosed by Warlow (C. Warlow, personal communication, 1993).

Risk Profile. A risk profile of 16 factors was recorded from 1988 to 1991 for the severely afflicted patients. Roughly one-third of the medical patients fell into each of the categories presenting with few (0–5), median (6), or many (7 or more) of these factors. The risk of stroke at 2 years rose from 17 percent for those with few, to 23 percent for those with the median of 6, to 39 percent for those with many.

Associated Conditions. Certain conditions made the medical but not the surgical outlook worse. Complete reports on these observations are in preparation but may be summarized as follows:

• The presence of ulceration in the involved carotid artery, particularly when it accompanied stenosis in the 10th decile, substantially worsened the likelihood of ipsilateral stroke. In total, the likelihood at 2 years of nonfatal stroke or death was 30 percent in the medical patients with ulcer and 17 percent in those without ulcer.
• The presence of brain infarction on computed tomography without a history of an event other than a TIA (so-

called silent brain infarction) increased the likelihood of ipsilateral stroke from 13 percent to 26 percent.
• Retinal TIA (amaurosis fugax) carried a much better prognosis than did hemispheric TIA. In the 59 medical patients entering NASCET with severe stenosis who had experienced only retinal transient events, the likelihood of ipsilateral stroke at 2 years was 17 percent. It was 44 percent in the 70 patients who entered the medical arm of NASCET with a history of solely hemispheric transient events.
• Contralateral occlusion but not contralateral stenosis added to the gravity of the outlook for the medical patients. A startling 54.6 percent of them experienced stroke or death at 2 years, as compared with 20 percent in the surgical group. The presence of contralateral occlusion added risk to the operation: 10 percent suffered a 30-day stroke or death, compared with the study average of 5.8 percent. Nevertheless, patients in this group treated surgically were substantially more likely to survive stroke free at 2 years than were patients in the medical group.

Thrombus. One small subset of patients had a worse outlook than their counterparts in the low-risk profile group that was not eliminated by surgery: those with thrombus visible in the carotid artery beyond the stenosis. The numbers were small (25 altogether; 9 randomized to surgery and 16 to medical care alone), but the 30-day ipsilateral stroke rate was high and similar (22% in the surgical group and 25% in the medical group). The high risk from surgery in this situation has been noted before[4] and was recently observed again in the survey of carotid endarterectomy being conducted in 12 academic centers by the Committee on Health Policy at Duke University (D. Matchar, personal communication).

Aspirin. The use of aspirin in the perioperative period interested the investigators. When the trial was planned, a dose of 1300 mg daily was recommended. Less was allowed in the event of side effects, and none was allowable in the case of intolerance. Because the study was not a randomized trial for aspirin dosage, the details of the aspirin doses actually taken in the perioperative period can only present an intriguing hypothesis about the relationship of aspirin use to stroke risk. A rigorous trial is planned to confirm or deny this dramatic differential favoring a higher dosage (Table 74–2).

REFERENCES

1. North American symptomatic carotid endarterectomy trial collaborators: Beneficial effect of carotid endarterectomy in symptomatic patients with high-grade carotid stenosis. *N Engl J Med.* 1991;325:445.
2. Rothwell PM, Warlow CP: The European carotid surgery trial (ECST). In Greenhalgh RM, Hollier LH, eds. *Surgery for Stroke.* Philadelphia: WB Saunders; 1993:369.
3. The EC/IC Bypass Study Group: Failure of extracranial-intracranial arterial bypass to reduce the risk of ischemic stroke. Results of an international randomized trial. *N Engl J Med.* 1985;313:1191.
4. Buchan A, Gates P, Pelz D, Barnett HJM: Intraluminal thrombus in the cerebral circulation. *Stroke.* 1988;19:681.

TABLE 74–2. Ipsilateral Stroke Rate* by Aspirin Dose

Day	0 mg (n = 51)	325 mg (n = 108)	650 mg (n = 94)	1300 mg (n = 74)
1	3.9	0.9	0	0
2–5	5.9	2.8	1.1	0
6–10	7.8	4.6	1.1	1.4
30	7.8	6.5	1.1	2.7

*Numbers represent a cumulative percentage from day 1 through day 30.

Prospective Randomized Trial of Symptomatic Patients with Carotid Artery Disease: Results of the European Carotid Surgery Trial

D. J. THOMAS

The European Carotid Surgery Trial[1] (ECST) is an ongoing, multicenter, randomized, controlled trial of best medical treatment versus best medical treatment plus carotid endarterectomy for patients with carotid stenosis and a recent relevant cerebral or retinal event. The trial was set up at a meeting at St. Mary's Hospital, London, in 1981. This was a fitting venue because the first reported carotid artery reconstruction to prevent stroke in a patient with a recurrent hemiplegia was reported by a group working at St. Mary's almost 30 years earlier.[2] The trial sprouted from the United Kingdom Transient Ischemic Attack (UK TIA) aspirin trial[3] that had started almost 2 years before and had in turn been inspired by the Canadian Antiplatelet Trial.[4] There was eventually free communication between the administration of the ECST and that of the North American Symptomatic Carotid Endarterectomy Trial (NASCET).[5] HJM Barnett, who was the prime investigator for NASCET, was on the monitoring committee of ECST.

The ECST was supported by the Medical Research Council of Great Britain. There are currently 80 centers in 14 countries enrolled in the trial. So far, 2920 patients have been randomly assigned to treatment. Interim results on the first 2200 patients available for study were reported in 1991 for patients with mild and those with severe carotid stenosis.[1] The trial continues for patients with moderate carotid stenosis, as it does for the similar group in NASCET.

PATIENTS AND METHODS

The mean age of the patients was 60 years; 70 percent of them were male. Patients were considered eligible if they had had an appropriate retinal or cerebral hemisphere event within the last 6 months. Most of the patients had had a transient cerebral ischemic attack or transient monocular blindness, but patients were also included if they had had a minor nondisabling completed stroke and embolic retinal infarction.

Patients were excluded if another likely cause for stroke existed; for example, rheumatic heart disease, atrial fibrillation, polycythemia, thrombocytosis, or leukemia. Patients were also excluded if they were known to have underlying cancer or if their general medical condition was precarious and they were unlikely to survive more than 12 months; for example, those with heart failure. On recruitment, patients underwent blood pressure measurement; height and weight measurements; electrocardiography; chest x-ray; full blood count; urea and electrolytes, blood glucose, and cholesterol assessments; and angiography, including intracranial views. Most patients also had computed tomography of the brain.

Risk Factor Modification

If indicated, patients were treated for hypertension. Antiplatelet treatment, usually with aspirin, was also encouraged. Patients were encouraged to stop smoking. A diet history was obtained in patients with high lipid levels and, if diet was inadequate, lipid-lowering agents were prescribed for patients with substantial, sustained hyperlipidemia.

There was no significant difference in baseline characteristics between the patients randomly assigned to medical treatment and those assigned to surgical treatment.

Patients were followed initially at 4 months and then yearly thereafter. Recruitment was initially slow, at a rate of approximately 100 patients per year. It then increased to approximately 400 patients per year. So despite the trial having been started 10 years before, the mean follow-up time was 3 years.

Endpoint

Further transient cerebral ischemic attacks were not considered to be endpoints but were recorded on the follow-up form. The important endpoints were stroke, myocardial infarction, and vascular death (mostly that caused by myocardial infarction or stroke, but some patients with, for example, ruptured aortic aneurysms were included). Soon after a patient reached any endpoint, the collaborator would submit to the Trial Office an endpoint form that gave clinical details and results of computed tomographic (CT) scanning or of autopsy. For patients who survived stroke, an assessment of the degree of disability was made at approximately 6 months.

Randomization Procedure

Ethical Committee approval was obtained at each randomizing center. Informed consent was also obtained from each patient included in the study before random assignment to a group.

There has been some confusion among people not involved with the trial about the randomization procedure used. Some observers have thought that patients and surgeons involved in the trial could choose which form of treatment they wished. This is emphatically not the case. All patients entered into the trial were randomly allocated via telephone to the Clinical Trials Service Unit in Oxford (Richard Peto). Randomization to treatment occurred within each center. Patients, not individual carotid arteries, were randomly assigned to two groups: immediate surgery or no immediate surgery.

At the time the ECST was established, there was resistance from some vascular surgeons to performing carotid endarterectomy on all degrees of stenosis. Some vascular surgeons felt they wanted to operate on patients with moderate and severe stenoses but not on those with mild stenoses. Others felt that they wanted to operate on patients with severe stenoses and not on those with mild stenoses, and they wished to randomly assign only those with the moderate stenoses to treatment.

The Concept of the Gray Area

Because of these differing surgical views among participating centers in 1981, the Steering Committee advised that because randomization was going to take place within each center, each center could choose the range of carotid stenoses that they were willing to randomly assign to treatment, provided they remained consistent. Some centers, including the author's center, randomly assigned all relevant patients with carotid stenoses from 10 percent to 99 percent. Other centers randomly assigned only patients with stenoses over 50 percent; still other centers, only those with stenoses between 30 and 80 percent; and others only those with stenoses under 70 percent. Of the 2200 patients reported in the interim result, approximately half were in the moderately stenotic group (30–69%). A total of 778 patients were in the severely stenotic group (70–99%), and 374 patients were in the mildly stenotic group (0–29%).

A further concession at the time to encourage surgeons to randomly assign their patients was to assign 60 percent of patients to immediate surgery and 40% to no immediate surgery. This was an unbiased but asymmetrical allocation.

RESULTS

The results for the mildly stenotic group (0–29% stenosis) and the severely stenotic group (70–99% stenosis) are reported here. For the moderately stenosed group (30–69% stenosis), statistical significance has not yet been reached in the study, and the trial continues.

Mild Carotid Stenosis

In the range of mild stenosis, 374 patients were randomly assigned to treatment. Very few of these patients developed ipsilateral stroke, at least in the mean follow-up period of 3 years. Not surprisingly, therefore, there was no significant or substantial difference between those who underwent surgery and those who received medical care alone. Therefore carotid endarterectomy on the side of the mild stenosis conferred no benefit over medical treatment.

Severe Carotid Stenosis

Carotid surgery was found to be very significantly better than medical treatment alone for patients with severe stenosis. The results are given in Table 75–1. These results mean that for every 20 endarterectomies performed on patients with tight carotid stenosis, two strokes are prevented and one stroke or vascular death is caused.

In the medical groups, three inter-related adverse risk factors, other than the degree of stenosis, were (1) history

TABLE 75–1. ECST Results for Severe (70–99%) Carotid Stenosis

	Treatment		
	Surgical	Medical	
Patients, n	455	323	
Disabling or fatal strokes			
Ipsilateral	5	27	2P < .0001
Others	6	5	NS
Minor stroke			
Ispilateral	9	44	2P < .0001
Others	9	14	2P = .03

NS, not statistically significant.

of stroke, (2) residual neurologic signs on initial examination, and (3) an infarct visible on CT scan at the time of randomization.

In the surgical group, the 30-day outcome was worse for patients whose baseline blood pressure revealed a systolic pressure exceeding 160 mm Hg and those who underwent a rapid carotid endarterectomy; that is, one lasting less than 1 hour in total. The timing of surgery is important, and it is worth emphasizing that all of these patients were operated on within 6 months of their last cerebral or retinal event and in many cases within 3 months of the last event. For disabling or fatal stroke, the risk to control subjects was greatest in the first year; therefore, delaying surgery by only a few months may render it ineffective.

At around the same time in 1991, NASCET published its results on patients with severely stenosed (greater than 70 percent) arteries.[5] A similar, highly significant benefit of surgery over medical treatment alone was demonstrated. NASCET did not assign patients with mild stenosis and is continuing to randomly assign patients with moderate stenosis.

What is sometimes not appreciated is that the methods of measuring the degree of stenosis in the ECST and the NASCET were different. In NASCET, the diameter of the stenosis, x, was divided by the diameter of the distal internal carotid artery, z. Therefore, the degree of stenosis according to NASCET equals x/z times 100. In the ESCT, the degree of stenosis was determined by dividing x by the estimated diameter of the carotid bulb. The diameter of the bulb was estimated from the general configuration of the carotid bifurcation, y. So in ESCT, the degree of stenosis equals x/y times 100. Since the diameter of the carotid bulb is approximately 1.15 times the diameter of the common carotid artery,[6] whereas the diameter of the internal carotid artery is approximately 0.55 of the common carotid artery, NASCET tends to underemphasize the degree of stenosis relative to ECST (Table 75–2).

TABLE 75–2. Difference Between ECST and NASCET in Percent Stenosis

ECST	NASCET
70	44.7
80	63.6
90	81.6
100	100.0

Risks by Decile

In the NASCET patients with more than 70 percent stenosis (equivalent to ECST's 84%), increased degrees of stenosis were associated with increasing risk of ipsilateral stroke and a greater benefit from carotid endarterectomy.

Similarly, in the ECST patients with more than 70 percent stenosis (equivalent to NASCET's 45%), the risk of ipsilateral stroke also increased with increasing degrees of stenosis.

Surgical Risk

The combined morbidity and mortality rate in the ECST for patients with over 70 percent stenosis was 7.5 percent for death, disabling stroke, or any other stroke producing symptoms for more than 7 days. However, if at 6 months only those who had died or had stroke severe enough to imply disability were considered, the perioperative risk was 3.7 percent. In the group with mild stenosis, the risks were lower, being 4.6 percent for death and any stroke and only 2.3% for death and stroke severe enough to cause disability. In NASCET, the perioperative death and stroke rates were somewhat less, at 5.8 percent and 2.7 percent for major stroke and death, respectively.

Interestingly, if the surgical risks are subdivided in the ECST tight stenosis group, patients with 84 percent to 99 percent stenosis (equivalent to NASCET's 70–99% stenosis) have an equivalent risk rate to that found in NASCET, approximately 5 percent. This is consistent with HHG Eastcott's aphorism about carotid endarterectomy: "the tighter they are, the safer they are." The pathophysiologic explanation for this might be that patients with extremely tight carotid stenoses by the time of surgery have already developed efficient collateral blood vessels and therefore are less vulnerable to perioperative clamping of the internal carotid artery and its threat to cerebral perfusion.

CONTINUED RANDOMIZATION IN THE MODERATELY STENOTIC GROUP

In order to achieve reliable results, particularly if subgroup analysis is needed, large numbers of patients are required. Every possible step must therefore be taken to avoid inhibiting clinicians from entering patients in the trial. As the trial has progressed, the randomization procedure has become much more simple. Collaborators are now presented with a randomization notepad for their own use. They no longer have to submit a fully completed two-page document; all the details are taken down by the clinical trial office at the time of randomization. Copies of angiograms and CT scans are still sent to the Trial Office. The trial will cease when the data monitoring committee is able to say that the results from one treatment arm are significantly better than those from the other.

THE ASYMPTOMATIC CAROTID SURGERY TRIAL

In view of the highly significant results of carotid surgery in patients with greater than 70 percent stenoses in both the NASCET and ECST trials, collaborating centers in Europe have now decided to start a trial on "asymptomatic" patients (ASCT). All patients who are found to have a unilateral or bilateral tight carotid stenosis with no symptoms relevant to a carotid artery and no previous major stroke and who are fit for carotid endarterectomy are considered for the trial. Tight carotid stenosis is not defined specifically, but most patients entered will have greater than 80 percent stenoses. Some will have unilateral occlusion. Some of the patients will already have had carotid surgery on the symptomatic contralateral side.

Patients will be randomly assigned to treatment based on the degree of stenosis as estimated by Doppler examination. Those patients who are assigned to surgical treatment will be examined by angiography in most centers. The main differences between the ASCT and the ongoing North American Asymptomatic Trial (ACAS) are that in ESCT, emphasis will be placed on plaque characterization because of the convincing preliminary work suggesting that echolucent plaques are more likely to produce ipsilateral stroke than are echogenic plaques. The ASCT has far fewer exclusion factors than the ACAS. The ASCT is essentially aiming to answer the questions about what to do with patients with tight carotid stenosis, those who would not have been included in either the ECST or the NASCET. Among other questions is whether carotid endarterectomy helps patients who present with vertebrobasilar ischemic attacks. The endpoints of ASCT will be stroke or death as opposed to transient ischemic attack, stroke, and death, as stipulated in ACAS. A total of 140 centers have been recruited around Europe for the ASCT.

It is hoped that when the results of all these trials on carotid endarterectomy are available, physicians and surgeons will have a better idea of how to manage the many different patients presenting to them with evidence of carotid stenoses.

REFERENCES

1. European Carotid Surgery Trialists' Collaborative Group: MRC European Carotid Surgery Trial: Interim results for symptomatic patients with severe (70–99%) or with mild (0–29%) carotid stenosis. *Lancet.* 1991;337:1235.
2. Eastcott HHG, Pickering GW, Rob CG: Reconstruction of internal carotid artery in a patient with intermittent attacks of hemiplegia. *Lancet.* 1954ii:994.
3. UK-TIA Study Group: The United Kingsdom transient ischemic attack (UKTIA) aspirin trial: final results. *J Neurol Neurosurg Psychiatry.* 1991;54:1044.
4. The Canadian Co-operative Study Group, Barnett HJM. A randomized trial of aspirin and sulfinpyrazone in threatened stroke. *N Engl J Med.* 1978;299:53.
5. North American Symptomatic Carotid Endarterectomy Trial Collaborators: Beneficial effect of carotid endarterectomy in symptomatic patients with high-grade carotid stenosis. *N Engl J Med.* 1991;325:445.
6. Williams MA, Nicolaides AN: Predicting the normal dimensions of the internal and external carotid arteries from the diameter of the common carotid. *Eur J Vasc Surg.* 1987;1:91.

CHAPTER 76

Veterans Affairs Cooperative Studies Program Trial for Carotid Endarterectomy in Patients with Symptomatic Carotid Stenosis

MARC R. MAYBERG, DAVID G. WEISS, FRANK YATSU, and S.E. WILSON

Clinical trials have an increasingly large role in the contemporary practice of medicine. The impetus for this trend originates from the advent of newer methodology for multicenter studies, increasing public awareness about the decision-making processes in health care, the role of clinical trials in determining reimbursement policies, and a general consensus in the medical community that any treatment administered should be proved effective according to rigorous scientific criteria. More recently, emphasis has been placed on the need to document the efficacy of surgical procedures by clinical trials. Prospective randomized trials have several distinct methodologic advantages in demonstrating *causality,* or the cause-and-effect relationship between treatment (eg, surgery) and outcome (eg, stroke). In addition, such trials have become (whether appropriately or not) the standard by which surgical procedures are judged and ultimately applied in clinical practice.

The Veterans Affairs Cooperative Studies Program #309 was a prospective, randomized, multicenter trial within the Veterans Administration (VA) health care system to examine the efficacy of carotid endarterectomy with best medical care versus best medical care alone.[1] The trial was designed to define a specific population at risk for stroke and to minimize the influence of extraneous factors that might otherwise affect this risk. Data from concurrent clinical trials[2, 3] demonstrating a profound benefit from carotid endarterectomy in similar patient cohorts prompted early termination of the trial and analysis of data prior to the anticipated completion date.

STUDY DESIGN

Planning for the VA trial was started in June, 1986.[4] An initial group of 13 VA Medical Centers was selected from 28 centers affiliated with major university training programs that were screened for participation in the trial. Each center was required to have performed 25 or more carotid endarterectomies annually in the previous 3 years, with overall morbidity and mortality rates for the procedure of less than 6 percent. Participating surgeons were required to have performed more than 10 endarterectomies annually within the same criteria. Principal investigators at each participating institution consisted of a surgeon and a neurologist. All angiograms for patients qualified for entry into the trial were reviewed locally and by an independent central reviewer. Detailed records for each treatment failure were evaluated by an independent Adjudication Committee. Ethical and procedural concerns were addressed annually by a Data Monitoring Board and a Human Rights Committee.

Men presenting to participating VA Medical Centers within 120 days of the onset of symptoms consistent with transient ischemic attack (TIA), transient monocular blindness (TMB), or recent small completed strokes underwent screening for multiple neurologic, medical, and cardiologic exclusionary factors. TIA was defined as the abrupt onset of unilateral motor or sensory disturbance, speech deficit, homonymous hemianopia, or constructional apraxia that completely resolved in less than 24 hours. TMB was defined as the abrupt onset of unilateral decreased visual acuity involving a portion or the entirety of the visual field that resolved in less than 24 hours. Recent completed small stroke was defined as symptoms and signs of focal unilateral cerebral ischemia as for TIA or TMB that were not disabling and did not fully resolve within 24 hours.

Exclusions

All potential patients were examined by a participating neurologist for determination of the neurologic exclusions, including global cerebral ischemia, focal seizures, vertebrobasilar ischemia, mass lesions, major strokes, potential cardiac source of emboli, subarachnoid or intracerebral hemorrhage, prior ipsilateral carotid endarterectomy, prior extracranial-intracranial bypass procedure or pre-existing incapacitating neurologic disease. Similarly, a designated cardiologist or anesthesiologist at each center determined cardiologic exclusions. These included chronic atrial fibrillation, myocardial infarction within 6 months, prosthetic heart valve, rheumatic heart disease with significant valvular involvement, mural thrombus as shown by echocardiography, congestive heart failure (class III or IV), resting ejection fraction less than 30 percent, ventricular ectopy more than 10 extrasystoles per minute, unstable angina, or evidence of cardiac ischemia as shown by thallium stress test or cardiac catheterization. General medical exclusions were defined as significant psychiatric illness or intellectual incapacity, poorly controlled diabetes mellitus, severe hypertension, renal failure, severe chronic obstructive pulmonary disease, malignancy with life expectancy less than 3 years, emergency medical condition requiring surgery or intensive care treatment, concurrent use of oral anticoagulants, and patient unreliability or noncompliance.

Radiologic and Noninvasive Assessment

After neurologic, medical, and cardiologic screening, all potential study patients underwent duplex ultrasonography of the carotid arteries, computed tomographic (CT) scan of the head, and three-vessel cerebral angiography. Additionally, transcranial Doppler ultrasonographic examination of the cerebral vasculature was performed at six participating centers. Exclusionary criteria from these tests included CT evidence of edema, hemorrhage, or nonvascular lesions potentially related to symptoms and duplex determination of stenosis less than 50 percent ipsilateral to the site of the presenting symptoms. Angiographic carotid stenosis was calculated from biplanar angiograms by local and central radiologists according to the formula used in the North American Symptomatic Carotid Endarterectomy Trial[3] and VA Asymptomatic Stenosis Trials.[5] Percent stenosis = $100 \times [1 -$ (diameter of narrowest segment of common or internal carotid artery at the bifurcation/diameter of normal internal carotid artery above lesion)]. Angiographic exclusions included ipsilateral internal carotid artery stenosis less than 50 percent, ipsilateral carotid artery occlusion, and ipsilateral internal carotid artery siphon or middle cerebral artery stenosis more severe than cervical internal carotid artery stenosis.

Stratification

Patients meeting the entry requirements for the study were randomized by central computer-generated lists for each center according to six (3 × 2) strata: presenting symptom (TIA, TMB, or small stroke) and the presence or absence of hemodynamically-significant internal carotid artery stenosis (or occlusion) contralateral to the symptomatic side. Qualified patients who refused entry were treated at the discretion of the referring physician and followed separately by telephone questionnaire for the primary outcome determinations. Surgery logs were made at each participating center to identify any potential study patients undergoing carotid endarterectomy outside of the trial.

Aspirin Therapy

Patients randomly assigned to both surgical and medical groups received enteric-coated aspirin (Ecotrin, Smith-Kline-Beecham Consumer Brands; Parsippany, NY), 325 milligrams orally once daily. Aspirin therapy was started at the time of initial screening and continued for the duration of the study. The degree of aspirin therapy compliance was determined by the pill-counting method at routine follow-up interviews. All patients entering the study were monitored and treated for the control of coexisting medical disorders, especially hypertension, diabetes mellitus, cardiopulmonary disease, and hyperlipidemia. Preoperative, intraoperative, and postoperative treatment protocols at participating institutions were not standardized.

Follow-Up

In the initial study design, all patients entering the trial were to be followed for a 36-month period. Routine follow-up, including history and physical examination by two principal investigators, determination of compliance with aspirin therapy, blood tests, and noninvasive testing, was performed at 4 weeks after randomization, at 13-week intervals in the first year, and at 26-week intervals in years 2 and 3. CT scans were performed at 1 year.

Endpoints

Primary endpoints (treatment failures) were defined exclusively as the following:

A. Cerebral or retinal infarction in the vascular distribution of the symptomatic carotid artery consisting of a neurologic deficit, including weakness, sensory loss, speech difficulty, homonymous hemianopia, constructional apraxia, or complete or partial loss of vision in one eye that persists for more than 24 hours.
B. Crescendo TIA, defined as recurrent transient cerebral or retinal ischemia in the distribution of the carotid artery under study, characterized by a definite change in pattern such as:
   1. Increased frequency: several episodes in a single day, or over several days, or clusters of spells over the course of several days, and/or
   2. Increased duration: spells lasting longer than the primary event, or several hours in duration, and/or
   3. Increased severity: spread in the distribution of ischemia with greater or new motor, sensory, speech, or visual deficits.
C. Death from any cause within 30 days of randomization or death related to ipsilateral stroke at any time in the follow-up period.

Secondary endpoints were defined as those events that eliminated patients from subsequent follow-up before the end of the 36-month period of observation. These included death from causes other than ipsilateral stroke, voluntary withdrawal from the study, severe adverse reaction to aspirin, or symptoms necessitating carotid endarterectomy on the contralateral side. Events that were not considered endpoints included stable persistent transient ischemic attacks in any vascular distribution, cerebral infarction in nonrandomized vascular distributions, and asymptomatic carotid occlusion.

Evaluation of Potential Treatment Failures

All patients experiencing potential treatment failure (primary endpoints) were hospitalized for evaluation by two principal investigators, CT scan, and duplex evaluation. If stroke or crescendo TIA was verified, patients in the nonsurgical group were offered surgical therapy at the discretion of the treating physician and followed outside of the study for the usual 36-month course. All treatment failures were subsequently reviewed by an independent Adjudication Committee.

Statistical Analysis

Predicted treatment failures were estimated at 5.4 percent from perioperative stroke or death plus 1.5 percent annual stroke rate in the surgical group (36 month total, 9.5%) versus 6.5 percent yearly stroke rate in the nonsurgical group (total, 19.5%). Based on these figures, the requisite sample size was estimated at 250 patients for each group (type I error = 0.05; $P = .90$), including an adjustment for estimated loss of follow-up at 15 percent. The data center was the VA Cooperative Studies Program Coordinating Center at Perry Point, Maryland. Comparisons were made for continuous variables (Student's t-test) and categorical variables (χ^2 procedures). Survival curves were estimated using the product limit method of Kaplan and Meier and statistically compared by the Mantel-Cox (log rank test) statistic. Subgroup analysis was not routinely performed owing to the limited sample size.

RESULTS OF THE TRIAL

Exclusions

Among 5000 patients screened for entry into the trial at 16 participating centers during the period of July, 1988 through February, 1991, 4807 were excluded according to one or more of the criteria listed earlier. Neurologic exclusions (n = 3011) were most commonly for nonfocal ischemia, major stroke, or potential cardiac source of embolus. The second most frequent exclusion was for ipsilateral duplex stenosis less than 50 percent (n = 2104). Medical exclusions (n = 951) were largely due to potential noncompliance or impaired intellectual capacity. Exclusions based on cardiologic criteria (n = 603) were most commonly due to chronic atrial fibrillation or unstable angina. Drug-related exclusions (n = 251) related mostly to concurrent use of oral anticoagulants or prior severe adverse reaction to aspirin. Among 414 patients excluded on the basis of angiographic findings, the majority had ipsilateral internal carotid artery occlusion or stenosis less than 50 percent. Forty-eight patients who were otherwise qualified for the trial refused entry. One participating center performed 10 carotid endarterectomies on patients who were not screened and may have been potential candidates for entry into the trial.

Demographic Characteristics of Patients Entered

After the appropriate patients were excluded, based on eligibility criteria and patient refusal, 193 men aged 35 to 82 years (mean, 64.8 years) were randomly assigned to surgical (n = 92) or nonsurgical (n = 101) treatment. Four patients (one surgical, three nonsurgical) were retrospectively excluded from analysis after central radiographic review demonstrated angiographic stenosis of less than 50 percent. The demographic characteristics of the two groups were similar, and no significant differences were observed between groups for any variable. Risk factors were prevalent in both groups, including tobacco use (91%), moderate to severe obesity (47%), hypertension (48%), and diabetes mellitus (30%). Concurrent cardiovascular disease was also prominent, especially angina (46%), significant peripheral vascular disease (43%), and prior myocardial infarction (36%). Family history was positive for cardiac disease (60%), hypertension (48%), stroke (37%), and diabetes mellitus (31%). History of cerebrovascular events preceding the event precipitating entry into the study was common, with 60 percent of patients reporting previous TIAs (78% of which were ipsilateral) or prior stroke (27% of all patients). Daily aspirin use prior to any vascular event was reported by 41 percent of patients entering the study.

Precipitating Event

Stroke was the event precipitating entry into the study in 24 percent of patients, compared with TIA in 38 percent, and TMB in 37 percent. The majority of precipitating events occurred in close temporal proximity to randomization (68% within less than 30 days; mean, 35 days), although there was a tendency for delayed entry among patients with completed stroke (mean, 49 days). Among transient events (TIA or TMB), most episodes were brief (66%, <10 minutes; 87%, <60 minutes) and frequently repetitive (73%, more than one event). Neurologic examination at the time of entry showed abnormal results in 52 percent of randomized patients, with the most frequent abnormal findings being hemiparesis (39%), sensory deficit (31%), and abnormal deep tendon reflexes (31%).

Arteriographic Findings

All 193 patients underwent cerebral arteriography, which was locally reviewed at participating centers; 184 angiograms were also reviewed centrally. Four patients were retrospectively excluded from the study by central determination of carotid stenosis less than 50 percent. The complication rate of cerebral angiography was low, with no permanent residual deficits and transient complications in 9 percent (3% local vascular, 4% transient neurologic, 2% minor allergic). Two thirds of randomly assigned patients demonstrated angiographic internal carotid artery stenosis greater than 70 percent.

Accuracy of Duplex Determinations

Comparisons between duplex scanning and angiography were made for 328 arteries, including both the symptomatic (>50% angiographic stenosis) and asymptomatic (variable degrees of stenosis) sides. Duplex sensitivity varied from 25 percent in the 30 to 49 percent stenosis range to 71 percent for the 80 to 99 percent stenosis range, and 92 percent for internal carotid artery occlusion (Fig. 76–1). Duplex readings underestimated the degree of stenosis in the 30 to 49 percent stenosis group in 50 percent of cases. No significant differences in duplex accuracy were observed among participating centers. There was no apparent relationship between carotid plaque morphology, external carotid artery stenosis,

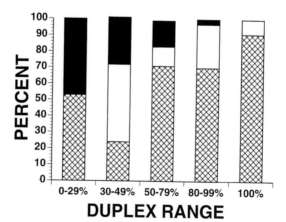

FIGURE 76–1. Duplex determinations for internal carotid artery stenosis compared with angiography. Data are expressed as percent of duplex determinations, showing accuracy *(hatched),* underestimation *(white),* or overestimation *(black)* in comparison with angiographic determinations for five categories of stenosis.

or the presence of plaque ulceration as shown by ultrasonography and the accuracy of duplex stenosis determinations.

Carotid Endarterectomy Procedure

Carotid endarterectomy was performed in 90 of 91 patients randomly assigned to surgical treatment. The mean elapsed time from randomization to surgery was 2.2 days. Intraoperative heparinization (98%), some type of monitoring of cerebral blood flow (94%), and intravascular shunt (44%), were commonly employed surgical techniques. Non-endpoint complications of surgery were relatively infrequent, including respiratory insufficiency requiring extended intensive care monitoring (5%), minor to moderate wound hematoma (5%), cranial nerve deficit (5%), myocardial infarction (2%), and pulmonary embolism (1%). None of these complications produced significant permanent deficit. Postoperative determination of carotid artery patency by duplex scanning or angiography showed good technical results, with minimal stenosis (less than than 25%) in 84 percent, mild stenosis (25–49%) in 7 percent, moderate stenosis (50–79%) in 7 percent, severe stenosis (80–99%) in 1 percent and occlusion in one patient who had intraoperative ligation of the carotid artery.

Secondary Endpoints

Follow-up was achieved in 188 of 189 patients entered into the trial, with a mean follow-up of 11.9 months. Secondary endpoints occurred in 23 patients evenly distributed between treatment groups (Table 76–1). There were three cross-overs from nonsurgical to surgical treatment, six late deaths unrelated to cerebrovascular causes, one patient with contralateral cerebral ischemia necessitating carotid endarterectomy, three patients with significant adverse reactions to aspirin, one patient lost to follow-up, and nine patients who withdrew from the study.

Primary Endpoints

Cumulative primary endpoints (ipsilateral stroke or crescendo TIA) for all patients in the two treatment groups based upon intent-to-treat are shown in Figure 76–2. At a mean follow-up of 11.9 months, there was a significant reduction in stroke or crescendo TIA in patients who under-

went carotid endarterectomy (7.7%) compared with nonsurgical patients (19.4%); the relative risk risk reduction was 60 percent ($P = .011$). Among patients with internal carotid artery stenosis greater than 70 percent (Fig. 76–2B), the benefit of surgery was more pronounced, with a 70 percent relative risk reduction ($P = .004$). Table 76–2 shows the distribution of primary endpoints by type between groups. In the nonsurgical group there were seven strokes (three major and four minor), two of which occurred within 30 days of randomization. Twelve of 19 primary endpoints in the nonsurgical group involved crescendo TIA, in which both investigators at the participating center determined that a distinct change had occurred in the frequency or severity, or both, of the transient ischemic spells (see earlier discussion). Non-endpoint transient ischemic events were similarly more frequent in the nonsurgical group (n = 36) compared with the surgical group (n = 3). In the surgical group, three deaths occurred after discharge from the hospital within 30 days of surgery (cerebral hemorrhage, ruptured aortic aneurysm, presumed pulmonary embolus). Two strokes occurred in the immediate postoperative period, one of which resolved within 72 hours. One stroke in the surgery group occurred at 13 months after surgery.

SIGNIFICANCE OF FINDINGS

The external validity for any clinical trial is determined in large part by the parameters used to define the population being studied. *Inclusion criteria* set forth parameters that determine the essential predictive variables to be studied, eg, carotid stenosis and transient ischemic attacks as risk factors for subsequent cerebral infarction. *Exclusion criteria*, on the other hand, define a set of variables that might otherwise confound the analysis, eg, atrial fibrillation in patients with carotid stenosis and transient ischemic attacks. A delicate balance between inclusionary and exclusionary criteria must be determined to provide a cohort that is selective and relatively uniform, yet large enough to provide adequate sample size and general enough to be applicable to larger populations. Patients in this study were men with relatively uniform predisposing risk factors for stroke. Although the VA patient population may differ somewhat from the general population in terms of demographic characteristics, the results of this study should be applicable to a comparable cohort of men in the United States. Risk factors for cerebral ischemia identified in this study were comparable to those described in previous retrospective cohort trials.[6, 7] Concurrent cardiac and vascular disease, hypertension, diabetes mellitus, cigarette use, and family history of cerebrovascular and cardiovascular disease were prevalent among patients in this study. In about one half of study patients, episodes of cerebral ischemia prior to the precipitating event were identified in the same or other vascular distributions. Inclusion criteria for this trial were established to utilize generally accepted indications for carotid endarterectomy. However, fewer than 1 in 25 patients referred for evaluation of cerebral ischemia fit the established criteria for surgical intervention. In light of the multiple exclusionary criteria employed, the efficacy of carotid endarterectomy demonstrated in this study was applicable to only a limited subset of patients with presumed cerebral ischemic symptoms.

TABLE 76–1. Secondary Endpoints

	Patients, n		
	Surgical	Nonsurgical	Total
Cross-over between groups	0	3	3
Withdrawal from trial	4	5	9
Significant reaction to aspirin	2	1	3
Nonstroke death > 30 days after randomization	4	2	6
Contralateral ischemia	0	1	1
Lost to follow-up	1	0	1
Total	11	12	23

From Mayberg MR, Wilson SE, Yatsu F, et al: Carotid endarterectomy and prevention of cerebral ischemia and symptomatic carotid stenosis. *JAMA*. 1991;266:3289; with permission. Copyright 1991, the American Medical Association.

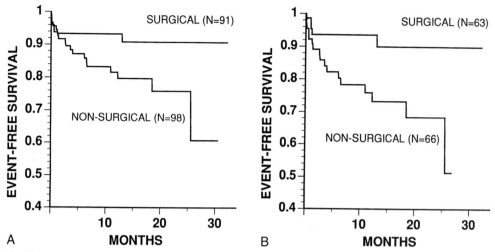

FIGURE 76–2. Kaplan-Meier survival curve analysis of cumulative event-free survival for ipsilateral stroke or crescendo transient ischemic attack in surgical versus nonsurgical patients. *A*, All patients (*P* = .028); *B*, patients with ipsilateral carotid stenosis greater than 70 percent (*P* = .010). (From Mayberg MR, Wilson SE, Yatsu F, et al: Carotid endarterectomy and prevention of cerebral ischemia and symptomatic carotid stenosis. *JAMA.* 1991;266:3289–3294; with permission. Copyright 1991, American Medical Association.)

In any clinical trial, extreme care must be taken to ensure that the study population is not biased by undefined selection criteria. To assess this issue, the VA Symptomatic Stenosis Trial and other contemporary clinical trials for cerebrovascular surgery[3, 5, 8] have incorporated follow-up of nonrandomized qualified patients to ensure against this potential deficit.

In the VA Symptomatic Stenosis Trial, for men with angiographic internal carotid artery stenosis greater than 50 percent, carotid endarterectomy provided significant protection from ipsilateral cerebral or retinal infarction or crescendo TIA. There was an 11.7 percent absolute risk reduction (60% relative risk reduction) for these outcomes among surgical compared with nonsurgical patients. The relatively small sample size, however, prevented direct comparison among these subgroups. The benefit for surgery was apparent early after randomization and persisted over the entire period of follow-up. The efficacy of carotid endarterectomy was durable, with only one ipsilateral stroke beyond the 30-day

perioperative period. Discounting one preoperative stroke, a perioperative morbidity of 2.2 percent and mortality of 3.3 percent (total, 5.5%) were achieved over multiple centers among relatively high-risk patients. No major perioperative strokes occurred. These figures compare favorably with previously published guidelines[9] and those reported in other North American trials for symptomatic[3] and asymptomatic[5] stenosis for patients in similar risk categories. In addition, nonstroke complications from surgery and angiographic morbidity were transient and relatively minor.

Comparison with Other Studies

The incidence of ipsilateral cerebral ischemia in the nonsurgical group considerably exceeded that reported from prior retrospective studies. In the current trial, stroke or crescendo TIA was noted in 6 percent of nonsurgical patients at 1 month and 19 percent at a mean of 1 year after initial presentation. By comparison, symptomatic patients in prospective multicenter trials for aspirin had annual stroke rates ranging from 3 to 7 percent.[10–12] A retrospective community analysis of patients with symptomatic carotid stenosis estimated annual stroke risk at 6 percent; this study suggested that stroke risk was greatest in temporal proximity to the presenting event.[13] The incidence of ipsilateral cerebral ischemia in nonsurgical patients in this trial was comparable to that reported for patients with high-grade carotid stenosis in NASCET[3] (26.6% at mean follow-up of 24 months) and ECST[2] (16.8% at mean follow-up of 32 months). Similarly, the persistent protection against ipsilateral stroke provided by endarterectomy was notable in all three studies, with subsequent annual stroke rates less than 2 percent in this group of patients.

Crescendo Transient Ischemic Attack

In the VA Symptomatic Stenosis Trial, a significant number of primary endpoints involved crescendo TIA. All such events were determined by both investigators at the participating institution and independently adjudicated according

TABLE 76–2. Primary Endpoints (Treatment Failures)

	Patients, n		
	Surgical	Nonsurgical	Total
First 30 days			
Minor stroke	2	2	4
Major stroke	1*	0	1
Crescendo TIA	0	4	4
Death	3†	0	3
More than 30 days			
Minor stroke	0	2	2
Major stroke	1	3	4
Crescendo TIA	0	8	8
Total	7	19	26

*One stroke occurred prior to surgery.
†Ruptured aortic aneurysm, pulmonary embolus, or cerebral hemorrhage after discharge from hospital.
TIA, transient ischemia attack.
From Mayberg MR, Wilson SE, Yatsu F, et al: Carotid endarterectomy and prevention of cerebral ischemia and symptomatic carotid stenosis. *JAMA.* 1991;266:3289; with permission. Copyright 1991, the American Medical Association.

to definitions established by an ad hoc committee. Although the association of crescendo TIA with impending stroke has not been well documented, this trial was designed to reflect practice patterns in the general medical community, in which crescendo TIA is generally considered to be a precursor to stroke. Patients in this trial who experienced crescendo TIA were offered surgery, with excellent results.[14] Since Sundt and colleagues[15] reported significant perioperative morbidity in the setting of crescendo TIA, a strategy to defer carotid endarterectomy until the development of crescendo TIA appears unwarranted.

Degree of Stenosis and Stroke Risk

Stroke risk has been previously associated with the degree of carotid stenosis for asymptomatic[16, 17] patients. Data from other prospective randomized trials for carotid endarterectomy have suggested a positive correlation between degree of stenosis and the surgical benefit[2, 3] In the current trial, there was a suggestion that surgery provided greater protection against stroke in those patients with carotid stenosis greater than 70 percent. The limited number of patients with 50 to 70 percent stenosis prevented subgroup analysis. The efficacy of carotid endarterectomy in preventing stroke among patients with lesser degrees of stenosis remains indeterminate pending the results of current prospective trials.

Acknowledgments

This study was supported by funding from Department of Veterans Affairs Cooperative Studies Program, Veterans Affairs Medical Research Service.

REFERENCES

1. Mayberg MR, Wilson SE, Yatsu F, et al: Carotid endarterectomy and prevention of cerebral ischemia and symptomatic carotid stenosis. *JAMA.* 1991;266:3289.
2. European Carotid Surgery Trialists' Collaborative Group: MRC European carotid surgery trial: Interim results for symptomatic patients with severe (70–99%) or with mild (0–29%) carotid stenosis. *Lancet.* 1991;337:1235.
3. NASCET Collaborators: North American Symptomatic Carotid Endarterectomy Trial. First results. *N Engl J Med.* 1991;325:445.
4. Wilson SE, Mayberg MR, Yatsu FR: Defining the indications for carotid endarterectomy. *Surgery.* 1988;104:932.
5. Hobson R, Weiss D, Fields W, et al: Efficacy of carotid endarterectomy for asymptomatic carotid stenosis. *N Engl J Med.* 1993;328:221.
6. Garraway WM, Whisnant JP: The changing pattern of hypertension and the declining incidence of stroke. *JAMA.* 1987;258:214.
7. Wolf PA, Kannel WB, McGee DL: Epidemiology of Strokes in North America. In Barnett HJM, Mohr JP, Stein BM, Yatsu FM, eds. *Stroke: Pathophysiology, Diagnosis and Management.* New York: Churchill Livingstone; 1986:3.
8. Asymptomatic Carotid Atherosclerosis Study Group: Study design for randomized prospective trial of carotid endarterectomy for asymptomatic stenosis. *Stroke.* 1989;20:844.
9. Callow AD, Caplan LR, Correll JW, et al: Carotid endarterectomy: What is its current status? *Am J Med.* 1988;85:835.
10. Barnett HJM: A randomized trial of aspirin and sulfinpyrazone in threatened stroke. *N Engl J Med.* 1978;299:53.
11. Bousser MG, Eschwege E, Hagvenau M, et al: "AICLA" controlled trial of aspirin and dipyridimole in the secondary prevention of atherothrombotic cerebral ischemia. *Stroke.* 1983;14:5.
12. Candelise L, Landi G, Perrone P, et al: A randomized trial of aspirin and sulfinpyrazone in patients with TIA. *Stroke.* 1982;13:175.
13. Whisnant JP, Matsomoto N, Elveback LR: Transient cerebral ischemic attacks in a community. *Mayo Clin Proc.* 1973;48:194.
14. Wilson SE, Mayberg MR: Crescendo transient ischemic attacks: A surgical imperative. *J Vasc Surg.* 1993;17:249.
15. Sundt TM, Whisnant JP, Houser OW, Fode NC: Prospective study of the effectiveness and durability of carotid endarterectomy. *Mayo Clinic Proc.* 1990;65:625.
16. Norris JW, Zhu CZ: Stroke risk and critical carotid stenosis. *J Neurol Neurosurg Psychiatry.* 1990;53:235.
17. Roederer GO, Langlois YE, Jager KA, et al: The natural history of carotid artery disease in asymptomatic patients with cervical bruits. *Stroke.* 1984;15:605.

XII

Surgical Management of the Vertebral Artery

CHAPTER **77**

Indications for Vertebral Artery Repair

RAMON BERGUER

The first recorded vertebral artery (VA) reconstruction was a thromboendarterectomy of the vertebral and subclavian arteries, performed in 1957 by Cate and Scott[1] and reported in the literature in 1959. Although further reports appeared sporadically,[2-6] surgery of the VA remained rare, devoid of pathophysiologic basis and haunted by a substantial percentage of failures. The surgical tools and techniques and the arteriography procedure of the 1960s were crude in comparison with today's standards. Vascular surgeons then were learning the fundamentals of carotid artery disease, which exposed them to patients with symptoms of vertebrobasilar ischemia (VBI), who traditionally were said to have vertebrobasilar "insufficiency." The word "insufficiency" implies that the ischemic symptoms are a consequence of decreased or tenuous flow as opposed to arterioarterial thromboembolization, a mechanism believed then to be rare in cerebrovascular disease. In general, patients with VBI were treated by neurologists with anticoagulant and vasodilating medication. By the late 1960s, surgeons had gained experience with bypass techniques on smaller vessels, such as coronary and posterior tibial arteries, selective angiography had become widely used, and the pathophysiology of brain ischemia was better and more widely understood by surgeons and physicians. Application of the bypass and transposition techniques to atherosclerotic disease of the VA made repair of this vessel easier and more successful and, gradually, VA operations became an integral part of cerebrovascular reconstructive surgery.[7-15] During the past decade, the pathophysiology of VBI has been redefined through pathologic studies, magnetic resonance imaging (MRI) and digital arteriographic images. The surgical treatment of VA disease has been streamlined, and longitudinal follow-up data of treated and untreated patients have become available.[16-18]

This chapter outlines the pathophysiology of VBI from the perspective of a surgeon, stressing the clinical and radiologic findings relevant to the selection of patients likely to benefit from a reconstruction of the VA.

The prime indication for VA surgery is the need to treat VBI in patients whose VA disease can be presumed to cause their symptoms. Reconstruction of the VA may also be indicated to increase total cerebral blood flow in symptomatic patients with occluded carotid arteries who have reconstructible disease of their VA. Finally, VA operations may be indicated for the treatment of arteriovenous fistulas or spontaneous intramural dissection of the VA with or without aneurysm formation and, exceptionally, to re-establish vascular continuity after extensive resection of tumors involving the cervical spine.

EVALUATION OF PATIENTS WITH VERTEBROBASILAR ISCHEMIA

Patients with VBI have one or more of the following symptoms: dizziness, syncope, vertigo, diplopia, blurring of vision, tinnitus, perioral numbness, and drop attacks. A detailed description of VBI is provided in Chapter 10.

Vertebrobasilar ischemia is common, as are lesions of the VA. But a cause-effect relationship between the syndrome and a diseased VA can only be established after the more frequent medical or cardiac causes of VBI have been ruled out and after certain anatomic criteria for VA disease have been satisfied.

The first step in selecting patients for arteriography and possible reconstruction is the elimination of the systemic causes of VBI. A neurologic evaluation, complemented by computed tomographic (CT) scanning, will rule out degenerative disease or tumor as a cause of VBI. A medical evaluation should focus on the detection of diabetes, hypoglycemia, orthostatic hypotension, anemia, or hyperventilation. Cardiac evaluation should seek the presence of arrhythmia or a malfunctioning pacemaker. The presence of vertigo associated with deafness or tinnitus necessitates an exploration of a labyrinthine function. Conversely, if positional vertigo or severe dizziness is associated with cranial nerve signs (tingling, diplopia, limb weakness), the etiology is likely to be hypoperfusion of the vertebrobasilar system rather than a vestibular or labyrinthine problem.

The etiologic mechanism for VBI can be hemodynamic, embolic, or mixed. The hemodynamic mechanism presumes a decrease in flow in the territory of the vertebrobasilar system not compensated by the contributions from the carotid system. The most common reason for hemodynamic symptoms is a severe plaque obstructing the vertebral, basilar, subclavian, or innominate artery. The plaque may have already caused the occlusion of the artery that bears it. Hemodynamic symptoms can also be caused by extrinsic compression of a dominant or of both vertebral arteries with different positions of the neck.

549

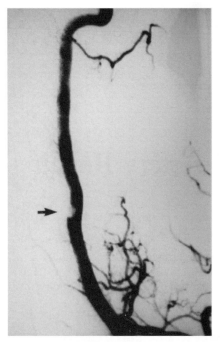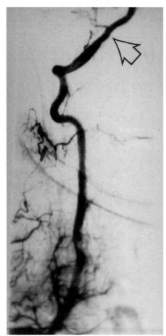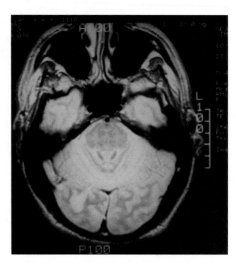

FIGURE 77–1. Extrinsic compression and repetitive trauma to the right vertebral artery resulted in an intraluminal thrombus *(solid arrow, left panel)* that embolized the right posteroinferior cerebellar artery *(open arrow, middle panel)* and resulted in an infarction of the right cerebellar lobe *(right panel)*. (From Berguer R, Kieffer E. *Surgery of the Arteries to the Head.* New York: Springer-Verlag; 1992; 35; with permission.)

The embolic mechanism presumes detachment of thrombotic or atheromatous material from the left side of the heart or from the innominate, proximal subclavian, vertebral, or basilar artery.

In some patients, it is not possible to determine whether the etiology is hemodynamic or embolic. Either mechanism could be responsible for symptoms when the problem is an extrinsic compression of the artery or an intramural dissection. In the case of extrinsic compression of the artery, the mechanism of compression can cause occlusion of the artery and can also traumatize its wall repeatedly, resulting in the formation of intramural thrombus capable of embolization (Fig. 77–1). In the case of an intramural dissection, the artery may be mechanically occluded by the dissecting intramural hematoma, or the latter may be a source of embolization.

The different symptoms experienced by patients with hemodynamic and embolic VBI have been well outlined by Rancurel[19] in a series of 402 patients with this syndrome. Patients who presented with hemodynamic VBI had symptoms usually prompted by positional changes that were repetitive and stereotyped. These patients had a low incidence of strokes during follow-up and the pathologic consequences of VBI were limited to the restrictions that the symptoms imposed in the patient's daily life (eg, driving, climbing stairs). Occasionally, patients with hemodynamic VBI have suffered serious traumatic injuries because of their loss of balance. MRI scans of patients with hemodynamic VBI usually show no abnormalities.

The other group, those patients with embolic VBI, have a different clinical course. The neurologic deficits are longer lasting, and they are varied and nonrepetitive. They do not generally depend on body or neck position and are not relieved when the patient lies down. MRI scans of patients with embolic VBI show infarctions of the cerebellum and brain stem, and such patients have a particularly bad prognosis in terms of further deterioration of neurologic function and eventual death.

In the case of patients with positional symptoms, the examining physician should trigger those symptoms clinically and during arteriography. The symptoms can usually be reproduced clinically by progressive slow rotation or extension of the neck into the trigger position. The patient should be seated and assisted during these examinations, since syncope may occur.

The demonstration of the compression of the VA in the arteriogram requires that the patient be positioned during arteriography in such a manner that symptoms can be triggered. This usually requires that rotation or extension of the head during injection be maintained while the patient is symptomatic. We place the patients in the reverse Trendelenburg position, with the head supported on a block, in order to mimic the longitudinal compression of the cervical spine that occurs during standing, which is when patients most often have hemodynamic symptoms. The technique in which the arteriogram is obtained while the patient is either sitting up or in the Trendelenburg position while the head and neck are rotated to the position that triggers symptoms is called dynamic vertebral arteriography.

ANATOMIC SEGMENTS OF THE VERTEBRAL ARTERY

The VA is divided into four segments, each with specific anatomic attributes (Fig. 77–2). The first segment (V1), or proximal VA, extends from the origin of this vessel, generally in the subclavian artery, to its entrance into the transverse process at the C6 level. In 6 percent of cases, the left VA originates in the aortic arch (Fig. 77–3). The right VA originates from the right common carotid artery in patients with a retroesophageal right subclavian artery. Although the entrance of the VA into the spinal column generally occurs at the C6 level, it may take place lower (C7) or higher (C5 or C4). When the left vertebral artery originates from the aortic arch, it often enters the spinal column above the C6 level.

The second segment (V2) of the VA comprises the intraspinal course between the transverse process of C6 and the top of the C2 transverse process. Here the artery travels in an osteomuscular conduit and is in relation posteriorly to the intervertebral joints and to the nerve roots at each vertebral level. The third (V3) segment (which together with the fourth segment is also referred to as the distal VA), extends from the top of the transverse process of C2 to the point where the artery crosses the atlanto-occipital membrane. The V4 or intracranial segment extends from the atlanto-occipital membrane to the point where the two VAs join to form the basilar artery.

The V1 segment gives no branches. The V2 segment has many small branching vessels exiting at each cervical vertebra, which supply the paravertebral musculature, bone, cervi-

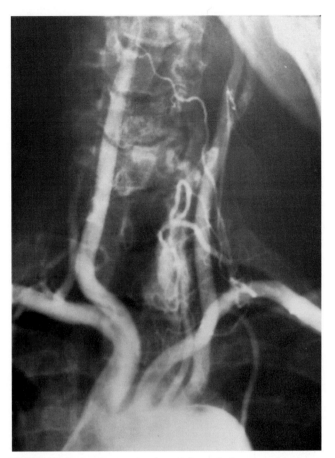

FIGURE 77–3. Arteriogram showing a left vertebral artery originating in the aortic arch. A thyroid or parathyroid stain is also seen.

cal joints, meninges, and cervical nerve roots (radiculomedullary branches). These branches of the VA to the deep musculature, the nerve roots, and meninges can maintain patency of the distal VA in the face of proximal occlusion and may also shunt blood from one VA to the other across the neck in cases of proximal VA or subclavian artery occlusion. This pattern is called segmental intervertebral anastomosis[21] (Fig. 77–4). The third segment (V3) has an important anastomosis (Fig. 77–5) to the occipital branch of the external carotid artery. In patients who have occlusion of the proximal VA, this collateral anastomosis becomes hypertrophic, particularly in individuals who have occlusion of one or both internal carotid arteries. This collateral also maintains patency of the distal VA and basilar arteries in cases of proximal VA occlusion. Collateral flow to the distal VA may also be supplied by branches of the ascending cervical artery.

This occipital connection between the external carotid and the distal VA is functionally analogous to the better known orbital connection between the external and internal carotid arteries. In some patients, both connections preserve intracranial flow. The occipital connection can become hypertrophic in cases of proximal VA or external carotid artery occlusion and may shunt blood in either direction, depending on which parent system is occluded (Fig. 77–6).

The right and left V4 segments join to form the basilar artery, which through the posterior communicating arteries connects with the internal carotid arteries. The most im-

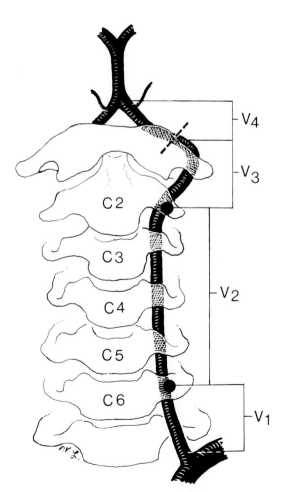

FIGURE 77–2. The four surgical segments into which the vertebral artery is divided.

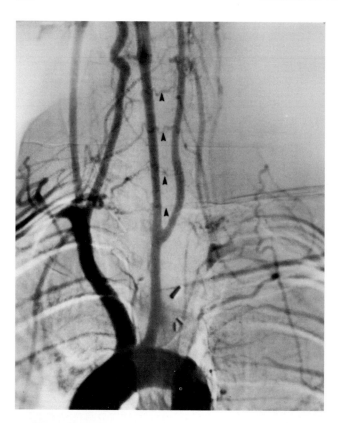

FIGURE 77–4. Arteriogram of a 14-year-old girl who had a coarctation of the aorta repaired as a child. She presented with vertebrobasilar ischemia secondary to a left-sided steal caused by the absence of the first portion of her left subclavian artery. The left vertebral steal was corrected by a transposition of the left vertebral artery to the left common carotid artery. The metameric intervertebral anastomoses derived from the radiculomedullary branches are still visible *(arrowheads)* and continue to supply blood to the left upper extremity across the neck.

FIGURE 77–5. Occipital connection *(between arrows)* feeding the V3 segment of the vertebral artery from the occipital artery. The internal carotid artery is occluded, and the origin of the external carotid artery is stenosed.

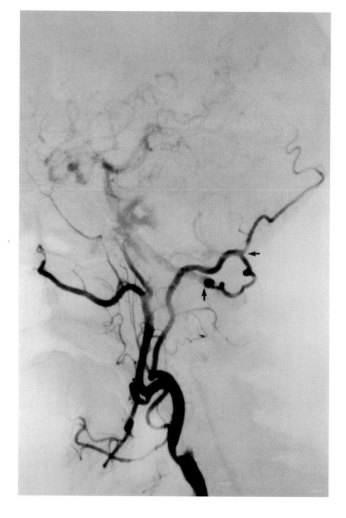

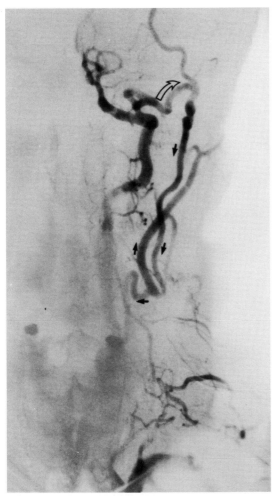

FIGURE 77–6. In this patient with occluded left common and internal carotid arteries, a large occipital connection *(open arrow)* supplies the external carotid territory. Blood flows *(solid arrows)* in a retrograde direction into the occipital artery and in an autograde direction into the branches of the external carotid artery.

portant branches of the V4 segment are the anterior and posterior spinal arteries and the posteroinferior cerebellar artery.

More often than not, one VA is larger than the other and is termed dominant. The concavity of the basilar artery when viewed in the anteroposterior Towne projection opens toward the side of the dominant VA, as seen in Figure 77–7.

We have already mentioned the unusual origin of the VA from the aortic arch or from the right common carotid artery and the different levels of entrance in the cervical spine. Other congenital abnormalities are a bifid origin from the subclavian artery and a fenestration, usually in its distal segment. In the latter case, the VA divides before entering one transverse process only to join again into a single trunk above it (Fig. 77–8). At the C1 level, the artery may also go around the transverse process rather than through it; in such cases, the bony orifice in the transverse process of C1 is absent.

Not infrequently (6% of cases), one of the two VAs is hypoplastic and does not join with the other to form the basilar trunk. These hypoplastic VAs terminate in the posteroinferior cerebellar artery.

ANGIOGRAPHIC CRITERIA AND FINDINGS

The arteriographic evaluation of patients with VBI requires an aortic arch injection with two oblique views and the selective injection of both proximal carotid and subclavian arteries. The arteriogram should display the vertebrobasilar system clearly from the origin of the VA to the top of the basilar artery. To accomplish this, additional views may be needed.

The completeness of both VAs must be assessed. When they are of different sizes, the examiner should determine which is dominant. Hypoplastic vertebral arteries that end up in the posteroinferior cerebellar artery do not contribute to vertebrobasilar perfusion. Dominance is generally identified by the caliber of the vessel; it is more common on the left side than on the right. If no VA is visualized, the potential reconstitution of one or both VAs at the level of C2 should be sought in delayed subtracted views.

A VA stenosis is arbitrarily called critical when it involves 75 percent of the lumen of two equivalent VAs. If one VA is hypoplastic or occluded, a 75 percent stenosis of the dominant or single VA is also considered critical. If one VA is normal, a severe stenosis of the contralateral artery would

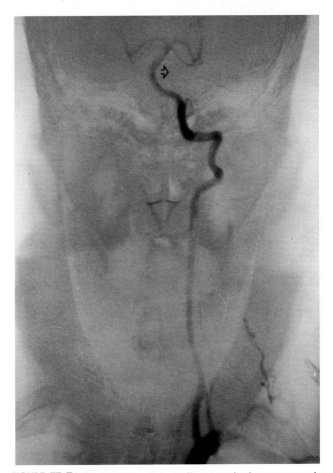

FIGURE 77–7. The concavity of the basilar artery in the anteroposterior Towne projection opens *(arrow)* toward the side of the dominant vertebral artery. (From Berguer R: The role of vertebral artery surgery after carotid endarterectomy. In Bergan JJ, Yao JST, eds. *Reoperative Arterial Surgery.* Orlando: Grune & Stratton; 1985; 555; with permission.)

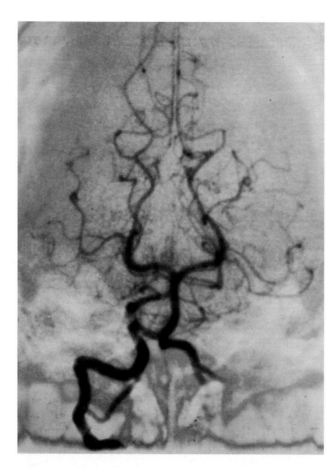

FIGURE 77–8. Vertebral arteriogram in anteroposterior Towne projection. Note the fenestration of the right vertebral artery around C1.

FIGURE 77–9. Arch injection showing two apparently normal vertebral arteries. The dominant left vertebral artery, however, has a very severe lesion *(arrow)* seen only after an additional selective oblique view. (From Berguer R: The role of vertebral artery surgery after carotid endarterectomy. In Bergan JJ, Yao JST, eds. *Reoperative Arterial Surgery.* Orlando: Grune & Stratton; 1985; 555; with permission.)

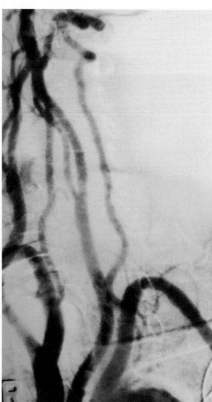
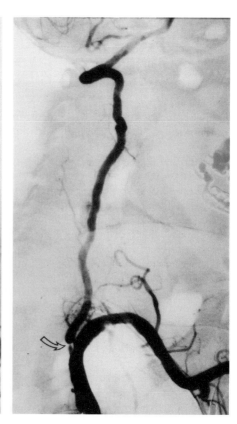
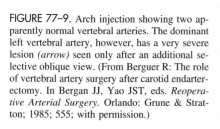

not be significant from a hemodynamic viewpoint: it is believed that one normal VA can supply the flow needed in the basilar artery. One must bear in mind that ulcerative or thrombotic lesions of a VA are a source of arterioarterial thromboembolization and may be responsible for VBI. In these cases, whether the opposite VA is normal is irrelevant in the need to surgically eliminate the source of embolization.

V1 Segment

By far the most common atherosclerotic lesion of the vertebrobasilar system is a stenosis of the origin of the VA. It is usually short and located at the ostium. Such lesions may be difficult to visualize (Fig. 77–9) because the VA originates in the posterior wall of the subclavian artery. The dye filling the subclavian artery in front of the VA obliterates the display of the origin of the VA; therefore, a severe stenosis at this location is often missed in standard arteriograms. Unless the origin is clearly displayed through additional oblique views, it may not be possible to discern severe lesions at this level.

Intraspinal (V2) Segment

It is important to notice an abnormal level of entry of the VA into the cervical spine because extrinsic compression of the artery is more likely in cases in which the artery has an ectopic origin. If, on the arteriogram, the first portion of the VA ascends parallel to the spine and then sharply turns into it, that is an abnormal entry. This is seen more often on the left side, where the artery arises directly from the aortic arch. More relevant to the surgeon are those instances in which the artery enters the spine below C6 (Fig. 77–10); in these cases, the V1 segment is generally too short to reach the common carotid artery for a transposition procedure. Unsubtracted views are often necessary to determine the level of entry into the spine. We have already mentioned that in patients with positional symptoms, compression of the V2 and V3 segments is studied by the technique of dynamic vertebral arteriography (Fig. 77–11).

V3 Segment

The V3 segment is generally free of atherosclerotic disease. In cases in which the VA is occluded proximally (segments V1 and V2), refilling of the V3 segment is achieved by collaterals fed by the occipital or cervical ascending arteries previously described. This collateral connection permits the surgeon to reconstruct the V3 segment in some patients in whom neither VA can be visualized by an arch injection arteriogram. This refilling is best shown in subtracted delayed views (see Fig. 77–5).

The V3 segment is naturally redundant in order to accommodate for the ample mobility of the atlanto-occipital and atlantoaxial joints. This redundancy is sometimes referred to

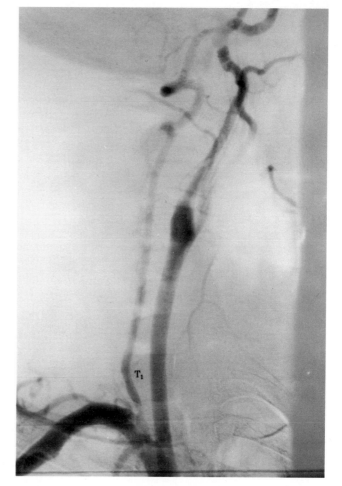

FIGURE 77–10. A single right vertebral artery, with a stenosis at its origin, entering the spine at the T1 level, an exceptionally low entry point. The very short V1 segment was inadequate for reimplantation, and a distal bypass from the external carotid to the V3 segment of the vertebral artery was performed to relieve this symptomatic stenosis. (From Berguer R: The role of vertebral artery after carotid endarterectomy. In Bergan JJ, Yao JST, eds. *Reoperative Arterial Surgery*. Orlando: Grune & Stratton; 1985; 555; with permission.)

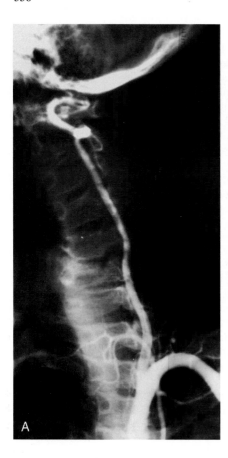

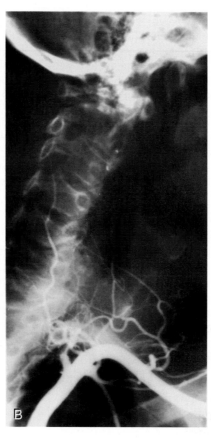

FIGURE 77–11. Arteriogram showing compression of the V2 segment with rotation of the neck. *A,* With the head turned to the right, there is minimal compression of the V2 segment. *B,* With the head turned to the left, there is complete occlusion of the vertebral artery.

FIGURE 77–12. Intramural dissection *(arrow)* of the vertebral artery in the C2-C1 segment. (From Berguer R: Aneurysms of the extra-arterial carotid and vertebral arteries. In Yao JST, Pearce WH, eds. *Aneurysms: New Findings and Treatments.* East Norwalk, CT: Appleton & Lange; 1994; 478; with permission.)

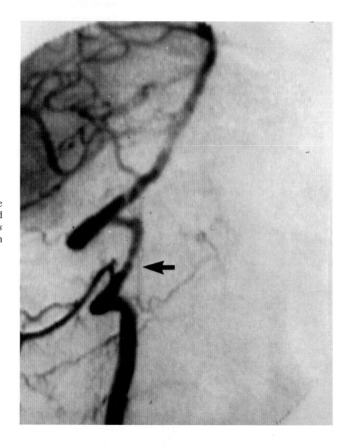

as the "safety loop." It should be remembered that roughly 50 percent of the neck rotation takes place in the atlantoaxial joint. The atlanto-occipital joint provides most of the flexion and extension of the head and neck segments.

These joints, already hypermobile, can be further stressed by trauma. The VA, attached by its adventitia to the periostium of the transverse processes of C1 and C2, can be stretched between these fixation points and suffer dissection (Fig. 77–12), rupture, and eventually occlusion. Intramural dissection is most common in the V3 segment and among patients who have evidence of fibromuscular dysplasia, although is by no means limited to arteries with the latter condition. A history of trauma is not available in many cases of intramural dissection. A dissection may heal or result in occlusion or stenosis or in a chronic dissecting aneurysm. The last condition has the same mechanics as the chronic dissecting aneurysms of the thoracic aorta. In cases of transmural acute rupture, a false aneurysm or, more commonly, an arteriovenous fistula or aneurysm may develop. Arteriovenous fistulization is a common complication of traumatic injury to the VA because of the multiple venae comitantes intimately surrounding the artery throughout most of its cervical course. Most of the dissections, false aneurysms, chronic dissecting aneurysms, and arteriovenous "aneurysms" and fistulas are seen in the V3 segment (Fig. 77–13). Rare anomalies such as fenestration or an extratransversarian course of the VA at the level of C1 may also be noted in the V3 segment.

V4 Segment and Basilar Artery

The VA may be stenosed at the point at which it perforates the atlanto-occipital membrane at the beginning of the V4 segment (Fig. 77–14). With the exception of a few reported cases,[22, 23] severe lesions at the V4 level of the vertebral artery or of the basilar artery are often inoperable and, generally (Fig. 77–15), preclude any reconstruction proximal to V4.

The basilar artery should be studied on subtraction films. The overlapping density of the temporal bone in the lateral projection may obscure the outline of the basilar artery. The anteroposterior view (Towne projection) poorly resolves short segmental lesions because of the foreshortening of the basilar artery in this projection. The presence of a posterior communicating artery at the top of the basilar artery should be noted, and the posterior cerebral arteries checked for evidence of atherosclerotic disease. Visualization of the posterior communicating arteries depends on the pressure differential existing between the top of the internal carotid artery and that achieved in the basilar artery at the time of contrast injection. Therefore, nonvisualization of the posterior communicating arteries is not necessarily evidence of their absence.

In some patients with a bilaterally occluded VA, the basilar artery can be observed to fill retrogradely through the posterior communicating arteries during selective injections of the common carotid artery (Fig. 77–16). Generally, the reflux into the basilar artery does not go beyond the level of the superior cerebellar arteries. This reflux is indirect evidence of hypotension in the vertebrobasilar system. Such reflux may be seen, however, in patients with no evidence of vertebrobasilar hypotension, if they have large posterior communicating arteries and if the carotid injection is done in the internal carotid artery, as is often the case in the evaluation of intracranial tumors.

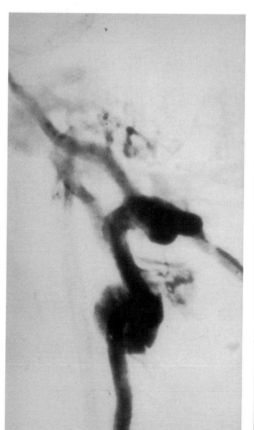

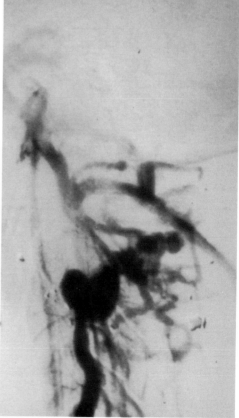

FIGURE 77–13. Chronic post-traumatic arteriovenous vertebral aneurysm. (From Berguer R: Aneurysms of the extra-arterial carotid and vertebral arteries. In Yao JST, Pearce WH, eds. *Aneurysms: New Findings and Treatments*. East Norwalk, CT: Appleton & Lange; 1994; 486; with permission.)

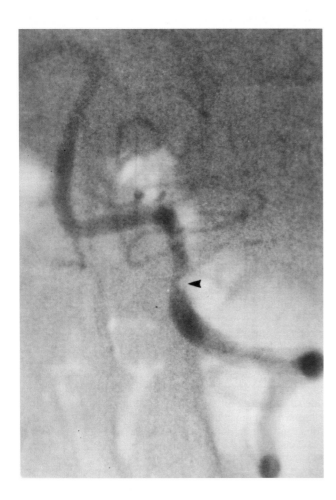

FIGURE 77–14. Severe plaque *(arrowhead)* in the V4 segment of the vertebral artery.

FIGURE 77–15. Severe occlusive disease of the basilar artery *(solid arrow)* naturally bypassed in this patient by anastomosis around the cerebellum *(open arrows)* from the posteroinferior cerebellar artery to the superior cerebellar artery. In this case, a severe proximal stenosis of a single left vertebral artery was corrected to improve perfusion around this distal collateral circuit.

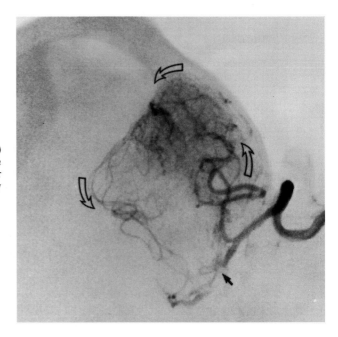

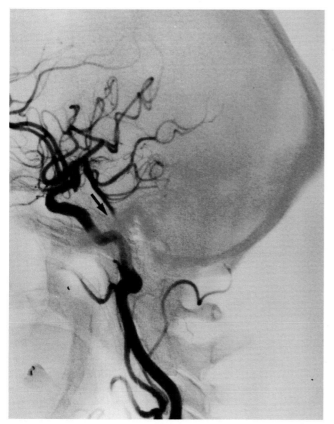

FIGURE 77–16. Retrograde filling of the basilar artery and its superior cerebellar branches *(arrow)* during a common carotid injection. This patient had a stenosis of the midbasilar artery.

PATHOLOGIC LESIONS OF THE VERTEBRAL ARTERY

Intrinsic Lesions

The most frequent lesion of the VA is an atherosclerotic plaque. This plaque is characteristically located at the ostium of the vessel (V1). Plaques may also be found at the level of the atlanto-occipital membrane and throughout the V2 segment. Although plaques in the VA are often described as fibrous and have less tendency to ulcerate than those found in the carotid bifurcation, there is little factual information on this subject. Most of what is known was published many years ago, before the relevance of plaque composition and surface characteristics was fully understood in relationship to disease of the carotid bifurcation. The classic autopsy study performed by Yates and Hutchinson[24] described a high incidence of VA plaques and correlated their presence with infarctions of the vertebrobasilar territory. They stated that "a not uncommon finding was hemorrhage into the base of the plaques of atheroma."

It is difficult to obtain specimens from patients because endarterectomy of the VA is hardly ever done, and most operations performed on the VA (transpositions, bypasses) exclude rather than remove the offending plaque (see Chapter 78). Since detailed visualization of these lesions by ultrasonographic imaging is also difficult or impossible, it is likely that this needed information will come mostly through autopsy studies.

Fibromuscular dysplasia of the VA is usually seen in the V3 segment and is frequently associated with similar pathology of the internal carotid artery. This is the segment in which the VA is bound to suffer stretch injuries from brusque torsion or flexion or extension movements, usually following motor vehicle and diving accidents, falls, chiropractic manipulation, and so on.[25, 26]

Dissections at this level, whether associated with fibromuscular dysplasia or not, may heal spontaneously, progress to occlusion, or result in a chronic dissecting aneurysm. Rupture of the arterial wall results in thrombosis or false aneurysm. The latter are usually fistulized into the vertebral veins that intimately surround the VA and are simultaneously damaged with it; hence the formation of arteriovenous aneurysms.

Some of these arteriovenous aneurysms in the V3 segment seem to appear spontaneously in children. Given that there is no associated arteriovenous malformation in the adjacent bone or skin in these cases, it is reasonable to think that these arteriovenous aneurysms are the consequence of unrecognized trauma, perhaps at birth.

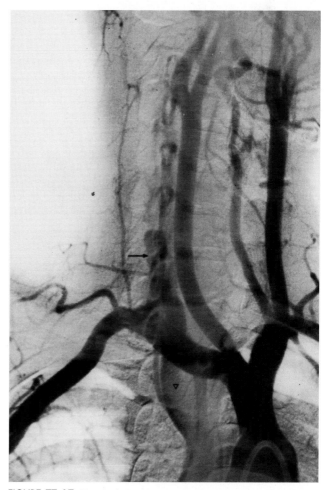

FIGURE 77–17. Vertebral arteriovenous fistula at the level of C1 from a stab wound to the neck. Right vertebral blood flow is shunted through the fistula *(arrow)* and renders the superior vena cava opaque *(triangle)*. The vertebral artery distal to the fistula is not seen. (From Berguer R, Feldman AJ, Wilner HI, Lazo A: Arteriovenous vertebral fistulae: Cure by combination of operation and detachable intravascular balloon. *Ann Surg.* 1982;196:65; with permission.)

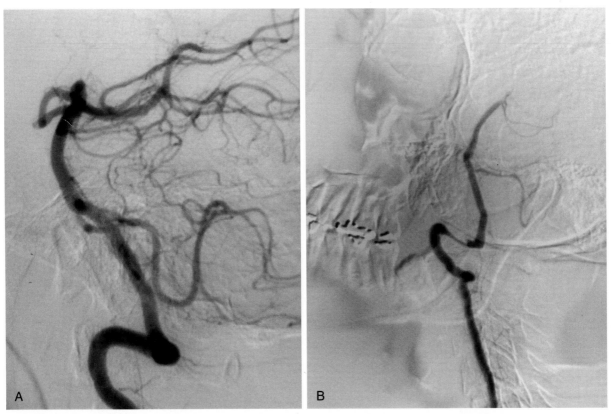

FIGURE 77–18. *A,* Normal appearance of the left distal vertebral and basilar arteries in neutral position in a patient who develops syncope when turning the head to the right. Her right vertebral artery was absent. *B,* With the head turned into the trigger position, the distal vertebral artery is compressed between the atlas and the occipital bone. Note the poor fillng of the basilar artery and branches.

The VA is characteristically spared in Takayasu disease, or its involvement is limited to its ostium. In cases of extensive Takayasu arteritis of the supraortic trunks, the VA is often hypertrophic and may be the only source of direct intracranial blood flow.

Extrinsic Disease

Open trauma to the VA is generally the result of a gunshot or stab wound (Fig. 77–17) and may be associated with cervical fractures. Its most common complication is the development of an arteriovenous fistula because of the intimate relationship between the VA and vertebral venous plexus in the V2-V3 segment.

Closed trauma may result in thrombosis or intramural dissection of the VA. Thrombosis of the vertebrobasilar arteries and sudden infarction of brain stem and cerebellar structures have been reported following chiropractic manipulation,[27] yoga, and other sports.

The most common extrinsic pathology of the VA[26] is its compression by an osteophyte in the V2 segment or, more rarely, compression by the longus colli prior to its entrance into the transverse foramen. Other structures can be demonstrated to cause VA compression, such as the lower sympathetic nerves (between the middle and lower cervical ganglion), the atlanto-occipital membrane, or the sharp upper edge of the posterior arch of the atlas (Fig. 77–18) when an elongated artery overhangs this bony ridge. Osteophyte compression is aggravated by specific movements of the neck, usually rotation or hyperextension. The bony spurs that compress the artery at the uncinate process may also press on the nerve roots, producing radicular signs such as pain, decreased tendon reflexes, and sensory changes.[27]

In infants, the atlanto-occipital joint may be unstable and cause pronounced arterial slippage of the atlas over the occipital bone. This anteroposterior dislocation may occlude the VA. This mechanism has been postulated in some cases of sleep apnea and sudden infant death syndrome. This subluxation of the atlanto-occipital joint has also been reported to cause VBI symptoms in patients with rheumatoid arthritis.[27]

REFERENCES

1. Cate WR, Scott HW: Cerebral ischemia of central origin: Relief by subclavian vertebral artery thromboendarterectomy. *Surgery.* 1959;45:19.
2. Imparato AM, Lin JPT: Vertebral arterial reconstruction: Internal plication and vein patch angioplasty. *Ann Surg.* 1967;166:213.
3. Natali J, Maraval M, Kieffer E: Surgical treatment of stenosis and occlusion of the carotid and vertebral arteries. *J Cardiovasc Surg.* 1972;13:4.
4. Labauge R, Thevenet A, Crouzet G, Nivolas M: Les insuffisances vertebro-basilaires d'incidence chirurgicale. *Rev Neurol.* 1967;117:373.
5. Rainer WG, Quianzon EP, Liggett MS, et al: Surgical considerations in the treatment of vertebrobasilar arterial insufficiency. *Am J Surg.* 1970;120:594.
6. Edwards WH, Wright RS: Current concepts in the management of arteriosclerotic lesions of the subclavian and vertebral arteries. *Ann Surg.* 1972;175:975.
7. Berguer R, Andaya LV, Bauer RB: Vertebral artery bypass. *Arch Surg.* 1976;111:976.
8. Berguer R, Bauer RB: Vertebral artery reconstruction: A successful technique in selected patients. *Ann Surg.* 1981;193:441.

9. Roon AJ, Ehrenfeld WK, Cooke PB, Wylie EJ: Vertebral artery reconstruction. *Am J Surg.* 1980;138:29.

10. Malone JM, Moore WS, Hamilton R, Smith M: Combined carotid-vertebral vascular disease. *Arch Surg.* 1980;115:783.

11. Edwards WH, Mulherin JL Jr: The surgical reconstruction of the proximal subclavian and vertebral artery. In Berguer R, Bauer RB, eds. *Vertebrobasilar Arterial Occlusive Disease.* New York: Raven Press; 1984;241.

12. Kieffer E, Rancurel G, Richard T: Reconstruction of the distal cervical vertebral artery. In Berguer R, Bauer RB, eds. *Vertebrobasilar Arterial Occlusive Disease.* New York: Raven Press; 1984;265.

13. Berguer R, Feldman AJ: Surgical reconstruction of the vertebral artery. *Surgery.* 1983;93:670.

14. Berguer R: Distal vertebral artery bypass: Technique, the ''occipital connection,'' and potential uses. *J Vasc Surg.* 1985;2:621.

15. Kieffer E: Chirurgie de l'artère vertébrale. Technique Chirurgicales. Chirurgie Vasculaire, 43130, 4.9.12, Encycl Méd Chir (Paris, France).

16. Branchereau A, Rosset ELD, Magnan PE, Espinoza CHA: Proximal reconstructions. In Berguer R, Caplan L, eds. *Vertebrobasilar Arterial Disease.* St Louis: Quality Medical Publishing; 1992;265.

17. Kieffer E, Koskas F, Rancurel G, et al: Reconstruction of the distal cervical vertebral artery. In Berguer R, Caplan L, eds. *Vertebrobasilar Arterial Disease.* St. Louis: Quality Medical Publishing; 1992;279.

18. Berguer R: Long-term results of reconstruction of the vertebral artery. In Yao JST, Pearce W, eds. *Long Term Results in Vascular Surgery.* Norwalk, CT: Appleton & Lange; 1993;69.

19. Rancurel G, Kieffer E, Arzimanoglou A, et al: Hemodynamic vertebrobasilar ischemia: Differentiation of hemodynamic and thromboembolic mechanisms. In Berguer R, Caplan L, eds. *Vertebrobasilar Arterial Disease.* St. Louis: Quality Medical Publishing; 1992;40.

20. Ruotolo C, Hazan H, Rancurel G, Kieffer E: Dynamic arteriography. In Berguer R, Caplan L, eds. *Vertebrobasilar Arterial Disease.* St. Louis: Quality Medical Publishing; 1992;116.

21. Baker RA, Rosenbaum AE, Robertson GH: Segmental intervertebral anastomosis in subclavian steal. *Br J Radiol.* 1975;48:101.

22. Allen GS, Cohen RJ, Preziosi TJ: Microsurgical endarterectomy of the intracranial vertebral artery for vertebrobasilar transient ischemic attacks. *Neurosurgery.* 1981;9:524.

23. Kodadad G: Occipital artery: Posterior inferior cerebellar artery anastomosis. *Surg Neurol.* 1976;5:225.

24. Yates PO, Hutchinson EC: *Cerebral infarction: The role of the extracranial cerebral arteries.* London: Medical Research Council Special Report 300; 1961.

25. Toole JF: Positional effects of head and neck on vertebral artery blood flow. In Berguer R, Caplan L, eds. *Vertebrobasilar Arterial Disease.* St. Louis: Quality Medical Publishing; 1992;11.

26. Koskas F, Comizzoli I, Gobin YP, et al: Effects of spinal mechanics on the vertebral artery: Anatomic basis of positional postural compression of the cervical vertebral artery. In Berguer R, Caplan L, eds. *Vertebrobasilar Arterial Disease.* St. Louis: Quality Medical Publishing; 1992;15.

27. Bauer RB: Mechanical compression of the vertebral arteries. In Berguer R, Bauer RB, eds. *Vertebrobasilar Arterial Occlusive Disease.* New York: Raven Press; 1984;45.

Surgical Exposure and Methods of Vertebral Artery Repair

RAMON BERGUER

APPROACH TO THE VERTEBRAL ARTERY

The standard anterior neck approach, along the anterior edge of the sternocleidomastoid muscle, gives access to the V1, V2, and proximal half of the V3 segments of the vertebral artery (VA). The supraclavicular approach is indicated for proximal VA reconstructions when the subclavian artery is the source of inflow. The VA can also be reconstructed in its proximal portion on either side through a median sternotomy incision brought up slightly into the neck. This is done when the VA repair is part of a multiple reconstruction of the branches of the aortic arch. Access to the VA as it courses over the arch of the atlas and toward the midline requires a suboccipital or posterior approach.

The Supraclavicular Approach

The supraclavicular approach (Fig. 78–1) is somewhat easier on the right than on the left, where the VA origin is generally deeper into the thoracic inlet. The incision is drawn a finger breadth above the clavicle from its head outward. The external jugular vein is ligated. The incision is deepened, exposing the omohyoid muscle, which is divided. The prescalene fat pad is entered, dissected, and reflected laterally, leaving a pedicle. The transverse cervical artery and vein that run through this fat pad are divided. The phrenic nerve, identified in the anterior surface of the anterior scalene muscle, is freed, isolated with an elastic loop, and gently retracted out of the way. The neurovascular bundle of the neck is then retracted medially.

The medial and lateral edges of the anterior scalene muscle are exposed; a dissector probe or a right-angle clamp is inserted below this muscle, as close as possible to its insertion in the first rib. Using the dissector as a guide, the muscle is divided.

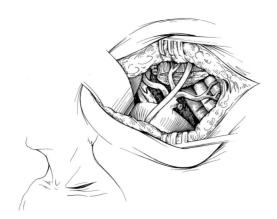

FIGURE 78–1. Supraclavicular approach to the proximal vertebral artery. The anterior scalene muscle has been cut. The phrenic nerve crosses the subclavian artery. The sympathetic nerves form a ring around the vertebral artery near its origin. The brachial plexus is seen lateral to the artery.

The subclavian artery lies behind the anterior scalene muscle. The dissection of the subclavian artery spares the thyrocervical trunk and the internal mammary artery. The vertebral vein runs on top of the VA and crosses the subclavian artery to empty into the subclavian vein. Once the vein is divided, the VA is found below it. The VA usually exits the posteromedial wall of the subclavian artery.

Dissection of the VA begins 2 cm from its origin, where it is easier to find, and is performed with the use of loupe magnification. The sympathetic trunks that cross the anterior surface of the proximal VA are preserved to avoid a Horner syndrome (Fig. 78–2). An intermediate ganglion may be lying next to or on top of the VA. The thoracic duct is identified and doubly ligated before it is divided. Transfixion sutures can result in lymphatic leaks that disturb the operative field and cause lymphoceles during the postoperative period. Single or multiple lymphatic ducts should be treated in this manner on both sides of the neck.

Distally, the dissection of the VA is carried up to the edge of the long muscle of the neck. Dissection of the proximal subclavian artery needs to be more extensive when an angioplasty or endarterectomy is planned to provide sufficient exposure and safe proximal control. Vertebral bypasses that originate in the subclavian artery do so distal to the origin of the VA, a segment that is easier to access. Palpation of the walls of the subclavian artery will give an indication of the location of plaques and the best place for an arteriotomy, if a transposition or a bypass graft is to be carried out.

Approach Through or Medial to the Sternomastoid Muscle

For a transposition of the VA to the common carotid artery, the most direct approach is between the two heads of the sternomastoid muscle (Fig. 78–3). Earlier accounts of this approach describe cutting the sternomastoid muscle, which is unnecessary.[1, 2] The two bellies of the muscle are separated, and the omohyoid muscle is cut. The carotid sheath is opened, and the dissection proceeds between the common carotid artery medially and the vagus nerve and jugular vein laterally, separating these structures with thin malleable retractors.

This direct approach can also be accomplished with an incision anterior to the sternomastoid muscle followed by lateral retraction of the latter. We use this approach when a VA transposition is done concomitant with an endarterectomy of the carotid bifurcation.

As the areolar and fat tissue over the thoracic inlet is dissected, attention is paid to the location of the thoracic duct that emerges from behind the carotid artery to empty into the confluence of the jugular and subclavian veins. More than one duct may be present. Once identified, the thoracic duct is ligated before it is divided. The inferior thyroid artery often crosses the field, and if that is the case, it is divided. The vertebral vein is a single vessel 3 to 4 mm in diameter.

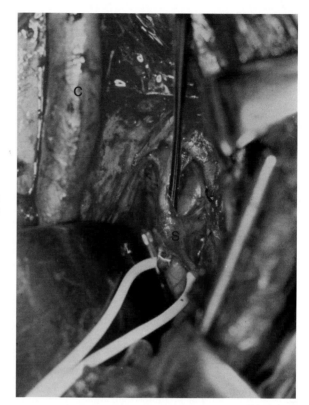

FIGURE 78–2. Anterior approach to the first segment of vertebral artery. A dissector lifts up the sympathetic trunks as they cross the vertebral artery approximately 1 cm from its origin. C, common carotid artery; S, sympathetic trunk.

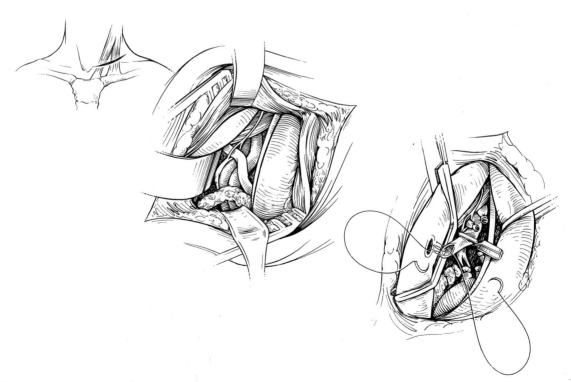

FIGURE 78–3. Anterior approach to the vertebral artery for its transposition to the common carotid artery. The thoracic duct can be seen at the bottom of the field. The inferior thyroid artery crosses the field, and the sympathetic trunks may form a ring around it. Below the inferior thyroid artery, the vertebral vein and artery run perpendicular to it. The anastomosis of the vertebral artery to the common carotid artery is performed in an open manner.

Once identified, the vein is divided. The VA is found below it.

The VA near its origin is crossed by sympathetic trunks. The trunks are protected (see Fig. 78–2) by being lifted with a nerve hook and dissected away from the underlying wall of the VA. Dissection of the VA continues proximally until its origin in the subclavian artery is identified. Eventually the VA is dissected above and below the sympathetic trunks that cross it. Once the V1 segment is dissected and its length is known, it is easy to determine the site in the common carotid artery wall to which it will be transposed.

Exposure of the V2 Segment

Exposure of the V2 segment is obtained through an incision that follows the anterior border of the sternocleidomastoid muscle. The muscle is freed from the carotid sheath medially. The neurovascular bundle of the neck and the esophagus are retracted medially, exposing the prevertebral fascia. In the lower neck, the inferior thyroid artery may need to be divided to permit this medial retraction.[3]

The anterior spinal ligament is exposed and incised. A periosteal elevator permits mobilization of the long muscles of the neck and head laterally until the anterior tubercle of the transverse process is exposed. With the bony surface of the transverse process exposed, its anterior wall may be removed with a rongeur, and the VA is exposed in its bony canal. The artery is dissected away from its accompanying vein or veins so that it, rather than the veins, is mobilized. Below the level of C2, the artery lies in front of the anterior rami of the cervical nerves. In the C2-C1 interval, the anterior ramus of C2 curves medially around and over the VA, crossing transversely in front of it. In the V2 segment, it is better to expose the artery in its bony canal than in the intertransverse space, where multiple veins surround it. The length of artery thus exposed in the V2 segment is considerably shorter than that obtained in the C2-C1 intertransverse space.

Exposure of the Proximal Segment of V3

To expose the V3 segment, an incision is made over the anterior edge of the upper two thirds of the sternocleidomastoid muscle (Fig. 78–4).[4–6] The tip of the parotid gland is lifted from the surface of the sternomastoid muscle. The greater auricular nerve is identified and a short length is freed anteriorly, to give it some mobility. The dissection proceeds between the jugular vein medially and the sternocleidomastoid muscle laterally, until the accessory spinal nerve is identified near its entrance into the latter. The nerve is slung with an elastic loop and dissected distally. The digastric muscle is identified, dissected, and retracted or cut. The accessory spinal nerve rests on the internal jugular vein as they both pass in front of the transverse process of C1. A finger following the top of the spinal nerve under the digastric muscle can easily feel the transverse process of C1; this prominent bony landmark is the upper limit of the exposure needed.

The next step is the identification of the levator muscle of the scapula by removing the fat pad covering it (Fig. 78–5). The location of the transverse process of C1 is kept in view,

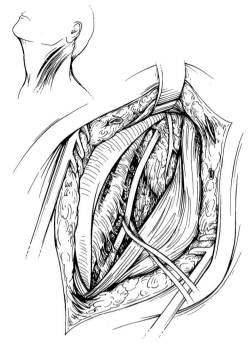

FIGURE 78–4. Exposure of the distal vertebral artery at the C2-C1 level. The approach is between the internal jugular vein and the sternomastoid muscle. A tape is shown looped around the vagus nerve. The accessory spinal nerve is shown as it travels from the top of the internal jugular vein at the top of the incision to the medial side of the sternomastoid muscle.

since the upper end of the levator muscle inserts there. Once the anterior edge of the muscle is freed, it is retracted posteriorly to expose the anterior ramus of C2 that emerges from beneath the muscle. This is a thick nerve trunk, about the size of a hypoglossal nerve; near the anterior edge of the levator muscle, it gives anastomotic loops to C1 and C3. The nerve is the guide to divide the levator muscle of the scapula and the underlying splenius muscle of the neck. These two muscles cover the C1-C2 intertransverse space in which the VA lies.

A dissecting spatula or an angled clamp is inserted between the nerve below and the muscle above, and the latter is cut. The proximal stump of the levator muscle is excised up to its tendinous insertion in C1 to improve exposure. As soon as this unroofing is done, the anterior ramus of C2 can be seen running transversely in the intertransverse space, closely hugging the VA as it crosses it. The sheath of the nerve is incised, and the nerve is lifted with a nerve hook and cut to expose the underlying VA (Fig. 78–6). Cutting this nerve does not result in a clinical deficit because of the abundant connections between the first three cervical nerves.

The VA is partially surrounded by thin-walled vertebral veins and must be freed from them (Fig. 78–7). It is the artery rather than the veins that is mobilized, lest the latter tear and bleed. In order to identify and precisely dissect these structures, the use of 3.5 loupe magnification and bipolar coagulation is recommended. As the artery is freed from these surrounding thin veins, blind maneuvers should be avoided, because an important collateral (the suboccipital anastomosis) may enter the posterior wall of the artery. If it is torn, bleeding can be difficult to control. The distal VA is now ready to be revascularized by bypass or transposition.

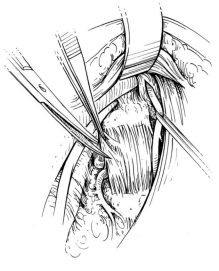

FIGURE 78–5. Identification of the levator muscle of the scapula. The spinal accessory nerve is slung with a Silastic loop. The anterior ramus of the second cervical nerve root is seen emerging below the anterior edge of the levator muscle. The levator muscle is cut.

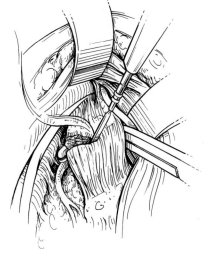

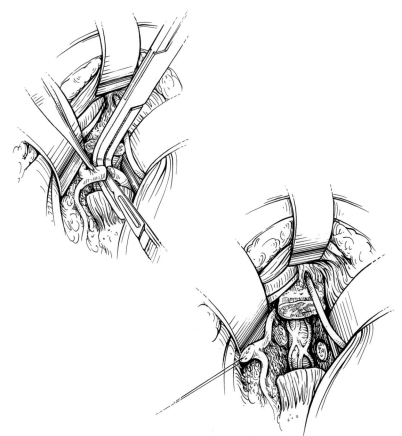

FIGURE 78–6. Cutting the anterior ramus of C2 exposes the vertebral artery below. The artery is partially covered by the vertebral veins.

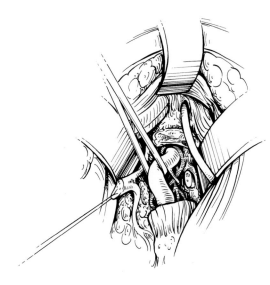

FIGURE 78–7. The vertebral artery is dissected free from the surrounding venous plexus.

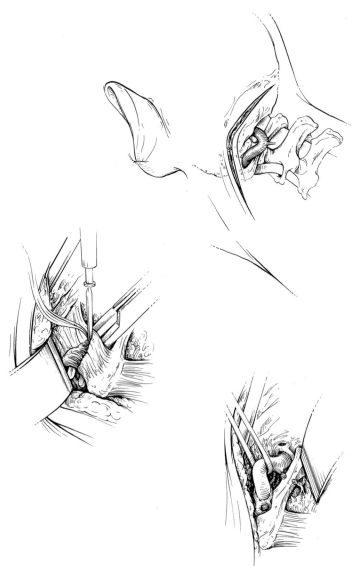

FIGURE 78–8. Exposure of the suboccipital segment of the vertebral artery. The splenius and superior oblique muscles of the head are cut. After freeing of the artery from its surrounding venous plexus, the artery is isolated. The posterior arch of the atlas is seen below the artery.

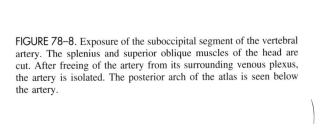

Suboccipital Exposure of the Distal Segment of V3

The suboccipital approach permits access to the distal segment of V3—the horizontal portion of the VA as it leaves the transverse foramen of C1 and rests on the posterior arch of C1 until it perforates the atlanto-occipital membrane to become intradural.

The patient is placed in the park-bench position. A racket-shaped incision is made, cutting horizontally below the occipital bone and downward along the posterior edge of the sternomastoid muscle for 4 cm (Fig. 78–8). The muscle layers that overlie the artery are cut in succession, first the splenius muscle of the head, then the superior oblique and the lateral straight muscles of the head. The transverse process of C1 is easily identified. After division of the muscle coverings, the VA is seen surrounded by a rich venous plexus. To extricate the artery from its accompanying veins, bipolar cautery is needed. The artery is looped. One or more posterior muscular branches are ligated and divided to mobilize the VA. The artery is dissected up to the level where it penetrates the dura. Part of the arch of the atlas is usually removed either to improve exposure during resection and grafting of an aneurysm or to eliminate a previously determined extrinsic compression of the artery by the atlas.

TECHNIQUES FOR RECONSTRUCTION

The VA is an artery of small caliber (3 to 4 mm) and, like its parent, the subclavian artery, has a thin wall. Its dissection requires fine instruments and loupe magnification, preferably of 3.5x. Anastomosis to the VA should be done with fine needles and fine monofilament sutures, generally 6–0 or 8–0. Heparinization is routinely used.

Use of an intraluminal shunt during VA reconstruction may damage the artery and is not needed. There is never a long static column of blood distal to a clamp (as happens in the internal carotid artery) because of the abundance of branches in the V2, V3, and V4 segments. The re-establishment of flow after a VA reconstruction should always be directed first into the vessel supplying noncerebral territory, such as the subclavian artery or the external carotid artery.

Direct Repair of Lesions in the V1 Segment

The direct approach to orificial stenoses of the VA by means of endarterectomy or angioplasty is rarely used today, although these direct techniques were the first ones used and the only ones reported for years.[7–10] The disadvantages of the direct techniques in treating stenosing disease of the V1 segment have been outlined by Kieffer[5]: (1) they require greater exposure of the subclavian artery, which may be difficult to obtain with a neck incision, especially on the left side; (2) once the subclavian wall is opened to perform the vertebral endarterectomy, one may be forced to continue the endarterectomy into adjacent subclavian lesions that by themselves would have not required any treatment; and (3) the subclavian artery tends to deteriorate with atherosclerosis, particularly on the left side, and is therefore a less

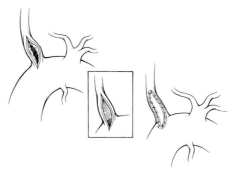

FIGURE 78–9. Endarterectomy and patch of the origin of the vertebral artery is hardly ever used.

desirable choice of inflow source for a long-term reconstruction.

Endarterectomy

There are two modalities for endarterectomy at the origin of the VA. The standard open endarterectomy (Fig. 78–9) requires a longitudinal arteriotomy along the VA and into the subclavian wall. It permits the surgeon to follow the VA plaque distally, should the latter not be limited to the ostium. The arteriotomy must always be closed with a patch, a maneuver that can be technically demanding, depending on the level and angle of takeoff of the VA from the subclavian artery.

For a stenosis limited to the orifice of the VA, a trans-subclavian endarterectomy can be used (Fig. 78–10).[5] After isolation of an appropriate segment of subclavian artery, a longitudinal incision is made, curving it slightly toward the VA orifice. The dissection plane is developed in the upper lip of the incision, much in the same way as it is done for the external carotid artery during the course of a standard carotid bifurcation endarterectomy. Slight proximal traction on the VA everts the orificial plaque into the lumen of the subclavian artery and permits its feathering. This technique is not suitable for plaques extending beyond the ostium, since it does not permit fixation of the distal intima should it not feather appropriately. The extent of the VA plaque should be determined by inspection and palpation before opening the subclavian artery. The subclavian artery must

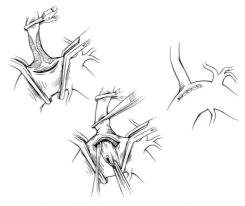

FIGURE 78–10. Trans-subclavian endarterectomy of the origin of the vertebral artery.

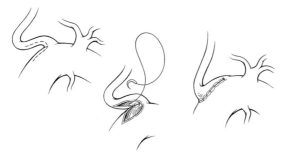

FIGURE 78–11. Plication angioplasty was used mostly in the early series of vertebral artery reconstruction. It is unnecessarily complex and requires specific and rare anatomic circumstances.

be relatively free of disease to accomplish a satisfactory endarterectomy.

Angioplasty

Angioplasty techniques are hardly ever used and are mostly of historical interest. On rare occasions, simple patch angioplasty has been used to enlarge the orifice of a stenotic VA. The feasibility of this technique depends on the characteristics of the VA plaque and the extent of subclavian involvement. Proper suture of the patch to the edges of the plaque may be difficult. When the VA exits the posterolateral wall of the subclavian artery at an open angle, one may need to shape the patch in a hockey-stick fashion to prevent its kinking.[5]

Plication angioplasty has been reported in cases in which the VA bends sharply after its takeoff and runs for a short length along the subclavian artery (Fig. 78–11). The opening is made over the VA, and the arteriotomy is continued over the adjacent wall. The walls of the VA arteriotomy are sutured to the corresponding lips of the subclavian arte-

riotomy to enlarge the VA orifice. This technique requires not only a specific configuration of the VA but also a soft and pliable wall in the subclavian artery. It is only of historical interest.

Transposition of the Vertebral Artery to the Subclavian Artery

If the V1 segment is long enough, stenosis of the origin of the VA may be treated by dividing the artery above the plaque and transposing it to another site on the subclavian artery (Fig. 78–12). This technique is used infrequently, since it requires enough redundancy of the VA for its transposition to a more lateral subclavian site and a reasonably normal subclavian artery. The subclavian artery is used as a donor vessel to revascularize the VA only if the contralateral internal carotid artery is occluded and one does not wish to clamp the ipsilateral carotid system for a conventional, and simpler, transposition of the VA to it.

The transposition site is always distal to the stenosed origin of the VA and is determined by palpation of the subclavian artery and by the available length of VA. The VA must be dissected up to the level of the tendon of the long muscle of the neck to obtain as much length as possible and also to allow it to settle without sharp bends after transposition. A microvascular Heifetz clip is used to control the VA at the level of the long muscle of the neck, and the chosen subclavian segment is isolated with a J-clamp. The arteriostomy is made in the superior wall of the subclavian artery with a 5 mm aortic punch. The VA is divided above the ostial stenosis and its stump is ligated with sutures. The free end of the VA is spatulated and anastomosed to the punch arteriostomy in the subclavian artery, preferably by open technique, using continuous 6-0 polypropylene suture. Before the anastomosis is completed, the vessels are back-

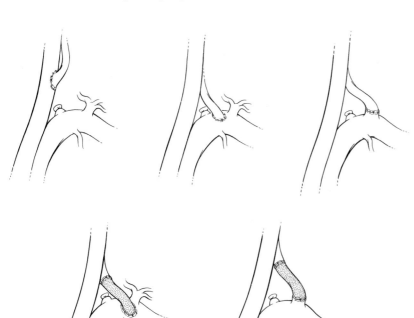

FIGURE 78–12. Common techniques used for reconstruction of the proximal vertebral artery. *Top row,* Transposition to the common carotid artery, the most frequently used technique *(left);* transposition to the second segment of the subclavian artery *(middle);* and transposition to the origin of the thyrocervical trunk *(right).* *Bottom row,* Subclavian to vertebral autogenous vein bypasses.

bled into the wound. Flow is re-established first into the distal subclavian artery and then into the VA.

Occasionally a short thyrocervical trunk of good caliber and free of disease offers a convenient site for transposition. Its suppleness and freedom from disease are determined by palpation. The branches of the thyrocervical trunk are amputated and ligated. The subclavian artery is clamped proximal and distal to the origin of the thyrocervical trunk. The trunk is amputated about 3 to 4 mm from its origin, and a small cut is made in its anterior wall. The VA is divided above the stenosis, and its stump is ligated with sutures. The free end of the artery is spatulated and anastomosed end to end to the thyrocervical stump with 6-0 polypropylene.

Bypass from the Subclavian Artery to the Vertebral Artery

The application of autogenous vein bypass techniques to the VA permitted the treatment of more extensive and diffuse lesions of this artery and extended the possibility of reconstruction throughout its extracranial course.[4, 11–13] For repair of lesions of the V1 segment, however, this technique (see Fig. 78–12) is used infrequently, since it is more complex than a standard transposition to the common carotid artery and requires the use of a vein graft. Nonetheless, there are specific indications for its use, such as when the VA atheroma extends through a substantial length of the V1 segment and when it is deemed unwise to clamp the ipsilateral carotid artery in order to anastomose the VA to it.

The V1 segment is exposed up to the level of the long muscle of the neck. If the VA origin is low and posterior, as is often the case on the left side, the dissection need not be pursued down to the origin of the artery, as long as a good segment of pliable VA is available higher up for the distal anastomosis of the bypass. This avoids disturbing the sympathetic trunks that cross the VA near its origin. An appropriate site is chosen in the subclavian artery for the proximal anastomosis of the bypass graft.

The bypass is always created from saphenous vein, chosen from either the thigh or the ankle, as dictated by the size of the VA and by preoperative ultrasonographic mapping. The distal anastomosis of the bypass graft is done in an end-to-side fashion after spatulation. Magnification, fine needles, and 6-0 polypropylene sutures are used. The distal anastomosis is done first. The graft is then cut to the appropriate size, bearing in mind that when the vein is distended by arterial pressure, it will lengthen and may kink.

The proximal anastomosis is done last. After appropriate backbleeding, the suture is completed and flow is re-established, first into the subclavian artery and then into the bypass graft. A hemoclip is then placed below the end-to-side anastomosis, making it function as an end-to-end anastomosis would.

Transposition of the Vertebral Artery Into the Common Carotid Artery

Transposition of the VA into the common carotid artery is the preferable technique for proximal VA reconstruction (see Fig. 78–3).[1, 6] It involves only one anastomosis, it does not require a valuable saphenous vein, and the artery is transposed to a large vessel that is usually of good quality.

Furthermore, the exposure for this approach is simple. The single drawback is the need to clamp the common carotid artery, which may be risky in a patient whose carotid system is occluded on the opposite side. Under normal circumstances, when both carotid systems are patent, clamping of the common carotid artery for the time needed to do an anastomosis has proved safe.

The VA is clamped first at the level of the long muscle of the neck with a microsurgical clip, and its origin is transfixed and divided above the plaque. The sympathetic fibers that cross the anterior surface of the VA are left undisturbed during dissection. After division of its distal end, the artery is drawn below those fibers and transposed anteriorly so that it can be brought to the site chosen for its transposition to the posterior wall of the common carotid artery. To expose the site in the common carotid artery, the clamp or clamps are placed pointing medially and then rotated to rest on the medial edge of the wound, exposing its posterolateral wall. During anastomosis, the common carotid clamp is held down near the thin-walled VA without tension. The anastomosis is done with an open technique to avoid tearing the wall of the VA. The proximal and distal carotid arteries, as well as the VA, are bled into the wound before the suture is tied and flow is re-established distally.

Bypass to the Distal Vertebral Artery

Once exposure of the VA is complete, (see Figs. 78–4 to 78–7), a 10 cm segment of saphenous vein is removed. Ideally, it should be a segment without valves, which facilitates backbleeding of the graft when the distal anastomosis is completed. The graft is prepared, and its distal end is spatulated appropriately. The distal VA is clamped with the use of a short baby J-clamp and opened with the use of a sharp coronary blade. The VA is thinner at this level than in its proximal segment, and its wall tears easily. The distal anastomosis is made with 8-0 polypropylene and 3.5 loupe magnification. The anastomosis is tested by temporarily opening the occluding clamp. The proximal end of the graft is then tunneled under the jugular vein alongside the common carotid artery. A Heifetz clip is placed on the proximal end of the graft, and the latter is allowed to distend to correct any rotation and to estimate the length required for its anastomosis to the common carotid artery.

The clip is then replaced distally, and the graft is washed with heparinized saline and spatulated for anastomosis. Clamps are placed above and below the selected anastomotic site in the common carotid artery. The arteriostomy in the common carotid artery is made with a 5-mm aortic punch, and it should be at least 2 cm below the bifurcation (Fig. 78–13). Care must be taken to keep the occluding carotid clamp clear of whatever plaque there may be at the carotid bifurcation. The site for anastomosis is chosen in the posterolateral wall of the common carotid artery. The common carotid artery is the preferred site for the proximal anastomosis of the bypass graft. When a graft is thus placed, it lies almost parallel to the carotid artery and does not kink.

Transposition Operations to Reconstruct the Distal Vertebral Artery

In patients with only one internal carotid artery open on the same side as the VA reconstruction, the surgeon must

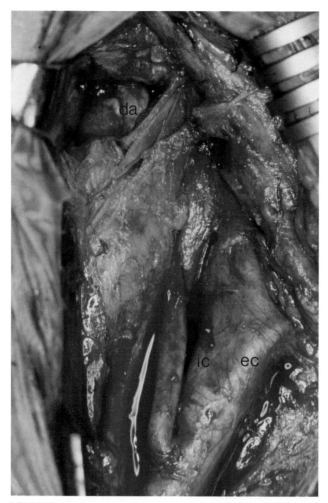

FIGURE 78–13. Intraoperative photograph of a completed common carotid–to–distal vertebral bypass. The carotid bifurcation has not been dissected. Distal anastomosis can be seen *(da)* above the internal jugular vein and accessory spinal nerve. ic, internal carotid artery; ec, external carotid artery.

avoid interrupting the carotid flow. In this specific instance, the external carotid artery may be isolated and transposed directly to the distal VA (Figs. 78–14 and 78–15). The main drawbacks of this alternative are that the orifice of the external carotid artery may be involved with bifurcation plaque and that the external carotid artery may have a short trunk that bifurcates early, leaving the surgeon with a terminal segment of external carotid artery too small to match the VA caliber.

In some patients, the internal carotid artery may be occluded above the bulb, leaving a stump that can be used for the proximal anastomosis. This is a rare occurrence, since carotid artery disease generally involves the entire bifurcation. I have also reported the use of the carotid bulb in patients with carotid aplasia, who characteristically have a normal carotid bulb that abruptly changes into a very thin internal carotid artery that does not reach the circle of Willis.[4] On such rare occasions, using the bulb for the proximal anastomosis permits maintenance of flow through the external carotid artery at all times during the procedure, a desirable precaution when the ipsilateral internal carotid artery is absent.

In a few patients, the occipital artery that supplies the

collaterals that keep the distal VA patent has hypertrophied to a size equivalent to that of the VA. In these patients, a direct occipital–vertebral anastomosis effectively revascularizes the distal VA (see Fig. 78–14). The occipital artery is isolated by the surgeon as it courses toward the mastoid muscle under the upper edge of the field.

Another technical solution to revascularize the distal VA is to transpose it to the internal carotid artery at the level of C1-C2 (see Fig. 78–14). The VA is divided above C2 and transposed to the internal carotid artery by means of an end-to-side anastomosis. This technique obviously requires an intact contralateral internal carotid artery system.

Access to the distal VA above the level of C1 is needed in one or two rare circumstances: in the course of resection and grafting of an aneurysm of the V3 segment or to relieve some mechanical compression demonstrated by arteriography.

Distal control of the VA near its entrance in the dura may be difficult, and temporary intraluminal balloon occlusion is an alternative. In the latter case, care should be taken not to advance the balloon into the intradural segment of the VA. It is easy to perforate or rupture the V4 segment of the VA, where the artery has only one elastic membrane and no adventitia.

OVERVIEW OF RECONSTRUCTION TECHNIQUES

Disease of the V1 segment is usually confined to the ostium and is best dealt with by transposing the proximal VA to the common carotid artery. This is the preferred technique and the one most often used today. If the VA does not easily reach the common carotid site of implantation, an interposition vein graft may be used. In the latter case, the distal anastomosis of the interposition graft to the VA is done before the common carotid artery is clamped.

Endarterectomy and angioplasty of the ostium of the VA have gradually fallen into disuse for the reasons mentioned. If it seems advisable in a particular patient not to use the common carotid artery as the VA inflow, either because it is the sole carotid supply to the brain or because it is severely diseased, the operations of choice are a transposition of the VA to another site of the subclavian artery or a subclavian–VA bypass graft. The feasibility of transposing the VA to another subclavian artery location is predicated on the availability of sufficient length of VA and on the quality of the neighboring subclavian wall. If the transposition does not appear technically feasible, a subclavian–VA bypass is preferred.

Dissection and reconstruction of the VA in the V2 segment have been reported, but distal VA bypass is preferable because it is easier and probably more durable. Reconstructions in the V2 segment involve removal of the anterior bony wall of the transverse process and result in less VA exposure than that obtained at the C2-C1 segment. In diffuse or multiple compression of the VA by osteophytes, reconstruction of the VA at the V3 level bypasses the usual points of bony compression. Furthermore, when the artery is involved by diffuse atheromatous disease, its quality is generally better above the level of C2.

A distal (V3) bypass with autogenous vein or a transposi-

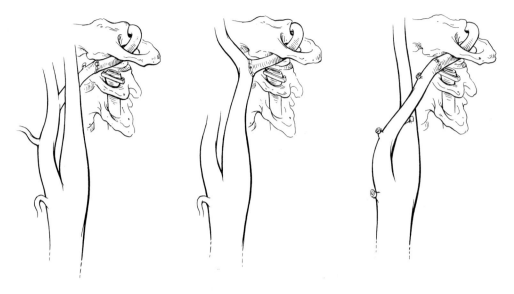

FIGURE 78–14. Three transposition procedures that can be used to revascularize the distal vertebral artery: transposition of a hypertrophic occipital artery to the distal vertebral artery *(left);* transposition of the distal vertebral artery to the internal carotid artery *(middle);* and, the most frequently used, transposition of the external carotid artery to the distal vertebral artery *(right).*

tion of the external carotid artery to the VA are the preferred techniques for extensive disease of the VA involving the V1 and V2 segments, as well as for VA occlusion with reconstitution at the level of C2.

An intraoperative digital arteriogram is obtained after every reconstruction. We have not had an immediate postoperative thrombosis since adopting this policy 4 years ago. We have, however, corrected technical defects shown by the arteriogram and not suspected by external inspection that might have resulted in thrombosis of the reconstruction.

RESULTS

Long-term follow-up data from my series[14] and from those of others[15, 16] show a similar pattern of complications and long-term patency rates and survival curves superior to those recorded after carotid operations.

Out of a total of 230 proximal VA reconstructions, there were two deaths, both in patients undergoing combined VA and carotid reconstruction.[17] There was no hospital death among the 191 patients undergoing single proximal VA

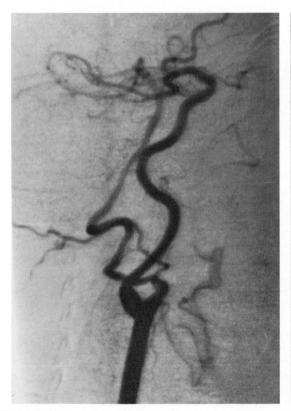
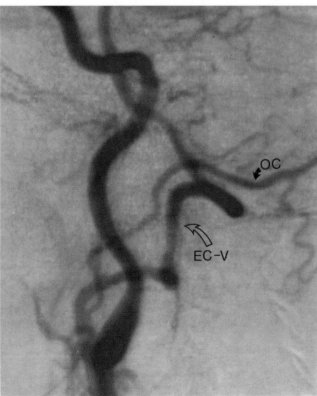

FIGURE 78–15. Two views of a transposition of the external carotid artery to the distal vertebral artery. EC-V, anastomosis site; OC, occipital artery.

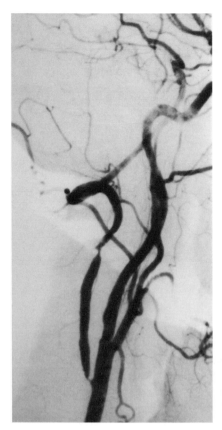
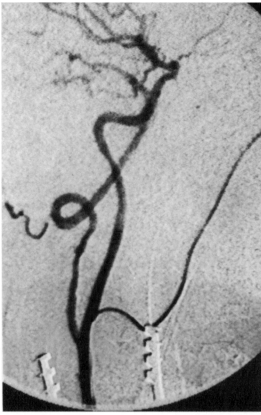

FIGURE 78–16. *Left,* Severe intimal hyperplastic lesions at both ends of an autogenous vein–distal vertebral bypass in a patient who presented with recurrent symptoms 1 year after surgery. *Right,* Intraoperative arteriogram after removal of the bypass graft and revascularization of the distal vertebral artery by transposition of the external carotid artery.

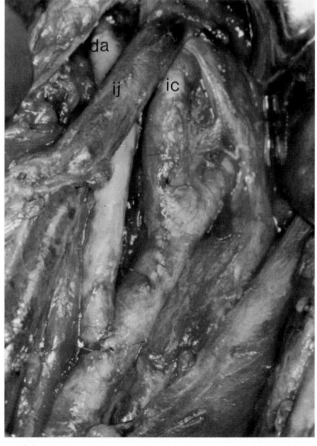

FIGURE 78–17. Intraoperative photograph following a combined carotid endarterectomy and distal vertebral bypass with autogenous vein. ic, internal carotid artery; da, distal anastomosis of the bypass; ij, internal jugular vein.

operations. The increased mortality of simultaneous carotid-vertebral reconstruction has also been reported in other series.[18] The morbidity of proximal VA reconstruction was higher in the first part of our experience, as expected. Table 78–1 shows the complications noted in the first 174 patients who underwent proximal VA reconstruction. Follow-up data of proximal VA reconstruction show secondary patency rates of 95 and 91 percent at 5 and 10 years, respectively. Life expectancy in these patients was 90 and 79 percent at 5 and 10 years. These are better figures than those reported in long-term follow-up of carotid endarterectomy series. Cure or substantial improvement of symptoms was achieved in 83 percent of patients; failure to relieve symptoms was noted in 17 percent.

Perhaps because of the more difficult dissection and anastomosis involved in reconstructions of the distal VA, there is a substantial rate of immediate thrombosis (6 of 75; 8%) and a much higher operative mortality (4%) in this group. The secondary patency rates of distal VA reconstructions were 87 and 82 percent at 5 and 10 years, respectively. Life expectancy at 5 years was 90 percent and at 10 years was 82 percent. Clinical assessment of patients who underwent distal VA reconstruction showed a cure or substantial improvement rate of 78 percent and a failure rate of 22 percent. As with the proximal vertebral operations, complications were more frequent and serious at the beginning of our experience, when these techniques were being developed. Of the six cases of early occlusion of a distal VA reconstruction, five occurred before intraoperative digital arteriography became routine. Since then, technical flaws noted during intraoperative arteriography have been corrected. Restenosis due to intimal hyperplasia, with recurrence of original symptoms, has been noted in three patients; two had had a bypass from the common carotid artery to the distal VA, and one had had an external carotid artery–to–VA transposition (Fig. 78–16).

The life expectancy of patients undergoing reconstruction of the VA is better than that observed following carotid reconstruction. This may be partly due to the fact that patients being operated on for extrinsic compression of the artery, although in the minority, are 10 to 20 years younger than those with symptomatic arteriosclerotic lesions.

The group of patients undergoing combined carotid and VA reconstruction (Fig. 78–17) showed an increased morbidity and mortality in our series and in those of others. We hypothesized that patients with combined disease had more advanced atherosclerosis. The causes of death in the two patients who died in our combined series were an atheromatous embolization (seen through a carotid shunt) in one and a myocardial infarction 3 days postoperatively in the other.[17]

In summary, the diagnosis of surgically reconstructible VA disease requires a detailed neurologic evaluation, special arteriographic techniques, and the use of magnetic resonance

TABLE 78–1. Complications in 174 Consecutive Patients Undergoing Proximal Vertebral Artery Reconstruction

Complication	Patients	
	n	%
Recurrent pharyngeal nerve palsy	3	2
Horner syndrome	26	15
Lymphocele	7	4
Chylothorax	1	.5
Immediate thrombosis*	2	1

*Both in vein grafts.

imaging. Once the diagnosis is established, the optimal techniques for reconstruction of the VA are those outlined earlier. These operations provide a reasonable chance of success with lower rates of mortality and morbidity than those reported for carotid operations. The rate for cure or substantial improvement is approximately 80 percent.

REFERENCES

1. Roon AJ, Ehrenfeld AJ, Cooke PB, Wylie EJ: Vertebral artery reconstruction. *Am J Surg.* 1980;138:29.
2. Edwards WH, Mulherin JL Jr: The surgical approach to significant stenosis of vertebral and subclavian arteries. *Surgery.* 1980;87:20.
3. Brink B: Approach to the second segment of the vertebral artery. In Berguer R, Bauer RB, eds. *Vertebrobasilar Arterial Occlusive Disease.* New York: Raven Press; 1984:257.
4. Berguer R: Distal vertebral artery bypass: Technique, the "occipital connection" and potential uses. *J Vasc Surg.* 1985;2:621.
5. Kieffer E: Chirurgie de l'artère vertébrale. Techniques Chirurgicales, Chirurgie Vasculaire, 43130, 4.9.12, Encycl Méd Chir (Paris, France).
6. Berguer R, Kieffer E: *Surgery of the Arteries to the Head.* New York: Springer-Verlag; 1992.
7. Cate WR, Scott HW: Cerebral ischemia of central origin: Relief by subclavian vertebral artery thromboendarterectomy. *Surgery.* 1959;45:19.
8. Crawford ES, DeBakey ME, Fields WS: Roentgenographic diagnosis and surgical treatment of basilar artery insufficiency. *JAMA.* 1958;168:509.
9. Natali J, Maraval M, Kieffer E: Surgical treatment of stenosis and occlusion of the internal carotid and vertebral arteries. *J Cardiovasc Surg.* 1972;13:4.
10. Labauge R, Thevenet A, Crouzet G, Nivolas M: Les insuffisances vertebrobasilaires d'incidence chirurgicale. *Rev Neurol.* 1967;117:373.
11. Berguer R, Andaya LV, Bauer RB: Vertebral artery bypass. *Arch Surg.* 1976;111:976.
12. Berguer R, Bauer RB: Vertebral artery reconstruction: A successful technique in selected patients. *Ann Surg.* 1981;193:441.
13. Kieffer E, Rancurel G, Richard T: Reconstruction of the distal cervical vertebral artery. In Berguer R, Bauer RB, eds. *Vertebrobasilar Arterial Occlusive Disease.* New York: Raven Press; 1984:265.
14. Berguer R: Long-term results of vertebral artery reconstruction. In Yao JST, Pearce WH, eds. *Long-Term Results in Vascular Surgery.* Norwalk, CT: Appleton & Lange; 1993:69.
15. Branchereau A, Rosset ELD, Magnan PE, Espinoza CHA: Proximal reconstructions. In Berguer R, Caplan LR, eds. *Vertebrobasilar Arterial Disease.* St. Louis: Quality Medical Publishing; 1992:265.
16. Kieffer E, Koskas F, Rancurel G, et al: Reconstruction of the distal cervical vertebral artery. In Berguer R, Caplan LR, eds. *Vertebrobasilar Arterial Disease.* St. Louis: Quality Medical Publishing; 1992:279.
17. McNamara M, Berguer R: Simultaneous carotid-vertebral reconstruction. *J Cardiovasc Surg.* 1989;30:161.
18. Bahnini A, Koskas F, Kieffer E: Combined carotid and vertebral artery surgery. In Berguer R, Caplan LR, eds. *Vertebrobasilar Arterial Disease.* St. Louis: Quality Medical Publishing; 1992:248.

CHAPTER 79

Surgery of the Vertebral Artery: Overview and Results

ANTHONY M. IMPARATO and THOMAS S. RILES

Although the syndromes of brain-stem ischemia secondary to basilar artery occlusion are well recognized[1, 2] and known to be dangerous, markedly shortening life expectancy,[3] less is known about similar ischemic syndromes associated with vertebral arterial lesions, although Caplan and associates[5] recently pointed out the potential for developing cerebellar and other brain stem infarcts from such lesions. This lack of knowledge is due in part to the reluctance to perform cerebral angiographic studies in patients who were overwhelmed by brain-stem strokes[6] in whom the infarct is more apt to be attributed to basilar artery thrombosis so that the possible role of vertebral arterial lesions in producing ischemia is likely to be overlooked. Added to this is the difficulty in delineating the condition of the vertebral arteries on conventional angiographic studies of the extracranial circulation,[7] and the fact that carotid lesions, more strikingly visualized, demand attention because of their often ominous appearance. In general, vascular surgeons have not intensively studied problems of transient brain-stem ischemia. Among the reasons for this lack are the facts that symptoms are often relieved by correction of serious carotid lesions[8] and that vertebral arterial lesions per se are thought by some to be associated with a benign course.[9] Another reason may be that a single, universally applicable corrective operative procedure similar to carotid bifurcation endarterectomy has not been available for atherosclerotic occlusive lesions or for other lesions described as producing vertebral artery compression. And yet, aside from the frequently quoted facts regarding the considerably lesser contributions of the vertebral arteries to total cerebral blood flow,[10] which imply that they have lesser significance in the etiology of strokes, their importance in pathologic states is impressive. Hutchinson and Yates[11] concluded that death from stroke was more apt to occur in the presence of combined carotid and vertebral arterial lesions. The Joint Study of Extracranial Occlusions revealed that lesions of vertebral artery origin were second in incidence only to lesions of the carotid bifurcation.[12] There are also patients, neurologically intact but severely symptomatic, who present with bilateral internal carotid arterial occlusions and vertebral arterial lesions and who have become almost totally dependent on the posterior circulation; these patients must be evaluated for possible corrective vertebral arterial surgery.[13]

What could well be premonitory symptoms of severe brain-stem ischemia may be nonspecific and so commonly encountered[14] (eg, vertiginous attacks, or "the dizzies," as they are referred to) that, in the absence of reliable noninvasive techniques, patients so afflicted are often not subjected to potentially hazardous invasive diagnostic angiographic study. Nevertheless, isolated vertiginous attacks associated with occlusive lesions of branches of the vertebrobasilar arterial system have preceded by several months frank infarction in the distribution of the anterior inferior cerebellar artery.[15]

Historically, there has been sporadic interest on the part of vascular surgeons in these problems.[16-18] Neurosurgeons have also become involved in attempts to prevent brain-stem strokes by performing microvascular anastomoses intracranially in patients whose vertebral arteries have become totally occluded.[19]

Since 1962, when participation in the prospective randomized Joint Study of Extracranial Arterial Occlusions[20] mandated that all surgically accessible extracranial "significant" arterial lesions found on four-vessel cerebral angiographic study be surgically corrected, these lesions have been carefully documented on our service. Until it became apparent that vertebrobasilar territory symptoms were frequently relieved by carotid procedures, all such lesions were operated on if both vertebral arteries were involved by flow-impeding lesions.[8] Thereafter, a more selective approach was used; the criteria for selection of patients for surgery are those that appear to be used by most groups that have reported significant series of vertebral operations, although the specific operative procedures performed have varied considerably among these groups.

ANATOMY

The significant fact about the anatomy of the vertebral artery relating to its surgical accessibility is that it can be divided into four parts.[6] The first part starts at the origin of the vertebral artery, which is located at the first portion of the subclavian artery at its upper posterior border between the medial edge of the anterior scalene muscle and the lateral border of the long muscle of the head. The vertebral artery passes upward, usually following a tortuous course for as much as 1½ inches (3.75 cm), to enter the foramen in the transverse process of the sixth cervical vertebra. Branches of the thyrocervical trunk usually pass anterior to the artery to reach the thyroid gland. The second part of the vertebral artery courses through the foramina of the transverse processes to the axis. This portion is surrounded by a dense plexus of small veins that join together to form the vertebral vein at the base of the neck and by sympathetic nerve fibers, which are less prominent than the veins. The third part extends from the upper border of the axis, from where it meanders upward and outward to enter the foramen in the transverse process of the atlas. It then winds backward behind the articular process, passing beneath the posterior occipitoatlantal ligament. The fourth part begins as the artery enters the skull through the foramen magnum and passes to the front of the medulla oblongata to join the vertebral artery from the other side, forming the midline basilar artery at the lower border of the pons.

Along its course, the vertebral artery lies anterior to the internal jugular and vertebral veins, is crossed by the inferior thyroid artery anteriorly, and lies on the seventh cervical vertebral transverse process and sympathetic nerves. On the left side, the thoracic duct lies anterior to the vertebral artery. Its course through the transverse foramina is ordinarily nearly a straight line. As it issues from the transverse process of the axis, it lies in proximity to the suboccipital nerve and the major posterior straight muscle of the head posteriorly.

Although there are no branches from the vertebral artery from its origin to its entrance to the foramen of the transverse process of C6, an important fact for identification of the artery at that level is the major cervical branches within the bony canal (lateral spinal and muscular) that help maintain its patency distal to ostial occlusions. There are several cranial branches, including the major, the posterior inferior cerebellar, and several smaller paired meningeal, spinal, and bulbar branches.

The vertebral artery is most easily surgically accessible at its first part[21]: its extraosseous location from its origin to its entrance into the bony canal at C6. It is also accessible at its third portion at C2, where it curves out of the foramen of the transverse process of the axis.[22] The bony canal can be unroofed for additional exposure of the second part at levels C4, C5, and C6, if careful control is kept of the bleeding from the plexus of veins surrounding the artery. Unroofing to as high as C2 has been described.[23]

In obtaining control of the origin of the vertebral artery, it is essential to expose the second part of the subclavian artery, which requires that the phrenic nerve be mobilized from its bed on the anterior scalene muscle. The muscle must then be divided and permitted to retract upward, and the internal mammary, intercostobrachial, and thyrocervical trunks must be controlled, usually after division of the transverse artery of the neck. On the right side, care must be exercised to protect the recurrent laryngeal nerve, which winds around the subclavian artery just medial to the origin of the vertebral artery. The vertebral artery's fourth, or intracranial, segment has also become accessible to neurosurgeons performing revascularization procedures.

PATHOLOGY

Most commonly, lesions that affect the first extraosseous portion of the vertebral artery are atherosclerotic, seemingly originating in the subclavian artery and impinging on the ostium of the vertebral artery, producing marked fibrous stenosis[24] (Fig. 79–1). Such is the case despite the assertions of Caplan and coworkers[5] that there exist "common myths that carotid arteries ulcerate and [vertebral arteries] do not . . . The essentially fibrotic nature of the vertebral artery origin plaque has been attested to by a number of observers, including Schwartz and Mitchell,[24] from post mortem studies . . . [T]hick but localized fibrous plaques . . . are the characteristic lesions found in these [vertebral] vessels." Imparato[7] holds the same view, which is based on observations made during operations at the subclavian vertebral junction. Ulcerations that may be the sources of embolization via the vertebral arteries are, when present, of the subclavian artery, a fact of major importance when surgical intervention on the subclavian vertebral junction is considered for the treatment of brain stem embolization. The subclavian artery may be either quite friable or buttery soft, with an almost gelatinous intima, although the ostial lesion, which rarely extends beyond the proximal 2 to 3 mm of the vertebral artery, is almost always pearly white and firm. Frequently there is marked tortuosity of the extraosseous first part of the vertebral artery, such that temporary total occlusion can

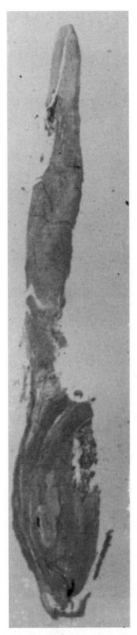

FIGURE 79–1. Longitudinal section of a subclavian plaque impinging on the origin of the vertebral artery, producing marked stenosis. (From Imparato AM, Lin JP-T: Vertebral artery reconstruction: Internal plication and vein patch angioplasty. *Ann Surg.* 1967;166:213; with permission.)

occur on the patient's turning the head[25] (Fig. 79–2). When the contralateral vertebral artery is occluded or is rudimentary, symptoms can be reproduced, including syncope. Rarely, ulceration has been encountered at the vertebral artery origin.

Other branches of the subclavian artery may share in the occlusive involvement. The thyrocervical trunk specifically, which is sometimes proposed as a site to which to transplant the vertebral artery, has been reported to have severe ostial stenosis[13] (Fig. 79–3).

Less frequently, atherosclerotic plaques have involved longer segments of both the extraosseous and the intraosseous portions, sometimes with thrombosis of the vessel extending various distances from its origin. Of particular

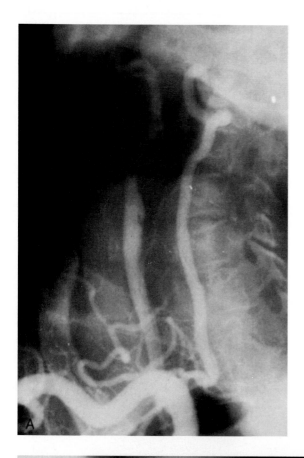

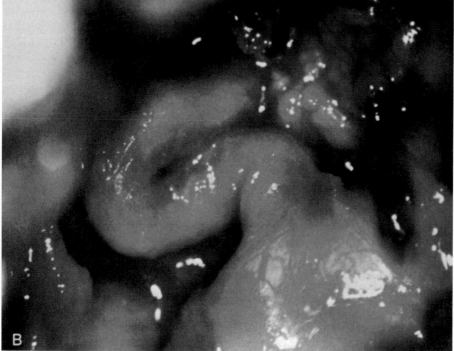

FIGURE 79–2. *A*, Angiogram of vertebral artery, demonstrating the marked tortuosity and kinking frequently found in association with ostial stenosis in symptomatic patients. (From Imparato AM, Lin JP-T: Vertebral artery reconstruction: Internal plication and vein patch angioplasty. *Ann Surg.* 1967; 166:213; with permission.) *B*, Photograph of tortuous first portion of the vertebral artery. (From Imparato AM, Riles TS, Kim GE: Cervical vertebral angioplasty for brain stem ischemia. *Surgery.* 1981;90:842; with permission.)

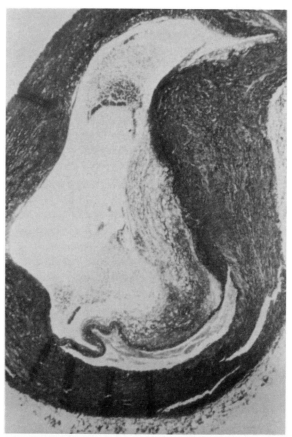

FIGURE 79-3. Microscopic cross section of the origin of the thyrocervical trunk, showing the marked intimal thickening similar to that found in the vertebral artery, which renders the thyrocervical trunk undesirable as a site to which to transpose the vertebral artery. (From Imparato AM, Lin JP-T: Vertebral artery reconstruction: Internal plication and vein patch angioplasty. *Ann Surg.* 1967;166:213; with permission.)

interest are lesions involving the most distal segments of the vertebral arteries such that the proximal vertebral artery terminates at the posterior inferior cerebellar artery rather than at the basilar artery (Fig. 79-4). Brain-stem perfusion has not been effectively restored when ostial lesions in such arteries have been corrected.

Other conditions that have resulted in marked vertebral arterial stenoses include bony spurs originating on the vertebral bodies,[26] varying degrees of cervical spondylolisthesis,[27] and herniations of the vertebral arteries between segments of the transverse foramina[28] (Fig. 79-5). Spontaneous vertebral artery dissections, although rare, can also result in a variety of brain-stem symptoms and mimic those caused by primarily occlusive disease.[29] In an identifiable group of patients, one vertebral artery may be unusually small, while the contralateral one may be unusually large, creating a situation in which there is only one effectively functioning vertebral artery and the patient loses the advantage of paired vessels.[30] Compression of the first part of the vertebral artery by the anterior scalene muscle and long muscle of the neck then produces cerebral ischemia.

Fibrodysplasia of vertebral arteries (Fig. 79-6) has been encountered and described. Although symptoms are recognizable when the condition involves the carotid arteries, symptomatic involvement of the vertebral arteries is not as obvious.[31, 32]

PHYSIOLOGY

The contribution of the vertebral arteries to total cerebral blood flow is calculated from direct flow measurements of the carotid and vertebral arteries using electromagnetic flowmeters, to be about 11 percent.[10] Blood flow in the vertebral arteries varies from 10 to 87 or more mL mean blood flow. There are reciprocal relationships among the four extracranial arteries through the circle of Willis such that occlusion of a common carotid artery may result in an immediate vertebral flow increase of as much as 100 percent, while occlusion in a vertebral artery may result in compensatory increase in carotid flow. The location of the vertebral arteries leads to variations in vertebral flow when the patient turns the head, which in some instances may be quite dramatic. These facts of the physiology of blood flow through the normal extracranial pathways, however, belie the ability of even a single vertebral artery to compensate for occlusion of the three other major extracranial vessels, which would indicate a potential for as much as a 10-fold increase in vertebral blood flow from an average flow of 45 mL/minute per artery to compensate for the 750 to 830 mL/minute total cerebral blood flow, which can be measured under physiologic conditions. This suggests an adaptability equal to that of muscular arteries under conditions of severe muscular exertion.

CLINICAL SYMPTOMS

Symptoms of carotid arterial insufficiency usually occur in the distribution of the middle cerebral arteries, resulting

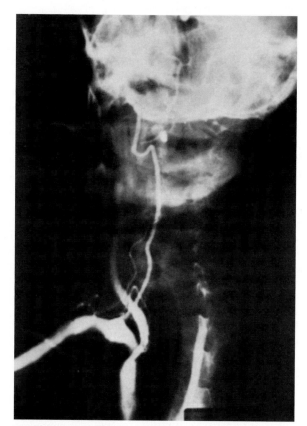

FIGURE 79-4. Angiogram of termination of the right vertebral artery at the posterior inferior cerebellar artery, a configuration that is unfavorable for revascularization of the brain stem by correcting vertebral ostial stenosis.

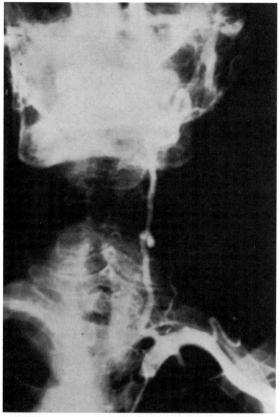

FIGURE 79–5. Angiogram showing marked tortuosity of the vertebral artery in its midportion, characteristic of herniation of the vertebral artery between segments of transverse foramina.

in contralateral motor and sensory disturbances, ipsilateral visual disturbances, and speech disorders if the dominant cerebral hemisphere is affected.

Vertebrobasilar insufficiency affecting the temporo-occipital areas of the cerebral hemispheres, the pons, thalamus, and mid-brain produces characteristically bilateral symptoms through involvement of long sensory tracts and both pyramidal tracts and cranial nerves III through XI.[2] Symptoms may be unilateral, however, and are sometimes difficult to ascribe to either anterior or posterior circulatory insufficiency, even by the most experienced neurologists.[33] Depending on the mechanism causing ischemia, be it embolization, intermittent compression of the cervical vertebral arteries, or disturbances in cardiac function in association with flow-impeding vertebral lesions, symptoms may be intermittent or progressive and, if infarction occurs, static. If associated with carotid lesions, combination cerebral lesions occur, producing various combinations of symptoms characteristic of insufficiency in both the anterior and posterior circulations.

It is not always possible to predict the arterial lesions that will be found with particular syndromes because of the great variability of the circle of Willis[34] and the ability of the circle to compensate for even multiple extracranial arterial occlusions. The joining together of the two vertebral arteries to form the basilar artery, from where the branches leading to the brain arise, makes possible asymptomatic occlusion of one vertebral artery. When the posterior communicating arteries are patent, as they are in approximately 75 percent of patients who undergo four-vessel angiographic studies,

even bilateral vertebral occlusions may fail to produce ischemic symptoms.[12]

Certain symptoms frequently reported are considered characteristic of vertebrobasilar insufficiency, whereas others are less convincing. These syndromes, however, were verified in the presence of basilar artery occlusion and may or may not express the full spectrum of disorders originating from vertebral arterial occlusive lesions, as there has not been a systematic evaluation of symptoms for other documented vertebral arterial lesions.[19] Table 79–1 lists symptoms and the diagnostic value ascribed to them based on the Millikan-Siekert classification.

Embolic occlusion of vessels of the posterior circulation may result in either very focal symptoms, such as inability to swallow, or catastrophic brain-stem strokes causing stupor and quadriplegia. Various syndromes of cerebellar infarction have been described.[35–37] Specific symptoms reflect the vascular territory involved and are caused either by embolization or possibly by regional hypoperfusion. Vertigo, headache, and gait imbalance are characteristic of posterior inferior cerebellar artery territorial ischemia, whereas with superior cerebellar artery territorial ischemia, gait disturbances predominate and vertigo and headache are less pronounced. Frequently these symptoms are ascribed to "benign labyrinthine disorder" yet may herald potentially fatal brain

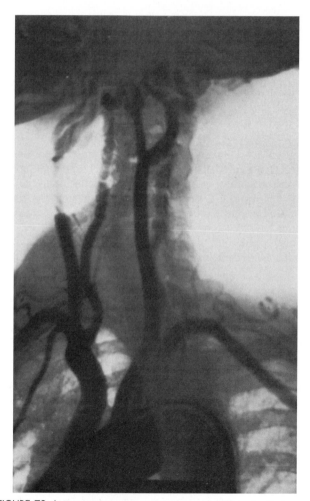

FIGURE 79–6. Beaded appearance of vertebral arteries on the angiogram, suggesting fibromuscular hyperplasia.

TABLE 79–1. Symptoms of Basilar Artery
Insufficiency

Diagnostic (two or more symptoms)
  Motor or sensory symptoms (bilateral) occurring during the
    same attack
  Ataxia of gait or clumsiness of both extremities
  Diplopia
  Dysarthria
  Bilateral homonymous hemianopia
Compatible with vertebrobasilar insufficiency but not diagnostic
  Vertigo
  Tinnitus
  Multiple cranial nerve involvement (opposite major sensory
    nerve of motor disturbances)
Not diagnostic if occurring alone
  Dizziness
  Drop attacks
  Syncope
  Transient global amnesia

stem compression if infarction and postinfarction edema should occur.[35–37]

Other symptoms usually not associated with occlusive cerebrovascular disease include cough syncope, which typically occurs in patients with chronic lung disease but has also been described as caused by critical carotid and vertebral occlusive disease and relieved by left subclavian to left common carotid artery bypass.[38]

DIAGNOSIS

Precise diagnosis of the vascular components contributing to cerebrovascular insufficiency neurologic syndromes depends on accurate assessment of the entire cerebral circulation from the origins of the cervical portions of the vertebral arteries to their terminations intracranially. Exclusion of other causes of brain-stem symptoms is mandatory. Most often patients present with combinations of cerebral hemispheric and either nonspecific or clear-cut brain-stem symptoms. Although ultimately radiographic visualization of the arteries combined with computed tomographic scanning of the brain in suspect patients is required for diagnosis, one or more noninvasive tests may help to differentiate those brain-stem symptoms that are related to vascular insufficiency from those that are related to primary end organ dysfunction.

Because dizziness, with or without hearing loss, is the single most common complaint reported by patients with confirmed vertebrobasilar arterial insufficiency,[7, 39, 40] an otologist may either see the patient initially or be consulted to help establish a differential diagnosis between an otologic cause and many other causes, including vertebrobasilar arterial insufficiency.

The precise nature of the "dizzies" may be quite variable and be variously described by the patient as giddiness, swimming, dropping, spinning, loss of balance, or true vertigo in which the surroundings appear to revolve or spin around the subject.

A battery of neuro-otologic tests examine oculomotor function for a possible central nervous system origin of symptoms. Among these are electronystagmography, which accurately characterizes existing nystagmus; caloric tests to detect vestibular weakness or semicircular canal paralysis,

thereby also differentiating between end organ and central origin of symptoms; and position testing, sinusoidal acceleration testing, and posturagraphy, which are useful tests for identifying the sites of lesions. None of these tests firmly establishes or rules out the diagnosis of vertebrobasilar arterial insufficiency, however, since there is no consistent pattern of electronystagmographic testing that is diagnostic.[40]

Auditory evoked potential responses alone, although the test is noninvasive, objective, and sensitive to brain stem infarctions that involve auditory pathways, are not helpful in the diagnosis of transient brain stem ischemic episodes because the patient's responses tend to be normal between attacks. How responses are affected during acute attacks of transient brain stem ischemia has not been defined.[41, 42]

Similarly, visual disturbances can be studied using visual evoked potentials.[43] Pattern shift or flashed visual evoked potential responses are normal in patients with intermittent attacks of vertebrobasilar arterial insufficiency; abnormal responses often denote coexistent ocular disease. The responses are complex and not easy to interpret but are used nevertheless in the differential diagnosis of established visual disorders, such as cerebral blindness, monochromatism (loss of color recognition), and visual fields defects. The tests are less useful in the differential diagnosis of transient symptoms for which results are negative between attacks.

Continuous-wave Doppler ultrasonographic studies, which yield ultrasonographic images and velocity waveforms in the supraclavicular areas at the origins of the vertebral arteries, along the courses of the vertebral arteries in the neck, and posteriorly at the base of the skull, have not been as rewarding as similar studies of the carotid bifurcations. The reasons for the inadequacy of Doppler for diagnosis include the tortuosity of the vertebral vessels, the overlap of many neighboring branch arteries, and the common problem of vertebral artery predominance in which one artery is considerably larger than the other. Establishing direction of flow in a vertebral artery may not be a reliable diagnostic tool because, in the presence of total vertebral arterial occlusion, steal can occur through branches of the subclavian artery other than the vertebral branch and can simulate retrograde flow in a patent vertebral artery. Nevertheless, when used by well-trained and dedicated technicians, duplex scanning can offer clues to the presence of occlusive vertebral arterial disease, although failure to detect abnormalities does not rule out its presence.

Computed axial tomography and magnetic resonance imaging of the brain can reveal areas of infarction in the vertebrobasilar watershed, but because most patients who present for evaluation have transient and possibly preinfarction symptoms, negative test results do not rule out the presence of severe occlusive arterial lesions of the vertebrobasilar system.

The computed tomographic scan of the brain has been useful in ruling out nonischemic space-occupying lesions and cerebral hemorrhages and in confirming, if posterior infarcts are encountered, the true nature and source of symptoms that otherwise might be considered noncharacteristic or even confusing.

Conventional arch angiographic study combined with selective injection of arch vessels has been the most reliable technique for assessing the entire cerebral circulation and especially the vertebrobasilar system. On occasion, when the vertebral artery origins are not clearly outlined, the studies are supplemented by retrograde brachial arterial injections with positioning of the patients in such a way as to project vertebral artery origins clearly (Fig. 79–7). Opacified subclavian arteries can sometimes obscure vertebral artery origins, since the origins are located at the posterior aspect of the subclavian arteries. Joining together of the two vertebral arteries to form the basilar artery must be particularly studied so that the surgeon can avoid reconstructing a vertebral artery that ends at the posterior inferior cerebellar artery. If one vertebral artery of acceptable dimension is free of obstructing lesions and is demonstrated to join the basilar artery, the contralateral one is often not studied unless embolization is suspected.[7]

Digital subtraction angiography with selective catheter injection of arch vessels has produced satisfactory diagnostic results, whereas intravenous digital subtraction angiography has been most unsatisfactory for delineation of the vertebrobasilar vessels. When the procedure is applied for suspected posterior circulatory insufficiency, often multiple studies employing retrograde brachial arterial injection must be performed before definitive information can be obtained.

In all cerebral studies, then, clear delineation of at least one vertebral artery is necessary; if that artery is found to be stenotic anywhere along its course, the contralateral vertebral artery is studied as well.

Magnetic resonance angiography (MRA), recently evaluated for use predominantly in carotid occlusive arterial disease,[44] has a similar use for the vertebrobasilar system[45] and exhibits similar limitations. Although all stenoses, occlusions, and aneurysms of the distal vertebrobasilar system were correctly identified and correlated well with the findings of extracranial and transcranial Doppler ultrasonographic studies, the degree of stenosis was difficult to evaluate with the use of MRA. In the region of the vertebral artery origins, where most lesions are to be found, MRA has yet to prove its superiority over conventional multiview contrast radioangiography. In combination with transcranial Doppler ultrasonography, however, it might prove useful in evaluating the need for vertebral arterial reconstruction in symptomatic patients with nonembolizing lesions, especially after stenotic carotid arteries have been repaired.

SELECTION OF PATIENTS FOR OPERATION

Symptoms

A review of a number of reported series of operations on the extracranial vertebral arteries in which symptoms were relieved shows the distribution of symptoms to be consistent. Dizziness, focal neurologic symptoms of either carotid or vertebrobasilar distribution, syncope, bilateral visual disturbances and diplopia, drop attacks, and headache are reported most often. Table 79–2 lists the characteristic symptoms encountered in our series as well as other series of direct vertebral operations in patients with intrinsic arterial lesions. Although some series report, as a primary indication for operation, incapacitating dizziness that confines the patient to bed, this symptom alone is not generally accepted as attributable to vertebrobasilar insufficiency and may not be totally relieved by vertebral operations, even when other classic vertebrobasilar symptoms are also present that may

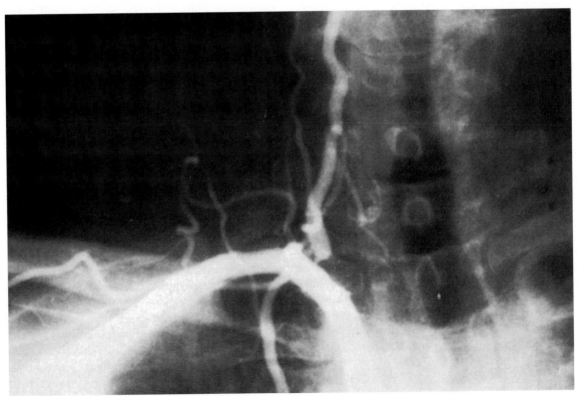

FIGURE 79–7. Angiogram of a typical stenotic lesion of the vertebral artery origin, often requiring selective injection for clear delineation. (From Imparato AM, Lin JP-T: Vertebral artery reconstruction: Internal plication and vein patch angioplasty. *Ann Surg.* 1967;166:213; with permission.)

TABLE 79–2. Selection of Patients for
Operation*

Symptoms†	Patients, n
Dizziness	51
Focal symptoms	41‡
Syncope	27
Diplopia	27
Drop attacks	22
Headache	15
Ataxia	14
Confusion	10
Generalized weakness	8
Global amnesia	4
Homonymous hemianopia	3
Aphasia	1

*n = 118.

†Symptoms are characteristic of those reported in a number of series in which vertebral arterial operations were performed for intrinsic or extrinsic vertebral arterial lesions.

‡Twenty-one had carotid and vertebral operations.

be relieved by surgery. Thus, although incapacitating dizziness may lead to the discovery of severe vertebral arterial compression or stenoses, operative intervention for its relief may be disappointing, especially since postural hypotension and sluggish vascular reflex responses to postural changes as well as middle and inner ear disturbances are so prevalent in the age group under discussion. As in the anterior circulation, fixed neurologic deficits cannot be expected to be relieved by vertebrobasilar revascularization. Rather, the ultimate aim beyond relief of incapacitating symptoms is to prevent cerebral infarction.

Syncope, which can be expected to be relieved by vertebral operation, must be differentiated from transient cardiac rhythm disorders such as transient heart block or sick sinus syndrome, from convulsive disorders, and from severe aortic valvular stenosis.

Headaches, too, although frequently reported in operative series, require extensive differential diagnostic investigation. Indeed, patients should be warned against expecting dramatic improvement in their headache patterns.

The notion that transient global amnesia results from vertebrobasilar insufficiency, when discussed with our neurologist colleagues, has evoked mixed reactions ranging from absolute skepticism to total agreement.[46] This suggests that this symptom must also be approached with great caution when it is the only presenting symptom without supporting and more easily recognized symptoms of brain-stem ischemia.

It is important to realize that mixed syndromes of cerebral hemispheric and brain-stem symptoms occur with great frequency and that associated symptoms whose cause is not clearly attributable to brain stem ischemia also occur and may be relieved by surgery, indicating the need for careful and thorough clinical evaluation. When angiographic studies are finally performed, they should delineate both the anterior and posterior circulations.

Radiographic Findings

It is generally agreed that patients subjected to vertebral reconstructive procedures should have evidence of bilateral flow-impeding vertebral lesions, since recognizable embolism carried to the brain stem via the vertebral arteries is relatively rare in the patient population referred for consideration for a vascular procedure. This is understandable, as ostial ulcerations occur rarely. In addition, those patients in whom embolism to brain-stem arteries occurs are rarely healthy enough to be considered for surgery. It is also clear that vertebrobasilar ischemic symptoms can be relieved by carotid operations, predictably so when the operation is for hemodynamically significant carotid lesions and a posterior communicating arterial system is radiographically visualized. The angiographic criteria for unilateral vertebral surgical intervention can be summarized as follows: Bilateral flow-impeding lesions must be present; one of them might be an atretic vertebral artery. Flow-impeding carotid lesions are corrected and symptoms persist or are inoperable. The vertebral artery to be operated on must be shown to join a relatively uninvolved basilar artery; those ending at the posterior inferior cerebellar artery are unsuitable to act as the only outflow tract to the brain stem.[7] These criteria are represented diagrammatically in Figure 79–8.

SURGICAL PROCEDURES

A number of surgical procedures have been used to relieve vertebrobasilar arterial insufficiency (Table 79–3), the greatest variety being for intrinsic lesions of the cervical vertebral arteries. Other procedures, directed at specific extrinsic lesions, are designed to correct kinks, to relieve bony or

TABLE 79–3. Surgical Procedures for
Vertebrobasilar Arterial Insufficiency

Direct-Intrinsic Lesions
  Cervical
    Subclavian vertebral endarterectomy
    Subclavian vertebral angioplasty
    Vertebral transposition to a new origin
      To thyrocervical trunk
      To subclavian artery
      To common carotid artery
    Carotid or subclavian vertebral bypass
      Proximal: to terminal first or proximal second portion of vertebral
      Distal: to vertebral artery at C1-C2 interspace
  Intracranial
    Occipital to PICA anastomosis
    Superficial temporal to superior cerebellar anastomosis
    Intracranial vertebral endarterectomy
    Other intracranial bypass procedures
      Anterior inferior cerebellar artery
      Superficial temporal artery to superior cerebellar artery
Indirect-Extrinsic Lesions
  Cervical
    Decompression
      Correction of tortuosity and kinking by scalene muscle and cervical fascial resection
      Subclavian traction
      Unroofing of transverse foramina
        To correct herniation of the vertebral artery
        To correct compression by bony spurs and spondylolisthesis
  Other
    Periarterial sympathectomy

PICA, posterior inferior cerebellar artery.

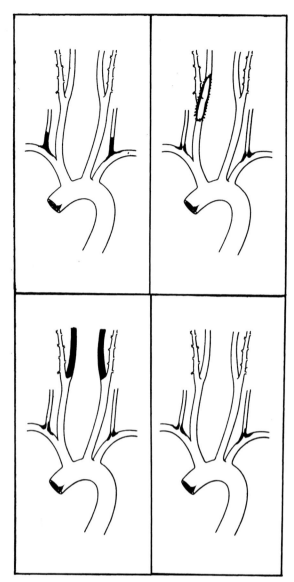

FIGURE 79–8. Diagrammatic summary of the angiographic patterns most often encountered that indicate the need for vertebral surgical intervention (see text for details). (From Imparato AM, Riles TS, Kim GE: Cervical vertebral angioplasty for brain stem ischemia. *Surgery*. 1981;90:842; with permission.)

muscular and ligamentous compressions, or to relieve herniations of the vertebral arteries between segments of the cervical transverse processes forming the transverse foramina.

Direct-Intrinsic Lesions

Cervical

Subclavian-Vertebral Endarterectomy

Since most intrinsic lesions involve the origins of the vertebral arteries and consist of atherosclerotic involvement of the subclavian arteries that impinge on the vertebral artery origins and rarely extend beyond their proximal few millimeters, direct ostial endarterectomy performed through subclavian arteriotomies is possible.[32] The surgical approach is supraclavicular, with exposure of the subclavian artery

and its branches by division of the anterior scalene muscle. On the left side, endarterectomy of the subclavian artery occasionally requires a median sternotomy incision. The subclavian artery is often friable and difficult to control following its endarterectomy, although endarterectomy has been used to great advantage by a number of surgical groups. The procedure suffers from another disadvantage in that it does not correct the rather marked kinking and tortuosity often found in the first portion of the vertebral artery, a condition that has been described as being a major factor in causing intermittent symptoms.

Subclavian-Vertebral Angioplasty

Recognizing the fact that the intima of the vertebral artery only just beyond its origin is usually involved by atherosclerosis and that ulceration in close proximity to the vertebral artery origin is rare, a procedure that corrects the ostial stenosis and the kink, without the need to perform the sometimes difficult subclavian endarterectomy or to enter the mediastinum, is termed subclavian vertebral angioplasty.[7, 47] It involves exposure of the subclavian artery and its branches through a supraclavicular incision, freeing up of the entire extraosseous segment of the vertebral artery, resection of the origin of the thyrocervical trunk with an ellipse of subclavian arterial wall, and extension of the arteriotomy longitudinally along the vertebral artery to within 1 cm of its entrance into the foramen of the transverse process of C6 (Fig. 79–9). The normal intima of the vertebral artery is sutured to the intima of the subclavian artery across the stenotic ostium, forming a plication of the vertebral artery that effectively covers the ostial plaque and eliminates the kink. The defect in the newly formed subclavian-vertebral juncture is closed with an autologous saphenous venous patch (Fig. 79–10). The resulting configuration of the vertebral origin is tapered, thereby avoiding the right-angle shape, which appears to predispose to intimal fibrous proliferation (Fig. 79–11).

Vertebral Transposition to a New Origin

Transposition to the subclavian artery is a variation of the angioplasty technique that entails incising the proximal 1 cm of the vertebral artery and an equal length of the upper border of the subclavian artery and then either performing in effect a side-to-side anastomosis between the subclavian and the vertebral arteries or, after suturing the posterior edge of the vertebral artery to the posterior edge of the subclavian artery, closing the defect with a roof patch. This procedure can be used to correct kinking as well as stenosis but has limited application in cases in which the wall of the subclavian artery is thick and calcified, making primary side-to-side anastomosis hazardous in terms of maintaining an adequate lumen of the vertebral artery.

The technique has been useful, however, in cases in which the wall of the subclavian artery was not thickened or calcified and in which the vertebral artery was unusually redundant. It therefore belongs (as a number of other procedures should) in the armamentarium of the surgeon wishing to deal with vertebral ostial lesions.

Transposition to the thyrocervical trunk involves transecting the vertebral artery distal to the area of stenosis at its origin and reanastomosing the distal segment to the thyrocer-

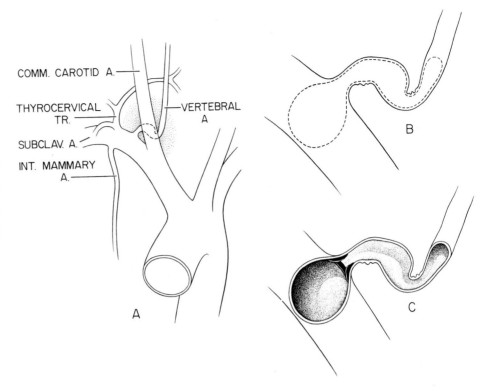

FIGURE 79–9. *A,* General relationships of the first part of the vertebral artery. *B, Dotted line* shows the extent of the arteriotomy in the subclavian artery obtained by excising the thyrocervical trunk, and extending the arteriotomy longitudinally to beyond the most distal kink in the vertebral artery. *C,* Appearance of stenosing plaque at the origin of the vertebral artery. (From Imparato AM, Lin JP-T: Vertebral artery reconstruction: Internal plication and vein patch angioplasty. *Ann Surg.* 1967;166:213; with permission.)

COMM. CAROTID A.

THYROCERVICAL TR.

VERTEBRAL A

SUBCLAV. A.

INT. MAMMARY A.

vical trunk. The technique is mentioned as an acceptable alternative, but has not been reported in any significant series of patients.[48] End-to-end anastomosis of these small arteries is difficult, and there is the added disadvantage that the origin of the thyrocervical trunk may have extensive atherosclerosis like the origin of the vertebral artery.[13]

Transposition to the common carotid artery apparently was first proposed as a technique for correcting subclavian steal syndrome.[49] The distal transected first portion of the vertebral artery is attached to the side of the common carotid artery.[31, 47, 50] The technique has gained considerable favor, since it, too, can be performed through a supraclavicular incision, does not require mobilization of the phrenic nerve or division of the anterior scalene muscle, and can be used effectively to correct the vertebral kink. It is widely employed by a number of surgeons, including our group on occasion, but suffers from two potential problems. First, clamping of the common carotid artery is required, with the risk of embolization and the relatively small though ever-present risk of producing carotid territory cerebral ischemia in those few patients with contralateral carotid occlusion or severe stenoses who do not even tolerate common carotid clamping without developing severe ischemic symptoms.[51] Second, the wall of the common carotid artery may be quite thick, resulting in minor or even severe ostial stenosis at the site of vertebral carotid anastomosis that may predispose to fibromuscular anastomotic thickening characteristic of the reaction seen where there is right-angle arterial branching. To overcome this latter problem, roof-patch angioplasty of the common carotid artery has been performed in our series, and the vertebral artery has been anastomosed to an opening made in the vein patch, thereby avoiding any pinching effect of the newly formed vertebral origin.

Carotid or Subclavian-Vertebral Bypass

Bypass procedures have been performed, usually with the use of reversed autologous saphenous vein from either the subclavian or the common carotid artery to the vertebral artery either at its first, second, or third portion.

For the few patients in whom the first segment of the vertebral artery is totally occluded, proximal bypass is performed. A patent segment of vertebral artery is exposed by unroofing one or more segments of the canal through the cervical transverse processes.[28] Unroofing C5-C6 is usually sufficient, and end-to-side anastomoses of the saphenous vein to the common carotid and patent vertebral arteries have been successfully performed. Dissection of the vertebral artery within the unroofed bony canal is tedious because of the plexus of minute veins surrounding the vertebral artery within the canal. A second potentially serious problem that led to rethrombosis in two patients is failure of the surgeon to perform the vertebral anastomosis beyond the most distal intimal thickening, which is often found in instances of proximal bypass. If such a procedure is contemplated, it is recommended that at least one segment be exposed beyond the level at which the artery looks and feels normal, to ensure anastomosis to an uninvolved vertebral artery.

Distal Vertebral Bypass

The difficult dissection of the artery within the bony canal can be avoided. Either carotid or subclavian reversed autologous saphenous vein bypass can be performed at the C2 level, where the vertebral artery can be exposed through an upper neck incision and then transected. End-to-end anas-

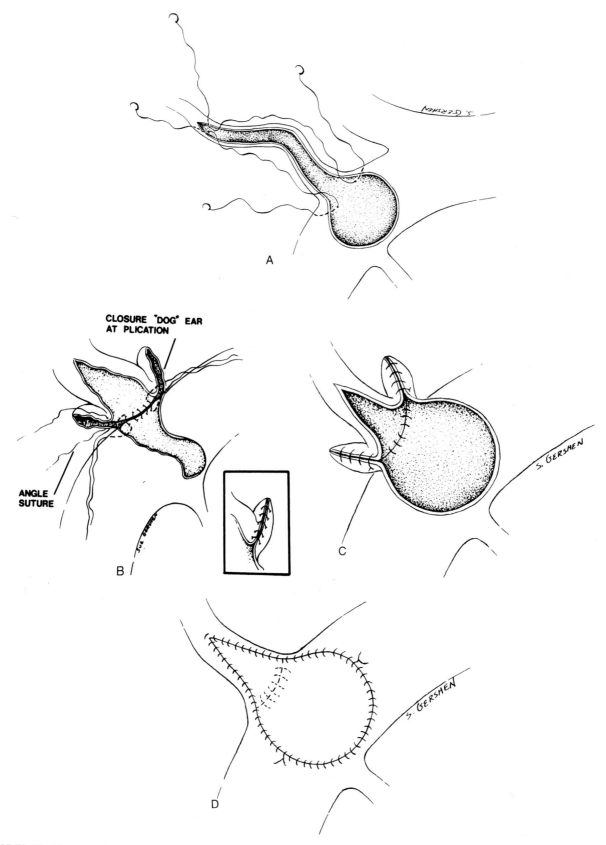

FIGURE 79–10. Plication and roof patch. *A*, Placing the plication sutures. *B and C*, Plication of the vertebral artery, covering the ostial plaque with normal vertebral intima and creating cul-de-sacs that must be sutured to prevent bleeding. *D*, Vein roof-patch closure of subclavian and vertebral arteries. (*A, C, D* from Imparato AM, Riles TS, Kim GE: Cervical vertebral angioplasty for brain stem ischemia. *Surgery.* 1981;90:842; with permission.)

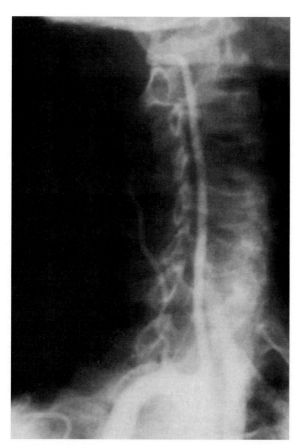

FIGURE 79–11. Angiogram of completed angioplasty, demonstrating the funnel-shaped tapering configuration of the newly formed vertebral origin.

tomosis between the distal transected end of the vertebral artery and the reversed saphenous vein receiving its inflow either from the carotid or subclavian artery can be done.[52, 53] The surgical approach is along the upper anterior border of the sternocleidomastoid muscle, dividing the external jugular vein, displacing the parotid gland, and mobilizing the internal jugular vein to permit its separation from the sternocleidomastoid muscle. The spinal accessory nerve is mobilized and, separating the muscles attached to the lower part of the C1 transverse process, the vertebral artery between transverse processes C1-C2 is exposed to permit either end-to-end or end-to-side anastomosis to a saphenous vein graft originating from either the common carotid or the subclavian artery or rarely from the internal carotid artery.

If exposure of the vertebral artery is limited and the end-to-end anastomosis to the collapsed vertebral artery is difficult, exposure can be improved by unroofing the bony canal at C2, requiring the tedious dissection of the periarterial veins but improving exposure sufficiently to perform end-to-side anastomoses, which is probably technically more reliable. For those patients in whom the occlusive process involves extensive section of the intraosseous second portion of the vertebral artery, this procedure is required for revascularization.

Series have been performed by Kieffer and coworkers[52] in Paris and Berguer and coworkers[53] in Detroit, who apparently now employ the procedure preferentially.

Balloon Dilatation of the Vertebral Artery and Basilar Artery

Balloon dilatations of the stenotic vertebral arteries are said to be done for ostial stenoses. Reports of such experiences are few but, if prohibitive embolization does not occur, it can be attributed to the fibrous nature of the plaque at that location. Judgment must be reserved as to whether this will become an acceptable procedure until such experiences are fully reported.[54, 55]

Intracranial Vertebral Revascularization

Occlusive lesions of the fourth portion of the vertebral artery, total occlusions of the vertebral arteries proximal to the posterior inferior cerebellar artery, and midbasilar artery occlusions have led to a number of intracranial revascularization procedures, including occipital to posterior inferior cerebellar artery bypass,[56] endarterectomy of the fourth portion of the vertebral artery,[57] and superficial temporal to superior cerebellar artery anastomoses.[58]

When the vertebral arteries are occluded proximal to the posterior inferior cerebellar artery, anastomoses of the occipital to the posterior inferior cerebellar artery have been performed with the use of microsurgical techniques. Because the amount of perfusion by way of the posterior inferior cerebellar artery to the basilar artery is sparse, Ausman's group,[56] which helped develop the procedure, has not done this operation since 1978, whereas Sundt and his group[57] have continued to perform such procedures.

For isolated occlusive lesions of the fourth portions of the vertebral arteries, localized intracranial vertebral endarterectomy procedures have been performed as first described by Allen and associates in 1981.[58]

Midbasilar artery stenosis has been treated (14 cases) by superficial temporal to superior cerebellar artery bypass.[59]

External carotid to posterior cerebral interposition graft of saphenous vein has been reported by Sundt and coworkers[57] in patients with extensive vertebrobasilar occlusive disease.

Indirect-Extrinsic Compressive Lesions

A number of extrinsic lesions have been operated on to relieve episodic basivertebral symptoms ascribed to kinking, musculofascial compression, bony spurs arising from vertebral bodies, spondylolisthesis, and herniations of the second portion of the vertebral arteries out of the vertebral canal.

Decompression

Correction of Tortuosity and Kinking. This was described by Husni and colleagues[30] as a new clinical concept, although the technique was reported 5 years earlier by Powers and colleagues.[60] Mechanical obstruction of a large vertebral artery opposite a hypoplastic one on the patient's turning the head was treated by clearing the transverse process of the sixth cervical vertebra of all tendinous attachments and interposing a portion of the scalene fat pad between the artery and bone to prevent reattachment. This was accomplished by resection of the anterior scalene muscle to the sixth cervical vertebra, attachment of the long muscle of the neck, clearing of the foramen in the transverse process of C6, and achievement of "absolute" hemostasis.

Variations of this operation have included completely freeing up the first part of the vertebral artery and correcting the kink by attaching the side of the subclavian artery to the clavicle.[61]

Correction of Extrinsic Compression. Intermittent extrinsic compression of the second portion of the vertebral artery within the transverse foramina has been described by Sheehan and coworkers[27] as producing a washboard appearance on angiogram and being caused by cervical spondylolisthesis, and by Hardin[26] as being caused by bony spurs. It has been treated surgically by Hardin by unroofing the transverse foramina from C6 to as high as C2.[26] In most instances, decompression at C6 and C5 was sufficient to relieve the intermittent obstruction. The series reported by Sheehan and colleagues[27] described nonsurgical treatment with bed rest and cervical traction.

Herniations of the Vertebral Artery. The intertransverse ligaments that join the transverse processes of the vertebral bodies consist of a few irregular fibers, unlike the dense cords attached to the lumbar transverse processes. Herniations of the vertebral arteries through these fibrous attachments are recognizable radiographically by the typical loop formed at the midcervical level. Drop attacks are produced on the patient's turning the head if involvement is bilateral or if the vertebral artery opposite an uninvolved artery is atretic. The technique of unroofing the bony canal at two or more levels and freeing fibrous bands that limit the excursions of the vertebral artery turns the kink into a gentle curve, correcting the intermittent compression of the artery.[28]

Periarterial Sympathectomy

In patients with intermittent obstruction produced by head-turning and caused by the artery's being trapped by the anterior scalene muscle, the long muscle of the neck, and the cervical fascia, periarterial sympathectomy, by which the vertebral artery is freed, has been claimed to have a beneficial effect on symptoms.[60] This effect is disputed, however,[30] and is mentioned here only for historical interest.

MEDICAL TREATMENT

The impetus for medical treatment of transient vertebrobasilar insufficiency resulted from the studies of Millikan and coworkers,[3] who administered coumadin to patients and reported improvement in symptoms. A thorough angiographic survey to document the locations and types of lesions was not performed. It was observed, however, that coumadin administered during the sixth to eighth decades of life increased the risk of intracranial hemorrhage three- to eightfold, depending on the particular age group treated, raising questions regarding the advisability of its use, in spite of the fact that the incidence of brain-stem strokes was reduced.

RESULTS

Interpretation of the results of surgical manipulations of the vertebrobasilar arterial system is difficult because of the lack of availability of control series of untreated patients for each pathologic entity. Symptomatic relief, late stroke incidence, and survival are reported in relatively few surgical series. These usually refer to a variety of conditions and operations.

For example, Rainer and coworkers[62] reported on a series of 54 operations, 20 (37%) performed for tortuosity, 13 (24%) for stenosis, 19 (35%) for extravascular compression, and 2 (4%) for aneurysms. Of these, 13 patients (24%) had fibromuscular decompression, 10 (19%) had reimplantation, 9 (17%) had bony decompression, 7 (13%) had endarterectomy and patch angioplasty, 4 (7%) had reimplantation to the thyrocervical trunk, 3 (6%) had subclavian vertebral angioplasty, and 2 (4%) had excision of aneurysm and reimplantation of the vertebral artery. Up to 7 years postoperatively, 86 percent of patients were reported to have become asymptomatic or improved.

Edwards and associates,[50] who favor vertebral reimplantation into the side of the common carotid artery, reported 244 operations performed in a series of 1700 patients operated on for extracranial cerebral occlusive disease, an incidence of 14 percent vertebral operations. Fifty-three (21.7%) had subclavian vertebral endarterectomy, 32 (13.1%) had bypass procedures, and 159 (65.2%) had reimplantation of the vertebral artery to the common carotid artery. Symptoms were relieved in 85 percent but late survival and stroke incidence were not reported.

Roon and coworkers[32] reported a series from the service of EJ Wylie, in which 43 patients were operated on between 1961 and 1978 for a variety of symptoms, including dizziness (51%), syncope (44%), visual symptoms (33%), motor symptoms (30%), vertigo (25%), drop attacks (12%), and a number of others, including headache, ataxia, and aphasia. A variety of operations, predominantly transcervical vertebral endarterectomy with or without vein patch (65%) but also left transthoracic vertebral endarterectomy (19%), vertebral reimplantation to the common carotid or subclavian artery (14%), and one resection of a kink with end-to-end anastomosis, were performed. One operative death (2.3%) and two neurologic deficits (4.7%) occurred. Of the survivors, 76 percent became asymptomatic and 17 percent improved in an average follow-up of 45 months; only three new strokes occurred in the late follow-up period. Survival calculated by the life-table method indicated 73 percent survival for the group at 5 years compared with 78 percent survival for an age-adjusted normal population.[32]

Reul and associates[47] reported 40 vertebral artery operations performed in a series of 3000 cerebrovascular operations. Indications for operation are given as vertigo and dizziness (73%), transient ischemic attack (43%), syncope (20%), and stroke (35%). Twenty-one (53%) vertebral reimplantations were performed, 15 (38%) patch grafts of the subclavian vertebral junction, and 3 (8%) bypass grafts. Follow-up was 1 to 12 years, with an average of 7.75 years. Survival at the twelfth year was 75.8 percent, eight patients having died between the first and ninth years postoperatively, free of vertebrobasilar symptoms. Of the 30 survivors at the twelfth year, 21 (70%) were asymptomatic, 7 (23%) remained stable, and 2 (7%) remained asymptomatic for 5 years and then had recurrences. Only one stroke (3.5%) occurred in the group at the seventh year.

Diaz and coworkers[48] reported 55 operations performed

for multiple repeated recognizable brain-stem events with five permanent deficits. Patients received treatment with antiplatelet agents or anticoagulants. Operations performed were 48 (87%) vertebral to carotid transpositions, two (4%) saphenous vein bypass grafts, and one (2%) subclavian artery graft. Fifty-three patients (96%) were rendered asymptomatic, one remained dizzy, and one experienced syncopal episodes. Postoperative complications included Horner syndrome in 30 of 55 patients (55%), of which 4 cases (7%) were permanent; three (5%) vocal cord paralyses; and two (4%) elevations of the hemidiaphragm. Long-term survival and late stroke rates were not given.

Our own series, performed between 1964 and June 1985, which consisted of 120 operations on vertebral arteries for the symptoms listed in Table 79–2, represents an incidence of 5 percent vertebral artery procedures as compared with carotid artery procedures. Of these, 108 patients had subclavian vertebral angioplasty with vertebral plication and roof patching, five had carotid vertebral reversed autologous saphenous vein bypass, five had reimplantation of the vertebral artery to the side of the common carotid artery, and two had unroofing of the vertebral bony canal for treatment of drop attacks. In 21 patients, carotid endarterectomy procedures preceded vertebral artery operations. Three deaths (2.5%) occurred during the early postoperative period, one of which was caused by acute myocardial infarction, one by a pulmonary embolus, and one probably by cerebral infarction occurring as coma. There was one asymptomatic occlusion of a vein bypass to the midcervical vertebral artery and one asymptomatic occlusion of a subclavian vertebral angioplasty. Follow-up of 2 months to 19 years revealed survival at 5 years of 88 percent, at 10 years of 69 percent, and at 15 years of 69 percent. Strokes occurred at the rate of one yearly between the second and ninth years, with an additional stroke occurring at the second and fifth years. Sixty-nine percent of patients were alive and essentially symptom-free, except for occasional mild dizziness, at the fifteenth year (Table 79–4). Only five patients were lost to follow-up. The two patients who had decompression of the vertebral canal for drop attacks were relieved of their attacks; they are not reported in the life table, however, which consists of patients with atherosclerotic lesions. Of those patients operated on for syncope, 20 were relieved of their syncopal episodes by cerebral revascularization, while seven required additional procedures. One had a cardiac pacemaker inserted prior to a vertebral procedure, four had pacemakers implanted during the same hospital admission, one required a pacemaker 9 years later, and one had aortic valve replacement for severe aortic stenosis.

TABLE 79–4. Results in 118 Patients Operated on for Intrinsic Vertebral Arterial Lesions

Time After Surgery	At Risk, n	Strokes, n	Deaths, Unrelated, n	Cumulative Success, %
0	118	0	0	n/a
1 mo	115	1(?)*	5	95
5 yr	36	6	15	88
10 yr	10	10	23	69
15 yr	7	0	26	69

*It is not certain that the patient died of a stroke.
n/a, not applicable.

One case of permanent Horner syndrome resulted; transient mild Horner syndrome occurred in 40 percent of cases. Transient elevation of the ipsilateral hemidiaphragm occurs in at least 30 percent of patients but has produced no instance of respiratory distress. No cases of vocal cord paralysis have occurred.

Bypass operations performed to the third portion of the vertebral artery at C2 or to the loop of vertebral artery between the axis and the atlas cannot be evaluated for long-term results as yet, although two relatively large series were performed by Kieffer and colleagues[52] (40 cases) and by Berguer[53] (31 cases). The anastomoses apparently remain patent in most patients. On short-term follow-up (average 2.5 years), Berguer reported that more than 80 percent could be considered "cured."

Surgical procedures performed on the intracranial segments of the vertebrobasilar system remain difficult to evaluate. Endarterectomy of the fourth portion of the vertebral artery,[58] bypass procedures to the posterior inferior cerebellar,[56, 57] to the anterior inferior cerebellar, to the superior cerebellar, and to the posterior cerebral[59] arteries are technically possible, with a gratifying incidence of early patency. There is a varying incidence of operative mortality and morbidity, ranging from 19 percent mortality for carotid-posterior cerebral artery bypass for basilar artery lesions to 5 percent mortality for occipital to posterior inferior cerebellar artery bypass, with 54 percent of patients enjoying an excellent immediate result and 29 percent satisfactory recovery. Duration of improvement in these often desperately ill patients is not reported, nor is protection from future stroke. The results justify continued investigation of the long-term efficacy of these procedures.

Among the series studying the effects of relief of extrinsic compression or of correction of kinks, in which the distribution of symptoms is similar to that reported in patients treated for atherosclerotic disease, dramatic symptomatic relief is reported. A review of the series finds complete relief or improvement occurring in up to 95 percent of patients.[20, 25, 43] The period of follow-up evaluation in these cases is not as long as in our series, however, and no mention is made of the effects on late stroke rates. Nor are there any reliable data from which the stroke incidence in these patients without intrinsic arterial lesions could be deduced.

CONCLUSIONS

A number of pathologic conditions, generally involving both vertebral arteries, can be associated with incapacitating symptoms of brain-stem ischemia. Those that produce extrinsic compression or kinking with interruption of vertebral flow are reported to be relieved by decompression of one artery. Although symptoms may be severe, there is no known stroke incidence associated with extrinsic compression. Careful differential diagnosis is required to exclude postural hypotension, sluggish vascular reflexes, and middle ear disturbances causing positional dizziness. Stokes-Adams syncope, convulsive disorders, aortic stenosis, migraine variants, and other causes of motor and sensory disturbances must be considered before vertebral arterial decompression or unkinking can be recommended as a treatment modality.

Those patients with intrinsic lesions of the vertebrobasilar system often have associated and severe involvement of the carotid circulation as well and, despite symptoms similar to those reported for patients with extrinsic lesions, they not infrequently have combined carotid and vertebrobasilar insufficiency symptoms, indicating that they are at risk of suffering catastrophic stroke. In this group, correction of carotid lesions that interfere with flow may relieve vertebrobasilar symptoms. If neurologic symptoms persist in spite of patent carotid arteries, or if the carotid arteries are inoperably occluded, restoration of one of the bilaterally involved vertebral arteries will often relieve symptoms and protect against future stroke, and perhaps against sudden death. The surgeon embarking on a project of vertebrobasilar revascularization must be prepared to perform a number of operative procedures, including subclavian vertebral angioplasty with or without endarterectomy, transposition of the vertebral artery origin to the common carotid artery, and venous bypass to various segments of the distal vertebral artery, and must be prepared as well to unroof the transverse foramina. Subclavian vertebral angioplasty with plication of the redundant vertebral artery and autologous saphenous vein roof patching of the subclavian vertebral junction has proved a durable reconstruction for approximately 90 percent of the lesions encountered and can be performed through a relatively simple supraclavicular incision. It is recommended that vertebral transposition to a thick-walled common carotid or subclavian artery be buffered with a vein roof patch of the thick host vessel in order to avoid constriction of the small lumen of the vertebral artery. The role of extracranial-intracranial bypass to the fourth part of the vertebral artery or to branches of the basilar artery is not yet clear as to either indications or long-term results.

REFERENCES

1. Kubick CS, Adams RD: Occlusion of the basilar artery: Clinical and pathological study. *Brain.* 1946;69:73.
2. Millikan CH, Siekert RG: Studies in cerebrovascular disease. I. The syndrome of intermittent insufficiency of the basilar arterial system. *Mayo Clin Proc.* 1965;3:61.
3. Millikan CH, Siekert RG, Shick RM: Studies in cerebrovascular disease. III. The use of anticoagulant drugs in the treatment of insufficiency or thrombosis within the basilar arterial system. *Mayo Clin Proc.* 1955;30:116.
4. Diaz FG, Ausman JI: Surgical reconstruction of vascular lesions of the vertebral basilar circulation. *Curr Concepts Cerebrovasc Dis Stroke.* 1984;19:19.
5. Caplan LR, Amarenco P, Rosengart A, et al: Embolism from vertebral artery origin occlusive disease. *Neurology.* 1992;42:1505.
6. Sahs AL, Hartman EC: *Fundamentals of Stroke Care.* DHEW Publ. (HRA) 76–14016. U.S. Department of Health Education and Welfare, Washington, DC, 1976.
7. Imparato AM: Vertebral artery surgery. *NeuroView.* 1986;2:6.
8. Blaisdell WF, Clauss RH, Galbraith JG, et al: Joint Study of Extracranial Arterial Occlusion: VA review of surgical considerations. *JAMA.* 1969;209:1889.
9. Mourfarrij NA, Little JR, Furlan AJ, et al: Vertebral artery stenosis: long term followup. *Stroke.* 1984;15:260–263.
10. Hardesty HW, Whitacre WB, Toole JF, et al: Studies on vertebral artery blood flow in man. *Surg Gynecol Obstet.* 1963;116:662.
11. Hutchinson EC, Yates PO: Carotid-vertebral stenosis. *Lancet.* 1957;272:2.
12. Hass WK, Fields WB, North RR, et al: Joint Study of Extracranial Arterial Occlusion: II. Arteriography, techniques, sites and complications. *JAMA.* 1968;203:96.
13. Imparato AM, Riles TS, Kim GE: Cervical vertebral angioplasty for brain stem ischemia. *Surgery.* 1981;90:842.
14. Whisnant JP, Cartlidge NEF, Elvebach LR: Carotid and vertebral transient ischemic attacks: Effects of anticoagulants, hypertension and cardiac disorders on survival and stroke—A population study. *Ann Neurol.* 1978;3:107.
15. Oas JG, Baloh RW: Vertigo and the anterior inferior cerebellar artery syndrome. *Neurology.* 1992;42:2274.
16. Cate WR, Scott HW Jr: Cerebral ischemia of central origin: Relief by subclavian-vertebral artery thromboendarterectomy. *Surgery.* 1959;45:19.
17. Myers KA: Reconstruction of vertebral artery stenosis. *Aust NZ J Surg.* 1977;47:41.
18. Imparato AM, Lin JPT: Vertebral arterial reconstruction: Internal plication and vein patch angioplasty. *Ann Surg.* 1967;166:213.
19. Ausman JI, Chou SN, Lee M, Klassen A: Occipital to cerebellar artery anastomosis for brain stem infarction from vertebral basilar occlusive disease. *Stroke.* 1976;7:6.
20. Fields WS, North RR, Hass WK, et al: Joint Study of Extracranial Arterial Occlusion. I. Organization of study and survey of patient population. *JAMA.* 1968;203:955.
21. Crawford ES, DeBakey ME, Fields WS: Roentgenographic diagnosis and surgical treatment of basilar artery insufficiency. *JAMA.* 1958;168:509.
22. Kornmesser TW, Bergan JJ: Anatomic control of vertebral arteriovenous fistula. *Surgery.* 1974;75:80.
23. Hardin CA, Poser CM: Rotational obstruction of the vertebral artery due to redundancy and extraluminal fascial bands. *Ann Surg.* 1963;158:133.
24. Schwartz CJ, Mitchell RA: Observations on localization of arterial plaques. *Circ Res.* 1962;11:63.
25. Imparato AM: Vertebral artery surgery: How I do it. In Chang J, ed. *Modern Vascular Surgery,* Vol 4. Costa Mesa, CA: PMA Publishing Corp; 1991;84.
26. Hardin CA: Vertebral artery insufficiency produced by cervical osteoarthritic spurs. *Arch Surg.* 1965;90:629.
27. Sheehan S, Bauer R, Meyer JS: Vertebral artery compression in cervical spondylosis. *Neurology (NY).* 1960;70:968.
28. Imparato AM, Riles TS: Surgery of vertebral and subclavian artery occlusions. In Bergan JJ, Yao STY, eds. *Cerebrovascular Insufficiency.* New York: Grune & Stratton; 1983;521.
29. Linden D, Steinke W, Schwartz A, Hennerici M: Spontaneous vertebral artery dissection initially mimicking myocardial infarction. *Stroke.* 1992;23:1021.
30. Husni EA, Bell HS, Storer J: Mechanical occlusion of the vertebral artery: A new clinical concept. *JAMA.* 1966;196:475.
31. Stanley JC, Fry WJ, Seeger JD, et al: Extracranial internal carotid and vertebral artery fibrodysplasia. *Arch Surg.* 1974;109:215.
32. Roon AJ, Ehrenfeld WK, Cooke PB, Wylie EJ: Vertebral artery reconstruction. *Am J Surg.* 1979;138:29.
33. Meda K, Toole JF, McHenry IC Jr: Carotid and vertebrobasilar transient ischemic attacks: Clinical and angiographic correlation. *Neurology (NY).* 1979;29:1094.
34. Fisher CM: The circle of Willis: Anatomical variations. *Vasc Dis.* 1965;2:99.
35. Kase CS, Norrving B, Levine SR, et al: Cerebellar infarction: Clinical and anatomic observations in 66 cases. *Stroke.* 1993;24:76.
36. Rubenstein RL, Norman DM, Schindler RA, Kaseff L: Cerebellar infarction: A presentation of vertigo. *Laryngoscope.* 1980;90:505.
37. Lehrich JR, Winkler GF, Ojemann RG: Cerebellar infarction with brain stem compression: Diagnosis and surgical treatment. *Arch Neurol.* 1970;22:490.
38. Linzer M, McFarland TA, Belkin M, Caplan L: Critical carotid and vertebral occlusive arterial disease and cough syncope. *Stroke.* 1992;23:1017.
39. Fields WS: Vertigo related to alterations in arterial blood flow. In Wolfson R, ed. *The Vestibular System and Its Diseases.* Philadelphia: University of Pennsylvania Press; 1966;472.
40. Cohn AM, Burres SA: Otologic considerations in vascular disorders of the vertebrobasilar system. In Berguer R, Bauer RB, eds. *Vertebrobasilar Arterial Occlusive Disease.* New York: Raven Press; 1984;99.
41. Rowe MJ: The brain stem auditory evoked response in neurologic disease: A review. *Ear and Hearing.* 1981;2:41.
42. Starr A: Correlation between confirmed sites of neurologic lesions and abnormalities of far-field auditory brain responses. *Electroencephalogr Clin Neurophysiol.* 1976;41:595.
43. Kaooi KA, Gilroy J: Alterations of visual evoked potentials associated with vertebrobasilar occlusive disease. In Berguer R, Bauer RB, eds. *Vertebrobasilar Arterial Occlusive Disease.* New York: Raven Press; 1984;95.
44. Riles TS, Eidelman EM, Litt AW, Pinto RS, Oldford F, Schwartzenberg GW: Comparison of magnetic resonance angiography, conventional angiography, and Duplex scanning. *Stroke.* 1992;23:341.
45. Rother J, Wentz KU, Rautenberg W, Schwartz A, Hennerici M: Magnetic resonance angiography in vertebrobasilar ischemia. *Stroke.* 1993;24:1313.
46. Mull M, Aulich A, Hennerici M: Transcranial Doppler ultrasound versus arteriography for assessment of the vertebrobasilar circulation. *J Clin Ultrasound.* 1990;18:539.
47. Reul GJ, Cooley DA, Olson SK, et al: Long term results of direct vertebral artery operations. *Surgery.* 1984;96:854.
48. Diaz FH, Ausmann JI, de los Reyes RA, et al: Surgical reconstruction of the proximal vertebral artery. *J Neurosurg.* 1984;61:874.
49. Clark K, Perry MD: Carotid vertebral anastomosis. An alternative technique for repair of subclavian steal syndrome. *Ann Surg.* 1966;163:414.
50. Edwards WH, Mulherin JL Jr: The surgical reconstruction of the proximal subclavian and vertebral artery. *J Vasc Surg.* 1985;2:634.
51. Imparato AM, Ramirez AA, Riles TS, Mintzer R: Cerebral protection in carotid surgery. *Arch Surg.* 1982;117:1073.
52. Kieffer E, Rancurel G, Richard T: Reconstruction of the distal cervical vertebral artery. In Berguer R, Bauer RB, eds. *Vertebrobasilar Arterial Occlusive Disease.* New York: Raven Press; 1984;265.
53. Berguer R: Distal vertebral by-pass: Technique, the "occipital connection," potential uses. *J Vasc Surg.* 1985;2:621.
54. Motarjeme A, Keifer JW, Zuska AJ: Percutaneous transluminal angioplasty of the vertebral arteries. *Radiology.* 1981;139:715.
55. Sundt TM Jr, Smith HC, Campbell JK, et al: Transluminal angioplasty for basilar artery stenosis. *Mayo Clin Proc.* 1980;55:673.

56. Ausman JI, Chow SN, Lee M, Klassen A: Occipital to cerebellar artery anastomosis for brain stem infarction from vertebral basilar occlusive disease. *Stroke.* 1976;7:6.

57. Sundt TM Jr, Piepgras DG, Houser OW, Campbell JK: Interposition saphenous vein grafts for advanced occlusive disease and large aneurysms in the posterior circulation. *J Neurosurg.* 1982;56:205.

58. Allen GS, Cohen RJ, Preziosi TJ: Microsurgical endarterectomy of the intracranial vertebral artery for vertebrobasilar transient ischemic attacks. *Neurosurgery.* 1981;8:56.

59. Ausmann JI, Diaz FG, de los Reyes RA, et al: Posterior circulation revascularization: Superficial temporal to superior cerebellar artery anastomosis. *J Neurosurg.* 1982;56:766.

60. Powers S, Drislane TM, Iandoli EW: The surgical treatment of vertebral arterial insufficiency. *Arch Surg.* 1963;86:60.

61. Wesolow A, McMahon JD, Cali JR, et al: Revascularization of the brain stem. *Conn Med.* 1979;43(5):269.

62. Rainer WG, Quainzon EP, Liggett MS: Surgical considerations in the treatment of vertebrobasilar arterial insufficiency. *Am J Surg.* 1970;120:594.

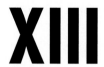

XIII

Surgical Management of the Brachiocephalic Trunks

Indications for Repair of the Brachiocephalic Trunks

THOMAS S. RILES and ANTHONY M. IMPARATO

OCCLUSIVE DISEASE OF THE ARCH VESSELS

Occlusive lesions of the arch vessels are encountered less frequently than carotid bifurcation lesions and account for fewer than 5 percent of the surgical procedures performed on the cerebral vasculature. Most of the lesions are atherosclerotic, although a number of other pathologic conditions are encountered, including dissections, emboli, compression syndromes, and occlusions resulting from vasculitis such as giant-cell arteritis and Takayasu disease.

Appreciation of the anatomy of the arch vessels is essential to an understanding of the various syndromes produced by pathologic changes of these vessels. On the right, the innominate artery gives rise to the right common carotid artery as well as the right subclavian artery. On the left, the common carotid and subclavian arteries generally arise as separate vessels off the aortic arch. The vertebral arteries arise distal to the origins of the subclavian arteries. The vertebrals unite to form a common basilar artery at the base of the skull and thus can serve as an important source of collateral circulation to the upper extremities in the presence of subclavian occlusions proximal to the origins of the vertebral arteries. Anomalies of the arch vessels are frequently encountered, the most common being the origin of the left common carotid artery from the innominate artery. Occasionally, the left vertebral artery will be found as a separate vessel originating at the aortic arch, ascending cephalad between the left common carotid and left subclavian arteries. In some instances, the right subclavian artery will be found to arise from a common trunk with the left subclavian artery. This and other anomalies may lead to misinterpretation of diagnostic tests. Awareness of the anomalies may also be important in planning operative procedures.

Occlusive disease of the brachiocephalic vessels is not uncommon among patients with arteriosclerosis. Unlike patients with carotid bifurcation disease or coronary artery disease, many patients with these lesions remain asymptomatic and undiagnosed. The only manifestation of the condition may be decreased blood pressure in one arm or a diminished common carotid pulse detected by an astute clinician. Of the arch vessel lesions, the most common is proximal left subclavian artery stenosis. In a review of more than 4000 arch angiograms for cerebrovascular disease reported by Hass and coworkers,[1] 12.4 percent of the patients had left subclavian stenosis. By comparison, 40 percent of the patients had a carotid bifurcation lesion of 30 percent or more.

The fact that most patients with brachiocephalic vessel lesions are asymptomatic is a reflection of the rich collateral circulation of the head and shoulder girdle. Although symptoms may result from plaque degeneration and distal embolization, in our experience, this is relatively uncommon.[2–4] When symptoms occur, they are usually flow related. Because of the collateral pathways, individuals with symptoms are often those with multiple brachiocephalic or extracranial lesions or cardiac disease resulting in arrhythmias or low cardiac output.

When patients with lesions of the arch vessels become symptomatic, the manifestations may be quite varied. Neurologic symptoms are most common. These symptoms may be indistinguishable from those of carotid bifurcation disease in the case of proximal left common and innominate artery lesions, or they may be related to the posterior cerebral circulation in patients with subclavian or innominate artery disease. Symptoms of posterior cerebral insufficiency include dizziness, vertigo, diplopia, ataxia, bilateral motor or sensory deficits, dysarthria, and drop attacks.

The term *subclavian steal syndrome* has been used to describe any condition in which there is reversal of vertebral blood flow distal to a subclavian artery lesion, irrespective of the clinical manifestations. The term may be properly applied when cerebral symptoms are produced by exercise of the affected upper extremity. It is presumed that under these circumstances, the collateral circulation to the arm becomes insufficient. The decrease in the blood pressure in the vertebral system results in a "steal" of blood from the intracranial circulation via the basilar artery. The decreased perfusion pressure in the intracranial circulation causes the transient neurologic symptoms. Cessation of the arm exercise results in an increase in the peripheral resistance, lessens the demand for blood flow through the vertebral–vertebral collateral pathway, raises the pressure at the vertebral–basilar junction, and stops or lessens the "steal" from the intracranial circulation. Understandably, the likelihood of symptoms increases if there are concomitant contralateral vertebral or carotid lesions (Fig. 80–1).

In lesions involving the innominate or the subclavian arteries, patients may present with upper-extremity ischemia. Ischemic symptoms in the upper extremity may be mild and intermittent, consisting of pain or weakness associated with the use of the arm, or they may be more persistent, with coldness, paresthesias, and discoloration of the hand. Embolization to the distal vessels of the forearm and hand may also occur, often resulting in severe ischemia of the fingers and sometimes in unilateral Raynaud phenomenon.

When the innominate artery that gives rise to the right common carotid and right subclavian arteries is involved by the occlusive process, symptoms may be described for the subclavian, common carotid, or both arteries. The physical examination may lead to the early diagnosis of brachiocephalic occlusive disease. Bruits in the upper chest or lower neck should alert the clinician to the possibility of arch vessel lesions, particularly if the sounds are asymmetric. Decreased pulses in the neck or upper extremities may be present. A comparison of the blood pressure of the two arms is often more valuable, since many individuals with severe lesions of the proximal subclavian artery have a good distal pulse if the collateral circulation is plentiful. A most interesting finding that may confirm the diagnosis of subclavian artery or innominate artery occlusion is the pulse lag de-

tected when simultaneous palpation of the radial pulses reveals a delayed pulse wave in the affected arm due to the increased transit time required for the pulse wave to travel through the vertebral collateral pathway.

SELECTION OF PATIENTS FOR OPERATION

Unlike carotid bifurcation lesions, little is known about the natural history of brachiocephalic stenoses and occlusions. In general, the selection of patients for surgery is based on a *presumed* risk of stroke, incapacitating transient ischemic attacks, ischemic arm symptoms, or prevention of distal embolization. Cerebral symptoms produced by occlusive lesions of the proximal arch vessels are neither unique nor characteristic, unless associated with upper-extremity ischemia or with brain-stem symptoms produced by arm exercise. Their frequent coincidence with carotid bifurcation and vertebral origin lesions makes it difficult to ascribe symptoms or the threat of stroke specifically to the more proximal lesions. Thus, in reported surgical series, operative indications have been nearly evenly distributed among cerebral hemispheric, basivertebral, exertional ipsilateral arm ischemia, or brain-stem symptoms (and constituting a subclavian steal syndrome) or have been asymptomatic. In general,

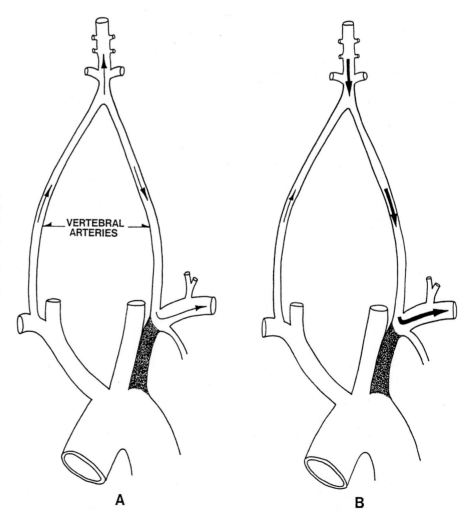

FIGURE 80–1. *A,* Collateral flow through the contralateral vertebral artery is sufficient to supply both the posterior cerebral circulation and the affected upper extremity at rest. *B,* With exercise, the flow to the affected upper extremity increases. If the contralateral vertebral artery is unable to provide the additional flow, the perfusion pressure to the posterior brain may decrease. The decreased perfusion pressure, with or without reversal of flow in the basilar artery, is referred to as the "steal" of blood from the cerebral circulation and may be associated with neurologic symptoms.

VERTEBRAL ARTERIES

A   B

most vascular surgeons would not recommend surgery for isolated asymptomatic arch vessel lesions. In patients with multiple lesions, there may indeed be a real risk of stroke due to impaired cerebral circulation. Considerable judgment is required in these cases because of the paucity of reliable data for making decisions.

If one becomes suspicious of a brachiocephalic lesion from the patient's history or the physical findings, the next step in the evaluation is often performed in the noninvasive vascular laboratory. An accurate comparison of Doppler-measured blood pressures of the upper extremities is helpful for the diagnosis of an isolated subclavian artery stenosis. Comparison of the pressures of both upper extremities to those of the lower extremities may reveal multiple arch vessel occlusions. The duplex scan is quite sensitive to the turbulence and decreased flow velocity in the common carotid and subclavian arteries that result from plaques near the origin of these vessels. Visualization of reversal of flow in the vertebral artery is considered diagnostic of a proximal subclavian artery stenosis or occlusion.

If a patient is symptomatic and has evidence of brachiocephalic occlusive disease, an angiogram with a contrast agent is the diagnostic procedure of choice. Whereas magnetic resonance angiography has been helpful in the preoperative evaluation of carotid bifurcation lesions,[5] in our experience, the resolution of the arch vessels has been unpredictable, particularly in the presence of severe occlusive disease. We prefer a catheter study via the femoral artery. It is important to discuss each case with a neuroradiologist and stress the need for selective studies and multiple views of the extracranial and intracranial vessels. Digital studies are generally used for the distal vessels. The great technical advances in cerebrovascular imaging over the past decade have greatly simplified the preoperative evaluation of these patients. With patience and careful technique, imaging of the extracranial vessels distal to completely occluded segments of the common carotid or subclavian artery is seldom a problem. One must always keep in mind, however, the possibility that vessels distal to an occlusion may simply be nonvisualized rather than occluded.[6]

In addition to the angiogram, other preoperative steps should include a thorough cardiac evaluation. In a patient with unusual neurologic symptoms, it is important to rule out the possibility that these symptoms are due to episodes of low cardiac output secondary to arrhythmias, hypotension, or valvular disease. The differential diagnosis should also include other systemic disorders such as hypoglycemia and seizure disorders. A magnetic resonance imaging study or computed tomographic scan of the head is useful to rule out intracranial pathology. Among patients who exhibit evidence of Takayasu disease or giant-cell arteritis, additional evaluation includes an erythrocyte sedimentation rate, selected serology, and possibly a distal aortogram looking for concomitant renal artery disease.

SURGERY

The first operations for correcting occlusive lesions of the arch vessels were performed through a sternotomy and used either endarterectomy of the lesion or bypass from the aortic arch.[7] In time, extra-anatomic procedures were introduced, permitting the surgeon to bypass the occluded vessel without a sternal-splitting incision. With these procedures, patent neck and shoulder vessels, or in some cases the femoral artery, are used for inflow to the extra-anatomic bypass. Devotees of these indirect approaches emphasize the lower rates of morbidity and mortality associated with the operation as well as satisfactory long-term results.[8] Those who prefer thoracic operations voice concern over the vulnerability of extra-anatomic grafts and the problems that may be encountered later, should other cardiovascular operations be required.[9] In our view, the decision to use one operation or another depends on the patient's general health and age and on other operations that may be required, such as myocardial revascularization. The vascular surgeon should be familiar with all the possible solutions to these problems.

Subclavian Artery

A variety of operative procedures have been used to correct subclavian artery lesions.[8–11] The procedures used for embolic symptoms are different from those used for flow-related symptoms. For embolic lesions, it is necessary to remove the plaque from the circulation by performing either an endarterectomy or a bypass and ligating the artery distal to the lesion. Most patients who come to surgery for subclavian artery stenosis or occlusion have flow-related symptoms. In this situation, a variety of bypass procedures has been described. The most widely used has been the carotid–subclavian bypass. Other procedures reported have been interposition of the subclavian artery into the ipsilateral carotid, subclavian–subclavian bypass, axillo–axillary bypass, carotid–axillary bypass, femoral–axillary bypass, and ascending aorta to subclavian or axillary artery bypass. Our preference has been for carotid–subclavian bypass in patients who do not have evidence of carotid bifurcation disease, although we have had excellent long-term results with axillo–axillary bypass. The advantage of this latter procedure is that it can be performed without interrupting any of the existing cerebral circulation. Details regarding the various operations used to correct subclavian artery lesions can be found in Chapters 81 and 82.

Common Carotid Artery

Indications for surgery of the common carotid artery may be quite varied. Certainly patients with high-grade stenosis of any portion of the common carotid artery and ipsilateral cerebral symptoms must be considered for reconstruction. Some surgeons also believe that severe stenosis in an asymptomatic patient is an indication for operation, although the natural history of these lesions is not well known. A more difficult problem is a patient with complete occlusion of the common carotid artery, particularly if the ipsilateral internal carotid artery is known to be patent. Some surgeons may argue that this lesion is unlikely to produce further emboli to the brain and therefore are reluctant to recommend surgery. On occasion, however, these patients are found to have continued ipsilateral hemispheric symptoms after the occlusion has been documented. These symptoms may be caused by emboli from the bifurcation (since the internal carotid artery is being supplied by retrograde flow from the external carotid artery) or by fluctuations in flow through this external–internal carotid system. Symptoms in these patients often stop once normal flow is restored to the endarterectomized bifurcation.

If the common carotid artery is occluded and totally asymptomatic, the decision to operate may depend on the status of the other extracranial vessels. If this is the only demonstrated lesion on a four-vessel angiogram, the patient usually has sufficient collateral flow that surgery is unnecessary. If, however, there are multiple extracranial lesions, restoration of flow to an internal or external carotid artery may be worthwhile to increase the cerebral blood flow as a prophylactic measure in the event of further occlusions. There are no large series of patients with these variations, so considerable judgment must be exercised to evaluate the risks and benefits of common carotid reconstruction for any individual patient.

Thromboendarterectomy is the procedure of choice for stenotic lesions of the distal two-thirds of the common carotid artery; it is performed in the same manner as a carotid bifurcation endarterectomy. Good exposure can be obtained proximally to the level of the clavicle by dividing the omohyoid muscle and sternal portion of the sternocleidomastoid muscle if necessary. Lesions of the proximal common carotid artery must be treated with extra-anatomic bypass[12–14] or an open sternotomy.

Occlusions of the common carotid artery present a challenge to the vascular surgeon, and the approach depends on a variety of circumstances. First, it is essential to establish the presence of an outflow vessel, that is, the external carotid or internal carotid artery, if reconstruction is to be performed successfully. If the distal vessels are not visualized either angiographically or by some other technique, exploration of the carotid bifurcation may be the only completely reliable means of deciding whether reconstruction is possible. In our series, out of 18 common carotid occlusions with nonvisualization of the distal vessels, nine were found to be reconstructible at the time of exploration.[6]

Once the vessel is judged to be operable, a decision must be made to use endarterectomy or bypass. If the occlusion is a recent thrombosis due to a distal common carotid stenosis after a bifurcation endarterectomy, disobliteration of the thrombus may be possible with a Fogarty balloon catheter, and flow may be restored directly through the vessels.[14] If there is concern that a proximal common carotid lesion may still exist, an intraoperative angiogram retrograde into the common artery may be necessary before establishing flow to the brain.

If the common carotid artery is chronically occluded or if a proximal lesion exists, a bypass may be the procedure of choice. Most surgeons prefer the subclavian–carotid bypass if the ipsilateral subclavian artery is a suitable vessel.[2, 6, 13] The procedure is essentially the same as that described for correcting a subclavian artery lesion, except that the bypass is usually attached to the bifurcation rather than the midportion of the common carotid artery and a thromboendarterectomy of the carotid bifurcation is generally necessary.

If a subclavian–carotid bypass is not possible, a carotid–carotid bypass may sometimes be performed if the contralateral carotid artery is preserved.[14] More often, the aorto-carotid reconstruction through a sternotomy is preferred to subclavian–carotid bypass, despite the higher rate of morbid-

ity associated with this procedure.[9, 12, 15] These procedures are discussed in Chapter 81.

Innominate Artery Stenosis or Occlusion

Although lesions of the innominate artery producing irregularity of its radiographic contour are frequently detectable by arch studies for cerebrovascular insufficiency syndromes, flow-impeding lesions or total occlusions are encountered infrequently. It is difficult to clearly recognize neurologic symptoms due to such lesions, since they are usually found in association with carotid bifurcation lesions; thus, clear-cut indications for their correction are difficult to describe. When associated with severe ischemia of the right upper extremity, their significance is apparent. If appropriate neurologic symptoms occur in the absence of carotid or vertebral lesions, stenotic lesions of the innominate artery can then be considered reparable; if hemodynamically significant lesions are found proximal to right carotid bifurcation lesions requiring surgical intervention, the need to deal with the innominate lesion becomes obvious. It is not known how often late strokes following ipsilateral carotid endarterectomy might be due to lesions in the innominate artery, whose pathologic changes have not been as carefully documented as those of carotid bifurcation and vertebral origin lesions. Steal phenomena, when observed, may be via the ipsilateral carotid and vertebral arteries.

Our own indications for operation on the innominate artery are as follows:

1. Innominate occlusion or hemodynamically significant stenosis proximal to an operable carotid bifurcation lesion.
2. Persistence or recurrence of ipsilateral cerebral hemispheric symptoms after successful ipsilateral carotid endarterectomy.
3. Symptomatic steal via the carotid, vertebral, or subclavian arteries brought on by right upper-extremity exertion.
4. Basivertebral symptoms in the presence of innominate stenosis and in the absence of other appropriate lesions.
5. Evidence of emboli or ischemia to the right upper extremity without other sources for these symptoms.

The operative procedures described to correct innominate artery lesions include endarterectomy, ascending aorto-carotid–subclavian bypass, and some procedures employed for correcting subclavian steal, which include subclavian–subclavian and axillo–axillary bypass.

CONCLUSION

Operations on the arch vessels appear to be most useful in correcting transient symptoms. The effect of these procedures on the prevention of stroke is unclear. Consequently, although these lesions are encountered relatively frequently during investigation of cerebrovascular symptoms, they are overshadowed by lesions in the carotid bifurcation whose role in the pathogenesis of stroke is more clearly defined. Operations on arch vessels are therefore performed for specific indications either to permit safe carotid bifurcation operations or to alleviate symptoms that persist after carotid bifurcation operations. Subclavian steal syndrome, when it occurs, is best relieved by an operative procedure that restores the normal pressure relationships between the basivertebral system and the involved carotid artery, correcting the steal. In the unusual situation in which the innominate artery is suspected of being the source of embolization to the brain, operation on that artery is indicated. Operations on the arch vessels in most series constitute fewer than 5 percent of the total number of operations performed for extracranial cerebrovascular insufficiency.

REFERENCES

1. Hass WK, Fields WS, North RR, et al: Joint study of extracranial arterial occlusion. II. Arteriography, techniques, sites and complications. *JAMA*. 1968;11:159.
2. Diethrich EB, Garrett HE, Ameriso J, et al: Occlusive disease of the common carotid and subclavian arteries treated by carotid–subclavian bypass. Analysis of 125 cases. *Am J Surg*. 1967;114:800.
3. Forestner JE, Ghosh SK, Bergan JJ, Conn J Jr: Subclavian bypass for correction of the subclavian steal syndrome. *Surgery*. 1972;71:136.
4. Reivich ME, Holling HE, Roberts B, et al: Reversal of blood flow through the vertebral artery and its effect on cerebral circulation. *N Engl J Med*. 1968;279:1413.
5. Riles TS, Eidelman EM, Litt AW, et al: Comparison of magnetic resonance angiography, conventional angiography and duplex scanning. *Stroke*. 1992;23:341.
6. Riles TS, Imparato AM, Posner MP, Eikelboom BC: Common carotid occlusion: Assessment of the distal vessels. *Ann Surg*. 1984;199:363.
7. DeBakey ME, Crawford ES, Cooley DA, Morris GC Jr: Surgical considerations of occlusive disease of innominate, carotid, subclavian, and vertebral arteries. *Ann Surg*. 1959;149:690.
8. Raithel D: Our experience of surgery for innominate and subclavian lesions. *J Cardiovasc Surg*. 1980;21:423.
9. Crawford ES, Stowe CL, Powers RW: Occlusion of the innominate, common carotid, and subclavian arteries: Long-term results of surgical treatment. *Surgery*. 1983;94:281.
10. Posner MP, Riles TS, Ramirez AA, et al: Axillo-axillary bypass for symptomatic stenosis of the subclavian artery. *Am J Surg*. 1983;145:645.
11. Thompson BW, Read RC, Campbell GS: Operative correction of proximal blocks of the subclavian or innominate arteries. *J Cardiovasc Surg*. 1980;21:125.
12. Ehrenfeld WK, Chapman RD, Wylie EJ: Management of occlusive lesions of the branches of the aortic arch. *Am J Surg*. 1969;118:236.
13. Collice M, DiAngelo V, Arena O: Surgical treatment of common carotid artery occlusion. *Neurosurgery*. 1983;12:515.
14. Moore WS, Malone JM, Goldstone J: Extrathoracic repair of branch occlusions of the aortic arch. *Am J Surg*. 1976;132:249.
15. Vogt DP, Hertzer NR, O'Hara PJ, Beven EG: Brachiocephalic arterial reconstruction. *Ann Surg*. 1982;196:541.

SUGGESTED READING

Crawford ES, DeBakey ME, Morris GC Jr, Howell JF: Surgical treatment of occlusion of the innominate, common carotid, and subclavian arteries: A ten year experience. *Surgery*. 1969;65:17.
Ekeström S, Liljequist I, Nordhus O: Surgical management of obliterative disease of the brachiocephalic trunk. Experience from 24 cases. *Scand J Thorac Cardiovasc Surg*. 1983;17:305.
Fields WS, Lemak NA: Joint study of extracranial arterial occlusion. VII. Subclavian steal: A review of 168 cases. *JAMA*. 1972;222:1139.
Hatner CD: Subclavian steal syndrome: A 12 year experience. *Arch Surg*. 1976; 111:1074.
Jacobson JH II, Mozersky DJ, Mitty HA, et al: Axillary–axillary bypass for subclavian steal syndrome. *Arch Surg*. 1973;106:24.
LeVeen HH, Picone VA Jr, Diza C, et al: A simplified correction of subclavian steal syndrome. *Surgery*. 1974;75:299.
Mozersky DJ, Sumner DS, Barnes RW, Strandness DE Jr: Subclavian revascularization by means of a subcutaneous axillary–axillary graft. *Arch Surg*. 1973;106:20.
Mozersky DJ, Sumner DS, Barnes RW, et al: The hemodynamics of the axillary–axillary bypass. *Surg Gynecol Obstet*. 1972; 135:925.
Najafi H, Javid H, Hunter JA, et al: Occlusive disease of the branches of the aortic arch. In Bergan JJ, Yao JST, eds. *Surgery of the Aorta and Its Body Branches*. New York: Grune & Stratton; 1979:191.
Selle JG, Cook JW, Elliott CM, et al: Simultaneous revascularization for complex brachiocephalic and coronary artery disease. *Surgery*. 1981;90:97.
Snider RL, Porter JM, Eidemiller LR: Axillary–axillary artery bypass for the correction of subclavian artery occlusive disease. *Ann Surg*. 1974;180:888.
Sproul G: Femoral–axillary bypass for cerebral vascular insufficiency. *Arch Surg*. 1971;103:746.
Williams CL, Woods LP, Clemmons EE: Carotid–subclavian bypass grafts for subclavian artery disease. *Am J Surg*. 1973;126:807.

CHAPTER 81

Transthoracic or Transmediastinal Repair of the Brachiocephalic Trunks

DAVID C. BREWSTER

Although far less common than stenotic or ulcerative lesions of the carotid bifurcation, atherosclerosis of the brachiocephalic vessels may be a source of cerebrovascular symptoms or otherwise threaten cerebral or upper-extremity circulation. On occasion, more unusual problems may require operative repair, such as aneurysmal disease, thromboemboli, or aortic dissection compromising the brachiocephalic trunks. Traumatic injuries to the great vessels in the mediastinum or base of the neck, caused by blunt or penetrating trauma, are being encountered more frequently. Nonatherosclerotic stenoses or occlusions of the great vessels may occur owing to Takayasu disease, other types of arteritis, or postradiation inflammatory changes. Iatrogenic problems or complications, such as tracheoinnominate fistula, may necessitate urgent operative repair.[1]

The nature of symptoms attributable to brachiocephalic lesions, as well as indications for surgical intervention for such problems, have been elucidated in other chapters. This chapter describes available methods for the direct operative repair of these lesions, as well as preferred surgical approaches to the various brachiocephalic trunks (right subclavian, right common carotid, innominate, left common carotid, and left subclavian arteries). Surgical management of vertebral artery lesions has already been considered in Chapters 77 and 78.

ADVANTAGES OF DIRECT REPAIR

Traditionally, brachiocephalic lesions were approached directly by transthoracic or transmediastinal procedures.[2–4] Concern regarding the often substantial morbidity and mortality rates reported following the initial experience with such direct repairs led, over the past several decades, to the development of a variety of indirect methods of remote bypass. Within recent years, however, improvements in patient care and surgical methods have made direct surgical reconstruction of the brachiocephalic arteries safer and more effective. In particular, the extensive experience with coronary artery revascularization has demonstrated that median sternotomy is remarkably well tolerated, even by elderly patients. Refinements in anesthesia and intraoperative monitoring and advances in postoperative intensive care have all contributed to the surgeon's ability to perform anatomic in-line reconstruction of the brachiocephalic trunks with low rates of morbidity and mortality and generally excellent and durable results.[1, 5–12]

In deciding between direct repair via median sternotomy or thoracotomy and indirect approaches using remote extrathoracic grafts, the surgeon must consider several factors. Obviously, the type of problem encountered often dictates the approach. Although occlusive lesions may often be handled by either direct or indirect means, other more unusual problems such as aneurysmal or traumatic lesions involving the brachiocephalic vessels demand direct surgical repair. For occlusive disease, the extent and location of atherosclerotic lesions, the pathophysiology of possible symptoms, the overall condition of the patient, and the surgeon's personal experience with the various techniques available must all be evaluated. Patients with multiple medical problems that considerably increase the risk of direct repair may be better served by extra-anatomic grafts. In patients with prior mediastinal operation, such as prior coronary bypass surgery, or other potential technical problems, a direct approach for brachiocephalic lesions may be more difficult and hazardous, thereby making remote methods of reconstruction preferable.

Other considerations may favor direct operation. Although extrathoracic grafts may augment cerebral or upper-extremity blood flow and alleviate symptoms attributable to overall decreased perfusion in these vascular beds, they may not eliminate the source of embolic phenomena from brachiocephalic lesions if this mechanism is indeed responsible for clinical manifestations, as is often the case. In such situations, the potential exists for continued symptoms despite a patent extrathoracic graft; anatomic reconstruction with resection, ligation, or bypass, with exclusion of the vessel responsible for atheroembolic events, is often preferable.

Similarly, although abundant experience has demonstrated generally satisfactory early function of extrathoracic grafts, long-term patency and clinical results of anatomic in-line reconstructions may be better, making such direct methods more desirable in younger, low-risk patients.

Finally, some patients do not have suitable cervical sites for the origin of extrathoracic grafts. This occurs most often in patients with multiple lesions of the brachiocephalic vessels that compromise potential donor arteries in more remote locations and possibly preclude extrathoracic grafts. In addition, symptomatic patients with multiple great-vessel lesions may be inadequately treated by more remote extrathoracic grafts and be more likely to require direct surgical correction of several proximal aortic branches.

SURGICAL ANATOMY

As with atherosclerotic lesions in most other major arteries, lesions in the great vessels are most prominent at their origin or major bifurcations (Fig. 81–1). Fortunately, most lesions are often strikingly segmental in nature, involving only the first several centimeters of the vessel (Fig. 81–2), unless superimposed total thrombosis of the vessel has occurred. Even in the event of total occlusion, the distal vasculature at or just beyond a major bifurcation is almost always patent. Therefore, the vast majority of brachiocephalic lesions are remarkably well suited to surgical repair.

Lesions of the left subclavian artery are most common,[3, 13–15] although many of these lesions may cause few, if any, symptoms. It is also important to realize that brachiocephalic lesions are often multiple—61 percent in Reul and coworkers' 1991 series.[12] For this reason, reconstructive procedures for great-vessel lesions must be highly individualized.

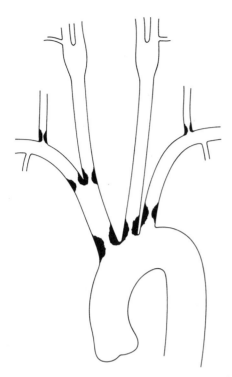

FIGURE 81–1. Usual locations of brachiocephalic trunk lesions.

Obviously, the major problem contributing to the morbidity and mortality of direct methods of brachiocephalic repair is the intrathoracic location of the aortic arch and its main branches. Although some more peripherally located great-vessel lesions, most commonly those involving the subclavian vessels, may be reached by transcervical incisions, most direct brachiocephalic repairs require a transthoracic or transmediastinal approach. The innominate, left common carotid, and left subclavian arteries arise right to left off the aortic arch in the mediastinum, beginning at approximately

the level of the second right costal cartilage. The innominate artery is located quite anteriorly in the mediastinum, passing beneath the crossing innominate vein for 4 to 5 cm before it divides into the right subclavian and right common carotid arteries at approximately the level of the right sternoclavicular joint. This anterior position allows easy access via a sternal splitting incision. Similarly, the left common carotid artery arises immediately adjacent or 1 to 1.5 cm to the left and slightly posterior to the innominate artery origin, from the highest aspect of the aortic arch. This location still affords good exposure via median sternotomy. Its proximity to the origin of the innominate artery may make application of vascular clamps between these two vessels difficult or impossible, however.[1, 10] Indeed, in approximately 10 percent of patients, a common brachiocephalic trunk may be present (Fig. 81–3), which may require modifications of direct operative repair of these vessels.

The origins of both the innominate and the left common carotid arteries are often obscured by the crossing left innominate vein, which traverses the anterior mediastinum in a horizontal plane, approximately 2.0 to 2.5 cm below the manubrium and sternal notch. Exposure of the proximal portions of the innominate and left common carotid arteries generally requires mobilization and retraction of the left innominate vein, which in turn frequently necessitates division of one or more venous branches, generally the inferior thyroid vein or thymic branches from the superior and inferior surfaces of the left innominate vein.

The anterior aspect of the ascending aorta, so useful for the site of proximal anastomosis of bypass grafts, is covered anteriorly by the medial pleural envelopes, anterior margins of the lungs, remains of the thymus, and pericardium. Adequate exposure of the ascending aorta for application of partial occluding vascular clamps requires opening of the upper pericardium, which can generally be loosely reapproximated at the time of wound closure.

The left subclavian artery arises from the aortic arch to the left of and considerably posterior to the left common

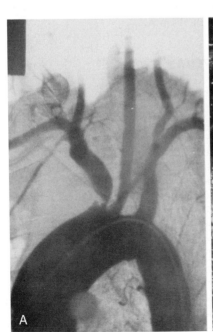
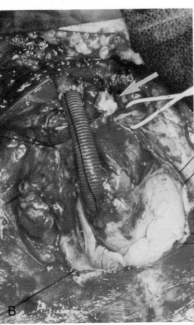

FIGURE 81–2. A, Tight atherosclerotic stenosis of proximal innominate artery causing repetitive episodes of amaurosis fugax. B, Ascending aorta–to–distal innominate artery bypass graft for operative correction of the lesion shown in A. Arrow indicates the oversewn stump of the proximal innominate artery just above the left innominate vein, which is surrounded by a Silastic loop. Pericardial edges are retracted by stay sutures.

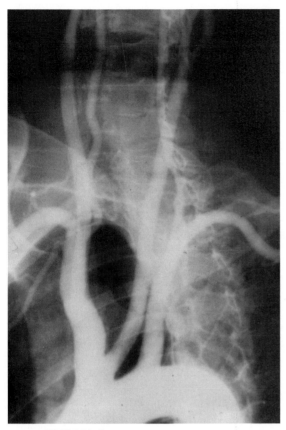

FIGURE 81–3. Common brachiocephalic trunk.

carotid artery, owing to the leftward oblique and posterior orientation of the aortic arch itself. The left subclavian origin is posterior enough to make adequate exposure and control of this vessel difficult with an anterior approach via a median sternotomy. For these reasons, direct repair of the proximal left subclavian artery generally requires left thoracotomy.

The right subclavian, right common carotid, and more distal left subclavian arteries can generally be reached adequately by a transcervical approach, working behind and somewhat below the sternoclavicular joint for exposure of the subclavian arteries at and just proximal to the vertebral artery origins. In some instances, resection of the medial one-third of the clavicle or partial sternal splitting incisions may facilitate exposure, but they are generally not necessary. Transcervical exposure requires care to identify the phrenic nerves on either side, running medially on the anterior surface of the anterior scalene muscle, which must be divided to expose the second portion of the subclavian artery immediately behind it. Similarly, the recurrent laryngeal branch of the right vagus nerve must be preserved in exposure of the innominate artery bifurcation and proximal right subclavian artery. On the left, the thoracic duct generally enters the confluence of the left internal jugular and subclavian veins and may require ligation during left transcervical dissection.

INNOMINATE ARTERY

Innominate artery lesions are particularly well suited to direct repair, being easily exposed by median sternotomy.

Because disease in the innominate artery may affect two of the four vessels contributing to cerebral circulation, as well as the right arm, such lesions are likely to be symptomatic and potentially catastrophic. In addition, ulcerated lesions are particularly common in the innominate artery (Fig. 81–4) and are often symptomatic owing to embolic phenomena to the eye, right cerebral hemisphere, or hand, even if they are not flow limiting.[1, 16]

Lesions other than arteriosclerotic occlusive disease may affect the innominate artery and require direct repair. Although traumatic lesions (Fig. 81–5) are seen relatively infrequently, owing in part to the high immediate mortality of many such injuries, the innominate artery seems to be the most vulnerable of all aortic arch branches.[1, 17, 18] True atherosclerotic innominate aneurysms are unusual and often asymptomatic; in many instances, they are first detected as a mediastinal mass on chest radiography (Fig. 81–6). The vascular nature of such lesions should be suspected and investigated by fluoroscopy, computed tomography scan with contrast, or preferably angiography prior to attempted needle biopsy or mediastinoscopy. Our experience also suggests that such aneurysmal disease often coexists with other aneurysms of the descending thoracic or abdominal aorta that should be investigated.

Conventional transfemoral arch aortography is generally preferred, although intra-arterial digital subtraction arteriography techniques usually provide satisfactory detail for diag-

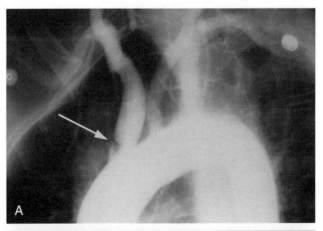

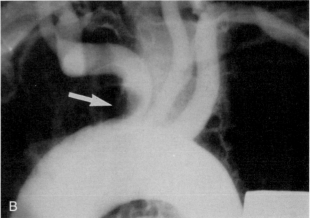

FIGURE 81–4. A and B, Examples of ulcerated atheromatous lesions of the proximal innominate artery (arrows). Neither was hemodynamically significant, but each caused symptoms by repeated embolic episodes.

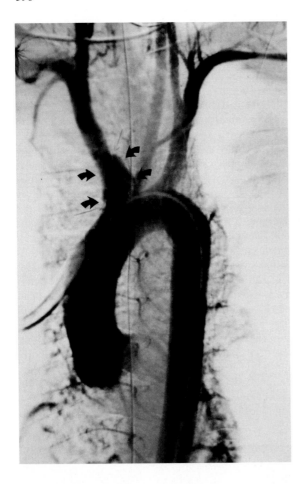

FIGURE 81-5. Traumatic pseudoaneurysm of the proximal innominate artery *(arrows)* after blunt trauma. An associated tracheal tear also required repair.

nosis and management decisions (Fig. 81-7). Intra-arterial digital subtraction arteriography has several potential advantages, such as lower contrast loads, less patient discomfort, and greater applicability to outpatient examination. In general, however, I have been relatively dissatisfied with intravenous digital subtraction images to date, because of lack of sufficient image clarity and detail in many instances.

Direct reconstruction of innominate artery lesions may be accomplished by endarterectomy, segmental graft replacement, or bypass grafting from the ascending aorta (Fig. 81-8). My own preference is for bypass grafting. Segmental graft replacement is often impossible, particularly in occlusive disease, as the plaque and calcification typically begin at the origin of the vessel or within the aortic arch itself,[5,]

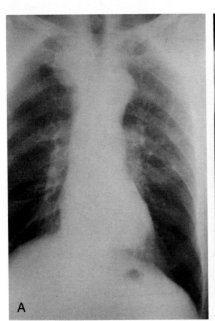
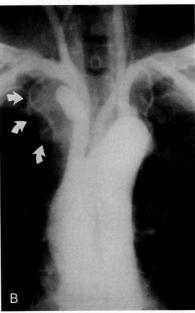

FIGURE 81-6. *A,* Aneurysm of the innominate artery, initially detected on chest radiograph as a right upper lobe mass. *B,* Arch aortogram demonstrating the aneurysm of the distal innominate artery, with a large amount of mural thrombus within the aneurysmal sac (edges indicated by *arrowheads).*

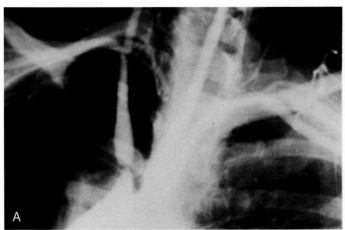
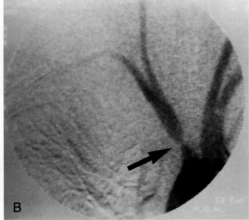

FIGURE 81-7. Innominate artery stenosis *(arrows)* shown on conventional arch aortogram *(A)* and by intra-arterial digital subtraction arteriography study *(B)*.

[19, 20] thereby precluding anastomosis of a replacement graft to the innominate origin. Similar problems may make endarterectomy difficult or hazardous, as the arteriotomy must usually be carried into the arch itself to remove the origin of the occluding or ulcerated plaque. In trying to accomplish this, it is sometimes difficult to place a partially occluding clamp that includes an adequate amount of aortic arch without compromising flow to the adjacent or sometimes contiguous left common carotid origin, even with the use of the specially designed Wylie J-clamp (Pilling). In addition, innominate endarterectomy requires clamp application in the area of the arch that is more often involved with calcification and atheromatous disease, more apt to cause embolization or prevent total hemostasis by the clamp because of plaque rigidity, and so forth.[1, 5, 10] Finally, secure closure of the arteriotomy following endarterectomy is occasionally prob-

lematic because of the thin and fragile adventitial and external elastic lamina layers remaining after endarterectomy. For these reasons, bypass grafting from the more proximal intrapericardial portion of the ascending aorta, which is infrequently involved with atheromatous disease, is usually safer and easier and is most often the preferred procedure.

Full median sternotomy (Fig. 81–9) is preferred to partial sternal splitting or trap-door incisions, which offer few, if any, advantages and often result in greater postoperative chest wall instability, pain, and respiratory compromise. As depicted in the inset of Figure 81–9, limited extension of the incision into the soft tissues of the neck is often desirable to enhance exposure of the distal innominate artery and its bifurcation. Such extension, with division of the sternal head of the sternocleidomastoid and proximal strap muscles, is mandatory if the proximal right subclavian and common

FIGURE 81-8. Surgical options for direct repair of innominate artery disease. *A,* Endarterectomy, *B,* interposition graft, and *C,* bypass from the ascending aorta to the distal innominate artery.

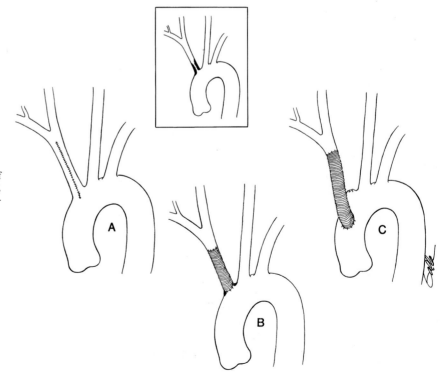

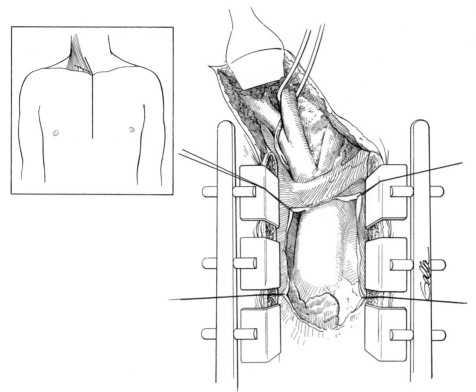

FIGURE 81–9. Exposure via median sternotomy. *Inset,* The full sternotomy incision is frequently extended into the soft tissues of the right neck *(dotted line)* to facilitate exposure of the innominate bifurcation or anterior to the sternocleidomastoid muscle if additional right common carotid exposure is required. Note the right vagus nerve passing anterior to the proximal right subclavian artery, with the recurrent laryngeal branch looping around and passing posterior to this vessel.

carotid arteries must be exposed. If more distal dissection is required, care should be taken to identify and protect the right vagus nerve and its recurrent laryngeal branch that usually passes anterior to, and then loops around, the proximal right subclavian artery to ascend in the posterior cervical region behind the carotid artery.

After sternal splitting, the sternal edges are gradually spread, pleural reflections are dissected from the midline, and remnants of thymic tissue are dissected off the ascending aorta and arch or divided between clamps. The innominate vein is then identified in the upper mediastinum and mobilized for retraction superiorly or inferiorly, as needed, to expose the proximal innominate artery. Although it is frequently stretched quite tautly, it is generally unnecessary to divide the innominate vein, although this may be done if required with minimal morbidity. The pericardium is then opened longitudinally over the ascending aorta and its edges retracted with stay sutures (see Fig 81–9).

Following systemic heparinization, a partial occluding tangential vascular clamp is applied to the anterolateral aspect of the ascending aorta (Fig. 81–10). It is often advisable to clamp the distal innominate or proximal right carotid and subclavian arteries first to minimize the chances of embolization at the time of proximal aortic clamping. In addition, the aortic clamp is often more easily and securely applied if systemic blood pressure is transiently lowered by use of systemic nitroglycerin or nitroprusside. Great care must be taken with clamp application and subsequent immobilization by a member of the operating team, as slipping or dislodgment of the clamp can obviously be disastrous. Selection of an appropriate clamp is also important; the partial occluding aortic clamp must be designed with jaws sufficiently long to allow an arteriotomy of approximately 2 cm in length. In

addition, it must be deep enough to obtain secure purchase of the aortic wall to prevent slippage from the pulsating aorta and expose adequate amounts of aortic wall following arteriotomy to enable anastomosis to be accomplished with good bites of the aortic wall edge.

Following proper application of the clamp, a small incision is made in the excluded portion of the aorta with a no. 11 scalpel blade to ensure adequate hemostasis. This is then enlarged with Pott's scissors. A small amount of aortic wall may be excised from each edge of the arteriotomy to create a slightly elliptical orifice, and the aortic wall edges can be held apart by placement of stay sutures on either side. A Dacron graft is then cut obliquely and anastomosed with an appropriate vascular suture. Use of a woven Dacron prosthesis is often preferable to limit blood loss through the graft interstices, or a polytetrafluoroethylene graft may be used.[11] In recent years, the availability of various biologically coated grafts offers an attractive alternative. Such grafts, impregnated with collagen, albumin, or gelatin, retain much of the desirable flexibility and handling characteristics of knitted Dacron grafts but have zero implant porosity, thereby avoiding the need for preclotting and limiting blood loss.

A continuous anastomosis using 4-0 or 3-0 polypropylene is generally used, but if the aorta is fragile or diseased, sutures may be interrupted and tied over Teflon pledgets. Following testing of the proximal anastomosis, the partial occluding aortic clamp is removed, the proximal prosthetic graft occluded, and clot evacuated from the distal graft. The innominate artery, which has been undisturbed to this point, is then clamped after the distal innominate or its branch arteries are first occluded to prevent embolization of atheromatous debris (Fig. 81–11). The graft may be passed either posterior or anterior to the innominate vein. My preference

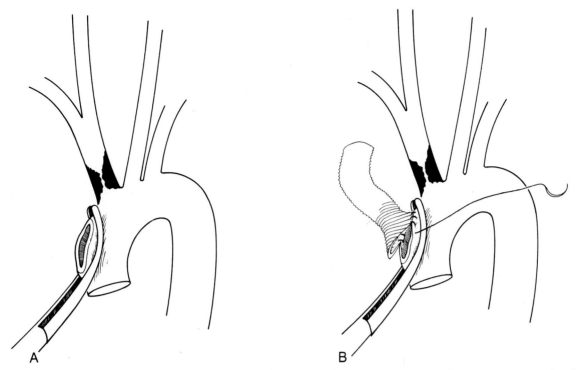

FIGURE 81–10. *A,* Partially occluding clamp on the anterolateral aspect of the intrapericardial ascending aorta, with an aortotomy approximately 2 cm in length. *B,* The graft is cut obliquely and the proximal anastomosis is performed with continuous suture.

is for end-to-end distal anastomosis, thereby excluding the atheromatous lesion and providing optimal hemodynamic flow. Attention must be directed to ensuring evacuation of all air, clot, or debris from the graft before restoration

of carotid flow. This is generally accomplished by careful antegrade and retrograde flushing through the almost-completed distal suture line and reclamping the right common carotid artery temporarily as flow is first restored to the right

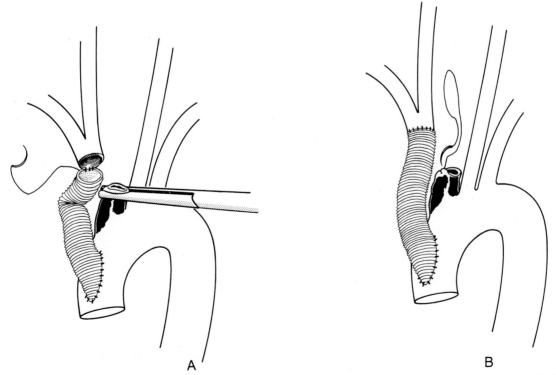

FIGURE 81–11. *A,* The innominate artery is clamped, and end-to-end anastomosis is carried out to the transected distal artery. *B,* The proximal innominate artery is oversewn to complete the operation (see also Fig. 81–2B).

subclavian artery. After a brief period, the carotid clamp is removed and cerebral perfusion restored.

At this point, reconstruction is completed by oversewing of the proximal innominate artery; I generally prefer to do this last, so as to minimize the clamp time of the carotid circulation. After protamine is administered and hemostasis ascertained, the sternotomy is closed routinely with wires over a single large mediastinal tube, which can usually be removed on the first postoperative day. If the pleural space on one or both sides has been inadvertently opened, an additional chest tube is generally recommended.

If the occlusive disease extends more distally, or if associated lesions involve the innominate bifurcation, distal anastomosis of the bypass graft must be done to both the right subclavian and common carotid arteries. This may be accomplished by either construction of a branched graft using a short side arm (Fig. 81–12A) or use of a bifurcation prosthesis similar to that utilized for aortobifemoral grafting (see Fig. 81–12B). My own preference is a bifurcation graft, usually 14 by 7 mm in size. Occasionally, such bifurcated grafts may prove too bulky, however, and cause tracheal or venous compression.[3, 10, 21] In such instances, use of a small 8 or 10 mm graft, with a short side arm originating higher up in the mediastinum or even in the cervical region, may be preferable. In such instances, it seems logical to graft preferentially to the right carotid artery, with a short branch extending to the right subclavian artery (Fig. 81–13).

Endarterectomy of innominate occlusive lesions is favored by some surgeons. Developed and promoted largely by Drs. Wylie, Stoney, and Ehrenfeld of San Francisco, this method has proved efficacious and durable in their experience and in that of other surgeons, including my own group.[1, 4, 5,]

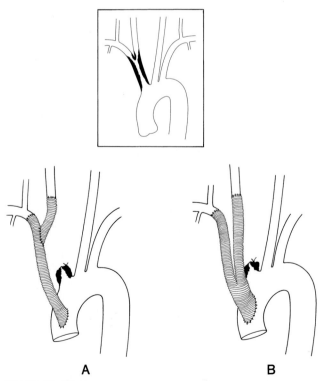

FIGURE 81–12. For reconstruction when the innominate bifurcation is involved, a branched graft may be fashioned with short side arm (A), or a bifurcation graft may be used (B).

[8, 10] However, occasional technical problems may limit its application.[1, 10, 20] Proper selection of patients is of paramount importance.[5, 8, 10] First, assessment of the extent of aortic arch atheroma is critical in determining if endarterectomy or bypass should be performed. If the occlusive lesion thins out or terminates within the innominate artery, permitting application of a partial occluding clamp on a relatively uninvolved arch, one may proceed with endarterectomy. Second, sufficient distance must exist between the innominate and left common carotid artery origins to permit application of a J-clamp to occlude the innominate origin without obstructing the left common carotid circulation. A longitudinal arteriotomy is made in the innominate artery and extended into the portion of the aorta within the jaws of the clamp (Fig. 81–14). The endarterectomy plane is identified, and endarterectomy carried out as customarily done in other locations, with the specimen transected proximally close to the clamp and distally as required by the disease process. Distal tacking sutures are generally unnecessary. Closure of the arteriotomy is then done carefully with fine suture material, as a patch is generally unnecessary.[5, 19]

Fortunately, shunting is rarely necessary during reconstruction of innominate or other brachiocephalic trunk vessels. This undoubtedly reflects the voluminous and complex patterns of collateral circulation generally available in this region. It is my preference to monitor the adequacy of cerebral blood flow during operation by means of intraoperative continuous electroencephalographic recording. The rare instances of ischemic electroencephalographic change have occurred when blood flow in the adjacent left common carotid artery was interfered with by clamps placed on the aortic dome or in several instances of relative hypotension in patients with multiple brachiocephalic occlusive lesions. Restoration of normotension alleviated these changes and permitted safe conduct of the procedure thereafter. Alternatively, many surgeons measure stump pressure in the common carotid artery. It is rare for this to be below 50 mm Hg, a level generally regarded as safely tolerable without risk of cerebral infarction.[8]

Should circumstances arise suggesting the need for temporary shunting to maintain adequate cerebral blood flow, a number of techniques may be used, but all are somewhat cumbersome. A Gott shunt or similar tubing may be inserted via a separate puncture site in some portion of the ascending aorta or aortic arch and inserted distally through the distal arteriotomy or separate distal site, but this may be awkward and could lead to troublesome bleeding or other difficulties. Wylie and coworkers[19] described use of a T-tube shunt from one carotid artery to the other or use of a bifurcation graft with a "temporary" limb to the right subclavian or axillary artery during innominate artery grafting. The subclavian anastomosis is done first, thereby providing flow to the right common carotid artery when the distal innominate artery is clamped. Following completion of the innominate graft and restoration of antegrade flow to the carotid artery, the subclavian limb is resected and the stumps of the graft simply oversewn. Undoubtedly, other ingenious maneuvers to achieve temporary blood flow to the cerebrum may be conceived by surgeons, but fortunately, this is rarely required.

COMMON CAROTID ARTERIES

Methods of direct repair of lesions involving the common carotid arteries vary, depending on the site of the principal

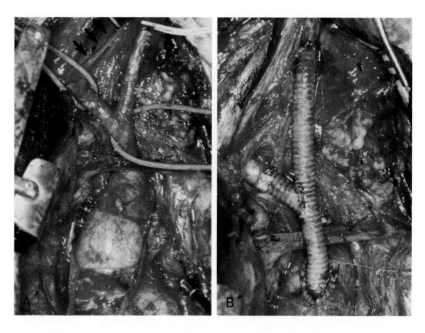

FIGURE 81-13. *A,* Wide exposure for occlusive disease involving the distal innominate artery and its bifurcation. The innominate vein crosses the innominate artery origin, while the right vagus and recurrent laryngeal nerves *(arrows)* have been mobilized lateral to the rubber tape around the proximal right subclavian artery. *B,* Graft from the ascending aorta to the middle right common carotid artery, with a short side branch constructed to the right subclavian.

disease (origin of carotid artery versus carotid bifurcation), side involved, and pathologic process involved (atherosclerosis versus nonatherosclerotic lesions). Most arteriosclerotic lesions, whether occurring proximally at the origin of the vessel or located principally at the bifurcation, are segmental in nature and suitable for thromboendarterectomy or bypass grafting. Various forms of arteritis, such as Takayasu disease, may involve more lengthy segments and are not generally manageable by endarterectomy. Lesions in the mid common carotid are unusual, except in patients with prior

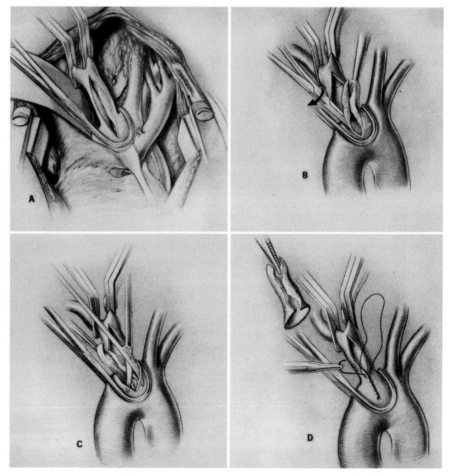

FIGURE 81-14. Steps in performing an innominate artery endarterectomy. *A,* Use of a Wylie J-clamp permits extension of the arteriotomy into the proximal arch, without impinging on the nearby left common carotid artery. *B,* Development of an endarterectomy plane to the confines of the clamp. *C,* Transection of the aortic intima. *D,* Primary closure of the arteriotomy. (From Carlson RE, Ehrenfeld WK, Stoney RJ, Wylie EJ: Innominate artery endarterectomy: A 16-year experience. *Arch Surg.* 1977; 112:1389; with permission. Copyright 1977, American Medical Association.)

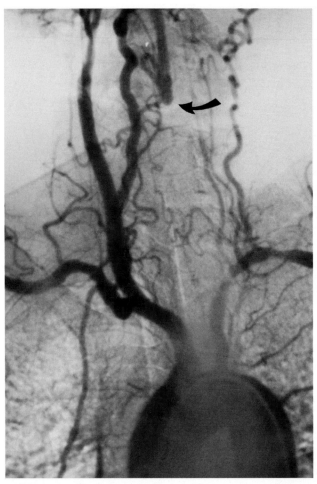

FIGURE 81–15. Occlusion of the left common carotid artery. Patency of the left carotid bifurcation *(arrow)* has been maintained by retrograde flow down the external carotid, permitting bypass grafting as illustrated in Figure 81–16.

quires a separate cervical incision to expose the carotid bifurcation. Any significant carotid bifurcation disease may be managed by standard carotid bifurcation endarterectomy; median sternotomy then permits anastomosis of an 8 or 10 mm prosthetic graft, which can then be tunneled to the left cervical incision for distal carotid anastomosis (Fig. 81–16).

If the left subclavian artery is free of significant associated disease, it may be used for extrathoracic subclavian–carotid bypass or serve as an implantation site for transfer of the left common carotid artery. In the latter procedure, dissection is carried down the common carotid artery through a cervical incision extending to the suprasternal notch. The proximal left common carotid artery is mobilized as far into the upper mediastinum as possible behind the head of the clavicle, transected caudal to the clavicle, and, after thromboendarterectomy, anastomosed end to side to the left subclavian artery beyond the thyrocervical trunk.[8, 19]

More often, the mechanism of common carotid artery occlusion involves progressive atheromatous occlusive disease at the carotid bifurcation as opposed to the origin of the common carotid artery, leading to retrograde thrombosis of the proximal common carotid artery. It is important that this pathophysiologic mechanism be recognized, because primary attention will have to be directed first at bifurcation endarterectomy. Following this, retrograde thrombectomy of the proximal common carotid artery may be possible, with restoration of adequate inflow. If this is unsuccessful, bypass grafting from a proximal mediastinal vessel, or use of an extrathoracic cervical donor site, will generally be feasible.

Lesions involving the proximal right common carotid ar-

neck irradiation.[8] These lesions are also poorly suited to endarterectomy and necessitate graft replacement or bypass.

If stenotic lesions involve the origin of the left common carotid artery from the aortic arch, direct exposure via median sternotomy is preferred. Attempts to manage such lesions by retrograde manipulations of ring strippers or similar instruments from limited cervical incisions without proximal exposure or vascular control are dangerous and ill advised. Limited origin stenoses may be managed by transmediastinal endarterectomy or bypass grafts from the ascending aorta to the mediastinal aspect of the left common carotid artery distal to the lesion, adhering to techniques and principles similar to those for innominate artery grafts, as previously described. Another method that has been reported is transection of the left common carotid artery distal to the occlusive lesion and transfer to the side of the neighboring innominate artery by end-to-side anastomosis within the mediastinum.

If total occlusion of the left common carotid artery develops owing to progressive origin disease, prograde propagation of the thrombus will occur, generally stopping at the carotid bifurcation in the cervical region. Retrograde flow in the external carotid artery is often sufficient to maintain patency of the carotid bifurcation and internal carotid artery and allow bypass grafting (Fig. 81–15). This generally re-

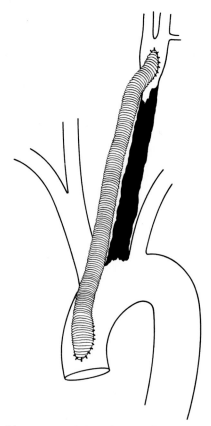

FIGURE 81–16. Bypass graft from the ascending aorta to the distal left carotid artery via median sternotomy.

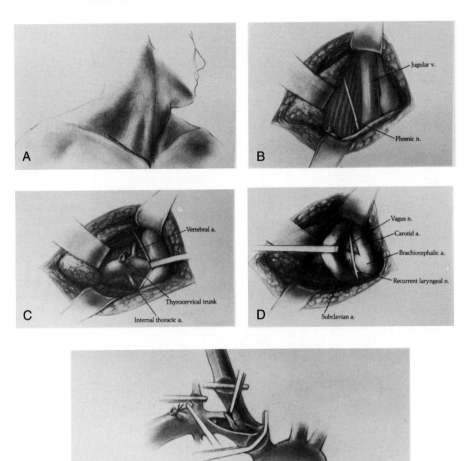

FIGURE 81-17. Steps in right subclavian artery exposure and repair by endarterectomy. *A,* Supraclavicular incision just above the clavicle from the suprasternal notch to the midsupraclavicular fossa. *B,* The phrenic nerve is identified medially on the anterior scalene muscle. *C,* Division of the anterior scalene muscle exposes the subclavian artery. The thyrocervical trunk has been divided to facilitate mobilization. *D,* Proximal dissection along the subclavian artery exposes the innominate bifurcation. *E,* Endarterectomy is carried out under direct vision. (From De Weese JA: Revascularization of proximal brachiocephalic, subclavian, carotid, and vertebral arteries. In Nyhus LM, Baker RJ, eds. *Mastery of Surgery,* Vol 2. Boston: Little, Brown; 1984:1334; with permission.)

tery are the least common of all brachiocephalic occlusive lesions.[22] When they do occur, they can often be managed by a cervical approach, owing to the higher origin of the right common carotid artery at the innominate bifurcation, usually just behind the right sternoclavicular joint. Most often, endarterectomy is preferred, with an approach similar to that used for right subclavian artery repair, described in the next section.

SUBCLAVIAN ARTERIES

Although the subclavian arteries, particularly the left subclavian, are the most frequent site of brachiocephalic trunk lesions, it is important to reemphasize that many such lesions are asymptomatic and do not require revascularization. Symptomatic lesions are often associated with other occlusive lesions in the brachiocephalic vessels or, more commonly, the carotid bifurcation. Surgical correction of these associated lesions often provides adequate symptom relief.

Nonatherosclerotic lesions of the subclavian artery are occasionally encountered and often require direct repair.

Atherosclerotic aneurysms are unusual, but post-traumatic aneurysmal changes secondary to thoracic outlet syndrome do occur; they usually present with thromboembolic complications involving the upper extremity or hand. Similar traumatic injuries following fractures, blunt trauma, or penetrating wounds may involve the subclavian vessels.

Most occlusive lesions of the right subclavian artery can be approached by cervical incisions and direct repair accomplished by endarterectomy (Fig. 81–17). Alternatively, the subclavian artery may be repositioned by end-to-side anastomosis to the common carotid artery, or extrathoracic bypass from the carotid to subclavian artery can be performed. The approach is similar to that used for vertebral artery procedures. If the cervical exposure proves inadequate, it can be enlarged by extension into a partial sternal splitting incision or by means of resection of the medial clavicle. These maneuvers are rarely required, however, except in instances of traumatic injuries with ongoing blood loss or other difficulties in exposure.

A transverse incision is made in the supraclavicular fossa, about one finger breadth above the clavicle, extending from the midline suprasternal notch 7 to 8 cm laterally. The

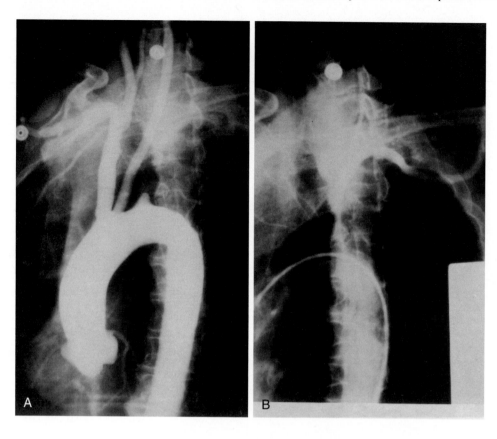

FIGURE 81–18. Occlusion of the proximal left subclavian artery just beyond its origin *(A)*, with later filling of the distal left subclavian *(B)* by retrograde left vertebral flow (''subclavian steal'' syndrome).

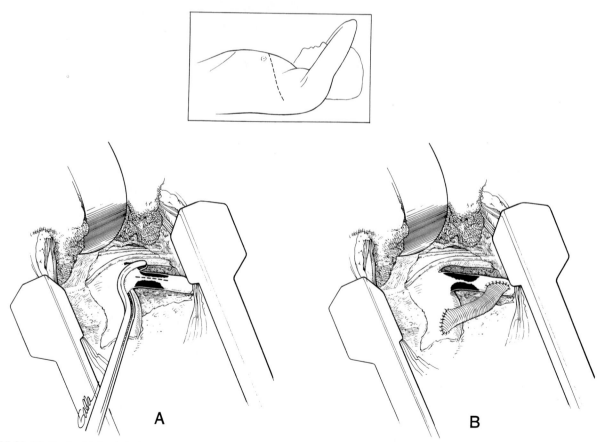

FIGURE 81–19. Proximal left subclavian artery lesions require thoracotomy *(inset)* for direct repair by endarterectomy *(A)* or grafting from the descending thoracic aorta to the subclavian artery distal to the lesion *(B)*.

sternocleidomastoid, sternohyoid, and sternothyroid muscles are divided, the scalene fat pad is mobilized upward and laterally, and the anterior scalene muscle is exposed. The phrenic nerve is carefully identified and protected; it is generally located toward the medial edge of the anterior scalene muscle, running in a lateral to medial downward oblique path, immediately on the anterior surface of the muscle (see Fig. 81–17). It is generally preferable to mobilize this to facilitate atraumatic retraction of the nerve in either direction during the subsequent dissection. The internal jugular vein is followed to its confluence with the subclavian vein, and both venous structures are freed to permit retraction. The subclavian artery is exposed by division of the anterior scalene muscle, with extreme care to avoid injury to the phrenic nerve. Dissection is then carried proximally along the subclavian artery; the thyrocervical and internal mammary branches may be sacrificed if this aids in dissection and mobilization of the subclavian artery. The vertebral origin is identified on the posterosuperior aspect of the proximal subclavian artery, and with a bit more proximal dissection behind the clavicular head, the innominate bifurcation and distal innominate artery itself can usually be sufficiently exposed to allow a small curved arterial clamp

to be placed for proximal control and to allow the endarterectomy to be carried out under direct vision.

Direct repair of proximal left subclavian artery lesions (Fig. 81–18) cannot be accomplished by either the cervical or transmediastinal approach because of the posterior origin of the left subclavian artery from the aortic arch at approximately the level of the fourth thoracic vertebra. For this reason, direct reconstruction requires left thoracotomy, usually employing an anterolateral incision through the third or fourth interspace. As illustrated in Figure 81–19, either endarterectomy or aortosubclavian grafting can be carried out. Although generally quite successful, the morbidity of such a transthoracic approach has led most surgeons to abandon direct repair of proximal left subclavian lesions in favor of other methods, usually employing extrathoracic routes of reconstruction.[3, 15, 23]

Direct subclavian–carotid transfer or repositioning procedures may be used for reconstruction of more proximal left subclavian lesions (Fig. 81–20). Although offering the advantages of a cervical approach and an autogenous tissue reconstruction, the procedure may be technically difficult and potentially dangerous if a technical mishap occurs during management of the proximally transected subclavian

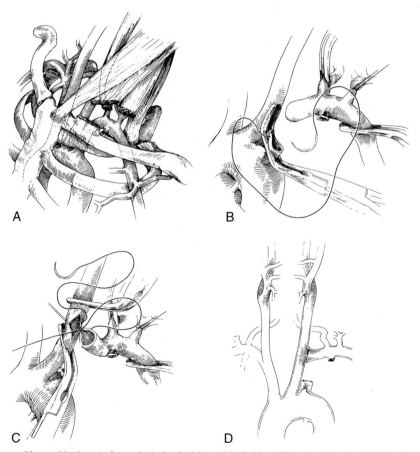

FIGURE 81–20. Subclavian–carotid repositioning. *A,* Supraclavicular incision, with division of the clavicular head of the sternocleidomastoid and anterior scalene muscles, enables the dissection to be carried into the thoracic inlet behind the sternoclavicular junction. *B,* The left subclavian artery is mobilized and divided caudal to the clavicle, and the proximal stump is oversewn. *C,* The transected end of the left subclavian artery is then anastomosed to the side of the adjacent left common carotid artery. *D,* Schematic of the transposition procedure. (From Diethrich EB, Koopot R: Simplified operative procedure for proximal subclavian arterial lesions: Direct subclavian–carotid anastomosis. *Am J Surg* 1981; 142:416; with permission.)

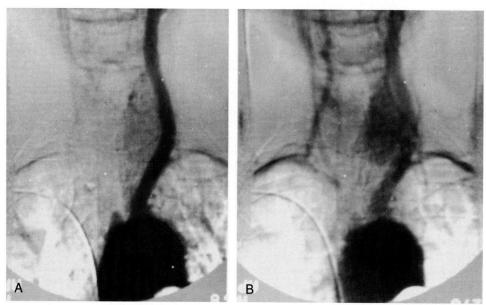

FIGURE 81–21. *A,* Digital subtraction angiography arch study demonstrating occlusion of both the innominate and the left subclavian arteries in a patient with repeated syncopal episodes and symptoms of global ischemia. *B,* On later films, bilateral "steal" is noted, with retrograde flow down the right common carotid and right vertebral arteries ("innominate steal"), and reversed left vertebral flow filling the left subclavian artery.

artery. Excellent results have been described by Diethrich and Koopot[24] and by Mehigan and coworkers.[25] A similar approach, using side-to-side anastomosis of the left common carotid and subclavian arteries through a cervical incision, has also been extensively described by Edwards and coworkers.[26–28]

MULTIPLE BRACHIOCEPHALIC OCCLUSIVE LESIONS

Frequently, there are multiple occlusive lesions affecting the brachiocephalic trunks.[12, 13, 29] These are generally atherosclerotic, but arteritis, particularly Takayasu disease, may involve multiple branches of the aortic arch.[30] Characteristically, the latter process is seen in young women, usually of Asian descent, with absent or reduced upper-extremity pulses (pulseless disease).

Symptomatology in such patients is often variable and severe, producing complex combinations of cerebral, ocular, brain-stem, and upper-extremity ischemic symptoms. "Steal" syndromes due to reversal of flow in one or both of the vertebral arteries, and even the right common carotid artery ("innominate steal" syndrome), may be seen, producing marked neurologic symptoms of a widespread or global nature (Fig. 81–21).

In many instances, reconstruction in patients with multiple brachiocephalic lesions requires direct repair, as proximal involvement of great-vessel trunks may preclude effective cervical extra-anatomic reconstruction or make single extrathoracic bypasses inadequate for sufficient symptom relief.[9, 10, 12]

Because of the almost infinite variety in the distribution of lesions in the brachiocephalic trunks, which may produce symptoms by distal embolization, flow reduction, flow reversal, or a combination of these pathophysiologic mechanisms, surgical reconstruction in patients with multiple lesions must

be highly individualized. Generally, however, priority is given to carotid territory revascularization, with emphasis on innominate and left common carotid circulation.[1, 31] In many instances, subclavian lesions can be left alone if carotid circulation is adequately restored.

The ascending aorta provides an optimal site of proximal anastomosis for bypass grafts when occlusive lesions in multiple arch branches reduce availability of cervical donor artery sites.[12, 21, 22, 31] Access is via a median sternotomy, similar to that previously described for isolated innominate artery repair. As illustrated in Figure 81–22, a branched graft can be constructed, or a bifurcated prosthesis can be used.

If more lengthy or peripherally located lesions are present, a median sternotomy may have to be combined with other appropriate cervical, supraclavicular, or infraclavicular incisions to permit simultaneous exposure of carotid, subclavian, or axillary vessels (Fig. 81–23). Grafts originating on the ascending aorta are then tunneled to these other sites for distal anastomosis. Quite often, it may be easier or advantageous to combine transmediastinal and extrathoracic methods, as with a cervical left carotid–subclavian graft originating from a bypass graft from the ascending aorta to the distal left common carotid artery (see Fig. 81–23*D*). A number of clinical examples are illustrated in Figures 81–24 through 81–26. Obviously, many lesions can be reconstructed by a variety of methods, depending on individual requirements, personal preferences, and the ingenuity of the surgeon.

CONCLUSIONS

Improvements in patient care and surgical methods have produced steady reduction of the morbidity and mortality of direct surgical reconstruction of lesions of the main branches of the aortic arch. Anatomic in-line repair achieves effective and durable results, excludes the source of embolic phenom-

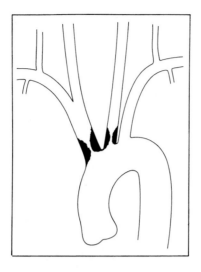

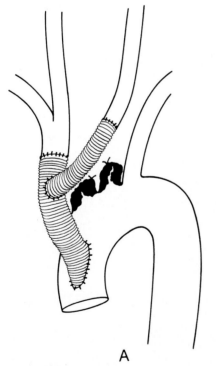

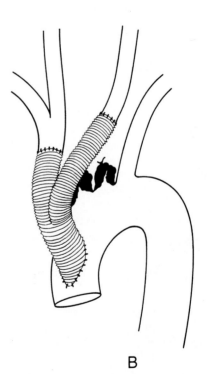

A

B

FIGURE 81–22. With multiple brachiocephalic trunk lesions, side branches may be attached to a single principal graft *(A),* or limbs of a bifurcated graft from the ascending aorta may be used *(B).*

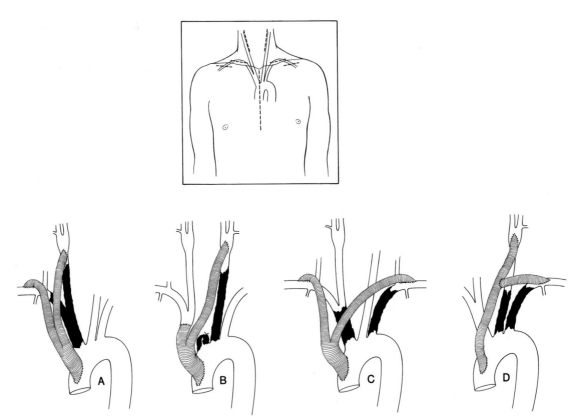

FIGURE 81–23. Examples of bypass grafts useful for reconstruction in patients with multiple brachiocephalic vessel involvement. For more extensive or more peripherally situated lesions, separate cervical, supraclavicular, or infraclavicular incisions must often be combined with median sternotomy *(inset)*.

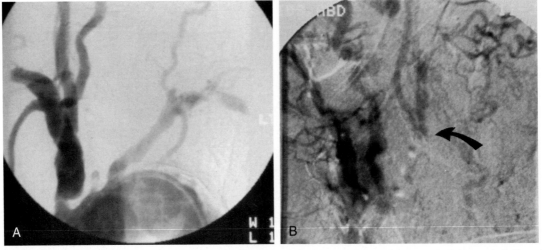

FIGURE 81–24. *A,* Stenosis of the proximal innominate artery and occlusion of the left common carotid artery. *B,* Later cervical views demonstrating patent left carotid bifurcation *(arrow).* The patient received a bifurcated graft from the ascending aorta to the innominate and left carotid arteries, as depicted in Figure 81–23*A.*

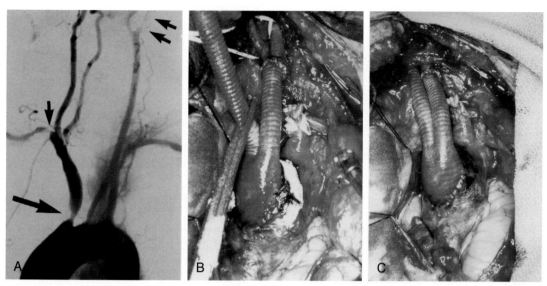

FIGURE 81–25. *A,* Arch aortogram demonstrating stenoses of the proximal innominate artery *(bold arrow)* and the second portion of the right subclavian artery *(single arrow)* distal to the right vertebral artery. There is total occlusion of the left internal carotid artery *(double arrows).* Reconstruction by bifurcation graft, with medial-limb to distal-innominate *(B)* is the first step, with subsequent tunneling of the lateral limb to the right axillary artery *(C),* exposed by separate infraclavicular incision.

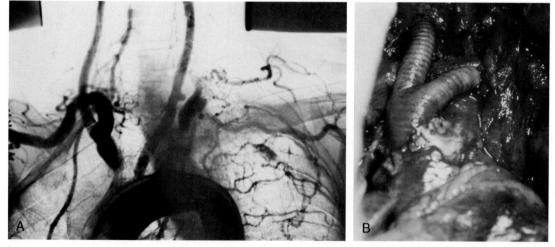

FIGURE 81–26. *A,* Preoperative study of a patient with failure of a previous left carotid–subclavian extrathoracic bypass for left subclavian occlusion. The stump of the prior graft can be seen on the lateral aspect of the middle left common carotid artery. Tight innominate origin stenosis is noted, with reconstitution of the left axillary artery just below the clavicle. *B,* Bifurcation graft from the ascending aorta to the innominate and left axillary arteries, similar to that shown in Figure 81–23C.

ena from the circulation, and achieves the most complete and definitive revascularization when multiple brachiocephalic vessels are involved.

REFERENCES

1. Brewster DC, Moncure AC, Darling RC, et al: Innominate artery lesions: Problems encountered and lessons learned. *J Vasc Surg.* 1985;2:99.
2. DeBakey ME, Morris GC Jr, Jordan GL Jr, Cooley DA: Segmental thrombo-obliterative disease of branches of aortic arch: Successful surgical treatment. *JAMA.* 1958;166:998.
3. Crawford ES, DeBakey ME, Morris GC Jr, Howell JF: Surgical treatment of occlusion of the innominate, common carotid and subclavian arteries: A ten year experience. *Surgery.* 1969;65:17.
4. Ehrenfeld WK, Chapman RD, Wylie EJ: Management of occlusive lesions of the branches of the aortic arch. *Am J Surg.* 1969;118:236.
5. Carlson RE, Ehrenfeld WK, Stoney RJ, Wylie EJ: Innominate artery endarterectomy: A 16-year experience. *Arch Surg.* 1977;112:1389.
6. Vogt DP, Hertzer NR, O'Hara PJ, et al: Brachiocephalic arterial reconstruction. *Ann Surg.* 1982;196:541.
7. Crawford ES, Stowe CL, Powers RW Jr: Occlusion of the innominate, common carotid, and subclavian arteries: Long-term results of surgical treatment. *Surgery.* 1983;94:781.
8. Ehrenfeld WK, Rapp JH: Direct revascularization for occlusion of the trunks of the aortic arch. From symposium on revascularization after thrombosis of the extracranial vasculature. *J Vasc Surg.* 1985;2:228.
9. Zelenock GB, Cronenwett JL, Graham LM, et al: Brachiocephalic arterial occlusions and stenoses: Manifestations and management of complex lesions. *Arch Surg.* 1985;120:370.
10. Cherry KJ, McCullough JL, Hallett JW Jr, et al: Technical principles of direct innominate artery revascularization: A comparison of endarterectomy and bypass grafts. *J Vasc Surg.* 1989;9:718.
11. Cormier F, Ward A, Cormier M-J, Laurian C: Long-term results of aortoinnominate and aortocarotid polytetrafluoroethylene bypass grafting for atherosclerotic disease. *J Vasc Surg.* 1989;10:135.
12. Reul GJ, Jacobs MJHM, Gregoric ID, et al: Innominate artery occlusive disease: Surgical approach and long-term results. *J Vasc Surg.* 1991;14:405.
13. Hass WK, Fields WS, North RR, et al: Joint study of extracranial arterial occlusion. II. Arteriography, techniques, sites, and complications. *JAMA.* 1968;203:159.
14. Fields WS, Lemak NA: Joint study of extracranial arterial occlusion. VII. Subclavian steal—a review of 168 cases. *JAMA.* 1972;222:1139.
15. Najafi H, Javid H, Hunter JA, et al: Occlusive diseases of the branches of the aortic arch. In Bergan JJ, Yao JST, eds. *Surgery of the Aorta and Its Body Branches.* New York: Grune & Stratton; 1979:191.
16. Hoyt WF: Ocular symptoms and signs. In Wylie EJ, Ehrenfeld WK, eds. *Extracranial Occlusive Cerebrovascular Disease: Diagnosis and Management.* Philadelphia: WB Saunders; 1970:64.
17. Johnston RH Jr, Wall MJ Jr, Mattox KL: Innominate artery trauma: A thirty year experience. *J Vasc Surg.* 1993;17:134.
18. Weaver FA, Suda RW, Stiles GM, Yellin AE: Injuries to the ascending aorta, aortic arch, and great vessels. *Surg Gynecol Obstet.* 1989;169:27.
19. Wylie EJ, Stoney RJ, Ehrenfeld WK: Manual of Vascular Surgery, Vol 1. New York: Springer-Verlag; 1980.
20. DeWeese JA: Revascularization of proximal brachiocephalic, subclavian, carotid, and vertebral arteries. In Nyhus LM, Baker RJ, eds. *Mastery of Surgery,* Vol 2. Boston: Little, Brown; 1984:1334.
21. Kieffer E, Natal J: Supraaortic trunk lesions in Takayasu's arteritis. In Bergan JJ, Yao JST, eds. *Cerebrovascular Insufficiency.* New York: Grune & Stratton; 1983:395.
22. Bergan JJ, Yao JST, Flinn WR: Brachiocephalic revascularization. In Najarian JS, Delaney JP, eds. *Advances in Vascular Surgery.* Chicago: Year Book Medical Publishers; 1983:125.
23. Wylie EJ, Ehrenfeld WK: Surgical techniques. In Wylie EJ, Ehrenfeld WK, eds. *Extracranial Occlusive Cerebrovascular Disease: Diagnosis and Management.* Philadelphia: WB Saunders; 1970:184.
24. Diethrich EB, Koopot R: Simplified operative procedure for proximal subclavian arterial lesions: Direct subclavian–carotid anastomosis. *Am J Surg.* 1981;142:416.
25. Mehigan JT, Buch WS, Pipkin RD, Fogarty TJ: Subclavian–carotid transposition for the subclavian steal syndrome. *Am J Surg.* 1978;136:15.
26. Edwards WH, Wright RS: Current concepts in the management of arteriosclerotic lesions of the subclavian and vertebral arteries. *Ann Surg.* 1972;175:975.
27. Edwards WH, Mulherin JL Jr: The surgical approach to significant stenosis of vertebral and subclavian arteries. *Surgery.* 1980;87:20.
28. Edwards WH, Mulherin JL Jr: The surgical reconstruction of the proximal subclavian and vertebral artery. *J Vasc Surg.* 1985;2:634.
29. Thompson JE, Patman RD, Talkington CM: Carotid surgery for cerebrovascular insufficiency. *Curr Probl Surg.* 1978;15:1.
30. Hall S, Barr W, Lie JT, et al: Takayasu arteritis: A study of 32 North American patients. *Medicine (Baltimore).* 1985;64:89.
31. Kozol RA, Bredenberg CE: Alternatives in the management of atherosclerotic occlusive disease of aortic arch branches. *Arch Surg.* 1981;116:1457.

CHAPTER 82

Extrathoracic Repair of the Brachiocephalic Trunks

WESLEY S. MOORE

The frequency of stenoses or occlusions involving the aortic arch trunks is relatively low as compared with carotid bifurcation disease. Occlusive disease of the aortic trunks represents about 6 percent of all extracranial arterial occlusive lesions.

The direct approach for repair of occlusive lesions involving the aortic arch trunks requires either mediastinal exposure of the aortic arch or transthoracic exposure of the left subclavian artery. These major operations carry a significant rate of morbidity and mortality. The alternative to a direct approach has been extrathoracic repair. Extrathoracic repair is made possible by the relative proximity of the three supra-aortic trunks and four cervical branches. Thus, when only one supra-aortic trunk is involved, an adjacent branch can be tapped to provide blood flow to the involved trunk, distal to the lesion. This is done without sacrificing blood flow to the donor vessel. Concerns that diverting blood from one aortic trunk to an adjacent vessel would cause a "steal phenomenon" are unjustified in the absence of proximal occlusive disease in the donor artery. This chapter deals with the surgical technique of extrathoracic repair for occlusive lesions involving each of the brachiocephalic trunks. The techniques are equally applicable to stenotic and occlusive lesions. It should be pointed out, however, that in patients who have symptoms secondary to embolic phenomena from stenotic lesions of an aortic arch trunk, their condition must be recognized and the source of emboli dealt with in addition to new blood flow being provided distal to the lesion. The most expeditious way of controlling this problem is a ligature distal to an ulcerated, stenotic lesion, or division and translocation of the artery distal to the lesion from which the emboli eminate.

LESIONS OF THE INNOMINATE ARTERY

Stenotic or occlusive lesions of the innominate artery (Fig. 82–1) compromise blood flow or provide a source of emboli to the right common carotid and subclavian arteries. As long as the innominate artery bifurcation is relatively free of disease, restoration of blood flow to the side of the right common carotid or right subclavian artery provides normal blood flow to both the right common artery and the right subclavian artery by bidirectional blood flow. Thus the options for restoring blood flow include a bypass graft from the left common to the right common carotid artery, from the left subclavian to the right subclavian artery, from the left axillary to the right axillary artery, and from the left subclavian to the right common carotid artery. It should be emphasized that if there is a suspicion that the patient is experiencing symptoms from emboli leaving the surface of a stenotic lesion of the innominate artery, a ligature must be placed proximal to the innominate artery bifurcation to prevent further emboli.

Carotid to Carotid Artery Bypass

This is the most direct approach to revascularization of the branches of the innominate artery. It has the theoretic disadvantage that it requires temporary alternate clamping of both carotid arteries. By contrast, if the left subclavian artery is used for a source of inflow and the right subclavian for the recipient artery, blood flow to the brain is not interrupted during the reperfusion process. Nonetheless, in my experience, carotid to carotid bypass is a safe operation when appropriate precautions are taken.

The patient is positioned supine on the operating table with the neck somewhat extended on the shoulders and the head placed in mid-position. Each common carotid artery is approached by a vertical incision placed anterior to the sternocleidomastoid muscle, below the carotid bifurcation. This presumes that an angiogram has shown absence of significant disease at the carotid bifurcation on both the donor and recipient sides. On the other hand, if significant carotid bifurcation disease is identified on either side, this can be dealt with by carotid bifurcation endarterectomy. It should be emphasized, however, that the graft anastomosis should be placed low in the neck so that the ultimate position of the graft assumes a retromanubrial course. After the vertical skin incisions are made, the platysmal layer is incised (Fig. 82–2). The sternomastoid muscle is mobilized off the carotid sheath. The carotid sheath is entered along

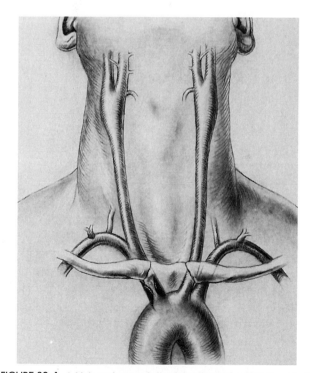

FIGURE 82–1. A high-grade stenosis involving the origin of the innominate artery shown in relationship to the aortic arch trunks and extracranial vessels.

613

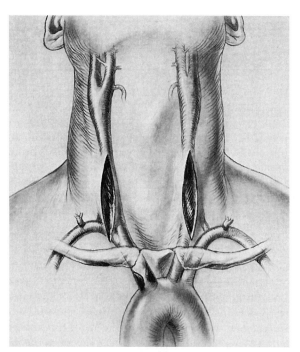

FIGURE 82–2. The common carotid arteries are approached by vertical incisions along the anterior of each respective sternocleidomastoid muscle.

the anterior medial border of the internal jugular vein, and the vein is retracted. Particular care is taken to look for the vagus nerve, in case it lies in an anterior rather than a posterior position. The common carotid artery is mobilized within its periadventitial plane for a sufficient length proximally and distally to permit clamping for an end-to-side

anastomosis. After the right and left common carotid arteries are isolated, the patient is ready for bypass grafting.

The selection of graft material is based on the surgeon's preference. In my experience, prosthetic grafts work better and last longer with respect to patency than do grafts of autogenous saphenous vein in this location. My personal preference is the use of an 8-mm polytetrafluoroethylene (PTFE) prosthesis. However, woven and knitted Dacron grafts work equally well. Five thousand U of heparin are administered intravenously prior to clamping of the carotid artery. The safety of clamping either common carotid artery can be ascertained by measuring the common carotid artery backpressure after placement of a proximal common carotid clamp. I have been willing to accept backpressures in excess of 25 mm Hg as a safe indication for satisfactory collateral blood flow to permit temporary clamping of the carotid artery during graft anastomosis. Alternatively, electroencephalographic monitoring provides equally reliable data. The common carotid artery is clamped proximally and distally. The graft is appropriately beveled and a longitudinal arterotomy of corresponding size is made. A suture is placed at the heel and toe of the prosthesis (as described in Fig. 82–3) and tied. The anastomosis is then completed in four quadrants. The carotid artery is backbled and forwardbled out the graft, and the prosthesis is clamped immediately distal to the anastomosis to permit restoration of blood flow through the common carotid artery. A tunnel is made between the right and left common carotid arteries behind the manubrium so that the graft will not press against the trachia. Once the opposite end of the graft is brought into contact with the left carotid artery, the second anastomosis is made in an identical fashion. Before completion of the anastomosis, the carotid artery is backbled and forwardbled, with care

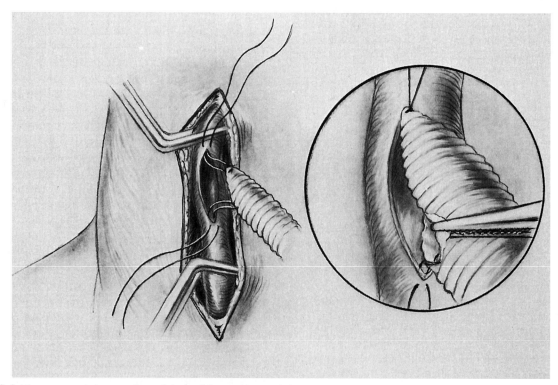

FIGURE 82–3. The anastomosis between the graft in the right carotid artery is begun by placement of a mattress suture at the heel and toe of the beveled graft. This is tied into position, and the anastomosis is constructed in quadrants.

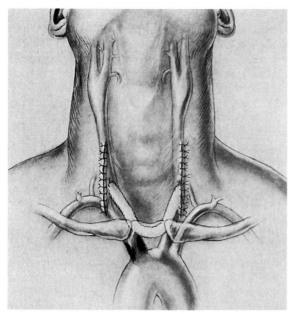

FIGURE 82–4. The completed carotid-to-carotid bypass graft. Note that the graft is placed in a retromanubrial position so as to avoid pressure on the trachea.

taken to prevent blood from filling the previously evacuated graft. This precaution avoids blood stasis in the graft as well as thrombosis and embolization. Immediately before completion of the anastomosis, the graft is backbled to remove all air, the anastomosis is completed and tied, and

blood flow is re-established first with the clamp on the distal right common carotid artery to retrogradely perfuse the subclavian artery and then with removal of the clamp providing bidirectional flow to the right common carotid artery and right subclavian artery. The final configuration of the prosthesis is illustrated in Figure 82–4. An alternative approach to tunneling between the carotid arteries is to use the retro-esophageal plane. Although I have no personal experience with this approach, its proponents point out two major advantages. First, the pathway is more direct, thus permitting a shorter graft to be used. Second, if the patient requires a sternotomy at a later date, the surgeon will not be encumbered with a graft in the retromanubrial position.

Subclavian to Subclavian Artery Bypass

This technique has the advantage that the branches of the innominate artery are reperfused without temporary interruption of blood supply to the brain. This is made possible by clamping the subclavian artery distal to the takeoff of the vertebral artery. The second advantage occurs with the placement of the prosthesis in a relatively remote and protected location. The major disadvantage of the technique concerns the somewhat difficult exposure of the subclavian artery and the relatively fragile nature of its wall, which must be handled with the utmost care to avoid injury.

The right and left subclavian arteries are exposed through corresponding supraclavicular incisions (Fig. 82–5). The incision is positioned over the lateral head of the sternocleidomastoid muscle approximately one fingerbreadth above the

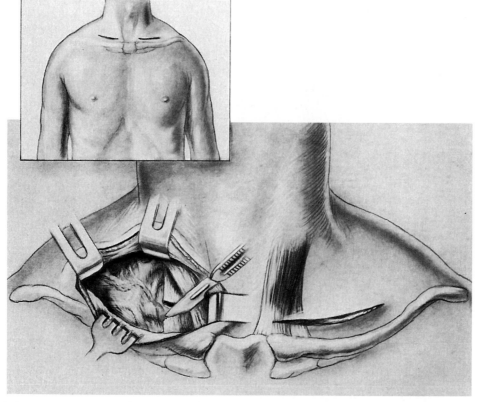

FIGURE 82–5. Each incision is placed in the supraclavicular region over the lateral head of the sternomastoid muscle. The lateral head of the sternomastoid muscle is divided.

clavicle. The dissection is carried down through the platysmal layer, and the lateral head of the sternomastoid muscle is encircled and divided. The dissection of the subclavian artery is carried out in the scalene triangle. The scalene triangle is bounded by the carotid sheath medially, by the subclavian vein as its base, and by the omohyoid muscle as the hypotenuse. The prescalene fat pad is mobilized inferiorly. The transverse cervical and transverse scapular vessels are divided between the ligature. The scalene fat pad is freed up from the carotid sheath along its medial aspect, with particular care taken to avoid injury to the thoracic duct on the left side and occasionally on the right side. The fat pad is mobilized superior to the omohyoid muscle and then held in place with a retractor. As the fat pad is mobilized off the omohyoid muscle, particular care must be taken to avoid injury to the phrenic nerve (Fig. 82–6). The phrenic nerve is carefully mobilized for its visible length off the anterior scalene muscle and retracted medially. A right-angle clamp is carefully passed between the anterior scalene muscle and the subclavian artery. The scalene muscle is then divided. This gives excellent exposure to the subclavian artery, which can now be mobilized carefully within the perivascular plane of Leriche. Mobilization of the subclavian artery can be made easier by division of several small branches, including the thyrocervical trunk. Once a sufficient length of the subclavian artery has been mobilized to permit proximal and distal clamping for an end-to-side anastomosis with a prosthetic graft, the identical maneuver is carried out on the opposite side.

I prefer to use an 8-mm PTFE graft for this procedure. The graft is appropriately beveled at approximately a 45- to 60-degree angle. The artery is clamped proximally and distally, and an end-to-side anastomosis is carried out. Following completion of the anastomosis, an occluding clamp is placed on the distal portion of the prosthesis adjacent to the anastomosis; flow is re-established through the subclavian artery. A tunnel connecting the two exposed portions of the subclavian arteries is made behind the sternomastoid muscle and behind the manubrium (Fig. 82–7). The graft is drawn through the tunnel, and an end-to-side anastomosis is constructed to the opposite subclavian artery (Fig. 82–8). This technique effectively establishes flow to the branches of the subclavian artery and to the right common carotid artery by retrograde flow using the principle of end-to-side anastomosis. Closure of the wound is carried out by replacing the scalene fat pad, followed by approximation of the platysmal layer and the skin.

Axillary to Axillary Bypass

An alternative method of reperfusion of the right subclavian and right carotid artery is to use the left axillary artery as a source of inflow to the right axillary artery and hence the subclavian and right carotid arteries via bidirectional blood flow. The axillary arteries are exposed by infraclavicular incisions placed approximately one fingerbreadth below each clavicle and centered over the coracoid process (Fig. 82–9). Dissection is carried down through the subcutaneous tissue to expose the greater pectoral muscle. The fibers between the sternal and clavicular heads of the greater pectoral muscle are separated and retracted. The clavipectoral fascia is incised and the underlying smaller pectoral muscle is exposed. The smaller pectoral muscle is encircled and divided through its tendinous portion. This provides exposure of the axillary neurovascular bundle. The axillary artery is then carefully separated from the axillary vein and mobi-

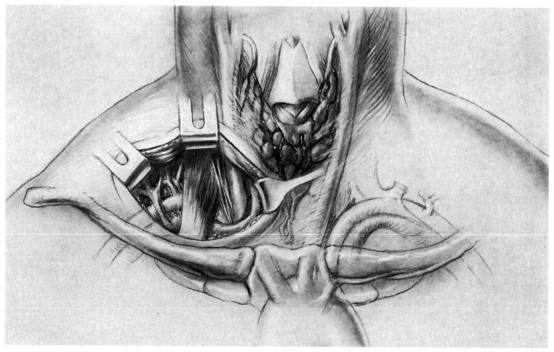

FIGURE 82–6. The anterior scalene muscle and the phrenic nerve are visualized covering the subclavian artery. The phrenic nerve is mobilized, and the anterior scalene muscle is divided.

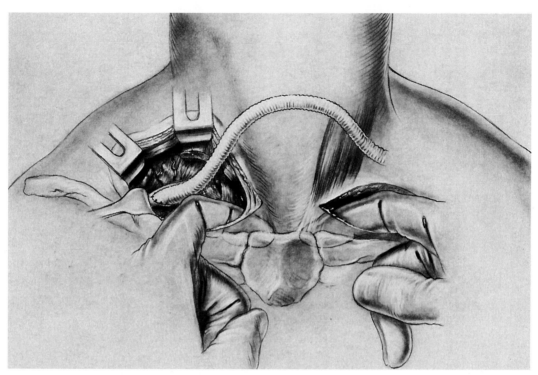

FIGURE 82–7. After completion of the anastomosis to the right subclavian artery, a tunnel is constructed between the right supraclavicular fossa and the left supraclavicular fossa behind the manubrium.

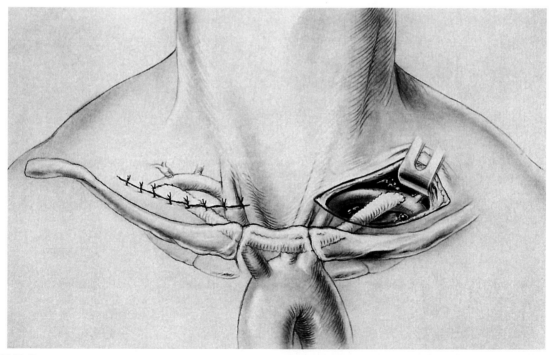

FIGURE 82–8. The prosthetic graft is drawn through the retromanubrial tunnel, and an anastomosis is constructed to the left subclavian artery.

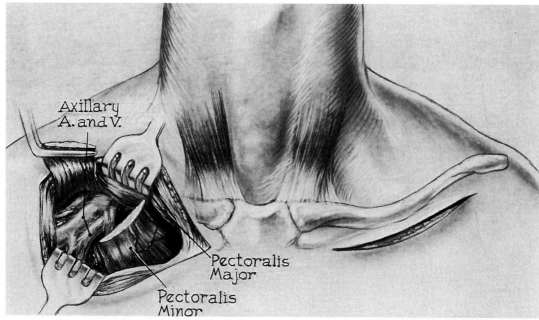

FIGURE 82–9. The right axillary artery is approached through an infraclavicular incision. After the heads of the pectoralis major muscle are split, the pectoralis minor muscle is divided to expose the axillary sheath.

lized. After a sufficient length of the axillary artery is prepared, the identical procedure is carried out on the opposite side. An 8-mm graft is appropriately beveled and anastomosed, end to side, to the axillary artery. A clamp is then placed on the distal portion of the graft next to the anastomosis; flow is re-established through the axillary artery. A subcutaneous tunnel, over the sternum, is developed. The graft is drawn through the tunnel in proximity to the opposite axillary artery (Fig. 82–10). An end-to-side anastomosis is

then constructed to the opposite end of the graft on the corresponding axillary artery, and blood flow is established (Fig. 82–11). The graft is protected by the greater pectoral muscle. The subcutaneous tissue and skin are closed in the usual fashion.

The major advantage of this bypass technique is the ease of exposing the axillary arteries, the relative strength of the axillary artery, and its usual freedom from atherosclerotic disease. The principal disadvantage of the technique involves

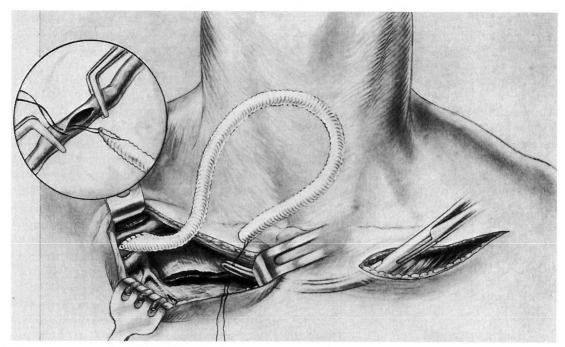

FIGURE 82–10. After the axillary artery is mobilized for a sufficient distance, it is clamped proximally and distally, an arteriotomy is made, and an end-to-side anastomosis is constructed between graft and artery. A heel and toe suture is placed and the anastomosis is constructed in quadrants. A tunnel is made from the left axillary incision to the right axillary incision over the sternum.

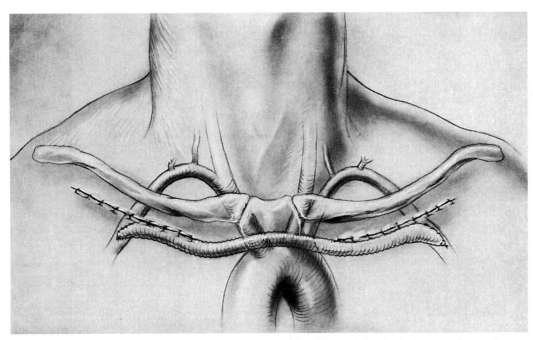

FIGURE 82–11. Demonstration of the completed axillary-to-axillary bypass graft as it is placed subcutaneously over the sternum.

the subcutaneous position of the graft over the sternum. Although this is usually well tolerated, there have been reported instances of graft erosion through the skin. Finally, in patients with diffuse atherosclerosis, it is not inconceivable that the patient may require coronary artery bypass grafting at some future date; the placement of this graft would be a problem for a medial sternotomy incision.

Left Subclavian to Right Common Carotid Artery Bypass

If it is the surgeon's preference to use a carotid to carotid bypass graft for innominate artery bypass, and if the left common carotid artery is diseased, an alternative technique is to use the left subclavian artery as an inflow source while preserving direct reperfusion of the right common carotid artery. The left subclavian artery is mobilized as described in Figures 82–5 through 82–8. The right common carotid artery is mobilized as described in Figures 82–2 through 82–4. An 8-mm graft is selected and appropriately beveled. An end-to-side anastomosis is constructed to the left subclavian artery. A clamp is placed at the distal portion of the graft, and flow is re-established through the subclavian artery. A retrosternomastoid retromanubrial tunnel between the left subclavian artery and the right common carotid artery is developed in a manner similar to that described in Figure 82–7. The graft is then brought into apposition with the right common carotid artery and an anastomosis is constructed as described in Figure 82–3. Before completion of the anastomosis, the common carotid artery is backbled and forwardbled. The graft is also flushed, the anastomosis completed, and blood flow begun first retrograde and then antegrade in the common carotid artery.

LESIONS OF THE COMMON CAROTID ARTERY

The common carotid artery can be affected by an atherosclerotic lesion at its origin from the aortic arch. Such a lesion may produce a high-grade stenosis with flow restriction, it may be the source of emboli, or it may produce a total occlusion by its progression with clot propagation to the carotid bifurcation. When this occurs, the clot may stop right at the bifurcation with the internal and external carotid arteries maintaining each other's patency by flow from the internal carotid to the external carotid or from the external carotid to the internal carotid arteries. This sequence is uncommon. The most common lesion of the left common carotid artery is total occlusion secondary to atherosclerotic plaquing at the carotid bifurcation, progressing to occlusion of the origin of both the internal and external carotid arteries with retrograde thrombosis down to the aortic arch. Surgical management for common carotid artery occlusion depends on the location of the atheromatous lesion initiating thrombosis.

Management of Lesions of the Origin of the Left Common Carotid Artery

When a lesion develops at the origin of the left common carotid artery (Fig. 82–12), symptoms may be generated in the ipsilateral hemisphere related to either flow reduction from high-grade stenosis or ulceration with embolization in the distribution of the left internal carotid artery. If the stenosis becomes critical, thrombosis of the common carotid artery with propagation to the carotid bifurcation can occur (Fig. 82–13). Options for repair include a left subclavian to common carotid artery bypass graft for restoration of blood flow or a left common to left subclavian transposition to restore blood flow and remove an embolic source.

Left Subclavian to Carotid Bypass

If the common carotid artery distal to the orifice lesion is patent, the operation can be performed entirely through a left supraclavicular incision. The incision is positioned one

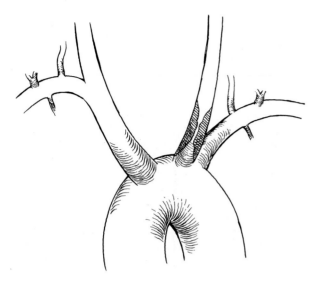

FIGURE 82–12. A stenotic lesion involving the origin of the left common carotid artery.

fingerbreadth above the clavicle and centered over the lateral head of the sternomastoid muscle. The incision is deepened through the platysmal layer, and the lateral head of the sternomastoid muscle is mobilized and divided. The scalene fat pad is mobilized superiorly, and the underlying scalenus anticus muscle and phrenic nerve are identified in a manner similar to exposure of the right subclavian artery (Fig. 82–6). The phrenic nerve is mobilized and the anterior scalene muscle encompassed and divided. This places the operator directly over the subclavian artery, which is carefully mobilized for a distance sufficient for an end-to-side anastomosis. Attention is then turned to the left carotid sheath, which is

approached posterior to the medial head of the sternocleido-mastoid muscle. The jugular vein is mobilized, with particular care taken to identify, clamp, and ligate the thoracic duct. Care is also taken to avoid injury to the vagus nerve. The left common carotid artery is then identified and mobilized for a distance sufficient for an end-to-side anastomosis. The short graft is then placed in a double end-to-side fashion, connecting the left subclavian with the left common carotid artery. The left subclavian artery then becomes a source of blood flow for the left common carotid artery as well as the left arm (Fig. 82–14).

Left Common to Subclavian Transposition

In the event that the clinician is suspicious that the lesion at the origin of the left common carotid artery may be a source of emboli, it is essential that this lesion be removed

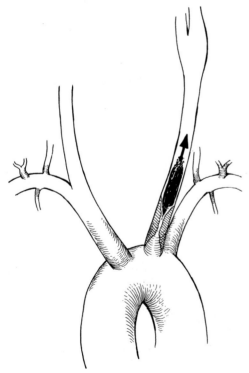

FIGURE 82–13. When the stenotic lesion of the left common carotid artery reaches a critical level, thrombosis will occur distal to the lesion, with propagation toward the carotid bifurcation.

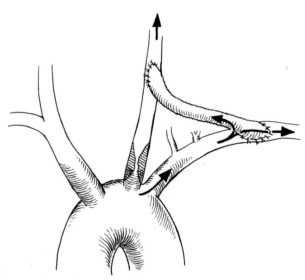

FIGURE 82–14. Demonstration of a functioning graft between the left subclavian artery and the left common carotid artery. Note that bidirectional blood flow takes place in the subclavian artery going to the arm as well as going to the left common carotid artery through the graft.

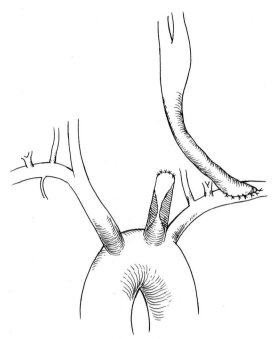

FIGURE 82–15. Completion of a left common carotid to left subclavian artery transposition. The left subclavian artery now provides blood flow to the arm as well as to the left common carotid artery in a manner similar to the innominate artery.

from the circulation to the carotid artery. The most direct means of accomplishing this end is a transposition of the left common carotid artery to the subclavian artery with a ligation of the proximal left common carotid artery. This is approached in an identical manner to a subclavian to carotid bypass grafting procedure. The left common carotid artery is mobilized as far proximal as possible. It is then clamped, ligated, and divided. The carotid artery is then transposed to the subclavian artery, and an anastomosis is constructed in an end-to-side fashion (Fig. 82–15).

Management of Carotid Artery Occlusion Secondary to Carotid Bifurcation Occlusion and Retrograde Thrombosis

Retrograde Thrombectomy and Bifurcation Endarterectomy of the Left Carotid Artery

When the mechanism of left common carotid artery thrombosis is retrograde propagation of clot secondary to atheromatous obstruction of the carotid bifurcation (as it usually is), restoration of blood flow can be accomplished by thrombectomy of the common carotid artery in conjunction with an endarterectomy of the carotid bifurcation. Under these circumstances, the internal carotid artery is usually occluded, but the external carotid artery will be patent immediately beyond the superior thyroid branch. The left supraclavicular fossa should be prepared in case it is not possible to carry out retrograde thrombectomy. Under these circumstances, a left subclavian to carotid bypass or carotid to subclavian transposition will serve equally well.

The procedure is begun after the left side of the neck

and left supraclavicular fossa are prepared. The field is appropriately draped for either operative procedure. An incision is placed along the anterior border of the sternocleidomastoid muscle and centered over the carotid bifurcation. Dissection is carried down through the platysmal layer, and the sternomastoid muscle is mobilized off the carotid sheath and held in place with self-retaining retractors. The carotid sheath is entered along the anterior border of the jugular vein. The common facial vein is identified, clamped, divided, and ligated. This then permits retraction of the jugular vein and exposure of the common carotid artery as well as the carotid artery bifurcation. The carotid artery and carotid bifurcation are fully mobilized. The internal carotid and external carotid arteries are also mobilized appropriately. At this point, it is usually possible to determine whether the internal carotid artery is patent or occluded. It is also possible to determine the presence of atheromatous plaque at the carotid bifurcation leading to retrograde thrombosis of the common carotid artery (Fig. 82–16). If the internal carotid artery is obviously occluded, it can be detached flush with the common carotid artery as the beginning of an arteriotomy on the common carotid artery. This arteriotomy can be extended proximally on the common carotid artery and distally onto the medial aspect of the external carotid in order to provide sufficient exposure for removal of the atheromatous lesion as well as retrograde thrombectomy. It is important to emphasize that the removal of the thrombus does not include removal of the intima in the common carotid artery. Thus it is mandatory to establish a dissection plane between the organized thrombus and the intima of the common carotid artery. An endarterectomy stripper can then be placed

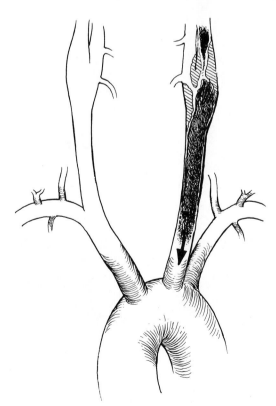

FIGURE 82–16. Retrograde thrombosis of the left common carotid artery secondary to an occlusive lesion of the carotid bifurcation involving the origins of the internal and external carotid arteries.

over the organized thrombus between the thrombus and the intima.

The stripper is gently advanced toward the aortic arch (Fig. 82–17). Once the thrombus is free down to the level of the aortic arch, arterial pressure will usually help propel the organized thrombotic plug out the arteriotomy, thus re-establishing arterial inflow (Fig. 82–18). Following establishment of inflow, an endarterectomy of the carotid bifurcation and origin of the external carotid artery can be carried out. The arteriotomy can be closed either with a prosthetic patch or with an autogenous patch made from a segment of occluded internal carotid artery (Fig. 82–19).

Should the internal carotid artery be patent, the arteriotomy is made on the common carotid artery and extended up onto the internal carotid artery in preparation for a stan-

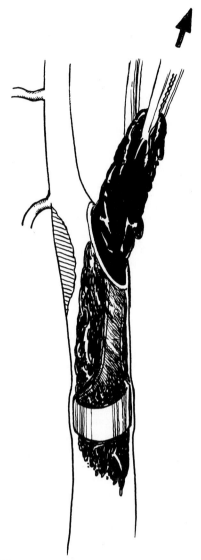

FIGURE 82–18. After the thrombus has been freed down to the level of the aortic arch, withdrawal of the thrombus through the orifice of the common carotid artery will permit re-establishment of normal blood flow.

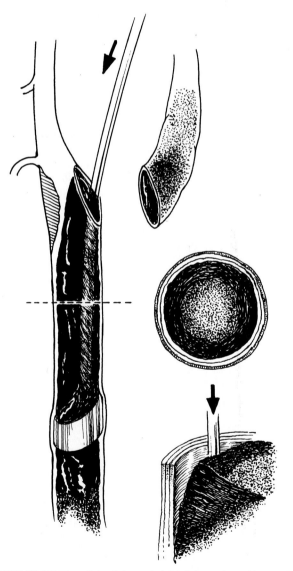

FIGURE 82–17. The origin of the occluded left internal carotid artery has been detached, allowing access to the left common carotid artery. This arteriotomy can be enlarged by extending it proximally and distally. Note the establishment of a plane between the chronic organized thrombus and the intact intima of the common carotid artery. It is this plane that is developed by passing an endarterectomy stripper to free up the thrombus from the intima.

dard bifurcation endarterectomy in conjunction with the retrograde thrombectomy procedure.

If it is not possible to achieve retrograde thrombectomy, the left subclavian artery is exposed, and either the common carotid artery is transposed to the left subclavian artery or an interposition graft is placed between the left subclavian and the proximal left common carotid artery for re-establishment of blood flow.

LESIONS OF THE LEFT SUBCLAVIAN ARTERY

The left subclavian artery is the aortic arch trunk most frequently involved with atheromatous disease at its origin (Fig. 82–20). Symptoms can occur from deprivation of blood flow to the left vertebral artery, from reversal of flow in the left vertebral artery (subclavian steal syndrome), and from compromised blood flow or embolization to the left arm.

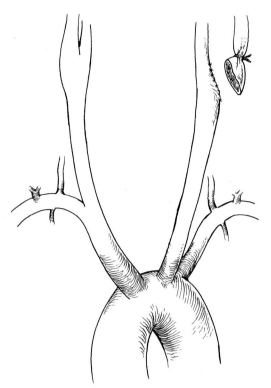

FIGURE 82–19. Primary closure of the arteriotomy after endarterectomy of the carotid bifurcation and retrograde thrombectomy of the common carotid artery.

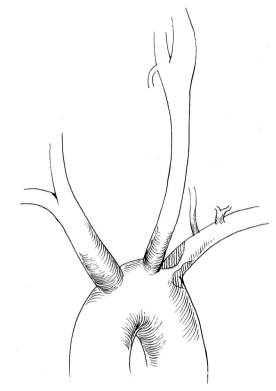

FIGURE 82–20. A lesion involving the origin of the left subclavian artery.

The operative procedures available for restoration of blood flow to the left subclavian artery include a left common carotid to left subclavian artery bypass and a left subclavian to left common carotid artery transposition.

If the objective of surgery is to increase blood flow to the left subclavian-vertebral system, no particular attention need be paid to the lesion of the origin of the left subclavian artery. By contrast, if the lesion of the left subclavian artery is generating emboli to the arm, the flow past that lesion must be interrupted either by clipping the left subclavian artery proximal to the vertebral takeoff or by transposing the left subclavian artery to the carotid artery.

Left Carotid to Subclavian Bypass

This operation can be accomplished through a left supraclavicular incision. The left subclavian and common carotid arteries are mobilized as described earlier. A graft of the surgeon's choice is selected. The choice of which anastomosis to perform first depends on the individual patient's anatomy. I usually prefer to do the subclavian anastomosis first. After the anastomosis is completed, a soft-jawed bulldog clamp can be placed in the most proximal portion of the graft; the common carotid artery is then clamped proximally and distally after the backpressure of the common carotid artery is measured. An arteriotomy is made, approximately 14 mm in length, and the graft is appropriately beveled. An end-to-side anastomosis is constructed with a running suture. Before completion of the anastomosis, the common carotid artery is backbled and forwardbled, and the subclavian artery is backbled through the graft. The anastomosis is completed.

Flow is restored to the subclavian artery by removal of clamps (Fig. 82–21).

If the patient was having symptoms secondary to emboli from the lesion of the left subclavian artery, it is necessary to interrupt flow from the proximal subclavian artery. The

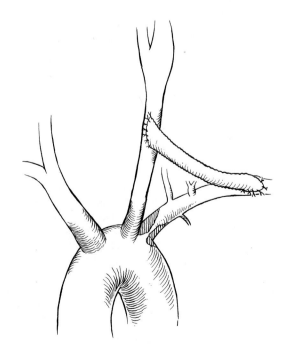

FIGURE 82–21. Completed graft, re-establishing blood flow to the left subclavian artery from the left common carotid artery.

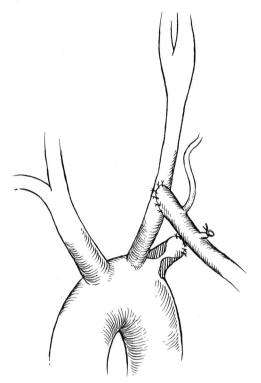

FIGURE 82–22. Completion of the anastomosis transposing the left subclavian artery to the left common carotid artery. Note sufficient mobilization of the left vertebral artery to avoid kinking of this vessel when the subclavian artery is repositioned.

simplest way to do this is to place a large clip proximal to the left vertebral artery or to clamp and oversew the subclavian artery proximal to the vertebral artery.

Left Subclavian to Common Carotid Artery Transposition

The advantage of this operation is that it is done entirely with autogenous tissue, obviating the need for prosthetic grafts. The disadvantage of the operation is that it requires extensive mobilization of the left subclavian artery, proximal to the left vertebral artery. The left vertebral artery often originates at a relatively proximal location, making mobilization of sufficient subclavian artery difficult at best. If the arteriogram demonstrates a relatively favorable location of the origin of the left vertebral artery, this surgical procedure is quite appropriate.

The approach is made through a left supraclavicular incision, as described earlier. After sufficient mobilization of the left subclavian artery, proximal to the left vertebral artery, the common carotid artery is also appropriately mobilized. The left subclavian artery is then clamped as far proximally as is feasible, and the left subclavian artery is divided with appropriate control of backbleeding from the vertebral and subclavian vessels distally. The clamp is oversewn, the vertebral artery is mobilized sufficiently to avoid kinking, and the left subclavian artery is brought into apposition with the left common carotid artery. The common carotid artery is clamped proximally and distally, and an arteriotomy is made. An anastomosis between the end of the subclavian artery

and the side of the common carotid artery is carried out (Fig. 82–22).

OCCLUSIVE LESIONS OF ALL THREE AORTIC ARCH TRUNKS

On occasion, a patient may present with major obstruction of all three trunks of the aortic arch, including the innominate artery, the left common carotid artery, and the left subclavian arteries. Under these circumstances, the optimum approach is a transmediastinal repair. On occasion, the patient may not be a surgical candidate for a direct approach. An extra-anatomic repair is feasible if the patient has intact blood flow to the aortofemoral system. A bypass graft from the right femoral artery to the right axillary artery and a secondary bypass from the right carotid artery to the left carotid artery will satisfactorily restore blood flow to both carotid arteries and the right vertebral artery.

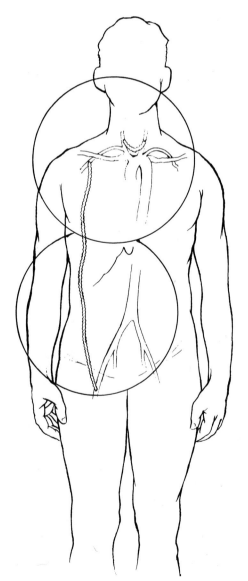

FIGURE 82–23. Large view perspective of a right femoral-to-axillary bypass graft in conjunction with a carotid-to-carotid bypass graft.

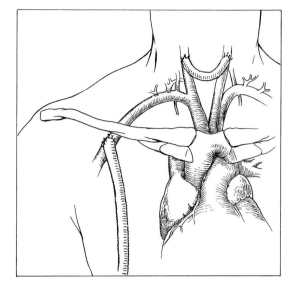

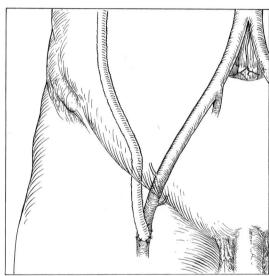

FIGURE 82–24. The upper view demonstrates the distal anastomosis to the right axillary artery, establishing new blood flow to the right subclavian or right common carotid artery. The left common carotid artery is perfused by connecting the right common carotid with the left common carotid artery. This effectively bypasses occlusive lesions of the innominate and left carotid arteries.

Femoral-Axillary and Carotid-Carotid Artery Bypass

The patient is prepared from the chin to the thighs and is appropriately draped. The operation is begun by exposure of the right axillary artery as described in Figure 82–9 and both common carotid arteries as described in Figure 82–2. The right femoral artery is then exposed in the usual fashion. I prefer to use an 8-mm ring-reinforced PTFE graft for the femoral to axillary bypass. I perform the femoral anastomosis in an end-to-side fashion in the usual manner. A tunneling instrument then connects the right axillary with the right femoral wound, and the graft is brought into position to the right axillary artery. An end-to-side anastomosis is constructed to the right axillary artery and flow is re-established. This will perfuse the right subclavian-axillary system as well as the right common carotid artery. Depending on the patient's symptoms, this may be sufficient to restore blood flow for correction of global ischemia. A carotid-to-carotid bypass can be performed at this time or during a second stage. The carotid-to-carotid bypass is performed as described in Figures 82–3 and 82–4. The end result is visualized in Figures 82–23 and 82–24.

Immediate and Long-Term Results of Brachiocephalic Repair: Direct Versus Extrathoracic Operations

ROBERT G. ATNIP and DAVID C. BREWSTER

The first detailed descriptions of brachiocephalic arterial occlusive disease were published by Martorell and Fabre in 1944 (atherosclerotic lesions)[1] and by Shimuzu and Sano in 1951 (Takayasu arteritis).[2] The first successful operative repairs were reported by Davis and coworkers in 1956[3] and by DeBakey and associates in 1958.[4] The first large series of patients treated surgically was subsequently reported by Crawford and colleagues in 1962.[5] These initial reconstructions consisted of either endarterectomy or direct bypass, performed through a transthoracic approach and attended by perioperative mortality rates (from ischemic heart disease) as high as 20 percent. In an effort to simplify the operative procedure and reduce the operative risk, a variety of extrathoracic procedures were developed,[6] beginning with the carotid-subclavian bypass in 1957.[7] In the ensuing decades, a number of centers have accumulated extensive experience in the management of brachiocephalic occlusive disease, using both intrathoracic and extracavitary techniques.

The methods of surgical repair of brachiocephalic vessels were extensively described in the preceding chapters of this book. The focus of this chapter is the examination and comparison of perioperative morbidity and mortality, as well as the early and long-term results of transthoracic versus extrathoracic reconstruction. The basis of the analysis in this chapter is a review of every major series of brachiocephalic reconstructions reported in the English literature since 1975 (Table 83–1). Some of these reports include groups of patients who were originally described in earlier publications, and thus the data include the vast majority of patients reported since 1956. All of these series are retrospective and exhibit all the limitations inherent in such case-control studies.

LIMITATIONS OF COMPARISONS

It is important to realize that brachiocephalic occlusive disease is characterized by imprecise correlation between symptoms and morbid anatomy. Although lesions of the brachiocephalic vessels may be detected by angiography or at autopsy in patients with diffuse atherosclerosis, patients with such lesions often lack any corresponding symptoms, probably because of the rich collateral networks of the brain and upper extremities.[8–10] When symptoms do occur, they can reflect ischemia of the arm, the cerebral hemispheres, the brain stem, or combinations of vascular beds, which creates a confusing clinical picture.[11] Furthermore, atherosclerosis can involve many sites and levels of the aortic arch branches, making it difficult or impossible to determine which lesion is responsible for which symptoms. It has been well demonstrated, for example, that carotid bifurcation endarterectomy may suffice to relieve ischemic neurologic symptoms in patients who also have more proximal innominate or carotid stenoses.[8, 12] Moreover, at least one investiga-

tor has reported spontaneous resolution of symptoms in patients managed nonoperatively.[13] Patients can suffer graft thrombosis and have no symptoms, or can exhibit nonspecific symptoms such as vertigo or headache in the absence of any arterial occlusion. For all the foregoing reasons, one must exercise caution when analyzing reported outcomes of treatment in a group of patients with brachiocephalic occlusive disease.

Any discussion of brachiocephalic occlusive disease must also include a careful consideration of the term "subclavian steal syndrome." Contorni in 1960[14] and Reivich and associates in 1961[15] were the first to demonstrate angiographically the presence of reversal of flow ("steal") in the vertebral arteries of a particular group of patients who had proximal subclavian stenosis or occlusion in association with brainstem ischemic neurologic symptoms (ataxia, vertigo, visual disturbances, and drop attacks). In 70 percent of such patients, the lesion is in the left subclavian artery and is more likely to be an occlusion than a stenosis. Yet there is no unequivocal evidence that the symptoms actually result from diminished intracranial flow,[16, 17] and in a large number of patients, the angiographic finding is not associated with any symptoms.[18, 19] Some investigators feel that the term "subclavian steal" should only be used if the neurologic symptoms are provoked by ipsilateral arm exercise,[20] but most use the designation loosely to apply to a constellation

TABLE 83–1. Brachiocephalic Reconstruction

Study*	Patients, n		Follow-up, years†
	T	E	
AbuRahma, et al[40]	—	67	6
Brewster et al[27]	29	8	4.2
Carlson et al[28]	34	—	6
Cherry et al[41]	26	—	3.6
Cormier et al[42]	53	—	4.2
Crawford et al[22]	43	99	7.5
Criado[6]	—	787	NA
DePalma and Broadbent[33]	9	16	Up to 13
Deriu and Ballotta[32]	7	27	3 to 8
Gross et al[36]	5	14	4
Liljeqvist et al[29]	85	—	6
Livesay et al[30]	—	31	3.6
Luosto et al[13]	63	58	3.5
Moore et al[31]	—	26	Up to 11
Raithel[23]	30	37	2
Reul et al[43]	38	16	Up to 10
Schroeder and Buchardt-Hansen[18]	30	35	3.6
Thompson et al[24]	16	78	Up to 17
Vogt et al[25]	34	66	4.3
Wylie and Effeney[26]	50	96	Up to 20
Zelenock et al[34]	17	—	2.6

*For full bibliographic information, see reference list at end of chapter.
†Reported as mean unless indicated.
E, extrathoracic approach; NA, information not available; T, transthoracic approach.

of symptoms associated with brachiocephalic occlusive disease, whether or not reversal of vertebral flow is seen angiographically. In any given report, one must carefully note which definition is in effect.

This chapter is divided into two major sections. The first section examines the major causes of perioperative morbidity and mortality for brachiocephalic arterial surgery and compares the operative risks of transthoracic and extrathoracic procedures. The second portion considers the late complications and long-term success of surgical therapy for this condition.

EARLY RESULTS

Operative Mortality

In the series reviewed, the major causes of early death after either thoracic or extra-anatomic surgery on the aortic arch branches were myocardial infarction, cerebrovascular accident (both infarction and hemorrhage), and technical complications (Table 83–2). In series in which both approaches were utilized by the same surgeons, the mortality rate was virtually always significantly higher in patients undergoing thoracotomy or sternotomy.[21–27] Mortality was generally 3 to 6 percent for patients undergoing direct repair, although figures as high as 15 percent[25] and 20 percent[24] were encountered. Surgeons who used the transthoracic ap-

proach exclusively did not achieve a lower mortality rate (death rates of 6–8%).[28, 29] By contrast, death was unusual after extrathoracic surgery, and in many series, there were no deaths in this group.[6, 13, 23–27, 30, 31] In isolated instances, the rate of mortality was higher in the extra-anatomic cohort,[18] or there were no deaths in either group.[32–34] It must be re-emphasized, however, that none of these reports was prospective or randomized.

Age and extent of concomitant medical problems were seldom specified for each group, except that ill-defined "poorer risk" patients were generally managed by extrathoracic methods if possible. To the extent that this was true, the patients at higher risk experienced a lower operative mortality by undergoing extrathoracic reconstruction. Most perioperative deaths were caused by myocardial infarction, stroke, or technical misadventures, as is discussed in the following sections.

Myocardial Infarction

Myocardial infarction was the leading single cause of death after transthoracic surgery, accounting for some 30 to 50 percent of early mortality in most series and 100 percent in some. Among patients with brachiocephalic occlusive disease, as among vascular surgical patients in general, there is a high incidence of coronary artery disease (CAD), as manifested by a history of angina pectoris, prior myocardial infarction, congestive heart failure, or the presence of elec-

Study*	Operation Type	Patients, n	Deaths, n	Fatal MI, n	Fatal CVA, n
AbuRahma et al[40]	E	67	2	2	0
Brewster et al[27]	T	29	1	0	0
	E	8	0	0	0
Carlson et al[28]	T	34	2	2	0
Cherry et al[41]	T	26	1	0	0
Cormier et al[42]	T	53	1	1	0
Crawford et al[22]	T	43	2	0	1
	E	99	1	0	1
Criado[6]	E	787	10	3	4
DePalma and Broadbent[33]	T	9	0	0	0
	E	16	0	0	0
Deriu and Ballotta[32]	T	7	0	0	0
	E	27	0	0	0
Gross et al[36]	Combined	21	2	0	0
Liljeqvist et al[29]	T	85	5	1	3
Livesay et al[30]	E	31	1	NA	NA
Luosto et al[13]	T	63	2	0	1
	E	58	1	1	0
Moore et al[31]	E	26	1	1	0
Raithel[23]	T	30	2	1	0
	E	37	0	0	0
Reul et al[43]	T	38	0	0	0
	E	16	0	0	0
Schroeder and Buchardt-Hansen[18]	T	30	0	0	0
	E	35	1	0	0
Thompson et al[24]	T	16	3	0	1
	E	78	0	0	0
Vogt et al[25]	T	34	5	2	1
	E	66	0	0	0
Wylie and Effeney[26]	T	50	2	1	1
	E	96	0	0	0
Zelenock et al[34]	T	17	0	0	0

TABLE 83–2. Early Mortality

*For full bibliographic information, see reference list at end of chapter.
NA, information not available; T, transthoracic; E, extrathoracic; CVA, cerebrovascular accident; MI, myocardial infarction.

trocardiographic changes.[18, 25, 31] Vogt and colleagues at the Cleveland Clinic[25] have suggested that patients with peripheral vascular disease be studied aggressively to define the extent of CAD and that patients with either symptomatic or anatomically severe CAD undergo coronary revascularization prior to or in conjunction with repair of the aortic arch branches. Other investigators have made similar recommendations.[35] In Vogt's series, however, the operative mortality rate was no higher in patients with clinically suspected coronary disease than in those without it.

Myocardial infarction was the most frequent cause of death after extrathoracic operation as well,[6, 13, 31] which simply underscores the prevalence of potentially lethal CAD in this patient population. Meticulous anesthetic management and postoperative care are required to minimize the risk of myocardial ischemia and its complications.

Cerebrovascular Accident

The second major cause of perioperative death in these series was cerebrovascular accident, both thromboembolic and hemorrhagic. The strokes usually occurred in the area of distribution of the operated vessels and could be attributed directly to the operation, although this was not uniformly the case.[6, 13, 22, 24–26, 29] Not surprisingly, Crawford and coworkers[22] found that stroke was more likely to occur in patients with atherosclerosis involving the distal vessels, particularly the internal carotid artery, or multiple arch branches. Fatal stroke was more common after thoracic surgery, probably because this approach was mandated in patients who had multiple-vessel disease and were thus more susceptible to cerebral ischemia. Wylie and Effeney[26] reported one fatal stroke in a patient whose left common carotid orifice was inadvertently included in the aortic clamp during innominate endarterectomy.

Strokes following extraanatomic reconstruction tended to be delayed and were usually due to either graft thrombosis or presumed embolism. Two cerebral hemorrhages in this group were probably not directly related to operation, but a third occurred in a patient on anticoagulant therapy as part of the surgeon's routine postoperative care.[29] Of interest, there were no fatal strokes in patients who underwent simultaneous carotid bifurcation endarterectomy, although several nonfatal strokes and transient deficits occurred after this procedure. In only one patient (who died of a stroke postoperatively) was it postulated that the use of an intraluminal shunt might have prevented the stroke.[13] This was a patient whose innominate artery was clamped for endarterectomy, but no further details were provided by the authors as to the status of the other vessels or of the carotid bifurcation.

The arguments for and against the use of shunts in brachiocephalic arterial surgery have been presented in previous chapters and will not be reiterated here. The authors of these reports discussed in this chapter used various methods for cerebral protection, including routine shunting,[13, 29] routine nonshunting,[25] and electroencephalographic monitoring.[27] Since most of the fatal strokes occurred more than 24 hours after surgery, it is unlikely that the method of cerebral protection was a major factor in stroke mortality.

Technical Difficulties

The third category of postoperative deaths consisted of those due to technical errors, which tended to occur early in the experience of the surgeons involved. Crawford and associates[22] reported on a patient who died of airway obstruction caused by compression by a bulky Dacron graft (with several limbs) that had been implanted in the mediastinum to bypass multiple vessel occlusions. Vogt and coworkers[25] performed simultaneous mitral valve replacement, aortoinnominate, and aortocoronary grafts on a patient who died several hours after surgery as a result of exsanguination from a tear in the left ventricle caused by a strut of the prosthetic valve ring. Another death by exsanguination occurred in a patient of Thompson and colleagues[24] and was caused by an aortic clamp injury at the level of the left subclavian origin. Finally, Raithel[23] reported a death from respiratory failure due to massive chylothorax, presumably caused by transection of the thoracic duct during a thoracotomy for subclavian artery reconstruction. Of note is that all of these fatal technical errors occurred in patients who underwent a trans-sternal or transthoracic operation.

Other Deaths

The remainder of the perioperative deaths were caused by a variety of unusual problems. Some of these were related to the type of arterial reconstruction being performed. These included pericardial tamponade after an innominate reconstruction,[25] early graft infection with ultimate death from hemorrhage after a subclavian-carotid graft,[18] and acute subclavian thrombosis following transthoracic repair, which eventually led to mural thrombosis of the aortic arch.[24] The other miscellaneous deaths were caused by conditions not peculiar to major arterial surgery, including bleeding ulcer,[13] uremia and liver failure,[6] pneumonia,[29] mesenteric infarction,[27] and pulmonary embolus.[36] The patients who died from uremia, liver failure, and graft infection had undergone extra-anatomic procedures, but the remainder were into the transthoracic category.

Early Complications

A number of complications occurred within the first 30 days after brachiocephalic reconstruction. The two most common problems were stroke and graft occlusion, but a variety of others were also reported, including bleeding, wound problems, nerve palsies, and graft infection.

Cerebrovascular Accident

Nonfatal cerebrovascular events were a major source of morbidity, occurring in up to 8 percent of patients in some series.[6, 13, 18, 22, 25, 27, 28, 30–32] A few affected patients recovered completely, but many were left with permanent neurologic deficits. These events were all caused by arterial thrombosis or embolism, and all except one occurred in the area of distribution of the operated vessel. In some patients, the deficits were immediately noted postoperatively, and in others, they developed hours to days later. Two of the strokes occurred as a result of technical error; one consisted of worsening of a pre-existing deficit caused by unavoidable clamping of both innominate and left carotid orifices to control bleeding at the origin of the innominate artery.[27] The other stroke occurred in a patient whose left common carotid artery had to be ligated to prevent exsanguinating hemorrhage after a complicated extra-anatomic procedure and several emergency reoperations.[12] Nonfatal strokes were numerically more common after extrathoracic procedures, but a significant correlation seems unlikely.

Crawford and colleagues[22] found that the risk of stroke was highest in those patients with either multiple-vessel or internal carotid artery disease. Criado,[6] Deriu and Ballotta,[32] Moore and colleagues,[31] and Vogt and colleagues[25] demonstrated a similar association in their series. Patients who sustained strokes after brachiocephalic repair in these series had either known occlusion of the ipsilateral internal carotid artery or a severe stenosis that was treated with a simultaneous carotid bifurcation endarterectomy. None of these patients received intraluminal shunts during operation, but as all of the deficits were delayed, shunting would probably not have influenced the outcome. This experience might seem to indicate an increased risk of stroke associated with simultaneous operation on the internal carotid artery, but this does not hold true when all patients' histories are analyzed. Crawford and associates[22] performed 28 simultaneous carotid endarterectomies, and none of the postoperative strokes that occurred among his patients occurred in this subgroup. Livesay and coworkers[30] and Schroeder and Buchardt-Hansen[18] had smaller numbers of concomitant procedures but similar stroke-free results. A more valid conclusion would be that untreated carotid bifurcation disease poses a significant hazard to patients undergoing operation on the proximal aortic arch branches and should be treated either before or at the same time as the proximal reconstruction is performed.

Early Graft Thrombosis

Early thrombosis following either endarterectomy or bypass of vessels other than the carotid artery was occasionally encountered. Its incidence ranged from 1 to 3 percent[6, 18, 23, 24, 30] to as high as 10 percent.[13, 36] Although both saphenous vein and prosthetic grafts (mostly Dacron) were used for bypass procedures, none of the authors specified which grafts thrombosed. The diagnosis was usually readily apparent on physical examination because of the absence of appropriate pulses, and immediate re-exploration was undertaken in all instances. Thrombectomy was successful except for two cases. These were patients with coexistent subclavian and distal upper extremity occlusive disease, whose subclavian reconstructions thrombosed, apparently owing to "poor runoff." Arm amputations were required in both cases.[36] In none of the other instances was any explanation offered as to the cause of thrombosis. There was no apparent difference in incidence according to whether transthoracic or extra-anatomic operation had been performed.

Other Early Complications

Other reported perioperative complications included bleeding, wound infection, graft infection, sternal dehiscence, nerve palsies, false aneurysm formation, pneumothorax, and chylothorax. Curiously enough, only one nonfatal myocardial infarction was reported, in a patient who had undergone a trans-sternal innominate endarterectomy. The number of these miscellaneous problems was approximately equal in the transthoracic and extra-anatomic categories, although obviously some problems such as sternal de-

hiscence were peculiar to one approach. One complication that occurred with disturbing frequency in some series was major nerve injury and palsy. Luosto and associates[13] reported two stellate ganglion injuries and two phrenic nerve palsies, all in patients operated on through the neck. Schroeder and Buchardt-Hansen[18] had four patients with nerve injuries, one phrenic and two recurrent laryngeal after extrathoracic procedures and one recurrent laryngeal nerve palsy after a thoracotomy. Thompson and colleagues[24] noted a vocal cord palsy after a left thoracotomy for subclavian endarterectomy. In Criado's review, there was a 10 percent incidence of median nerve dysfunction after axilloaxillary bypass.[6] Several lymph fistulas were also reported, most occurring after cervical operation in the region of the thoracic duct. This experience emphasizes the necessity of meticulous surgical technique and thorough knowledge of the anatomy, especially in the supraclavicular region where vessels lie deep and exposure can be limited.

LATE RESULTS

Patients who survived the perioperative period remained susceptible to a variety of late complications. A significant number succumbed, either to progressive atherosclerosis or to other intercurrent diseases.

Long-Term Survival

The mean age of patients undergoing repair of aortic arch branches in these series ranged from 50 to 60 years—somewhat younger than that of patients with lower extremity atherosclerosis, but still advanced enough that a significant late mortality would be expected. When actuarial survival was plotted in these series, it was lower than expected for a population of this age. The 5-, 10-, and 15-year actuarial survival rates in the series of Crawford and coworkers[22] were 85, 58, and 25 percent, respectively. Among patients in the group of Vogt and coworkers,[25] 5- and 10-year survival rates were 84 and 45 percent, respectively. Moore and associates[31] calculated a crude 5-year survival of only 47 percent, and only 62 percent of patients treated by Gross and colleagues[36] were alive at 5 years. Among investigators who did not compute interval survival rates, 10 to 25 percent of patients died over mean follow-up periods of 2 to 6 years, confirming a substantial late death rate in this population.[6, 13, 18, 23–25, 27–33] However, it is of interest that 5-year survival rates among patients undergoing brachiocephalic repair are substantially better than those of patients undergoing carotid bifurcation endarterectomy.[37]

Myocardial Infarction

Myocardial infarction was the chief cause of late death, just as it was the primary cause of perioperative death. Myocardial infarction accounted for 50 to 80 percent of late mortality in most reports and 100 percent in some. Although clinical evidence of CAD was not a useful predictor of early myocardial infarction, it *was* accurate in predicting late death, at least in the Cleveland Clinic experience.[25] In those patients with suspected CAD, 60 percent of late deaths were caused by myocardial infarction. By contrast, only 12 percent of patients with no clinical evidence of CAD eventually succumbed to myocardial ischemia.

Unfortunately, none of the reports segregated late deaths according to whether the operation was transthoracic or extrathoracic; thus, no valid conclusions can be drawn as to the influence of operative approach on late mortality.

Stroke and Malignancy

The next two most common causes of death were cancer and stroke, in that order. The location of the cancer malignancies was usually not specified. Similarly, information about stroke deaths was often obtained from family members or death certificates; thus the site or cause of the stroke was seldom known. Crawford and associates[22] reported the largest number of late deaths from stroke (11 of 140 patients), probably because they had the longest mean follow-up period (7.5 years). These deaths occurred a mean of 9 years after surgery. Whether any of them was caused by complication of the vascular reconstruction is not known. The single late stroke mortality in Vogt's group[25] was a patient who died of a midbrain infarction several years after a vertebral artery reconstruction, but again, the actual cause of the stroke was undetermined.

Other Late Deaths

Two other causes of death deserve special mention. Criado[6] reported two deaths that occurred as a result of infection of extra-anatomic Dacron grafts. One of these was a carotid to axillary artery graft that became infected from skin erosion where it had been tunneled *over* the clavicle. Another catastrophe that claimed several lives was mesenteric infarction,[13, 18, 28] a complication well known among vascular surgical patients.

The remainder of late deaths resulted from an assortment of conditions common to individuals of this age group. Several patients expired of chronic pulmonary disease, an expected finding in a population in which 80 to 100 percent of patients are current or former cigarette smokers. Other lethal conditions included renal failure, intestinal perforation, gastrointestinal bleeding, pulmonary embolus, pneumonia, and peritonitis.

Late Complications

The three most frequent late complications seen after brachiocephalic reconstruction were graft occlusion, graft infection, and stroke.

Graft Thrombosis

Graft occlusions occurred as early as 2 months after surgery and as late as 8 years. There was a definite predominance of this complication in patients who underwent extra-anatomic procedures, and the great majority of failed grafts were saphenous vein carotid-subclavian bypasses. Late thrombosis occurred in 10 to 25 percent of vein grafts over periods of 2 to 6 years,[6, 22–27, 29–31] similar to developments seen in femoropopliteal vein grafts.[38] Thrombosis of Dacron grafts in both the chest and the neck was occasionally seen, but much less often. Late occlusion of innominate and

subclavian endarterectomies was rare, except in the series by Liljeqvist and associates,[29] in which 9 of 83 vessels eventually occluded after endarterectomy.

The symptomatic status of most of the patients with graft occlusion was not recorded. Among those in whom symptom status was noted, two thirds had no symptoms resulting from graft thrombosis, and one third had recurrence of the original symptoms for which the operation had been performed. Five of these eight symptomatic patients underwent successful thrombectomy or graft revision. Asymptomatic graft thrombosis was not treated, nor was any mention made of reoperation among the large group for whom symptom status was not reported. It is of interest that all patients who underwent surgery for brachiocephalic occlusive disease presented originally with either arm or neurologic symptoms, yet most with failed reconstructions had no recurrence of those symptoms. This is in marked contrast to what occurs following lower extremity arterial repair, failure of which usually results in return or actual worsening of ischemic symptoms.[38]

The suspected cause of graft failure was generally not mentioned, but at least in the case of saphenous vein grafts, it is reasonable to postulate that proliferative changes in the graft and at the anastomoses played a significant role. Such changes were thoroughly studied in femoropopliteal grafts by Szilagyi and coworkers.[39] Gross and colleagues[36] maintain that graft failures are less common in upper extremity reconstructions, but little has been written about the pathology of brachiocephalic vein graft failure. Wylie and Effeney[26] believe that the acute angulation and consequent redirection of blood flow that occur at the proximal anastomosis of most cervical extra-anatomic grafts may contribute to both immediate and delayed thrombosis. Length and location of grafts may influence the late failure rate as well. Among these series, there were several reported occlusions of Dacron axillo-axillary grafts, which of necessity are long and must be tunneled anterior to the sternum. One half of the failures in this group were strongly suspected to have resulted from compression of the graft against the sternum during sleep.[6, 24]

On the basis of this experience, most vascular surgeons would agree that a Dacron graft is preferable to a saphenous vein graft in brachiocephalic reconstruction, unless there are mitigating circumstances, such as infection, that preclude the use of synthetic graft material. Most of these grafts are short in length and high in flow, and the vessels involved are often substantially larger than the average saphenous vein. In addition, the use of Dacron obviates the need to harvest vein from a remote operative field and spares the saphenous vein for potential use in coronary or lower extremity revascularization.

Graft Infection

In spite of the advantages of prosthetic material, its use does introduce the risk of infection. Fortunately, this was an unusual complication in the experiences reviewed here. Most investigators reported no late graft infections, and only Thompson and associates[24] had a significant number, with three infections among 76 patients. All of these were carotid-subclavian grafts and each patient was treated with graft excision and axilloaxillary bypass, with good results. In contrast, two patients in Criado's review died of carotid-subclavian graft infection.[6] Also, Criado and Thompson each reported instances of erosion of the presternal skin overlying an axillo-axillary graft, again highlighting a significant disadvantage of this particular type of extra-anatomic bypass.[6, 24]

Cerebrovascular Events

The third category of late morbidity was that caused by central nervous system ischemia. Three investigators reported late strokes among their patients. Brewster and associates[27] had two patients who suffered nonfatal strokes among 38 innominate reconstructions. One of these strokes affected the contralateral hemisphere and was presumably unrelated to the operation. The other was an embolic right hemispheric stroke that occurred 1 year after surgery. Vogt and colleagues[25] had one patient who developed a left hemispheric stroke due to thrombosis of a left aorto-carotid graft 1 year after surgery. They reported a total of 12 late neurologic complications, consisting of six transient ischemic attacks and six completed strokes among 95 patients. Although no direct link could be established, seven of these events affected areas of the central nervous system supplied in part by vessels that had been operated on. In contrast to this experience, Crawford and coworkers[22] considered only one of thirteen nonfatal central nervous system ischemic events as directly related to the operation. These 13 events (among 142 patients) consisted of five transient ischemic attacks, three strokes with progressive complete recovery, and five completed strokes with residual deficit. All except one were either not in the distribution of the operated artery or were associated with new or progressive atherosclerotic lesions.

In none of these series was the incidence of stroke related to the operative approach used. Vogt and associates[25] analyzed their patients to determine whether complete correction of all atherosclerotic lesions yielded better results than repair of only symptomatic ones. The "complete correction" group included a number of patients with asymptomatic but anatomically worrisome carotid bifurcation atheromas, which were removed by endarterectomy at the time of other brachiocephalic repair; however, symptomatic relief rate, perioperative or late stroke rate, and operative mortality rate were not statistically different in the two groups. This contrasts with data cited earlier regarding the higher incidence of perioperative strokes in patients with uncorrected internal carotid lesions.[18, 22, 30]

Other Late Complications

Several miscellaneous late complications were reported as well. The only serious one of these was a false aneurysm after a carotid-subclavian bypass. This apparently required several reoperations for correction.[25]

Symptom Relief and Clinical Outcome

The diversity of reporting methods used by the authors of these numerous series makes it impossible to assimilate the data into one large pool and quantitatively determine the success rates of all the operations performed. Nonetheless, it is possible to draw general conclusions regarding the efficacy of surgery in relieving symptoms of central nervous system and upper extremity ischemia caused by occlusive

lesions of the brachiocephalic vessels. Patients who survived surgery, as the vast majority did, usually experienced immediate relief of symptoms, and remained symptom-free throughout the follow-up period or until death. Late deaths were unrelated to the reconstructive surgery, except in a very few cases of graft infection and possibly stroke. Many investigators reported total relief of symptoms in 90 to 100 percent of patients (Table 83–3). The remainder listed the majority as either totally relieved or improved. This category included several patients who required reoperation, either for graft occlusion or for new lesions, but who had subsequent good results. Among those patients classified as unchanged were those whose symptoms persisted and those who were symptomatic after graft occlusion but who did not undergo further surgery.

Patients whose condition was classified as worse than before surgery constituted 4 to 8 percent of the total and included living patients with residual neurologic deficits, graft infections, and, in two cases, arm amputations.

Three investigators made note of patients who developed new symptoms during the follow-up period. Crawford and associates[22] described 21 such patients, 15 of whom underwent angiography. Reconstructions were patent in all cases, but 11 showed new or progressive occlusive lesions in previously unoperated vessels. These lesions were repaired, and all patients apparently became asymptomatic. Vogt and associates[25] mention eight patients who subsequently required a total of 12 carotid bifurcation endarterectomies at intervals following brachiocephalic repair. Finally, Raithel[23] described 14 patients who presented with new cerebral ischemic symptoms, eight of whom went on to have carotid endarterectomy performed, resulting in relief of symptoms. These reports underscore the multilevel and multivessel nature of this disease process and the need for ongoing close follow-up.

CONCLUSIONS

This chapter has reviewed the experience of the past 35 years with brachiocephalic arterial reconstruction and compared, when possible, the risks and results of the transthoracic and extra-anatomic methods of operation. We believe that the information available in the literature, supported by our own personal experience, justifies the following conclusions.

Reconstruction of the branches of the aortic arch is technically feasible and is indicated for patients with disabling symptoms of upper extremity or central nervous system ischemia in the face of occlusive or ulcerated lesions in these vessels. Surgery is probably not justified in asymptomatic patients.

Either transthoracic (synonymous with trans-sternal) or extrathoracic repair can be used. The choice of procedure should be made on the basis of careful evaluation of the patient's general condition and thorough angiographic documentation of all lesions, from the arch of the aorta to the base of the skull. Lesions of the innominate artery or involvement of multiple vessels is more likely to dictate the necessity for a transthoracic approach. Endarterectomy, transposition, and bypass graft are all suitable methods of reconstruction, with the proviso that any lesion thought to

TABLE 83–3. Long-Term Results

Study*	Operation Type	Patients in Follow-up, n	Effect on Symptoms, n				Late Deaths, n
			Relieved†	Improved	No Change	Worse	
AbuRahma et al[40]	E	67	59		6		9
Brewster et al[27]	T	25	22	—	1	2	NA
	E	8	6	—	2	—	2
Carlson et al[28]	E	32	30	—	2	—	8
Cherry et al[41]	T	26	21	—	3	—	1
Cormier et al[42]	T	53	45	—	—	1	6
Crawford et al[22]	T	40	33	—	2	1	59
	E	96	80	—	6	3	(combined)
DePalma and Broadbent[33]	T	9	9	—	—	—	0
	E	16	16	—	—	—	0
Deriu and Ballotta[32]	Combined	28	12	13	3	—	4
Gross et al[36]	Combined	17	15	—	—	—	5
Liljeqvist et al[29]	T	80	70%‡		30%‡		9
Livesay et al[30]	E	31	70%‡		30%‡		5
Luosto et al[13]	Combined	118	42%	51%	—	7%	15
Moore et al[31]	E	25	21	—	3	1	9
Raithel[23]	Combined	64	56	—	8	—	4
Reul et al[43]	T	38	46	—	—	1	7
	E	16	(combined)				(combined)
Schroeder and Buchardt-Hansen[18]	Combined	59	42	—	16	1	7
Vogt et al[25]	T	29	24	4	—	1	>20
	E	66	43	11	9	3	
Wylie and Effeney[26]	T	50	50	—	—	—	NA
	E	96	90	—	6	—	NA
Zelenock et al[34]	T	17	17	—	—	—	0

*For full bibliographic information, see reference list at end of chapter.
†Includes patients asymptomatic at the time of death.
‡Values do not differentiate between "relieved" and "improved" or between "no change" and "worse."
E, extrathoracic; NA, information not available; T, transthoracic.

be the source of emboli must be excluded or excised from the circulation.

In the experience of most vascular surgeons, transthoracic surgery carries a higher operative mortality, primarily because of myocardial infarction. This approach should thus be avoided, if possible, in older patients with significant coronary artery disease or multiple medical problems. For other patients, with careful anesthetic management and perioperative monitoring, it is a safe, anatomic (ie, the resulting configuration of the grafts resembles normal anatomy), and highly durable method of arterial repair. Because of the proximity and number of vital structures in the mediastinum, technical errors are likely to have grave consequences; thus, these procedures should be performed only by vascular surgeons who are well versed in complex reconstructive techniques.

Extra-anatomic reconstruction, although not free of risk, is better suited to patients who are deemed high operative risks. This form of repair may be somewhat less durable than direct transthoracic reconstruction, primarily because of the higher incidence of late thrombosis of extra-anatomic bypass grafts. Thus, transthoracic surgery is generally preferable for younger patients. Although patients with brachiocephalic atherosclerosis do not generally survive as long as age-matched control subjects, their longevity is sufficient that a durable form of reconstruction should be used.

The most durable forms of extra-anatomic repair are endarterectomy, transposition, and bypass graft with prosthesis. In most reports, Dacron has been the material of choice. Reported experience with expanded polytetrafluoroethylene has been scant. Saphenous vein has proved less reliable than

prosthesis in this location. Endarterectomy and transposition carry less risk of infection because no prosthesis is introduced. No bypass graft should be tunneled over the clavicle, and axilloaxillary grafts should be avoided, if possible, because of their superficial location and high failure rate.

Coronary artery disease is the leading cause of late death among patients who undergo brachiocephalic arterial repair. Patients should be screened carefully for overt or covert CAD and should be offered coronary revascularization in appropriate cases.

Stroke is also a significant cause of early and late morbidity and mortality. In evaluating patients for surgery, surgeons should give particular attention to disease of the carotid bifurcation. Carotid endarterectomy alone may alleviate symptoms. If proximal reconstruction is definitely indicated for cerebrovascular symptoms, simultaneous ipsilateral carotid endarterectomy should probably be performed if significant occlusive or ulcerated carotid artery lesions are present. All patients should be carefully followed for the development of new or progressive extracranial cerebrovascular disease in order to minimize the risk of late stroke, death, or disability.

REFERENCES

1. Martorell F, Fabre J: El sindrome de obliteracion de los troncos supraarticos. *Med Clin.* 1944;2:26.
2. Shimuzu K, Sano K: Pulseless disease. *J Neuropathol Clin Neurol.* 1951;1:37.
3. Davis JB, Grove WJ, Julian O: Thrombotic occlusion of branches of the aortic arch. Martorell's syndrome: Report of a case treated surgically. *Ann Surg.* 1956;144:124.
4. DeBakey ME, Morris GC Jr, Jordan GL Jr, Cooley DA: Segmental thrombo-obliterative disease of branches of the aortic arch. *JAMA.* 1958;166:988.

5. Crawford ES, DeBakey ME, Morris GC Jr, Cooley DA: Thrombo-obliterative disease of the great vessels arising from the aortic arch. *Thorac Cardiovasc Surg.* 1962;43:38.

6. Criado FJ: Extra-thoracic management of aortic arch syndrome. *Br J Surg.* 1982;69(Suppl):545.

7. Lyons C, Galbraith G: Surgical treatment of atherosclerotic occlusion of the internal carotid artery. *Ann Surg.* 1957;146:487.

8. Blaisdell WF, Clauss RH, Galbraith JG: Joint study of extracranial arterial occlusion. IV. A review of surgical considerations. *JAMA.* 1969;209:1889.

9. Fields WAS, Lemak NA: Joint study of extracranial arterial occlusion. VII. "Subclavian steal": A review of 168 cases. *JAMA.* 1972;222:1139.

10. Schwartz CJ, Mitchell JRA: Atheroma of the carotid and vertebral arterial systems. *Br Med J.* 1961;2:1057.

11. Najafi H, Javid H, Hunter JA, et al: Occlusive diseases of the branches of the aortic arch. In Bergan JJ, Yao JST, eds. *Surgery of the Aorta and Its Body Branches.* New York; Grune & Stratton; 1979;191.

12. Hewit RL, Weichert RF, Drapanas T: Centrifugal cerebral ischemia. *Arch Surg.* 1970;101:155.

13. Luosto R, Jarjola PT, Kefonen P, Tala P: Operative treatment of atherosclerotic lesions in innominate, subclavian, vertebral arteries. *Ann Chir Gynecol.* 1976;65:153.

14. Contorni L: Il circolo collaterale vertebravertebrale nella obliterazione dell'ateria succlavia alla sue origine. *Minerva Chir.* 1960;15:268.

15. Reivich M, Holling HE, Roberts B, Toole JF: Reversal of blood flow through the vertebral artery and its effect on cerebral circulation. *N Engl J Med.* 1961;265:878.

16. Solti F, Iskum M, Papp S: The regulation of cerebral blood circulation in subclavian steal syndrome. *Circulation.* 1970;42:1185.

17. Hardesty WH, Whitacre WB, Toole JF, et al: Studies on vertebral artery blood flow in man. *Surg Gynecol Obstet.* 1963;116:662.

18. Schroeder T, Buchardt-Hansen HJ: Arterial reconstruction of the brachiocephalic trunk and the subclavian arteries: Ten-years' experience with a follow-up study. *Acta Chir Scand.* 1980;502:122.

19. Ehrenfeld WK, Chapman RD, Wylie EJ: Management of occlusive lesions of the branches of the aortic arch. *Am J Surg.* 1968;118:236.

20. Piccone VA, LeVeen HH: The subclavian steal syndrome. *Ann Thorac Surg.* 1970;9:51.

21. Edwards WH, Mulherin JL: The surgical approach to significant stenosis of vertebral and subclavian arteries. *Surgery.* 1980;87:20.

22. Crawford ES, Stowe CL, Powers RW Jr: Occlusion of the innominate, common carotid, and subclavian arteries: Long term results of surgical treatment. *Surgery.* 1983;94:781.

23. Raithel D: Our experience of surgery for innominate and subclavian lesions. *J Cardiovasc Surg.* 1980;21:423.

24. Thompson BW, Read RC, Campbell GS: Operative correction of proximal blocks of the subclavian or innominate arteries. *J Cardiovasc Surg.* 1980;21:125.

25. Vogt DP, Mertzer NR, O'Hara PJ, Beven EG: Brachiocephalic arterial reconstruction. *Ann Surg.* 1982;196:541.

26. Wylie EJ, Effeney DJ: Surgery of the aortic arch branches and vertebral arteries. *Surg Clin North Am.* 1979;59:669.

27. Brewster DC, Moncure AC, Darling RC, et al: Innominate artery lesions: Problems encountered and lessons learned. *J Vasc Surg.* 1985;2:99.

28. Carlson RE, Ehrenfeld WK, Stoney RJ, Wylie EJ: Innominate artery endarterectomy. *Arch Surg.* 1977;112:1389.

29. Liljeqvist L, Ekestrom S, Nordhus O: Intrathoracic approach for subclavian and innominate artery reconstruction. *Scand J Thorac Cardiovasc Surg.* 1979;13:309.

30. Livesay JJ, Atkinson JB, Baker JD, et al: Late results of extra-anatomic bypass. *Arch Surg.* 1979;114:1260.

31. Moore WAS, Malone JM, Goldstone J: Extra-thoracic repair of branch occlusions of the aortic arch. *Am J Surg.* 1976;132:249.

32. Deriu GP, Ballotta E: The surgical treatment of atherosclerotic occlusion of the innominate and subclavian arteries. *J Cardiovasc Surg.* 1981;22:532.

33. DePalma RG, Broadbent RV: Management of occlusive disease of the subclavian and innominate arteries. *Am J Surg.* 1981;142:197.

34. Zelenock GB, Cronenwett JL, Graham LM, et al: Brachiocephalic arterial occlusions and stenoses: Manifestations and management of complex lesions. *Arch Surg.* 1985;120:370.

35. Salle JG, Cook JW, Elliot CM: Simultaneous revascularization for complex brachiocephalic and coronary artery disease. *Surgery.* 1981;90:97.

36. Gross WAS, Flanigan DP, Kraft RO, Stanley JC: Chronic upper extremity arterial insufficiency: Etiology, manifestations, and operative management. *Arch Surg.* 1978;113:419.

37. Hertzer NR, Lees DC: Fatal myocardial infarction following carotid endarterectomy: 335 patients followed six to eleven years after operation. *Ann Surg.* 1981;194:212.

38. Brewster DC, LaSalle AJ, Robison JG, et al: Femoropopliteal graft failures: Clinical consequences and success of secondary reconstruction. *Arch Surg.* 1983;118:1043.

39. Szilagyi DE, Elliot J, Hageman JH, et al: Biologic fate of autogenous vein implants as arterial substitutes: Clinical, angiographic, and histopathologic observations in femoropopliteal operations for atherosclerosis. *Ann Surg.* 1973;178:232.

40. AbuRahma AF, Robinson PA, Khan MZ, Khan JH, Boland JP: Brachiocephalic revascularization: A comparison between carotid-subclavian artery bypass and axilloaxillary artery bypass. *Surgery.* 1992;112:84.

41. Cherry KJ Jr, McCullough JL, Hallett JW Jr, Pairolero PC, Gloviczki P: Technical principles of direct innominate artery revascularization: a comparison of endarterectomy and bypass grafts. *J Vasc Surg.* 1989;9:718.

42. Cormier F, Ward A, Cormier J-M, Laurian C: Long-term results of aortoinnominate and aortocarotid polytetrafluoroethylene bypass grafting for atherosclerotic lesions. *J Vasc Surg.* 1989;10:135.

43. Reul GJ, Jacobs MJHM, Gregoric ID, et al: Innominate artery occlusive disease: Surgical approach and long-term results. *J Vasc Surg.* 1991;14:405.

XIV

Extracranial–Intracranial Bypass Surgery

Indications for Extracranial–Intracranial Bypass Surgery

JOHN R. LITTLE

In 1963, Woringer and Kunlin[1] first described an extracranial–intracranial (EC–IC) bypass procedure in a patient with proximal internal carotid artery (ICA) occlusion. These investigators used a saphenous vein graft that extended from the common carotid artery to the intracranial segment of the ICA. Donaghy and Yasargil[2] subsequently reported in 1967 the first superficial temporal artery to middle cerebral artery (STA–MCA) bypass operation. The latter procedure stimulated considerable interest in the neurologic and neurosurgical communities; by the mid-1970s, it was being widely applied to the treatment of symptomatic patients with inaccessible occlusive lesions of the ICA and MCA. Later reports indicated that a similar approach could be used in the posterior circulation. EC–IC bypass was also adopted as a means of potentially reducing the risk of stroke with the therapeutic occlusion of a major brain artery for an inaccessible or unclippable aneurysm.

The main unresolved question regarding EC–IC bypass is not Can it be done? but Should it be done? The objective of this chapter is to discuss the current indications for EC–IC bypass in the treatment of cerebral ischemia and to identify areas for further investigation.

INDICATIONS FOR EC–IC BYPASS BEFORE THE EC–IC BYPASS STUDY

Initially, the criteria used to determine whether to recommend surgery were very broad. Similar criteria were subsequently used for entry into the EC–IC bypass study[3] that began in 1977. They included cerebral transient ischemic attacks or monocular blindness (amaurosis fugax) within 3 months before entry or minor completed stroke or strokes in the carotid distribution within 3 months before entry, or both. The angiographic criteria included inaccessible atherosclerotic stenosis or occlusion of the ICA or atherosclerotic stenosis or occlusion of the trunk of the MCA, or both. Patients with an acute ischemic neurologic deficit (ie, stroke) were not entered into the study until at least 8 weeks after the event. In addition, patients without symptoms after the angiographic demonstration of ICA or MCA occlusion were included and constituted a large subgroup. Indeed, ICA occlusion without symptoms after angiography constituted the

largest subgroup by far for which EC–IC bypass was done in most series.

The EC–IC bypass study failed to confirm the hypothesis that STA–MCA bypass is effective in preventing cerebral infarction in the group of patients studied.[4] This international multicenter trial evaluated 1377 adult patients, with 714 randomized to best medical care and 663 randomized to STA–MCA bypass together with best medical care. The bypass patency rate was 96 percent. No patients were lost to follow-up, which averaged 55.8 months (range, 28 to 90 months). The overall analysis, as well as separate analyses of angiographic subgroups, showed no reduction in stroke and stroke-related death with surgery.

The EC–IC bypass study clearly demonstrated that an STA–MCA bypass is not beneficial in the broad clinical and angiographic groups studied, but it did not preclude the need for an EC–IC bypass in all patients. The dilemma is the clinical identification of those patients, if any, who might benefit from this approach.

INDICATIONS FOR EC–IC BYPASS AFTER THE EC–IC BYPASS STUDY

Focal cerebral ischemia is caused by embolization or hemodynamic insufficiency. Although these two mechanisms might act together in some cases, a gathering body of information indicates that embolization is usually the dominant factor. EC–IC bypass surgery is designed to improve circulation in ischemic brain and thereby reduce the likelihood of infarction from hemodynamic insufficiency. It is unlikely that EC–IC bypass benefits those patients who are symptomatic as a result of embolization. Consequently, the initial challenge is to identify which patients are having symptoms primarily on the basis of hemodynamic insufficiency.

Clinical recognition of patients at high risk of cerebral infarction from hemodynamic insufficiency is difficult. Some clinical features are helpful in differentiating symptoms of hemodynamic insufficiency from embolization. For example, patients with classic amaurosis fugax, either alone or in combination with cerebral symptoms, are far more likely to be having embolization. Often, embolic material can be seen in the retinal arteries of these patients. Ocular symptoms are more likely to be hemodynamic in origin if there is low retinal artery pressure or signs of ischemic retinopathy. Patients with hemodynamic monocular visual loss usually describe a "camera shutter" or "gray-out" of vision as opposed to sudden complete blindness or a "shade" dropping to obscure part or all of the visual field.

Some patients with cerebral symptoms from hemodynamic insufficiency are "pressure sensitive." In this setting, symptoms recur with the overzealous use of antihypertensive agents. In other cases, elevation of systemic arterial blood pressure with hypertensive agents may abolish the ischemic symptoms.

Symptoms of focal cerebral ischemia that invariably develop when the patient is standing suggest a hemodynamic mechanism. Such attacks are probably related to a slight drop in systemic arterial blood pressure. Weakness of the contralateral lower extremity is often a prominent component in patients with unilateral ICA occlusion and reflects ischemia in the border zone between the MCA and anterior cerebral artery territories. Patients with bilateral ICA occlusion can experience episodic weakness of both lower extremitites while standing. This is often accompanied by feelings of light-headedness or confusion.

Unfortunately, most cerebral ischemic attacks have no telltale features indicating their pathogenesis. Nor can one easily differentiate those attacks that are benign from those that are ominous in terms of stroke risk. It is generally accepted that ischemic symptoms of recent onset (ie, 1 to 2 months) are more dangerous than those that have occurred remotely. Increasing frequency, duration, and severity of these symptoms are also considered to be worrisome features.

Angiographic Factors

Patients being considered for cerebral revascularization should undergo complete angiography, with visualization of both the anterior and posterior circulations. A complete study is essential in evaluating both the occlusive lesion and the collateral circulation. Although angiography does not provide a measurement of cerebral blood flow, it does serve as an index of circulation in the region normally supplied by the occluded artery and is an important factor in the decision-making process. Those patients with limited collateral input and very slow filling and washout of the arterial system distal to a major artery occlusion are likely to have hemodynamic insufficiency.

Surgery for an EC–IC bypass has been recommended most often for inaccessible severe stenosis or occlusion of the ICA or MCA. In cases of stenosis, ulceration is often present at the site of stenosis as well as at other locations proximally and distally (ie, tandem lesions). In cases of occlusion, the main site of origin of emboli has been eliminated by the closure of the pre-existing stenotic lesion, although emboli may still arise from the ICA stump or from atherosclerotic lesions in the external carotid artery.

The timing of the major artery occlusion in relationship to symptoms is also an important factor. For example, recurrent ipsilateral ischemia after ICA occlusion is uncommon. Consequently, bypass surgery should be considered only for those patients who are clearly symptomatic after the angiographic demonstration of the occlusion.

Occlusion of the ICA or MCA has a more profound effect on cerebral perfusion pressure than stenosis of the same arteries.[5, 6] Normally, cortical artery pressure approaches the systemic arterial pressure, with the ratio of cortical to systemic arterial pressure being 0.90 or greater. In one series,[5] 22 percent of patients undergoing EC–IC bypass for an occluded ICA or MCA had a cortical-to-systemic ratio of 0.25 or less. Such low cortical artery pressure would barely permit perfusion of the capillary bed. These patients may be at high risk of stroke from hypoperfusion and might be appropriate candidates for bypass surgery. Unfortunately, there is no technique available that allows the noninvasive measurement of cortical artery pressure. However, one report indicates that in patients with ICA occlusion, retinal artery pressure might be predictive of cortical artery pressure.[5] In such patients, the intracranial segment of the ICA (including the ophthalmic artery origin) is usually patent, thereby preserving continuity between the retinal and cortical arterial systems.

Patients With Stenotic Lesions

Treating patients with inaccessible severe stenosis of the ICA or MCA has proved more difficult than treating patients with occluded arteries. Many of these patients are symptomatic on the basis of embolization and must be treated accordingly. The stenotic lesion itself can change.[7, 8] Repeat angiography has shown that some stenotic lesions improve with time. This improvement could be the result of dissolution of thrombus or resolution of a dissection. In other cases, the stenosis progresses to occlusion. In our unit, symptomatic patients found to have severe, inaccessible stenosis are usually treated with antiplatelet agents. If symptoms recur, they are treated with anticoagulants for a 3-to 6-month period. Failure of anticoagulant therapy leads to consideration of surgery, but angiography is repeated before making a final decision because of the changes that may have occurred at the site of the stenotic lesion.

Patients Who Fail Medical Therapy

EC–IC bypass surgery can be considered for patients who continue to have ischemic symptoms despite best medical therapy. Such medical therapy includes the use of medication to reduce the likelihood of embolization as well as to control systemic arterial blood pressure, diabetes mellitus, cardiac dysrhythmias, and other potential risk factors. Overzealous treatment of hypertension in patients with suspected hypoperfusion should be avoided. Other lesions seen on angiography, such as contralateral ICA stenosis or an ipsilateral ICA stump, might have to be treated surgically before EC–IC bypass is considered. Presently, clear-cut failure of best medical therapy in patients with appropriate clinical and angiographic findings is the strongest indication for consideration of this surgical approach.

Patients With Ischemic Retinopathy

Ischemic retinopathy or low perfusion pressure retinopathy occurs most commonly with ICA occlusion. A number of these patients also exhibit symptoms of cerebral ischemia in the territory of the occluded carotid artery. Retinal artery pressure is markedly reduced in this setting (retinal-to-systemic ratio ≤ 0.25). The condition can progress to retinal infarction with complete blindness if not treated.

Cerebral revascularization has been used to treat patients with ischemic retinopathy secondary to ICA occlusion. Many of these patients have had resolution of their ocular symptoms and findings with surgery. Retinal artery pressure and retinal fluorescein circulation have been shown to improve significantly in many patients after surgery.[9]

Patients With Impending Cerebral Infarction

The role of emergency EC–IC bypass in the setting of evolving cerebral infarction has not been determined. Clinical experience with this approach is limited,[10] and experimental studies have not uniformly supported its use.[11, 12] A period of time exists between symptom onset and irreversible tissue injury. This period can range from minutes to hours. Revascularization before infarction has occurred might be beneficial, but revascularization after infarction could increase swelling or induce hemorrhage in the necrotic tissue. Currently, there is no technique available to reliably predict which situation exists in a given patient. In addition, considerable time is usually lost as the patient undergoes the various examinations and tests. It is also possible that the neurologic event being evaluated during its early phase might represent only a transient ischemic attack and not an evolving cerebral infarct.

CEREBRAL BLOOD FLOW MEASUREMENT AND PATIENT SELECTION

The application of techniques to measure cerebral blood flow and metabolism is essential if patients with hemodynamic insufficiency are to be accurately identified. Our knowledge and technology appear to be reaching a point where measurement of cerebral blood flow and metabolism can be an important component in the evaluation of patients with cerebrovascular occlusive disease.

Cerebral blood flow is not static in the normal setting but continually changes with the level of brain activity. In the resting state, it is in the 50 to 60 mL/100 g/minute range. Neurologic function and electroencephalographic activity are not altered with mild to moderate reduction of cerebral blood flow. However, when it is reduced to the 18 to 22 mL/100 g/min level, neurologic function and electroencephalographic activity are lost. If cerebral blood flow drops below 16 to 18 mL/100 g/min (ie, the ischemic threshold) for a sustained period, brain infarction occurs. The rapidity with which irreversible injury takes place has been correlated with the degree of cerebral blood flow reduction below the ischemic threshold.[13] For example, infarction may take hours to develop if the flow is in the 14 to 16 mL/100 g/min range but may occur within minutes below 5 mL/100 g/min. Those patients with a flow reduction approaching, but not below, the ischemic threshold (ie, decreased perfusion reserve) are at high risk for infarction and might benefit from bypass surgery.

A situation in which cerebral blood flow is below the functional threshold but above the threshold for structural integrity has been described, but its frequency in the clinical setting is unclear. During this state, called the ischemic penumbra,[14] neurologic function is lost, but infarction does not occur. Increasing the cerebral blood flow in these areas could result in restoration of neurologic function. Improvement of neurologic deficits, reported in some patients shortly after EC–IC bypass,[6] might reflect the resolution of a chronic state of ischemic penumbra.

Theoretically, the ideal candidate for bypass surgery is a symptomatic patient with severely reduced cerebral blood flow but preserved tissue viability. Therefore, cerebral metabolism and cerebral blood flow must be evaluated. Positron emission tomography is being used to identify patients with various hypoperfusion profiles. The technique provides a tomographic measurement of cerebral blood flow as well as other important parameters such as cerebral blood volume, oxygen metabolism, oxygen extraction fraction, and glucose metabolism. Powers and coworkers[15] reported on a small group of patients with reduced cerebral blood flow, slightly reduced oxygen metabolism, increased oxygen extraction fraction, and increased cerebral blood volume. The increase in oxygen extraction fraction is thought to be indicative of retained tissue viability. Patients with this combination of findings, termed ''misery perfusion,'' might be appropriate candidates for revascularization, provided they fulfill the clinical criteria.

Positron emission tomography is generally viewed as a research tool. It is a very expensive and sophisticated technology. The nature of positron emission tomography has limited its application to small numbers of patients, and it is unlikely to become a widely available clinical tool.

Xenon[133] clearance is the measurement technique used most frequently in evaluating the cerebral blood flow of bypass candidates. In most studies, xenon[133] has been administered by inhalation or intravenously; the measurements are performed using arrays of sodium iodide crystal detectors applied to the scalp. The wide variability of results and poor sensitivity, however, seriously limit its usefulness.[16] This method does not provide tomographic data, and areas of focal ischemia are not well demonstrated. Furthermore, it does not provide any information about brain metabolism. Consequently, this technique is not useful for identifying patients who might benefit from surgery.

Stable xenon-enhanced computed tomographic flow measurements provide quantitative tomographic cerebral blood flow data.[17] This technique appears to be well suited to the evaluation of patients with suspected brain ischemia. Critical reduction of cerebral blood flow can be detected in relatively small cortical or subcortical regions. The distribution of cerebral blood flow changes can be correlated with morphologic changes on the computed tomographic scan, thereby providing some information about structural integrity in areas of cerebral blood flow measurement. This technique holds considerable promise, as it is safe and can be applied to large numbers of patients.

Selection of patients for surgery on a clinical basis alone is imprecise. The application of cerebral blood flow measurement techniques is essential if patients with hemodynamic insufficiency are to be accurately identified.

TECHNICAL CONSIDERATIONS

Surgery for STA–MCA bypass is by far the most frequently performed EC–IC bypass procedure. Concern has arisen, however, regarding the ability of the STA–MCA bypass operation to correct cerebral hypoperfusion. Although early postoperative cerebral blood flow studies have demonstrated improved cerebral circulation, repeated studies during the months and years after STA–MCA bypass have failed to confirm significant or sustained improvement.[18, 19]

The failure of STA–MCA bypass to improve cerebral blood flow and to reduce the occurrence of subsequent stroke might be partly related to the arteries used in the standard procedure. For example, the luminal diameters of the STA–MCA cortical branches used are very small, usually less than 2 mm. The STA is frequently severely arteriosclerotic.[20] Extensive mural fibrosis, a major component of the arteriosclerotic process, probably prevents substantial increases in luminal size after surgery in many cases. In addition, many of the diabetic and chronically hypertensive patients undergoing the procedure have considerable atherosclerotic changes in the MCA cortical branches.

Alternative approaches should be considered. Long or short vein grafts have been used in a few cases of cerebral revascularization and provide a much larger input channel than the STA.[21, 22] Anastomosis to the MCA trunk or one of its major branches lying within the sylvian fissure has been described and is a much larger recipient than the cortical branches.[23] Such a large conduit seems a prerequisite in correcting a state of hypoperfusion in the brain.

CONCLUSION

The ultimate role for EC–IC bypass surgery in treating cerebral ischemia remains elusive. The EC–IC bypass study clearly demonstrated that the standard STA–MCA bypass operation has been overutilized and that our expectations were excessive.

The theory that some patients are symptomatic on the basis of hemodynamic insufficiency and that a subgroup of patients exists that would benefit from EC–IC bypass with augmentation of cerebral perfusion remains viable. How to identify such patients and reverse symptomatic cerebral hypoperfusion effectively remain important and challenging areas for future investigation.

REFERENCES

1. Woringer E, Kunlin J: Anastomose entre la carotide primitive et la carotide intracranienne ou la sylvienne par greffon selon la technique de la suture suspendice. Neurochirurgie. 1963;9:181.
2. Donaghy RMP: Patch and bypass in microangional surgery. In Donaghy RMP, Yasargil MG, eds. Microvascular Surgery. St. Louis: CV Mosby; 1967:75.
3. EC-IC bypass study group: The international cooperative study of extracranial–intracranial arterial anastomosis: Methodology and entry characteristics. Stroke. 1985;16:397.
4. EC-IC bypass study group: Failure of extracranial–intracranial arterial bypass to reduce the risk of ischemic stroke. N Engl J Med. 1985;313:1191.
5. Little JR, Tomsak RL, Ebrahim ZY, Furlan AJ: Retinal artery pressure and cerebral artery perfusion pressure in cerebrovascular occlusive disease. Neurosurgery. 1986;18:716.
6. Spetzler RF, Roski RA, Zabramski J: Middle cerebral artery perfusion pressure in cerebrovascular occlusive disease. Stroke. 1983;14:552.
7. Awad IA, Furlan AJ, Little JR: Changes in intracranial stenotic lesions after extracranial–intracranial bypass surgery. J Neurosurg. 1984;60:771.
8. Day AL: Indications for surgical intervention in middle cerebral artery obstruction. J Neurosurg. 1984;60:296.
9. Standefer MJ, Little JR, Tomsak RL, et al: Improvement in retinal circulation after superficial temporal artery to middle cerebral artery bypass. Neurosurgery. 1985;16:525.
10. Diaz FG, Ausman JI, Mehta B, et al: Acute cerebral revascularization. J Neurosurg. 1985;63:200.
11. Crowell RM, Olsson Y: Effect of extracranial–intracranial vascular bypass graft on experimental acute stroke in dogs. J Neurosurg. 1973;38:26.
12. Diaz FG, Mastri AR, Ausman JI, et al: Acute cerebral revascularization after regional cerebral ischemia in the dog. Part 2. Clinicopathological correlation. J Neurosurg. 1979;51:644.
13. Jones TH, Morawetz RB, Crowell RM, et al: Thresholds of focal cerebral ischemia in awake monkeys. J Neurosurg. 1981;54:773.
14. Astrup J, Siesjo BK, Symon L: Thresholds in cerebral ischemia—the ischemic penumbra. Stroke. 1981;12:723.
15. Powers WJ, Martin WRW, Herscovitch P, et al: Extracranial–intracranial bypass surgery: Hemodynamic and metabolic effects. Neurology (NY). 1984;34:1168.
16. Awad IA, Little JR, Furlan AJ, et al: Correlation of clinical and angiographic findings in brain ischemia with regional cerebral blood flow measured by the xenon inhalation technique. Neurosurgery. 1982;11:1.
17. Yonas H, Wolfson SK, Gur D, et al: Clinical experience with the use of xenon-enhanced CT blood flow mapping in cerebral vascular disease. Stroke. 1984;15:443.
18. Halsey JH, Morawetz RB, Blauenstein VW: The hemodynamic effect of STA–MCA bypass. Stroke. 1982;13:163.
19. Meyer JS, Nakajima S, Okabe T, et al: Redistribution of cerebral blood flow following STA–MCA bypass in patients with hemispheric ischemia. Stroke. 1982;13:774.
20. Diaz FG, Chason J, Shrontz C, et al: Histological structural abnormalities of superficial temporal arteries used for extracranial–intracranial anastomosis. J Neurosurg. 1982;57:328.
21. Little JR, Furlan AJ, Bryerton BB: Short vein grafts for cerebral revascularization. J Neurosurg. 1983;59:384.
22. Spetzler RF, Rhodes RS, Roski RA, et al: Subclavian to middle cerebral artery saphenous vein bypass graft. J Neurosurg. 1980;53:465.
23. Diaz FG, Umansky F, Mehta B, et al: Cerebral revascularization to a main limb of the middle cerebral artery in the sylvian fissure. J Neurosurg. 1985;63:21.

CHAPTER 85

Technique for Extracranial–Intracranial Bypass Grafting

FERNANDO G. DIAZ

It is even conceivable that someday vascular surgery will find a way to bypass the occluded portion of the artery during the period of ominous fleeting symptoms. Anastomosis of the external carotid artery or one of its branches, with the internal carotid artery above the area of narrowing should be feasible.[1]

The first surgical procedure intended to increase the collateral circulation directly to the brain was the application of the temporalis muscle over the cerebral convexity described by Kredell[2] in 1942. Few other attempts were performed in the following two decades to revascularize the ischemic brain. Chou[3] reported the first successful middle cerebral artery (MCA) embolectomy without the aid of a microscope in 1963. A rather innovative and revolutionary procedure was reported by Pool and Potts[4] in 1965. While attempting to clip a large anterior cerebral artery aneurysm, Pool and Potts realized that they could not do it without sacrificing the parent vessel. To prevent the ligation of the anterior cerebral artery, they placed a plastic tube connecting the superficial temporal artery (STA) to the anterior cerebral artery; however, angiographic occlusion was demonstrated 10 days later. In 1963, Woringer and Kunlin[5] performed a saphenous vein graft between the common carotid artery and the supraclinoid internal carotid artery; the patient died, but the anastomosis was found to be patent at autopsy.

However brave and innovative, the early procedures suffered from the limitations imposed by the small size of the intracranial cerebral vessels. The difficulty in handling vessels smaller than 3 mm prevented a more aggressive approach to revascularizing the ischemic brain, and surgical procedures to treat cerebral ischemia were thus restricted to reconstruction of the cervical vasculature. A breakthrough in cerebrovascular surgery occurred in 1960, when Jacobsen and Suarez[6] described their experience with vascular anastomoses of small vessels performed through a surgical microscope. Through the efforts of Donaghy[7] and Yasargil,[8] the first microvascular anastomoses were completed in the laboratory; the first two anastomoses of the STA to the MCA in humans were completed on June 7, 1967, in Vermont and Zurich.[8] From this point, we have witnessed the rapid development of a variety of surgical procedures, all of which have been based on the principle of re-establishing flow to a specific area of the brain by developing an anastomosis that has its source in the extracranial circulation.

Since most early procedures were done with microinstruments used for eye surgery, the early years of microneurosurgery were dedicated to perfecting the surgical technique and developing better suture material and microinstruments.[8]

As previously noted, Worringer and Kunlin[5] attempted the first extracranial–intracranial (EC–IC) bypass with a saphenous vein graft in 1963, but the patient died. Late in 1970, Lougheed and coworkers[9] finally succeeded with this type of vein graft, and many have reported similar success.[10, 11] Prosthetic grafts have also been tried since very early in the management of intracranial cerebrovascular disease[4]; Story

and associates[12] are the only investigators to report any success with this procedure.

CLINICAL CONSIDERATIONS

Patients with cerebrovascular disease present in different ways, and their symptoms have different causes. The most typical types of presentation include transient ischemic attacks, reversible ischemic neurologic deficits, progressing stroke, and completed stroke.[13, 14]

The diagnosis of patients with transient cerebral ischemia must be prompt and aggressive, since once transient ischemic attacks develop, there is a 35 percent probability that the patient will develop a cerebral infarction within 4 to 5 years from the onset of symptoms.[15] The diagnosis of patients with transient ischemic attacks or reversible ischemic neurologic deficits is based mostly on clinical suspicion, since there is usually no residual neurologic dysfunction. In patients with progressing stroke or established stroke, the deficit is usually evident to the clinician, and the diagnosis can be promptly established. Evaluation of patients with stroke in evolution should be aggressive and prompt; as we have reported, a surgically correctable lesion may be encountered, and the progression of the infarct may be arrested or reversed.[16]

These patients should have comprehensive medical and neurologic tests. Sources other than vascular disease should be excluded as possible causes of cerebrovascular ischemic events. A computed tomographic scan of the brain will rule out an intracranial space-occupying lesion that could be responsible for symptoms similar to transient ischemic events. In patients with cerebral infarctions, the scan will provide an evaluation of the state of the cerebral parenchyma, but computed tomography is effective in demonstrating cerebral infarction only 2 or 3 days after the event. Isotope brain scanning is also effective in demonstrating a brain tumor or a cerebral infarction but is seldom used since the advent of computed tomography. Positron emission tomography and nuclear magnetic resonance imaging are two newer diagnostic modalities that could be useful in deciding whether a cerebral infarction has occurred and whether any viable tissue remains that might benefit from a vascular reconstructive procedure. However, since these modalities are still not widely available, their value in detecting tissue viability and providing a prognostic indication of recovery has not been explored.

The definitive diagnostic evaluation of patients with cerebrovascular disease is by means of cerebral angiography. The introduction of digital subtraction angiography has facilitated the evaluation of these patients. Intravenous digital subtraction angiography provides a picture similar to that obtained by arch angiography, but it fails to identify most ulcerative problems, underestimates the severity of stenotic lesions, and is generally inadequate to evaluate intracranial vessels. Arterial digital subtraction angiography provides accurate and sharp images, with minimal contrast injection. Magnetic resonance angiography (MRA) is a promising new technique for noninvasive evaluation of the cerebral circulation. Spatial resolution and detailed small vessel acquisition are being developed.

Precise diagnostic accuracy can be obtained only with selective catheterization of the greater vessels as they originate from the arch of the aorta.[17] Selective cerebral angiography with detailed evaluation of the extracranial and intracranial circulation avoids the possibility of missing extracranial or intracranial lesions capable of producing symptoms. The risks of this procedure are well under 1 percent in competent hands and should not deter clinicians from evaluating these patients completely.

OPERATIVE CRITERIA

Our selection criteria for EC–IC bypass depend on the clinical presentation, angiographic findings, and cerebral blood flow studies.[15, 19–21] At our center, a patient presenting with transient ischemic attack, reversible ischemic neurologic deficit, or cerebral infarction is thoroughly evaluated.[16, 22–24] After other nonvascular causes of the symptoms have been eliminated, a complete four-vessel angiogram is performed. In patients with hemodynamically significant angiographic lesions, we then obtain a regional cerebral blood flow study to determine the possible effect of the lesion.

If stenosis or occlusion in the extracranial or intracranial arteries is found that is consistent with the patient's ischemic events, is inaccessible by other surgical means, and demonstrates ipsilateral focal hemodynamic changes on cerebral blood flow studies, the patient is considered a candidate for cerebral revascularization. Patients with bilateral internal carotid artery occlusion generally have a dismal long-term prognosis and are excellent candidates for EC–IC bypass.[18, 20, 25] However, unilateral internal carotid artery occlusion by itself may be compensated by the collateral cerebral circulation; some of these patients may not be clinically at risk or require a bypass.[26] In our practice, patients with MCA stenosis or occlusion are advised to have bypass surgery regardless of symptoms, because we believe that the collateral supply to these areas is usually poor. Patients with severe neurologic deficits are excluded from surgery, because past experience indicates that they are not helped by reconstructive vascular surgery.[15, 26–31]

For posterior circulation ischemia, no treatment is of proven value. Cerebral revascularization of the distal vertebral or basilar circulation has been developed for patients with symptomatic brain-stem ischemia.[11, 15, 32–43]

Contraindications to the procedure are generally relative. The procedure is discouraged in patients with severe neoplastic disease who have a limited life expectancy. Patients with multiple and advanced medical problems such as severe cardiovascular disease, chronic obstructive pulmonary disease, or severe diabetes mellitus are generally considered unsuitable candidates for the procedure.[14, 15, 18, 20–22, 44, 45] The only definite contraindication to cerebral revascularization is the presence of an acute established cerebral infarct, because of the potential risk of developing a hemorrhagic infarction.[16, 32]

Results of the use of nuclear magnetic resonance and positron emission tomography in the evaluation of patients considered candidates for cerebral revascularization have not been published to date. Since these two studies provide an accurate assessment of tissue viability, they may help in determining the possibility of reversible ischemia. Therefore, any studies that do not consider these two diagnostic modalities in the evaluation of the value of EC–IC bypass should be considered largely inadequate and incomplete.[26]

SURGICAL PROCEDURES

Anterior Circulation

Encephalomyosinangiosis

Different procedures have been designed to revascularize the anterior circulation. The oldest was described by Kredell,[2] who used a portion of the temporal muscle applied directly to the brain through a temporal craniectomy. The muscle is placed in direct contact with the brain after the dura mater has been reflected away from the cerebral surface. This procedure does not establish a direct, immediate anastomosis with the cerebral circulation and depends entirely on the eventual development of neovascularization from the muscle surface to the brain. The procedure has been used preferentially for patients with moyamoya disease, especially for young children in Japan.[46]

Another variation of the same procedure is the direct placement of omentum over the cortical surface.[14, 29] The omentum may be brought to the cerebral surface through a subcutaneous tunnel placed from the abdomen, leaving it attached to the greater epiploic vessels. Alternatively, it may be excised entirely from the abdomen, anastomosing its vascular pedicle to the superficial temporal or cervical vessels and then placing the omentum over the cortical surface. A lipid substance with angiogenetic properties has been isolated from omental tissue and is currently under investigation.

The advantage of these two procedures is that a microanastomosis is not necessary for either; therefore, in those cases in which no suitable cortical vessel can be found to receive a microanastomosis, one can proceed with either of these methods. Another option, described by Spetzler and colleagues,[45] is the direct application of the STA to the cortical surface without microanastomosis. For this procedure, it is important to preserve flow through the artery by maintaining continuity at the proximal and distal ends of the vessel. The eventual success of these procedures rests on the anticipated demand for blood of the ischemic brain, which should result in the development of neovascularization.

Superficial Temporary to Middle Cerebral Artery Anastomosis

The most common procedure to revascularize the anterior cerebral circulation is anastomosis of a branch of the external carotid artery to a branch of the internal carotid artery, most commonly anastomosis of the STA to the MCA.[7, 15, 20, 22, 24, 27, 28, 30, 32, 44, 47] After the patient has been anesthetized and placed in a supine position with the ipsilateral shoulder elevated approximately 30 degrees, the head is turned later-

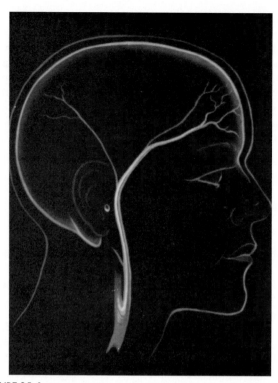

FIGURE 85–1. Diagram demonstrating the location of the superficial temporal artery on the scalp. The posterior temporal branch is usually the smaller of the two branches, but in general it is 1 to 1.5 mm in diameter and therefore of sufficient caliber for most anastomoses.

to that used to expose the posterior branch. However, since the anastomosis with the MCA is best accomplished with one of the branches emerging in the angular or posterior parietal area, it is necessary to either extend the incision or make a new incision to reach the angular region. A separate incision can be placed directly over the angular region, and the anterior branch of the STA can then be brought to it through a subgaleal tunnel. Otherwise, the incision can be extended back diagonally from the preauricular area in front of the tragus to approximately 2 or 3 cm behind the pinna of the ear. One of these two incisions is usually required when the anterior branch of the STA extends low on the forehead and does not have an ascending branch that curves up into the superior frontal region. In patients in whom the anterior branch has a more superior direction or in whom the main trunk or a large branch of the vessel extends into the superior frontal area, the incision can be extended back in the manner of a reverse question mark to approximately 1 or 2 cm behind the posterior margin of the ear. This incision is preferable to the V-type incision because it provides a broad pedicle for the flap and prevents the development of a sharp corner at the apex of the V, which could become an area of necrosis.

With any of these incisions, the idea is to expose the posterior and midparietal areas, placing the center of the operative area 6 cm directly above the external auditory meatus.[18] The muscle incision is started just below the proximal portion of the STA, extending posteriorly to the superior temporal crest and then following the crest to develop anterior and posterior muscle flaps, which are then reflected off the bone. When hemostasis is completed and the muscle

ally so that the surgical surface is parallel to the floor. The anterior and posterior branches of the STA are traced on the scalp with an ultrasonic Doppler and marked on the scalp surface (Fig. 85–1). Different approaches have been designed to expose the STA. In the earliest approach, a broad scalp flap centered on the ear was turned, extending anteriorly to the edge of the anterior branch of the STA at the level of the superior temporal line and posteriorly toward the dorsal border of the mastoid, thus developing a semicircular flap with an inferior base.[27] Once the flap had been elevated, the STA could be dissected on the undersurface of the flap beneath the galea. This lengthy procedure required extensive mobilization of the scalp and was frequently associated with scalp necroses, poor healing, and subgaleal hematomas. This approach has, for the most part, been abandoned.

The surgical approach now used involves dissection of the STA by an incision made directly over the vessel.[48] In general, the posterior or parietal branch of the artery is used; occasionally, however, when the posterior branch is small or nonexistent, the anterior or frontal branch is used. The STA is exposed immediately below the subcutaneous tissue along its entire length from the inferior temporal region to the midparietal region. Once the necessary length has been exposed, an incision is made along the anterior and posterior edges of the vessel to provide a 2 to 3 mm cuff around the STA. All side branches are individually cauterized or ligated with fine sutures and then transected; continuity is maintained only at the proximal and distal end of the STA.[16]

The anterior branch of the STA is exposed and dissected with an incision directly over the vessel in a manner similar

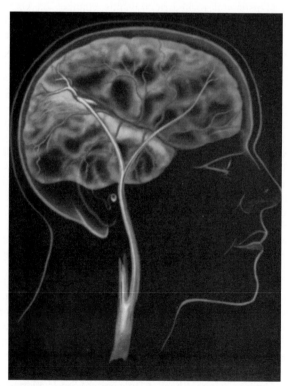

FIGURE 85–2. Diagram demonstrating the anastomosis of the posterior branch of the superficial temporal artery to the angular branch of the middle cerebral artery. To locate the angular branch, it is necessary to center the craniotomy on a point 6 cm directly above the external auditory meatus.

flaps are retracted, a free bone flap can be raised with a craniotome, or a craniectomy can be developed so that the margins of the skull opening have an approximate diameter of 5 cm, and the area of exposure is centered in the sylvian fissure. The dura is fixed to the bone with fine sutures to control any epidural bleeding, and it is then opened in a cruciate manner, exposing the middle and posterior portion of the sylvian fissure. When the craniotomy is placed properly, the sylvian fissure bisects the exposed area, the angular branch is located on the central and posterior portion of the flap, and the principal branches of the MCA are readily apparent (Fig. 85–2). The largest of the exposed vessels is dissected under the microscope, and as few cortical perforators as possible are cauterized and transected to expose an 8 mm segment of dissected vessel; a small rubber dam is placed under the vessel to facilitate the anastomosis. We prefer using the MCA branches with the greatest diameter and as close to the sylvian fissure as possible.

At this point, a temporary clip is placed on the proximal section of the STA, the distal end of which is cauterized and transected. The STA is then irrigated with a 10 percent heparinized saline solution. A section of approximately 1.5 cm is then freed of adventitia, and a fish-mouth stoma is prepared at the required length (Fig. 85–3). It is important to leave sufficient slack on the vessel so that both anterior and posterior walls can be anastomosed without tension. The segment of MCA that was previously dissected is then isolated between temporary clips, and a longitudinal arteriotomy equal in length to the STA stoma is made by

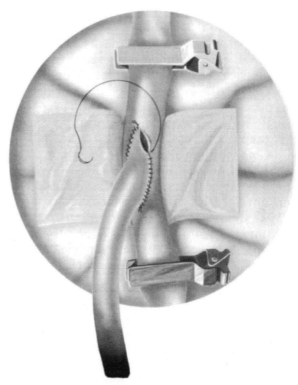

FIGURE 85–4. Diagram illustrating the technique for continuous or running suture. The most proximal portion of the superficial temporal artery stoma is fixed first to the middle cerebral artery. We then prefer to close the distal wall of the anastomotic surface first, since it is usually the more difficult of the two walls, anchoring the suture at the commissure opposite to the one where the anastomosis was started. We would then complete the anastomosis with a new suture on the anterior wall.

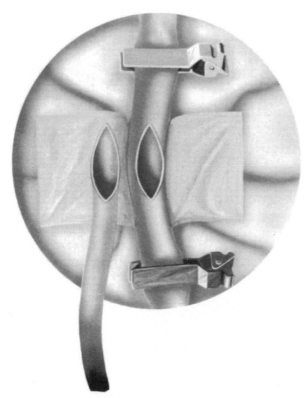

FIGURE 85–3. Diagram showing a microscopic view of the distal end of the superficial temporal artery after it has been fashioned into a fish-mouth stoma. A segment of the middle cerebral artery has been isolated with two soft temporary arterial clips, and a longitudinal arteriotomy has been made equal in length to the superficial temporal artery stoma.

removing a small elliptical section of the vessel. A small polyethylene stent is placed inside the MCA, and an end-to-side anastomosis is completed between the STA and the MCA with either interrupted or continuous 10-0 nylon sutures.

The anastomosis with interrupted sutures is started by fixing the heel of the STA stoma to one of the commissures of the MCA. The opposite end of the stoma is then sutured to the other commissure, and two more anchoring sutures are placed in the midportion of either anastomotic surface. In this manner, the anastomotic surface is divided in four quadrants; the spaces in each quadrant are then closed with interrupted sutures.[8] Another alternative is to place the two corner sutures as previously described and then insert a row of individual sutures on either anastomotic surface, leaving these sutures untied until they have all been placed correctly.[19] The advantage of this method is that the entire suture line is open as each of the two surfaces is sutured; therefore, the potential for placing a suture incorrectly is minimized. However, this method is inconvenient because there are so many loose sutures in the operative field at one time, which can make the area confusing for the surgeon trying to tie each suture individually.

The anastomosis with running sutures (Fig. 85–4) can also be started by first securing the corners with two individual sutures and then running a through-and-through suture on either side of the anastomotic surface.[49] Extreme care has to be exercised when running the suture so that the suture line does not become loose as the needle is passed through each new point. It is also important not to tie the two ends of the two different sutures together, as this would make the suture line a rigid purse string.

There is no difference in results with either the interrupted or the running suture anastomosis (Fig. 85–5).

When the anastomosis is completed, the temporary clips are removed serially; a small amount of bleeding usually develops after the clips are removed, but it can be controlled by packing the anastomotic surface gently with cotton. Occasionally, if the bleeding does not stop spontaneously, one or two additional sutures are required to stop it. Whenever possible, it is best not to add any extra sutures, because strictures may develop on the anastomosis.

Occipital to Middle Cerebral Artery Anastomosis

When the STA was unavailable for EC–IC anastomosis, other procedures were developed. Spetzler and Chater[50] introduced anastomosis of the occipital artery to the MCA in 1974. The occipital artery originates from the external carotid artery, passes under the posterior border of the mastoid muscle, pierces the superficial cervical fascia, and is directed cranially toward the occipital convexity, lying on the galea to its point of termination in the parietal occipital region. The vessel can be dissected from its point of penetration through the occipital muscle to its most distal extent. The dissection is generally tedious and difficult because the occipital artery is more tortuous and deeper than the STA. When the dissection is completed, the incision is extended anteriorly to expose the middle and posterior parietal areas (Fig. 85–6).

A free bone flap is placed as described for the STA anastomosis, centered approximately 6 cm above the external auditory meatus. In most cases, however, the bone flap ends up being a little more posterior than for the STA exposure, and the angular branch of the MCA is usually in the anterior part of the craniotomy. It is important to dissect sufficient length of occipital artery, since the angular artery, which is the most posterior branch of the MCA, is frequently far from the occipital artery. The preparation of the occipital artery and the anastomosis to the MCA are the same as that described for the STA–MCA anastomosis (Fig. 85–7).

Deep Superficial Temporal–Middle Cerebral Artery Anastomosis

It is sometimes necessary to perform an EC–IC anastomosis to a more proximal branch of the MCA (Fig. 85–8). We have found it necessary to anastomose directly to the primary divisions of the MCA in cases in which immediate high flow was needed.[24] To reach the proximal portion of the MCA, it is necessary to open the sylvian fissure, facilitated by the

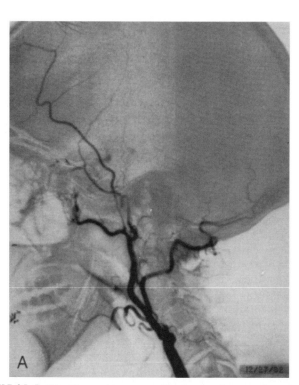 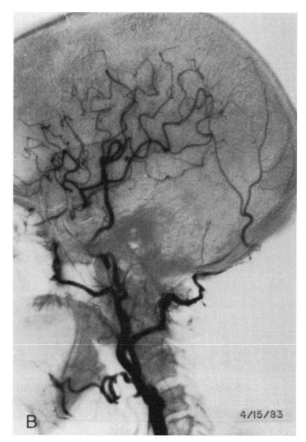

FIGURE 85–5. This 62-year-old woman suffered repeated events of transient cerebral ischemia on the left hemisphere. *A*, Cerebral angiogram revealed a complete occlusion of the right internal carotid artery; a cerebral blood flow study indicated a 20 percent flow deficit on the left side. *B*, Postoperative angiogram of the left common carotid artery shows complete filling of the entire middle cerebral artery territory through a patent anastomosis between the superficial cerebral artery and the middle cerebral artery.

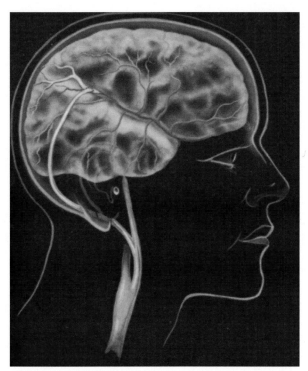

FIGURE 85–6. Diagram illustrating the anastomosis of the occipital artery to the angular branch of the middle cerebral artery.

administration of intravenous furosemide and mannitol. The dissection of the sylvian fissure is also easier when spinal fluid is removed through a spinal drain inserted in the lumbar subarachnoid space at the beginning of the procedure. The actual anastomosis is the same as that described for the cortical STA–MCA anastomosis, but the procedure is much more challenging because the anastomosis is carried out deep within the cranium. Because of the direct manipulation of the brain, the more extensive dissection of the MCA trunks and primary divisions can be associated with significant cerebral edema and postoperative seizures (Fig. 85–9).

Saphenous Vein Grafts: Extracranial to Middle Cerebral Artery

Another alternative to an extracranial arterial anastomosis is a graft of saphenous vein interposed between an extracranial vessel and the MCA. Although vein grafts were introduced for cerebral revascularization by Worringer and Kunlin[5] in 1963, their successful application did not occur until 1975, when Tew[51] reported using a saphenous vein graft to create an anastomosis from the common carotid artery to the supraclinoid internal carotid artery in four patients. The more common anastomosis to a cortical branch of the MCA was reported by Story and coworkers[10] in 1978.

The saphenous vein graft is obtained from the distal portion of the leg and should be long enough to extend from the subclavian or common carotid artery to the MCA without tension. The graft is obtained in a conventional manner, and care should be taken to cauterize or ligate side branches without damaging the vein wall. It is also important not to strip the vein clean of all periadventitial tissue, since this could damage the vasa vasorum and result in endothelial necrosis.[23]

To preserve the normal venous wall structure, I prefer to infiltrate the venous bed with a 10 percent papaverine and normal saline solution, which is injected around the vein prior to its actual manipulation. Once the vein has been removed, it is irrigated with heparinized warm blood and is gently distended with a calibrated balloon to no more than 300 cm H_2O pressure. This maneuver permits the identification of small leaking points, which are then obliterated with fine sutures. Gentle distention prevents the unwanted development of venous spasm, which may precipitate separation of the endothelial layer. As the preparation of the vein is completed, it is important to mark the end that was closest to the foot, since this end must be anastomosed most proximally on the arterial tree. Although the physical characteristics of the venous wall may make it seem more desirable for the foot end to be anastomosed distally on the cerebral vessels, since this end is smaller, the presence of venous valves makes the proximal orientation necessary. The arterial flow would be blocked by the valves if the vein were placed with the foot end distally on the arterial tree. Once the correct end is marked, the vein is stored in cold heparinized blood or saline until it is used.[23]

The proximal anastomosis can be completed on the third portion of the subclavian artery, on the common carotid artery, on the external carotid artery, or directly on the most proximal portion of the STA in front of the tragus. An end-to-side anastomosis is generally completed on any of these vessels with 6-0 or 7-0 monofilament nylon. The distal portion of the sylvian fissure is exposed as described above for the STA–MCA anastomosis; the vein is then tunneled subcutaneously and oriented properly without any kinks. After the MCA has been dissected and temporarily occluded in the manner previously outlined for the STA–MCA anastomosis, the distal anastomosis is completed end to side with continuous or interrupted 10-0 nylon sutures (Fig. 85–10). It is extremely important to use the largest available cortical vessel and to create a wide stoma on the MCA wall, since the saphenous vein and the MCA differ considerably in size. Because of the large size discrepancy, it is sometimes better to complete the anastomosis to a more proximal branch of the MCA (Fig. 85–11).[24]

Many pitfalls are associated with the use of saphenous vein grafts; the success of the procedure depends on careful and compulsive attention to minor details. As previously mentioned, occlusion of the graft may occur because of the incorrect orientation of the venous valves in the arterial flow. Endothelial damage may also result from vigorous removal of the adventitia or from the development of spasm when the vein is not dilated carefully prior to storage. This manual dilatation of the vein can also result in endothelial separation or endothelial tears when the vein is distended too much. The disruption of the endothelial layer may result in the formation of intraluminal thrombi and vessel occlusion. The ligation of small branches with sutures or cautery and the occlusion of small bleeding points on the vein wall with sutures may cause local stenosis if it is not done carefully. Torsion or angulation of the vein with subsequent occlusion may result from incorrect placement of the graft in the subcutaneous tunnel.[23]

Synthetic grafts were first tried in 1965, although unsuccessfully, by Pool and Potts.[4] The first successful synthetic graft (polytetrafluoroethylene) was reported by Story and

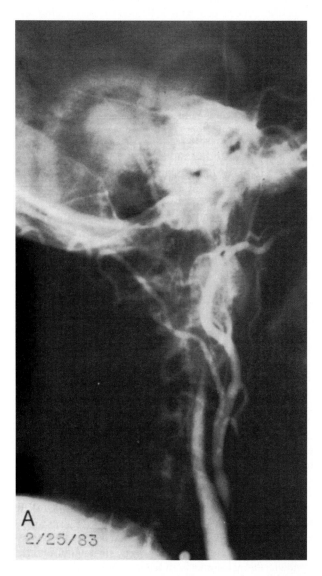

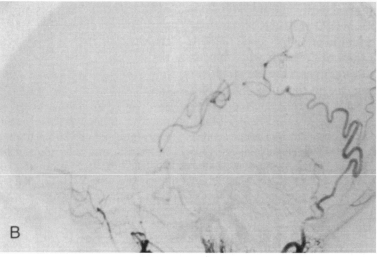

FIGURE 85–7. This 52-year-old woman presented with numerous events of right hemiparesis and expressive dysphasia. *A*, Preoperative angiogram of the left common carotid artery demonstrates a complete occlusion of the left internal carotid artery and a hypoplastic superficial temporal artery. *B*, Postoperative angiogram of the left common carotid artery demonstrates a patent occipital to middle cerebral artery anastomosis.

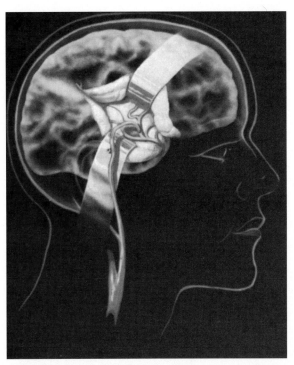

FIGURE 85–8. Diagram illustrating the exposure of the proximal portion of the middle cerebral artery (MCA) in the sylvian fissure. The frontal and temporal lobes are retracted to expose the area of the MCA trifurcation. An anastomosis is then completed deep within the sylvian fissure from the superficial temporal artery or a saphenous vein graft to one of the proximal trunks of the MCA.

associates[12] in 1978, anastomosed between the external carotid artery and cortical MCA.

Posterior Circulation

Different procedures have been designed to revascularize the vertebrobasilar circulation. Cerebral revascularization of the vertebrobasilar circulation began with the report of the anastomosis of the occipital artery to the posterior inferior cerebellar artery (PICA) by Ausman and colleagues[34] and then by Khodadad[40] in 1976. Since then, numerous procedures have been developed.

Intracranial Vertebral Endarterectomy

In 1980, Sundt and coworkers[43] reported the use of transluminal angioplasty for basilar artery stenosis, although their results were poor. In 1981, Allen and associates[33] reported a successful distal vertebral artery endarterectomy for selective focal stenosis in the third and fourth portions of the vertebral artery. The vertebral artery is approached through a suboccipital craniectomy performed with the patient lying in a three-quarter prone position with the side to be operated on closest to the table (Fig. 85–12). A midline incision is made from the inion to the C5 spinous process and is carried down and extended laterally until the vertebral artery is exposed as it arises from the first transverse foramen. The artery is then dissected from its exit from the first transverse process to its entry into the dura through the atlanto-occipital membrane. The vertebral artery is surrounded by a venous plexus that

must be carefully dissected, cauterized, and transected. A standard unilateral suboccipital craniectomy is then performed ipsilateral to the stenotic artery, and the dura is opened from the midline in the direction of the vertebral artery entry.

The perimedullary portion of the vertebral artery is dissected to expose the origin of the PICA. At this point, the patient receives an intravenous bolus of 250 mg thiopental, 100 mg lidocaine, and 5000 units of heparin. The artery can be clipped proximally at C1 and distally prior to the PICA. A longitudinal arteriotomy is made (Fig. 85–13), and the plaque is dissected under the microscope. After the plaque is removed, the arteriotomy is closed with running 6-0 or 7-0 polypropylene sutures.

Occipital to Posterior Inferior Cerebellar Artery Anastomosis

For occlusive lesions of the vertebral artery proximal to the PICA, the vertebrobasilar circulation can be reconstructed by an anastomosis of the occipital artery to the PICA itself.[40–42, 45, 52] The patient is placed in a park-bench or lateral position with the surgical side up. The occipital artery is traced on the scalp with the ultrasonic Doppler, and the incision is marked in a lazy S shape, outlining first the vertical portion of the occipital artery and then curving the incision from the point of perforation of the artery through the posterior cervical fascia, toward the posterior edge of the mastoid; the incision is then extended vertically down to the C3 level. Dissection of the occipital artery is carried out in the same way as previously outlined for the anterior circulation, but it is extended to the level of the mastoid muscle to obtain sufficient vessel length. The suboccipital muscles are then incised and retracted; a unilateral suboccipital craniectomy is completed from the foramen magnum to the transverse sinus and from the edge of the mastoid to the midline. Generally, it is not necessary to remove the arch of C1. After the dura is opened, the cerebellum usually falls away by its own weight once the cisterna magna has been drained of spinal fluid. When the perimedullary portion of the PICA has been identified on the lateral medullary area and either the rostral or the caudal branches of the PICA have been dissected, a section of the vessel devoid of any branches is isolated and temporarily clipped. A longitudinal arteriotomy is made on the isolated segment of PICA; an end-to-end anastomosis of the occipital artery to the perimedullary portion of the PICA is then completed (Fig. 85–14).

Occipital to Anterior Inferior Cerebellar Artery Anastomosis

When the vertebral arteries are occluded distal to the PICA or when a high-grade stenosis of the vertebral artery is distal to the level of the PICA, the EC–IC anastomosis must be to the anterior inferior cerebellar artery (AICA).[35] The exposure is essentially the same as that for anastomosis to the PICA; the dissection of the occipital artery is completed in a similar manner. The cerebellum must be gently retracted laterally to expose the area of the seventh and eighth cranial nerves. The prepontine portion of the AICA is identified as it extends from in front of the foramen of

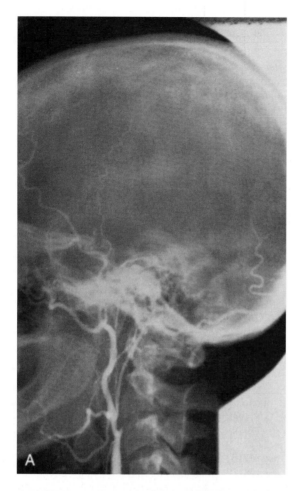

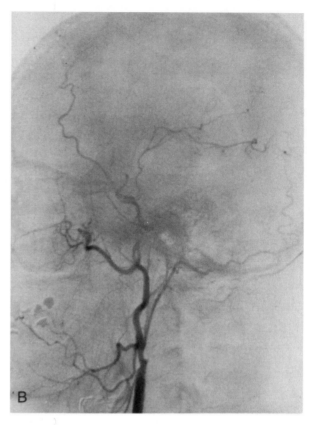

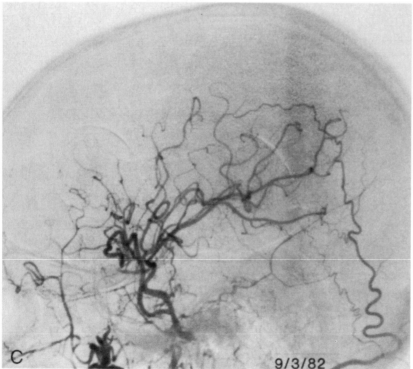

FIGURE 85–9. This 64-year-old man presented with repeated events of right hemiparesis, expressive dysphasia, and amaurosis fugax of the left eye. *A,* Preoperative angiogram of the left common carotid artery demonstrates a complete internal carotid artery occlusion. *B,* First postoperative angiogram demonstrates a patent anastomosis of the left superficial temporal artery (STA) to the middle cerebral artery (MCA) filling only two cortical branches of the MCA. The patient's symptoms persisted for several weeks after surgery in spite of oral antiplatelet agents. *C,* Second postoperative angiogram performed after an anastomosis of the anterior branch of the STA to a proximal trunk of the MCA reveals complete filling of the MCA territory through a patent anastomosis.

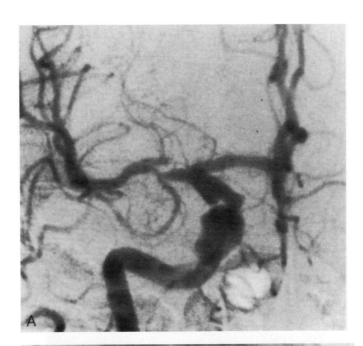

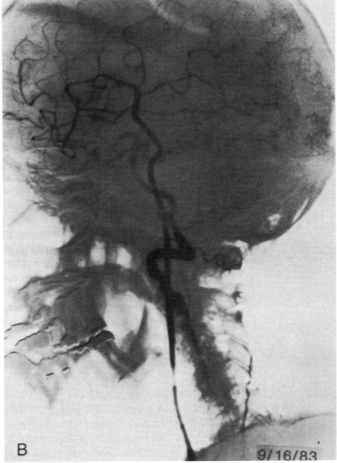

FIGURE 85–10. This 53-year-old woman presented with multiple events of left hemiparesis and left facial palsy. *A*, Preoperative angiogram of the right internal carotid artery revealed a high-grade middle cerebral artery (MCA) stenosis proximal to the origin of the lenticulostriate vessels. *B*, Postoperative angiogram of the right common carotid artery demonstrates complete filling of the MCA territory through a patent saphenous vein graft from the subclavian artery to the angular branch of the MCA.

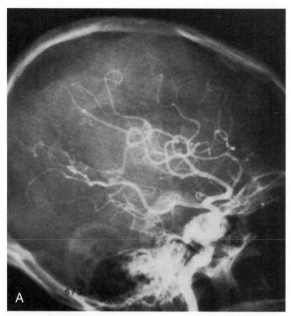

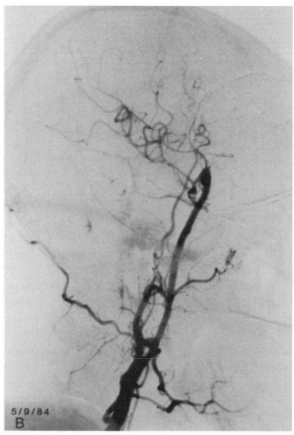

FIGURE 85–11. This 54-year-old woman developed progressive diplopia, ptosis, and retro-ocular pain on the right side. *A*, Preoperative angiogram of the right internal carotid artery demonstrates a large area of contrast material pooling in the region of the cavernous sinus, compatible with a giant aneurysm of the internal carotid artery and rapid flow of contrast agent into the cavernous sinus, suggestive of a carotid cavernous fistula. Since it is not surgically possible to approach these ruptured aneurysms directly, the fistula was embolized with muscle pledgets through an arteriotomy in the internal carotid artery in the neck, after the intracranial internal carotid artery was occluded with a clip. When the embolization was completed, the proximal internal carotid artery was ligated in the neck, and a saphenous vein graft was anastomosed from the common carotid to a proximal trunk of the middle cerebral artery. *B*, Postoperative angiogram of the right common carotid artery demonstrates complete occlusion of the internal carotid artery, no filling of the carotid cavernous fistula, and a patent saphenous vein graft filling the entire distribution of the middle cerebral artery.

Luschka and is directed toward the anterior surface of the cerebellum; at this point, the vessel has already divided in its rostral and caudal branches. When choosing the anastomosis site, it is preferable to use the branch without collateral branches to the brain stem. In some patients, the AICA may be confused with a high branch of the PICA; to prevent this confusion, it is important to follow the branch selected for the anastomosis to its level of origin. After the chosen branch is dissected and carefully isolated, an anastomosis is completed from the occipital artery to the AICA in a manner

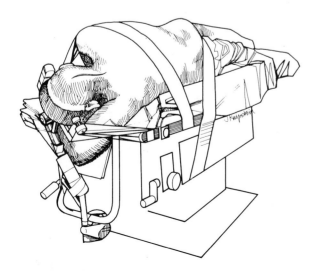

FIGURE 85–12. Diagram illustrating the three-quarter prone position. The patient is lying on the side intended for the endarterectomy. This position facilitates dissection of the vertebral artery: the horizontal position of the artery places it in direct line of vision for the surgeon, and the operating microscope can easily be used.

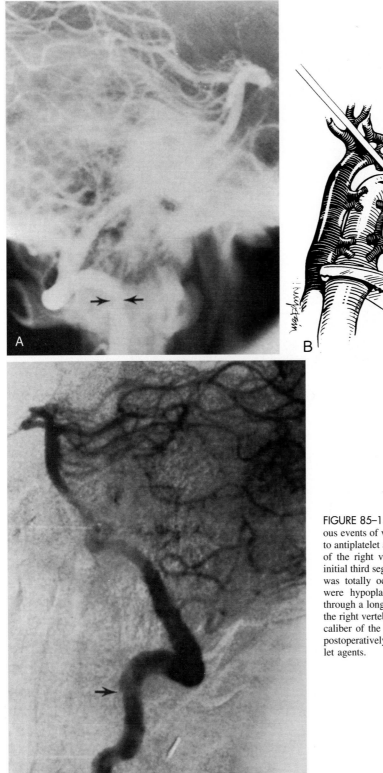

FIGURE 85–13. This 62-year-old man was admitted with numerous events of vertigo, dysarthria, diplopia, and ataxia unresponsive to antiplatelet and anticoagulant agents. *A*, Preoperative angiogram of the right vertebral artery shows a high-grade stenosis of the initial third segment of the artery. The contralateral vertebral artery was totally occluded, and the posterior communicating arteries were hypoplastic. *B*, Removal of the vertebral artery plaque through a longitudinal arteriotomy. *C*, Postoperative angiogram of the right vertebral artery reveals full anatomic reconstitution of the caliber of the vertebral artery. The patient became asymptomatic postoperatively and his health is maintained only with antiplatelet agents.

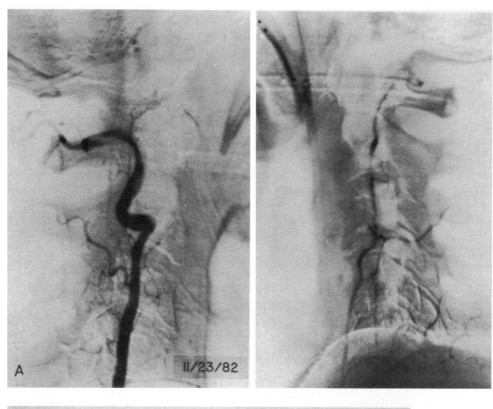

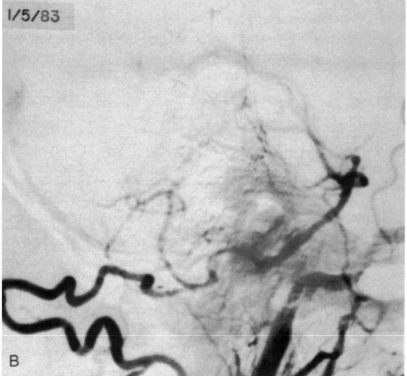

FIGURE 85–14. This 57-year-old man was admitted with multiple events of dysarthria, diplopia, and ataxia. *A*, Preoperative angiography demonstrates an occlusion of the right vertebral artery at C2 and a hypoplastic left vertebral artery. Partial filling of the distal basilar artery was observed via the right internal carotid artery. *B*, Postoperative angiogram of the right external carotid artery demonstrates complete filling of the basilar artery and its branches through a patent anastomosis of the occipital to the posterior inferior cerebellar artery.

similar to that described for other EC–IC microanastomoses (Fig. 85–15).

Superficial Temporal to Superior Cerebellar Artery Anastomosis

In patients who have stenosis or occlusion of the proximal or midportion of the basilar artery without collaterals from the anterior circulation, the previously described procedures would be ineffective. These patients require an anastomosis to the superior cerebellar artery[34, 36, 37, 39] or to the posterior cerebral artery.[11] In either case, the patient is positioned supine with the ipsilateral shoulder elevated and the operative area oriented horizontally in relation to the floor. The STA is traced on the scalp with a Doppler. A minimum of 15 cm is required to reach the perimesencephalic area from

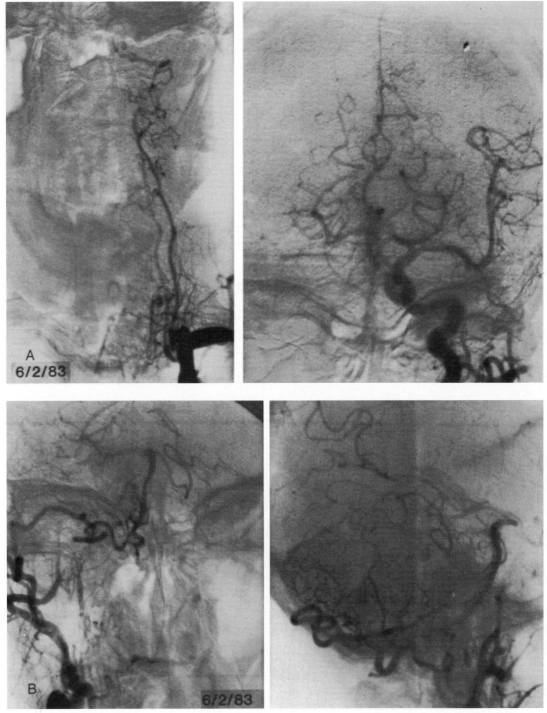

FIGURE 85–15. This 71-year-old man developed recurring events of vertigo, ataxia, dysmetria, and diplopia unresponsive to treatment with anticoagulants. *A*, Preoperative angiogram shows a hypoplastic left vertebral artery with numerous muscular collaterals. The right vertebral artery was totally occluded at its origin. The distal basilar artery was filled partially by the left internal carotid artery. *B*, Postoperative angiogram of the right internal carotid artery demonstrates total filling of the basilar artery and its branches through a patent anastomosis of the occipital to anterior inferior cerebellar artery.

the scalp surface; the largest of the two branches of the STA is therefore dissected, gaining as much length as possible. Centered on the ear, a temporal craniotomy is completed flush with the middle cranial fossa. It is necessary to extend this craniotomy a minimum of 3 cm in front and 3 cm behind the external auditory meatus to have enough room to manipulate the instruments for the anastomosis. A lumbar subarachnoid drain is mandatory in these anastomoses to ensure that the pressure exerted on the temporal lobe during retraction is minimal. After the dura has been opened, the temporal lobe is elevated. Care must be taken to preserve the temporal veins; otherwise, postoperative swelling and postoperative cerebral contusions are common. The superior cerebellar artery is exposed by incising the tentorium; this is accomplished by exposing first the fourth cranial nerve under the tentorial incisura and extending the incision toward the petrous apex approximately 2 cm from the insertion of the tentorium on the posterior clinoid process. The two flaps of the tentorium are then retracted laterally and sutured back to the dura. This approach permits exposure of the peri-mesencephalic portion of the superior cerebellar artery, which at this point usually has no branches and divides into its rostral and caudal branches. The largest of the two branches is carefully dissected and isolated. At this point, the distal end of the STA is transected, and a temporary clip is placed at the base. A fish-mouth stoma is prepared, and an end-to-side anastomosis is completed from the STA to the superior cerebellar artery in a manner similar to that previously described (Fig. 85–16). It is important to use the maximum available length of the STA for the anastomosis; otherwise, the procedure is practically impossible.

Superficial Temporal to Posterior Cerebral Artery Anastomosis

When the superior cerebellar artery is of insufficient caliber, the posterior cerebral artery is used.[11] The posterior cerebral artery is found in the perimesencephalic area just beneath the edge of the uncus of the hippocampus; the vessel is usually large and easy to isolate, although much more retraction is needed to identify and separate the posterior cerebral artery. The vessel has less mobility than the superior cerebellar artery, and the cortical perforators cannot be cauterized, since they are usually large. Once the vessel has been isolated and temporarily clipped, an anastomosis is completed with the STA or a saphenous vein graft to the posterior cerebral artery in a manner similar to that described previously. Use of the posterior cerebral artery is not the optimal choice, because its collateral circulation is not as extensive as that of the superior cerebellar artery, and the risk of a cortical injury with secondary cortical blindness is greater than that of a cerebellar deficit when the superior cerebellar artery is used.

To complete a cerebral revascularization of the posterior circulation successfully, it is mandatory to have adequate exposure and complete cerebral relaxation. A lumbar subarachnoid drain is a useful adjunct and must be considered in all patients who undergo any of these procedures. The intravenous administration of furosemide and mannitol is also useful in providing cerebral relaxation, but the drugs must be administered at least 1 hour before the brain is exposed. Mannitol may also have a protective effect during the period of cross-clamping of any major cerebral vessel. These anastomoses are difficult to perform because of the depth at which they are done. They require the use of long instruments and require considerable skill to complete.

CURRENT CLINICAL APPLICATIONS

Cerebral revascularization became popular because it offered a surgical option to patients with severe and generally diffuse cerebrovascular disease for whom there was no other available treatment. The success of the procedure was predicated on the existence of an area of hypoperfused but viable brain that could be improved by an extracranial to intracranial bypass. An international cooperative study was conducted to demonstrate whether an STA anastomosis to a cortical

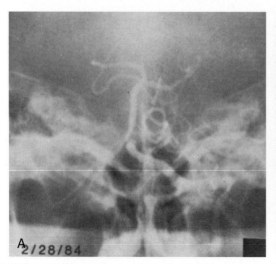
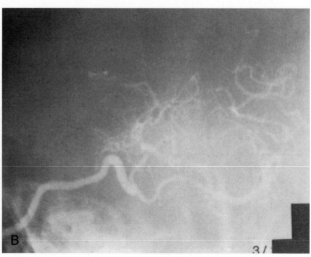

FIGURE 85–16. This 73-year-old man presented with daily events of diplopia, dysarthria, ataxia, and vertigo unresponsive to antiplatelets and anticoagulants. *A*, Preoperative angiogram of the left vertebral artery demonstrates a severe midbasilar stenosis. No distal basilar artery filling was observed through either carotid artery injection. *B*, Postoperative angiogram of the right external carotid artery shows filling of the distal basilar artery through a patent anastomosis of the superficial temporal artery to the superior cerebellar artery.

branch of the MCA would reduce the risk of stroke or stroke-related death compared with aspirin treatment in patients with specific, otherwise surgically inaccessible cerebrovascular occlusive lesions in the carotid or middle cerebral circulation. The conclusion was that EC–IC bypass surgery was no better than aspirin in reducing stroke or stroke-related death in the patients in this study. But based on the following observations, this conclusion cannot be accepted.

There was no demonstration of a perfusion deficit by any physiologic study to document that these patients had abnormalities in their hemispheric blood flow and that they needed surgery. The collateral circulation through the circle of Willis was not determined, as selective bilateral vertebral angiography was not required; therefore, not even angiographic perfusion deficits could be shown by the international study.

Fifty-eight percent of the patients entered in the study had internal carotid artery occlusions, which would be the least likely to benefit from any form of cerebral revascularization, since the collateral circulation through the brain would most likely be sufficient without operation. At least 38 percent of the patients were asymptomatic at the time of admission to the study.

A clinical and angiographic correlation was inappropriately made at the end of the study. All patients underwent angiography prior to entry into the study, but only the surgical patients had repeat angiography in the first few weeks after surgery. No patients had any further angiography over the 5 years of follow-up. It is therefore impossible to determine whether the progression of symptoms or the occurrence of infarction was related to the original angiographic lesion, was secondary to another newly developed lesion, or was a result of bypass failure.

The bypass procedure used to reperfuse the brain may not have provided sufficient immediate flow, since approximately 30 percent of these patients required 6 months or more for the bypass to reach satisfactory caliber. It is possible that a much larger afferent vessel or an anastomosis to a more proximal portion of the MCA would be needed to evaluate this problem.[24]

Patients with MCA stenosis did not benefit from the procedure. However, there was an insufficient number of patients with pure MCA stenosis to reach statistical significance. To achieve statistical validity, the investigators mixed patients with MCA lesions and patients with combined lesions (a lesion of the MCA plus a proximal stenosis of the internal carotid artery at the siphon or the bifurcation). These combinations are not scientifically valid because the pathophysiologic mechanisms involved in the development of cerebral ischemia in these two cases are not likely to be the same. Therefore, no valid statistical conclusion can be made regarding these subgroups.

As a result of the international cooperative study, the use of cerebral revascularization to treat patients with cerebral ischemia has basically disappeared. There has been no other study to date that can counter the findings of the international cooperative study. Today, the only indications for a cerebral revascularization procedure are the presence of cerebral ischemic symptoms that are refractory to medication, a vascular occlusion in the territory of distribution of the ischemic area, a normal computed tomographic or nuclear magnetic resonance scan or absence of a significant ischemic infarct, or a perfusion deficit on cerebral blood flow studies performed with Diamox that demonstrate limited or no reserve.

Cerebral revascularization has been used to treat surgically induced areas of cerebral ischemia, such as those that occur when acute internal carotid artery occlusion is used to remove large skull-base tumors, or during planned occlusions of any intracranial vessel in the course of aneurysm or arteriovenous malformation surgery. Excellent results have been achieved with this combined technique of acute vascular occlusion and immediate cerebral revascularization. Since surgically induced acute vessel occlusion works well to treat patients with brain tumors and aneurysms, it does not make intuitive sense that patients who develop otherwise acute carotid occlusions caused by arteriosclerosis should not be candidates for cerebral revascularization and respond equally as well.

CONCLUSIONS

It is unknown whether cerebral revascularization by anastomosis of the STA to the MCA prevents cerebral infarction or death in patients with a demonstrated cerebral perfusion deficit and with viable residual cerebral tissue in the area of ischemia. A randomized study must be conducted to identify individuals among the population with cerebral ischemic symptoms who have both perfusion deficits and preserved cerebral tissue. The random allocation to surgical and medical groups with adequate follow-up by clinical, angiographic, blood flow, and metabolic criteria would then allow the value of EC–IC bypass to be determined. Until then, the EC–IC bypass study indicates that not all patients seen in daily clinical practice who have unilateral internal carotid artery or MCA occlusive lesions should be subjected to cerebral revascularization. However, the EC–IC bypass study does not exclude the value of cerebral revascularization for patients with focal cerebral perfusion deficits associated with viable cerebral tissue. Furthermore, the findings of the EC–IC bypass study cannot be generalized to other bypass procedures such as proximal MCA anastomosis or posterior fossa revascularization.

REFERENCES

1. Fisher M: Occlusion of the internal carotid artery. *Arch Neurol Psychiatry.* 1951;65:346.
2. Kredell FE: Collateral cerebral circulation by muscle graft technique of operation with report of three cases. *South Surg.* 1942;11:235.
3. Chou S: Embolectomy of middle cerebral artery. *J Neurosurg.* 1963;20:161.
4. Pool L, Potts DG: *Aneurysms and Arteriovenous Anomalies of the Brain.* Hagerstown, MD: Harper & Row; 1965.
5. Woringer E, Kunlin J: Anastomose entre la carotide primitive and le carotide intra-craniene ou le silicene par greffon elon le technique de la suture suspendue. *Neurochirurgie.* 1963;9:181.
6. Jacobsen JH, Suarez EL: Microsurgery in anastomosis of small vessels. *Surg Forum.* 1960;11:243.
7. Donaghy P: Evaluation of extracranial–intracranial blood flow diversion. In Austin GM, ed. *Microneurosurgical Anastomoses for Cerebral Ischemia.* Springfield, IL: Charles C Thomas; 1976:256.
8. Yasargil MG: *Microsurgery Applied to Neurosurgery.* Stuttgart: Georg Thieme-Verlag; 1969.
9. Lougheed WM, Marshal BM, Hunter M, et al: Common carotid to intracranial internal carotid bypass venous graft. Technical note. *J Neurosurg.* 1971;34:114.
10. Story JL, Brown WE, Eidelberg E, et al: Cerebral revascularization: Common carotid to distal middle cerebral artery bypass. *Neurosurgery.* 1978;2:131.
11. Sundt TM, Piepgras DG, Houser OW, et al: Interposition saphenous vein grafts

for advanced occlusive disease and large aneurysms in the posterior circulation. *J Neurosurg*. 1982;56:205.

12. Story JL, Brown WE, Eidelberg E, et al: Cerebral revascularization: Proximal external carotid to distal middle cerebral artery bypass with a synthetic tube graft. *Neurosurgery*. 1978;3:61.

13. Gowers WR: *A Manual of Diseases of the Nervous System*, Vol 2. London: J & A Churchill; 1888.

14. Karasawa J, Kikuchi H, Kawamura J, et al: Intracranial transplantation of the omentum for cerebrovascular moya moya disease: A two year follow-up study. *Surg Neurol*. 1980;14:444.

15. Sundt TM, Siekert RG, Piepgras DG, et al: Bypass surgery for vascular disease of the carotid system. *Mayo Clin Proc*. 1976;51:677.

16. Diaz FG, Ausman JI, Mehta B, et al: Acute cerebral revascularization. *J Neurosurg*. 1985;63:200.

17. Ojemann RG, Crowell RM: *Surgical Management of Cerebrovascular Disease*. Baltimore: Williams & Wilkins; 1983.

18. Chater N: Neurosurgical extracranial–intracranial bypass for stroke: With 400 cases. *Neurol Res*. 1983;5:1.

19. Reichman OJ: Extracranial to intracranial arterial anastomosis. In Yeoumans JR, ed. *Neurological Surgery*, Vol 3. Philadelphia: WB Saunders; 1982:1584.

20. Samson DS, Boone S: Extracranial–intracranial arterial bypass: Past performance and current concepts. *Neurosurgery*. 1978;3:79.

21. Spetzler RF: Extracranial–intracranial arterial anastomosis for cerebrovascular disease. *Surg Neurol*. 1979;11:157.

22. Ausman JI, Lee MC, Klassen AL, et al: Stroke: What's new? Cerebral revascularization. *Minn Med*. 1976;59:223.

23. Diaz FG, Pearce J, Ausman JI: Complications of cerebral revascularization with autogenous vein grafts. *Neurosurgery*. 1985;17:271.

24. Diaz FG, Umansky F, Mehta B, et al: Cerebral revascularization to a main limb of the middle cerebral artery in the sylvian fissure. An alternative to conventional anastomosis. *J Neurosurg*. 1985;63:21.

25. Boone SC: The surgical management of bilateral carotid artery occlusive disease. In Peerless SJ, McCormick CW, eds. *Microsurgery for Cerebral Ischemia*. New York: Springer-Verlag; 1980:297.

26. Barnett HJM: Is there a place for cerebral revascularization? *Clin Neurosurg*. 1979;26:314.

27. Chater N, Popp J: Microsurgical vascular bypass for occlusive cerebrovascular disease: A review of 100 cases. *Surg Neurol*. 1976;6:115.

28. Deruty R, Bret P, Lecuire J, et al: L'anastomose arterielle extra-intracranienne. Bilan d'une expérience clinique de 40 cas. *Neurochirurgie*. 1978;24:355.

29. Goldsmith HS, Saunders RL, Reeves AG, et al: Omental transposition to brain of stroke patients. *Stroke*. 1979;10:471.

30. Guegan R, Deruty R, Rey A, et al: EICA in transient ischemic attacks and neurological deficits. *Acta Neurochir*. 1979;28(suppl):304.

31. Spetzler RF, Zabramski J: Revascularization of anterior and posterior circulation ischemia. *Clin Neurosurg*. 1982;29:575.

32. Agnoli A, Maira G, Pola P, et al: Extra-intracranial arterial anastomosis in ischemic completed stroke (abstract). *Acta Neurochir*. 1981;57:131.

33. Allen GS, Cohen RJ, Preziosi TJ: Microsurgical endarterectomy of the intracranial vertebral artery for vertebrobasilar transient ischemic attacks. *Neurosurgery*. 1981;8:56.

34. Ausman JI, Chou SN, Lee M, et al: Occipital to cerebellar artery anastomosis for brain stem infarction from vertebral basilar occlusive disease. *Stroke*. 1976;7:13.

35. Ausman JI, Diaz FG, de los Reyes RA, et al: Anastomosis of occipital artery to anterior inferior cerebellar artery for vertebrobasilar junction stenosis. *Surg Neurol*. 1981;16:99.

36. Ausman JI, Diaz FG, de los Reyes RA, et al: Posterior circulation revascularization: Superficial to superior cerebellar artery anastomosis. *J Neurosurg*. 1982;56:766.

37. Ausman JI, Diaz FG, de los Reyes RA, et al: Superficial temporal to proximal superior cerebellar artery anastomosis for basilar artery stenosis. *Neurosurgery*. 1981;9:56.

38. Ausman JI, Diaz FG, Pearce JE, et al: Endarterectomy of the vertebral artery from C2 to posterior inferior cerebellar artery intracranially. *Surg Neurol*. 1982;18:400.

39. Ausman JI, Lee MC, Chater N, et al: Superficial temporal artery to superior cerebellar artery anastomosis for distal basilar artery stenosis. *Surg Neurol*. 1979;12:227.

40. Khodadad G: Occipital artery–posterior inferior cerebellar artery anastomosis. *Surg Neurol*. 1976;5:225.

41. Khodadad G: Short and long-term results of microvascular anastomosis in the vertebrobasilar system, critical analysis. *Neurol Res*. 1981;3:33.

42. Sundt TM, Piepgras DG: Occipital to posterior inferior cerebellar artery bypass surgery. *J Neurosurg*. 1978;48:916.

43. Sundt TM, Smith HC, Campbell JK, et al: Transluminal angioplasty for basilar artery stenosis. *Mayo Clin Proc*. 1980;55:675.

44. Merei TF, Bodosi M: Microsurgical anastomosis for cerebral ischemia in 90 patients. In Schmiedek P, ed. *Microsurgery for Stroke*. New York: Springer-Verlag; 1977:264.

45. Spetzler RF, Roski RA, Kopaniki DR: Alternative superficial temporal artery to middle cerbral artery revascularization procedure. *Neurosurgery*. 1980;7:484.

46. Kikuchi H, Karasawa J: Extra–intracranial arterial anastomosis in ten patients with moya moya syndrome (occlusion of the circle of Willis). In Schmiedek P, ed. *Microsurgery for Stroke*. New York: Springer-Verlag; 1977:260.

47. Donaghy RMP: What's new in surgery? Neurological surgery. *Surg Gynecol Obstet*. 1972;134:269.

48. Peerles SJ: Technique of cerebral revascularization. *Clin Neurosurg*. 1976;23:258.

49. Little JR, Salerno TA: Continuous suturing for microvascular anastomosis: Technical note. *J Neurosurg* 1978;48:1042.

50. Spetzler RF, Chater N: Occipital artery–middle cerebral artery anastomosis for cerebral artery occlusive disease. *Surg Neurol* 1974;2:235.

51. Tew JM: Reconstructive intracranial vascular surgery for prevention of stroke. *Clin Neurosurg*. 1975;22:264.

52. Ausman JI, Nicoloff DM, Chou SN: Posterior fossa revascularization. Anastomosis of vertebral artery to PICA with interposed radial artery graft. *Surg Neurol*. 1978;9:281.

CHAPTER 86

Immediate and Late Results of Extracranial–Intracranial Bypass Surgery

JOHN R. LITTLE

Superficial temporal artery to middle cerebral artery (STA–MCA) anastomosis is a procedure designed primarily to bypass atherosclerotic occlusion or inaccessible stenosis of the internal carotid artery (ICA) or middle cerebral artery (MCA). This is the only type of extracranial-intracranial bypass surgery that has been performed on a sufficient number of patients and for which some control data exist to permit meaningful interpretation of results. Results of other procedures, such as posterior circulation bypass or bypass surgery done for nonatherosclerotic disease (eg, moyamoya syndrome), are therefore not considered.

Before the international extracranial-intracranial (EC–IC) bypass study was performed,[1, 2] scant data were available regarding long-term stroke risk in patients with ICA occlusion or inaccessible ICA stenosis who did not undergo surgery. Virtually no data were available regarding long-term stroke risk in patients with MCA stenosis or occlusion. It is useful to review briefly what was known about the natural history of angiographic lesions amenable to STA–MCA bypass before the international EC–IC study was undertaken. It is important to emphasize that such natural history data should not be used as a historical control to assess the outcome of bypass surgery in individual surgical series. Rather, natural history data serve to help estimate appropriate sample sizes when multicenter prospective randomized trials are designed.

OCCLUSION OF THE INTERNAL CAROTID ARTERY

In most series, ICA occlusion, often asymptomatic in the period following its documentation by angiography, constitutes by far the most common lesion for which bypass surgery has been performed. For example, in the EC–IC bypass study,[2] 38 percent of randomized patients had an ICA occlusion that had been asymptomatic since angiography, 21 percent had asymptomatic ICA occlusion, 15 percent had inaccessible ICA stenosis, 14 percent had MCA stenosis, and only 12 percent had MCA occlusion.

It has often been reported anecdotally that recurrent ischemic events ipsilateral to an ICA occlusion are uncommon. However, recurrent events ipsilateral to an established ICA occlusion do occur and by several mechanisms, including stump emboli, external carotid stenosis, and hypoperfusion. Studies that have examined the natural history of ICA occlusion have not considered these different mechanisms of ischemia, only some of which may be correctable by bypass surgery.

Although at least 11 studies have addressed the prognosis following ICA occlusion, few have followed a sizable group of patients with an established ICA occlusion while excluding patients who suffered a severe initial stroke or who underwent some form of cerebrovascular surgery. Follow-up studies should also provide ipsilateral recurrent stroke rates and long-term mortality rates. In a retrospective study of 138 patients with ICA occlusion followed for an average of 5 years, Furlan and coworkers[3] found a 3 percent per year subsequent stroke rate, and two thirds of the strokes were ipsilateral to the ICA occlusion. The observed stroke rate for patients 35 years old or over was eight times the expected rate for a matched normal population. The relative risk of stroke was greatest in the youngest patients with ICA occlusion, which implies that once a certain degree of atherosclerosis is present, the long-term stroke risk is relatively independent of age. The 5-year survival rate on an actuarial basis was 77 percent compared with an expected rate of 85 percent, and coronary artery disease was the cause of death in 57 percent of patients.

In a prospective study, Cote and associates[4] followed 47 patients with ICA occlusion for an average of almost 3 years. The overall recurrent stroke rate was 8 percent per year, and the ipsilateral recurrence rate was 5 percent per year. The mortality rate was about 3 percent per year, which is comparable to the 4 percent per year in the retrospective series. Fifty percent of the deaths resulted from cardiac events. Whereas Furlan and associates[3] concluded that the risk of recurrent stroke following ICA occlusion was higher than expected but lower than that in patients with transient ischemic attacks (TIAs), Cote and associates[4] concluded that the recurrence rate in their population with ICA occlusion was comparable to that of populations of patients with TIAs. If minor strokes were excluded from the smaller prospective series, there was a 3 percent per year ipsilateral recurrence rate that was similar to the 2 percent per year ipsilateral rate found in the larger retrospective study.

INTRACRANIAL STENOSIS OF THE INTERNAL CAROTID ARTERY

Three retrospective studies have examined the long-term prognosis for patients with intracranial ICA stenosis, all with remarkably similar results. Marzewski and colleagues[5] followed 66 patients with 50 percent stenosis of an intracranial ICA for almost 4 years. Ten patients (15.2%) experienced a stroke, and 8 patients (12.1%) had isolated TIAs. The annual ipsilateral stroke rate was 4.9 percent. The observed stroke rate was 13 times the expected infarction rate for a normal population. Patients with tandem extracranial ICA stenosis appeared to have a greater stroke risk than patients with isolated intracranial stenosis. Thirty-three patients (50%) died, and 55 percent of all deaths were related to cardiac events. The observed 5-year survival rate was 60 percent, compared with an expected rate of 87 percent.

Craig and coworkers[6] followed 58 patients with at least 33 percent stenosis of an intracranial ICA. Seventeen patients (29%) suffered a stroke, and 8 patients (14%) experienced TIAs. Forty-three percent of the patients died during follow-up, 44 percent of the deaths being related to cardiac events. The annual ipsilateral stroke rate was 7.6 percent in this series.

Wechsler and colleagues[7] followed 15 patients with isolated intracranial ICA stenosis for an average of 51 months and reported a 13 percent (3.1%/year) ipsilateral stroke rate. These studies indicate that intracranial ICA stenosis carries a significant long-term risk of stroke and death and that this lesion is a marker of widespread atherosclerotic disease, especially coronary artery disease.

STENOSIS OR OCCLUSION OF THE MIDDLE CEREBRAL ARTERY

Stenosis or occlusion of the MCA related to atherosclerosis rather than embolism is rare, although it appears to be more common among Asian peoples. Hinton and associates[8] accumulated 16 patients over 7 years with atherosclerotic MCA stenosis. During the follow-up period, two patients (12%) experienced a stroke, both ipsilateral to the stenosis. The authors considered this a favorable outcome and suggested that patients with MCA stenosis may do well with medical therapy. Corston and colleagues[9] questioned whether MCA stenosis is truly a benign lesion. They reported a 24 percent stroke rate and a 48 percent mortality rate among 21 patients with MCA stenosis followed for 82 months. Unfortunately, the vascular territory in which the strokes occurred is unclearly reported in this study.

A few studies have addressed the natural history of MCA occlusion. Most of these studies deal with initial clinical presentation and immediate prognosis, and many include both embolic and atherosclerotic occlusions, as well as main trunk and branch lesions. Kaste and Waltimo[10] noted a 5-year survival rate of 78 percent among 78 patients with MCA occlusion. Death was related to a stroke twice as frequently as to cardiovascular disease, although specific details were not provided in the report. Sacquegna and coworkers[11] reported a 2 percent per year ipsilateral stroke recurrence rate among 70 patients with MCA occlusion. The observed 5-year survival rate was 82 percent, compared with an expected rate of 94 percent.

In summary, natural history data available prior to the EC–IC study suggested that, of the lesions for which STA–MCA bypass is usually performed, intracranial ICA stenosis carries the worst long-term prognosis for both stroke and mortality. Preliminary analysis of natural history data from the EC–IC bypass study corroborates this finding (HJM Barnett, personal communication, 1985). As many as 25 percent of patients with intracranial ICA stenosis will die of heart disease within 5 years of diagnosis. ICA occlusion is not a completely benign lesion and carries at least a 2 percent per year risk for ipsilateral stroke. A single prospective study suggested that the annual ipsilateral stroke rate following ICA occlusion may be as high as 5 percent. Younger patients with atherosclerotic ICA occlusion have a relatively higher risk of subsequent stroke. The natural history of MCA stenosis or occlusion was uncertain. One small retrospective series indicated a relatively good prognosis for MCA stenosis treated with anticoagulant therapy, but another study suggested a worse outlook.

PERSONAL SURGICAL SERIES

Perhaps the best single large surgical series appearing before the prospective EC–IC Study was that from the Mayo Clinic.[12, 13] The 30-day postoperative stroke morbidity and mortality rates from that and other early representative series are given in Table 86–1.[14–17] In the Mayo series, after the first month following surgery, the mortality rate, judged on an actuarial basis, was 3 percent per year; two thirds of all deaths resulted from cardiac events. Strokes occurred at a rate of 2.5 percent per year, with two thirds of the strokes occurring ipsilateral to the surgical site. With regard to stroke risk, this surgically treated group compared favorably with populations of patients with TIAs due to a mixture of causes and vascular lesions. However, the ratio of observed to expected stroke rate for this surgical group was higher than that for the previously reviewed series of patients with ICA occlusion or inaccessible ICA stenosis who did not undergo surgery. Thus, although these series are not strictly comparable, the Mayo Clinic results suggested that STA–MCA bypass did not improve the risk of stroke in patients with suitable angiographic lesions and clinical symptoms. By contrast, a number of early uncontrolled surgical series claimed excellent results for bypass surgery.

THE EXTERNAL CAROTID–INTERNAL CAROTID BYPASS STUDY

Given this background, the results of the prospective multicenter EC–IC bypass study were eagerly anticipated.[1] The design of the EC–IC bypass trial has been discussed in detail elsewhere.[2] The key feature that distinguishes this study from all other studies of STA–MCA bypass is the use of concurrent prospective randomized controls. The study achieved 100 percent follow-up with a bypass patency rate of 96 percent (median time to postoperative angiogram, 32 days). The perioperative stroke rate was 12.2 percent (81 patients). Seven of 30 major perioperative strokes were fatal, and 10 of 30 perioperative strokes occurred after randomization but before the surgery was actually performed. Importantly, however, the negative conclusions of the study are not altered even if the postrandomization presurgical strokes are deleted from the data analysis.

The long-term results of the EC–IC bypass study were clearly negative. For this group of 1377 patients, bypass surgery did not lower stroke risk or improve mortality during an average follow-up of 55.8 months. A number of patient subgroups were analyzed, with similar negative findings (Table 86–2). An attempt was also made to correlate out-

TABLE 86–1. Stroke Morbidity and Mortality Within 30 Days After Superficial Temporal Artery–Middle Cerebral Artery Bypass Operation for Cerebral Ischemia

Study*	Patients, n	Strokes, %	Deaths, %	Strokes + Deaths, %
Yasargil and Yonekawa[14]	84	5	5	6
Samson et al[15]	50	6	4	10
Lee et al[16]	40	0	0	0
Chater[17]	400	2	3	5
Whisnant et al[13]	239	3	0	3

*For full bibliographic information, see reference list at end of chapter.

Modified from Whisnant JP, Sundt TM Jr, Fode NC: Long-term mortality and stroke morbidity after superficial temporal artery–middle cerebral artery bypass operation. *Mayo Clin Proc.* 1985; 60:241, with permission.

TABLE 86–2. Fatal and Nonfatal Stroke Among Clinically Interesting Subgroups

	Medically Treated Group			Surgically Treated Group			Mantel-Haenzel χ^2 Test
Subgroup	n	Observed*	Expected†	n	Observed*	Expected†	
All patients	714	205	218.3	663	205	191.7	1.72
Excluding those with ICA occlusion, no symptoms	438	133	148.0	418	148	133.0	3.23
Including only those with							
ICA occlusion, no symptoms‡	276	72	69.9	245	57	59.1	0.13
ICA occlusion, symptoms§	147	51	61.7	140	64	53.3	4.04
Including only those with severe¶							
ICA stenosis	72	26	27.1	77	29	27.9	0.10
MCA stenosis	59	14	20.5	50	22	15.5	4.74
Including only those with							
Bilateral carotid occlusion	43	17	17.4	31	14	13.6	0.02
MCA occlusion	79	18	16.9	80	16	17.1	0.15
First TIA within 3 months of entry and total TIAs >3	87	27	31.5	109	41	36.5	1.32
Center size							
Smaller (<25 patients)	350	98	112.1	337	113	98.9	3.81
Larger (>25 patients)	364	107	105.9	326	92	93.1	0.02
Geographic region							
North America	352	115	126.8	327	120	108.2	2.37
Europe	247	60	64.9	230	63	58.1	0.77
Asia	115	30	26.8	106	22	25.2	0.78

*Values indicate the observed number of patients in each treatment group who had a stroke.

†Values indicate the number of patients in each treatment group who would be expected to have a stroke if surgery had no effect, taking into account difference in sample size and duration of follow-up.

‡No symptoms were experienced between angiographic demonstration of occlusion and randomization.

§Symptoms were experienced between angiographic demonstration of occlusion and randomization.

¶Severe stenosis is stenosis of 70 percent or more of the luminal diameter.

From the EC–IC Bypass Study Group: Failure of extracranial–intracranial arterial bypass to reduce the risk of ischemic stroke. Results of an international randomized trial. N Engl J Med. 1985; 313:1191, with permission.

come with the angiographic adequacy of the bypass, again with negative results.

Patients with symptomatic ICA occlusion and MCA stenosis actually fared worse with bypass surgery. The reasons for this are unclear in the group with ICA occlusion. In the group with MCA stenosis, a patent bypass actually precipitated MCA occlusion in 14 percent of cases, a hazard previously documented with high-grade ICA siphon stenosis.[18]

Two other interesting results of the EC–IC bypass study deserve comment. First, STA–MCA bypass did not appear to improve neurologic recovery after a stroke occurred, although the study was not specifically designed to address this issue. There have been scattered reports of dramatic reversal of chronic ischemic neurologic deficits following bypass surgery. Second, in nearly identical proportions of patients (80% in the medically treated group and 70% in the surgically treated group), the frequency of TIAs at 1 year was nearly halved. This finding emphasizes that a decrease in TIA frequency is a poor indicator of treatment efficacy.

CONCLUSIONS

Although STA–MCA bypass is a technically safe procedure with a high patency rate, it has not been shown to prevent stroke or improve mortality among patients with occlusive cerebrovascular disease. Identification of subgroups who might benefit from revascularization surgery remains an active area of investigation. This identification is a formidable task, however, since any such group, if it exists, likely constitutes only a small fraction of the patients who were previously considered for a bypass operation.

REFERENCES

1. The EC/IC Bypass Study Group: Failure of extracranial-intracranial arterial bypass to reduce the risk of ischemic stroke. Results of an international randomized trial. N Engl J Med. 1985;313:1191.
2. EC/IC Bypass Study Group: The International Cooperative Study of Extracranial/Intracranial Arterial Anastomosis (EC/IC Bypass Study): Methodology and Entry Characteristics. Stroke. 1985;16:397.
3. Furlan AJ, Whisnant JP, Baker HL Jr: Long-term prognosis after carotid artery occlusion. Neurology (NY). 1980;30:986.
4. Cote R, Barnett HJM, Taylor DW: Internal carotid occlusion: A prospective study. Stroke. 1983;14:898.
5. Marzewski DJ, Furlan AJ, St Louis P, et al: Intracranial internal carotid artery stenosis: Long-term prognosis. Stroke. 1982;13:821.
6. Craig DR, Meguro K, Watridge C, et al: Intracranial internal carotid artery stenosis. Stroke. 1982;13:825.
7. Wechsler LR, Kistler JP, Davis KR: The prognosis of carotid siphon stenosis. Neurology (NY). 1984;34(suppl 1):200.
8. Hinton RC, Mohr JP, Ackerman RH, et al: Symptomatic middle cerebral artery stenosis. Ann Neurol. 1979;5:152.
9. Corston RN, Kendall BE, Marshall J: Prognosis in middle cerebral artery stenosis. Stroke. 1984;15:237.
10. Kaste M, Waltimo O: Prognosis of patients with middle cerebral artery occlusion. Stroke. 1976;7:382.
11. Sacquegna T, De Carolis P, Andreoli A, et al: Long-term prognosis after middle cerebral artery occlusion. Br Med J. 1984;28:1490.
12. Sundt TM, Whisnant JP, Fade NC, et al: Results, complications, and follow-up of 415 bypass operations for occlusive disease of the carotid system. Mayo Clin Proc. 1985;60:230.
13. Whisnant JP, Sundt TM, Fade NC: Long-term mortality and stroke morbidity after superficial temporal artery-middle cerebral artery bypass operation. Mayo Clin Proc. 1985;60:241.
14. Yasargil MG, Yonekawa Y: Results of microsurgical extra-intracranial arterial bypass in the treatment of cerebral ischemia. Neurosurgery. 1977;1:22.

15. Samson DS, Hodosh RM, Clark WK: Microsurgical treatment of transient cerebral ischemia: Preliminary results in 50 patients. *JAMA*. 1979;241:376.

16. Lee MC, Ausman JI, Geiger JD, et al: Superficial temporal to middle cerebral artery anastomosis: Clinical outcome in patients with ischemia or infarction in internal carotid artery distribution. *Arch Neurol*. 1979;36:1.

17. Chater N: Results of neurosurgical microvascular extracranial-intracranial bypass for stroke: A decade of experience. *West J Med*. 1983;138:531.

18. Furlan AJ, Little JR, Dohn DF: Arterial occlusion following anastomosis of the superficial temporal artery to middle cerebral artery. *Stroke*. 1980;11:91.

Therapeutic Perspective

The Social, Economic, and Personal Impact of Stroke and Its Prevention

ALLAN D. CALLOW and WILLIAM C. MACKEY

Stroke is the third leading cause of death in the United States. It is the underlying cause of approximately 8 percent of all deaths reported in this country.[1] Because the majority of patients survive their first stroke and remain disabled, the personal, social, and economic impact of stroke is greatly underestimated by mortality statistics alone. Among stroke patients who survive for 1 month, two-thirds are permanently disabled to some degree.[2] Approximately half of 30-day stroke survivors will survive for at least 5 years, and one-third will require prolonged inpatient rehabilitative services.[2] Thus, the quality of life is grossly impaired for many stroke survivors.

Because stroke causes premature death and disability, its economic impact includes not only direct medical costs but also costs of lost productivity or self-sufficiency in stroke patients.[3] These indirect costs, though more difficult to measure, may exceed direct medical costs.[4]

The personal, social, and economic impact of stroke in our society mandates the development of effective programs for stroke prevention. Because of the unique sensitivity of the central nervous system to ischemia and the lack of effective anatomic neural regeneration after ischemic insult, stroke prevention is far more likely to reduce the impact of stroke in our society than are stroke treatment and rehabilitative programs. However, stroke prevention programs remain embryonic, and the optimal means for preventing stroke remain controversial. A comprehensive multidisciplinary stroke prevention program would reduce the devastating impact of stroke and therefore should be a national health priority. This chapter is devoted to a description of the profound impact of stroke and to a discussion of the available means of lessening this by effective stroke prevention.

INCIDENCE, MORTALITY, AND PREVALENCE: THE SOCIAL IMPACT OF STROKE

The incidence and prevalence of stroke have been discussed elsewhere, and only a summary is presented here. The National Survey of Stroke, which covered the years 1970 to 1976, reported an incidence of approximately 407,000 for each of the 5 years surveyed.[5] Of these, approximately 299,000 strokes a year were initial strokes; the remaining 108,000 represented recurrent strokes. Figure 87–1,

taken from the National Survey of Stroke, shows the age-specific stroke incidence in three major surveys.[5–7] The major impact of stroke is in those 65 years of age or older. The age-adjusted stroke incidence was 152.1 per 100,000 in 1971 and declined to 137.9 by 1976, the last year of the survey. This decline of 9.3 percent was significant only in those over 65. The age-adjusted and age-specific incidence of initial strokes during the years of the National Survey of Stroke is shown in Table 87–1. More recent data are not available, because the National Center for Health Statistics compiles stroke prevalence data only.

The age-adjusted stroke mortality was just under 90 per 100,000 in 1950; by 1982, it had fallen to 35.8 per 100,000.[1] In the years 1979 to 1982 alone, the age-adjusted stroke mortality rate fell 13.9 percent.[1] Age-specific and age-adjusted mortality rates are shown for 1979, 1981, and 1982 in Table 87–2. This decline in stroke mortality appears to be most significant in the older age groups, and although the decline is almost certainly real, its exact magnitude and significance are difficult to interpret. Death certificates are unreliable, with high false-negative (40%) and false-positive (21%) rates in stroke reporting. The importance of stroke in causing the death of elderly individuals with multiple medical problems may be difficult to ascertain.[8] The decline in stroke mortality may be related to declining stroke incidence, declining fatality rates, or both.[9] The ongoing Rochester, Minnesota, study suggests that declining stroke incidence is primarily responsible.[10]

Sacco and coworkers[11] demonstrated in the Framingham study population that stroke mortality may be determined by the same factors that correlate with initial stroke incidence. Hypertension and cardiac comorbidity, especially congestive heart failure, are both significant risk factors for stroke and for mortality following stroke. Declining stroke incidence and declining fatality rates may both be related to improved control of significant risk factors and may together account for the observed decline in stroke-related mortality.

Stroke prevalence data from the 1981 Health Interview Survey identified 2,192,000 surviving stroke patients in the United States, a prevalence rate of 9.7 per 1000 population.[12] Age-specific prevalence rates from the 1981 survey are shown in Table 87–3 and are compared with the prevalence rates from the 1977 survey. Of note is the moderate decline in stroke prevalence in all age groups during this 5-year period. The Health Interview Survey data probably overesti-

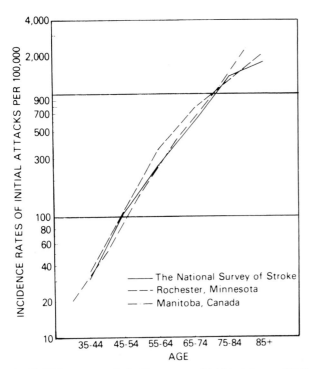

FIGURE 87–1. Age-specific incidence rates of initial stroke per 100,000 population in three community-based stroke surveys. (From Robins M, Baum HM: The national survey of stroke: Incidence. *Stroke.* 1981;12(I):45; with permission.)

TABLE 87–2. Age-Adjusted and Age-Specific Cerebrovascular Disease Mortality Rates per 100,000 Population

Age, y	1979	1981	1982
All	75.5	71.3	68.0
<1	4.6	9.7	3.7
1–4	0.3	0.3	0.3
5–14	0.3	0.3	0.3
15–24	0.9	0.9	0.7
25–34	2.6	2.6	2.4
35–44	9.1	8.4	7.7
45–54	26.4	24.9	23.7
55–64	68.1	62.9	58.9
65–74	226.9	206.3	193.5
75–84	793.8	715.6	675.1
>85	2264.9	2126.8	2000.8
Age adjusted	41.6	38.1	35.8

From National Center for Health Statistics: *Monthly Vital Statistics Report.* 1984; 33:9; with permission.

than 30 days after acute stroke was concomitant cardiovascular disease.

These incidence, mortality, prevalence, and survival data represent the total figures for strokes of all diagnostic categories—large artery thrombosis, lacunar infarction, embolic infarction, intracerebral hematoma, and subarachnoid hemorrhage. In the Harvard Stroke Registry, large artery thrombosis accounted for 34 percent of strokes, lacunar infarction for 19 percent, embolism for 31 percent, intracerebral hematoma for 10 percent, and subarachnoid bleeding for 6 percent.[14] Early mortality rates are higher for patients with intracerebral hematoma and subarachnoid hemorrhage than for infarction (59% vs. 25% 30-day mortality in the National Stroke Survey), but after 30 days, the survival curves are parallel.[13] In addition to type of stroke and concomitant cardiovascular disease, age at onset of stroke is a strong determinant of survival. Survival data by age group and etiology are shown in Table 87–4, taken from the National Stroke Survey.[13]

Incidence, mortality, prevalence, and survival data identify the demographic impact of stroke in our society, qualifying stroke as a major public health problem.

ECONOMIC IMPACT

The economic impact of stroke is determined by both direct costs for stroke care (ie, direct outlay of money for diagnosis, treatment, rehabilitation, and chronic care) and indirect costs related to lost productivity due to premature disability (morbidity costs) or death (mortality costs).[3] Indi-

mate the true prevalence of stroke, but the trend seen in the data is unmistakable.[12]

Age-specific survival rates for patients suffering acute stroke are shown in Figure 87–2. The 1-year survival rate in the National Survey of Stroke was 52 percent and the 5-year survival rate was 30 percent. The highest mortality occurred in the first 6 months following the stroke, so survival rates for patients who survived at least 6 months were much higher (approximately 90% at 1 year and 56% at 5 years).[13]

Surviving stroke patients are at continued risk for recurrent stroke and for other fatal or disabling cardiovascular events. In the Framingham study population of 394 stroke patients, 84 (21.3%) had second strokes and 27 (6.9%) had third strokes.[11] In this study, both hypertension and cardiac disease adversely affected both survival and recurrence rates following stroke. The leading cause of death occurring more

TABLE 87–1. Age-Adjusted and Age-Specific Initial Stroke Incidence per 100,000 Population

Age, y	1971	1973	1975	1976
All	152.1	144.0	144.1	137.9
<35	5.1	3.3	3.3	3.3
35–44	8.9	17.9	13.4	48.6
45–54	77.1	126.9	114.4	98.0
55–64	265.7	297.1	233.6	290.4
65–74	640.9	637.2	614.5	551.2
75–84	1682.8	1269.0	1569.1	1214.3
>85	3076.9	2275.5	1814.3	1834.9

From Robins M, Baum HM: The national survey of stroke: *Stroke.* 1981;12(I):45; with permission.

TABLE 87–3. Overall and Age-Specific Prevalence of Stroke per 1000 Population

Age, y	1977	1981
<45	3.9	1.7
45–64	20.7	13.0
>65	70.0	45.4
Overall	12.4	8.3

From National Center for Health Statistics: *Health Interview Survey.* 1982; with permission.

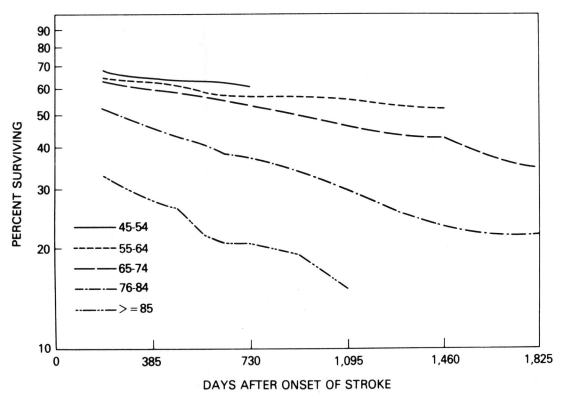

FIGURE 87–2. Age-specific incidence of survivorship by interval since the onset of an initial stroke requiring hospitalization, based on life-table methodology. (From Baum HM, Robins M: The national survey of stroke: Survival and prevalence. *Stroke.* 1981;12(I):59; with permission.)

rect costs are determined by calculating the present dollar value of future anticipated earnings of disabled or dying stroke victims. Detailed surveys of the direct and indirect costs of stroke are available for 1972 and 1976.[3, 4] More recent data are less detailed but permit estimation of direct and indirect costs by extrapolation, assuming that the relationship between direct and indirect costs has remained constant.[15]

Cooper and Rice[3] reported the direct cost of stroke in 1972 as $2.03 billion and the indirect costs as $624 million for morbidity and $3.43 billion for mortality, giving a total cost of $6.1 billion. Corrected to 1985 dollars, the total cost of stroke in 1972 was $15.3 billion, of which $5.0 billion represented direct costs. The 1976 costs as estimated by the National Survey of Stroke were direct costs, $3.26 billion; morbidity, $438 million; and mortality, $2.9 to $4.8 billion. The total 1976 cost was $12.8 to $16.5 billion (1985 dollars), of which $6.2 billion represented direct costs.[4] Stroke costs for 1980 as estimated by Hodgson and Kopstein[15] were direct costs, $5.1 billion; and total costs, $11.2 to $15.5 billion. Corrected to 1985 dollar values, the total 1980 cost was $15.9 to $20.6 billion, with $6.8 billion in direct costs.

Table 87–5 summarizes the economic data for 1972, 1976, and 1980, corrected for inflation to 1985 dollars. There appears to be a trend toward an increase in direct costs. Direct costs were attributable to acute hospital charges, nursing home charges, physicians' services, or miscellaneous costs (nonphysician medical and social services, aids, appliances, and drugs). The 1972 data revealed that 45.9 percent of the $2.03 billion was spent on acute hospitalization, 32.0 percent on nursing home care, 4.1 percent on physicians' services, and the remaining 18 percent on miscellaneous

TABLE 87–4. Stroke Survival by Diagnosis and Age at Onset

| Category | Cases, n | Survival, & | | | | |
		30 Days	180 Days	1 Year	3 Years	5 Years
Diagnosis						
All	1365	69.7	56.9	52.4	39.4	30.2
Hemorrhage	199	40.7	32.1	30.6	26.0	20.1
Infarction	1166	75.0	61.1	56.1	41.2	31.9
Age						
<65	409	73.7	65.9	63.2	54.8	49.2
65–74	369	75.6	63.1	59.4	46.1	34.5
75–84	425	68.1	52.4	45.7	30.0	21.9
>85	162	52.4	33.0	27.8	15.1	7.4

From Baum HM, Robins M: The national survey of stroke: Survival and prevalence. *Stroke.* 1981;12(I):59; with permission.

TABLE 87–5. Stroke Costs

Study*	Year	Direct Costs†	Total Costs†
Cooper and Rice[3]	1972	5.04	15.3
Adelman[4]	1976	6.28	12.8–16.5‡
Hodgson and Kopstein[15]	1980	6.78	14.9–20.6§

*Full full bibliographic information, see reference list at end of chapter.

†In billions of dollars, corrected for inflation to 1985 dollar values.

‡Range dependent on which discounting rate (2.5–10%) used in determining present value of anticipated future earnings.

§Range based on extrapolation from relationship between direct and total costs in 1972 and 1976 studies, employing a discounting rate that yielded indirect costs representing the mean of those estimated using 2.5 and 10% as the discounting rates.

items.[3] The 1976 data revealed that 42.2 percent of the $3.26 billion was spent on acute hospital care, 31.6 percent on nursing home care, 3.9 percent on physicians' services, and the remaining 22.3 percent on miscellany.[4] The 1980 data, however, showed that 52 percent of the $5.1 billion was spent on acute hospitalization, 35 percent on nursing home care, and the remaining 13 percent on professional services and miscellany.[15] The cost of acute hospital care for stroke patients represents a large and increasing percentage of the total cost of stroke care. Rising hospital costs, therefore, may account for the overall increase in direct costs for stroke care.

The method used for calculating costs in these studies attributes all costs for stroke patients to the year of the initial stroke. Thus, per patient costs can be derived by dividing total costs by the incidence of initial strokes. Thus, for 1976, the total cost per initial stroke patient was between $22,160 and $28,569 ($42,680 to $55,024 in 1985 dollars). Of this total cost per patient, $10,903 ($20,999 in 1985 dollars) was spent for direct costs; the per patient cost of time lost from work due to illness (morbidity costs) was $1,464 ($2,820 in 1985 dollars), and the per patient cost of lost earnings due to premature mortality was between $9,795 and $16,200 ($18,865 to $31,200 in 1985 dollars).

These costs per patient data are supported by a 1975 study from Massachusetts, which found a total cost per initial stroke patient of $28,540 ($58,079 in 1985 dollars).[16] Direct costs totaled $15,460 ($31,461 in 1985 dollars) per patient in this study, and indirect costs totaled $13,080 ($26,681 in 1985 dollars) per patient. The higher direct costs noted in this study when compared with the national data are attributable to the fact that in 1975, hospitalization costs in Massachusetts exceeded the national mean by 50 percent.[16]

Age-specific comparisons of direct and indirect costs are instructive, as illustrated by the 1975 Massachusetts data.[16] Over 95 percent of all direct costs for stroke in this study accrued to patients over 55 years of age, but only 53 percent of the indirect costs accrued to this group. Thus, although patients under age 55 accounted for less than 5 percent of direct stroke costs, they accrued approximately 47 percent of the indirect costs and 24 percent of the total costs. Sex-specific comparisons reveal that men age 35 to 54 account for only 2.6 percent of direct costs but 30.8 percent of indirect costs and 15.6 percent of total costs. Such data emphasize that the economic impact of stroke burdens all segments of the population. The elderly, who suffer a high incidence of stroke, account for most of the direct and total costs. The young and middle-aged, who account for only a small fraction of direct costs due to the low incidence in this group, bear a large portion of the indirect costs due to significant loss of earning power from premature death or disability. In Massachusetts in 1975, the per patient cost of stroke for those age 35 to 54 was $78,600, of which over $70,000 was in the indirect costs.[16] In males in this age group, the figures were even more staggering: the total cost per stroke patient rose to over $92,400, of which almost $84,000 represented indirect costs.[15] Conversion of these figures to 1985 dollar values predicts a current cost of over $188,000 per male stroke patient age 35 to 54, with over $170,000 representing indirect costs.

Stroke represents an enormous economic burden to the government, to private insurers that cover most of the direct costs, and to patients and their families who must absorb and overcome the indirect costs. These demographic and economic data provide ample evidence of the importance of stroke as a public health problem. Such data, however, still do not accurately reflect the overall impact of stroke.

PERSONAL IMPACT

The impact of stroke is most devastating to its survivors, whose quality of life is markedly diminished. Although diminution in quality of life is difficult to measure, the extent of the impact of stroke cannot be understood without appreciating the personal suffering that follows the acute event.

In a Rochester, Minnesota, study, Matsumoto and colleagues[6] found that of 610 survivors evaluated 6 months after an acute stroke, 29 percent were functionally normal, 36 percent were working or able to work, 18 percent were capable of providing self-care, and 4 percent required total care. Aphasia compounded other disabilities in 10 percent of the patients in this study. In 12 percent of the 6-month survivors, functional status could not be determined.

In a more detailed survey of stroke-related disability and recovery, Kotila and colleagues[17] catalogued the evolution of neurologic, neuropsychologic, and activities of daily living (ADL) disabilities in stroke patients in Finland during the acute event and at 3- and 12-month follow-up. Their findings are summarized in Table 87–6. They found that 31 and 22 percent of their patients were not able to return home by 3 and 12 months, respectively. This study not only clearly documents improvement in neurologic, neuropsychologic, and ADL performance in the aftermath of stroke but also provides a discouraging list of residual long-term disabilities in acute stroke survivors.

TABLE 87–6. Stroke-Related Disabilities

Disability	Patients, %		
	Acute Stage	3 Months	12 Months
Neurologic			
Hemiparesis	73	50	37
Coordination	86	73	61
Dysphasia	36	29	28
Dysarthria	57	29	21
Dysphagia	13	4	4
Incontinence	29	11	9
Neuropsychologic			
Visuoperceptual	—	60	41
Aphasia	—	33	30
Dyslexia, dysgraphia, dyscalculia	—	61	37
			39
Intelligence	—	63	
Memory	—	55	31
Depression	—	44	29
Inadequate emotional responses	—	30	32
Activities of daily living			
Independent	32	62	68
Needs some help	31	19	18
Needs much help	25	12	8
Totally disabled	12	7	7

From Kotila M, Waltimo O, Marjaiisa N, et al: The profile of recovery from stroke and factors influencing outcome. *Stroke.* 1984;15:1039; with permission.

Return to work is an important endpoint evaluated in the Finnish study. By 3 months after a stroke, 11 percent of the total study group had returned to work, and 31 percent of the 58 patients under age 65 who had been working prior to their strokes had returned to work. After 1 year, 20.8 percent of the total group and 55 percent of the less than age 65 previously employed group had resumed gainful employment.[17]

In a similar study in the United States, of 379 stroke patients previously employed and surviving for 1 year, only 73 (19%) returned to work within 1 year of their strokes.[18] Even in the subgroup of patients less than 65 years of age, less than 30 percent returned to work. The reasons for the differences in the rate of return to work in the Finnish and American studies are not evident. Together, the studies suggest that at most one half of stroke victims employed prior to their acute events will return to gainful employment.

The Finnish and American studies examined factors that appeared to influence the likelihood of return to work. In the Finnish study, age over 65, severity of hemiparesis, and impairment of intelligence all had a significant negative influence on outcome, as measured by return to work.[17] In the American study, age, race, functional capacity at admission, occupation, and education significantly influenced return to work.[18] Patients 65 years of age or younger were five to seven times more likely to return to work than those 65 and over. Not surprisingly, functional capacity on admission strongly influenced the likelihood of working after a stroke. Professional and managerial workers and patients with a college education were more than twice as likely to resume working as blue-collar workers, farmers, or patients with less than a college education.

An interesting finding in the American study was that the side of hemispheric infarction did not influence return to work unless race was taken into account. Whites with left hemispheric infarctions were slightly less likely to return to work than whites with right hemispheric infarctions; however, nonwhites with left hemispheric infarctions were much more likely to return to work than nonwhites with right hemispheric infarctions.[18] The authors proposed that this finding may be attributed to the social profile of the white and nonwhite patients in this study population from the southeastern United States. Whites in this group were more likely to hold professional or managerial positions in which verbal skills (left hemisphere) are of paramount importance; nonwhites were more likely to hold blue-collar or farming positions in which visuospatial skills (right hemisphere) are paramount.[18] The extent of work disability caused by a stroke-related deficit appears to be a function of both the type and severity of the deficit and the impact of that particular deficit on each patient's ability to meet the demands of his or her specific career.

Although return to work is a critical endpoint in stroke recovery, it is an unrealistic goal for many patients. Many stroke patients can hope only to return home and avoid long-term institutionalization. In a study of stroke-related disabilities and their influence on return home, Feigenson and colleagues[19] from the Burke Rehabilitation Center found that 80 percent of stroke patients could return home after a coordinated rehabilitation program averaging 43 days in duration. These investigators found that severe weakness, long interval from onset of stroke to rehabilitation center

admission, perceptual or cognitive dysfunction, poor motivation, combined hemianopia and motor deficit, and age over 80 predicted a need for long-term institutionalization. Age less than 80, dysphasia, hemisensory deficit, or associated medical problems (heart disease, hypertension, and diabetes) were unrelated to prognosis for discharge home. Thus, stroke results in the need for chronic institutionalization in at least 20 percent of patients, even with state-of-the-art rehabilitative efforts.

Kotila and associates[17] stressed the importance of neuropsychologic disturbances in determining a patient's ability to return home. Inadequate emotional responsiveness such as lability, indifference, euphoria, and anosognosia had a significant negative influence on the ability to return home and to remain independent in ADL. By 3 months after their strokes, 100 percent of patients with appropriate emotional responses were home and independent in ADL; among patients with impaired emotional responsiveness, only 64 percent were home, and only 50 percent were fully independent in ADL. Although impaired physical functioning may be the most apparent and estimable disability resulting from stroke, emotional impairment may contribute significantly to decline in the quality of life.

Clinically evident depression is the most common emotional impairment seen in stroke patients. It affects 26 to 60 percent of stroke patients, as compared with approximately 4.2 percent of the general population.[20-23] Despite the prevalence of depression in the poststroke population, the use of antidepressant medication or psychiatric consultation is rare in the stroke setting. Lack of effective treatment for poststroke depression continues to be one of the substantial unmet needs of stroke patients.[24] Depression may have a profound effect on recovery. In fact, poor recovery from stroke, poor cooperation in rehabilitative efforts, or unexpected deterioration after a period of neurologic stability may all be manifestations of depression.

The etiology of poststroke depression is almost certainly multifactorial, resulting from both neurophysiologic and neurochemical malfunctions and psychological factors. Robinson and colleagues[25] found that location of the infarct in the left frontal area resulted in a higher incidence and greater severity of depression in the immediate poststroke period than did lesions in other areas. Quality of social functioning, functional physical impairment, intellectual impairment, and age influenced the incidence and severity of depression. Young patients with more severe physical, social, or intellectual impairment were the group at highest risk for severe depression. The increased incidence and severity of depression in younger patients with more severe impairments suggests that acute poststroke depression may represent an appropriate, though exaggerated, grief response. However, its association with left frontal lesions suggests a neurophysiologic basis.

The neurophysiologic basis for depression in stroke patients is supported by a follow-up study by the same investigators. Prevalence and severity of depression were greatest between 6 months and 2 years following stroke. Again, patients with left hemispheric lesions were more frequently and more severely depressed than patients with right hemispheric or brain-stem lesions. In contrast to their findings in acute stroke victims, the extent of functional physical and cognitive impairment did not correlate with the prevalence or severity of depression in the late poststroke period. It appeared, therefore, that neurophysiologic abnormalities were a more important etiologic factor in late poststroke depression than were psychologic reactions and that this abnormality was most commonly and severely manifest during the 6- to 24-month period after stroke.[26] Additional evidence for a neurophysiologic and neurochemical mechanism in poststroke depression stems from the finding that abnormalities in the single-dose dexamethasone suppression test correlate well with mood and vegetative disturbances in stroke patients. Finkelstein and coworkers[22] demonstrated moderate to severe mood and vegetative (appetite and sleep) disturbances in 48 and 52 percent, respectively, of stroke patients undergoing inpatient rehabilitation, and in 0 and 8 percent of control patients in the same setting. Of the stroke patients with mood or vegetative disturbances, 70 percent of those with depressed mood, 88 percent of those with diminished appetite, and 13 percent of those with sleep disturbance had abnormal dexamethasone suppression tests ($P<.02$ when compared with patients without clinical mood or vegetative disturbances). In addition, this study confirmed a higher incidence of depression in patients with left hemispheric lesions (69% vs. 25%).[22] These data suggest that poststroke depression is at least in part neurochemically mediated and associated with measurable neuroendocrine abnormalities. Thus, depression may be viewed as one more stroke-related disability that is especially devastating in its personal impact.

Cognitive impairment may also add significantly to the burden of stroke-related disability. Studies of invalid stroke patients confined to bed or chair have shown that physical disability often contributes little toward these patients' incapacity. Rather, it is more readily attributable to impaired comprehension, difficulty in communication, inattentiveness, and lack of effort.[27]

Frank dementia is not usually attributable to stroke alone, but cerebral infarction may play some role in up to 36 percent of demented patients.[28] Alzheimer's disease accounts for more than 50 percent of cases of dementia and is certainly far more important than multiple cerebral infarcts in causing dementia.[29] Many authors have cautioned that although Alzheimer's disease is a more frequent primary etiologic agent in dementia, vascular disease and cerebral infarction should not be ignored.[30, 31] Alzheimer's-type dementia and cerebral infarction may coexist in many older patients, and the sequelae of stroke might add to the morbidity of degenerative dementias.

A detailed discussion of cognitive impairments resulting from infarction of specific anatomic areas of the brain is beyond the scope of this chapter. Table 87–7, however, provides a brief summary of the more common cognitive deficits resulting from stroke.

Physical, emotional, and cognitive deficits following stroke are devastating in their impact on the quality of life. Their influence is heightened by inadequate interpersonal responses. Family life may be seriously stressed by the presence of a disabled stroke patient in the household, and if such an individual is demanding, depressed, or lacking in appropriate emotional responses, the stress may lead to resentment and anger.[32] Frustration over lack of improvement in the patient's disabilities may lead to disappointment and heightened anger. Right hemispheric stroke patients are more often the cause of serious family problems than aphasic

TABLE 87–7. Cognitive Deficits Accompanying Stroke

Dominant hemisphere
  Broca's nonfluent aphasia
  Fluent aphasia (Wernicke type, conductive, anomic)
  Agraphia
  Acalculia
  Alexia
  Finger agnosia
  Right-left confusion
Nondominant hemisphere
  Anosognosia
  Hemisomatognosia
  Unilateral neglect
  Unilateral spatial agnosia
  Dressing apraxia
  Constructional apraxia
  Visual illusions
  Impaired comprehension or expression of emotion (aprosodias)

patients because such patients often lack emotional sensitivity. Yet because of intact speech, their families have high expectations for normal interpersonal relationships.[32]

Sexual disability may compound family and interpersonal difficulties. Bray and associates[33] found that 88 percent of males and 73 percent of females reported little change in their sexual desire following stroke. Only 46 percent of the males, however, could consistently achieve stable erections after their strokes, although 75 percent had had normal erections before their strokes.[33] Eighty-eight percent of the males were able to ejaculate prior to their strokes, but only 29 percent were able to do so afterward. Of the females in this series, 45 percent experienced orgasm during their prestroke sexual experiences, but only 9 percent did so after their strokes.[33] The women interviewed described their poststroke sexual encounters as pleasant but noted diminished sensation in comparison with their prestroke experiences. Thus, although the majority of stroke survivors have continued sexual desire, most experience sexual dysfunction, which can provide another significant source of frustration in their personal and family lives.

In a similar study of sexual behavior in stroke patients, Goddess and colleagues[34] found that dominant hemisphere damage was more often associated with a decrease in libido than nondominant lesions, which were occasionally associated with increased libido. Regardless of the location of the infarct, the majority of patients experienced little change in sexual desire. Almost one-third of their patients who were sexually active prior to their strokes, however, discontinued sexual activity following the stroke, despite expressing continued interest in sexual activity when interviewed.[34] The personal impact of stroke as measured by loss of ability to work or even to return home; physical, perceptual, cognitive, or emotional disability; and disruption of family and sexual ties is devastating. Although social agencies and insurers measure the demographics and economics of stroke to determine its impact, only the stroke patient can fully illustrate its tragic implications in diminishing the quality of life.

STROKE PREVENTION

The impact of stroke clearly indicates the need for the development of effective programs in stroke prevention.

Nevertheless, stroke prevention programs that coordinate the skills and efforts of internists, neurologists, vascular surgeons, neurosurgeons, nutritionists, pharmacologists, and public health officials are almost unknown. Several studies, some large-scale, have shown that by altering risk factors in the population at large, stroke prevention is feasible. In fact, there is evidence to suggest that the decline in stroke incidence, mortality, and prevalence is due in large part to control of a single risk factor—hypertension. However, despite evidence suggesting that stroke is a preventable disease, there are no large-scale multidisciplinary stroke prevention programs. The remainder of this chapter is devoted to discussing what is currently known about stroke prevention, ideas for translating this knowledge into an effective program for stroke prevention, and the potential influence of such a program.

Stroke prevention might be achieved either by identification and modification of risk factors in the population at large or by identification and effective treatment of high-risk subgroups. To be most effective, a stroke prevention program must incorporate both approaches.

Risk Factors for Stroke and Their Modification

The Subcommittee on Risk Factors and Stroke of the Stroke Council of the American Heart Association reviewed the suspected risk factors for stroke and classified them according to their documented association with stroke risk and their treatability (Table 87–8).[35] To be most effective, a stroke prevention program should focus first on those known risk factors that are amenable to treatment and whose treatment is of established value in decreasing stroke risk.

TABLE 87–8. Risk Factors for Stroke

Well documented
  Treatable
    Hypertension
    Cardiac disease
    Transient ischemic attacks
    Elevated hematocrit
    Sickle cell disease
  Not treatable or treatment value not established
    Age and gender
    Family history
    Race
    Diabetes mellitus
    Prior stroke
    Asymptomatic carotid bruit
Less well documented
  Treatable but treatment value not established
    Elevated cholesterol and lipids
    Cigarette smoking
    Alcohol consumption
    Oral contraceptive use
    Physical inactivity
    Obesity
  Not treatable
    Geographic location
    Season and climate
    Socioeconomic factors

Modified from Dyken ML, Wolf PA, Barnett HJM, et al: Risk factors in stroke. *Stroke.* 1984;15:1105; with permission.

Hypertension

Hypertension is the best established risk factor for stroke and is readily treatable. Furthermore, effective treatment of hypertension has been shown to reduce the risk of stroke. The Veterans Administration Cooperative Study, a randomized placebo-controlled study, demonstrated a significant reduction in stroke incidence and stroke death in treated hypertensive patients when compared with a control group.[36] The Hypertension Detection and Follow-Up Program study randomized over 10,000 patients into a comprehensive management program that achieved blood pressure goals in over 65 percent of patients versus a customary care group in which goals were achieved in only 43 percent. There was a 45 percent reduction in stroke incidence in the comprehensive care group.[37] Moser reviewed data on stroke prevention and cited five separate studies demonstrating reductions in stroke mortality from 44 to 100 percent by the effective treatment of mild to moderate hypertension.[38] Furthermore, effective control of hypertension lessens stroke risk in all age groups; it is as effective in stroke prevention for those in their eighth and ninth decades as it is in younger patients.[39] Clearly, any comprehensive prevention program must begin with the detection and effective treatment of hypertension in the general population.

Current evidence strongly suggests that control of hypertension has already played a major role in the reduction of stroke incidence, prevalence, and mortality in the general population. Control of hypertension has improved dramatically since 1960. Surveys of hypertension control done in the 1960s showed that less than 20 percent of hypertensive patients had adequately controlled blood pressure. Data from the early 1970s suggested that less than 40 percent were adequately controlled.[38] Two studies from 1982, however, showed that almost 75 percent of hypertensive patients had their blood pressure under control.[28] This improved hypertension control was associated with a 40 percent reduction in age-adjusted stroke mortality between 1968 and 1982.[38] Although the relationship between improved blood pressure control and declining stroke mortality may be coincidental, the 20 percent decline in age-adjusted death rates for hypertension-related cardiovascular disease between 1972 and 1978—when compared with the 9 percent decline in nonhypertension-related cardiovascular disease mortality during the same period—argues for improved control of hypertension as a major factor in the decline in stroke mortality.[35]

Cardiac Disease

The presence of occult or symptomatic cardiac disease is a significant risk factor for stroke and results in a twofold increase in stroke prevalence.[35] Coronary artery disease, congestive heart failure, arrhythmias, and electrocardiogram or chest radiograph evidence of left ventricular hypertrophy all result in an increase in stroke risk.[40] In addition, coronary disease with myocardial infarction remains the leading cause of death in stroke survivors and in patients with transient ischemic attacks (TIAs) or carotid bruits.[41] Arrhythmias, especially atrial fibrillation, increase the risk of stroke more than fivefold, even after adjustment for age and blood pressure.[42] Reduction in the incidence of heart disease by risk factor control and effective treatment of existing heart disease should reduce the incidence of stroke. The prevention of all associated cardiovascular disease and the treatment of existing disease will become both desirable by-products and fundamental goals of stroke prevention programs.

Blood Disorders

Elevated hematocrit and homozygous sickle cell anemia are both known to increase stroke risk significantly by altering blood viscosity. Elevated hematocrit is not often associated with cigarette smoking, hypertension, and significant cardiopulmonary disease in this setting, so it may not be an independent risk factor.[43] Nevertheless, correction of primary or secondary polycythemia can significantly increase cerebral blood flow.[44] The association of sickle cell disease and stroke is well established, and adequate control of the hemorrheologic abnormalities associated with crises may result in a decrease in stroke incidence in this population.[45]

Other Factors

Additional risk factors that are less well documented or for which the value of treatment is less well documented are those associated with generalized atherosclerosis, hypertension, and cardiac disease. Cigarette smoking, hyperlipoproteinemias, excessive alcohol use, obesity, and physical inactivity are all treatable. Reduction in the prevalence of these risk factors has probably played a role in lowering cardiovascular morbidity in general. Additional reduction cannot help but lower the incidence of stroke as one manifestation of generalized vascular disease.

Diabetes mellitus is clearly associated with accelerated atherosclerosis and increased stroke risk, especially in women and especially in the presence of coexisting hypertension.[46] Data are not available, however, to suggest that effective control of diabetes alters stroke risk, and the role of diabetes management in stroke prevention remains ill defined.[35] Similarly, the influence of oral contraceptives as an independent risk factor remains controversial.[35] Their use may increase stroke risk, but possibly only in the presence of cofactors such as hypertension, migraine, age over 35, diabetes, hyperlipidemia, and cigarette smoking.

Although identification and elimination of risk factors for stroke in the general population may reduce stroke incidence and mortality, identification and effective treatment of a stroke-prone population subset should yield a more substantial reduction in stroke morbidity and mortality.

Identification and Management of the Stroke-Prone Population

TIAs clearly identify individuals at high risk for stroke. In one study, 23 percent of untreated patients who suffered TIAs went on to have completed strokes within 1 year of the TIA, and 45 percent suffered stroke within 5 years.[47] In other surveys, stroke was preceded by TIA in approximately 26 percent of all patients[14] and in slightly over 50 percent of patients with carotid territory stroke.[48] Prompt recognition and effective treatment of TIAs may well be essential in the prevention of significant numbers of strokes.

Prompt recognition of signs and symptoms of transient cerebral ischemia depends on improved public and physician awareness. Educational programs such as those used by the American Heart Association for hypertension and myocardial infarction, and by the American Cancer Society for early detection of cancer, should be helpful.

Once recognized, symptoms of transient cerebral ischemia must be evaluated and effectively treated. Optimal treatment for TIAs related to ipsilateral carotid stenosis of 70 percent or more includes carotid endarterectomy. The results of the North American Symptomatic Carotid Endarterectomy Trial and the European Carotid Surgery Trial clearly support the efficacy of endarterectomy in stroke prevention in this population.[49, 50] Ulceration of an atherosclerotic plaque with 30 to 70 percent stenosis ipsilateral to carotid territory TIA symptoms may also constitute an indication for carotid endarterectomy, but randomized controlled trials confirming benefit in this subgroup are incomplete.[49, 50] It has been suggested that even microscopic irregularities of the arterial wall can be the source of embolic TIAs and strokes,[51] but the significance of minimal arterial wall irregularities remains unclear.[52] The European Carotid Surgery Trial showed that carotid endarterectomy is not beneficial in patients with less than 30 percent ipsilateral stenosis.[50]

Optimal treatment for patients with carotid territory TIA symptoms, minimal ipsilateral carotid disease, and no other source of emboli remains unknown, although a trial of antiplatelet agents in such patients seems reasonable. Carotid territory TIAs ipsilateral to carotid occlusion may be managed initially with medical therapy. Recurrent symptoms of threatened stroke in these patients are difficult to manage, especially since the results of a controlled, prospective, randomized study of medical therapy versus extracranial–intracranial bypass do not support surgical intervention.[53]

Still less well defined is the management of posterior circulation TIAs. The coexistence of nonhemispheric symptoms and bilateral high-grade carotid stenoses may be an indication for carotid endarterectomy, ostensibly to improve total cerebral perfusion.[54, 55] Patients with nonhemispheric symptoms not associated with flow-limiting carotid lesions and patients with pure vertebrobasilar disease and TIAs are most often treated initially with antiplatelet agents or anticoagulation. Direct reconstruction of vertebral arteries is gaining acceptance, but as yet, no randomized controlled trials support vertebral reconstruction over medical therapy.

Although there is growing consensus regarding appropriate means of stroke prevention in symptomatic patients, no such consensus exists for the identification, let alone the management, of asymptomatic high-risk patients. The fact that almost 50 percent of acute carotid territory strokes may not be preceded by TIAs illustrates the problem and should give urgent impetus to its study.[48] The presence of an asymptomatic carotid bruit may identify an individual as being at high risk for stroke. In the Framingham study, the risk of stroke in males with asymptomatic bruits was increased more than twofold and in females more than threefold over their cohorts.[56] Carotid bruits also predict an increased risk for myocardial infarction and for death, usually from cardiovascular disease.[56] Furthermore, in this study, less than a third of the observed strokes were referable to the involved carotid territory. The authors concluded that an asymptomatic bruit was indicative of systemic atherosclerosis, with all its attendant risks, but did not in and of itself predict an inordinate risk for stroke in the distribution of the involved carotid territory.[56] This conclusion was further supported by an Evans County, Georgia, epidemiologic study in which a carotid bruit appeared to be a reliable marker for systemic atherosclerosis but a rather poor predictor of stroke risk in the ipsilateral carotid territory.[57] Although a carotid bruit by itself may not be indicative of high stroke risk in the ipsilateral cerebral territory, certain bruits may be. A bruit produced by a hemodynamically significant lesion may place an individual at high risk. Busuttil and coworkers[58] and Kartchner and McRae[59] reported that hemodynamically significant carotid lesions as detected by ocular plethysmography were associated with a higher stroke risk (10–12%) than were lesions that were hemodynamically insignificant (2%). They recommended that hemodynamically significant lesions be evaluated arteriographically and be considered for surgical correction even in asymptomatic patients.

Theoretically, at least, high-grade carotid stenoses, especially when bilateral, may be associated with increased stroke risk. They can be easily detected and measured by noninvasive techniques. Many, if not most, carotid territory strokes appear to be the result of emboli originating in ulcerated plaques rather than the consequence of flow reduction secondary to high-grade stenosis.[60] Thus it may be the morphologic character of the plaque itself rather than its hemodynamic effects that determines stroke risk.

Moore and associates[61] claimed that asymptomatic individuals with large or compound ulcerated plaques as depicted by angiography are at high risk for stroke, compared with individuals with small plaques and minimal ulceration. They recommended surgical treatment for asymptomatic patients with large or compound ulcers and nonsurgical management of those with minimal ulcers. Noninvasive duplex ultrasonographic examination detects plaque ulceration and may provide a satisfactory screening tool for the identification of asymptomatic patients at high risk for nonstenotic but ulcerated plaques.[62, 63] Because it provides the best available indirect assessment of plaque morphology, duplex ultrasonography is a substantial improvement in noninvasive assessment and is replacing noninvasive techniques based on pressure, flow, and pulse arrival measurements.

Intraplaque hemorrhage may be another plaque characteristic associated with high risk. Lusby and colleagues[64] demonstrated an association between intraplaque hemorrhage and cerebrovascular symptoms, finding hemorrhage in 92.5 percent of plaques from symptomatic patients and in only 27 percent of plaques from asymptomatic patients. Imparato and coworkers[65] and Persson and associates[66] confirmed this correlation. Hemorrhage into a carotid plaque with sudden acute plaque expansion may explain the abrupt conversion of a silent plaque into a symptomatic one. Eruption through the plaque surface causes ulceration, embolization, and the possibility of immediate symptoms. Angioneogenesis within the plaque may result in a plaque that is mechanically unstable and prone to additional intraplaque hemorrhage and delayed ulceration, with subsequent production of symptoms.[64–66] Intraplaque hemorrhage may be detected by duplex ultrasonographic evaluation and in some asymptomatic individuals may warrant consideration of carotid endarterectomy.[62, 67]

Although accurate documentation is lacking, certain asymptomatic patients with high-grade stenosis, large or compound ulcers, or evidence of intraplaque hemorrhage may be candidates for prophylactic carotid endarterectomy. Still, the role of surgery in the management of asymptomatic patients remains controversial. There is a small, highly variable, but definite risk associated with angiography and cerebrovascular surgery. The goal of stroke prevention cannot be advanced by surgery in either symptomatic or asymptomatic high-risk individuals if the risk of complications of angiography and operation exceeds the risk associated with the natural history of a particular cerebrovascular lesion left untreated or treated medically.

The VA Cooperative Trial, a randomized, controlled, prospective trial of surgery versus medical therapy in patients with 50 percent or greater asymptomatic carotid stenosis, failed to determine conclusively the efficacy of carotid endarterectomy in asymptomatic patients.[68] In this study, the patients treated surgically fared better than medically treated patients when the endpoints of TIA, transient monocular blindness, and stroke were combined (17 of 211 surgical vs. 48 of 233 medical; $P < .001$), but the difference in stroke incidence in the two groups (10 of 211 surgical vs. 22 of 233 medical; $P = .056$) failed to reach statistical significance.[68] Interpretation of the data was further complicated by an unexpectedly high mortality in both the surgical and the medical groups. Subgroup analysis by degree of stenosis was unrevealing because of the small number of patients in the subgroups with the greatest degree of stenosis. Although endarterectomy in asymptomatic patients in this study seemed to be beneficial, its efficacy in stroke prevention must be considered unproved.

The Asymptomatic Carotid Atherosclerosis Study, which will randomize over 1500 patients with 60 percent or greater carotid stenosis, should determine the role of endarterectomy in patients with asymptomatic stenosis.[69] Until the results of this trial are available, asymptomatic patients considered to be at high risk for stroke should be approached conservatively. Surgical intervention, if entertained at all, should be considered only for very high-grade stenoses or large, compound ulcers. There must be full understanding of the risks implicit in both surgical and nonsurgical management. In addition, if the goal of stroke prevention is to be served, surgical management of asymptomatic patients should be permitted and performed only in centers with documented mortality and neurologic morbidity rates well below 5 percent.[70]

Stroke Prevention: An Overview

Based on the preceding discussions of risk factor reduction and management of the stroke-prone population, a protocol for stroke prevention can be outlined (Fig. 87–3). At their initial evaluation, patients are clinically evaluated and classified according to stroke risk. Classification of patients according to overall stroke risk is feasible according to the Framingham study. Hypertension, elevated cholesterol levels, glucose intolerance, cigarette smoking, and left ventricular hypertrophy by electrocardiogram findings identified 10 percent of the population in which over 33 percent of all strokes occurred.[71] Paffenberger and Williams[72] found an eightfold increase in stroke mortality among patients with hypertension, smoking, and obesity. Other factors such as carotid bruits may influence stroke risk and must be considered in the initial classification.

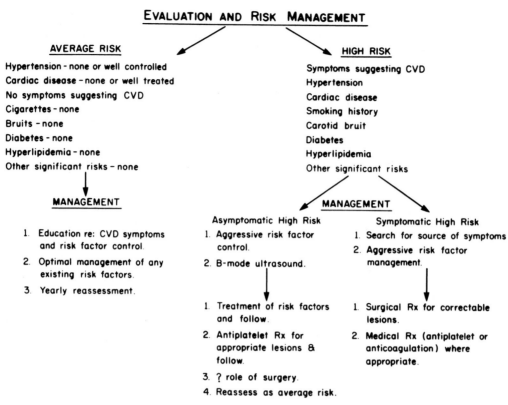

FIGURE 87–3. Protocol for a stroke-prevention program.

Patients classified as being at low or average risk are instructed in risk factor management and in the early symptoms of cerebral ischemia. They should receive appropriate management of their existing risk factors and yearly reassessment. Patients classified as high risk are further classified as being symptomatic or asymptomatic. Symptomatic patients are more intensely studied for risk factor management and for evaluation of symptoms. Specific management should be based on the source of the cerebrovascular symptoms as determined by clinical, noninvasive, and neuroradiologic data. Asymptomatic patients judged to be at high risk should undergo aggressive outpatient management of their risk factors along with duplex ultrasonographic examination of the carotid arteries. Management of these patients should be designed to diminish their stroke risk by early appropriate management of those factors leading to their high-risk classification.

Moser[38] estimated that the decline in stroke incidence and stroke deaths noted from 1976 to 1983 resulted in savings of $2 billion to $3 billion per year in direct and indirect stroke-related costs. This decline in incidence, mortality, and cost probably stemmed from better risk factor control, especially hypertension, and from improved health consciousness and subsequent behavior modification by the American public. It is likely that a simple but organized stroke prevention protocol, including both risk factor management and thorough evaluation and management of stroke-prone patients, could result in a much greater reduction in stroke incidence and mortality, with an even greater reduction in stroke-related costs. Such a program may well be economically self-justifying. A greater benefit is the enhanced well-being of our older population.

Our current approach to stroke prevention is too passive. Modification of risk factors has reduced the incidence of stroke in the population at large, but little has been done for those at high risk. Internists, neurologists, and surgeons must take an active role in the identification, evaluation, and management of these stroke-prone patients.

CONCLUSION

Despite recent declines in incidence and associated mortality, stroke remains a serious public health problem. Currently, almost 1 out of every 100 living Americans has suffered a stroke. In the over 65 age group, prevalence approaches 5 per 100. The direct cost of caring for stroke patients exceeds $6 billion per year, and this appears to be rising at a rate faster than inflation. The cost of lost productivity due to stroke-related disability and mortality exceeds the direct cost of caring for stroke patients and probably exceeds $10 billion per year. In addition, stroke is a huge personal tragedy for its victims and their families. The bewildering array of stroke-related disabilities leaves stroke patients physically, mentally, and emotionally crippled. Often, no amount of physical therapy or counseling can overcome these handicaps.

Stroke prevention is feasible. It has been practiced for years in the guise of blood pressure control and public education regarding smoking and other cardiovascular risk factors. Even these fragmented efforts at stroke prevention by risk factor control have had significant results, as measured by stroke incidence, prevalence, and mortality data. By combining risk factor control with aggressive management of stroke-prone patients in an organized multidisciplinary program, a much greater reduction in stroke incidence and impact might be achieved. Pilot programs to test this hypothesis are desperately needed, both for their potential to provide data on optimal stroke prevention techniques and for their potential benefit to our patient population.

Acknowledgment

The authors acknowledge with gratitude the assistance of Drs. Louis Caplan, Michael Pessin, and William S. Fields, who reviewed the manuscript and offered helpful suggestions. Source material was identified and provided by Drs. Robert Levy, Dorothy Rice, Carl Granger, Seth Finkelstein, Manning Feinleib, Richard Shader, and Dallas Anderson.

REFERENCES

1. National Center for Health Statistics: *Monthly Vital Statistics Report.* 1984;33:9.
2. American Heart Association Stroke Council: Statement on stroke rehabilitation. Sept. 14, 1984.
3. Cooper BS, Rice DP: The economic cost of illness revisited. *Soc Secur Bull.* 1976:21.
4. Adelman SM: The national survey of stroke: Economic impact. *Stroke.* 1981;12(I):69.
5. Robins M, Baum HM: The national survey of stroke: Incidence. *Stroke.* 1981;12(I):45.
6. Matsumoto N, Whisnant J, Kurland LT, et al: Natural history of stroke in Rochester, Minnesota, 1955–1969. *Stroke.* 1973;4:20.
7. Abu-Zeid HAH, Choi NW, Nelson NA: Epidemiological features of cerebrovascular disease in Manitoba: Incidence by age, sex, and residence, with etiologic implications. *Can Med Assoc J.* 1975;113:379.
8. Corwin LI, Wolf PA, Kannel WB, McNamara PA: Accuracy of death certification of stroke: The Framingham study. *Stroke.* 1982;13:818.
9. Nicholls ES, Johansen HL: Implications of changing trends in cerebrovascular and ischemic heart disease mortality (editorial). *Stroke.* 1983;14:153.
10. Anderson GL, Whisnant JP: A comparison of trends in mortality from stroke in the United States and Rochester, Minnesota. *Stroke.* 1983;13:804.
11. Sacco RL, Wolf PA, Kannel WB, McNamara PA: Survival and recurrence following stroke: The Framingham study. *Stroke.* 1982;13:290.
12. National Center for Health Statistics, US Department of Health and Human Services: *Health Interview Survey.* 1982.
13. Baum HM, Robins M: The national survey of stroke: Survival and prevalence. *Stroke.* 1981;12(I):59.
14. Mohr JP, Caplan LF, Melski JW, et al: The Harvard cooperative stroke registry: A prospective registry. *Neurology.* 1978;28:154.
15. Hodgson TA, Kopstein AN: Health care expenditures for major disease. In *Health: United States—1983.* Public Health Service Pub. no. (PHS) 84–1232. Washington, DC: US Government Printing Office; 1983.
16. Mills E, Thompson M: The economic costs of stroke in Massachusetts. *N Engl J Med.* 1978;299:415.
17. Kotila M, Waltimo O, Marjaiisa N, et al: The profile of recovery from stroke and factors influencing outcome. *Stroke.* 1984;15:1039.
18. Howard G, Till JS, Toole JF, et al: Factors influencing return to work following cerebral infarction. *JAMA.* 1985;253:226.
19. Feigenson JS, McDowell FH, Meese P, et al: Factors influencing outcome and length of stay in a stroke rehabilitation unit. *Stroke.* 1977;8:651.
20. Feibel JH, Springer CJ: Depression and failure to resume social activities after stroke. *Arch Phys Med.* 1982;63:276.
21. Robinson RG, Szetela B: Mood change following left hemisphere brain injury. *Ann Neurol.* 1981;9:447.
22. Finkelstein S, Benowitz LI, Baldessarini RJ, et al: Mood, vegetative disturbance, and dexamethasone suppression test after stroke. *Ann Neurol.* 1982;12:463.
23. Boyd JH, Weissman MM: Epidemiology of affective disorders: A reexamination and future directions. *Arch Gen Psychiatry.* 1981;38:1039.
24. Feibel JH, Berk S, Joynt RJ: The unmet needs of stroke survivors. *Neurology.* 1979;29:592.
25. Robinson RG, Starr LB, Kubos HL, Price TR: A two year longitudinal study of post-stroke mood disorders: Findings during the initial evaluation. *Stroke.* 1983;14:736.
26. Robinson RG, Price TR: Post stroke depression disorders: A follow-up study of 103 patients. *Stroke.* 1982;13:635.
27. Lishman T: *Organic Psychiatry.* London: Blackwell; 1980.
28. Tomlinson BE, Blessed G, Roth M: Observations on the brains of demented old people. *J Neurol Sci.* 1970;11:205.
29. Wells CE: Role of stroke in dementia. *Stroke.* 1978;9:1.
30. Tomlinson BE: Morphological changes and dementia in old age. In Smith WL, Kinsbourne M, eds. *Aging and Dementia.* New York: Spectrum; 1977:25.
31. O'Brien MD: Vascular disease and dementia in the elderly. In Smith WL, Kinsbourne M, eds. *Aging and Dementia.* New York: Spectrum; 1977.
32. Binder L: Emotional problems after stroke. Curr Concepts *Cerebrovasc Dis.* 1983;18:17.
33. Bray GP, DeFrank RS, Wolfe TL: Sexual functioning in stroke survivors. *Arch Phys Med Rehabil.* 1981;62:286.
34. Goddess ED, Wagner NN, Silverman DR: Poststroke sexual activity of CVA patients. *Med Aspects Human Sexuality.* 1979;13:16.
35. Dyken ML, Wolf PA, Barnett HJM, et al: Risk factors in stroke. *Stroke.* 1984;15:1105.
36. Veterans Administration cooperative study group on antihypertensive agents: Effects of treatment on morbidity in hypertension. II. Results in patients with diastolic blood pressure averaging 90–114 mmHg. *JAMA.* 1980;231:1143.
37. Hypertension detection and follow-up program cooperative group: Five year findings of the hypertension detection and follow-up program: Reduction in mortality of persons with high blood pressure, including mild hypertension. *JAMA.* 1979;242:2565.
38. Moser M: Social and economic implications of stroke prevention. *J Public Health Policy.* 1984;5:228.
39. Kannel WB, Wolf PA, Verter J, McNamara PM: Epidemiologic assessment of the role of blood pressure in stroke: The Framingham study. *JAMA.* 1970;214:301.
40. Wolf PA, Kannel EB, Verter J: Current status of risk factors for stroke. *Neurol Clin.* 1983;1:317.
41. Toole JF, Janeway R, Choi K, et al: Transient ischemic attacks due to atherosclerosis: A prospective study of 160 patients. *Arch Neurol.* 1979;32:5.
42. Tanaha H, Veda Y, Hayashi N, et al: Risk factors for cerebral hemorrhage and cerebral infarction in a Japanese rural community. *Stroke.* 1982;13:62.
43. Kannel WB, Gordon T, Wolf PA, McNamara P: Hemoglobin and the risk of cerebral infarction: The Framingham study. *Stroke.* 1972;3:409.
44. Thomas DJ, Marshall J, Russell RWR, et al: Effect of hematocrit on cerebral blood flow in man. *Lancet.* 1977;2:941.
45. Portway BA, Herion JC: Neurologic manifestations in sickle-cell disease, with a review of the literature and emphasis on the prevalence of hemiplegia. *Ann Intern Med.* 1972;76:643.
46. Schoenberg BS, Schoenberg DG, Pritchard DA, et al: Differential risk factors for completed stroke and transient ischemic attacks (TIA): Study of vascular diseases (hypertension, cardiac disease, peripheral vascular disease) and diabetes mellitus. In Duvoisin RC, ed. *Transactions of the American Neurological Association,* Vol 105. New York: Springer; 1980:165.
47. Whisnant JP, Matsumoto N, Eluebach LR: The effect of anticoagulant therapy on the prognosis of patients with transient cerebral ischemic attacks in a community. *Mayo Clin Proc.* 1973;48:844.
48. Pessin M, Hinton RC, Davis HR, et al: Mechanisms of acute carotid stroke. *Ann Neurol.* 1979;6:245.
49. North American symptomatic carotid endarterectomy trial collaborators: Beneficial effect of carotid endarterectomy in symptomatic patients with high grade carotid stenosis. *N Engl J Med.* 1991;325:445.
50. European carotid surgery trialists collaborative group: MRC European surgery trial: Interim results for symptomatic patients with severe (70–99%) or mild (0–29%) carotid stenosis. *Lancet.* 1991;337:1235.
51. Hertzer NR, Beven EG, Benjamin SP: Ultramicroscopic ulcerations and thrombi of the carotid bifurcation. *Arch Surg.* 1977;112:1394.
52. Harrison MJG, Marshall J: Prognostic significance of carotid atheroma in early manifestations of cerebrovascular disease. *Stroke.* 1982;13:567.
53. EC–IC bypass study group: Failure of extracranial–intracranial arterial bypass to reduce the risk of ischemic stroke. *N Engl J Med.* 1985;313:1191.
54. Rosenthal D, Cossman D, Ledig CB, Callow AD: Results of carotid endarterectomy for vertebrobasilar insufficiency. *Arch Surg.* 1978;113:1361.
55. Ford JJ, Baker WH, Ehrenhaft JL: Carotid endarterectomy for nonhemispheric transient ischemic attacks. *Arch Surg.* 1975;110:1314.
56. Wolf PA, Kannel WB, Surlie P, McNamara P: Asymptomatic carotid bruit and risk of stroke. *JAMA.* 1981;245:1442.
57. Heymin A, Wilkinson WE, Heyden S, et al: Risk of stroke in asymptomatic persons with cervical arterial bruits: A population study in Evans County, Georgia. *N Engl J Med.* 1980;302:838.
58. Busuttil RW, Baker JD, Davidson RK, Machleder HI: Carotid artery stenosis: Hemodynamic significance and clinical course. *JAMA.* 1981;245:1438.
59. Kartchner MM, McRae LP: Noninvasive evaluation and management of the asymptomatic carotid bruit. *Surgery.* 1977;82:840.
60. Thiele BL, Young JV, Chikos PM, et al: Correlation of arteriographic findings and symptoms in cerebrovascular disease. *Neurology.* 1980;30:1041.
61. Moore WS, Boren C, Malone JM, et al: Natural history of nonstenotic, asymptomatic ulcerative lesions of the carotid artery. *Arch Surg.* 1978;113:1352.
62. O'Donnell TF, Erdoes L, Mackey WC, et al: Correlation of B-mode ultrasound imaging and arteriography with pathological findings at carotid endarterectomy. *Arch Surg.* 1985;120:443.
63. Johnson JM: Angiography and ultrasound in the diagnosis of carotid artery disease: A comparison. *Contemporary Surg.* 1980;20:79.
64. Lusby RJ, Ferrell LD, Ehrenfeld EK, et al: Carotid plaque hemorrhage: Its role in production of cerebral ischemia. *Arch Surg.* 1982;117:1479.
65. Imparato AM, Riles TS, Mintzer R, Baumann FG: The importance of hemorrhage in the relationship between gross morphologic characteristics and cerebral symptoms in 376 carotid artery plaques. *Ann Surg.* 1983;197:195.

66. Persson AV, Robichaux WJ, Silverman M: The natural history of carotid plaque development. *Arch Surg.* 1983;118:1048.

67. Reilly LM, Lusby RJ, Hughes L, et al: Carotid plaque histology using real time ultrasonography: Clinical and therapeutic implications. *Am J Surg.* 1983; 146:188.

68. Hobson RW, Weiss DG, Field WS, et al: Efficacy of carotid endarterectomy for asymptomatic carotid stenosis. *N Engl J Med.* 1993;328:221.

69. Asymptomatic Carotid Atherosclerosis Study Group: Study design for randomized prospective trial of carotid endarterectomy for asymptomatic atherosclerosis. *Stroke.* 1989;20:844.

70. Chambers BR, Norris JW: The case against surgery for asymptomatic carotid stenosis. *Stroke.* 1984;15:964.

71. Wolf PA, Kannel WB, Verter J: Current status of risk factors for stroke. *Neurol Clin.* 1983;1:317.

72. Paffenberger RS, Williams JF: Chronic disease in former college students. V. Early precursors of fatal stroke. *Am J Public Health.* 1967;57:1290.

CHAPTER 88

Cost-Benefit Analysis of Carotid Endarterectomy: A Surgical Perspective

HUGH H. TROUT III, RICHARD L. FEINBERG, and LOUIS KOZLOFF

Until 1970, health care costs consumed less than 7 percent of the gross domestic product. Moreover, the overall cost of care of the markedly ill was relatively modest, since those in critical condition tended to get better or die relatively quickly. Now, because of improved technology and advances in scientific understanding, most of these severely ill patients survive or die after prolonged and expensive health care. Because of this phenomenon, and also because of the ever-increasing costs of both technology and caring for an aging population, the percentage of gross domestic product devoted to health care is now in excess of 14 percent and continues to grow at a rate at least twice that of inflation.

For all these reasons, it is obvious that allocation of health care resources will be necessary. To date, the allocation that has occurred has been on the basis of race, gender, geographic location, wealth, insurance coverage, or some other inequitable method. Now, however, it is apparent that our ability to provide unlimited care, even to favored subgroups, exceeds our ability to pay for it. Accordingly, there will be an increased emphasis on looking at a more rational allocation method such as value received per health care dollar or, in current jargon, cost-effectiveness. Indeed, it has been stated that "leaders of health reform would do well to set two goals for the medical system: the care provided should be proved effective by good science; and among effective services, those that bring the most health for the resources spent should be given the highest priority."[1]

In brief, like it or not, efforts at measuring the cost-effectiveness of treatments will increase and are likely to have a substantial impact on what services will be provided in the future. For carotid endarterectomy (CEA), the efficacy of the operation has been established,[2] the range of appropriate indications is being determined, and the need to evaluate the cost-effectiveness of CEA is now becoming apparent. That is the goal of this chapter.

Estimates of the cost of CEA vary considerably, based primarily on the region of the country being considered, the extent of preoperative evaluation and postoperative surveillance employed, whether or not perioperative complications are encountered, and whether treatment for coronary artery disease, discovered as part of the preoperative evaluation, is included in the cost. Although the length of the hospital stay incurred by patients undergoing CEA has been reduced considerably over the past decade, the diagnosis-related group method of reimbursement for Medicare patients has lessened the impact of this factor on the overall cost of CEA.

Similarly, a reliable assay of the overall societal cost of stroke rehabilitation requires a reasonably accurate knowledge of, among other things, the expected incidence of ischemic stroke among both surgically and medically treated patients; the average severity of such strokes caused by extracranial carotid artery ulceration, stenosis, or occlusion (as distinguished from hemorrhagic stroke and cerebral infarction resulting from cardiogenic embolization); the average life expectancy of stroke patients; and the costs of providing long-term care for patients with stroke.

As is readily apparent, such an endeavor is difficult at best, for many reasons. The many variables involved (merely alluded to in the preceding paragraphs) make a precise analysis virtually impossible. Further confounding the problem is the lack of uniformity with which both surgically and medically treated patients are managed. For example, many centers perform CEA based on the findings of duplex ultrasonography alone, thus obviating the need for preoperative angiography, with its attendant expense (as well as avoiding the small but obligate risk of angiographic complications, with their own attendant costs).[3-5] Questions regarding the cost-effectiveness of such alternative approaches to patient management, however, are currently insoluble. In laboratories in which the accuracy of noninvasive cerebrovascular testing is rigorously validated, angiography may be eliminated in many cases without sacrificing diagnostic reliability, and significant savings can be expected. But such a policy in less reliable vascular laboratories may introduce the potential for inappropriate CEA, and the savings in preoperative testing may be exceeded by the expenses of suboptimal medical practice.

Further adding to the difficulty of such an analysis is the fact that much of the available natural history data on stroke did not classify patients according to the type of stroke (eg, ischemic cerebral infarction caused by cardiogenic embolization, extracranial carotid atheroma, or intracranial occlusion, as well as subarachnoid or intracerebral hemorrhage) or location of stroke (eg, ipsilateral or contralateral to an extracranial carotid artery lesion). Moreover, few studies are methodologically complete, making them difficult to interpret and compare. Despite the continuing evolution of accepted standards for the evaluation and treatment of patients who are candidates for CEA or have already sustained a stroke, our knowledge base is increasing, and the cost of much of the relevant technology is becoming more standardized.[6, 7] Consequently, our ability to perform cost-benefit analyses is improving.

Given the considerations outlined earlier, and in view of the current environment of cost-consciousness in medical decision making, it seems reasonable to undertake a reasoned inquiry into the cost-effectiveness of CEA and its overall impact on the societal cost of caring for patients at risk for ischemic stroke. It must be emphasized at the outset that the techniques of analysis employed here are crude, and much of the data upon which this evaluation is based are imprecise and flawed. Accordingly, throughout this chapter, we attempt to make clear what assumptions have been made and how costs have been calculated so that refinements can be made as the "art" of medical cost analysis becomes more of a science.

STROKE

Stroke is the third leading cause of death in the United States and accounts for 5 percent of all acute care bed days.[8]

Stroke mortality is about 31 per 100,000 population among white males and 27 per 100,000 among white females; the corresponding figures are 59 per 100,000 for black males and 48 per 100,000 for black females.[9] It is postulated that this difference between the races is related primarily to the higher incidence of untreated hypertension among black patients. Interestingly, however, despite the higher incidence of stroke among black patients, there is a much lower incidence of stroke as a result of extracranial carotid artery occlusive disease among these patients, compared with their white counterparts.

The overall incidence of ischemic stroke in Rochester, Minnesota, from 1980 to 1984 was 112 per 100,000 population (compared with 14 per 100,000 population for hemorrhagic stroke).[10] The incidence of and rate of mortality from stroke have declined significantly since 1950: the decreasing incidence has been attributed to better control of atherosclerotic risk factors, especially hypertension, and the decline in mortality is thought to result either from improvements in the treatment of patients suffering strokes or from a decrease in the severity of those strokes.[11, 12] The rates of decline in stroke incidence and mortality appear to have slowed, however, perhaps because of an aging population combined with an increase in detection of milder strokes with imaging studies such as computed tomography (CT) and magnetic resonance imaging (MRI).[9, 10, 13]

Approximately half of all strokes occur as a result of atherothrombotic brain infarction.[14] One study of 1000 patients with first-time stroke, using CT and Doppler ultrasonography, demonstrated that 89 percent had infarction and that the carotid territory was involved in 68 percent of those with infarcts.[15] Of those patients with carotid territory infarcts, 34 percent had greater than 50 percent stenosis (or occlusion) of the ipsilateral internal carotid artery. Thus, in 206 of the 1000 patients with first-time stroke, infarction was caused by a lesion that a carotid endarterectomy might have prevented (and this does not consider the possibility that some patients with less than 50 percent stenosis and significant ulcerative bifurcation lesions may also benefit from CEA).

The incidence of stroke increases with age, doubling in each decade of life from 45 to 85 years (1440 per 100,000 population for those between 75 and 84 years of age).[13] In addition, the percentage of strokes caused by infarction increases with the age of the patient.[16] Among those patients over age 65 at the time of their strokes, only 35 percent were subsequently independent in five acts of daily living; about 50 percent remained totally dependent on others for the remainder of their lives.[16]

Prognosis after stroke is related to race (blacks have a higher mortality from stroke and seem to have a worse prognosis if they survive the initial stroke period.[17] It is also related to the type of stroke (hemorrhagic or ischemic) and to the level of consciousness at the time of hospitalization.[18]

The pertinent questions about stroke for the purposes of this analysis are (1) what are the range and distribution of stroke caused by lesions in the extracranial carotid arteries (ie, those strokes that would presumably be prevented by CEA), (2) what happens to these patients, and (3) what are the costs associated with caring for them?

The 30-day mortality for patients suffering ischemic stroke is about 15 percent: half of the 30-day survivors will live 5 years, but a third of them will require prolonged inpatient rehabilitation. Strokes caused by hemorrhage are generally more severe and have a worse short-term prognosis than strokes caused by embolus or occlusive disease.[7] Given that 15 percent of all strokes are hemorrhagic, with a mortality rate of roughly 30 percent, then approximately 13 percent of the total stroke population eligible for rehabilitation comprises patients with hemorrhagic infarction (this assumes a mortality of 15 percent in patients with ischemic stroke). In a recent community-based study of the outcome following stroke, 58 percent of patients suffering ischemic infarction were discharged home, another 27 percent required extended institutional care, and 15 percent died. In contrast, of patients sustaining hemorrhagic stroke, 43 percent went home, 14 percent were institutionalized, and 43 percent died.[18] These data suggest that, although there are considerable short-term prognostic differences between patients with hemorrhagic infarction and those with ischemic infarction, the difference in long-term rehabilitation prognosis for patients surviving 30 days is not large. Indeed, surviving hemorrhagic stroke patients appear to have a better prognosis than their ischemic stroke counterparts, possibly as a result of the gradual improvement in cerebral perfusion and metabolism as intracerebral blood is resorbed and the initial increase in intracerebral pressure subsides. Thus, rehabilitation statistics based on data from stroke patients of all types may slightly overestimate the degree of recovery that can be anticipated following ischemic stroke, since the 30-day survivors of hemorrhagic stroke have fewer disabilities and seem to recover better.

In a study of 539 stroke patients admitted to a rehabilitation unit at a mean of 19 days after their strokes, 70 percent were eventually discharged to the community, 8 percent required additional acute inpatient care, 17 percent required extended nursing home care, 4 percent were transferred to other rehabilitation units, and 6 percent died.[19] At 6 months' follow-up, another 14 percent had died, and 80 percent of the original cohort were living in the community; however, 12 percent were receiving home care services, and only 21 percent were classified as unlimited in performing their daily activities.

The costs of stroke care are primarily one-time costs, except for the 15 to 20 percent of patients who require nursing home care. Postdischarge care, in the form of either home physical therapy or treatment provided in an outpatient rehabilitation unit, is frequently required shortly after discharge; however, this utilization drops considerably after 3 to 6 months as the incremental benefits of such care diminish and the availability of transportation and insurance coverage becomes a limiting factor. Stroke care for younger patients tends to be more expensive than that for older patients, probably for two reasons. First, younger patients are more likely to have had a hemorrhagic stroke and thus are more severely compromised in the acute phase. Second, their potential for substantive recovery and the enormous financial incentive to return them to home living are strong inducements for prolonged rehabilitation efforts.

Of 61 ipsilateral strokes among the patients receiving medical therapy in the North American Symptomatic Carotid Endarterectomy Trial (NASCET), 29 were classified as major (defined as causing a functional deficit persisting 90 or more days) and 32 as minor.[2] These data (as well as data from asymptomatic patients with high-grade carotid stenoses

TABLE 88–1. Outcome and Cost Estimates for Stroke

Factor	Estimate	Cost ($)/Unit	Total Cost per Patient, $
30-day death rate, %	15	—	—
Average acute hospitalization for those who die*	14 days	3000/day	42,000
First-year death rate (excluding first 30 days), %	15	—	—
Average acute hospitalization for survivors*	19 days	2500/day	47,500
Percent transferred to nursing home†	17	—	—
Average duration in nursing home*	3 years	3500/mo	126,000
Percent transferred to rehabilitation unit	20	—	—
Average duration in rehabilitation unit*	28 days	1100/day	30,800
Percent transferred directly home	48	—	—
Percent eventually sent home†	68	—	—
Percent receiving home care	20	—	—
Average duration of home care*	60 days	150/day	9000
Yearly death rate after first year, %	9	—	—

*Includes all professional fees.
†Includes those sent directly and those who went to a rehabilitation unit first.

that show a 15 to 20 percent incidence of previous stroke on CT or MRI) suggest that at least half of all strokes caused by high-grade carotid stenosis will be mild.

We have chosen not to consider what impact additional strokes (beyond the first) may have on the overall cost of care, as the available data are inadequate to allow credible estimation. But unless a second stroke results in a higher short-term mortality (thus effectively lowering the cost of care for these patients by virtue of early death), it seems logical to expect that the inclusion of this contingency in our cost analysis would increase the disparity between the cost of nonoperative management and the cost of CEA (in favor of endarterectomy), since it is likely that the incidence of subsequent stroke would be higher in patients not having CEA. Also not included in this analysis are the indirect costs associated with stroke (although they may be substantial), such as loss of personal income and loss of tax revenue and the cost of disability payments to stroke patients. These costs affect primarily those patients who are younger than 65 years of age and are exceedingly difficult to estimate.

Summary of Assumptions About Stroke

1. Approximately 20 percent of all strokes are secondary to extracranial carotid artery disease. This is the population group that is likely to benefit from CEA.

2. It is probable that, in patients with carotid artery stenosis, the majority of strokes occur without antecedent transient ischemic attacks (TIAs).

3. Factors associated with an increased risk of stroke include advanced patient age, history of hemispheric TIA, recent TIA, increased frequency of TIA, severe carotid artery stenosis (at least 70 to 99%), and echolucent carotid artery plaques.

4. About half of first strokes from carotid artery disease are mild.

Although the data on which our calculations are based are admittedly imprecise, the figures in Table 88–1 seem to be a reasonable estimate of the outcome of patients who have strokes from carotid artery disease. For purposes of cost calculations, the assumptions in the table are based on those

patients who have strokes from extracranial carotid occlusions (assuming that the ipsilateral stroke was from progression of a tight stenosis to an occlusion) or stenosis of greater than 50 percent. Table 88–2 shows the total estimated costs for 100 stroke patients.

CAROTID ENDARTERECTOMY

The costs of CEA generally include preoperative evaluation, preoperative surgical consultation, consultation with the patient's primary care physician, noninvasive carotid duplex scan, cerebral imaging study (CT or MRI), cerebral arterial imaging study (magnetic resonance angiography, digital subtraction angiography, or formal cerebral arteriogram), preoperative laboratory studies, hospital fee, anesthesiologist's fee, surgeon's fee, postoperative office visit to a primary care physician, and whatever postoperative surveillance is deemed appropriate. Other costs that may accrue during the preoperative preparation of a patient for CEA include neurologic consultation, cardiologic consultation, noninvasive and invasive studies for cardiac evaluation (thallium myocardial scintigraphy or coronary angiography), and, if

TABLE 88–2. Total Estimated Costs for 100 Stroke Patients

Factor	Calculation, % × $	Total Cost, $
Average cost of acute hospitalization for those who die	15 × 42,000	630,000
Average cost of acute hospitalization for survivors	85 × 47,500	4,037,500
Average cost of nursing home	17 × 126,000	2,142,000
Average cost of rehabilitation unit	20 × 30,800	616,000
Average cost of home care	20 × 9000	180,000
Total cost of care for 100 stroke patients		7,605,500
Average cost of care for one stroke patient		76,055

indicated, myocardial revascularization (percutaneous trans-luminal coronary angioplasty or coronary artery bypass). Additionally, for patients not insured by Medicare, the type of anesthesia, whether electroencephalographic monitoring is used (and if so, whether a neurologist is present), length of stay in the intensive care unit, length of hospital stay, and surgeon's fee can all alter the total cost of CEA. A brief look at these component costs follows.

Preoperative Surgical Consultation. This is usually a mid-level consultation lasting 30 to 40 minutes (CPT codes 99242–4 for office consultations; codes 99252–4 for inpatients). Decisions are made regarding the need for additional consultations and evaluation.

Consultation with Primary Care Physician. Since most CEAs are performed on the same day as hospital admission, the admitting history and physical are usually provided by the patient's primary care physician.

Cardiologic Consultation and Evaluation. Most anesthesiologists request that patients be evaluated by a cardiologist before they administer anesthesia. Coronary disease is often present in CEA patients, and significant perioperative blood pressure lability is common and potentially hazardous. Occasionally, cardiologic consultation is not indicated, for example, in a patient with frequent TIAs and a tight internal carotid artery stenosis detected by duplex scan. In this setting, the urgency of CEA takes precedence over cardiac evaluation. Overall, however, approximately 80 percent of patients undergoing CEA require preoperative cardiac evaluation.

Most patients have at least one cardiac study before undergoing CEA. If the patient can exercise, an exercise stress test is done; if the patient is unable to exercise, a dipyridamole thallium scan is usually done. If either is negative, cardiac clearance is usually given, and no further workup is required. If either is positive, a coronary angiogram generally follows. Coronary angiography reveals lesions that should be addressed by either percutaneous transluminal coronary angioplasty or coronary artery bypass in roughly one third of cases.

Neurologic Consultation. A neurologic opinion is frequently obtained when an explanation for the patient's symptoms is sought by the patient or the primary care physician. If a patient has focal symptoms appropriate to a tight carotid stenosis detected by noninvasive testing, neurologic consultation is usually not indicated. A neurologic evaluation can be useful as a baseline in the event of postoperative neurologic symptoms, but since the appropriateness of CEA in this setting is apparent, neurologic consultation will not alter patient management. Also, patients with asymptomatic carotid bruits frequently do not see neurologists preoperatively. About 30 percent of patients have neurologic evaluations prior to CEA.

Cerebral Imaging Studies. All patients have at least one study performed prior to CEA to provide information on the cerebrovascular anatomy and possibly the brain itself. Most have two imaging studies, and some have three. Almost all patients considered for CEA undergo duplex ultrasonography of the carotid bifurcation. An exception to this might be a patient who has recent onset focal TIAs. Even in this setting, however, a duplex scan is frequently performed to assess for patency of the distal internal carotid (and if it is patent, a CEA without further study is likely). Although an increasing

number of surgeons are performing CEA on the basis of duplex scanning alone, this test is highly operator dependent and is subject to inaccuracy or misinterpretation unless rigorous internal quality control is maintained by individual laboratories. Consequently, this practice is not yet our routine and, for the purposes of this analysis, is not adopted as the standard in assessing the cost of CEA.

Ocular pneumoplethysmography is an excellent physiologic test. It is particularly useful in those patients who have about a 70 percent stenosis detected by duplex scanning. If the ocular pneumoplethysmogram is positive, this suggests that the stenosis is hemodynamically significant and CEA is appropriate. This test is usually not necessary, however, except for the less than 5 percent of patients whose degree of stenosis is borderline.

CT and MRI scans are frequently obtained to evaluate patients with neurologic symptoms. These studies may also provide some information as to whether an asymptomatic patient has had a previous silent cerebral infarction. They play little role, however, in determining whether a patient should undergo CEA.[20] They are obtained equally frequently in patients who do not undergo CEA as in those who do. Consequently, although the cost of obtaining these studies contributes to the overall cost of medical care, it does not alter the relationship between the cost of CEA and that of nonoperative management of patients with cerebrovascular disease.

After duplex ultrasonography, magnetic resonance angiography is the cheapest and safest method of evaluating the degree of stenosis of a carotid lesion. In those settings in which a tight stenosis with a patent distal internal carotid artery has been identified, magnetic resonance angiography is a good objective confirming study. It is not, however, reliable enough to serve as the standard imaging test because of a consistent tendency to overread the degree of stenosis. Digital subtraction angiography remains the standard imaging technique that should be used. It is expensive and has some risks (about a 0.5% complication rate), but in general, it is a superb imaging test. It should be obtained in about 90 percent of patients who undergo CEA.

Formal cerebral arteriography gives more complete information about cerebral blood flow than any other imaging study. It is, however, associated with more risks and is more expensive to perform than other techniques. Fewer than 10 percent of carotid imaging studies should use this method, provided digital subtraction angiography is available.

Using the fees listed in Table 88–3, the cost of an uncomplicated, simple CEA (including preoperative surgical consultation, consultation with the primary care physician, cardiologist's consultation with a negative stress test, noninvasive carotid duplex scan, magnetic resonance angiogram, preoperative laboratory studies, hospital fee, anesthesiologist's fee, surgeon's fee, postoperative office visit to a primary care physician, and five postoperative duplex scans for yearly surveillance) would be about $11,538.

The cost of a complex CEA (including preoperative surgeon's consultation, consultation with the primary care physician, cardiologist's consultation, neurologist's consultation, dipyridamole thallium scan and coronary artery angioplasty, noninvasive carotid duplex scan, digital subtraction angiogram, preoperative laboratory studies, hospital fee, anesthesiologist's fee, surgeon's fee, postoperative office visit to a primary care physician, and five postoperative duplex scans for yearly surveillance) would be about $18,848.

Finally, the cost of a complicated CEA (including preoperative surgeon's consultation, consultation with the primary care physician, neurologist's consultation, cardiologist's consultation, dipyridamole thallium scan and coronary artery angiogram, coronary artery bypass, noninvasive carotid duplex scan, digital subtraction angiogram, preoperative laboratory studies, anesthesiologist's fee, surgeon's fee, 7-day hospitalization because of a mild myocardial infarction from which the patient recovers sufficiently so as not to need posthospitalization rehabilitation, three postoperative office visits to a primary care physician, and five postoperative duplex scans for yearly surveillance) would be about $34,848.

COST ANALYSIS

A number of assumptions regarding CEA must be made in order to analyze costs in various settings:

1. The figures modified from Gelabert and Moore[21] in Table 88–4 are generally correct.
2. The indications for CEA are generally distributed as follows[22, 23]: asymptomatic patients, 30 percent; TIA patients, 55 percent; mild to moderate stroke patients, 15 percent. Amaurosis fugax patients are included in the TIA group, with the understanding that although amaurosis fugax may reflect small strokes, the prognosis is probably better than for patients with hemispheric TIAs.[24]
3. The endpoint of death is not a major factor in assessing the costs of CEA. CEA is thought to prolong the stroke-free

TABLE 88–4. Stroke Rates

Group	First Year, %	Annual, %	5 Year, %
Asymptomatic patients			
Medical treatment	5.0	5.0	25.0
Surgical treatment	1.3	0.5	3.3
TIA patients			
Medical treatment	8.5	5.0	28.0
Surgical treatment	3.0	1.5	9.0
Stroke patients			
Medical treatment	9.0	9.0	45.0
Surgical treatment	7.0	2.2	15.8

Modified from Gelabert HA, Moore WS: Carotid endarterectomy: Current status. *Curr Probl Surg.* 1991;28:181; with permission.

interval but not prolong life; in the NASCET study,[2] after 2 years there were seven deaths—including during the perioperative period—in the surgical group (2.1%) and nine deaths in the medical group (2.7%).
4. Regardless of whether a patient has had a CEA, strokes cost the same whether they occur spontaneously or within the 30-day perioperative period (ie, the severity of a stroke is not influenced by whether a patient has had a CEA, nor is the severity of a stroke in a patient who has had a CEA influenced by when it occurs after the CEA).
5. Including a cost analysis of patients who have had two or more strokes would not substantially alter the cost relationship between the CEA group and the non-CEA group.
6. Ninety percent of patients have uncomplicated CEAs, 5 percent have complex CEAs, and 5 percent have complicated CEAs.

The average cost of stroke care and rehabilitation is $76,055 per patient (see Table 88–2). Using the assumptions enumerated previously, the cost of 100 carotid endarterectomies (90 uncomplicated [90 × $11,538 = $1,038,420]; 5 complex [5 × $18,848 = $94,240]; 5 complicated [5 × $34,848 = $174,240]) would be $1,306,900 ($1,038,420 + $94,240 + $174,240).

The cost of stroke care over 5 years in the surgical group with asymptomatic carotid bruits (see Table 88–4) is $75,294 (3.3 strokes × $76,055 × 0.30, since asymptomatic patients account for 30% of the total). Using this same approach, the cost of stroke care in the TIA group is $376,472 (9 × $76,055 × 0.55), and the cost of stroke care in the group of patients undergoing CEA for prior cerebral infarction is $180,250 (15.8 × $76,055 × 0.15). Thus, the total cost for stroke care in the surgical group over 5 years would be $632,016 ($75,294 + $376,472 + $180,250).

The cost of stroke care in an identical group of 100 patients treated medically would be $570,413 in the asymptomatic group (25 × $76,055 × 0.30), $1,171,247 in the TIA group (28 × $76,055 × 0.55), and $513,371 in the stroke group (45 × $76,055 × 0.15). Thus, the total cost for stroke care in the medically treated group of patients would be $2,255,031 ($570,413 + $1,171,247 + $513,371).

Adding the total cost of CEA ($1,306,900) to the total cost of stroke care that the patients with CEA incur ($632,016) gives a total cost over 5 years in 100 patients of $1,938,916, compared with stroke costs of $2,255,031 for the medical group. Thus, if the assumptions listed are

TABLE 88–3. Fees for Carotid Endarterectomy

Service	Fee, $
Preoperative surgeon's consultation	90
Consultation with primary care physician	140
Cardiologist's consultation	140
Neurologist's consultation (no lab tests)	140
Noninvasive and invasive studies for cardiac evaluation	
Dipyridamole thallium	700
Exercise stress test	500
Coronary angiography	2800
Cardiac procedure to enhance coronary blood flow	
Angioplasty (includes hospital charge, cardiology fee)	3200
Coronary artery bypass (includes hospital charge, cardiology fee, surgeon's fee)	15,000
Noninvasive carotid duplex scan	223
Cerebral imaging study	
Magnetic resonance angiography	1000
Digital subtraction angiography	2000
Formal cerebral arteriogram	2000
Preoperative laboratory studies	
Electrocardiogram	30
Chest radiographs (posteroanterior, lateral)	150
Complete blood count	20
Urinalysis	10
SMA-6	20
Prothrombin time, partial thromboplastin time	20
Carotid endarterectomy (includes hospital charge, anesthesiologist's fee, surgeon's fee)	8000
Postoperative office visit to primary care physician	50

generally correct, CEA, in addition to prolonging stroke-free life, appears to be of slight economic advantage.

If the cost of caring for a stroke patient is $61,650, as suggested by Ahn and coworkers[25] (rather than the $76,055 used in our cost analysis), the total cost of CEA ($1,306,900) added to the total cost of stroke care that patients with CEA incur ($512,310) gives a total cost over 5 years in 100 patients of $1,819,210. The stroke costs of the medical group (based on $61,650 per patient with stroke) would be $1,827,922.

If the cost of stroke care were $50,000 per patient, the total cost of CEA ($1,306,900) added to the total cost of stroke care that patients with CEA incur ($415,500) would yield a total cost over 5 years in 100 patients of $1,722,400. The stroke costs of the medical group (using the $50,000) would be $1,482,500.

SCREENING

Patients with neurologic symptoms present few dilemmas regarding screening tests: a patient with a definite focal TIA or a discrete mild to moderate stroke is likely to have a single duplex scan that will add little to the cost of care. The issue of who should be given screening tests is not trivial. Screening for asymptomatic disease (whether it involves the breast, the uterus, the prostate, the heart, or the carotid artery) is expensive, and demonstrating cost-effectiveness can be difficult.

Who, then, should be surveyed for the presence of hemodynamically significant carotid artery disease? Carotid bruit is a notoriously poor predictor of carotid artery stenosis greater than 50 percent; conversely, a bruit may be missing in as many as one third of patients with severe carotid stenosis. We know that stroke incidence doubles in every decade of life. Should all patients over 67 years of age who have peripheral vascular disease be screened, as has been suggested by Ahn and colleagues?[25] Although the cost of a carotid duplex scan is relatively low (current Medicare reimbursement is probably below the actual cost of the study; JD Baker, personal communication), the uncertainty as to which asymptomatic patients are likely to have hemodynamically significant stenosis means that many scans would be required to detect a small number of patients who would be likely to benefit from CEA. Thus, any money saved by preventing stroke and its attendant costs would likely be negated by the costs of widespread screening. It is therefore apparent that the total cost of screening asymptomatic patients would be a prime determinant of how enthusiastic paying agencies would be about reimbursing for screening tests. This highlights the importance of keeping screening costs low and of identifying subsets of patients at increased likelihood of having carotid stenosis. The lower the screening costs, the higher the incidence of discovered disease; the greater the health consequences of a missed sign in the population under study, the greater the likelihood of the treatment being cost-effective.

LOWERING COSTS

Stroke Care

A perusal of the component costs of stroke care reveals that the greatest opportunity to reduce the cost of caring for a patient with a completed stroke (aside from preventing the stroke in the first place) is to reduce the time the patient spends in institutions. Savings in the initial acute care facility, however, will probably be modest, as stroke patients seem to require care that is reasonably intense in quality and duration before they improve enough to be sent to nursing homes, rehabilitation units, or home. The greatest savings are likely to be in reducing the number of patients requiring nursing home care. The challenge for rehabilitation facilities, therefore, is to determine whether a patient requires nursing home care or can be discharged back to his or her community with the aid of the rehabilitation unit. The sooner this assessment can be done accurately, the more cost-effective it will be, keeping in mind that the cost of a few extra days in a rehabilitation unit are well worth the expenditure if permanent custodial care in a nursing home can be avoided.

Carotid Endarterectomy

A reduction in the costs of CEA itself can be achieved by reducing the frequency and duration of intensive care unit use (using step-down units instead) and minimizing hospitalization time. One potentially important step toward cost reduction is to better define which patients will benefit from cardiac imaging and treatment before CEA and to restrict cardiac evaluation to those who are likely to have significant cardiac disease. Also, magnetic resonance angiography and duplex scanning are cheaper and safer than angiography, whether by digital subtraction or formal cut-film techniques. As a consequence, once acceptable levels of reliability (reduction of operator dependency for duplex scans, refinement of image for magnetic resonance angiography) are achieved, one or the other of these imaging tests should supplant arteriography, thus lowering the costs of CEA. The greatest savings, of course, will be realized by ensuring that CEA is performed with strict adherence to appropriate indications and by minimizing the perioperative morbidity associated with the procedure.

COST-EFFECTIVENESS ANALYSIS: PRO AND CON

If CEA and best medical therapy were compared and CEA was found to result in a better clinical outcome and lower resource requirements (as the data presented here suggest for patients with TIA and greater than 70 percent ipsilateral carotid stenosis), experts in the field of cost-effectiveness analysis would deem CEA to be "dominant" and recommend its adoption without further economic analysis (assuming, of course, that there was consensus that the data were correct).[26] If there were a better clinical outcome but *increased* resource requirements (as in the case of CEA for asymptomatic carotid artery disease with greater than 70 percent stenosis, because of the considerable costs of screening), the decision whether to adopt the better treatment would be more complicated and uncertain. Experts use several methods to make such determinations, including computing cost-effectiveness ratios, cost-utility ratios (which include estimates of quality of life—referred to as quality-adjusted life years), and cost-benefit ratios (which calculated the amount patients are willing to pay in order to avoid the pain or disability caused by the disease in question).[26]

These analyses are complex and fraught with limitations. Nonetheless, an entire field of study is being developed to perform these analyses, and the results are already having an impact on public policy.[27, 28] For instance, no cost savings can be documented by vaccinating for pneumococcal pneumonia or influenza or screening for cervical cancer, colorectal cancer, or hypercholesterolemia.[1] This does not mean that these procedures are not of considerable value, just that they are not "dominant." This situation of procedures improving the quality or duration of life at some additional cost is at the core of clinical decision making and cost-effectiveness analysis: are the tests and procedures providing sufficient value to justify the additional resources necessary?

The frequency of screening can also have a major impact on the value of a test as determined by cost-effectiveness analysis. For instance, it is believed that screening for cervical cancer is highly effective in preventing death and is indisputably of good value if done at a reasonable frequency.[29] It has been estimated that such screening costs only $22,000 per year of life gained if the screening is done every 3 years; the cost increases to $440,000 if the screening is performed every 2 years, and to $1,800,000 if the screening is performed yearly.[1]

Examples such as these indicate that preventive care "usually increases medical expenditures."[1] This should give pause to those who believe that health care costs will be lowered by increasing the amount of preventive care given.

Con

Cost analysis of medical procedures is often (and not inappropriately) threatening to the medical profession because important policy decisions may be made on the basis of flawed, misinterpreted, or manipulated data. Moreover, policy makers tend to use data that are accessible only in government publications. Although these publications are available to the public, the clinicians who are profoundly affected by them rarely know of their existence or importance.

Policy planners, epidemiologists, and clinicians tend to have divergent views of health care delivery. Most policy planners would like to construct a health care system that provides excellent care at an affordable price, but their primary goal at present is to control costs. Epidemiologists have a greater sense of the realities of health care delivery, but they too are focused on the overall picture and often have little experience with or knowledge of the issue of daily clinical medicine. Clinicians, although intimately knowledgeable about the problems they confront on a frequent basis, are generally uninformed about broader health care issues. Clinicians are usually confident of the efficacy of treatment regimens, but close scrutiny often fails to support this confidence.

Confounding the disparity of insights among these three groups is the fact that each has a major impact on the others, yet communication among them, whether written or verbal, is often disjointed. For instance, data from Medicare for 1991 (a sample of 20% of all Medicare data) indicate that among all patients admitted to acute care hospitals in 1991, there were 51,537 strokes caused by cerebral in-

farction. The mean length of hospital stay for these stroke patients was 9.7 days, the average hospital and physician charges totaled $7,155.53, and 73.3 percent of the patients were cared for in urban hospitals. These data also indicate that the mean hospital stay after CEA was 7.4 days. For a clinician who works in a hospital with more than 200 beds, these data appear flawed. Our impression is that stroke patients stay longer than 10 days and cost far more than $7,155 to care for. CEA patients are hospitalized for 3 to 4 days at most, except for the small minority who suffer complications. Can these Medicare numbers be correct? Certainly one has to suspect a certain amount of misclassification—CT and MRI are not good tests for acute stroke, and duplex ultrasonography is highly operator dependent and not available in many hospitals. Since classification has proved difficult for stroke data banks, it can be assumed that family physicians and hospital coding clerks might misallocate many patients who present with mild neurologic dysfunction. Also, clinicians tend to see and remember patients with major stroke. If, as we defined earlier, roughly 50 percent of patients with ischemic cerebral infarction present with minor neurologic deficits (and thus will have short hospital stays), an average stay of 10 days for all stroke patients may be generally correct. As for the average hospitalization of 7.4 days for CEA patients, this is probably correct for the large referral clinics whose patients come from afar or for those hospitals with a high percentage of indigent patients. In addition, the Rand study[30] showed a 9.8 percent major complication or death rate in 1302 Medicare patients undergoing CEA in 1981. If the average CEA is still associated with a high complication rate, the average hospital stay of 7.4 days cited in the 1991 Medicare data may be generally accurate because of the much longer hospitalization needed as a result of this excessive complication rate.

The point is, health policy planners look for ways to control costs; they see averages and may draw erroneous conclusions. (Recall the 6-foot weather forecaster who drowned in a flood despite an average 4-foot depth of water.) Clinicians see the microcosm of their own clinical experience and may miss the meaning of the bigger picture. For instance, a health policy guru might conclude from an average hospital stay of 7.4 days that CEA is a difficult, expensive procedure. A clinician, in contrast, might dismiss the 7.4 number as obviously incorrect and typical of government ineptitude. But both groups, if they were knowledgeable about the other's work, would deduce that CEA is an excellent operation when done properly (based on multiple retrospective studies as well as prospective studies such as NASCET), that large clinics should devise a way to expedite their pre-CEA evaluations, and that the rest of the surgical community had best focus on reducing the complication rate of CEA. (Clinicians are now doing this but have only belatedly and reluctantly done so. Had they understood the ramifications of the national statistics, more concerted efforts to improve care and contain costs might have been made earlier.)

Pro

Because of escalating costs, health care is in a state of crisis in the United States. Changes are mandatory, and rational allocation of limited resources will be a high priority. This cannot be done without an understanding of the costs of therapeutic regimens as well as an understanding of the value received from these therapies. Thus, the importance of accurate and comprehensive data collection is apparent, as is the need for health care policy to be based on scientific analysis rather than political whim. Cost analysis, therefore, is essential if health policy is to have any logical basis.

Clinicians will become more amenable to cost analysis being included in the assessment of treatment protocols as the importance of cost containment becomes apparent. We will be able to move from the sort of intuitive clinical cost analysis employed in this chapter to a more rigorous analytic format. The importance of clinical impression and judgment should not be underestimated, however. Without this input, the frequency of unintended and unanticipated adverse consequences is likely to be high.

DIRECTIONS FOR THE FUTURE

One of the frustrations surgeons have is that many neurologists have long discounted what is, to surgeons, the obvious benefit of CEA. Of all the available methods to prevent stroke in patients with atherosclerotic risk factors, CEA is by far the most potent weapon in our therapeutic arsenal. Similarly, those who are skeptical about the benefits of CEA have claimed that perioperative morbidity and mortality are too high and that many operations have been performed for questionable or inappropriate indications. Both the advocates and the skeptics regarding CEA are correct. The NASCET study has done much to narrow the gap between these two groups. It demonstrated overwhelming efficacy for CEA when done for proper indications by surgeons with proven track records of few operative complications and deaths. Thus, it is obvious that the greatest cost-effectiveness will be achieved by continued efforts to define proper indications for CEA as well as by restricting the performance of CEA to those surgeons who demonstrate low morbidity and mortality rates.

Another less obvious way to reduce costs is to obtain better information about the causes of stroke. With the availability of better and cheaper imaging techniques, it becomes important for those taking care of stroke patients to obtain this anatomic information and for stroke registries to record it. Although we have estimated in this chapter that 20 percent of all strokes are potentially preventable by the appropriate utilization of CEA, this figure is, at best, speculative. Before substantial efforts can be made to reduce costs, information must be available about the latitude as well as the magnitude of the problem. For instance, advanced age and a history of prior stroke are negative predictors for efficacy of rehabilitation. What is the correlation between advanced age and prior stroke and the incidence of extracranial carotid artery disease? If 50 percent of all strokes are caused by cerebral infarction and carotid stenosis accounts for 20 percent, what causes the other 30 percent? With better data collection, it may be shown that emboli from the heart play a larger role than is now thought.

Randomized clinical trials and complicated data collection are expensive and should not be undertaken frivolously. Nonetheless, with regard to stroke prevention, both have a lot to offer in determining how best to direct future efforts. A disease that causes so much devastating, prolonged, and expensive morbidity and ranks third as a cause of death in the United States warrants the allocation of considerable resources to allow accurate characterization so that appropriate prevention and treatment can be promoted.

CONCLUSIONS

Although great effort should be made to collect accurate data, absolute precision in cost analysis will never be possible, nor is it essential. Data that are generally accurate allow a reasonable assessment of the cost-effectiveness of different treatment strategies. Because the costs of all CEAs are approximately equal to all the costs associated with taking care of those patients whose strokes are likely to have been prevented by CEA, analysis shows substantial improvement in the quality of life at little or no cost for those who are symptomatic and have a greater than 70 percent carotid artery stenosis. In contrast, it may be difficult to document high cost-effectiveness for general screening for carotid disease in asymptomatic patients because of the added costs of screening. Cost-effective screening may require the identification of a subgroup of the asymptomatic population that has a fairly high prevalence of hemodynamic carotid artery stenosis.

REFERENCES

1. Russell LB: The role of prevention in health reform. N Engl J Med. 1993;329:352.
2. North American symptomatic carotid endarterectomy trial collaborators: Beneficial effect of carotid endarterectomy in symptomatic patients with high-grade carotid stenosis. N Engl J Med. 1991;325:445.
3. Goodson SF, Flanigan DP, Bishara RA, et al: Can carotid duplex scanning supplant arteriography in patients with focal carotid territory symptoms? J Vasc Surg. 1987;5:551.
4. Gelabert HA, Moore WS: Carotid endarterectomy without angiography. Surg Clin North Am. 1990;70:213.
5. Wagner WH, Treiman RL, Cossman DV, et al: The diminishing role of diagnostic arteriography in carotid artery disease: Duplex scanning as definitive preoperative study. Ann Vasc Surg. 1991;5:105.
6. Baker JD, Rutherford RB, Bernstein EF, et al: Suggested standards for reports dealing with cerebrovascular disease. Subcommittee on Reporting Standards for Cerebrovascular Disease, Ad Hoc Committee on Reporting Standards, Society for Vascular Surgery/North American Chapter, International Society for Cardiovascular Surgery. J Vasc Surg. 1988;8:721.
7. Foulkes MA, Wolf PA, Price TR, et al: The stroke data bank: Design, methods, and baseline characteristics. Stroke. 1988;19:547.
8. Weingarten S, Bolus R, Riedinger MS, et al: The principle of parsimony: Glasgow coma scale score predicts mortality as well as the APACHE II score for stroke patients. Stroke. 1990;21:1280.
9. Cooper R, Sempos C, Hsieh SC, Kovar MG: Slowdown in the decline of stroke mortality in the United States, 1978–1986. Stroke. 1990;21:1274.
10. Broderick JP, Phillips SJ, Whisnant JP, et al: Incidence rates of stroke in the eighties: The end of the decline in stroke? Stroke. 1989;20:577.
11. Howard G, Toole JF, Becker C, et al: Changes in survival following stroke in five North Carolina counties observed during two different periods. Stroke. 1989;20:345.
12. Wolf PA, D'Agostino RB, O'Neal MA, et al: Secular trends in stroke incidence and mortality: The Framingham study. Stroke. 1992;23:1551.
13. Kuller LH: Incidence rates of stroke in the eighties: The end of the decline in stroke? Stroke. 1989;20:841.
14. Wolf PA: An overview of the epidemiology of stroke. Stroke. 1990;21(9 suppl):II4.
15. Bogousslavsky J, Van Melle G, Regli F: The Lausanne stroke registry: Analysis of 1,000 consecutive patients with first stroke. Stroke. 1988;19:1083.
16. Kojima S, Omura T, Wakamatsu W, et al: Prognosis and disability of stroke patients after 5 years in Akita, Japan. Stroke. 1990;21:72.
17. Gillum RF: Stroke in blacks. Stroke. 1988;19:1.
18. Coull BM, Brockschmidt JK, Howard G, et al: Community hospital-based stroke programs in North Carolina, Oregon, and New York. IV. Stroke diagnosis and its relation to demographics, risk factors, and clinical status after stroke. Stroke. 1990;21:867.

19. Granger CV, Hamilton BB, Gresham GE, Kramer AA: The stroke rehabilitation outcome study: Part I. General description. *Arch Phys Med Rehabil.* 1988; 69:506.

20. Martin JD, Valentine RJ, Myers SI, et al: Is routine CT scanning necessary in the preoperative evaluation of patients undergoing carotid endarterectomy? *J Vasc Surg.* 1991;14:267.

21. Gelabert HA, Moore WS: Carotid endarterectomy: Current status. *Curr Probl Surg.* 1991;28:181.

22. Sundt TM Jr, Whisnant JP, Houser OW, Fode NC: Prospective study of the effectiveness and durability of carotid endarterectomy. *Mayo Clin Proc.* 1990;65:625.

23. Healy DA, Clowes AW, Zierler RE, et al: Immediate and long-term results of carotid endarterectomy. *Stroke.* 1989;20:1138.

24. Amaurosis fugax study group: Current management of amaurosis fugax. *Stroke.* 1990;21:201.

25. Ahn SS, Baker JD, Walden K, Moore WS: Which asymptomatic patients should undergo routine screening carotid duplex scan? *Am J Surg.* 1991;162:180.

26. Detsky AS, Naglie IG: A clinician's guide to cost-effectiveness analysis. *Ann Intern Med.* 1990;113:147.

27. Laupacis A, Feeny D, Detsky AS, Tugwell PX: Tentative guidelines for using clinical and economic evaluations revisited. *Can Med Assoc J.* 1993;148:927.

28. Eddy DM: Clinical decision making: From theory to practice. Three battles to watch in the 1990s. *JAMA.* 1993;270:520.

29. Eddy DM: Screening for cervical cancer. *Ann Intern Med.* 1990;113:214.

30. Winslow CM, Solomon DH, Chassin MR, et al: The appropriateness of carotid endarterectomy. *N Engl J Med.* 1988;318:721.

CHAPTER 89

A Health Policy Perspective on Carotid Endarterectomy: Cost, Effectiveness, and Cost-Effectiveness

DAVID B. MATCHAR, JOHN PAUK, and JOSEPH LIPSCOMB

In an era of constrained resources, medical interventions are coming under increasing scrutiny. It is not sufficient that a diagnostic or treatment strategy provide a clearer view of some anatomic structure or an improvement in some intermediate outcome such as blood pressure or degree of arterial stenosis. A medical intervention must be able to produce improvements in health that are important to individuals (eg, survival and quality of life) and must be able to do so at reasonable cost. In current health policy parlance, a medical intervention must be demonstrably effective *and* cost-effective.

Ischemic stroke is the third leading cause of death in the United States and is a major cause of chronic disability. The annual incidence of ischemic stroke in the United States has been estimated to be 500,000 cases.[1] The average cost for each of these strokes is substantial. Including acute and long-term care, the medical expenditures associated with an average stroke typically range from $15,000 to $45,000, which suggests an aggregate annual cost to the U.S. health care system of $7.5 billion to $22.6 billion. When the dollar cost of lost productivity of the stroke victim is added in, the total U.S. cost may be as great as $25 to 30 billion per year.[2] With the aging of the population, both the human and economic burdens of ischemic stroke will substantially increase, making medical interventions aimed at stroke prevention of tremendous importance.

Carotid endarterectomy is one stroke prevention strategy that has attracted considerable health policy interest. This procedure is intended to reduce the risk of stroke in patients with carotid occlusive disease. Indeed, three recently published trials indicate that carotid endarterectomy can reduce the incidence of stroke and death in symptomatic patients with high-grade carotid stenosis (>70%).[3-5] It has also been suggested that this procedure is of benefit in asymptomatic patients with significant carotid occlusive disease.[6] However, the procedure has risks and is costly.

The policy question raised by these studies is whether the benefits of carotid endarterectomy are always (or ever) worth the risk and the cost. More precisely, for what types of patient is the decision to perform the procedure appropriate, inappropriate, or equivocal?

In this chapter we describe the measures frequently used by clinical policy analysts to evaluate alternative medical interventions. Then we illustrate how these measures can be applied by constructing a decision model to investigate, in turn, the appropriateness of carotid endarterectomy in (1) patients with symptoms of anterior circulation transient ischemic attack (TIA) or minor completed stroke (*symptomatic*); (2) patients without cerebrovascular symptoms (*asymptomatic*); and (3) patients with carotid bruit (*asymptomatic with bruit*). For each of these patient types, we examine the sensitivity of our base-case results to variations in both the clinical and economic parameters in the model. We conclude by considering the implications for clinical practice.

DEFINING COST, EFFECTIVENESS, AND COST-EFFECTIVENESS

Although there are many variations on the theme, the concepts of cost, effectiveness, and cost-effectiveness are central ingredients in most clinical policy evaluations. We consider them in turn.

Cost

The cost of a disease is defined in terms of the economic burden it imposes, measured in monetary terms; similarly, the cost of a disease intervention is its economic burden, again expressed in monetary terms. In either case, the concept of "cost" takes on concrete meaning only after we specify the perspective from which the evaluation is being conducted.

For example, from a patient's perspective, cost is measured in terms of out-of-pocket losses. For the third-party payer (medical insurance carrier), the cost of disease and treatments is measured in terms of the dollar volume of claims that must be paid (net of patient cost-sharing). A third perspective for defining cost—and the one adopted in this chapter and in many other clinical studies—is that of "society." Operationally, this requires that we attempt to measure the actual economic value (the social opportunity cost) of the resources that are consumed by the disease and by treatments to combat it. That is, societal cost is measured in terms of the value of these resources in their next best alternative use, as indicated by what must be paid for them in viable economic markets. For example, if the going wage rate for a registered nurse is $10/hour, the social opportunity cost of an hour of this nurse's time in treating a given patient is typically assumed to be $10/hr, since that is evidently what someone else in society is willing to pay for that hour if it were available for reallocation; the social opportunity cost of all other inputs absorbed by a disease and its treatments can be conceptualized and measured in an analogous manner.

Regardless of perspective, costs can be usefully divided into direct costs, reflecting the dollar burden of the medical care and also the nonmedical expenditures made in response to disease, and indirect costs, reflecting the dollar value of the lost productivity induced by disease.[7]

Although certain approaches to cost-benefit analysis include both direct and indirect costs in the decision calculations, the standard practice in cost-effectiveness analysis (of the type illustrated here) is to include only direct costs.[8] The rationale is that indirect cost is often so highly correlated with the chosen measure of effectiveness that to include it would amount to double-counting the benefits. We adopt this convention and thus ignore the indirect cost of stroke and the corresponding indirect cost benefits of preventing stroke.

Moreover, our calculations focus entirely on direct medical costs, thus ignoring such nonmedical costs as the construction of special stairs or ramps for the stroke victim. In doing so, we understate the total direct cost of stroke and, in effect, impart a conservative bias in our calculations bearing on the appropriateness of carotid endarterectomy.

Effectiveness versus Efficacy

Most clinical trials seek to identify whether a medical intervention has a statistically demonstrable impact. When this impact is limited to only a few important aspects of outcome such as stroke incidence or mortality, this is an evaluation of *efficacy*. The *effectiveness* of an intervention is more broadly defined to include its impact on all outcomes of importance to the patient. (Some analysts distinguish effectiveness from efficacy in a somewhat different way, with the latter referring to the intervention's impact in idealized or controlled circumstances [like a trial] and the former, its impact in everyday medical practice. For the type of analyses presented here, we find our distinction more compelling.)

There are several broad categories of effectiveness measures. The simplest, and perhaps most common, are unidimensional indicators of program output, for example, life-years saved, disability days averted, or swollen joints reduced (eg, for arthritis).

Next, for a richer, more detailed measure of effectiveness, one can choose among a number of existing instruments designed to capture the impact of disease, and treatment, along a number of outcome dimensions (eg, physical, social, and mental functioning). Examples include the Barthel index for activities of daily living, the Medical Outcome Study (MOS)-36 scale, and the National Institutes of Health scale.[9] Typically, the patient being evaluated receives an overall score based on his or her responses to a series of questions about functional ability or capacity. Usually, the scoring algorithm reflects the instrument developer's judgments about the relative importance of the individual items, not the respondent's own preferences about their importance.

A given unidimensional or multidimensional effectiveness measure may be either disease-specific (eg, motor performance, judged on the National Institutes of Health scale) or generic, implying that it could be applied in cross-disease comparisons (eg, life-years saved, or improvement in the MOS-36).

A third category of effectiveness measure differs from either of the first two in only one respect (but a very important one): there is an effort to incorporate the decision maker's own *preferences* for the alternative outcomes of the intervention. In a decision analysis pertaining to the individual patient, it is that patient's preferences that are to be used to assign value to the functional outcomes associated with the intervention. How this is done will be illustrated in the decision analysis following, in which we employ one especially attractive value-weighted measure of program effectiveness, the Quality-Adjusted Life-Year (QALY).

The QALY captures two aspects of outcome typically perceived by patients as important: quantity of life and quality of life. If an individual could live his or her entire (expected) lifetime in excellent health, the QALY score would be equivalent to life expectancy. If the individual experiences an undesirable event, such as a disabling stroke, the QALY score is basically life expectancy reduced by the value-weighted amount of time the individual suffers the effects of the stroke. The value associated with being in the stroke state (per unit of time)—often termed the "disutility" of the stroke state—should reflect individual preferences. In most analyses, if the health state being evaluated is deemed to be as good as the best state (excellent health, presumably), it is assigned a value of 1.0. If it is deemed to be as undesirable as the worst state (typically assumed to be death), it is assigned a value of zero. States that are interjacent in preference to the best and worst are accordingly assigned a number along the interval from 0 to 1.

Practically speaking, the analyst has three basic sources for the preference information required for computing QALYs: (1) solicit it directly from the patient whose alternatives are being analyzed; (2) employ a "standard" set of preference weights available from the literature, which have been derived on the basis of values rendered by "representative" respondents in well-conducted surveys; and (3) simply select reasonable base-case preference values for the patient being analyzed, then conduct extensive sensitivity analysis to test the robustness of the decision model's conclusions to these "modeled" preference weights.

When a physician is working with actual patients one-on-one to determine a treatment strategy, source (1) is preferred, of course. Moreover, an increasing number of clinical trials are starting to collect health outcome preference data on subjects across treatment arms. However, the great majority of cost-effectiveness analyses to date focus not on real, identifiable patients, nor do they pertain to clinical trials in which the preferences of relevant patients have been sampled. Rather, these studies focus on "statistical" patients, defined operationally in terms of a set of baseline risk characteristics and analyzed in some general clinical context (eg, treated by a neurologist and surgeon in a tertiary hospital). In fact, the decision analysis that follows is of this type.

In these cases, the only available options are (2) and (3). Prominent examples of survey-based preference weights are those found in the Quality of Well Being (QWB) scale[10] and the EuroQol index.[11] The former, in particular, has been applied extensively.[12] However, in a number of well-known evaluations, the analysts have elected to "model" patient preferences, then mathematically test the reasonableness of their initial assumptions.[13] This strategy is the one adopted in the decision analyses described in the following paragraphs.

Cost-Effectiveness

Although the term "cost-effective" is often applied haphazardly in the discussion of medical interventions, its meaning is quite specific: When one of two interventions is more effective and is more expensive than the other, it is cost-effective if the additional effectiveness is worth the additional cost. Similarly, if one intervention is less effective and less costly than a second, it is cost-effective if the loss in effectiveness is judged to be more than offset by the reduction in cost. In this light, the index of cost-effectiveness is the marginal cost-effectiveness ratio:

$$\frac{COST_A - COST_B}{EFFECTIVENESS_A - EFFECTIVENESS_B}$$

where A is the more (or less) expensive *and* more (or less) effective treatment strategy. When costs are measured in dollars and effectiveness in QALYs, the ratio expresses the additional cost per QALY by using intervention A instead of B. Recall that, by convention, only direct costs (medical plus any nonmedical) are included in the numerator.

Within this cost-effectiveness framework, under what circumstances will intervention A turn out to be "worth it" relative to B? That is, when will we actually be led to choose A over B? First, note that if A is both more effective and less costly than B, it is unambiguously preferred to B; likewise, if A is both less effective and more costly than B, then B is preferred to A. Under such circumstances, no ratio is even computed; the decision is clear.

But the issue becomes more difficult when the ratio is positive, as first assumed. Basically, there are two paths to reaching a decision about A and B. First, if the decision context involves an explicit budget targeted to the disease that A and B are "competing" to treat, then one should select that intervention with the lower cost-effectiveness ratio, for it will produce the greater total volume of QALYs. This holds true, of course, for any number of interventions competing to treat the target population.

However, for virtually all cost-effectiveness analyses reported in the literature (produced typically by clinicians and other analysts from the research community), there is no decision context involving an actual budget and therefore no simple way to determine whether an intervention A is worth it relative to B. In response, some analysts have constructed, and many others make reference to, what has become known as "league tables," which typically display the range of cost-effectiveness ratios (from low to high) found in selected portions of the clinical evaluation literature.[14] Any analyst can then compare the ratio from a cost-effectiveness study of interest with those found in the table.

Although there are major empirical and methodologic problems in drawing valid comparisons, because the studies reported in the table are rarely comparable, analysts nonetheless frequently draw such comparisons. Cost-effectiveness ratios roughly in the range from $50,000 to $100,000 per QALY (current U.S. dollars) are typically judged to demonstrate that A is "cost effective" relative to B.

COST-EFFECTIVENESS OF CAROTID ENDARTERECTOMY

The methodology for evaluating the cost-effectiveness of carotid endarterectomy for a number of (statistically defined) patient types has been demonstrated in a previously published paper.[15] In what follows, we build upon and empirically extend this work to investigate the cost-effectiveness of the procedure for three selected patient types:

Symptomatic: A 65-year-old man presents with a recent TIA or minor completed stroke in the anterior circulation.
Asymptomatic: A 65-year-old man with no history of cerebrovascular symptoms arrives for a health maintenance visit. His history and physical examination are unremarkable.
Asymptomatic with Bruit: A 65-year-old man presents with the same characteristics as an asymptomatic patient,

except he is found on physical examination to have a carotid bruit.

For each of the three "patients," the two alternative options for intervention are to consider carotid endarterectomy, or not to consider carotid endarterectomy. When the carotid endarterectomy is chosen, the patient can be screened with the use of a noninvasive test (eg, carotid Doppler or duplex ultrasonography). If a high-grade stenosis is identified, carotid angiography is recommended. If a high-grade stenosis is confirmed, carotid endarterectomy is recommended.

In this section, we discuss both the structure of the decision model used for the cost-effectiveness analysis and the derivation of the base-case values for its clinical and economic parameters.

Decision Model

A decision model provides a convenient way to represent and evaluate alternative interventions. This is especially the case when each intervention is associated with a variety of possible outcome scenarios, and each scenario itself is a complex, multiperiod stream of events—a common situation for many chronic diseases.

However, decision modeling is important to clinical policy analysis not simply because it allows us to picture complex treatment choices in an organized, coherent fashion. In many studies, the decision model becomes the "analytic arena" within which relevant clinical and economic data, from a variety of sources, are brought to bear synergistically to analyze management options in ways not possible if one had to rely on data from single treatment sites (or even single clinical trials). For most clinical problems, there is no single source for data on the natural history of disease, the effectiveness of different treatments, the costs of disease conditional on treatment, and patient preferences for possible health outcomes. This is certainly the case for our evaluation of carotid endarterectomy. Accordingly, we have used data from a variety of sources to estimate effectiveness and cost, then integrated these within a decision model to study the cost-effectiveness of this procedure for each of our three patient types.

It is useful to present this decision model in two parts, or stages, although in reality there is but one, fully integrated model generating the cost-effectiveness results.

In the first stage, shown in Figure 89–1, the overarching choice is whether or not to embark on a screening and treatment strategy, which begins with a noninvasive test to check for high-grade stenosis and can lead to the patient's undergoing a carotid endarterectomy. If a noninvasive test is performed, the likelihood of having a high-grade carotid stenosis, together with the characteristics of the test (that is, its sensitivity and specificity), determine the probabilities that the test will generate true positive, false negative, false positive, or true negative results regarding the stenosis. We assume that all patients with positive screens proceed promptly to angiography and that the latter examination yields only true positive and true negative results. With angiography there is some small risk of death and of a nonfatal stroke. If angiography confirms the stenosis (and there is no fatal complication), the patient is referred for a carotid endarterectomy.

In general, this second stage, shown in compressed form in Figure 89–2, is a Markov model representation of the outcome options facing the patient in each succeeding time period once the first stage is exited. In the period immediately following the first stage, the patient referred for a carotid endarterectomy faces some risk of dying (entering Dead state) or suffering a nonfatal stroke (entering Stroked state) in the perioperative period. If he survives, he faces some reduced probability of stroke, with the amount of reduction depending on the "efficacy" of the procedure. The latter is defined here as (1 − relative risk). But if stroke does occur, there is some probability of immediate death.

If the patient entering the second stage Well does not receive a carotid endarterectomy, he will enter the Stroked state if there was a stroke in stage one of the model, or the Well state if no stroke has occurred. In either case, the patient is at risk for a new stroke and early death from such a stroke on entering the second stage, as can be seen in Figure 89–2. In a similar fashion, the patient continues to move through the decision model by recycling, period after period.

More formally, the decision structure shown in Figures 89–1 and 89–2 can be characterized as a Markov simulation model. In the analyses here, a hypothetical cohort of 1000 statistically identical patients is sent through the model, the actual path each "patient" takes being governed by the model's probabilities. Each of our three patient types is analyzed in a distinct simulation, with the decision model's parameters specified accordingly. The length of each period in this model is 1 month, and all probability and cost parameters are calibrated to reflect this.

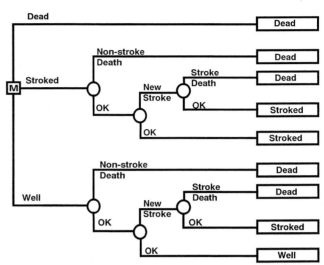

FIGURE 89–2. Stage 2 of the decision model (Markov). The second stage of the decision model is shown in compressed form as a Markov model, representing the outcome options facing the patient at the end of the first month and in each succeeding time period once the patient has exited the first stage. In the period immediately following the first stage, the patient referred for carotid endarterectomy faces some risk of dying (Dead) or suffering a nonfatal stroke (Stroked) in the perioperative period. If he survives, he faces some reduced probability of stroke, with the amount of reduction depending on the efficacy of the procedure. But if stroke does occur, there is some probability of immediate death.

If the patient entering the second stage at Well does not receive a carotid endarterectomy, he will enter the Stroked state if there was a stroke in stage 1 of the model, or the Well state if no stroke has occurred. In either case, the patient is at risk for a new stroke and early death from such a stroke on entering the second stage. The patient moves through the decision model by recycling, period after period.

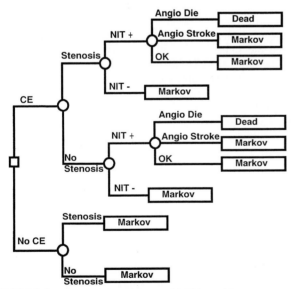

FIGURE 89–1. Stage 1 of the decision model. This model represents events that are assumed to occur in the first month following the choice to consider carotid endarterectomy (CE) or not (No CE). The CE strategy begins with a noninvasive test (NIT) to check for high-grade stenosis and may lead to the patient's undergoing a carotid endarterectomy. All patients with positive results on their screening tests promptly undergo angiography, which yields only true positive and true negative results. With angiography there is some risk of death (Angio Die) and of a nonfatal stroke (Angio Stroke). If angiography confirms the stenosis (and there is no fatal complication), the patient is referred for a carotid endarterectomy. At the end of the first month, the patient either is dead or is at the threshold for entry into stage 2 of the decision model (Markov).

The decision model can be thought of as a simulated clinical trial in which a hypothetical cohort of identical patients is sent one-by-one through the model, the actual path each patient takes being governed by the model's probabilities. As the simulation proceeds, patients accumulate cost and QALYs (or months). When all patients in the simulation are "dead," the cumulative costs and QALYs for the screening and treatment intervention relative to the nonscreening alternative can be computed. A symbolic representation of how an individual patient can move through the Markov model, period by period, is shown in Figure 89–3.

Parameter Estimates for the Model

The parameters that must be estimated before the cost-effectiveness analysis can proceed fall into three broad categories: the probabilities of various events (eg, of stroke, with and without carotid endarterectomy); the costs of disease and of treatment; and patient preferences for the outcomes represented in the model. In addition, there is a fourth type of parameter, termed the discount factor, that determines how the various future streams of costs and health outcomes should be valued from a present-time perspective (the here-and-now). This is, in fact, the perspective assumed for the decision maker as he or she "stands poised" at the choice node (the square) in Figure 89–1, attempting to determine whether the carotid endarterectomy strategy is advisable.

In Table 89–1 we define each model parameter and, for each of our three patient types, report both the base-case

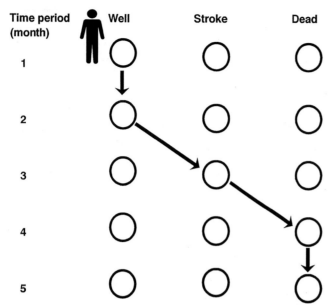

FIGURE 89–3. Hypothetical patient traversing the decision model. The decision model may be thought of as a simulated clinical trial in which a hypothetical cohort of identical patients is sent one-by-one through the model, the actual path each patient takes being governed by the model's probabilities. As the simulation proceeds, patients accumulate cost and quality-adjusted life-years or life-months (QALYs). When all patients in the simulation are dead, the cumulative costs and QALYs for the screening and treatment intervention relative to the nonscreening alternative can be computed.

value of the parameter and the range over which it was varied in subsequent sensitivity analyses to test the robustness of base-case conclusions. Recall that all analyses are for a 65-year-old male, with the patient type distinction hinging on the risk for carotid stenosis and for stroke.

In what follows, we briefly note the various event probabilities and the published sources from which they were drawn. Then we discuss in more detail the parameters related to cost, preferences, and discounting to present value, both because they may be less familiar to the reader and because they led the authors to piece together data from diverse sources.

Event Probabilities

For each of the probabilities in the decision model, the base-case value and the plausible range were determined from published sources to the extent possible; otherwise, they were specified by the authors. As indicated in Table 89–1, estimates were required for the following parameters (with supporting literature noted where applicable): the probability of high-grade stenosis (>70%[16, 17]); the probability of stroke, with and without stenosis[18–21]; the efficacy of carotid endarterectomy[3–6]; the duration of the efficacy[22, 23]; carotid endarterectomy mortality and stroke risk[24–30]; the risks of stroke and death related to angiography[31, 32]; the risk of mortality in the general population of 65-year-old men and the nonstroke-related increase in this risk in the subpopulation with stenosis[33]; the probability of death, given stroke[34–36]; and the true positive and false positive rates for noninvasive testing.[37] Recall, finally, that in the decision model, angiography is assumed to be completely accurate.

Costs

The costs reported in Table 89–1 were calculated from the societal perspective, include only direct medical costs (as discussed earlier), and were adjusted to 1993 U.S. dollars via the medical care component of the Consumer Price Index.[38] The major components of costs will be considered now in turn.

Acute Care for Stroke. The acute costs of treating a stroke reflect expenditures for inpatient hospitalization, rehabilitation services, and home health care following discharge.

The costs associated with the initial hospitalization were computed two alternative ways. First, the institutional costs were estimated from the 1993 Medicare reimbursement rates for diagnosis-related group 014 (cerebrovascular disorders), and the associated professional charges for the admission were based on the Medicare physician fee schedule for an average 7-day stay. The sum of hospital costs ($4525) and physician payments ($456) is $4981.[39, 40] In the second approach, a 20 percent sample of Medicare inpatient admissions for cerebral infarction was used to estimate the actual hospital and physician costs associated with this type of admission; the result was approximately $7000. In light of these estimates, we adopted $6000 as the base-case value for the cost of acute hospitalization.

Medicare data on the use of posthospital care and inpatient medical rehabilitation were used to estimate the cost of rehabilitation for stroke survivors. Using an estimate that 6.8 percent of patients will require inpatient rehabilitation after a stroke,[41] and that the average cost for these services is $25,000 (1984 dollars), the cost of rehabilitation is approximately $3000 in 1993 terms.[42]

About 22 percent of stroke patients use home health services following discharge from the hospital, according to Medicare data. Assuming that stroke patients, in 1984, received the same number of visits as all patients who have postdischarge home health care, the total cost of home health services would be approximately $1360 in 1993 dollars (14 visits × $54 [1984]). This would be about $300 per case ($1360 × 0.22).

By combining the costs of these three phases of treatment and assuming that Medicare reimbursement rates are adequate proxies for true costs, we compute the total acute care cost for treating a stroke to be $9300.

Chronic Care for Stroke. There is an ongoing cost of caring for the survivors of stroke involving skilled nursing home care, professional services, medical equipment purchases, and many other miscellaneous expenses. Unfortunately, comparatively little information is published on these costs for specifically defined populations of stroke victims; consequently, our estimates rely on several key observations from the published studies, plus some strategic assumptions.

The cost of caring for patients who need permanent skilled nursing home care represents a large portion of the long-term cost of stroke. We assumed that approximately 35 percent of patients remain functionally dependent after experiencing a stroke, based on studies of stroke outcome.[43–46] In addition, we estimated that 26 percent of all functionally dependent stroke victims reside in nursing homes,[47] implying that about 9 percent of these patients will require long-term skilled nursing home care. This proportion is consistent

TABLE 89–1. Parameters for Decision Model: Base-Case Values and Ranges, by Patient Type

Parameters	Patient Type*		
	Symptomatic	Asymptomatic with Bruit	Asymptomatic
Probabilities,† %			
P(High-Grade Stenosis)	50 (20–70)	20 (5–40)	5 (2–20)
P(Stroke, Given Stenosis)‡ (Annual Rate)	7 (0–10)	5 (0–10)	5 (0–10)
P(Stroke, without Stenosis) (Annual Rate)	2 (0–5)	0.8 (0–3)	0.8 (0–3)
P(Early Stroke Death)	17 (10–35)	17 (10–35)	17 (10–35)
P(Nonstroke Death, without Stenosis)§ (Annual Rate)	—	—	—
Excess Annual Mortality Rate Due to Stenosis (Nonstroke Causes)	3 (0–10)	3 (0–10)	3 (0–10)
Efficacy of Carotid Endarterectomy¶	0.43 (0.20–0.80)	0.40 (0.20–0.80)	0.40 (0.20–0.80)
Duration of Efficacy, yr	10 (2–20)	10 (2–20)	10 (2–20)
P(Operative Death)	1.5 (0–3)	1.5 (0–3)	1.5 (0–3)
P(Operative Stroke, Nonfatal)	5 (0–7.5)	5 (0–7.5)	5 (0–7.5)
P(Angiography-Related Death)	0.1 (0–1)	0.1 (0–1)	0.1 (0–1)
P(Angiography-Related Stroke, Nonfatal)	1 (0–2)	1 (0–2)	1 (0–2)
Noninvasive Test True Positive Rate (Sensitivity)	90 (80–100)	90 (80–100)	90 (80–100)
Noninvasive Test False Positive Rate (1-Specificity)	10 (0–20)	10 (0–20)	10 (0–20)
Cost, 1993 US$			
Acute Care for Stroke	9300 (2000–20,000)	9300 (2000–20,000)	9300 (2000–20,000)
Chronic Care for Stroke (Monthly Rate)	410 (200–1000)	410 (200–1000)	410 (200–1000)
Carotid Endarterectomy	10,000 (5000–15,000)	10,000 (5000–15,000)	10,000 (5000–15,000)
Angiography	1500 (800–3000)	1500 (800–3000)	1500 (800–3000)
Noninvasive Testing	450 (50–1000)	450 (50–1000)	450 (50–1000)
Patient Preferences**			
Value (disutility) of Stroked State	0.70 (0–1)	0.70 (0–1)	0.70 (0–0.10)
Disutility of Surgery Event	0.02 (0–0.10)	0.02 (0–0.10)	0.02 (0–0.10)
Discount Rate,†† % (annual)	5 (0–10)	5 (0–10)	5 (0–10)

*All parameters pertain to 65-year-old male, whose patient type classification is based solely on risk of carotid stenosis and of stroke.

†In general, P(X) means the probability of event X, where probability is expressed here on the 0–100 scale.

‡For symptomatic patients, the risk of stroke given stenosis is assumed to be about 0.117 in the first year of the model, 0.082 in the second year, and 0.07 in all remaining years.

§Obtained from standard life tables; varies by year as patient "ages" in the model.

¶Efficacy is defined as (1 − Relative Risk of Stroke, given carotid endarterectomy [CE]), which equals (1 − [P(Stroke, given CE) / P(Stroke, without CE)]).

**Expressed along the [0, 1] interval, where 1 is the value of the best possible state of health and 0 is the value of the worst state, as defined by the patient.

††Costs and effectiveness are discounted at the same rate in the decision model.

with results from a community-based study in Australia that reported that 10 percent of stroke victims were in a nursing home 2 years following the event.[48]

A 1985 nursing home survey reported that the average 1985 monthly charge for patients residing in nursing homes after discharge from the hospital was $1627 (or $2734 in 1993 terms).[49] Assuming a 10 percent utilization rate, the average monthly skilled nursing home cost per stroke victim is about $275. (Because of data limitations here, we use charges rather than direct measures of economic costs and assume that the former provide a reasonable estimate of the latter.)

Next, from a Swedish community-based cohort study that examined the direct costs of treating strokes in the second year following the accident, we calculated that outpatient medical expenses are approximately $150 per patient per month.[50] Assuming that 90 percent of stroke patients are not in a skilled nursing home and thus incur such outpatient costs on a regular basis, the expected chronic care cost per patient is about $275 + 0.90($150) = $410 per month.

Carotid Endarterectomy. The cost of carotid endarterectomy was estimated from the Medicare diagnosis-related group data and physician fee schedules for 1993. Reimbursement for professional services was based on the initial procedure charges, ancillary (anesthesia) professional charges, and

in-hospital follow-up for an average 5-day stay. The sum of the diagnosis-related group reimbursement and professional charges for carotid endarterectomy is $8117.

To account for the costs of outpatient postoperative follow-up and the treatment of nonfatal complications, it was assumed that the average patient would require two postdischarge clinic evaluations at a total cost of $250. From available estimates of nonstroke, nonfatal complication rates, an associated cost of $1250 was estimated.[43–47] Consequently, the cost of outpatient care and treatment of complications is about $1500, and the total estimate for carotid endarterectomy is $9617.

This is in line with two earlier carotid endarterectomy cost estimates, which implied a range of $8000 to $10,000 (1993 dollars).[51, 52] But Medicare cost data from 1991 yielded a cost estimate for the carotid endarterectomy procedure alone of about $11,500. In response, a base-case value of $10,000 was adopted. The cost of treating strokes arising as complications of carotid endarterectomy was computed separately from the cost of the procedure, by assigning value to the acute and chronic care resources consumed by the stroke as outlined earlier.

Angiography and Noninvasive Testing. The costs for both of these procedures, as reported in Table 93–1, were derived from the Medicare physician fee schedule for 1993.

Patient Preferences

Value (Disutility) of Stroked State. In the absence of empirical data on how a 65-year-old man of the clinical type portrayed in the decision model would assess the disutility of the stroked state, we assigned it a value of 0.70. Because this is an arbitrary (though, we think, reasonable) assignment, our sensitivity analysis will focus on the range of stroke state preference values for which the carotid endarterectomy screening and treatment strategy is preferred.

Disutility of Surgery. To acknowledge that carotid endarterectomy, as an event to be anticipated and endured, is associated with a certain amount of pain, functional limitation, and anxiety, we assigned a disutility value to the procedure itself. In the base case, we assumed that undergoing carotid endarterectomy generated an extra disutility "debit" equivalent to 1 week in the worst possible health state (here, assumed to be death). Arithmetically, this amounts to deducting $(1/52) = 0.02$ QALYs from the patient's total QALY score for the period in the decision model when the surgery occurs. For a similar approach, see Matchar and Pauker.[15]

Discount Rate

A prominent recommendation in the literature on cost-effectiveness methods is that both future costs and future health-related outcomes be calculated in "present value" terms so that the decision maker—who must make a choice in the here-and-now—can properly weigh the treatment options from a current-time perspective.[53]

However, there is currently much controversy about how this should be accomplished.[54] There is virtually no debate about whether costs should be discounted to present value, or about the mathematical formula for doing it; but there is ongoing disagreement about how to select the appropriate discount rate for converting future costs to present value, especially when the evaluation is being carried out from the societal perspective. Currently, the most common rates for discounting costs are 5 percent and 3 percent (in real, not nominal, terms).

Perhaps the most debated question is whether, and how, health-related outcomes (which, by definition, are not valued in monetary terms) should be stated in present value terms. The most common approach currently, and the one adopted here, is to discount QALYs using the same formula and same discount rate as employed for costs. This is in keeping with the "consistency argument," put forth by Weinstein

and Stason,[8] that costs and effectiveness should be discounted identically so as to maintain over time in the decision model the same value relationship between them that is posited to exist in the initial period.

This is the approach adopted in the discussion following, with both costs and QALYs discounted at 5 percent in the base case.

Results

The cost, effectiveness, and cost-effectiveness of a screening and treatment strategy involving carotid endarterectomy are reported in Table 89–2 for our three patient types, each defined as a 65-year-old man with some suspected level of carotid artery stenosis. Recall from Figures 89–1 and 89–2 that the No CE option implies standard medical management of the patient over the rest of the life cycle. For the calculations in Table 93–2, all parameters in the decision model were set at their base-case values, as reported in Table 89–1.

To test the robustness of these base-case conclusions to reasonable variations in the model parameters, we conducted extensive sensitivity analyses, whose results are summarized in Table 89–3.

Base-Case Conclusions

Symptomatic. Although the carotid endarterectomy strategy is more costly than No CE by $4285, it is also more effective in producing quality-adjusted life-years: 8.50 vs. 8.39, for a difference of about 0.11 QALY, or about 5.7 quality-adjusted life-weeks. This means that the effectiveness of carotid endarterectomy, relative to medical management, for this patient is the equivalent of gaining about 5.7 weeks of excellent health over the remaining portion of the life cycle.

If we accept the current "standard" that cost-effectiveness ratios in the range from $50,000 to $100,000 per QALY suggest that an intervention is cost-effective, then carotid endarterectomy for the symptomatic 65-year-old man—which costs about $39,000 per QALY gained—clearly passes the test.

Asymptomatic with Bruit. For this patient, the carotid endarterectomy strategy is very slightly more effective (9.72 vs. 9.71 QALYs). But with a ratio of about $247,500 per QALY gained, it is not cost-effective by the current standard.

Asymptomatic. For the typical asymptomatic 65-year-old man, carotid endarterectomy is neither effective nor (thus) cost-effective. Indeed, the carotid endarterectomy strategy

TABLE 89–2. Cost, Effectiveness, and Cost-Effectiveness of Carotid Endarterectomy: Base-Case Results for 65-Year-Old Man by Patient Type

Patient Type	CE		No CE		Cost-Effectiveness of CE, Δ$/ΔQALY
	Cost, 1993 US$	Effectiveness, QALY	Cost, 1993 US$	Effectiveness, QALY	
Symptomatic	17,288	8.50	13,003	8.39	4,285/0.11 = 38,955
Asymptomatic with Bruit	7854	9.72	5379	9.71	2,475/0.01 = 247,500
Asymptomatic	5141	10.1535	4029	10.1541	Ratio Not Operative*

*Since CE is both more costly and less effective, the No CE option dominates, and the standard ratio (which would be negative in this case) is not required. The effectiveness calculations are carried to four decimal places here simply to indicate the (very slight) decline in QALYs with CE.

CE, carotid endarterectomy; QALY, quality-adjusted life-year.

TABLE 89–3. Sensitivity Analyses to Test Robustness of Base-Case Recommendations to Variations in Decision Model Parameters*

Parameters	Patient Type		
	Symptomatic	Asymptomatic with Bruit	Asymptomatic
Probabilities			
P(High-Grade Stenosis)	Yes†	No‡	No
P(Stroke, Given Stenosis) (Annual Rate)	Yes if > 4.6%§	Yes if > 6.6%	No
P(Stroke, without Stenosis) (Annual Rate)	Yes	No	No
P(Early Stroke Death)	Yes	Yes if > 34%	No
Excess Annual Mortality Rate Due to Stenosis (Nonstroke Causes)	Yes	No	No
Efficacy of Carotid Endarterectomy	Yes if > 30%	Yes if > 50%	Yes if > 71%
Duration of Efficacy, yr	Yes if > 4.6%	No	No
P(Operative Death)	Yes¶	Yes if < 0.39%	No
P(Operative Stroke, Nonfatal)	Yes	Yes if < 1.6%	No
P(Angiography-Related Death)	Yes	No	No
P(Angiography-Related Stroke, Nonfatal)	Yes	No	No
Noninvasive Test True Positive Rate (Sensitivity)	Yes	No	No
Noninvasive Test False Positive Rate (1 − Specificity)	Yes	No	No
Cost			
Acute Care for Stroke	Yes	No	No
Chronic Care for Stroke (Monthly Rate)	Yes	No	No
Carotid Endarterectomy	Yes	No	No
Angiography	Yes	No	No
Noninvasive Testing	Yes	No	No
Patient Preferences			
Value (Disutility) of Stroked State	Yes	No	No
Disutility of Surgery Event	Yes	No	No
Discount Rate (Annual)	Yes	Yes if < 0.8%	No

*The option involving carotid endarterectomy (CE) is deemed to be "cost-effective" if the corresponding cost-effectiveness ratio comparing this option to (No CE) is less than $100,000 per quality-adjusted life year (QALY) gained.

†"Yes" implies that CE is cost-effective for all values of this parameter within the range specified in Table 89–1, assuming all other parameters are at their base-case values.

‡"No" implies that CE is not cost-effective for any values of that parameter within the range specified in Table 89–1, assuming all other parameters are at base-case values.

§Conditional "Yes" implies that CE is cost-effective for all values of that parameter meeting the specified inequality condition, assuming all other parameters are at base-case values.

¶If operative stroke and death are considered together, the combined rate must be less than 10% for the marginal cost-effectiveness ratio for surgery to remain less than $100,000/QALY.

leads to a very slight decrease in QALYs, reflecting that the small increase in risks of death and stroke from testing and surgery outweigh the small positive impact of these interventions on preventing stroke.

Sensitivity Analyses

Virtually all of the parameters in the decision model were determined by the authors either from secondary data of greatly varying quality and precision or by simple assumption. Therefore, it is particularly important to investigate how sensitive our base-case conclusions are to possible variation in the values of these parameters. Consequently, we conducted extensive sensitivity analyses, which are reported in Table 89–3 by patient type. For illustration, we adopted a cost-effectiveness ratio cut-off value of $100,000 per QALY gained; for any model run in which the ratio was lower than this, carotid endarterectomy was regarded as "cost-effective" relative to the No CE strategy.

In each instance, we performed what is termed a "one-way" sensitivity analysis, in which we vary the (one) parameter of interest along its plausible range while fixing all other parameters at their base-case values. We then determine those values of the parameter of interest for which carotid endarterectomy is deemed to be cost-effective, those values for which it is not cost-effective, and hence that one value

for which the choice is a toss-up; the latter is often referred to as the "switchpoint" value of the parameter. In addition to performing one-way sensitivity analysis, we examined the effect of considering all possible combinations of surgical mortality and stroke rate (termed "two-way" sensitivity analysis).

We now consider the robustness of our base-case conclusions:

Symptomatic. As indicated by the pattern of "Yes" responses in Table 89–3, the carotid endarterectomy strategy was cost-effective over the entire plausible range of the great majority of parameters (tested, of course, one at a time). There were three characteristics of surgery and one patient feature that could strongly influence the cost-effectiveness of carotid endarterectomy.

The efficacy of carotid endarterectomy (defined as [1 − relative risk of stroke given surgery versus no surgery]) must remain above 30 percent for this option to be cost-effective. Interestingly, the assumed length of time over which carotid endarterectomy is assumed to remain clinically effective is an important factor: the surgery must be durable beyond about 4.6 years for it to be cost-effective, all other factors being equal. Evidence regarding long-term patency rates[22, 23] suggests that the duration of carotid endarterectomy effectiveness may be considerably longer than this switchpoint value; indeed, based on these reports, we designated 10 years as the base-case value of this parameter. Also, the combined surgical mortality and morbidity must be less than approximately 10 percent for these symptomatic patients.

Finally, the stroke rate for patients with high-grade stenosis (without surgery) must exceed 4.6 percent for carotid endarterectomy to be cost-effective (by the criteria adopted here).

Asymptomatic with Bruit. For this 65-year-old man, the carotid endarterectomy strategy would not be cost-effective unless the annual rate of stroke for patients with stenosis exceeds 6.6 percent (base-case value is 5%); surgical efficacy exceeds 50 percent; the probability of early stroke death exceeds about 34 percent (double the base-case rate); the probability of operative death drops below 0.39 percent (base-case is 1%); the probability of operative nonfatal stroke is less than 1.6 percent (base-case is 4%); or the discount rate for converting costs and effectiveness to present value falls below 1 percent (base-case rate is 5%).

Asymptomatic. As indicated in Table 89–3, only if the efficacy of carotid endarterectomy were to exceed 70 percent would this strategy be recommended on cost-effectiveness grounds (all else being equal). Given that the base-case efficacy rate is 40 percent, it is not credible that carotid endarterectomy is a cost-effective intervention for the average 65-year-old man.

IMPLICATIONS FOR CLINICAL PRACTICE

In light of evidence demonstrating benefit from carotid endarterectomy for symptomatic patients with high-grade stenosis, it is reassuring to note that carotid endarterectomy is also cost-effective compared with other accepted clinical interventions.

Although this conclusion is robust over a wide range of cost estimates, several factors were seen to substantially diminish the cost-effectiveness of carotid endarterectomy: reduced surgical efficacy and durability, elevated surgical risk, and low underlying stroke risk. This suggests that enthusiasm for carotid endarterectomy should be tempered by two important caveats. First, the procedure must be performed by a surgeon in a setting in which surgical risk is minimized. Although many centers have documented low risk, evidence from Medicare data indicates a wide range of risk, with average 30-day mortality and stroke rates of 3 percent and 6.6 percent, respectively.[30] Second, patients selected for the procedure should be at significantly elevated stroke risk. Patients who have had cerebrovascular symptoms in the distant past are at significantly less risk for stroke than are those with more recent symptoms.[55] Performance of carotid endarterectomy in this setting may be modestly efficacious but would not likely be cost-effective.

Strategies involving carotid endarterectomy for asymptomatic patients are difficult to justify. In our baseline analysis, stroke risk was assumed to be relatively high (5% per year) and surgery was assumed to be highly efficacious (reducing the rate of stroke by 40 percent). Even with these estimates favoring the strategy, carotid endarterectomy is not likely to be effective when the risks of angiography and carotid endarterectomy are taken into account.

If carotid endarterectomy does reduce stroke rate in asymptomatic individuals—an issue not yet resolved by published clinical trials—there may be patient types for which carotid endarterectomy would be cost-effective. However, it is difficult to identify those patients. Carotid bruit is a marker for both carotid stenosis and increased stroke risk, but even if this is taken into account in an analysis favoring the surgical strategy, this intervention is not cost-effective. If we could inexpensively and accurately identify clinical features that mark asymptomatic individuals as having an unusually high stroke risk (greater than 6.6% per year) and a low surgical risk, then carotid endarterectomy would be cost-effective. Unfortunately, characteristics that place patients at increased stroke risk also mark them as individuals at high surgical risk.[24] Thus, the subset of asymptomatic patients for whom carotid endarterectomy is appropriate is at best a small fraction of all asymptomatic individuals. The identification of this subgroup presents a substantial challenge to stroke research.

REFERENCES

1. American Heart Association: 1991 Heart and Stroke Facts. Dallas, 1991.
2. Adelman SM. Economic Impact. *Stroke.* 1981;12(Suppl):I–69.
3. North American Symptomatic Carotid Endarterectomy Trial: Beneficial effect of carotid endarterectomy in symptomatic patients with high grade carotid stenosis. *N Engl J Med.* 1991;325:442.
4. European Carotid Surgery Trialists' Collaborative Group: MRC European Carotid Surgery Trial: Interim results for symptomatic patients with severe (70–99%) or mild (0–29%) carotid stenosis. *Lancet.* 1991;337:1235.
5. Mayberg MR, Wilson SE, Yatsu F, and the VA Symptomatic Carotid Stenosis Group: Carotid endarterectomy and prevention of cerebral ischemia in symptomatic carotid stenosis. *JAMA.* 1991;266:3289.
6. Hobson RW II, Weiss DG, Fields WS, et al, and the VA Asymptomatic Carotid Stenosis Group: Efficacy of carotid endarterectomy for asymptomatic carotid stenosis. *N Engl J Med.* 1993;328:221.
7. Hodgson TA, Meiners MR: Cost-of-illness methodology: A guide to current practices and procedures. *Milbank Q.* 1982;60:429.
8. Weinstein MC, Stason WB: Foundations of cost-effectiveness analysis for health and medical practices. *N Engl J Med.* 1977;296:716.
9. Goldstein LB, Bertels C, Davis JN: Interrater reliability of the NIH stroke scale. *Arch Neurol.* 1989;46:660.
10. Kaplan RM, Bush JW: Health-related quality of life measurement for evaluation research and policy analysis. *Health Psychol.* 1982;1:61.
11. EuroQol Group: EuroQol: a new facility for the measurement of health-related quality of life. *Health Policy.* 1990;16:199.
12. Kaplan RM, Anderson JP, Wu A, et al: The Quality of Well-Being Scale: Applications in AIDS, cystic fibrosis, and arthritis. *Med Care.* 1989;27(suppl 3):S27.
13. Naglie IG, Detsky AS: Treatment of chronic nonvalvular atrial fibrillation in the elderly. *Med Decis Making.* 1992;12:239.
14. Mason J, Drummond M, Torrance G: Some guidelines on the use of cost-effectiveness league tables. *Br Med J.* 1993;306:570.
15. Matchar DB, Pauker SG: Endarterectomy in carotid artery disease: a decision analysis. *JAMA.* 1987;258:793.
16. Pessin MS, Duncan GW, Mohr JP, Poskanzer DC: Clinical and angiographic features of carotid transient ischemic attacks. *N Engl J Med.* 1977;296:358.
17. O'Donnell TF, Erodes L, Mackey WC, et al: Correlation of B-mode ultrasound imaging and arteriography with pathologic findings at carotid endarterectomy. *Arch Surg.* 1985;120:443.
18. Norris JW, Zhu CZ, Bornstein NM, Chambers BR: Vascular risks of asymptomatic carotid stenosis. *Stroke.* 1991;22:1485.
19. Dennis MS, Bamford JM, Sandercock PAG, Warlow CP: Incidence of transient ischemic attacks in Oxfordshire, England. *Stroke.* 1989;20:333.
20. Cartlidge NEF, Whisnant JP, Elveback LR: Carotid and vertebral-basilar transient cerebral ischemic attacks. *Mayo Clin Proc.* 1977;52:117.
21. Hennerici M, Hulsbomer H, Hefter H, et al: Natural history of asymptomatic extracranial arterial disease. Results of a long-term prospective study. *Brain.* 1987;110(pt3):777.
22. Bernstein EF, Torem S, Dilley R: Does carotid restenosis predict an increased risk of late symptoms, stroke or death? *Annals of Surgery.* 1990;212:629.
23. DeGroote RD, Lynch TG, Jamil Z, Hobson RW II: Carotid restenosis: Long-term non-invasive follow-up after carotid endarterectomy. *Stroke.* 1987;18:1031.
24. McCrory DC, Goldstein LB, Samsa GP, et al: Predicted complications of carotid endarterectomy. *Stroke.* 1993;24:1285.
25. Easton JD, Sherman DG: Stroke and mortality rate in carotid endarterectomy: 228 consecutive operations. *Stroke.* 1977;8:565.
26. Moore DJ, Modi JR, Finch WT, Sumner DS: Influence of the contralateral carotid

artery on neurologic complications following carotid endarterectomy. *J Vasc Surg.* 1984;1:409.

27. Brott T, Thalinger K: The practice of carotid endarterectomy in a large metropolitan area. *Stroke.* 1984;15:950.

28. Brott TG, Labutta RJ, Kempczinski RF: Changing patterns in the practice of carotid endarterectomy in a large metropolitan area. *JAMA.* 1986;255:2609.

29. Fisher ES, Malenka DJ, Solomon NA, et al: Risk of carotid endarterectomy in the elderly. *Am J Public Health.* 1989;79:1617.

30. Brook R, Park E, Chassin M, et al: Carotid endarterectomy for elderly patients. Predicting complications. *Ann Intern Med.* 1990;113:747.

31. Mani RL, Eisenberg RL, McDonald EJ, Pollock Mani JR: Complications of catheter cerebral angiography: Analysis of 5000 procedures: I. Criteria and incidence. *AJR Am J Roentgenol.* 1978;131:861.

32. Earnest F IV, Forbes G, Sandok BA, et al: Complications of cerebral angiography: Prospective assessment of risk. *AJR Am J Roentgenol.* 1984;142:247.

33. Norris JW, Zhu CZ, Bornstein NM, Chambers BR: Vascular risks of asymptomatic carotid stenosis. *Stroke.* 1991;22:1485.

34. Walker EA, Robins M, Weinfeld FD: The results of the NINCDS national survey of stroke: Clinical Findings. *Stroke.* 1981;12(Suppl 1):113.

35. Sacco RL, Wolf PA, Kannel WB, McNamara PM: Survival and recurrence following stroke: The Framingham Study. *Stroke.* 1982;13:290.

36. Bamford J, Sandercock P, Dennis M, Burn J, Warlow C: A prospective study of acute cerebrovascular disease in the community: The Oxfordshire Community Stroke Project 1981–1986. 2. Incidence, case fatality rates, and overall outcome at one year of cerebral infarction, primary intracerebral and subarachnoid hemorrhage. *J Neurol Neurosurg Psychiatr.* 1989;53:16.

37. Feussner JR, Matchar DB: When and how to study the carotid arteries. *Ann Intern Med.* 1988;109:805.

38. Bureau of Labor Statistics: Consumers Price Index Report 1993: Washington, DC: Bureau of Labor Statistics Publication.

39. Health Care Financing Administration: Medicare Program: Changes to the hospital inpatient prospective payment systems and fiscal year 1993 rates. *Federal Register.* 1992;57(108):23618.

40. Health Care Financing Administration: Fee schedule for Physician Services for calendar year 1993. *Federal Register.* 1992;57(228):55895.

41. Gornick M, Hall MJ: Trends in Medicare use of post-hospital care. *Health Care Financing Review.* 1988; Annual Suppl:27.

42. McGinnis GE, Osberg JS, Seward ML, et al: Total charges for inpatient medical rehabilitation. *Health Care Financing Review.* 1988;9:31.

43. Wade DT, Hewer RL: Functional abilities after stroke: Measurement, natural history, and prognosis. *J Neurol Neurosurg Psychiatr.* 1987;50:177.

44. Aho K, Harmsen P, Hatano S, et al: Cerebrovascular disease in the community: Results of a WHO Collaborative Study. *Bull WHO.* 1980;58:113.

45. Gresham GE, Phillips TF, Wolf PA, et al: Epidemiological profile of long-term stroke disability: The Framingham study. *Arch Phys Med Rehabil.* 1979;60:487.

46. Sorenson PS, Boysen G, Jensen G, Schnohr P: Prevalence of stroke in a district of Copenhagen. *Acta Neurol Scand.* 1982;66:68.

47. U.S. Department of Health and Human Services: Use of long-term care. Vital and Health Statistics 1990; Series 13: Data from the National Health Survey No. 104:26.

48. Christie D: Prevalence of stroke and its sequelae. *Med J Aus.* 1981;2:182.

49. Hing E: Nursing home utilization by current residents: United States, 1985. Vital and Health Statistics 1989; Series 13: Data from the National Health Survey No. 102:1.

50. Persson U, Silverberg R, Lindgren B, et al: Direct costs of stroke for a Swedish population. *Int J Technol Assess Health Care.* 1990;6:125.

51. Gableman CG, Gann DS, Ashworth CJ, Carney WI: One hundred consecutive carotid reconstructions: Local versus general anesthesia. *Am J Surg.* 1983;145:477.

52. Green RM, McNamara J: Optimal resources for carotid endarterectomy. *Surgery.* 1987;102:742.

53. Drummond MF, Stoddart GL, Torrance GW: Methods for the Economic Evaluation of Health Care Programmes. New York: Oxford University Press; 1987.

54. Lipscomb J: Time preference for health in cost-effectiveness analysis. *Med Care.* 1989;27:S233.

55. Whisnant JP, Matsumoto N, Elveback LR: Transient cerebral ischemic attacks in a community: Rochester, Minnesota, 1955 through 1969. *Mayo Clin Proc.* 1973;48:194.

Index

Note: Page numbers in *italics* indicate illustrations; those followed by t indicate tables.